A PRACTICE OF

ANAESTHESIA

(WYLIE AND CHURCHILL-DAVIDSON)

A PRACTICE OF ANAESTHESIA

EDITED BY

H. C. CHURCHILL-DAVIDSON
M.A., M.D. (Cantab.), F.F.A.R.C.S.

*Consultant Anaesthetist, St. Thomas's Hospital and
The Chelsea Hospital for Women*

Fourth Edition

W. B. SAUNDERS COMPANY
PHILADELPHIA · LONDON · TORONTO
1978

Distributed in the United States, Canada, Central and South America by the

W. B. SAUNDERS COMPANY

through arrangement with

LLOYD-LUKE (MEDICAL BOOKS) LTD.

FIRST EDITION . . .	1960
Reprinted . . .	1960
Reprinted . . .	1962
Polish translation . .	1962
SECOND EDITION . . .	1966
Spanish translation . .	1969
Italian translation . .	1969
Reprinted . . .	1970
THIRD EDITION . . .	1972
Portuguese translation . .	1974
FOURTH EDITION . . .	1978

Library of Congress Catalog Card Number:
78-58497

PRINTED IN ENGLAND BY
HAZELL WATSON AND VINEY LTD
AYLESBURY, BUCKS
ISBN 0 85324 131 7

ASSOCIATE EDITORS

PREFACE TO THE FOURTH EDITION

WITH the passing of each quinquenium the need arises to look back over the field of anaesthesia and try to pick out especially those areas where new knowledge may lead to improvement in the skills of the anaesthetist and greater safety for the patient. Nearly twenty years ago Dr. Wylie and I set out to try to provide in a single manual the broad spectrum of that ill-defined subject—Anaesthesia. The success of this venture has been proved by the succeeding editions and translations. It is sad for me, therefore, to have to record that due to the intense pressure of work as Dean of our Medical School, Dr. Wylie (founder, author and editor) no longer felt able to participate in this Fourth Edition. His tolerance, fair-mindedness and meticulous attention to detail, coupled with a long-lasting friendship, have been a hall-mark of previous editions, so it is very reassuring to know that he is still around and willing to advise.

Any textbook (like a business) either improves or falters and it is in this context that I have approached the Fourth edition. The format of attempting to provide the physiological and pharmacological basis of a safe practice for anaesthesia has been preserved.

In this new edition there have been many changes. Foremost of these has been the expansion of the list of Associate Editors. Each has chosen a special area of interest, but all have met regularly and interchanged manuscripts in an attempt to get an up-to-date yet balanced viewpoint of a particular topic. Any success of this edition will be due to their tireless efforts. Every chapter has been thoroughly revised and many completely re-written. New chapters on paediatric anaesthesia (Dr. John Mathias) and placental transmission (Dr. Felicity Reynolds) have been introduced.

Our task has not been made easier by the adoption of the Système International d'Unités (S.I. units) in Europe. This has created many problems because the large majority of our readership does not use this nomenclature. The art of good teaching lies in the simplicity of communication and nothing is better designed to interrupt this dialogue than a sudden change of the rules. Because it seems doubtful if the kilo-pascal (kPa) will replace the millimetre of mercury (mm Hg) for many years to come and as pressure measurements play such an integral part in modern anaesthesia, the board of editors has decided to give the millimetre of mercury pride of place with the kilo-pascal in parenthesis. The purist may be offended but the student will be grateful!

I am truly indebted to Dr. Robert Linton who has not only carefully checked each manuscript but has assumed the awesome task of providing all the necessary S.I. unit equivalents.

The advent of 1978 marks the centenary of the appointment of the first anaesthetist (Dr. Samuel Osborn, 1848–1936) to this hospital. Since that time anaesthesia throughout the world has made great progress and it seemed appropriate that some mention should be made of this history through the principles of the development of anaesthetic apparatus. It is difficult to be truly international and pay tribute to the architects of new ideas in every country because apparatus was designed to suit particular needs (within the limitations of cost and availability of servicing), yet the principles remain universal. I am very grateful to Dr. Charles Foster for providing (in the final chapter) a brief outline of some of the highlights of this development.

Any book of this magnitude requires a guiding light and all concerned will freely admit that our secretary—Mrs. Coral Feltham—is owed a debt of gratitude, for without her efforts it is unlikely that the stage of publication would ever have been reached. Others that must be mentioned are Professor I. Phillips for advice on sterilisation of anaesthetic equipment and Professor G. W. Bisset for help with the role of prostaglandins in uterine physiology. I am also grateful to Mrs. J. L. W. Wynn for the medical illustrations and, as throughout all previous editions, Mr. Brandon for his photographic skills, and Mrs. Kathleen McKay and Mrs. Dorothy Daly for their versatile assistance with illustrations, diagrams and typing of manuscripts.

Finally, I would like to thank our Publisher—Douglas Luke—for his most helpful advice, unfailing courtesy and patience throughout the long preparation of this manuscript.

H. C. CHURCHILL-DAVIDSON

May, 1978

PREFACE TO THE FIRST EDITION

PHYSIOLOGICAL and pharmacological principles now govern the choice of anaesthetic drugs and techniques; and, although many patients can be safely dealt with by routines born of experience, a sound understanding of the background of a particular patient enables the proper and best choice to be made.

In a sense anaesthesia is simply the application of a knowledge of the pharmacological action of drugs to known physiology and pathology, and for this reason the student of anaesthesia must be well-versed in the basic sciences and their application to anaesthesia. Moreover, he must be aware of the modern trends in the medical and surgical care of patients.

We have deliberately assumed that our readers are familiar with the elementary practice of anaesthesia, and practical methods are not always dealt with in great detail, unless they are either of special value though rarely performed, or likely to be required by only a small proportion of practitioners. By the addition of a little more than the bare requirements for competent anaesthesia in the operating theatre, and in some places by the description of a particular disease, pathological process or therapeutic measure, it is hoped to give the reader a broader view of the subject and a better foundation from which to assess the value of the specialty.

The preparation of a book of this nature has necessitated frequent reference to standard and specialised texts and papers in the world literature. These are acknowledged in the relevant parts of this work, but we wish to express our indebtedness to their authors since they have been the foundations upon which we have built, and to crave indulgence should any acknowledgement—through oversight—have been omitted.

A very special word of thanks must be made to Dr. M. D. Nosworthy, who first interested and instructed us in the art and science of anaesthesia. Not only has he read and corrected the greater part of the manuscript, and contributed a foreword to it, but he has never failed to give us helpful advice. We are very grateful to the contributors of special chapters, and to Dr. C. A. Foster for his continuous industry and unstinted aid during each stage of the preparation of the book.

It is a very great pleasure to acknowledge the help of Mr. Douglas Luke, our publisher, who, despite the many years that have passed during the preparation of this work, has never failed to understand the difficulties that beset medical authors.

Finally, without the expert secretarial care and continuous aid of Miss Jean Davenport and her assistants, it is very doubtful whether this book could ever have been completed.

W. D. WYLIE
H. C. CHURCHILL-DAVIDSON

May, 1959

ACKNOWLEDGEMENTS

WE wish to express our thanks to the many individuals, editors, publishers and manufacturers who have so kindly helped us in numerous ways, but principally by allowing reproduction of their own illustrations or materials, and by supplying photographs or blocks.

The following grateful acknowledgements are made in detail for each chapter.

Section One

Chapter 1—Figs. 2 and 3, Dr. J. D. K. Burton and the Editor of the *Lancet*; Fig. 5, The Bird Corporation; Fig. 6, Dr. P. Herzog, Dr. O. P. Norlander and Dr. C. G. Engstrom and the Editor of *Acta Anaesthesiologica Scandinavica*; Fig. 9, based on two illustrations in a chapter by W. J. Hampton and R. J. Hamilton in *Disease of the Ear, Nose and Throat*, Vol. 1, by W. B. Scott-Brown, published by Butterworth and Co.; Fig. 15, Dr. G. H. Bush and John Sherratt and Son, publishers of the *British Journal of Anaesthesia*; Fig. 16, photographs of the original drawings belonging to Mr. M. Meredith Brown; Fig. 18, based on two figures in the *Anatomy of the Bronchial Tree* by Lord Brock and published by the Oxford University Press; Fig. 20, reproduced from William Snow Miller's *The Lung*, courtesy of Charles C. Thomas, publisher, and Fig. 21, based on reconstruction models illustrated in the same book; Fig. 23, Dr. J. A. Clements and *Scientific American*; Fig. 24, Dr. R. E. Brooks; Table 7, from *Lung Function* by Dr. S. E. Cotes, published by Blackwell Scientific Publications.

Chapter 2—Fig. 2, Professor B. Delisle Burns and the Editor of the *British Medical Bulletin*; Figs. 3 and 6, Professor J. W. Severinghaus and the American Physiological Society; Fig. 4, Dr. J. Weldon Bellville and the Editors and publisher, J. B. Lippincott Company, of *Anesthesiology*; Figs. 5(a) and (b), Drs. C. P. Larson, Jr., E. I. Eger II, M. Muallem, D. R. Buechel, E. S. Munson and J. H. Eisele, and the Editors and publisher, J. B. Lippincott Company, of *Anesthesiology*; Fig. 8, based on a figure in *Anatomy for the Anaesthetist*, by Professor H. Ellis and Miss McLarty and published by Blackwell Scientific Publications; Fig. 9, based on anatomical dissections made available by Professor R. J. Last of the Royal College of Surgeons of England; Fig. 10, Dr. B. R. Fink and John Sherratt and Son, publishers of the *British Journal of Anaesthesia*; Fig. 11, from *Respiration in Health and Disease* by R. M. Cherniack and L. Cherniack, published by W. B. Saunders Co.; Fig. 18(c), Dr. H. A. Fleming and the Editors of *Thorax*; Figs, 21, 22, 23 and 24, Dr. H. J. V. Morton and the Editor of *Anaesthesia*; Figs. 25 and 26, are adapted from illustrations in *Physics for the Anaesthetist* by Sir Robert Macintosh, Professor W. W. Mushin and Dr. H. G. Epstein, published by Blackwell Scientific Publications; Fig. 27 is reproduced from the same work; Figs. 28, 29 and 30, Dr. E. S. Munson and the Editors and publisher, J. B. Lippincott Company, of *Anesthesiology*; Fig. 32, Dr. M. L. Kain and Professor J. F. Nunn and the Honorary Editors of the *Proceedings of the Royal Society of Medicine*.

Chapter 3—Fig. 1, from *Respiration in Health and Disease* by R. M. Cherniack and L. Cherniack, published by W. B. Saunders Co.; Table 1 and Fig. 2, Professor M. K. Sykes; Figs. 3(a) and (b), Professor J. B. West and the Editor of the *Lancet*; Fig. 3(c), Professor J. B. West, Professor C. T. Dollery and Dr. A. Naimark and the Editor of the *Journal of Applied Physiology*; Table 3, adapted from *Applied Respiratory Physiology* by Professor J. F. Nunn and published by Butterworth and Co.; Fig. 4, Dr. J. Panday and Professor J. F. Nunn and the Editor of *Anaesthesia*; Fig. 9, Dr. B. E. Marshall and the Editor of the *Journal of Applied Physiology*; Figs. 11 and 13, are adapted from two figures in *The Physiological Basis of Medical Practice* by C. H. Best and N. B. Taylor, published by Williams and Wilkins Co.; Fig. 14, from a *Textbook of Medical Physiology* by A. C. Guyton published by W. B. Saunders Co.; Fig. 15, from *The ABC of Acid-Base Chemistry* by H. W. Davenport published by the University of Chicago Press; Fig. 16, Professor T. C. Gray and John Sherratt and Son, publishers of the *British Journal of Anaesthesia*; Fig. 18, J. & A. Churchill Ltd.; Fig. 20, the Editor of the *Scandinavian Journal of Clinical and Laboratory Investigation*.

Chapter 4—Fig. 1, adapted from a figure in *The Physiological Basis of Medical Practice* by C. H. Best and N. B. Taylor, published by Williams and Wilkins Co.; Fig. 2, from a chapter by Group Captain J. Ernsting in *Oxygen Measurements in Biology and Medicine*, edited by Professor J. P.

Payne and Dr. D. W. Hill and published by Butterworth and Co.; Fig. 4, Bakelite Xylonite Ltd.; Fig. 5, Oxygenaire Ltd.

Chapter 5—Fig. 3, from Brown I. W., *et al.*; Hyperbaric Oxygenation (Hybaroxia): Current Status, Possibilities and Limitations. In: *Advances in Surgery*, Vol. I, ed. by Claude E. Welch and by permission of the Year Book Medical Publishers, Inc.,; Fig. 4, reproduced from an illustration in a chapter by the Rev. Edward Lanphier, M.D. and Dr. I. W. Brown in *Fundamentals of Hyperbaric Medicine*, and with the permission of the National Academy of Sciences; Figs. 5, 6 and 7, Vickers Ltd.; Figs. 8 and. 11, are reproduced from *The Physiology and Medicine of Diving and Compressed Air Work*, edited by P. B. Bennett and D. H. Elliott and published by Baillière Tindall; Fig. 9, Professor P. M. Winter and Dr. G. Smith and J. B. Lippincott Company, publisher of *Anesthesiology*; Fig. 10, reproduced from a chapter by Dr. B. Chance, Dr. Dana Jamieson and Dr. J. R. Williamson in *Proceedings of the Third International Conference on Hyperbaric Medicine*, edited by Dr. I. W. Brown, Jr. and Dr. Barbara G. Cox, and reproduced with the permission of the National Academy of Sciences; Fig. 12, is reproduced from a chapter by Rev. E. H. Lanphier M.D. in *Proceedings of the Underwater Physiology Symposium*, edited and reprinted with the permission of the National Academy of Sciences.

Chapter 6—Figs. 2 and 3, are reproduced from *Physics for the Anaesthetist* by Sir Robert Macintosh, Professor W. W. Mushin and Dr. H. G. Epstein, published by Blackwell Scientific Publications; Fig. 4, Dr. G. W. Black, Dr. L. McArdle, Dr. H. McCullough and Dr. V. K. N. Unni and the Editor of *Anaesthesia*; Fig. 5, is reproduced from *Trichlorethylene Anaesthesia* by Gordon Ostlere, published by E. & S. Livingstone Ltd.; Fig. 6(*a*) Cyprane Ltd.; Fig. 6(*b*) is reproduced from *Understanding Anesthesia Equipment* by Drs. J. A. and S. E. Dorsch, published by Williams and Wilkins Co.; Fig. 7, Dr. G. M. Paterson, Dr. G. H. Hulands and Professor J. F. Nunn and John Sherratt and Son, publishers of the *British Journal of Anaesthesia*.

Chapter 7—Figs. 3, 4, 5, 6, 12, 13, 14, 16 and 17 are reproduced from *Anesthetic Uptake and Action* by Dr. E. I. Eger II, and published by Williams and Wilkins Co.; Fig. 11, is based on a figure by Dr. J. G. Bourne and published in *Anaesthesia*.

Chapter 8—Figs. 2 and 3, the United States Bureau of Mines.

Chapter 9—Fig. 1, Dr. V. Goldman and Dr. P. W. Thompson and John Sherratt and Son, publishers of the *British Journal of Anaesthesia*; Fig. 2, Medical and Industrial Equipment Ltd.

Chapter 10—Fig. 1, Dr. M. H. Brook and the Editor of the *British Medical Journal*; Figs. 2 and 5, Medical and Industrial Equipment Ltd.; Fig. 3(*a*), British Oxygen Company Ltd.; Fig. 3(*b*), Ambu International; Fig. 4, The Laerdal Resusci Folding Bag is marketed by Vickers Limited Medical Engineering who kindly supplied the illustration; Figs. 6 and 7, Dr. W. H. Kelleher; Fig. 9, Portex Ltd.; Fig. 14, Mr. G. Kent Harrison; Fig. 16, Littlemore Engineering Co., Oxford.

Chapter 12—Fig. 9, Longworth Scientific Instrument Co. Ltd.; Fig. 10, Professor W. E. Spoerel and Dr. P. A. Grant and the Editor of the *Canadian Anaesthetists' Society Journal*; Fig. 24(*d*), British Oxygen Company.; Fig. 26, Professor T. C. Gray and the Editors of *Thorax*; Fig. 28, is adapted from a diagram in *Thoracic Surgery for Physiotherapists* by Miss G. M. Storey, published by Faber and Faber Ltd.

Section Two

Chapter 13—Figs. 1 and 10, are adapted from figures in *Principles of Clinical Electrocardiography* by Mervyn J. Goldman, published by Lange Medical Publications; Fig. 3, Dr. Peter Stock and the Editor of the *British Journal of Hospital Medicine*; Fig. 4, the Editor of the *British Medical Bulletin*; Fig. 9, is reproduced from *Unipolar Lead Electrocardiography and Vectorcardiography* by E. Goldberger, published by Lea and Febiger; Figs. 14 and 17, are adapted from *A Primer of Electrocardiography* by G. E. Burch and T. Winsor, published by Lea and Febiger; Fig. 16, reproduced from *Electrocardiography* by M. Bernrieter, published by J. B. Lippincott Co.; Fig. 18, is reproduced from *Applied Physiology* by Samson Wright, published by Oxford Medical Publications.

Chapter 14—Fig. 9(*a*), is adapted from an illustration in *The Lung* by J. H. Comroe, Jr., R. E. Forster II, A. B. Dubois, W. A. Briscoe and E. Carlson, published by the Year Book Medical Publishers, Inc.; Fig. 11, Dr. I. C. W. English, Dr. R. M. Frew, Dr. J. F. Pigott, Dr. M. Zaki and the Editor of *Anaesthesia*.

Chapter 16—Figs. 1, 2, 3, 4, 5, 6, 7 and 9, Dr. J. S. Fleming, Mr. M. V. Braimbridge and Blackwell Scientific Publications; Fig. 8, Dr. G. Melrose and Honeywell Controls Ltd.

Chapter 19—Fig. 1, is adapted from a figure in a paper by Dr. M. A. Hayes, published in the *New England Journal of Medicine*; Tables 3 and 4, Dr. G. Dobb.

Section Three

Chapter 21—Fig. 4 is adapted from a figure previously printed in the *British Journal of Pharmacology*; Fig. 7, Professor W. D. M. Paton and the Honorary Editors of the *Proceedings of the Royal Society of Medicine*; Fig. 8, is adapted from a table in a paper by N. F. Paxson published in *Anesthesia and Analgesia, Current Researches*.

Chapter 22—Fig. 2, Dr. T. H. Gawley and the Editor of the *British Medical Journal*.

Chapter 24—Figs. 2 and 4(*a*) and (*b*), Professor Sir Bernard Katz and the Editors of the *Journal of Physiology*; Fig. 3, the Editors of the *Journal of Biophysical and Biochemical Cytology* and the Pergamon Press Ltd.; Fig. 5, Professor W. D. M. Paton and Dr. D. R. Waud and the Cambridge University Press, publishers of the *Journal of Physiology*; Fig. 6, the Honorary Editors of the *Proceedings of the Royal Society of Medicine*; Figs 8(*a*) and (*b*), Dr. S. Page and the Editor of the *British Medical Bulletin*; Fig. 9, Dr. P. Furniss and the Honorary Editors of the *Proceedings of the Royal Society of Medicine*; Fig. 12(*b*), Dr. C. Collier and the Honorary Editors of the *Proceedings of the Royal Society of Medicine*.

Chapter 25—Figs. 7, 9, 10, 11, 15 and 16, Dr. C. L. Hewer and J. & A. Churchill Ltd.; Fig. 13, Drs. H. H. Ali, R. S. Wilson, J. J. Savarese and R. J. Kitz and Macmillan Journals Ltd., publishers of the *British Journal of Anaesthesia*; Fig. 18, the Honorary Editors of the *Proceedings of the Royal Society of Medicine*; Figs. 20(*a*) and (*b*), Dr. V. A. Goat, Dr. M. L. Yeung, Dr. C. Blakeney and Dr. S. A. Feldman and Macmillan Journals Ltd., publishers of the *British Journal of Anaesthesia*; Figs. 23(*a*) and (*b*) Drs. E. N. Cohen, H. W. Brewer, D. Smith and J. B. Lippincott Company, the publishers of *Anesthesiology*; Fig. 24, the Editors and publisher, J. B. Lippincott Company, of *Anesthesiology*.

Chapter 26—Figs. 1, 13 and 15, Dr. E. N. Cohen, Dr. N. Hood and Dr. R. Golling and the Editors and publisher, J. B. Lippincott Company, of *Anesthesiology*; Fig. 3, Dr. H. H. Birch and the Editor of the *Journal of the American Medical Association*; Fig. 4, Professor G. A. Gronert and Professor R. A. Theye and the Editors and publisher, J. B. Lippincott Company, of *Anesthesiology*; Fig. 5, Professor J. Crul; Fig. 9, the Editors and publisher, J. B. Lippincott Company, of *Anesthesiology*; Fig. 14, Dr. S. A. Feldman and the Editors and publisher, J. B. Lippincott Company, of *Anesthesiology*.

Chapter 28—Fig. 2, Professor D. Elmquist, Drs. W. W. Hofman, J. Kugelburg and D. M. J. Quastel and the Editors of the *Journal of Physiology*; Fig. 6, is reproduced from a chapter by Dr. E. H. Lambert in *Myasthenia Gravis*, courtesy of Charles C. Thomas, publisher.

Chapter 29—Fig. 3, Professor P. R. Bromage and the Honorary Editors of the *Proceedings of the Royal Society of Medicine*; Appendix, is reprinted with the kind permission of the Editor of the *British Medical Journal*.

Chapter 30—Figs. 1 and 6, Dr. E. H. Burrows and the Wessex Neurological Centre; Fig. 7, the late Dr. Christine John; Fig. 8, Sir Wylie McKissock and the Editor of the *British Medical Journal*.

Chapter 31—Fig. 1, Dr. C. L. Hewer and A. K. Hawkins & Co. Ltd.

Chapter 32—Fig. 1, Charles C. Thomas, publisher; Fig. 3, Dr. J. C. White and the Williams and Wilkins Company; Fig. 4, Professor R. Melzack and Professor P. D. Wall.

Chapter 33—Figs. 2 and 3, are redrawn from originals in *Regional Block* by D. C. Moore, published by Charles C. Thomas; Fig. 5, from *Functional Neuroanatomy*, edited by N. B. Everett and published by Lea and Febiger.

Chapter 34—Fig. 2, Dr. P. R. Bromage and the Editor and publisher, Macmillan Journals Ltd., of the *British Journal of Anaesthesia*; Fig. 3, Dr. L. Ekblom and Dr. B. Widman and the Editors of *Acta Anaesthesiologica Scandinavica*.

Chapter 35—Figs. 1, 2 and 3, are reproduced from *Anatomy for the Anaesthetist* by Professor H. Ellis and Miss M. McLarty published by Blackwell Scientific Publications.

Chapter 36—Fig. 2, is adapted from an illustration in *A Method of Anatomy: Descriptive and Deductive*, by J. C. Boileau Grant, published by the Williams and Wilkins Co.; Fig. 7(*a*) is from *Lumbar Puncture and Spinal Analgesia* by Professor Sir Robert Macintosh and Dr. J. Alfred Lee and published by Churchill Livingstone; Fig. 7(*b*), Professor Sir Robert Macintosh and Dr. R. Bryce Smith and E. & S. Livingstone; Fig. 9, Lloyd-Luke (Medical Books) Ltd.

Section Four

Chapter 37—Parts of the section on regurgitation and vomiting are reprinted from articles by Dr. H. J. V. Morton and one of us, and are published here by kind permission of Dr. Morton and the Editor of *Anaesthesia*. Other parts are based on an article by one of us in the *British Journal of Anaesthesia* and are reproduced by kind permission of John Sherratt and Son, publishers of this journal.

Chapter 38—Tables 1 and 2, Professor A. P. Waterson and Macmillan Journals Ltd., publishers of the *British Journal of Anaesthesia*.

Chapter 39—Professor H. E. de Wardener, author of *The Kidney*, and published by Churchill Livingstone.

Section Five

Chapter 40—Figs. 1 and 2, are adapted from figures in a chapter by Drs. J. J. Brown, A. F. Lever and J. I. S. Robinson, in *Recent Advances in Medicine* (15th edit.) by kind permission of J. & A. Churchill Ltd.

Section Six

Chapter 41—Figs. 1 and 4, Lloyd-Luke (Medical Books) Ltd.; Fig. 5, from a chapter by Dr. E. H. G. Hon in *Principles and Practice of Obstetric Analgesia and Anesthesia*, edited by Dr. J. J. Bonica and published by F. A. Davis Company.

Chapter 42—Figs. 2, 3 and 4, British Oxygen Company Ltd.; Fig. 5, Medical and Industrial Equipment Ltd.; Figs. 6 and 7, Cyprane Ltd.; Fig. 8, first published in *Anaesthesia* and reproduced with the permission of the Editor.

Chapter 43—Table 1, H.M. Stationery Office; Fig. 1, Lloyd-Luke (Medical Books) Ltd.; Figs. 2 (*a*) and (*b*) and 6, Professor M. G. Kerr, Dr. D. B. Scott and Dr. E. Samuel and the Editor of the *British Medical Journal*; Figs. 3 and 5, Drs. M. M. Lees, D. B. Scott, M. G. Kerr and S. H. Taylor and Blackwell Scientific Publications Ltd., publishers of *Clinical Science*; Fig. 4, Dr. D. B. Scott and John Sherratt and Son Ltd., publishers of the *British Journal of Anaesthesia*.

Chapter 44—Fig. 1, is an adaptation of a figure in *The Physiology of the Newborn Infant* by C. A. Smith, published by Blackwell Scientific Publications Ltd.; Fig. 2, Drs. G. Levinson, S. M. Shnider, A. A. Lorimer and J. L. Steffenson and the Editor and publisher, J. B. Lippincott Company, of *Anesthesiology*.

Chapter 45—Fig. 1, Professor G. V. R. Born, Dr. G. S. Dawes and the Editor of *Cold Spring Harbor Symposia on Quantitative Biology*; Fig. 5, H. G. East and Co. Ltd. of Oxford; Figs. 8(*a*) and (*b*), Dr. H. B. Sandiford; Fig. 10, Dr. G. J. Rees.

Section Seven

Chapter 46—Figs. 1, 5, 9, 10, 18 and 19, are from *The Development of Anaesthetic Apparatus*, by Dr. K. Bryn Thomas and published by Blackwell Scientific Publications; Fig. 2, Dr. B. Duncum and the Editor of the *British Medical Bulletin*; Figs. 3(*a*) and (*b*) and 8, are taken from Dr. John Snow's book on *The Inhalation of the Vapour of Ether*; Figs. 6, 11(*a*) and (*b*), Dr. H. G. Epstein and the Editor of the *British Medical Bulletin*; Fig. 7, British Oxygen Company Ltd.; Fig. 14, from *Essays on the First Hundred Years of Anaesthesia* by W. Stanley Sykes and published by E. & S. Livingstone Ltd.

Appendices

Appendix I—Table 1, reproduced from *The Sterilisation of Plastics*, Portex Ltd.

CONTENTS

Section Two—THE CARDIOVASCULAR SYSTEM

Section Three—THE NERVOUS SYSTEM

Section Four—THE METABOLIC, DIGESTIVE AND EXCRETORY SYSTEMS

Section Five—THE ENDOCRINE SYSTEM

Section Six—THE REPRODUCTIVE SYSTEM

Section Seven—HISTORY

APPENDICES

Section One

THE RESPIRATORY SYSTEM

Chapter 1

STRUCTURE AND FUNCTION OF THE RESPIRATORY TRACT IN RELATION TO ANAESTHESIA

THE NOSE

Functions

The nose has five important functions to perform:—

1. The adult patient breathes through his nose, unless there is some form of obstruction caused, for example, by nasal polypi or a severe catarrhal condition. In normal subjects the resistance created by breathing through the nose is $1\frac{1}{2}$ times greater than mouth breathing. Deflection of the nasal septum may diminish the lumen of the respiratory airway and in some cases it is sufficiently severe to prevent the passage of all but the smallest of endotracheal tubes. Before attempting nasal intubation it is advisable to test the patency of each nostril in turn by listening for the sound that indicates a free flow of air. The side where the obstruction is greatest anteriorly (due to deflection of the nasal septum) often proves the easiest to intubate. One of the disadvantages of nasal intubation as compared with the oral route it that in adults it usually necessitates using an endotracheal tube of small diameter.

2. The stiff hairs in the anterior part of the nasal fossa together with the spongy mucous membrane and the ciliated epithelium comprise a powerful defence against the invasion of any organism. In reserve lie the flushing action of the watery secretions, the bactericidal properties of these secretions, and the extensive lymph drainage of the whole area.

3. Warming and humidifying the inspired air or gases is probably the most important work the nose performs. The enormity of the task can only be realised if it is recalled that 10,000 litres of air pass through every twenty-four hours. The great vascularity of the mucosa helps to maintain a constant temperature: inspired air at 17° C is heated to approximately 37° C during its passage through the nose and variations in external air temperature ranging from 25–0° C produce less than 1° C change in the temperature of air reaching the laryngeal inlet.

The supply of moisture comes partly from transudations of fluid through the mucosal epithelium and to a lesser extent from secretions of glands and goblet cells in the nasal mucous membrane. The daily volume of nasal secretions is about 1 litre, of which about three-quarters is utilised in saturating the inspired air.

The optimum relative humidity of air is 45–55 per cent but the bronchi and alveoli require 95 per cent for adequate function. As a result of endotracheal intubation, or after tracheostomy, only relatively dry gases or air reach the lower part of the trachea, thus compelling the mucosa in this area to perform the duties of the nasal mucous membrane. Although in time the mucosa can adapt itself to the changed conditions, to begin with it becomes dry, and the absence of moisture, even for a few minutes, leads to a cessation of ciliary activity. When adaptation is slow there may be degeneration of the mucosal cells. Endotracheal anaesthesia is in fact frequently followed by a mild tracheitis; this incidence is accentuated when gases, which have had almost all their moisture removed before storage in cylinders, are used in an anaesthetic system that has a relatively low humidity. Even the nasal inhalation of dry gas can be dangerous if it is prolonged, and when oxygen therapy is ordered the gas should always be humidified.

4. Vocal resonance is influenced by the patency of the nasal passages.

5. The nose detects smells.

The blood supply to the nasal mucosa is controlled by an elaborate autonomic reflex which enables the mucosa to swell or shrink on demand. There is a dual nerve supply to this area. Parasympathetic fibres pass via the facial, greater superficial petrosal and vidian nerves to relay in the sphenopalatine ganglion. Sympathetic fibres reach the ganglion from the plexus surrounding the internal carotid artery, via the vidian nerve.

The sensory nerve supply to the nasal mucosa is derived from the first and second divisions of the trigeminal nerve. The anterior third of both the septum and the lateral wall are supplied by the anterior ethmoidal branch of the nasociliary nerve (first division) and the posterior two-thirds by the nasopalatine nerves via the sphenopalatine ganglion (second division). For operations on the nasal septum local analgesia can be produced either by topical analgesia or by blocking the maxillary and anterior ethmoidal nerves on both sides.

In animals a notable reflex from this area is that known as the "Kratschmer" reflex in which stimulation of the anterior part of the nasal septum leads to constriction of the bronchioles. When a patient's nose is plugged with gauze after a nasal operation, intense restlessness often occurs during the recovery period even though the oral airway is adequate and there is no pain. This situation is frequently encountered in adolescents who have had a fractured nasal septum remodelled. It suggests a reflex from the nasal mucous membrane.

CILIARY ACTIVITY

Throughout the respiratory tract the continuous activity of the cilia is probably the most important single factor in the prevention of the accumulation of secretions. In the nose the flow of material is swept towards the pharynx, whereas in the bronchial tree the flow is carried towards the entrance to the larynx.

Each cilia consists of a very fine hair-like structure approximately $7\mu m$ long and $0\cdot3\mu m$ thick, in which the tip is always bent towards the direction of the flow of mucus (Fig. 1). The co-ordinated movement of numerous cilia is capable of moving large quantities of material but their activity is greatly assisted by their mucous covering, which consists of two layers: an outer layer of thick viscous mucus which is designed to entrap particulate matter such as dust, soot, or micro-organisms, and an inner layer of thin serous fluid designed to lubricate the action of the ciliary mechanism. The tips of the cilia come just in contact with the outer layer with each beat. Acting in unison, they set the outer mucous layer in motion and with gathering momentum this flows towards the pharynx and larynx.

Ciliary movement consists of a rapid forward thrust followed by a slow recoil which occupies about four-fifths of the cycle. At 30° C the cilia of the nasal mucosa beat about 10–15 times per second. The streaming movement of

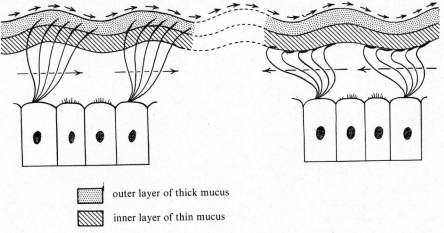

▦ outer layer of thick mucus

▨ inner layer of thin mucus

1/Fig. 1.—Ciliary movement.

the overlying mucus has been estimated at 0·25–1·0 centimetre per minute, the slowest speeds being in the bronchioles. The entire contents of the nose can thus be emptied into the pharynx every 20–30 minutes.

Factors Influencing Ciliary Activity

Temperature.—The optimum range of temperature for ciliary movement in excised human nasal mucosa is 28°–33° C, while the average nasal temperature is about 32° C. Ciliary activity ceases when the temperature of the mucosa falls to 7°–10° C and is depressed by temperatures rising above 35° C; however, only these extreme variations in temperature have much effect on ciliary action and any changes that do occur are largely caused by alterations in the amount of mucus secreted rather than by any direct influence on the ciliated epithelium.

Mucus.—Cilia cannot work without a blanket of mucus. Negus (1949) has compared their action to that of a conveyor belt system in which the platform on which the packages rest corresponds to the blanket of mucus and the propulsive force underneath is represented by the cilia. In all probability the volatile general anaesthetics not only slow the propelling mechanism but also limit the production of suitable secretions. If a patient has an inadequate secretion of mucus after the use of atropine, or breathes dry gases for a long period, then evaporation will result in drying of the mucosa and ciliary activity will cease.

Changes in pH.—Cilia prefer a dilute alkaline solution and are readily paralysed by acid solutions with a pH of 6·4 or less. A rise of pH to 8·0 or more leads to swelling of the columnar cells bearing the cilia and thus to depression of their activity.

Sleep.—Natural sleep has little effect on ciliary activity and even several hours after death the cilia may still be found moving.

Drugs.—In low concentrations all volatile general anaesthetic agents stimulate ciliary activity, but in high concentrations they are directly depressant. Nitrous oxide has no effect on ciliary activity. The opiates have a direct depressant action, whereas atropine weakens ciliary activity only indirectly by altering the viscosity of the secreted mucus.

1/TABLE 1
EFFECTS OF VARIOUS AGENTS ON CILIARY ACTIVITY

Drugs		Low concentrations	High concentrations
Nitrous oxide		0	0
Ether		+	− −
Chloroform		+	− −
Cyclopropane		+	− −
Morphia		−	− −
Atropine		−	− −
Cocaine	10 per cent		− − −
,,	5 per cent		− −
,,	2½ per cent	+	
Ephedrine	½ per cent	+	
Adrenaline	(1 : 10,000)	− − −	

− = inhibition of ciliary movement.   0 = no effect on ciliary movement.
+ = stimulation of ciliary movement.

Posture.—Gravity appears to have no effect on ciliary action and the flow always continues in the same direction whatever the patient's position.

ANAESTHESIA AND HUMIDITY

Importance of humidity.—The importance of humidifying the inspired gases is well-known to all those responsible for the management of patients on intermittent positive-pressure respiration. The anaesthetised patient undergoing a routine operation usually breathes virtually dry gases for long periods of time. With an artificial airway in position the gases tend to flow through the mouth so that the functions of the nose are largely short-circuited, while with an endotracheal tube, the whole role of providing adequate humidification falls on the lower respiratory tract. This situation may influence the incidence of tracheitis, bronchitis and pulmonary collapse in the post-operative period.

Physical principles.—The quantity of water needed to saturate air with water vapour increases with the temperature (Fig. 2).

Thus, the warmer the air becomes the more vapour it can hold. For example, if warm air is breathed out on to the surface of a mirror (at room temperature) then this air is cooled and can no longer hold so much water vapour, consequently the water vapour condenses on the glass. On the other hand, if a mirror is warmed to body temperature or above (as in indirect laryngoscopy) then condensation does not occur.

At a room temperature of 17° C the air contains 2 volumes per cent of water when fully saturated. At a body temperature of 37° C the air in the trachea contains 6 volumes per cent of water vapour. The nose and respiratory tract, therefore, not only have the task of warming the inspired air but also of adding large

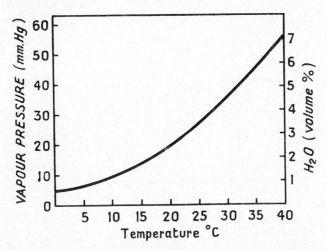

1/Fig. 2.—The relationship of water vapour tension in air to temperature.

quantities of water vapour. The value of this mechanism is appreciated to the full by anyone who runs rapidly on a cold, dry morning. The increased inhalation of air through the mouth leads to drying of the tracheal mucous membrane and an uncomfortable "soreness" in the chest.

Anaesthetic Apparatus

In most anaesthetic systems the temperature of the gases reaching the patient is approximately the same as the room temperature. This is because the gases are cooled or warmed during their passage through a long length of flexible rubber breathing tubing. The principal exception to this rule is in the to-and-fro' system where the temperature of the cannister (near the patient's mouth) may rise to as high as 45° C and in which no time is available for the cooling of gases en route to the patient. This system, therefore, provides very efficient humidification but it has other disadvantages (see p. 117).

Two other principal types of anaesthetic system should be considered:

(a) The non-rebreathing valve system (Fig. 3).

The inspired air is always at room temperature (17° C) and therefore even if fully saturated it can only hold about 2 volumes per cent of water. Because there is no rebreathing the expired air (at 37° C and fully saturated) passes out through the valve and is lost to the atmosphere.

In this type of system anaesthetic gases are usually supplied direct from source without passing through a humidifier, and therefore are completely dry.

(b) The circle absorption system.

Here the inspired mixture consists not only of fresh dry gases but also of

some expired gases containing water vapour at room temperature. The latter
leave the patient at body temperature, but by the time they have traversed the
apparatus they will have cooled to room temperature and so have lost the major
part of their water content in the apparatus. Dry fresh gas is also added to the
system.

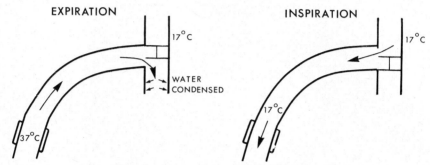

1/Fig. 3.—The non-rebreathing valve system.

Approximate values for the humidity of gases using various anaesthetic
systems are shown in Table 2.

1/Table 2

The Relative Humidity of Gases in the Various Anaesthetic Systems

Anaesthetic system	Percentage humidity of gases
Non-rebreathing valve	0
T-piece	0
To and fro'	40–100
Closed circle	40–60
Human nose	100

Effect of Premedication, Intubation and Dry Gases

Burton (1962) studied the effects of premedication, the endotracheal tube,
and dry anaesthetic gases on ciliary activity by observing the movement of an
ink marker placed at the carina of anaesthetised dogs. Under pentobarbitone
anaesthesia alone the ink passed up the trachea and out through the vocal cords
within 20–30 minutes.

After atropine premedication, the rate of movement of the ink was slowed
to 10 cm in 30 minutes and normal movement was not resumed for some 4–5
hours. The endotracheal tube by itself had little untoward action if the gases
were humidified, but the inflation of a cuff immediately produced a complete
barrier to the passage of the marker ink. Dry anaesthetic gases, as delivered
direct from a cylinder, produced gross reduction in ciliary movement. Thus,
after 4½ hours anaesthesia using a Rubens non-rebreathing valve the maximal
movement of the marker was only 2·5 cm in 30 minutes.

It is hardly surprising, therefore, that after a prolonged period of anaesthesia the mucosa of the trachea and lower respiratory tract shows evidence of dryness and an inflammatory reaction.

The whole process may be summarised as follows:

$$\left.\begin{array}{c}\text{Atropine}\\+\\\text{Dry gas}\end{array}\right\} \to \text{Dry mucosa} \to \text{Inflammatory reaction} \to \text{Excessive mucus}$$

$$\text{Tracheitis} \qquad \text{? Pulmonary collapse}$$
$$\&$$
$$\text{Bronchitis}$$

Methods of Humidification

1. **Direct installation.**—Normal saline can be administered by direct instillation into an endotracheal tube or tracheostomy. Though not used much these days as a method of humidification in adults the method is still useful in the management of nasotracheal tubes in babies and children, and in adults may be effective in aiding the removal of plugs of dried mucus during long-term intubation.

2. **Water-bath.**—The gas mixture is passed across the surface of a heated, thermostatically controlled, water-bath. This may be used in conjunction with an artificial ventilator, when the humidifier must be placed on the inspiratory side of the system, and the gases led to the patient by the shortest possible route. The tubing should be insulated to prevent heat loss, with consequent condensation. By raising the temperature in the humidifier slightly above body temperature it is possible to deliver gases to the patient which are at 37° C and completely saturated with water vapour. The exact temperature setting of the water-bath will depend on the surface area of water exposed to the gases, the flow rate of these gases and the amount of cooling and condensation taking place in the inspiratory tubing. Sterility of the water in the humidifier is greatly aided if the temperature is maintained at 60° C.

This type of humidifier, when combined with a fan to blow air through it, can be used to humidify a tracheostomy. The attachment to the tracheostomy is of a T-piece design which allows the moistened air to flow freely across the opening. The weight of the tubing can be a serious disadvantage to the patient.

3. **Moisture exchanger.**—The heat and moisture exchanger offers a light and moderately efficient method of humidification for a patient breathing spontaneously through a tracheostomy or endotracheal tube. The modern version consists of a replaceable condenser that can be taken out and cleaned (Fig. 4). As it is at a lower temperature than the body, part of the water vapour of expiration is condensed on its inner surface where it is available to humidify the inspired air. It cannot, of course, achieve full saturation owing to the lower temperature. Nevertheless such a device can considerably improve the humidity of inspired air, especially if this already contains a little water vapour. Two problems are encountered with the use of an "artificial nose". First is colonisation by bacteria and the other is increasing airway resistance as the condenser becomes moisturised. These disadvantages can largely be overcome if the condenser unit is changeable and sterilisable.

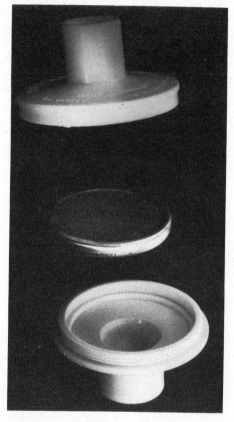

1/FIG. 4.—Artificial nose with replaceable heat and moisture exchanger. The central metal filter can be removed, sterilised and replaced.

4. **Mechanical nebuliser.**—This is a pneumatic device which breaks up a liquid into small particles. Water, when placed in the nebuliser passes up a capillary tube at the summit of which it is nebulised by a jet of gas. The droplet leaving the capillary tube then crashes into the side of a ball where it is fractured into numerous small particles. Most particles of 5 microns and above cling to the ball, coalesce, and fall back into the reservoir. Those particles of 4 microns or less tend to float out and join the inspired gases. In this type of nebuliser 80 per cent of the particles are in the range 2–4 microns and the remainder are smaller. Most of these particles are deposited around the pharynx, and only a small percentage reach the bronchial level, but for many patients this is sufficient. Because it is compact this nebuliser can conveniently be placed in close proximity to the patient's airway (Fig. 5). It can also be used pre- or post-operatively with a face mask for the improvement of lung function, or it can be attached directly to a tracheostomy tube.

5. **Ultrasonic nebuliser.**—All the methods so far described have various disadvantages, and they may interfere with ventilator treatment.

In 1964 Herzog and his colleagues introduced to clinical practice an ultrasonic nebuliser consisting of a plexiglass container to hold 150 ml of fluid and with a vibrating transducer head at its base. The transducer head is activated by

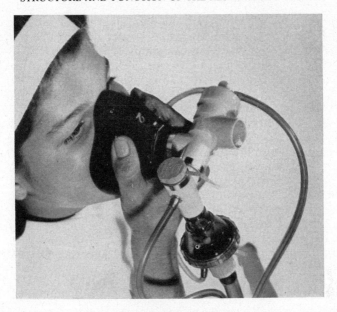

1/Fig. 5.—Mechanical nebuliser (Bird).

a high-frequency (3 MHz) generator and is fed with drops of fluid by a capillary tube which passes through the top of the container. The nebuliser should be connected to the inspiratory side of a ventilator (Fig. 6).

Each drop of fluid is completely nebulised to an aerosol in which 70 per cent of the particles have a size of 0·8 to 1 micron, the actual size being dependent on the frequency of the transducer head. Most particles of 1 micron or less are deposited in the lower airways and alveoli of the lungs. At the maximum rate

1/Fig. 6.—Diagram of an ultra-sonic nebuliser (Herzog *et al.*, 1964).

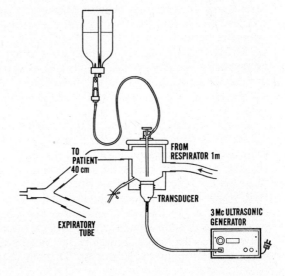

of 12 drops per minute dripping on to the transducer head and with a ventilator delivering 10 litres of gas per minute, 72 mg water are provided with each litre of gas. This corresponds to a relative humidity of 164 per cent at 37° C.

Ultrasonic nebulisers produce satisfactory humidification in patients who have very dry airways at the start of treatment (e.g. children with tracheobronchitis) and they can be used for the administration of water-soluble aerosol drugs, but they are not without dangers. Their extreme efficiency makes overhydration possible, especially in children, and they are difficult to sterilise by conventional methods. Ringrose and his colleagues (1968) have described how outbreaks of infection can follow inadequate cleaning of ultrasonic nebulisers. When used for a long time continuously on the same patient an ultrasonic nebuliser will increase the airway resistance (Cheney and Butler, 1968), and may cause pulmonary collapse (Modell et al., 1968).

Variations on the design of Herzog's nebuliser are in production, their main difference being the frequency of the transducer head and hence an alteration in the size of the particles of fluid produced.

An ultrasonic nebuliser can be used to sterilise a ventilator by producing an aerosol of alcohol (Spencer et al., 1968).

PHARYNX

The pharynx extends from the posterior aspect of the nose at the base of the skull down to the level of the lower border of the cricoid cartilage where it becomes continuous with the oesophagus, and the respiratory tract through the larynx. The soft palate partially divides the pharynx into two—an upper nasopharyngeal portion and a lower orolaryngeal portion.

In the nasopharyngeal part a collection of lymphoid tissue—the nasopharyngeal tonsil or "adenoids"— lies embedded in the mucous membrane at the junction of the roof with the upper and posterior part of the pharynx. Lying close to the base of the nasopharyngeal tonsil is a small recess—the pharyngeal bursa. These structures often impede the passage of an endotracheal tube; if force is used the tube may penetrate the mucosa and create a false passage which can lead to trouble from sepsis and collection of secretions during the postoperative period.

The lymph drainage of the pharynx is often of clinical importance because enlargement of the lymphatic glands and swelling of the overlying mucosa may, in some instances, lead to partial obstruction of the airway. These lymph glands are numerous and are arranged in a circular fashion—the ring of Waldeyer (Fig. 7).

In essence the ring consists of the large palatine tonsils (P) lying between the pillars of the fauces; the smaller lingual tonsil (L) at the base of the tongue on each side of the middle line and in front of the vallecula, the Eustachian tonsil (E) which is an accumulation of lymphoid follicles sometimes found on the posterior lip of the orifice of the Eustachian tube, and the nasopharyngeal tonsil (NP) which is a group of follicles united in one mass on the posterior wall of the nasopharynx. On the posterior wall of the pharynx at the level of the large palatine tonsils some small lymph nodes are often found. These are of particular importance when sepsis occurs in this neighbourhood because they swell up to form a retropharyngeal abscess. This may occur either in conjunction with sepsis tracking inwards from the spinal column or with a peritonsillar abscess ("quinsy"). The presence of a large retropharyngeal abscess makes nasal intubation extremely difficult and dangerous because the endotracheal tube may be deflected sharply forwards or it may impinge on and rupture the abscess.

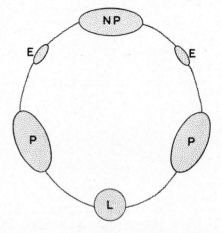

1/FIG. 7.—PHARYNGEAL AND TONSILLAR
       GLANDS (RING OF WALDEYER)

P = Palatine tonsil.
L = Lingual tonsil.
E = Eustachian tonsil.
NP = Nasopharyngeal tonsil or "adenoids".

Pharyngeal obstruction and the airway.—One of the principal duties of an anaesthetist is to learn the art of maintaining a completely unobstructed airway in an unconscious patient. The introduction of endotracheal intubation enables the lazy anaesthetist to circumvent this duty. Nevertheless, the fact that intubation may lead to a sore throat, infection, or—rarely—laryngeal lesions is a reason why it should only be used when indicated.

The principal difficulty in maintaining a perfect airway in an unconscious patient is the tendency of the tongue to fall backwards and obstruct the laryngeal opening. This occurs as soon as consciousness is lost and the muscles supporting the tongue start to relax. If the tongue is brought forward then the laryngeal opening once again is cleared.

Various manoeuvres may be used to attain this object.

1. The head should be extended (Fig. 8). In the supine unconscious subject flexion of the neck, such as occurs when the head is resting naturally on a pillow, is almost invariably associated with respiratory obstruction. The simple manoeuvre of extending the neck will clear the airway in about 75 per cent of cases by causing a forward movement of the mandible, to which the tongue is attached, and by stretching the anterior tissues of the neck, rather like straightening a washing line.

2. Extension of the neck causes the mouth to fall open due to the downward pull of the neck tissues. Simply closing the mouth will often improve the airway by straightening the tissues of the neck still further.

3. If the airway is still not perfect the mandible can be drawn forward by placing the fingers behind the angles of the jaw and exerting a forward pressure.

4. An oropharyngeal airway can be inserted. In neonates and infants a satisfactory airway is most often achieved if the mouth is allowed to fall open

because the tongue is relatively large in this age group and closing the mouth tends to push the soft palate against the posterior wall of the nasopharynx and to obstruct the nasal airway.

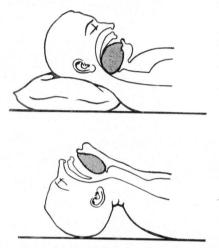

1/FIG. 8.—Maintenance of a clear airway.

An unconscious patient is safest in the lateral position. Unless there is a specific surgical contra-indication, an unconscious patient following anaesthesia should be nursed on his side. In this position the tongue tends to fall away from the posterior pharyngeal wall and foreign material is less likely to enter the larynx.

LARYNX

The larynx lies at the levels of the 3rd–6th cervical vertebrae and comprises a number of articulated cartilages surrounding the upper end of the trachea (Fig. 9.). The laryngeal cavity extends from the inlet at the top to the lower level of the cricoid cartilage below, where it becomes continuous with the trachea. The inlet is bounded anteriorly by the upper edge of the epiglottis, posteriorly by a sheath of mucous membrane stretched between the two arytenoid cartilages, and on each side by the free edge of a fold of mucous membrane—the aryepiglottic fold—which joins the apex of the arytenoid cartilage to the side of the epiglottis. When this fold is viewed down a laryngoscope the underlying cartilages protrude through the mucous membrane, making a ridge which appears to form the entrance to the larynx on each side. These projections are formed posteriorly by the arytenoid cartilages with the corniculate cartilages lying in close proximity; anteriorly the cuneiform cartilages can be seen.

The next structures in the laryngeal cavity are the vestibular folds which run on either side as narrow bands of fibrous tissue passing from the antero-lateral surface of the arytenoid cartilages to the angle of the thyroid cartilage at the point of attachment of the epiglottis. These folds are usually called the false vocal cords and are separated from the true vocal cords which lie below by the laryngeal sinus.

The vocal cords are two pearly-white folds of mucous membrane stretching from the angle of the thyroid cartilage to the vocal processes of the arytenoid cartilages. Beneath their outer lining of stratified squamous epithelium lies the tough fibrous vocal ligament. Since there is no true submucosa with the usual network of blood vessels, the vocal cords have a characteristic pale appearance.

In the adult the narrowest part of the laryngeal cavity is the area between the vocal cords, whereas in children under about ten years of age it is just below the vocal cords at the cricoid ring. The clinical significance of this anatomical difference is to be found when small children are intubated, since an endotracheal tube which can pass between the vocal cords may yet be too large to pass beyond the cricoid ring.

Movements of the Vocal Cords

It is not intended to give a detailed description of the actions of the intrinsic muscles but certain brief details of the laryngeal mechanism may be recalled. In each case the focal point of movement is the arytenoid cartilages which rotate and slide up and down on the sloping shoulders of the cricoid cartilage.

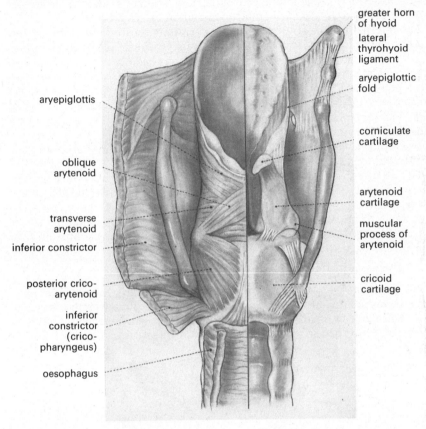

1/FIG. 9.—The larynx, showing muscles and cartilages.

The muscles concerned are most conveniently thought of as pairs having opposing actions controlling three parts of the larynx:

First, the laryngeal inlet which is closed by the aryepiglottic and opened by the thyro-epiglottic muscles.

Secondly, the rima glottidis which is dilated by the posterior crico-arytenoid muscles assisted by the lateral crico-arytenoid muscle, and is closed by the inter-arytenoid muscles which approximate the arytenoids without rotation.

Thirdly, those acting on the vocal cords—the cricothyroid muscles which lengthen the vocal cords and the thyro-arytenoid muscles which shorten them.

The tension of the vocal cords is altered by the vocales, which are a part of the thyro-arytenoid muscles.

Nerve Supply to the Larynx

The mucous membrane receives its nerve supply from both the superior and recurrent laryngeal nerves. The superior laryngeal nerve arises from the inferior ganglion of the vagus but receives a small branch from the superior cervical sympathetic ganglion. This nerve descends in the lateral wall of the pharynx, passing posteriorly to the internal carotid artery, and at the level of the greater horn of the hyoid divides into an internal and an external branch.

The internal laryngeal branch, which is entirely sensory apart from a few motor filaments to the arytenoid muscles, descends to the thyrohyoid membrane, pierces it above the superior laryngeal artery and then divides again into two branches. The upper branch supplies the mucous membrane of the lower part of the pharynx, epiglottis, vallecula and vestibule of the larynx. The lower branch passes medial to the pyriform fossa beneath the mucous membrane and supplies the aryepiglottic fold and the mucous membrane of the posterior part of the rima glottidis.

The external laryngeal branch carries motor fibres which innervate the cricothyroid muscle.

The recurrent laryngeal nerve accompanies the laryngeal branch of the inferior thyroid artery and travels upwards, deep to the lower border of the inferior constrictor muscle of the pharynx immediately behind the cricothyroid joint. Apart from sensory fibres which supply the mucous membrane of the larynx below the level of the vocal cords, this nerve innervates all the muscles of the larynx except the cricothyroid, and a small part of the arytenoid muscles.

Cord Palsies

The cords can be visualised either indirectly by means of a mirror or—and this is the more familiar method for the anaesthetist—directly with a laryngoscope. This description of normal and abnormal cord movements is, therefore, written and illustrated from the point of view of direct laryngoscopy.

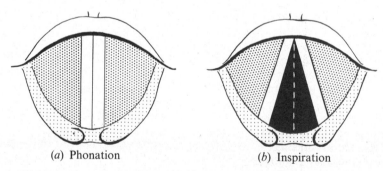

(a) Phonation   (b) Inspiration

1/Fig. 10.—The vocal cords.

During phonation the vocal cords meet in the mid-line (Fig. 10a). On inspiration they abduct (Fig. 10b), returning to the mid-line on expiration, but leaving a small gap between them. The opening into the trachea between the vocal cords is maximal at the end of a deep inspiration. In order, therefore, to minimise the risk of any possible trauma to the cords, intubation and extubation should be carried out during inspiration. When laryngeal spasm is present, both the false and the true cords are held tightly in apposition.

Topical analgesia of the throat and larynx blocks the sensory nerve endings of the superior and recurrent laryngeal nerves. Following this procedure, an occasional patient is unable to phonate clearly and develops a "gruff" voice—an effect which is probably due to some local analgesic solution reaching and blocking the external branch of the superior laryngeal nerve. This nerve carries motor fibres to the cricothyroid muscle, which is the principal tensor of the cords. Paralysis of the cricothyroid muscle produces visible alterations in the shape of the glottis and vocal cords—effects that must be remembered should they follow topical analgesia for diagnostic laryngoscopy. The superior laryngeal nerve itself may be traumatised during thyroidectomy when the superior thyroid artery is tied. Since the only motor fibres of the nerve are those that run on into its external branch, exactly similar effects to those just described will follow.

Damage to the recurrent laryngeal nerve may take the form of complete section or merely bruising. This nerve carries both the abductor and the adductor motor fibres of the vocal cords. The abductor fibres, however, are more vulnerable so that moderate trauma usually leads to a pure abductor paralysis. Severe trauma or section of the recurrent laryngeal nerve causes both abductor and adductor paralysis. A pure adductor paralysis does not occur as a clinical entity.

It is not always easy to differentiate between the various types of cord palsy but the main points are illustrated diagrammatically below. Unilateral lesions are assumed to exist on a patient's left side. The position of the cords during both phonation and inspiration is diagnostic.

Pure abductor palsy—left.—On phonation both cords meet in the mid-line because the adductor fibres on the left (damaged) side are still active. It will be noticed, however, that the right false cord tends to lie slightly anterior to that on the left (Fig. 11a). On inspiration the cord on the side of the injury remains in approximately the same position, but the cord on the unaffected side moves into full abduction (Fig. 11b).

Abductor and adductor palsy—left.—In this case both types of fibre are no longer functioning on the left, so that the cord tends to rest in a slightly more abducted position. On phonation, the right cord crosses the mid-line in an attempt to meet its opposite number (Fig. 12a). As it is forced to move in the arc of a circle, the right false cord appears to lie in front of the left. On inspiration, the unaffected cord moves back again into full abduction (Fig. 12b).

Bilateral damage to the recurrent laryngeal nerves.—This may occur during removal of the thyroid gland. The position of the vocal cords will depend upon the severity of the damage.

When the trauma is mild on both sides, then a bilateral abductor paralysis may result. Severe trauma, or complete section, on both sides affects both abductor and adductor fibres. It is important to differentiate between these two conditions because they have differing effects on the laryngeal airway. After partial damage the vocal cords lie near the mid-line because the adductor fibres are still functioning, and the airway is reduced to a mere chink (Fig. 13a). A patient in this condition usually rapidly shows signs of severe respiratory

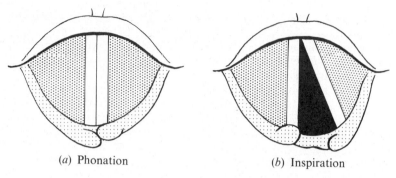

(a) Phonation   (b) Inspiration

1/Fig. 11.—Pure abductor palsy—Left.

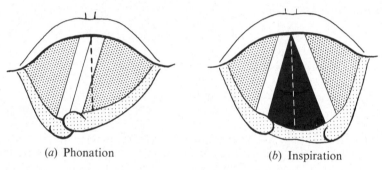

(a) Phonation   (b) Inspiration

1/Fig. 12.—Abductor and adductor palsy—Left.

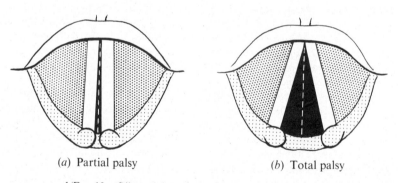

(a) Partial palsy   (b) Total palsy

1/Fig. 13.—Bilateral damage to the recurrent laryngeal nerve.

1/Fig. 14.—Bilateral palsy of the recurrent laryngeal nerves with palsy of the external branch of the superior laryngeal nerve.

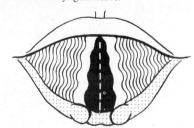

obstruction, particularly when respiration is active due to fear or other causes. When both nerves are severely damaged, or cut across, the vocal cords lie stationary in the mid position with a fair-sized lumen between them (Fig. 13b). Now, the airway is fairly adequate unless respiratory effort is very marked, when the cords tend to be sucked in with each inspiration.

Bilateral palsy of the recurrent laryngeal nerves with palsy of the external branch of the superior laryngeal nerve.—Total paralysis of the cords is now associated with paralysis of the cricothyroid muscles. The vocal cords are no longer tensed and the antero-posterior diameter of the glottis is reduced. This is the true cadaveric position. With complete relaxation, such as may be obtained by one of the muscle relaxants, exactly the same position is seen (Fig. 14).

Laryngeal Trauma and Oedema

Trauma to the larynx during intubation of the trachea may lead to oedema (particularly in small children) and to a granuloma of the cords at a later date.

TRACHEA AND BRONCHIAL TREE (Figs. 16 and 17)

The trachea is a tube formed of rings of cartilage which are incomplete posteriorly. It is about 10–11 cm long, extending downwards from the lower part of the larynx opposite the level of the 6th cervical vertebra to the point of its bifurcation into a right and left main bronchus at the carina, about the upper border of the 5th thoracic vertebra. It is lined by ciliated columnar epithelium.

The trachea moves with respiration and with alterations in the position of the head. Thus on deep inspiration the carina can descend as much as 2·5 cm. Extension of the head and neck—the ideal position in which to maintain an airway in an anaesthetised patient—can increase the length of the trachea by as much as 23 to 30 per cent. Clinically, if a patient is intubated with the head in a flexed position at the atlanto-occipital joint, and the endotracheal tube is so short that it just reaches beyond the vocal cords, the subsequent hyperextension of the head may withdraw the tube into the pharynx.

A variety of names has been given to the divisions of the bronchial tree and this has for many years past been a constant source of confusion. In 1948 an international committee agreed on a generally acceptable nomenclature which is shown in diagrammatic and schematic form in Fig. 16 and Table 3. In the description that follows the English nomenclature will be used throughout.

Right Bronchial Tree

The *right main bronchus* is wider and shorter than the left, being only 2·5 cm long. As it is more nearly vertical than the left main bronchus there is a much greater tendency for either endotracheal tubes or suction catheters to enter this lumen. In small children under the age of three years the angulation of the two main bronchi at the carina is equal on both sides (Fig. 15). In the event of an endotracheal tube being inserted too far a further complication is that the bevel-led end of the tube (as usually cut) may become blocked off by its lying against the mucosa on the medial wall of the main bronchus. The short length of this bronchus also makes the lumen difficult to occlude when this is required in thoracic anaesthesia.

The right main bronchus gives off branches to the upper and middle lobes before becoming continuous with the lower lobe bronchus.

The *right upper lobe bronchus* passes in an upward and lateral direction at 90° to the right main bronchus for 1 cm before dividing into its three main divisions.

The apical bronchus runs upwards with a lateral inclination and after about 1 cm usually gives off a lateral branch and then almost immediately divides into anterior and posterior branches.

The posterior bronchus runs in a backward, lateral, and slightly upward direction. After about 0·5–1·0 cm it gives off an important lateral branch and then ends by dividing into superior and inferior divisions.

The anterior bronchus runs in a downward, forward and slightly lateral direction. Soon after its origin it also gives off a lateral branch.

Each of these bronchi supplies a segment of the upper lobe. The posterior segment of the upper lobe, together with the apical segment of the lower lobe,

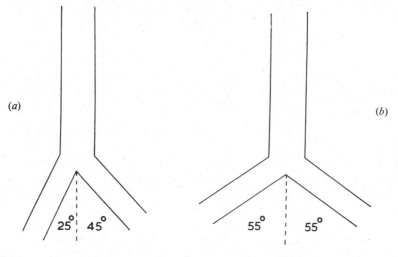

(a)   (b)

1/Fig. 15.—Angle of the Main Bronchi. (After Bush, 1963)
(a) In the adult.   (b) In children.

is one of the common sites for the development of a lung abscess. When a patient is lying wholly or partly on his side, inhaled material tends to gravitate into the lateral portion of the posterior segment of the upper lobe—particularly on the right side (Fig. 18a). Alternatively, if the patient lies on his back the material accumulates in the apical segment of the lower lobe (Fig. 18b). The incidence of lung abscess is nearly twice as high in the upper lobes as in the lower ones. Surgery offers some of the most favourable conditions for aspiration of infected material, since if the anaesthetised patient is placed on his side either during or after operation then the upper lobe bronchus acts as the most dependent drain. The accumulation of secretions here, together with an inadequate cough reflex, results in an area of pulmonary collapse which may later suppurate to form a lung abscess. Although the posterior segment of the upper lobe is the commonest to be involved, it is the most difficult segment to examine radiographically or

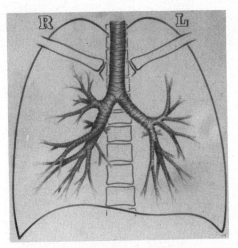

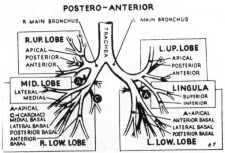

POSTERO-ANTERIOR

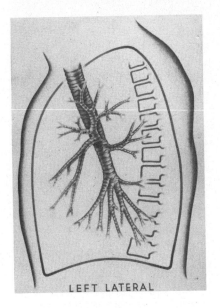

LEFT LATERAL

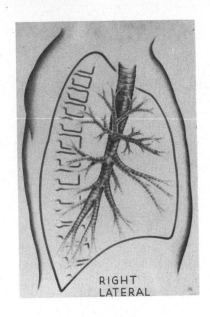

RIGHT LATERAL

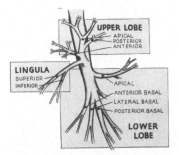

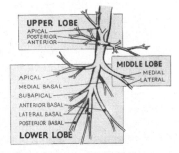

1/Fig. 16

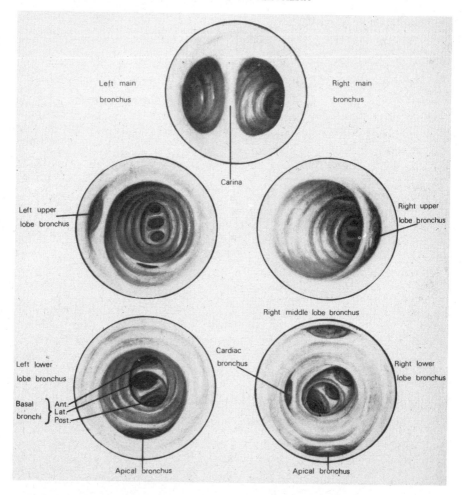

1/Fig. 17.—The normal bronchial tree as seen down a bronchoscope.

clinically, because being situated in the upper part of the axilla, it is almost completely hidden by the scapula.

In an attempt to avoid this complication the following measures may be used. (*a*) The main bronchi, trachea and nasopharynx should be cleared of mucus by suction at the end of a long operation; (*b*) the patient should be placed in the lateral position with a slight head down tilt after operation, thus encouraging mucus to flow into the pharynx rather than accumulate in a lobe of a lung. Frequent changes from side to side should be made in the early post-operative period; (*c*) the anaesthetic technique chosen should be such that the patient has an adequate cough reflex soon after the surgery has ended. On recovery of consciousness he should be urged to cough.

The *right middle lobe bronchus* springs from the anterior aspect of the right bronchus about 3 cm from its origin. It arises just above the apical branch of the right lower lobe. After 1–1·5 cm the middle lobe bronchus divides into lateral and medial branches. The medial branch runs downwards and forwards with a convex curve following the contour of the right side of the heart. The patency of the middle lobe bronchus is particularly vulnerable to glandular swelling because it is closely related to the right tracheobronchial groups of glands.

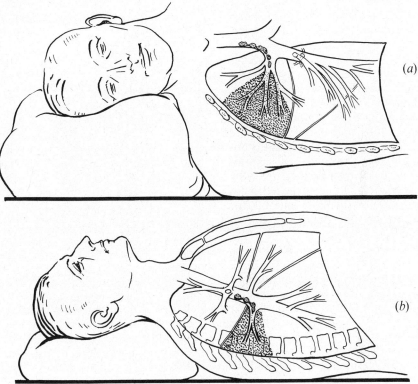

1/Fig. 18.—Diagrams to Illustrate the Relationship between Posture and the Focal Incidence of Lung Abscess

(a) Patient lying on side: inhaled material collects in posterior segment of right upper lobe.
(b) Patient lying on back: inhaled material collects in apical segment of right lower lobe.

The *right lower lobe bronchus* is the continuation of the right main bronchus and has five, or occasionally six, divisions. The apical branch comes off 0·5–1·0 cm below the origin of the middle lobe but slightly more laterally (Fig. 16). About 1·5 cm below the apical bronchus the cardiac or medial basal branch arises from the medial side of the lower lobe stem and passes downwards for 2·5 cm before dividing into its two terminal branches—anterior and posterior. Sometimes there is a subapical branch which comes off the posterior wall of the main bronchus just below the cardiac branch. After giving off these branches the main stem divides into the basal bronchi—the anterior, lateral and posterior branches—to supply the appropriate segments.

The apical segment of either of the lower lobes is particularly vulnerable to inhaled material when the patient lies supine (Fig. 18b), and the right and left sides provide an approximately similar incidence of lung abscess. When a patient is propped up in bed in the post-operative period, secretions tend to gravitate to the lower lobes (Fig. 19).

Left Bronchial Tree

The *left main bronchus* is narrower than the right and is nearly 5 cm long. It terminates at the origin of the upper lobe bronchus becoming the main stem to the lower lobe. It should be noted that this is in direct contrast to the right lung, where the branches to the upper lobe and middle lobes are offshoots of the parent main bronchus. The presence of 5 cm of bronchial lumen uninterrupted by any branching makes the left main bronchus particularly suitable for intubation and "blocking" during thoracic surgery.

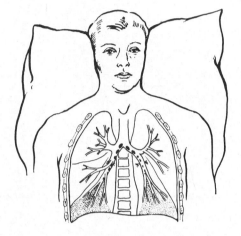

1/Fig. 19.—Figure to show the accumulation of secretions in the lower lobes of a patient in the sitting position.

The *left upper lobe bronchus* is unlike that of the right upper lobe, for it does not arise as an offshoot of the left main bronchus but as one part of the bifurcation of the main trunk. After its origin it begins to curve rapidly to the lateral side. The angle that it forms when visualised from within the main bronchial lumen often makes it possible to insert in it a very small bronchial blocker. The upper lobe bronchus continues for 1–1·5 cm before bifurcating into an upper and a lower division. The upper division curves upwards in line with the main stem bronchus before dividing into apical, posterior and anterior branches. The lower division descends as the *lingular bronchus*.

The *left lower lobe bronchus* arises as a continuation of the left main bronchus and runs in a downward, backward and lateral direction. About 1 cm below its origin it gives off the apical branch from its posterior wall. This branch is important because, when the patient is lying on his back, inhaled material tends to flow through it into the apical segment of the lower lobe. The apical branch runs backwards as a short stem before dividing into three branches.

Sometimes, the left lower lobe bronchus gives off a subapical branch from its posterior wall about 1–1·5 cm below the origin of the apical branch before finally dividing into its main terminations—the basal bronchi. The anterior basal branch arises from the antero-lateral aspect of the lower lobe stem and runs downwards, forwards and slightly laterally. About 1 cm below its origin it may give off a small branch from its medial side which corresponds to the cardiac bronchus on the right side. The lateral basal bronchus runs in a downward and lateral direction. The posterior basal bronchus is the largest of three and sometimes appears as a continuation of the main stem running downwards, backwards and slightly laterally.

All three basal bronchi may give off lateral branches soon after their origin. These branches are often found to play an important part in the surgical anatomy of lung abscess.

Bronchioles

Before the introduction of the new nomenclatures shown in Table 3 considerable confusion existed in any description of this area.

1/TABLE 3

B.N.A.	English
Bronchioli	Bronchiole (incl. terminal bronchiole)
Bronchioli Respiratorii	Respiratory bronchiole
Ductuli Alveolares	Alveolar ducts; alveolar passages
Atria	Atria
Sacculi Alveolares	Air sacs
Alveoli Pulmonum	Air cells

As a bronchiole is traced distally the cartilaginous rings gradually recede, forming irregular plates which occur sporadically until the diameter of the bronchiole is approximately 0·6 mm, when they disappear completely. Continuing the progress down the bronchial tree the tubular outline of the bronchiole wall changes and small projections in increasing numbers appear on all sides. This area is now termed a respiratory bronchiole and the small projections are alveolar ducts leading to the air sacs (Fig. 20). The name "terminal bronchiole" has arisen in the English nomenclature and usually denotes that area of the bronchiole not containing cartilage which lies just before the origin of the respiratory bronchiole.

The Bronchial and Bronchiolar Musculature

As long ago as 1822 Reisseissen, using a small hand-lens, dissected fresh material to show that a muscle-layer could be traced down to the finer bronchioles. So great was his contribution to the anatomy of the lung that later investigators often refer to the bronchial musculature as the "muscle of Reisseissen."

The fundamental purpose of this muscle is to permit alterations in the length and width of the bronchial tube with the various phases of respiration. The particular arrangement of the muscle fibres is of great importance, for the muscle-pattern is best described as a "geodesic network" (a geodesic line on any curved surface is the one of shortest distance between two points, e.g. an arc of a great circle on a sphere). A geodesic pattern, therefore, is the ideal method of withstanding or producing pressures in a tubular structure without there being a tendency for the fibres to slip along the surface (Fig. 21).

As the muscle layer is followed down the bronchial tree so it becomes thinner, but the relative thickness of this layer in relation to that of the wall as a whole increases. Thus in a bronchiole of 1 mm diameter the muscle bands are relatively five times as strong as in a bronchus of 10 mm. The terminal bronchiole, which has the narrowest lumen, has therefore relatively the thickest muscle layer.

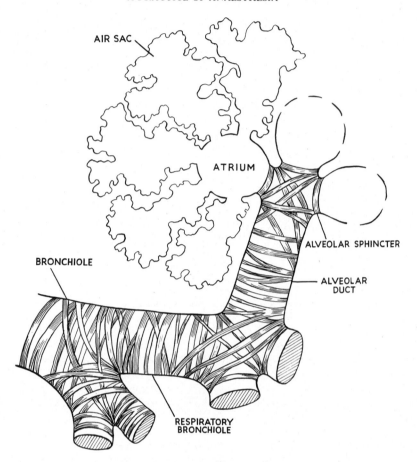

1/Fig. 20.—Diagram of alveoli and bronchiole.

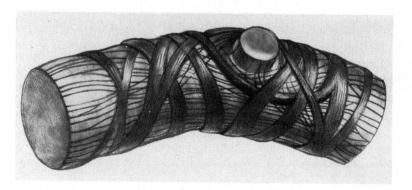

1/Fig. 21.—Diagram to show the geodesic arrangement of the musculature in a bronchiole.

Elastic fibres run lengthwise between the mucosal and muscle layers. In general their course is longitudinal, but at the points where branching of the bronchioles occur the fibres swing over and encircle each branch as it leaves (Fig. 21). Since the smooth muscle fibres also undergo this arrangement the origin of each branch is reinforced by a series of interlacing fibres. So close is the admixture of elastic and muscle fibres that some authorities refer to this layer as a "myo-elastic layer".

Bronchial and Bronchiolar Epithelium

The trachea down to the beginning of the respiratory bronchiole is lined by ciliated columnar epithelium freely interspersed with goblet cells lying on an intermediate layer of spindle-shaped cells; these are derived from the basal cells with round nuclei found in the deepest layer. In the lower part of the bronchial tree the ciliated cells far outnumber the other forms, but at the beginning of the respiratory bronchiole they give way to a cuboidal cell without any cilia.

Bronchial Vessels

There are usually three bronchial arteries, one for the right and two for the left lung, each taking its origin from the ventral side of the aorta, although occasionally they arise as a common trunk.

On entering the lung the bronchial arteries embed themselves in the layer of connective tissue surrounding the bronchus. Usually two or three branches of the bronchial artery run with the larger bronchi and bronchioli until finally each bronchial subdivision is accompanied by a corresponding division of the artery. In this manner the arteries continue until the distal end of the terminal bronchiole is reached.

Anastomotic branches from the bronchial artery pierce the outer fibrous coat of the bronchi and form an arterial plexus in the adventitia around the muscle layer. From this outer arterial plexus, branches pierce the muscle layer to enter the submucosa. The vessels run for a short distance parallel with the muscle fibres before splitting up into a fine capillary plexus which supplies the mucous membrane. From this capillary network venous radicles arise which in their turn pierce the muscle layer to reach a venous plexus in the outer adventitia. From this second plexus veins arise and form one of the sources of the pulmonary vein. It is evident, therefore, that an arterial and venous plexus lies on the outside of the muscle layers, whilst a capillary plexus lies on the inside (Fig. 22). A point of great importance is that blood must pass through the muscle layer in its passage between the various plexuses.

Therefore, when the muscle layer contracts, it is probable that whilst the arterial plexus with its higher pressure can maintain a flow to the capillary plexus, the latter is unable to empty into the outer venous plexus. This must lead to swelling of the mucosa with a further narrowing of the lumen.

When the respiratory bronchiole is reached the bronchial arteries disappear as a distinct set of vessels. The internal capillary plexus, however, fuses with that of the pulmonary artery in the walls of the alveoli. It appears that the pulmonary artery supplies the respiratory bronchiole in a similar manner to the bronchial artery supplying the terminal bronchiole.

True bronchial veins are only seen at the hilum of the lung and do not play a significant part in the venous drainage of the bronchioles. They arise at the level of the first divisions of the main bronchial tree and usually drain into the azygos, hemi-azygos and intercostal veins. The pulmonary vein arises from the venous plexus in the terminal bronchiole wall, from that in the wall of the respiratory bronchiole down to and including the alveoli, and finally from the plexus underlying the pleura.

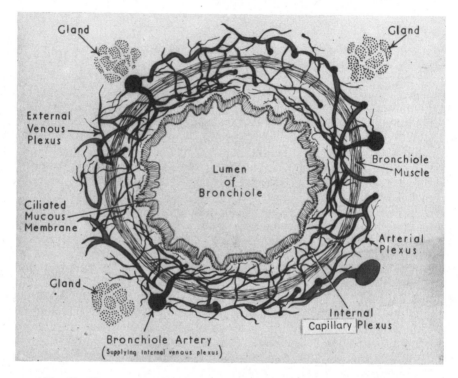

1/Fig. 22.—Diagrammatic Representation of the Blood Supply of a Respiratory Bronchiole.

Below the ciliated mucous membrane lies a capillary plexus. The arterial supply reaches it by piercing the muscle layer. Venous drainage also has to pass back through this muscle layer.

Innervation of the Bronchial Tree

The lung receives innervation from both sympathetic and parasympathetic sources. The sympathetic nerve fibres are derived from the 1st–5th thoracic ganglia along with branches from the inferior cervical ganglion, though some fibres may also be received from the middle cervical ganglion. The vagus nerve supplies the parasympathetic fibres, joining with the sympathetic fibres to form the posterior pulmonary plexus at the root of the lung. Fibres from this plexus pass round the root of the lung to form the anterior pulmonary plexus.

The posterior pulmonary plexus divides into a peri-arterial and peri-bronchial plexus. The latter again divides into an extrachondrial and intra-chondrial plexus in relation to cartilaginous plates in the bronchial wall. On reaching the non-cartilaginous parts of the lung the two plexuses again unite and continue distally as one. Ganglia are to be found at all levels of the bronchial tree so that short post-ganglionic fibres reach the bands of smooth muscle in which they break up into individual fibres. These fibres give off twigs to supply the individual smooth muscle fibres of the geodesic network and, at the distal end of the alveolar duct, delicate motor terminals pass to the muscle fibres of the sphincter at the atrial openings.

In all probability the mucous glands are innervated solely by the vagus. As regards the nervous control of the vessel walls, recent evidence suggests that the vagus carries cholinergic dilator fibres whilst the thoraco-lumbar nerves carry predominantly adrenergic constrictor fibres to the bronchial arterial system.

Control of Bronchial Calibre

The bronchi dilate and retract passively with each phase of respiration. On inspiration the pressure in the air ducts is greater than that in the pleural cavity—consequently the bronchi are dilated by the pull of the negative intrapleural pressure. As the lung expands, therefore, the bronchial tree is dilated and lengthened, and as it diminishes in size the bronchi shorten and contract due to the retraction of the elastic tissue in their walls. In man, it is known that most sympathomimetic drugs produce bronchial relaxation whilst cholinergic drugs lead to constriction.

Bronchomotor Tone

Bronchomotor tone is a continuous and variable state of contraction of the bronchial musculature which is present during both phases of respiration. In the dog, section of the sympathetic nerves has no effect on bronchial calibre, while vagal section produces considerable alterations. In fact, bilateral vagal section results in the bronchi opening more widely during inspiration and narrowing to a greater degree than normal during expiration. These facts strongly suggest that it is predominantly the vagi that carry impulses influencing the diameter of the bronchial lumen and that they are responsible for normal bronchial tone.

Apart from the vagi, there is evidence that the baroceptors in the carotid sinus and aortic arch, together with reflexes from other vasosensory areas, play an important role in this matter. Thus—in dogs under chloralose anaesthesia—a severe and rapid haemorrhage leading to a fall in blood pressure to 40 mm Hg (5·3 kPa) will be accompanied by bronchodilatation. This will change to constriction as the pressure rises again (Daly and Schweitzer, 1952).

On the other hand the chemoreceptors do not appear to play any role in controlling bronchomotor tone and their inactivation leaves the bronchial lumen unaffected in size. Carbon dioxide does, however, play some part in the maintenance of normal tone, but probably through an entirely central effect. Perfusion of a dog's brain with blood containing a high concentration of carbon dioxide causes bronchoconstriction but, when a low concentration is used, bronchodilatation follows (Daly et al., 1953). The role of oxygen is imperfectly understood, but hypoxia leads to bronchial dilatation.

Respiratory Tract Reflexes

Because of the immense difficulties involved, most of the studies of respiratory reflexes have been made in animals rather than in man, yet these reflexes play a significant role in the control of the respiratory and the cardiovascular systems. This subject is well reviewed by Widdicombe (1974 *a* and *b*).

(**a**) **Inflation.**—Hering and Breuer in 1868 showed that the inflation of the lungs inhibited the spontaneous contraction of the diaphragm in anaesthetised animals, and Adrian (1933) concluded that the pulmonary stretch receptors were responsible for this inflation reflex. These receptors are unencapsulated, and are found in the airway smooth muscle without end-organs. They are generally believed to be responsible for signalling changes in the mechanical state of the lungs to the brain.

Barbiturate anaesthesia depresses the inflation reflex, but only abolishes it completely with very high doses (May and Widdicombe, 1954).

A weak inflation reflex has been demonstrated in man, but it may be absent in the anaesthetised subject (Widdicombe, 1961). It may be responsible for the apnoea produced on inflation of the newborn baby's lung, though this response only persists for the first few days of life.

(**b**) **Deflation.**—During expiration the tonic discharge of the stretch receptors diminishes so that soon inspiration can start again. Nevertheless, there is evidence that a deflation reflex exists in its own right; the receptors are sited differently in that they lie principally in the alveoli and terminal bronchioles. Sensitisation of these receptors leads to an increase in the rate and force of the inspiratory effort and its role may be designed primarily to protect the individual by increasing ventilation in the event of pulmonary collapse. Paintal (1964) has shown that these receptors are stimulated by inhalational anaesthetics.

(**c**) **Paradoxical reflex.**—This reflex was described by Head in 1889 and can only be demonstrated when the vagus nerve is *partially* blocked. Inflation of the lungs under this condition leads to a strong diaphragmatic contraction. It does not occur if the vagus nerve is intact or completely blocked, and because it is the opposite response of the normal inflation reflex it has been termed "paradoxical". This reflex may account for the primitive gasp observed in newborn babies when the lungs are first inflated (Cross, 1961).

(**d**) **Irritant receptors.**—Afferent nerve endings responding to both mechanical and chemical irritants have been described lying in the epithelium of the airways from the trachea to the respiratory bronchioles. They are concentrated mainly at the carina and at the points of branching of the bronchial tree. These nerve endings are excited by particulate matter and are paralysed by ether and local analgesic sprays (Widdicombe *et al.*, 1962).

Aspiration of fluid, whether it be fresh-water, sea-water, or vomit with a hydrochloric acid content, always leads to reflex closure of the glottis and bronchoconstriction. Animal experiments have demonstrated that even after both vagi have been sectioned atropine, neostigmine and isopropyl-noradrenaline are all capable of influencing the bronchial response (Colebatch and Halmagyi, 1962). This suggests that aspiration of fluid invokes a reflex response of the parasympathetic nervous system, but there is not only a central component acting via the vagus nerve, but also a peripheral fraction which is intrinsic within the bronchial wall.

(**e**) **J-receptors.**—J-receptors (or juxta-pulmonary capillary receptors) lie in the walls of the alveoli and possibly of the smaller airways. Like the other lung receptors their afferent pathway is vagal. They are stimulated by pulmonary congestion and oedema, pneumonia, some irritants (including halothane) and emboli. The chief effect of their stimulation is tachypnoea, but there is some evidence that bronchoconstriction and contraction of the adductor muscles of the larynx are also produced.

1/TABLE 4

SUBSTANCES INFLUENCING BRONCHIAL SMOOTH MUSCLE TONE

Bronchodilatation

1. β_2 Sympathomimetics.	Salbutamol, isoprenaline, adrenaline, ephedrine.
2. Xanthine derivatives.	Aminophylline.
3. Volatile anaesthetics.	Halothane, diethyl ether.
4. Nitrites.	Amyl nitrite, glyceryl trinitrate.
5. Prostaglandins E1 and E2.	Allergic response, infusion.
6. Muscarinic cholinergic receptor blockers.	Atropine, hyoscine.

Bronchoconstriction

1. Muscarinic cholinomimetics.	
(a) Anticholinesterases.	Neostigmine, pyridostigmine, physostigmine, edrophonium.
(b) Choline esters and alkaloids.	Carbachol, pilocarpine.
2. β_2 Adrenergic blockers.	Propranolol, etc.
3. Autacoids.	Histamine, 5-hydroxytryptamine, kinins, prostaglandin F2α.
	(a) Histamine-releasing drugs: *d*-tubocurarine, morphine, thiopentone.
	(b) Allergic response.
	(c) Carcinoid tumours.
	(d) Prostaglandin infusion.

The response to some of these agents may be minimal in the normal and enhanced in the presence of abnormal bronchial smooth muscle tone or in susceptible individuals, e.g. asthmatics.

Bronchospasm

This condition is occasionally encountered during anaesthesia. The term denotes spasm of the bronchi, but a better name would be bronchiolar spasm, as this is the area of the respiratory tree which is mainly involved. Stimulation can be initiated by chemical, mechanical or neurogenic methods. It is most commonly encountered in patients who have an "irritable" bronchial tree, i.e. chronic bronchitics. The constriction of the bronchiole is greater during expiration than inspiration. The unfortunate patient rapidly shows signs of respiratory embarrassment with his chest fixed in a position of inspiration, while an inspiratory and expiratory wheeze can be heard on auscultation. In anaesthetised patients, progressively increasing resistance to positive-pressure inspiration occurs, but before a presumptive diagnosis of bronchospasm is made it is essential to eliminate a mechanical obstruction of the airway due to kinking of an endotracheal tube or the presence of secretions. A tension pneumothorax can readily simulate severe bronchospasm, and Galloon and Rosen (1965) have shown how the use of a negative phase during intermittent positive pressure ventilation for patients with normal lungs may lead to bronchiolar narrowing and wheezing. Bronchospasm is a diagnosis that only should be made when all other causes of ventilatory difficulty have been excluded. The treatment of this condition is broadly the same as the treatment of an attack of asthma in an unanaesthetised patient (see p. 38).

THE ALVEOLI

The respiratory tree terminates at the alveoli, 15–20 of which arise from each air sac. Gas exchange occurs not only at alveolar level but also in the respiratory bronchioles, alveolar ducts and air sacs, so that from the functional aspect the exact anatomical differences between these structures are not of great importance. The average diameter of an alveolus is about 0·2 mm at functional residual capacity, though the size obviously varies with the state of inflation of the lung. It is also affected by gravity, the alveolar diameter being smallest within the most dependent parts of the lung and largest in the uppermost parts. This is due to the weight of the lung tissue itself compressing the lowermost alveoli, and has important functional implications.

Within the alveoli, blood and air are separated by a thin layer of tissue about 1–2 microns thick and which is built up of four layers:

(1) **Alveolar lining fluid.**—This is a very thin fluid layer lining the alveolar surface and which tends to collapse them due to surface tension effects. This surface tension is very much reduced by a lipoprotein contained in the fluid, termed "surfactant", so that alveolar collapse does not occur so readily.

(2) **Alveolar epithelium.**—Three types of cell have been described in this layer, and are designated by Roman numerals. Type I cells are the real alveolar lining. They consist of nuclei with thin cytoplasmic extensions which spread out to line the majority of the alveolar surface. Type II are cuboidal and their main feature is that their cytoplasm contains characteristic granules which consist of layers of osmophyllic material built up rather like the layers of an onion. The material is believed to be a phospholipid and these granules may give rise to surfactant. The evidence for this theory is mostly circumstantial, the most important fact being that these granules appear in the fetal lung at the same time as dipalmitoyl lecithin and about the same time as the fetus becomes viable. Dipalmitoyl lecithin is thought to be surfactant. Type III cells are very rare and are called alveolar brush cells. They resemble the brush cells found in the conducting airways, especially the trachea. Their function is unknown.

(3) **Interstitial layer.**—This is a very thin layer separating the alveolar epithelium and the capillary endothelium and about half of it consists only of the fused basement membranes of the capillary and alveolar lining cells.

(4) **Capillary endothelium.**—The alveolar septa between adjacent alveoli consist of mirror images of layers (1), (2) and (3) described above placed back-to-back with the capillary network inserted between them. The capillary network is dense and in places may form continuous sheets in the alveolar wall, although on average they underlie about 75 per cent of the alveolar surface. The spaces between adjacent alveolar lining layers and between adjacent capillaries are filled with interstitial tissue and contain elastic and collagen fibres, smooth muscle and nerves.

Collateral Ventilation

Kohn (1893) described the presence of fibrinous threads running through the walls of the alveoli in cases of lobar pneumonia but many investigators considered these pores were only artefacts occurring in a pathological state. More recently, however, the demonstration of collateral respiration has supplied confirmatory evidence of the normal presence of these pores. Adams in 1930 found that if the bronchus of a dog was permanently obstructed by painting the mucosa with silver nitrate, collapse of the distal pulmonary tissue only occurred when the main bronchus was occluded. Obstruction of a secondary bronchus was not followed by collapse. He concluded that there must be a communication between adjacent lobules at alveolar level. Since then collateral ventilation has been demonstrated and confirmed in man (Macklem, 1971), and may occur not only at alveolar level but also between small bronchioles and nearby alveoli, and even between slightly larger bronchioles. Recent evidence indicates that the pores of Kohn may close at the lower degrees of lung inflation and collateral ventilation therefore ceases.

Surfactant.—It was originally believed that retraction of the lungs during passive expiration was due entirely to their elastic tissue. However, Von Neergaard (1929) noted that when lungs were distended to peak capacity with air, the transpulmonary pressure was two to three times as great as when they were distended to the same volume with fluid. Because the only difference was the presence of an air-liquid interface in the air-filled lung, he concluded that up to two-thirds of the elastic recoil of the lung could be ascribed to surface forces. Mead *et al.* (1957) confirmed this, and also noted that the contribution of surface forces to the elastic recoil was less at low lung volumes. This was surprising in view of the formula of Laplace (an 18th century mathematician) which states that the pressure across a curved surface is equal to twice the surface tension at the air-liquid interface divided by the radius.

$$\text{Pressure} = \frac{2\,(\text{Surface Tension})}{\text{Radius}}$$

For the average alveolus, with its minute size, a very considerable pressure could thus be exerted by the fluid lining it; in fact, if pure water lined it, this pressure would equal 20,000 dynes per cm, or 20 cm of water.

Laplace's formula implies that as the alveoli decrease in size during expiration, the pressure tending to collapse them increases and a vicious circle is established. The fact that this does not happen must mean that the surface tension has, in some way, altered during expiration.

Measurement of surface tension.—The simplest method of measuring the surface tension of a liquid is with the aid of a Maxwell frame (Fig. 23). This is a U-shaped wire with the open end of the U closed by a cross-wire that can slide along the edges of the frame. A film of liquid placed in the frame tends to pull the cross-wire downwards so that the force necessary to resist this pull is a measure of surface tension. The surface tension of a liquid varies with temperature, that of pure water at 37° C being about 70 dynes per centimetre $(7 \times 10^{-2}\,\text{Nm}^{-1})$.

Clements (1962) used a surface balance that permitted the measurement of surface tension at different surface areas (which is not possible with the Maxwell frame). He studied washings of minced lungs, and found that a reduction of the surface area to 20 per cent was associated with a reduction in surface tension from about 40 dynes per cm (4×10^{-2} Nm^{-1}) to about 30 dynes per cm (3×10^{-2} Nm^{-1}). This is due to an increase in the concentration of surfactant on the surface of the fluid as the surface area is reduced. Within the lungs, therefore, the action of surfactant becomes more effective as the alveoli decrease in size. Ordinary biological fluids such as plasma show very little change in surface tension with change in area.

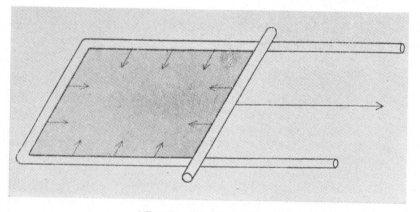

1/Fig. 23.—The Maxwell frame.

He concluded that the change in surface tension, as well as the ability to achieve a very low tension, was essential to the stability of the alveoli; in other words, the substance at the alveolar-air interface (surfactant) is a kind of anti-atelectasis factor.

Nature of surfactant.—Chemical analysis has shown that surfactant is a lipoprotein, which is a compound molecule made up of protein and fatty constituents. Only the phospholipid fraction is strongly active, the other constituents—neutral lipids and protein—playing no part. One particular phospholipid, namely dipalmitoyl lecithin, has been isolated from the lung fluid (Brown, 1962) and made synthetically. This is known to produce high surface activity and is probably the principal surface-acting material in human lung.

Production of surfactant.—Recent studies, particularly with the electron microscope, have demonstrated that the vacuolated alveolar lining cells contain peculiar osmophilic inclusions, and the evidence suggests that these inclusions are a storage site for surfactant. In addition the use of isotopically tagged glucose has indicated that these large vacuolated cells may also be the site of the synthesis of phospholipids, an important component of surfactant. Macklin (1954) postulated that the large alveolar cells were secretory, and he showed, on electron micrographs, osmophilic inclusions entering the airspace (Fig. 24). This process may be the way in which surfactant is secreted into the alveoli.

Clinical significance.—Absence of this material in the infant at birth is believed to be one of the primary causes of the"respiratory distress syndrome"

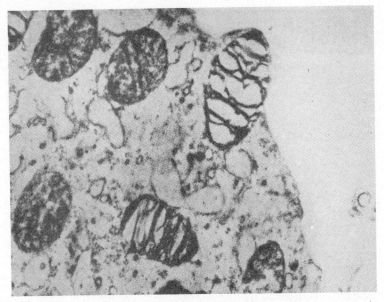

1/Fig. 24.—Osmophylic granules found in the Type II alveolar lining cells. One appears to be passing into the alveolar space.

(see p. 1418). Attempts have been made to aerosolise one component of the surfactant (dipalmitoyl lecithin) into the airways of infants with the syndrome but these have not proved of value.

Oxygen therapy may lead to a reduction in surfactant (Norlander, 1968), and hence it should be used in the lowest possible concentration, and for the shortest time, necessary to achieve the desired effect. Hill (1967) found that intermittent positive-pressure ventilation at normal pressures and volumes did not produce a fall in surfactant, but when abnormally high pressures were used there was a marked reduction, with consequent atelectasis.

Pulmonary collapse, whether occurring on its own or in association with a reduction in the pulmonary circulation—as from embolism or ligation (Chernick et al., 1966)—may well be associated with too little surfactant (see p. 38). Deficiency of it may also account for some of the respiratory difficulties that are encountered in patients who have been artificially perfused with a pump oxygenator (Tooley et al., 1961). Guest et al. (1966) investigating humans and dogs following such perfusion found an absent or decreased surfactant level in many cases. In the humans this was always associated with valve replacement procedures. Evidence of the action of anaesthetic drugs on surfactant is scanty. Nishimura and Metori (1967) examined the effects of halothane, methoxyflurane and ether on rabbits and humans. In the former they found there was definite evidence of increased surfactant action, but in the latter the changes were extremely variable. On balance they concluded that such agents will lower surface tension in clinically used concentrations.

1/TABLE 5
DIFFUSION RATES OF GASES RELATIVE TO OXYGEN (Cotes, 1968)

Substance	Molecular weight	Solubility at 37° C	Partition coefficient	Rate of diffusion
Oxygen	32	0·0239	5·0	1·00
Acetylene	26	0·749	—	34·8
Argon	40	0·0259	5·3	0·97
Carbon dioxide ..	44	0·567	1·6	20·3
Carbon monoxide ..	28	0·0184	—	0·83
Ethylene	28	0·0784	14·4	3·43
Helium	4	0·0085	1·7	1·01
Krypton	85*	0·0449	9·6	1·15
Nitrogen	28	0·0123	5·2	0·55
Nitrous oxide	44	0·388	3·2	13·9
Xenon	133*	0·085	20·0†	1·75

* Radioactive isotope.
† Fat-to-blood partition coefficient 8·0–9·8 : 1.

Pulmonary Collapse and Gas Absorption

The rate of absorption of gases in pulmonary collapse is affected by many factors. This probably explains the wide variations in the literature describing the time taken for the entrapped gases to become absorbed. Coryllos and Birnbaum (1928), working on dogs, reported that it took six hours for the lung to collapse after obstruction of the main bronchus, but others have reported, also in dogs with an open chest, an almost phenomenally rapid speed of gas absorption (Table 6).

1/TABLE 6

Carbon dioxide	..	1 min 6 seconds
Oxygen	.. ..	1 min 20 seconds
Nitrous oxide	..	1 min 42 seconds
Air ..	.. ..	9 min 21 seconds
Nitrogen	.. ..	12 min 6 seconds

(Lemmer and Rovenstine, 1935)

One lung is filled with 600 cc of the gas to be tested and the animal is respired on the other lung. The time taken for the lung to collapse to $\frac{7}{8}$ of its original size is recorded.

The rate of gas absorption can be varied more than 60-fold by alteration in the partial pressures of the blood gases as well as by changes in the initial gas composition. If the composition of the gases in the occluded lobe is analysed it will be found that a state of constant composition between the blood and alveolar gases is rapidly attained (Dale and Rahn, 1952).

In man there are no figures available but clinical observation suggests that such rapid rates of absorption are only applicable to the condition of the open chest. In the closed chest the negative intrapleural pressure opposes the elastic recoil of the lung and thus tends to retard the rate of collapse. During anaesthesia for thoracic surgery it is often necessary to occlude one of the main bronchi before commencing a thoracotomy. If the affected lung is filled with oxygen by hyperventilation prior to the introduction of the "blocker" it can be assumed that the entrapped gases contain a high percentage of oxygen, which will be rapidly absorbed, but at the moment of opening the chest twenty minutes or so later, no evidence of gross pulmonary collapse will be seen. Two to three minutes later partial collapse becomes evident and very quickly the whole process becomes complete. However, Nilsson *et al.* (1965) have shown that, in spite of an apparently total collapse obtained in such circumstances, the circulation is still partly maintained through the collapsed lung. This is shown by a marked reduction in the patient's systemic arterial oxygen tension which indicates a shunt of from 20 per cent to 40 per cent. When the branch of the pulmonary artery supplying the collapsed lung was clamped, there was an immediate rise in systemic arterial oxygen tension. Thus the occlusion of a main bronchus may impair the oxygenation of vital organs, and there is a case for clamping the supplying artery of the collapsed lung as soon as possible when this is feasible. Otherwise the inspired oxygen concentration should be maintained at as high a level as possible to compensate for the shunt.

The following factors are concerned in the rate of progress of pulmonary collapse:

Intrapleural pressure.—This opposes the elastic recoil of the lung and also any attempt on the part of the pulmonary tissue to reduce its volume. It is to a certain degree offset by movement of the mediastinum and falling-in of the surrounding soft tissues.

Position of the obstruction in the bronchial tree.—"Collateral respiration" makes it necessary for the obstruction to be present in the main bronchus.

Respiratory movements.—The abolition of the cough reflex and impairment of respiratory movements as in profound anaesthesia or in the presence of large abdominal tumours greatly accelerate the speed of pulmonary collapse.

Partial pressure of the entrapped gases.—Assuming that at the moment the block occurs the entrapped gases are in equilibrium with those in the blood stream, then the process begins by oxygen or some other rapidly diffusible gas —such as an anaesthetic agent—being taken up by the circulation. This is because the gas in the alveolus is at a higher partial pressure than that in the mixed venous blood returning to the lung. As the gas enters the circulation so the elastic tissue of the lung retracts to fill this hypothetical space and the total pressure of the retained gases thus remains the same. Each individual gas is, however, now at a slightly higher pressure than that in the circulation, so that the process is repeated again, and indeed repeatedly, until finally the alveolar walls are in apposition and the lung completely collapsed. The rate of collapse will be rapid if the lung is filled with oxygen and very slow if filled with nitrogen.

Several attempts have been made to reduce the incidence of post-operative atelectasis by ventilating the lungs with a gas of low solubility (such as air) at the end of anaesthesia, in order to wash out oxygen which, because of its rapid rate of absorption, has been thought to predispose to this condition. Results are conflicting, and different workers have reached diametrically opposite conclusions (Dery *et al.*, 1965; Stevens *et al.*, 1966).

Ciliary activity.—Little is known of the force that can be exerted by ciliary activity in man, but the isolated trachea and bronchi of the hen are capable of pushing a bolus of mucus towards the larynx with a propulsive force of 30 to 40 mm of water (0·4 kPa). Baetjer (1967) has shown that the rate of removal of mucus by cilia ranges from 7–17 mm per minute, being increased by ventilation with warm moist air (as occurs in a closed or semi-closed system), and decreased with cold, dry air (as occurs with a high-flow open system). If, therefore, a plug of mucus obstructs the lumen of a bronchiole, the affected area will rapidly become collapsed, but during this time the cilia in the region of the plug will constantly be trying to push the plug towards the larger bronchi, thereby creating a negative pressure in its wake which will increase the rate of the collapse.

Circulation through the collapsed lung.—Under normal conditions about half the output of the right side of the heart passes through each lung, and continues to do so for the first few hours after blockage of the main bronchus, provided the chest wall remains intact and the lung inflated. By twenty-four hours this flow of blood to the blocked lung has begun to diminish, and at the end of the first week it represents only a very small proportion of the output from the right heart. This circulation of blood is important since on it depends the absorption of gases from an affected lung. If the lung contains air, the oxygen is rapidly removed, leaving the nitrogen to be slowly absorbed. In this state the affected lung represents a large venous shunt, as nearly half the output of the right side of the heart is no longer oxygenated. The patient may develop cyanosis. When the pleural cavity is opened the lung collapses, the pulmonary circulation diminishes rapidly and the arterial saturation improves again. It is advisable, therefore, to attempt to wash out the nitrogen and replace it with oxygen before placing a "blocker" in the main bronchus.

Surface tension of the alveolar epithelium.—As explained on p. 33, the presence of surfactant is essential to prevent alveoli progressively collapsing as they periodically decrease in size during ventilation. A reduction in surfactant would, therefore, be a potent predisposing cause of pulmonary collapse. Imrie *et al.* (1966) described a case of acute massive collapse of one lung seen during thoracotomy. The lung was completely airless, like a lobe of the liver, which suggests a primary alveolar collapse rather than one secondary to an obstruction when some air-trapping would have taken place. Their patient suffered from a disordered pulmonary capillary circulation (known to affect the production of surfactant) which was probably made worse by surgical manipulation, thus accounting for the sudden massive collapse. Re-expansion of the lung was very slow and required inflation pressures far in excess of normal.

Ball-valve action.—If the obstruction in the bronchus is arranged in such a manner that the entrapped gases can partially escape with each expiration but no fresh gases can enter again on inspiration, the affected part of the lung will collapse rapidly.

ANAESTHESIA AND BRONCHIAL DISEASE

Asthma

Asthma is a condition characterised by attacks of bronchospasm often with a precipitating factor such as allergy—usually in the summer months, although a variety of allergens are commonly associated with an attack, such as house dust and domestic animals, or bronchial infections and concurrent chronic bronchitis. The cardinal symptoms are breathlessness and an expiratory wheeze though there may be inspiratory difficulty as well. Except when associated with chronic bronchitis the disease usually appears in attacks between which the sufferer is completely or relatively symptom free. The mainstays of treatment are avoidance of contact with precipitating factors and the use of broncho-dilator drugs when necessary. Aerosol preparations of isoprenaline or sal-butamol will often relieve the immediate distress of the patient. A tachycardia following systemic absorption of these drugs almost invariably occurs, but tolerance to this side-effect develops with continued use. The use of sympatho-mimetic drugs relieves a high Pco_2 caused by the decreased alveolar ventilation, but usually lowers the arterial Po_2 to some extent, due to changes in the ventila-tion-perfusion relationships in the lungs. The increase in the mortality of acute asthmatic attacks which followed the introduction of the isoprenaline inhaler was probably due to the isoprenaline increasing the irritability of the myo-cardium at the same time as causing a further reduction in Pao_2. Disodium cromoglycate (Intal) is often used in the prevention of allergic attacks of asthma. In severe and intractable cases the use of steroids may be the only method of affording relief.

Until recently, there has been no clear indication of just how commonly bronchospasm or asthma developed during routine anaesthesia. Shnider and Papper (1961), however, report that an incidence of wheezing of 6·5 per cent was found in a group of unselected patients with a clear chest pre-operatively. The only incriminating factor appeared to be endotracheal intubation. Regional analgesia in the conscious subject was associated with the same incidence of wheezing as general anaesthesia without endotracheal intubation. Simonsson et al. (1967) have found that the intravenous administration of atropine prior to irritation of the bronchial tree by a catheter or a chemical dust prevents bronchoconstriction in patients with obstructive airway disease. This may not appear in accord with the clinical experience of many anaesthetists, but it is possible that an adequate dose of atropine given in advance of stimulation is more valuable than one given after the bronchial constriction has been produced.

Pre-operative preparation.—The prevention of an attack of asthma, or im-provement of ventilation in a patient suffering from asthma, requires careful pre-operative treatment. Whenever possible, elective surgery should be per-formed only under optimum conditions, i.e. in the summer months for bron-chitics, and in the absence of a high pollen count for those patients with an allergic response, or a season when chest infections are rare. Bronchodilator drugs combined with active physiotherapy can considerably improve the patient's ventilation; isopropyl noradrenaline given as an aerosol is particularly useful and the effectiveness of this therapy can be observed by such routine tests as maximal expiratory flow rate or timed vital capacity. Antihistamines, especi-ally promethazine, may be found effective in producing bronchodilatation, dry-ing of secretions, and general sedation. In very severe cases the adrenal cortical steroids may relieve wheezing where other agents fail. Several cases of sudden death have been recorded following the use of aerosols, and they should not be prescribed indiscriminately (Committee on Safety of Drugs, 1967). For pre-medication of these patients pethidine, promethazine and atropine are particu-larly useful as they all tend to have a bronchodilator action. Aminophyline sup-positories (250 mg) may be useful given at the same time as the premedication, or alternatively one puff of an aerosol spray, such as salbutamol, half an hour before operation. Every effort should be made to reassure the patient. With these measures and with good anaesthetic technique asthma patients seldom give much trouble during surgery.

Anaesthesia.—Intravenous induction is the best method to employ. Thiopentone in particular has a tendency to lead to bronchospasm and it is usually better to use some other agent such as methohexitone. Halothane is probably the agent of choice for the maintenance of anaesthesia because it is relatively non-irritating to the respiratory tract and also produces some bronchodilatation. Anaesthesia must be adequately deep to avoid reflex bronchospasm. Relaxants should be used discreetly in the presence of bronchospasm for two reasons. Firstly reversal with neostigmine may precipitate bronchospasm even if the patient has been well atropinised, and secondly respiratory failure may occur in the immediate post-operative period due to the fact that it is seldom possible to reverse completely the effect of non-depolarising relaxants, and the slight residual paralysis remaining, although not enough to embarrass pulmonary ventilation in the patient with normal lungs, may be sufficient to precipitate ventilatory failure until the relaxant has had time to wear off. For operations requiring abdominal relaxation it is therefore better to employ less relaxant and a deeper level of anaesthesia than usual. Before intubation the trachea should be thoroughly sprayed with a local analgesic solution to avoid reflex bronchospasm. During artificial ventilation it may be necessary to use a long expiratory period in order to allow as complete exhalation as possible especially in view of the fact that the natural expiratory effort of the patient will have been abolished by the use of relaxants.

In the event of a severe attack of bronchospasm developing during anaesthesia the *slow* intravenous injection of 250 to 500 mg of aminophylline (i.e. given over five minutes) will often improve ventilation and this should be combined with assisted respiration. It should be remembered, however, that the rapid injection of aminophylline may increase the rate and amplitude of contraction of cardiac muscle in the same manner as an injection of adrenaline; thus, in combination with hypoxia the result might prove fatal. An intravenous injection of hydrocortisone (100 mg) remains the most effective treatment of a severe and protracted attack of bronchospasm. Recently, an intravenous preparation of salbutamol has become available and may prove to be effective. The dose, when given intravenously for bronchospasm, is 4 mcg/kg body weight, given slowly.

REFERENCES

ADAMS, W. E. (1930). Further studies in obstructive pulmonary atelectasis. *Proc. Soc. exp. Biol. (N.Y.)*, **27**, 982.

ADRIAN, E. D. (1933). Afferent impulses in the vagus and their effects on respiration. *J. Physiol. (Lond.)*, **79**, 332.

BAETJER, A. M. (1967). Effect of ambient temperature and vapor pressure on cilia-mucus clearance rate. *J. appl. Physiol.*, **23**, 498.

BROWN, E. S. (1962). Chemical identification of a surface-active agent. *Fed. Proc.*, **21**, 438.

BURTON, J. D. K. (1962). Effects of dry anaesthetic gases on the respiratory mucous membrane. *Lancet*, **1**, 235.

BUSH, G. H. (1963). Tracheo-bronchial suction in infants and children. *Brit. J. Anaesth.*, **35**, 322.

CHENEY, F. W., and BUTLER, J. (1968). The effects of ultrasonically produced aerosols on airway resistance in man. *Anesthesiology*, **29**, 1099.

CHERNICK, V., HUDSON, W. A., and GREENFIELD, L. J. (1966). Effect of chronic pulmonary artery ligation on pulmonary mechanics and surfactant. *J. appl. Physiol.*, **21**, 1315.

CLEMENTS, J. A. (1962). Studies of surface phenomena in relation to pulmonary function. *Physiologist*, **5**, 11.

COLEBATCH, H. J. H., and HALMAGYI, D. F. J. (1962). Reflex airway reaction to fluid aspiration. *J. appl. Physiol.*, **17**, 787.

CORYLLOS, P. N., and BIRNBAUM, G. L. (1928). Obstructive massive atelectasis of the lung. *Arch. Surg. (Chicago)*, **16**, 501.

CROSS, K. W. (1961). Respiration in the new-born baby. *Brit. med. Bull.*, **17**, 163.

DALE, W. A. and RAHN, H. (1952). Rate of gas absorption during atelectasis. *Amer. J. Physiol.*, **170**, 606.

DALY, M. de B., LAMBERSTEN, C. J., and SCHWEITZER, A. (1953). The effects upon the bronchial musculature of altering the oxygen and carbon dioxide tensions of the blood perfusing the brain. *J. Physiol. (Lond.)*, **119**, 292.

DALY, M. de B. and SCHWEITZER, A. (1952). The contribution of the vasosensory areas to the reflex control of bronchomotor tone. *J. Physiol. (Lond.)*, **116**, 35.

DERY, R., PELLETIER, J., JACQUES, A., CLARET, M., and HOUDE, J. (1965). Alveolar collapse induced by denitrogenation, *Canad. Anaesth. Soc. J.*, **12**, 531.

GALLOON, S., and ROSEN, N. (1965). Changes in airway resistance and alveolar trapping with positive-negative ventilation. *Anaesthesia*, **20**, 429.

GUEST, J. L., SEKULIC, S. M., YEH, T. J., ELLISON, L. T., and ELLISON, R. G. (1966). Role of atelectasis in surfactant abnormalities following extracorporeal circulation. *Circulation* (Suppl. I), **33–34**, 65.

HERING, E., and BREUER, J. (1868). Die Selbsteuerung der Athmung durch den Nervus Vagus. *S.-B. Akad. Wiss. Wien*, **57**, 672.

HERZOG, P., NORLANDER, O. P., and ENGSTROM, C. G. (1964). Ultrasonic generation of aerosol for the humidification of inspired gas during volume-controlled ventilation. *Acta anaesth. scand.*, **8**, 79.

HILL, D. W. (1967). *Physics Applied to Anaesthesia*, p. 87. London: Butterworth.

HOWELL, J. B. L. and ALTOUNYAN, R. E. C. (1967). A double-blind trial of disodium cromoglycate in the treatment of allergic bronchial asthma. *Lancet*, **2**, 537.

IMRIE, D. D., McCLELLAND, R. M. A., and SHARDLOW, W. B. (1966). Massive pulmonary collapse during thoracotomy. *Brit. J. Anaesth.*, **38**, 973.

KOHN, H. N. (1893). Zur Histologie der indurirenden fibrinösen Pneumonie. *Münch. med. Wschr.*, **40**, 42.

LEMMER, K. E. and ROVENSTINE, E. A. (1935). Rate of absorption of alveolar gases in relation to hyperventilation. *Arch. Surg. (Chicago)*, **30**, 625.

MACKLEM, P. T. (1971). Airway obstruction and collateral ventilation. *Physiol. Rev.*, **51**, 368.

MACKLIN, C. C. (1954). The pulmonary alveolar mucoid film and the pneumonocytes. *Lancet*, **1**, 1099.

MAY, A. J., and WIDDICOMBE, J. G. (1954). Depression of the cough reflex by pentobarbitone and some opium derivatives. *Brit. J. Pharmacol.*, **9**, 338.

MEAD, J., WHITTENBERGER, J. L., and RADFORD, E. P. (1957). Surface tension as a factor in pulmonary volume-pressure hysteresis. *J. appl. Physiol.*, **10**, 191.

MODELL, J. H., MOYA, F., RUIZ, B. C., SHOWERS, A. V., and NEWBY, E. J. (1968). Blood, gas and electrolyte determinations during exposure to ultrasonic nebulised aerosols. *Brit. J. Anaesth.*, **40**, 20.

NEGUS, V. E. (1949). Ciliary action. *Thorax*, **4**, 57.

NILSSON, E., SLATER, E. M., and GREENBARG, J. (1965). Cost of the quiet lung: fluctuations in PaO_2 when Carlens tube is used in pulmonary surgery. *Acta anaesth. scand.*, **9**, 49.

NISHIMURU, N., and METORI, S. (1967). Effect of gaseous anaesthetic agents on pulmonary compliance. *Anesth. et Analg.*, **46**, 187.

NORLANDER,O. P. (1968). The use of respirators in anaesthesia and surgery. *Acta anaesth. scand.*, (Suppl. 30), p. 35.

PAINTAL, A. S. (1964). Effects of drugs on vertebrate mechano-receptors. *Pharmacol. Rev.*, **16**, 341.

REISSEISSEN, R. D. (1822). Ueber den Bau der Lungen (Thesis), Berlin. (Quoted by Macklin, C. C. (1929). *Physiol. Rev.*, **9**, 1.)

RINGROSE, R. E., MCKOWN, B., FELTON, F. G., BARCLAY, B. O., MUCHMORE, H. G., and RHOADES, E. R. (1968). A hospital outbreak of serratia marcescens associated with ultrasonic nebulizers. *Ann. intern. Med.*, **69**, 719.

SHNIDER, S. M., and PAPPER, E. M. (1961). Anesthesia for the asthmatic patient, *Anesthesiology*, **22**, 886.

SIMONSSON, B. G., JACOBS, F. M., and NADEL, J. A. (1967). Role of autonomic nervous system and the cough reflex in increased responsiveness of airways in patients with obstructive airways disease. *J. clin. Invest.*, **46**, 1812.

SPENCER, G. T., RIDLEY, M., EYKYN, S., and ACHONG, J. (1968). Disinfection of lung ventilators by alcohol aerosol. *Lancet*, **2**, 667.

STEVENS, W. C., GOSSETT, J. A. HAMILTON, W. K., and MOORHEAD, R. T. (1966). Relation of postoperative atelectasis to solubility of gases filling lungs at termination of anaesthesia. *Anesthesiology*, **27**, 163.

TOOLEY, W. H., FINLEY, T. N., and GARDNER, R. (1961). Some effects on the lungs of blood from a pump oxygenator. *Physiologist*, **4**, 124.

VON NEERGAARD, K. (1929). Neue Auffassungen ueber einen Grundbegriff der Atemmechanik, abhaengig von der Oberglaichen spannung in der Alveolen. *Z. ges. exp. Med.*, **66**, 373.

WIDDICOMBE, J. G. (1961). Respiratory reflexes in man and other mammalian species. *Clin. Sci.*, **21**, 163.

WIDDICOMBE, J. G. (1963). Respiratory reflexes from the lung. *Brit. med. Bull.*, **19**, 19.

WIDDICOMBE, J. G. (1974a). Reflex control of breathing. In: *International Review of Science, Respiratory Physiology*, pp. 273–301. Ed. by J. G. Widdicombe. London: Butterworth & Co.

WIDDICOMBE, J. G. (1974b). Reflexes from the lungs in the control of breathing. In: *Recent Advances in Physiology*, No. 9, p. 239. Ed. by R. J. Linden. Edinburgh: Churchill Livingstone.

WIDDICOMBE, J. G., KENT, D. C., and NADEL, J. A. (1962). Mechanism of bronchoconstriction during inhalation of dust. *J. appl. Physiol.*, **17**, 613.

Chapter 2

PULMONARY VENTILATION

NERVOUS CONTROL OF BREATHING

The Respiratory Centres (Karczewski, 1974)

Situated in the pons and medulla are nerve cells which are responsible for the automatic rhythm of breathing. These cells are arranged in functional groups called respiratory centres. The concept of a single respiratory centre is untenable because of the multiplicity of factors and parts of the brain which can influence respiratory activity.

The medullary centres.—Section of the brain stem at the lower end of the medulla (Fig. 1, Section 4) results in the complete cessation of respiration. A section across the junction between the pons and the medulla (Fig. 1, Section 3) does not abolish breathing but instead leads to a gasping type of respiration which is irregular both in depth and rhythm, and which is not influenced by vagal afferent impulses. Therefore, somewhere in the medulla there must be a group of neurones which is capable of maintaining a primitive type of respiratory rhythm. These cells are the medullary centre and have been localised to an area in the reticular formation beneath the caudal end of the floor of the IVth ventricle. The medullary centre has been divided into two different parts, the inspiratory and expiratory centres. The most important evidence for this is as follows:—(1) Records of neuronal activity in various parts of the medulla have

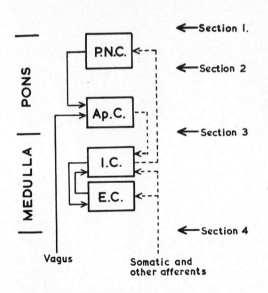

2/Fig. 1.—Schematic diagram of the possible organisation of the respiratory centres.

revealed electrical activity which coincides with either inspiration or with expiration. (2) Electrical stimulation of these two areas causes either inspiration or expiration, and indeed rhythmic respiration can be produced by stimulating them alternately. Anatomically the expiratory centre has been described as being

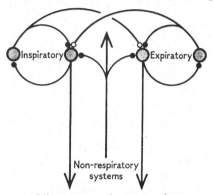

Efferents to respiratory muscles

● : excitatory synaptic functions
○ : inhibitory synaptic functions

2/FIG. 2.—Brain stem respiratory system (see text).

situated in the reticular substance under the floor of the IVth ventricle, the inspiratory centre lying more caudal and deep to the expiratory centre (Fig. 3) (Pitts, 1946), although other workers have not been able to locate anatomically separate centres (Burns and Salmoiraghi, 1960). The medullary centres have connections with the higher respiratory centres, the reticular activating system and the hypothalamus.

Records of neuronal activity within the inspiratory or expiratory centres indicate that stimulation of one part of the centre results in a spread of activity throughout the whole group of cells, and that activity in one group causes reciprocal inhibition of the other. Alter-

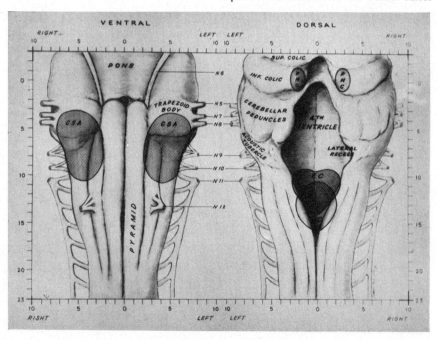

2/FIG. 3.—The ventral and dorsal surfaces of the brain in the region of 6th–12th cranial nerves. The central chemoreceptor (CSA) is seen lying superficially on the ventral surface. The respiratory centre (EC & IC) lies deep in the medulla oblongata in the floor of the 4th ventricle.

nating activity of the two centres can be explained by a system such as that shown in Fig. 2 (Burns, 1963). The respiratory neurones belong to one of two different classes concerned either with the act of inspiration or of expiration. They are so arranged that when excitation starts in one class it spreads to all members of that class. The activity of the whole system depends on initial excitation from both respiratory and non-respiratory sources, and possibly from chemical stimuli such as the arterial carbon dioxide tension. Inspiration begins with the activity of a few neurones which rapidly spreads through the network of inter-connecting inspiratory neurones. At the same time there is inhibition of the ex-piratory neurones. After a while the activity of the inspiratory neurones wanes and inhibition of the expiratory neurones then ceases. The whole process is then repeated for expiration. Other workers have suggested that expiration is merely a passive process and that, during quiet breathing, occurs because of the absence of inspiratory activity (Pitts, 1946).

The apneustic centre.—Section of the brain stem at the junction of the upper third and lower two-thirds of the pons (Fig. 1, Section 2) leads to slower and deeper breathing. If the vagus nerves on both sides are also divided a state of inspiratory spasm appears (Apneusis), which is interrupted by expiratory gasps (Apneustic Breathing). The inference is that uninhibited action of the apneustic centre causes prolonged activation of the inspiratory centre in the medulla, but that its action can be interrupted by afferent vagal impulses, and to a lesser extent by the pneumotaxic centre (see below) (Wang *et al.*, 1957). These workers have also suggested that it acts as a central station for vagal inhibitory impulses. Pitts (1946) held that apneusis arises from uninhibited activity of the inspiratory centre in the medulla. Although afferent stimuli can influence apneustic breath-ing, its origin almost certainly lies in the pons. It has been suggested that the apneustic centre provides the initial stimulus which begins inspiratory activity in the medulla.

The pneumotaxic centre.—Section of the brain stem at the upper limit of the pons (Fig. 1, Section 1) has no effect on respiration, so that in the upper third of the pons must lie a further respiratory centre which is capable of inhibiting the apneustic centre. Stimulation of this centre—the pneumotaxic centre—results in tachypnoea. The pneumotaxic centre has no inherent rhyth-micity, but seems to act by controlling the other centres.

The Origin of Respiratory Rhythm

Although a primitive rhythmicity lies in the medullary centres, in the intact animal respiration probably arises as a result of outside influences acting upon them. Inspiration is initiated by the action of the apneustic centre and somatic afferent impulses exciting the inspiratory centre. Once inspiration is in progress the activity of the inspiratory centre is inhibited by the action of impulses from the pneumotaxic centre and from the pulmonary stretch receptors via the vagus nerves. A series of feedback loops probably exists. For example, inspiratory activity causes nerve impulses to pass up the brain stem to the pneumotaxic centre. These excite the pneumotaxic centre which in turn causes inhibition of inspiration and allows expiration to take place. A similar negative feedback loop involving the vagus nerve also tends to terminate inspiration. The relative importance of the pneumotaxic centre and the vagus varies from species to species, and indirect evidence suggests that vagal inhibitory reflexes are of little importance in man.

The Stimulant Effect of Wakefulness on Respiration

Hyperventilation in the anaesthetised patient will lead to apnoea. This occurs at various levels of carbon dioxide tension in the blood and is partly dependent on the anaesthetic technique used. Thus with thiopentone and nitrous oxide a Pa_{CO_2} of approximately 38·5 mm Hg (5·1 kPa) may be obtained before apnoea occurs in contrast to 33·0 to 37·0 mm Hg (4·4–4·9 kPa) with halothane (Fink *et al.*, 1960; Hanks *et al.*, 1961). Fink (1961*a*), however, found that in *conscious* healthy volunteers the Pa_{CO_2} could be reduced to a mean of 22 mm Hg ± 4 (2·9 kPa ± 0·5) without apnoea developing at the end of the period of hyperventilation. On the contrary in the first minute of recovery, ventilation was usually greater than before the test. Subsequently the minute volume fell to about two-thirds of the control value. Thus wakeful subjects do not develop apnoea but continue to breathe rhythmically. It would appear from these observations that rhythmic respiration can be maintained by wakefulness in the presence of a reduced blood carbon dioxide, or by an increased carbon dioxide level in the blood in an anaesthetised patient, but not when both wakefulness and the carbon dioxide level of blood are below normal.

The stimulant effect of wakefulness on respiration can be ascribed tentatively to the brain stem reticular system. The depression of respiration at the onset of natural sleep may be due to lack of wakefulness.

Other Centres Affecting the Respiratory Centre

Many of the higher centres exert some influence on respiration—for example, the acts of swallowing, speaking and coughing require a careful integration of the mechanical systems. These changes are due to impulses arising in the cerebral cortex. Similarly, impulses from the cortical and thalamic areas influence the respiratory pattern during crying and laughing.

Effect of Anaesthetic Agents on the Respiratory Centres

Little is known of the effects which anaesthetic agents have on the respiratory centres, although it seems likely that their activity is depressed in common with other parts of the brain. Katz and Ngai (1962) observed in decerebrate cats that the inhalation of ether raised the electrical intensity required to produce inspiration on stimulation of the inspiratory centre, and that deepening the level of anaesthesia raised the threshold. This finding suggests that the medullary centres are depressed by ether. The possibility that trichloroethylene stimulates the pneumotaxic centre, thus producing tachypnoea, has also been suggested (Ngai *et al.*, 1961). Reports that other areas of the brain associated with respiration in animals are depressed during anaesthesia have also been published.

THE CHEMICAL CONTROL OF BREATHING

The Response to Carbon Dioxide

Since the primary function of the respiratory system is to maintain satisfactory partial pressures of O_2 and CO_2 in the arterial blood, it is not surprising to find that these pressures exert an influence on ventilation. The volume of ventilation is affected by both the arterial Po_2 and Pco_2, and is especially responsive to changes in carbon dioxide. When a subject is presented with a steep increase in inhaled CO_2 concentration, the arterial Pco_2 rises, but takes some minutes to reach a steady value. This is because the body can absorb large volumes of CO_2 and it therefore takes a little time for a new equilibrium to be reached. Both the rate and depth of ventilation increase steadily, and after about 10 to 20 minutes reach constant values. Similarly, after the withdrawal of inhaled CO_2 ventilation takes some minutes to return to control values.

Carbon Dioxide Response Curve

The ventilatory response to CO_2 is usually measured using either the steady-state method or the rebreathing method (Read, 1967). In the steady-state method the subject inspires three different concentrations of CO_2 (e.g. 2 per cent, 4 per cent, 6 per cent) each for about 20 minutes or until ventilation is steady. Towards the end of each period the ventilation and end-tidal CO_2 concentrations are measured. Points relating ventilation to end-tidal Pco_2 are derived and the line of best fit is obtained. This is the carbon dioxide response curve. The slope of the line (1 min^{-1} kPa^{-1}) is a measure of the subject's ventilatory sensitivity to CO_2. In the rebreathing method, the subject rebreathes from a 1-litre bag which is filled initially with 7 per cent CO_2, 50 per cent O_2, 43 per cent N_2. During the first half-minute equilibration occurs between the CO_2 in the bag and the subject. During the next 3–5 minutes there is a linear increase in Pco_2 and consequent increase in ventilation; a line relating ventilation to end-tidal Pco_2 is derived from measurements made during this time. For comparable levels of Po_2 the rebreathing and steady-state methods give similar results for the CO_2 sensitivity except during metabolic acidosis and alkalosis. The advantages of the rebreathing method are that it is rapid, less distressing to the subject and so can more readily be repeated.

The carbon dioxide response curve is a sensitive index of respiratory depression and as such has been used in the study of respiratory effects of narcotic drugs (Bellville and Seed, 1960).

Factors Influencing the Carbon Dioxide Response Curve

Alterations in the CO_2 response curve may be of two types. (a) The *slope* may be increased or decreased, sometimes termed as an alteration in CO_2 sensitivity, or (b) the curves may be displaced either to the left or to the right. Both types may of course be seen together. Some of the factors which influence the CO_2 response are as follows:

(1) *Individual responses* vary widely from person to person, and in the same individual from time to time (*Environmental Factors*).

(2) *Hypoxia*. In the presence of hypoxia the CO_2 response curve becomes steeper. Hypoxia therefore reinforces the ventilatory response to CO_2 (Lloyd *et al.*, 1958).

(3) *Metabolic acidosis and alkalosis*. Metabolic acidosis shifts the curve to the left and alkalosis shifts it to the right, although the slopes remain unchanged. When the ventilation is plotted as a function of CSF pH, however, no displacement occurs (Fencl *et al.*, 1969).

(4) *Chronic bronchitis*. In chronic bronchitis or other lung diseases causing

chronic diffuse airway obstruction the slope of the curve is flattened, and is displaced to the right in the presence of CO_2 retention. If the increase in respiratory *work*, rather than the ventilation, is plotted against the PCO_2, in some patients the increase in work when breathing CO_2 is close to normal, and in others it is reduced. It has been suggested that these different responses may characterise "blue bloaters" (reduced work response) and "pink puffers" (normal work response) (Lane, 1970).

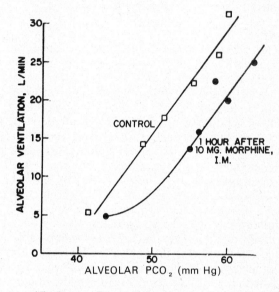

2/Fig. 4.—Carbon dioxide response curve after 10 mg of morphine sulphate.

(5) *Drugs.* Two methods have been used to assess the effect of drugs on respiration. One is to measure the arterial PCO_2 and/or the ventilation before and after the administration of the drug under study. A rise in PCO_2, or a fall in ventilation indicates that respiration has been depressed. Alternatively, a full CO_2 response curve can be performed. The latter is more sensitive than the former, and may show a depressed response to CO_2 inhalation in spite of there having been no change in the resting arterial PCO_2. Analgesic drugs depress the ventilatory response to CO_2. For example, morphine shifts the response curve to the right, but its slope is not usually affected (Fig. 4). Pethidine depresses the slope as well as moving it to the right, although the dose of the drug which has been administered is probably important as regards its precise effect. In Table 1 are

2/TABLE 1

DOSES OF SOME ANALGESIC DRUGS WHICH HAVE THE SAME RESPIRATORY DEPRESSANT EFFECT AS MORPHINE 10 MG. (COMPILED FROM VARIOUS SOURCES)

Pethidine	— 75 mg	Oxymorphone	— 0·68 mg
Dihydrocodeine	— 60 mg	Phenazocine	— 1·5 mg
Codeine	— 100 to 120 mg	Pentazocine	— 20 mg
Methadone	— 10 mg	Phenoperidine	— 2 mg
		Fentanyl	— 0·1 mg

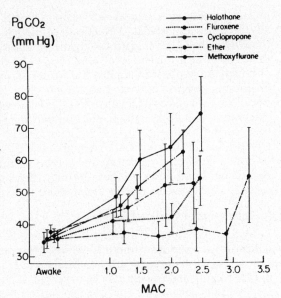

2/FIG. 5(a).—Alterations in P_{CO_2} with increasing depth of anaesthesia, the latter expressed as multiples of the Minimum Alveolar Anaesthetic Concentration (MAC). Note that with diethyl ether the P_{CO_2} remains around normal until deep levels of anaesthesia, and the wide variations in P_{CO_2} about the mean values. P_{CO_2} plotted as means $\pm$ one Standard Deviation. (Larson *et al.*, 1969).

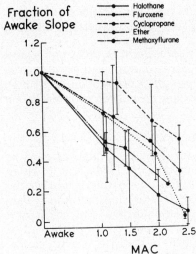

2/FIG. 5(b).—Alterations in the response to CO_2 inhalation with deepening anaesthesia. The slope of the ventilatory response to administering CO_2 in the inspired gases is plotted as a fraction of the slope obtained before the induction of anaesthesia. Note that as anaesthesia is deepened the response to CO_2 progressively falls and that, as in the conscious subject, there is a wide variation in the individual response. CO_2 response plotted as mean values $\pm$ one Standard Deviation. (Source: as for Fig. 5a)

listed the doses of a number of analgesic drugs which depress the CO_2 response curve an equivalent amount to 10 mg of morphine.

(6) *Inhalation anaesthetics.* A number of studies into the effects of anaesthetic agents on the ventilatory response to inhaled CO_2 have appeared in the literature (Munson *et al.*, 1966; Dunbar *et al.*, 1967; Larson *et al.*, 1969). The use of the Minimum Alveolar Anaesthetic Concentration (MAC) to describe the depth of anaesthesia has enabled several different agents to be compared. Cyclopropane, halothane, fluroxene and methoxyflurane all cause a fall in ventilation and a rise in arterial P_{CO_2}, these changes increasing with the depth of anaesthesia (Fig. 5). The ventilatory response to inhaled CO_2 is also pro-

gressively reduced as anaesthesia becomes deeper with these agents, and eventually becomes almost flat. The effects of diethyl ether are slightly different to those described above. With this agent ventilation and arterial P_{CO_2} are maintained at or near normal levels until deeper levels of anaesthesia are obtained, although the response to inhaled CO_2 progressively diminishes as with the other anaesthetic agents, even at light levels of anaesthesia. In a study on dogs Muallem et al. (1969) concluded that this effect was due to a central effect of the drug rather than to its irritant effect on the lining of the respiratory tract, as has been suggested in the past. The alterations in CO_2 response curves during anaesthesia are probably due to depression of the medullary H^+ chemoreceptor, or of its influence in regulating the activity of the respiratory centres. d-Tubocurarine in small doses has been found to have no effect on the CO_2 response curve in conscious man (Rigg et al., 1970).

Inhalation of Carbon Dioxide

A concentration of 5 per cent carbon dioxide, though unpleasant, can be inhaled for long periods without ill-effects. However, unconsciousness inevitably supervenes when the concentration is raised to 15 per cent or above. At this level, muscle rigidity and tremor may be observed. If 20–30 per cent carbon dioxide is inspired then generalised convulsions can be produced. Thus, the acidosis produced by a high P_{CO_2} probably plays a part in deepening anaesthesia produced by other agents and may also be responsible for part of the delay in recovery from narcotic poisoning.

About three-quarters of the ventilatory response to CO_2 is due to central chemoreceptor stimulation and the remainder is due to peripheral chemoreceptor activity. The peripheral chemoreceptor discharge is reduced by high levels of P_{O_2} and increased by low levels, providing the only drive to ventilation in response to hypoxia.

THE CENTRAL H^+ CHEMORECEPTOR

The pioneer studies by Leusen first suggested the possible importance of the cerebrospinal fluid in the control of ventilation (Leusen, 1954 a and b). Using anaesthetised animals he showed that perfusion of the ventriculo-cisternal system with mock CSF containing either a high P_{CO_2} or a low bicarbonate concentration (low pH) caused an increase in ventilation. In 1963 Mitchell and his colleagues located a bilateral superficial chemoreceptor on the ventro-lateral surface of the medulla in the region of the origins of the IXth and Xth cranial nerves, extending partially towards the mid-line (Fig. 3). These areas are termed the Medullary H^+ Chemoreceptor. The topical application to these sites of pledgets soaked in cerebrospinal fluid with a raised H^+ concentration leads to an almost immediate increase in ventilation which is proportional to the increase in H^+ concentration above normal. Furthermore, the application of a pledget containing a very low concentration of procaine causes apnoea even when the arterial P_{CO_2} is high. The area of the medullary respiratory centre below the floor of the IVth ventricle does not react to any of these manoeuvres.

In a series of most elegant experiments Pappenheimer and his colleagues (1965) examined the responses mediated by the medullary chemoreceptor. They used normal unanaesthetised goats into which had been chronically implanted nylon catheters leading to the lateral ventricles and the cisterna magna. The ventriculo-cisternal system could then be perfused with artificial CSF of any desired composition. The goats were trained to tolerate masks for long periods, and samples of arterial blood could be withdrawn at will from carotid artery loops. The respiratory responses of the animals to various alterations in the H^+ concentration of both blood and CSF could then be studied. The main conclusions they reported were: (1) The sensitivity of the chemoreceptor in normal animals to changes in CSF pH was two to seven times that found when the animals were anaesthetised. (2) The P_{CO_2} in the outflow of CSF was constantly about 10 mm Hg (1·3 kPa) higher than that in the arterial blood, irrespective of the P_{CO_2} in the infused artificial CSF. The P_{CO_2} of the CSF is therefore controlled by the P_{CO_2} in the brain tissue adjacent to the walls of the ventricular cavities. (3) During the inhalation of CO_2 the difference between the P_{CO_2} in CSF and arterial blood decreased, and this effect was thought to be secondary to an increase in cerebral blood flow at this time. (4) CO_2 response curves were slightly more linear when referred to CSF P_{CO_2} than when referred to arterial blood P_{CO_2}. (5) Ventilation was increased when the CSF H^+ concentration was raised by perfusing the cerebral ventricles with mock CSF containing a low bicarbonate concentration. This response to a "metabolic acidosis" within the CSF was much reduced if the increase in ventilation was allowed to cause a reduction in the P_{CO_2} of the CSF outflow. (6) During CO_2 inhalation it was estimated that about 40 per cent of the ventilatory response was due to the alteration of the CSF H^+ concentration, the remaining 60 per cent being the result of changes in P_{CO_2} or H^+ concentration elsewhere. Other estimates of the contribution of the medullary H^+ chemoreceptors to the response to the inhaled CO_2 vary from 30 per cent to over 80 per cent.

From these and other experiments there has emerged the concept of the medullary H^+ chemoreceptor and the factors which affect it. It is situated superficially near the surface of the medulla, and is sensitive to the H^+ concentration of the interstitial fluid bathing it. Because CO_2 combines with water to form H^+, it also reacts to changes in P_{CO_2} via this reaction. There is no convincing evidence that it is sensitive to changes in P_{CO_2} *per se*. The H^+ concentration of the all-important interstitial fluid is determined by its P_{CO_2} and bicarbonate concentration. These in turn are influenced by the P_{CO_2} of the CSF and the cerebral capillary blood and by the bicarbonate concentration of the CSF. The bicarbonate concentration in the blood has no immediate effect on the medullary H^+ chemoreceptor due to the diffusion barrier for bicarbonate ions which exists between blood and CSF and between blood and brain, although there appears to be free diffusion of bicarbonate between the CSF and the interstitial fluid bathing the receptor. Carbon dioxide, being rapidly diffusible throughout blood, tissues and CSF, provides the means whereby rapid changes in the H^+ concentration of the CSF and the fluid surrounding the receptor can be produced. Slower adjustments are mediated through alterations in the CSF bicarbonate concentration and the processes involved are probably more than diffusion alone. The evidence suggests that there is an active transport mechanism between blood and CSF which is capable of adjusting the CSF pH, although whether this involves the transport of bicarbonate or hydrogen ions is not clear (Severinghaus *et al.*, 1963; Mitchell, 1966).

The normal values for the pH, P_{CO_2} and bicarbonate concentration in arterial plasma and cerebrospinal fluid in man are shown in Table 2 (Bradley and Semple, 1962). Because the bicarbonate system is the only buffer in the cerebrospinal fluid, its chemical buffering power is small, and for a given rise in P_{CO_2} the CSF pH will, therefore, fall more than that of blood. Because of this the influence of the CSF on the activity of the medullary H^+ chemoreceptors is increased in response to changes in CO_2 in the body. In spite of this poor buffering capacity the CSF pH is kept remarkably constant in a wide variety of acid-base disturbances. Thus, it is normal or near normal in patients with chronic metabolic acidosis and alkalosis, moderate long-standing respiratory acidosis, and following acclimatisation to high altitude (respiratory alkalosis). Only in severe

2/TABLE 2

NORMAL VALUES FOR pH, P_{CO_2}, AND $[HCO_3^-]$ IN ARTERIAL
PLASMA AND CSF IN MAN. MEANS AND STANDARD DEVIATIONS

	pH	P_{CO_2} mm Hg (kPa)	$[HCO_3^-]$ mmol/l
Arterial Plasma	7·397 (0·022)	41·1 (5·5) 3·6 (0·5)	25·3 (1·8)
CSF	7·307 (0·027)	50·5 (6·7) 4·9 (0·7)	23·3 (1·4)

(Modified from Bradley and Semple, 1962)

respiratory acidosis is the CSF pH below normal, and also in acute respiratory changes before compensation has had time to occur.

FACTORS REGULATING CSF pH

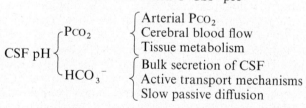

CSF pH
P_{CO_2} — Arterial P_{CO_2} / Cerebral blood flow / Tissue metabolism
HCO_3^- — Bulk secretion of CSF / Active transport mechanisms / Slow passive diffusion

As CO_2 is rapidly diffusible throughout the brain and CSF, and because the CSF P_{CO_2} is controlled by the P_{CO_2} of adjacent brain tissue, changes in arterial P_{CO_2} are followed by only slightly less rapid changes in CSF P_{CO_2}, and therefore in its pH. Bradley *et al.* (1965) have studied the changes in P_{CO_2} in blood and CSF following the sudden administration of 5 per cent CO_2 to anaesthetised patients for a period of 20 minutes. The arterial P_{CO_2} rose rapidly over 4–6 minutes and then became stable. There was a delay of 2–3 minutes before the CSF P_{CO_2} began to increase, and thereafter the rise was rather slower than that which occurred in the arterial blood so that after 20 minutes the CSF P_{CO_2} and pH lagged behind those in arterial and jugular venous blood, the time difference being measured in minutes. During the time of these experiments the plasma and CSF bicarbonate rose by the amount expected from the rise in P_{CO_2}. In conscious man Bradley et al. (1965) found that ventilatory changes lagged behind the rising P_{CO_2} in arterial and jugular venous blood, so that after 15 minutes ventilation was still increasing slowly, although both blood P_{CO_2} values were now constant. Opposite, but equally rapid changes in P_{CO_2} and pH occur in both blood and CSF following the institution of hyperventilation. However, if alterations in P_{CO_2} in either direction are maintained beyond the acute stage, the CSF bicarbonate slowly alters so that the changes in CSF pH are minimised even though there is no further change in the blood bicarbonate. In contrast to the changes in P_{CO_2} this change in bicarbonate is slow, and its time course can be measured in hours. McDowell and Harper (1970) have reported on the changes occurring in the CSF during hyperventilation to an arterial P_{CO_2} of 19–20 mm Hg (2·5–2·7 kPa) in baboons. They found that the CSF pH rose rapidly from an average value of 7·32 to 7·49 following the institution of hypocapnia. Over the next 3 hours the CSF pH fell slowly to an average value of 7·41, and during this time the CSF bicarbonate concentration fell from 21·4 mEq/litre (mmol/l) to 17·5 mEq/litre (mmol/l). The CSF P_{CO_2} remained stable at 29 ± 2 mm Hg (3·9 ± 0·3 kPa) during the whole period.

Practical Implications

When a patient inspires a high concentration of carbon dioxide, the raised P_{CO_2} of the blood reaching the brain causes an increased number of CO_2 molecules to diffuse into the extracellular fluid and stimulate respiration. If this inhalation continues for a time, the H^+ ion concentration of the cerebrospinal fluid is decreased by a compensatory rise of HCO_3^-. A sudden withdrawal of the inhaled CO_2 will be accompanied by a diminution of ventilation below normal because the stimulus of a high H^+ ion content is no longer present in the cerebrospinal fluid.

The practical significance of this mechanism can best be illustrated by taking a few hypothetical examples:

Normal patient breathing air:

	BLOOD			CSF	
P_{CO_2} mm Hg (kPa)	pH	Bicarb mEq/l (mmol/l)	Bicarb mEq/l (mmol/l)	pH	P_{CO_2} mm Hg (kPa)
40 (5·3)	7·4	25	23	7·32	48 (6·4)

N.B. Under resting conditions the P_{CO_2} of CSF is about 8 mm Hg (1·1 kPa) higher than that found in blood.

Patient hyperventilated for 30 minutes under anaesthesia:

20 (2·7)	7·60	19·5	22	7·55	28 (3·7)

N.B. The time interval is too short for any significant change to have occurred in the bicarbonate level of the CSF.

After 6 hours of hyperventilation:

20 (2·7)	7·55	17·0	14	7·32	28 (3·7)

N.B. The pump mechanism is now in full force in an attempt to return the CSF pH to normal.

Return to spontaneous respiration:

23 (3·1) | 7·51 | 18·0 ‖ 14 | 7·28 | 31 (4·1)

N.B. At first the large amount of H^+ ions together with the low level of bicarbonate in the CSF stimulates ventilation, but soon the bicarbonate level starts to creep up as the pump mechanism reduces the amount of H^+ ions in the CSF. There is less stimulus to breathe so the P_{CO_2} of the blood rises. This cycle of events repeats itself over and over again until normal values for both blood and CSF have been reached. However, in the anaesthetised patient who has been on positive-pressure ventilation for, say, six hours, it may take at least that period of time again before the blood level of arterial P_{CO_2} has returned to the normal level of 40 mm Hg (5·3 kPa).

The effect of this central chemoreceptor reflex is probably of even greater significance in the patient who is underventilating during anaesthesia for a long time. For example:

At start of anaesthesia:

BLOOD			CSF		
P_{CO_2}	pH	Bicarb mEq/l (mmol/l)	Bicarb mEq/l (mmol/l)	pH	P_{CO_2}
40 (5·3)	7·4	25	23	7·32	48 (6·4)

After 30 minutes of hypoventilation:

80 (10·7) | 7·20 | 30 ‖ 26 | 7·07 | 88 (11·7)

After 6 hours of hypoventilation:

80 (10·7) | 7·20 | 30 ‖ 32 | 7·19 | 88 (11·7)

N.B. The pump mechanism now attempts to raise the bicarbonate level of the CSF so that the pH may return to its normal level.

At the end of anaesthesia (patient breathing on room air):

BLOOD			CSF		
P_{CO_2}	pH	Bicarb mEq/l (mmol/l)	Bicarb mEq/l (mmol/l)	pH	P_{CO_2}
52 (6·9)	7·33	26	32	7·35	60 (8·0)

N.B. At this time, although the P_{CO_2} of the blood is falling, the patient's central chemoreceptor mechanism has ceased to act due to the low level of H^+ or the high level of HCO_3^- ions in the CSF. In these circumstances, the patient will continue to underventilate despite the fact that the level of blood P_{CO_2} appears to be improving towards normal. The activity of the respiratory centre is influenced purely by hypoxic drive acting through the peripheral chemoreceptors. The sudden administration of oxygen may abolish this drive and lead to apnoea.

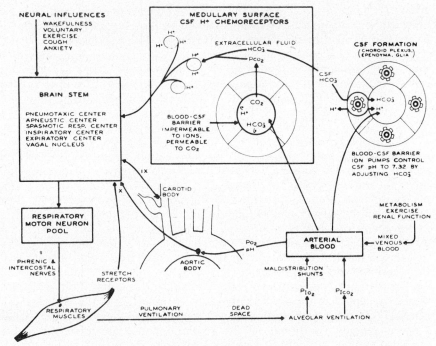

2/Fig. 6.—Diagram of the Theory of the Chemical Control of Respiration.

The medullary surface CO_2 chemoreceptor responds to the extracellular hydrogen ion concentration. The latter is controlled by (a) the local P_{CO_2}, which, in turn, is determined by arterial P_{CO_2}, local blood flow and metabolism; and (b) by the bicarbonate ion concentration in the CSF which is unaffected by sudden changes in the P_{CO_2} of arterial blood, but is determined by active transport in the formation of CSF and is adjusted in an attempt to keep the pH of the CSF constant (Severinghaus and Larson, 1965).

Such an example helps to emphasise the dangers of hypoventilation under anaesthesia, because the hypoxia may be avoided during the administration by increasing the inspired oxygen concentration, but when the reduced ventilation persists in the post-operative period with the patient breathing room air, then hypoxia may supervene. In the presence of a metabolic acidosis the patient may have a normal blood level of P_{CO_2} yet be underventilating. Though such a state of affairs must be highly unusual, it can only arise if the hypoventilation during anaesthesia has been very prolonged. The only satisfactory treatment is a period of normal ventilation on a mechanical ventilator to allow the homeostatic mechanisms to regain control.

The theory of the chemical control of respiration is shown diagrammatically in Fig. 6.

Effects of Anaesthetic Agents on the Medullary H^+ Chemoreceptor

Although the ventilatory response to inhaled CO_2 is depressed during general anaesthesia, the mechanism of this phenomenon is unknown. Experiments in which the central chemoreceptor have been stimulated by the application of pledgets to the medulla have shown that the ventilatory response to a given pH change is much less in anaesthetised animals than has been found in other experiments in conscious animals and man. This suggests that the chemoreceptor itself may be depressed by anaesthesia. The response of the central respiratory mechanisms to chemoreceptor activity may also be depressed. In total spinal analgesia the action of the local analgesic at this site may well explain the cessation of respiration which occurs. It has also been observed that the direct application of d-tubocurarine to this site stimulates respiration.

THE PERIPHERAL CHEMORECEPTORS

The peripheral chemoreceptors, the carotid and aortic bodies, consist of small masses of glandular-looking cells, richly supplied with blood vessels and nerves. The carotid bodies are located between the origins of the external and internal carotid arteries. They lie adjacent to the carotid sinus, but are completely different both in structure and function. They receive a lavish blood supply from the carotid arteries, and the afferent nerve fibres leaving them run first in the carotid and then in the glossopharyngeal nerve. The aortic bodies are situated next to the arch of the aorta, between it and the pulmonary artery, and their afferent nerve fibres enter the vagosympathetic trunks, usually with the recurrent laryngeal nerves.

The peripheral chemoreceptors respond to changes in Po_2, Pco_2 and pH of the blood supplying them. Of these the most important is the Po_2. A fall in arterial Po_2, or in the supply of oxygen to the peripheral chemoreceptors, causes a rise in pulmonary ventilation. The respiratory response to oxygen lack is mediated entirely through the peripheral chemoreceptors, although the mechanism whereby a fall in Po_2 is converted into nervous impulses is unknown.

The Ventilatory Response to Oxygen Lack

At sea level about 20 per cent of the total respiratory drive arises in the carotid and aortic bodies. This drive can be eliminated by raising the arterial Po_2 to 200 mm Hg (26·7 kPa) or over. The ventilatory response to hypoxia differs from that due to a rise in Pco_2 in a number of ways. The peripheral chemoreceptors are not very sensitive to a fall in arterial Po_2. Thus, no change in ventilation is seen until the inspired oxygen concentration falls to about 16 per cent and then the increase in breathing is only marginal. Obvious increases in ventilation are not seen until the inspired oxygen concentration falls to about 10 per cent, but at concentrations below this, ventilation increases steeply as the oxygen concentration falls. At these low inspired oxygen percentages there is a marked individual variation in the response to hypoxia. If the arterial Pco_2 is kept constant while breathing low oxygen mixtures, ventilation is approximately doubled at an arterial Po_2 of 45 mm Hg (6·0 kPa). However, if the arterial Pco_2 is allowed to fall naturally as a result of increasing ventilation, the full hypoxic response is masked by the change in Pco_2, and at a Po_2 of 45 mm Hg (6·0 kPa) only a 10 per cent increase in ventilation is seen. The response to hypoxia is more sensitive in the presence of acidaemia, hypotension or sympathetic activity. Ventilatory responses which arise in the peripheral chemoreceptors are rapid, the full response being seen almost from breath to breath. Also, unlike the respiratory response to a high Pco_2, the response to hypoxia is relatively unaffected by narcotic drugs, barbiturates or by anaesthetic agents.

REFLEX CONTROL OF RESPIRATION

Pulmonary Reflexes

Although physiology has made great strides in the past few years, many of the present-day views on the nervous control of respiration are based on observations made many years ago in animals. Prominent amongst these is the concept of the automatic control of the rhythm of respiration postulated by Hering and Breuer in 1868, who showed in cats that a sudden inflation immediately made the lungs come to rest in the position of expiration, while a sudden deflation led to a sharp inspiratory effort. From this it was concluded that there are stretch receptors in the lung which signal the volume changes in the alveoli to the respiratory centre. Later in 1933, Adrian, also working with cats, demonstrated a stream of nerve impulses passing up the vagus nerve as the lungs increased in size. The number of these impulses passing at any one moment bore a direct relationship to the degree of distension of the lung. This evidence, while emphasising the importance of the inflation receptors, left deflation as a purely passive movement. Later writers drew attention to the role of deflation receptors. It was generally agreed that the vagus nerve played a vital part in the control of respiration, since section of it resulted in slow deep respiratory activity, whilst stimulation of the central end led to apnoea.

In man, despite the fact that numerous nerve filaments are known to exist in the lungs and can be traced right down to the bronchial tree to their final terminations, nerve fibres have never been successfully demonstrated in the alveolar walls. Widdicombe (1961) studied the inflation and deflation reflexes in a number of mammalian species, including conscious and anaesthetised man, and concluded that in man the reflexes were relatively weak when compared to the other species which he studied. In conscious man bilateral vagal blockade causes no change in the pattern of respiration, making man unique in this respect, but has been found to effect the sensation of breathlessness. In patients anaesthetised with nitrous oxide and halothane Guz *et al.* (1964) found that (i) Bilateral vagal blockade caused no alteration in the respiratory pattern, arterial P_{CO_2}, heart rate or blood pressure. (ii) Sudden lung inflation only caused a period of apnoea when large volumes (1 litre or more) were used. This effect was abolished by vagal block. (iii) Vagal stimulation, when intense, was capable of causing apnoea. They concluded that, although vagal afferent impulses were able to affect respiration in anaesthetised man, their influence was weak and probably of little physiological importance. In 1968 Paskin *et al.* attempted to excite the inflation reflex in humans during the administration of various anaesthetic agents—halothane, methoxyflurane, fluroxene and cyclopropane—but were unable to find any evidence that the reflex was active under these conditions. The action of diethyl ether on the respiration is also unaffected by vagal blockade in dogs, and Ngai *et al.* (1961) showed that the tachypnoea caused by trichloroethylene in decerebrate cats continued even after division of the vagi. It appears, therefore, that the suggestion made by Whitteridge and Bülbring (1946) that anaesthetic agents lead to sensitisation of the inflation reflex cannot be applied to man.

The cause of the tachypnoea which is so often seen under anaesthesia remains undecided, although many suggestions have been put forward. These include sensitisation of the pulmonary stretch receptors, irritation of the respiratory tract, stimulation of extrapulmonary receptors, mobilisation of catecholamines and the development of acidosis in either blood or CSF. Studying the effects of diethyl ether on respiration in the dog Muallem *et al.* (1969) found no change in the pattern of breathing following vagal blockade, high spinal analgesia (up to cervical level), carotid body denervation or a combination of all three, and neither could they detect any difference in the acid-base status of the CSF between halothane and ether anaesthesia, although the respiratory effects of the two drugs were quite different. They concluded that ether asserts its characteristic action on breathing through a central action on respiratory control.

There are, however, instances during anaesthesia when the lung receptors may influence the character of the respiratory pattern: for example, if a patient's breathing is depressed by too much cyclopropane or pethidine, apnoea will follow. On manual compression of the breathing bag, as the lung starts to become inflated the patient may suddenly check the inspiration and then go on to make a full deep inspiratory movement of his own accord. The slightest increase in intratracheal pressure appears to trigger-off a complete inspiration, yet, without some manual assistance, the patient remains in apnoea for long periods. This type of respiration is often believed to be due to stimulation of the stretch receptors, but this seems an inadequate explanation. Stimulation would be expected to arrest rather than to complete respiration.

Another variation, which may well be concerned with the lung receptors, is sometimes seen in conscious patients placed in a tank ventilator. Despite a normal arterial oxygen saturation, a low carbon dioxide tension, and a raised pH, the patient may feel inadequately ventilated, frequently requesting greater ventilation—which only results in a further rise in the pH. Also, if respiration becomes severely depressed in the cat or dog under nembutal or chloroform anaesthesia, it is often possible to initiate a full deep inspiration by squeezing the thoracic cage tightly. Similarly on rewarming an animal, after a period of hypothermia with cessation of respiratory activity, either compression of the thorax or inflation of the lung may initiate rhythmical activity. In all probability both these mechanisms act by stimulating either the stretch or deflation receptors.

Other reflex pathways.—Apart from reflex afferent impulses from the respiratory tract, stimulation of the respiratory centre may arise from the cardiovascular system, abdominal and pelvic viscera, skeletal muscle and joints, skin, and other places (Fig. 7). One of the commonest reflex arcs of this type is the increase in pulmonary ventilation that occurs on cutting the skin of a patient under light anaesthesia.

In animal experiments, alterations in the systemic blood pressure are transmitted to the respiratory centre through the medium of the pressor receptors (carotid sinus and aortic arch). A rise in blood pressure causes a fall in pulmonary ventilation and vice versa. However, in anaesthetised patients a large pressor response to adrenaline leads to stimulation rather than depression of respiration (Young, 1957). It seems, therefore, that in anaesthetised man the pressor receptors do not play an important part in the control of respiration.

The Effects of Anaesthetic Agents on Respiration

Qualitatively the actions of different anaesthetic agents on breathing are very

similar. They produce a fall in tidal volume associated with an increase in the
rate of breathing. The result on the minute or alveolar ventilation is variable,
depending on the relative changes in rate and tidal volume. Thus, halothane
cyclopropane and methoxyflurane cause a fall in tidal volume which is not
completely compensated for by a rise in respiratory rate, with the result that
alveolar ventilation is reduced and the arterial PCO_2 rises. Trichloroethylene

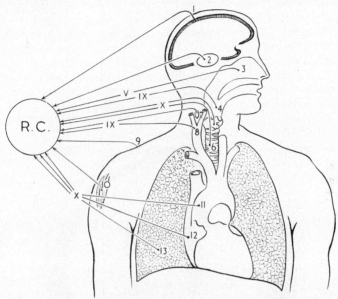

2/FIG. 7.—NERVOUS PATHWAYS INFLUENCING THE RESPIRATORY CENTRES.

1. Cerebral cortex; 2. Hypothalamus; 3. Nasal mucous membrane; 4. Pharyngeal mucous
membrane; 5. Laryngeal mucous membrane; 6. Tracheal mucous membrane; 7. Carotid body;
8. Carotid sinus; 9. Skin; 10. Muscle; 11. Aorta; 12. Right atrium; 13. Lung.

often causes a marked rise in respiratory rate, and it is generally considered that
this is detrimental to the efficiency of gas exchange. However, measurements of
the arterial PCO_2 under these circumstances show that it is normal or low
(Severinghaus and Larsen, 1965). The administration of intravenous pethidine
or a similar agent in order to reduce the tachypnoea only results in depression
of the respiratory centre and a rise in the arterial PCO_2. This effect has been
demonstrated during halothane anaesthesia (Davie et al., 1970). Similarly,
tachypnoea during anaesthesia with all anaesthetic agents is reduced by premedication with opiates. Surgical stimulation reduces the respiratory depression
caused by anaesthetic agents.

THE RESPIRATORY MUSCLES

THE diaphragm is the principal muscle of respiration, but many other muscles,
including the intercostals, the abdominals, the scalenes, the sternomastoids and
even some of the back muscles, have their part to play. All of these muscles
have one thing in common—they are attached to the thoracic cage. Each group
will now be considered in turn.

THE DIAPHRAGM

Anatomy

The diaphragm (Fig. 8) consists of a central tendon which is arched on both sides to form a cupola. Muscle fibres radiate from each portion of the tendon and can be traced to their origin in three distinct regions. First, the spinal or crural portion in which the fibres arise from the upper three or four lumbar vertebrae and from the arcuate ligaments. This division is inserted into the posterior margin of the central tendon. Secondly, the costal portion which arises by a series of digitations from the inner surface of the lower six ribs and cartilages. Finally there is a small contribution arising from the back of the ensiform process. The central or tendinous part of the diaphragm is domed upwards into the chest, partly due to the higher intra-abdominal pressure and partly due to the negative pressure pull exerted by the elastic recoil of the lung.

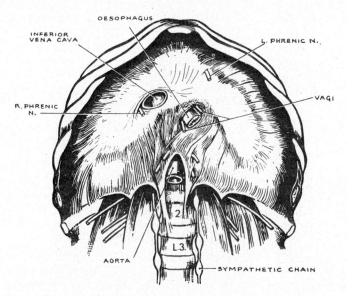

2/FIG. 8.—The diaphragm.

The motor innervation of the diaphragm is largely supplied by the phrenic nerves whose fibres are 90 per cent motor and 10 per cent sensory and autonomic. The two crura receive a motor supply from the 11th and 12th intercostal nerves. Peripheral parts of the diaphragm receive a sensory and autonomic innervation from the lower six intercostal nerves.

Movements

The diaphragm moves in a vertical plane and in quiet respiration it is almost wholly responsible for the tidal exchange, thus fully deserving the title of the principal muscle of respiration. The exact extent to which it moves has been studied radiologically. Wade (1954) gives it a range of about 1·5 cm upwards or downwards during quiet respiration, but this distance may be extended to 6–

10 cm with deep breathing. Extension of the spine and lifting of the whole thoracic cage are associated with maximal respiratory effort and account for part of this extended movement.

Contrary to popular belief, the range of movement of the diaphragm does not alter with a change of posture from the standing to the supine position. The resting level, however, is higher when the subject is lying down.

It is sometimes claimed that diaphragmatic excursion can be aided by nursing patients in the upright position after an operation, thus avoiding undue pressure on the muscle from the abdominal contents. There is no truth in this assertion.

In normal circumstances a movement of 1 cm downwards of the diaphragm causes about 350 ml of air to enter the lungs and thus the normal tidal exchange of 500 ml per breath is attained by a movement of about 1·5 cm (Wade, 1954). This figure does not take into account the effects of any of the other muscles of respiration but it emphasises the fact that in quiet breathing the diaphragm is probably the only muscle taking part. During deep breathing the contraction of the diaphragm increases the volume of the thorax by an amount equal to 75 per cent of the volume of gas which is inhaled; the remaining 25 per cent is attributable to the movement of the ribs. Thus total paralysis of the diaphragm, as when both phrenic nerves are cut, greatly reduces the ability to ventilate the lungs, though adequate tidal exchange for rest and light activity can still be maintained. Unilateral phrenic crush produces little more than a 15–20 per cent reduction in Maximum Breathing Capacity (MBC) with a normal tidal exchange. The paralysed half of the diaphragm moves paradoxically by rising in the thorax during inspiration and falling during expiration, thus reflecting the differences in pressure between the thorax and the abdomen during the two phases of the respiratory cycle. Paralysis of the diaphragm may be diagnosed on X-ray screening of the chest by asking the patient to sniff (see also Hiccup, p. 98).

It is interesting to reflect that morphologically all vertebrates except mammals use the principle of body-wall compression to provide an expiratory force. For them this is the fundamental act of breathing. In mammals, however, the demands for oxygen cannot be met by this type of inspiration and a new principle of active respiration is introduced and carried out by an entirely new structure—the muscular diaphragm—situated below the heart and lungs. The diaphragm thus provides mammals with a new and more efficient form of ventilation than that of other vertebrates. Primrose (1952) takes the view that the need for this new muscle is evidence that the existing body wall musculature—namely the intercostals—is unable to provide sufficient respiratory function and that they are therefore relatively unimportant as muscles of respiration.

INTERCOSTAL MUSCLES

Anatomy

The *external* intercostal muscle fibres, which are mostly in the posterior part of the intercostal space, run obliquely *downwards* and *forwards* from the lower and outer border of one rib to the upper and outer border of the rib below. Contraction of these fibres tends to draw the ribs closer together, but by virtue of their articulations the ribs move upwards and outwards. The result is that in the upper part of the chest the antero-posterior diameter and in the lower part the transverse diameter, is increased.

The *internal* intercostal muscle fibres, which are mostly in the anterior part of the intercostal space, run from the floor of the costal groove and corresponding costal cartilages *downwards* and *backwards* and are finally inserted into the upper and inner border of the rib below. It will be noted, therefore, that both types of intercostal muscles run downwards and their fibres cross obliquely in opposite directions, the one set going forward and the other backwards.

Both groups of muscles are supplied by the intercostal nerves.

Movements

Throughout the years the part played by the intercostal muscles in respiratory movement has been strongly debated. Some believed that they were merely a relic of the past and did little more than regulate the tension in the intercostal spaces. Others felt that they had some part to play, but no general agreement on this could be reached. Campbell (1955) has shown that the external intercostals, with the aid of those parts of the internal intercostals which run between the cartilaginous portions of the ribs, raise the ribs. They also contract during inspiration in both quiet and strenuous respiration. These muscles, therefore—particularly those lying in the fifth to ninth spaces—play an important part in inspiration. Campbell's studies prompt him to suggest that the external intercostals are second only in importance to the diaphragm as muscles of inspiration. He found, however, no evidence that they play any part in expiration.

Green and Howell (1955) have made similar studies and are in agreement with these findings. In addition they note that although the external intercostal muscles in the fifth to ninth space contract during inspiration, this contraction persists into the first part of the expiration, especially during vigorous breathing: this has the effect of smoothing the transition between the two phases of the respiratory cycle. They found little evidence of activity in the other intercostal spaces.

The function of the intercostal muscles is in doubt. Campbell (1958) believes that their action is determined by the incline of the structures to which they are attached. Thus those fibres which are parasternal lie between costal cartilages and slope upwards, paralleling therefore the external intercostal muscles in both direction and action during inspiration, while the fibres that lie between the ribs slope backwards as well as downwards and contract during expiration. These inter-osseous fibres also contract during speech.

Abdominal Muscles

There are four principal groups of abdominal muscles that influence respiration—namely the external and internal obliques, the transversi and the recti muscles (Fig. 9).

Anatomy

The *external oblique* muscle arises from the outer surface of the lower eight ribs and the fibres pass downwards in a fan-shape to be inserted into the iliac crest posteriorly and into a fibrous aponeurosis blending with the rectus sheath anteriorly. The lower border of this aponeurosis forms the inguinal ligament.

In contrast, the *internal oblique* arises from the iliac crest, lumbar fascia and inguinal ligament, and the fibres pass vertically upwards to be inserted into the lower three ribs posteriorly and into the aponeurosis forming part of the rectus sheath anteriorly. The *transversus abdominis* muscle arises from the costal cartilages of the lower six ribs, the lumbar fascia, the iliac crest and a small portion of the inguinal ligament. The fibres run horizontally and are attached to the aponeurosis forming part of the rectus sheath. Finally, the *rectus abdominis* muscle arises from the pubic symphysis and crest and the fibres pass vertically upwards to become attached to the 5th, 6th and 7th costal cartilages. During their passage these fibres are enclosed in an aponeurosis or sheath which is closely related to the three abdominal muscles already mentioned.

2/Fig. 9.—The muscles of the abdominal wall.

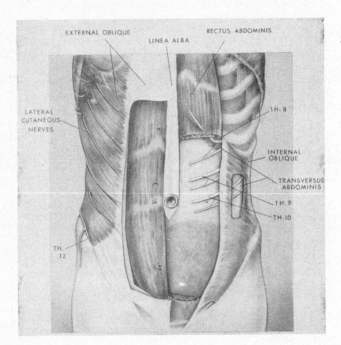

Movements in Conscious People

During quiet respiration, and any increase in ventilation up to 40 l/min (i.e. about five times the resting minute volume), the abdominal muscles remain inactive in the conscious subject when supine, and often even when the body is erect (Campbell and Green, 1953). As the volume of respiration increases further so the abdominal muscles gradually start to take an active part. By the time forceful abdominal contractions can be seen, ventilation will have risen to 90 l/min—the equivalent of strenuous exercise. These muscles also contract when a forced expiratory effort is made.

The time at which abdominal muscle activity starts in relation to the respiratory cycle is interesting, for the earliest movements are seen at the end of expiration. This finding may be connected with their function, and may perhaps be explained as follows:—The maximum intra-abdominal pressure that can be maintained by a conscious patient for more than a few seconds is 110 mm Hg (14·7 kPa), yet Gordh and Silferkiold (1943) found that intra-abdominal pressures of 150–200 mm Hg (20·0–26·7 kPa) were reached during electro-convulsive therapy. Campbell (1958) believes that the function of the abdominal muscles in the conscious subject is to preserve a steady intra-abdominal pressure and that, for this purpose, there are reflex pathways which tend to prevent too rapid or too great a rise. Thus, during inspiration the diaphragm descends and causes an increase in intra-abdominal pressure; then early in expiration it starts to ascend again, due to the elastic recoil of the lungs. This leads to a fall in pressure in the abdomen and the muscles of the abdomen now start to contract in a reflex attempt to keep the intra-abdominal pressure stable. These facts help to explain why the abdominal muscles start to contract at the end of expiration. The abdominal muscles, therefore, play no part in inspiration. In expiration they maintain the stability of the intra-abdominal pressure and thus indirectly assist the ascent of the diaphragm.

In the past various people have argued that the abdominal muscles have an inspiratory function on the basis that they contract during inspiration, so fixing the lower ribs and allowing the diaphragm a greater range of movement. Campbell (1958) made electromyographic studies of the abdominal muscles in over thirty subjects during increased breathing and found an inspiratory contraction in only two patients. He feels that the elastic property of the abdominal wall, rather than muscular contraction, is the more important factor in producing the intra-abdominal tension of inspiration.

To summarise, the abdominal muscles are muscles of expiration. Essentially they have two functions during expiration—one to raise the intra-abdominal pressure, and the other to draw the lower ribs downwards and medially. In normal quiet respiration they play no part at all, but when ventilation becomes more vigorous, they contract during expiration and thus aid the ascent of the diaphragm. They are the major muscles concerned in developing the enormously high expulsive pressures of defaecation and coughing.

Movements in Anaesthetised Patients

Fink (1961b), using an electromyographic technique, has studied the movements of both the abdominal muscles and the diaphragm during anaesthesia. Under all types of light anaesthesia some electrical activity can always be detected in the abdominal musculature (oblique-transverse group) during expiration. This can be abolished by the use of a muscle relaxant.

In anaesthetised patients under light anaesthesia the diaphragm contracts with inspiration and the abdominal muscles with expiration (see Fig. 10a). On the other hand, if the patient is now ventilated manually until spontaneous respiration is abolished, then activity ceases in the diaphragm during the period of apnoea but persists as continuous activity in the abdominal muscles (Fig. 10b). Such an observation does not support Campbell's theory that the role of the abdominal muscles is to preserve an even intra-abdominal tension because there is no obvious reason why such a reflex should be abolished by light anaesthesia. Fink favours the view that the diminished abdominal activity during a spontaneous inspiration is due to a direct inhibition of these muscles brought about by the respiratory centre. During apnoea this inhibition is removed, so that they enter a state of continuous activity.

Other Accessory Muscles of Respiration

The *scalene muscles* contract during quiet inspiration and as such are almost entitled to be considered as a principal muscle of respiration. Their total contribution to the amount inspired, however, is not considered to be great. They also are believed to contract during violent expiratory motions such as coughing, presumably in an attempt to support the apex of the lung.

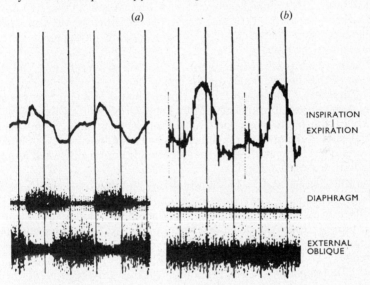

(*a*)   (*b*)

INSPIRATION
EXPIRATION

DIAPHRAGM

EXTERNAL
OBLIQUE

2/Fig. 10.—Electromyogram of diaphragmatic and abdominal muscle activity in an anaesthetised patient.
   (*a*) Spontaneous respiration under halothane/nitrous oxide/oxygen anaesthesia.
   (*b*) Controlled respiration (i.e. apnoea) under same anaesthesia.

The *sternomastoid muscles,* on the other hand, are inactive during quiet breathing but become vigorous as ventilation increases. They then contract during inspiration and are regarded as important accessory muscles and their action can be seen well in patients with dyspnoea.

There are many other muscles attached to the thoracic cage which have, at one time or another, been considered as important accessory muscles of respiration. Campbell (1954), using electromyography, has studied many of them, including the trapezius, serratus anterior, latissimus dorsi and pectoralis muscles. He failed to find any evidence that they play a significant part in respiration. Many of them contract during the act of coughing. The latissimus dorsi is important in this respect as it may become paralysed following section of its nerve supply at a radical amputation of the breast or division of the muscle fibres at a thoracotomy incision. As a result there is sometimes a serious limitation of the power to expel sputum. A posterior incision for thoracotomy alone may, by dividing the latissimus dorsi, cause a permanent reduction of lung function.

NORMAL LUNG MOVEMENTS

Those parts of the lung lying in direct relation to the mobile or expansile parts of the thoracic cage—i.e. the ribs and diaphragm—are expanded in direct contact with their neighbouring wall. The peripheral parts of the lung thus undergo a greater degree of expansion than those nearer the hilum. There are three areas of the lung which are not expanded directly, the mediastinal surface in contact with the pericardium, the dorsal surface in contact with the spinal segments of the ribs, and the posterior apical surface lying close to the deep cervical fascia of Sibson. At each inspiration the capacity of the chest is increased in its transverse, antero-posterior and vertical diameters; the converse applies during expiration. As the chest wall expands, so the glottis opens more widely and air enters the lungs.

The movements of the lungs are best considered in relation to the change in position of the chest wall and diaphragm.

I. *The apex.*—The thoracic inlet, formed by the first two ribs, the vertebral column, and the manubrium sterni, moves upwards and forwards on inspiration to increase the antero-posterior diameter of the chest wall. In this manner the anterior part of the apex of the upper lobe is expanded directly. In later life (60 years and over) the manubrio-sternal junction becomes ankylosed and this part of the lung ceases to expand.

II. *The thoracic cage.*—This is best divided into two parts, the upper stretching from the second to the sixth ribs and the lower from the seventh to the tenth. The ribs move outwards and upwards on inspiration; in the upper portion it is the antero-posterior diameter of the thoracic cage that is chiefly increased, whereas in the lower portion the main enlargement lies in the transverse diameter.

III. *The diaphragm.*—The diaphragm has already been mentioned as the principal muscle of respiration. In quiet breathing it can account for the whole of the inspired air, whilst in a maximal inspiratory effort it can still claim over 60 per cent. It is hardly surprising, therefore, that the bases of the lung are the parts which undergo the greatest movement. Radiographically the position of the diaphragm can be seen to vary markedly with changes in posture. In the supine position the abdominal muscles are relaxed and the intestines push the diaphragm up to its highest level. In this position, therefore, the diaphragm possesses its greatest potential powers of contraction. In the erect posture, on the other hand, the weight of the intestines falls away and the level of the diaphragm descends. Frequently, however, the abdominal muscles are contracted, presumably in an attempt to maintain an even intra-abdominal pressure. A similar set of circumstances prevails in the sitting position because the cupola lies at a low level and the abdominal muscles may be contracting if the ventilation is large.

Patients with severe dyspnoea adopt the sitting posture for comfort. This is not due to any change in position of the diaphragm, which would tend to be detrimental rather than beneficial, but to a reduction in the pulmonary congestion and also an improved action of the accessory muscles of respiration. The most satisfying position is often found to be with the trunk bent forward and the head and arms fixed on a support.

IV. *Other factors.*—Vertical movements of the thoracic cage occur in some subjects, mainly at the end of deep inspiration, and are usually most marked in the standing position. These movements are caused by flexion and extension of the vertebral column, but they do not appear to play an important part in ventilating the lungs. They are especially marked during voluntary hyperventilation and thus may aid the contractions of the diaphragm (Wade, 1954).

To summarise, during normal ventilation those parts of the lung near the diaphragm are better ventilated than their relatively static cousins near the apex.

LUNG VOLUMES

The terminology used in this chapter to describe the lung volumes and capacities was introduced by a group of American physiologists in an attempt to simplify the subject, and has now gained general acceptance (Table 3 and Fig. 11) (Pappenheimer, 1950).

Tidal Volume and Minute Volume

The tidal volume is the amount of air passing in and out of the lungs and respiratory passages during each respiratory cycle. The quantity, therefore, varies with the size and age of the individual and the depth of respiration. It ranges from 19 ml in the average newborn infant (less in premature infants) to between 450 and 750 ml in resting adults. The tidal volume multiplied by the respiratory rate (breaths per minute) gives the minute volume.

2/TABLE 3

NOMENCLATURE FOR LUNG VOLUMES AND CAPACITIES, with normal values in adults. Normal values have been taken from Needham *et al.* (1954). The figures are mean values, with the standard deviation in brackets. 98 per cent of the population will lie within ± two standard deviations of the mean.

Terminology	Explanation	Normal Values M.	Normal Values F.
Tidal volume	Volume of air inspired or expired at each breath.	660 (230)	550 (160)
Inspiratory reserve volume	Maximum volume of air that can be inspired after a normal inspiration.	2240	1480
Expiratory reserve volume	Maximum volume of air that can be expired after a normal expiration.	1240 (410)	730 (300)
Residual volume	Volume of air remaining in the lungs after a maximum expiration.	2100 (520)	1570 (380)
Vital capacity	Maximum volume of air that can be expired after a maximum inspiration.	4130 (750)	2760 (540)
Total lung capacity	The total volume of air contained in the lungs at maximum inspiration.	6230 (830)	4330 (620)
Inspiratory capacity	The maximum volume of air that can be inspired after a normal expiration.	2900	2030
Functional residual capacity	The volume of gas remaining in the lungs after a normal expiration.	3330 (680)	2300 (490)

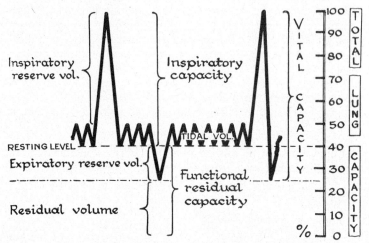

2/Fig. 11.—Spirometer record showing lung volumes and capacities.

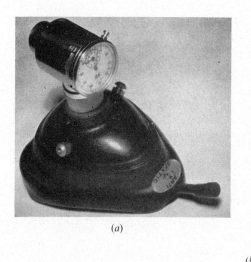

(a)

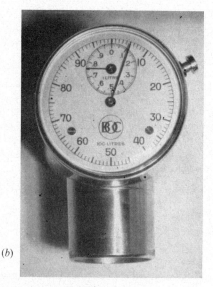

(b)

2/Fig. 12.—The Wright respirometer.

The tidal volume is of particular importance in anaesthesia, for almost every anaesthetic can depress respiration. There is, moreover, no simple device for ensuring that it is adequate for the respiratory needs of the patient, so that the anaesthetist must judge on clinical grounds whether ventilation is satisfactory. At times this decision may be a difficult one.

Measurement of tidal and minute volumes during anaesthesia.—Of the various methods of measuring minute volume, the Wright respirometer has been found the most satisfactory (Fig. 12). After allowing the instrument to record for one minute, the minute volume can be read directly, and the tidal volume then calculated from this reading and the respiratory rate. A rough estimate of the tidal volume can also be made for each breath. The instrument is compact and light; it under-reads at low flow rates and over-reads at high flow rates, but in practice the respiratory waveform and the nature of the anaesthetic gases tend to minimise these errors. For clinical purposes the instrument offers an accurate assessment of the patient's minute volume ($\pm$ 10 per cent) within the range of 3·7 to about 20 l/minute (Nunn and Ezi-Ashi, 1962). A falsely high reading (+ 10 to 20 per cent) will be obtained if the instrument is connected directly to the catheter mount unless the baffled connecting piece provided by the manufacturers is also inserted into the circuit. This is done to avoid channelling of gases.

Some Abnormalities of Ventilation

Tachypnoea.—Tachypnoea means an increase in the rate of respiration. The rate of respiration in any given situation is such that the work of breathing is at a minimum.

Hyperpnoea.—Hyperpnoea means an increase in ventilation which is in proportion to an increase in carbon dioxide production. The arterial P_{CO_2} therefore remains near normal. The commonest example of this situation is the hyperpnoea which occurs on exercise. In hyperthyroid states the general body metabolism is raised, and the pulmonary ventilation may be increased by as much as 50–100 per cent.

Hyperventilation.—Hyperventilation is an increase in ventilation out of proportion to carbon dioxide production. It is a common occurrence during controlled ventilation. Another example is the hyperventilation which accompanies a metabolic acidosis, such as occurs in renal failure and especially in diabetic coma. It can also be due to psychological factors or it may follow brain damage.

Hypoventilation.—This means a decrease in ventilation so that the arterial P_{CO_2} rises. Some degree of hypoventilation is the rule rather than the exception during anaesthesia with spontaneous respiration.

Dyspnoea.—Dyspnoea is a subjective sensation which is difficult to define. It is best described as an awareness of respiration which is unpleasant or distressing. This description does not include "breathlessness", which is not distressing, and may indeed be mildly pleasurable, such as is experienced after mild or moderate exercise.

The physiological mechanisms leading to dyspnoea are not well defined, and the most satisfying theory is that of Campbell and Howell (1963), who have suggested that the sensation arises when there is an inappropriate result (i.e. volume of inspiration) for a given muscular effort, or that a greater effort than expected is required to produce a given ventilation. They describe this as "length-tension inappropriateness", the normal situation being "learnt" by experience. The abnormal sensation of dyspnoea can then be recognised.

Dyspnoea is a common symptom of disease, and is the presenting symptom in many pulmonary and cardiac abnormalities. Its severity is very variable from person to person, so that in two patients with disease of apparently similar severity one may complain of crippling dyspnoea while it is of much less importance to the other.

Increased ventilation during anaesthesia.—During anaesthesia with spontaneous respiration, an increase in ventilation is usually due to one of four causes; (1) Oxygen lack; (2) Carbon dioxide excess; (3) Irritation of the respiratory tract by an anaesthetic vapour or other stimulating procedure; (4) Reflex surgical stimulation.

Carbon dioxide, acting through the medium of a change in the acid-base balance of the blood bathing the respiratory centre, brings about an increase mainly in the depth of respiration. In the past some anaesthetists deliberately added 5 per cent of carbon dioxide to produce a hyperpnoea when inducing with an agent such as ether. Provided this practice is only continued for a short time, and that once a physiological response has been obtained the concentration is gradually diminished, then little harm can follow in normal subjects. The danger, however, of the ill-advised use of carbon dioxide has led some people to dispense with it entirely, except through the medium of rebreathing. The continued increase in concentration that follows its prolonged use leads to an alteration in the response of the respiratory centre so that a sudden withdrawal of the stimulus causes a depression of the centre, possibly resulting in Cheyne-Stokes respiration or apnoea.

Ether brings about an increase in respiratory rate and depth together with the production of copious secretions in the respiratory tract. Premedication and induction with such respiratory depressants as the short-acting barbiturates tend to diminish all these effects.

Hyperventilation as a result of *reflex stimulation* from the operation site or stimulation of bronchial mucosa has already been discussed. Pulling on the mesentery, or dilating the anal sphincter under too light anaesthesia—in other words, inadequate reflex suppression—results in an increase in the depth of respiration. If the stimulus is even more severe or the depth of anaesthesia totally inadequate, then laryngeal spasm may result.

The tidal volume and minute volume are made up from two components, the dead space and the alveolar ventilation.

Dead Space

1. **Anatomical dead space** (VD anat) comprises the volume of the respiratory passages, extending from the nostrils and mouth down to (but not including) the alveoli. The term "dead space" is used since in it there is no exchange of gases between blood and air. Its capacity varies with age and sex, the figure normally quoted being 150 ml, but in young women it may be as low as 100 ml, whereas in old men it can rise to as much as 200 ml. The position of the lower jaw can influence dead space. Depression of the jaw with flexion of the head (a common cause of respiratory obstruction in the anaesthetised patient) reduces dead space by 30 ml. On the other hand, protrusion of the jaw with extension of the head increases dead space by 40 ml (Nunn *et al.*, 1959). Pneumonectomy or tracheostomy clearly reduces the volume of dead space.

2. **Physiological dead space** (VD phys) is defined as that fraction of the tidal volume which is not available for gaseous exchange. It includes therefore not only the anatomical dead space, but also the volume of gas which ventilates alveoli that are not being perfused, as in these alveoli gaseous exchange does not occur. This ventilation is therefore wasted, appearing as an increase in physiological dead space. This second component is called "alveolar dead space". The

actual situation is not so clear-cut as has been outlined above, because if areas of lung are overventilated, although normally perfused, they also contribute to an increase in dead space. The relationships between ventilation and perfusion of alveoli are further discussed on page 133. In normal man, anatomical and physiological dead space are numerically almost equal, and amount to about one-third of the tidal volume. Because the relationship between physiological dead space (V_D phys) and tidal volume (V_T) remains fairly constant when tidal volume is altered, the physiological dead space is often expressed as a fraction of the tidal volume (V_D/V_T ratio; normal 0·25 to 0·4).

Physiological dead space is increased in old age, in the upright position when compared with supine subjects, with large tidal volumes or high respiratory rates, after the administration of atropine, when inspiratory time is reduced to 0·5 seconds or less during controlled ventilation, and in the presence of lung disease whenever ventilation-perfusion relationships are altered. For instance, in chronic bronchitis or asthma the physiological dead space may rise to 50–80 per cent of the tidal volume; it is also found to be high following pulmonary embolism. It is increased following haemorrhage (Freeman and Nunn, 1963) and during controlled hypotension, especially if the patient is tilted head up (Askrog et al., 1964).

The effect of anaesthesia on the physiological dead space appears to be very variable, but as a general rule it can be taken that both V_D phys and V_D/V_T are increased during anaesthesia, after taking into account any changes due to apparatus dead space. During intermittent positive pressure respiration, this increase in V_D phys is approximately compensated for by intubation (which reduces dead space by about 70 ml); thus for ventilated, intubated and anaesthetised patients V_D/V_T is found to be 0·3–0·45, but if the effect of intubation is corrected for, then V_D/V_T appears to be in the 0·4–0·6 range. In one study the effects of intubation on total functional dead space during halothane anaesthesia during spontaneous ventilation has been studied (Kain et al., 1969). These workers found that, using a mask and Frumin valve, the total dead space was increased considerably (mean V_D/V_T = 0·68; SD = 0·062), being reduced by intubation (mean V_D/V_T = 0·51; SD = 0·073), representing in absolute terms an average difference in total functional dead space of 82 ml between intubated patients and those anaesthetised with a mask. These subjects were able to compensate for changes in dead space by altering their tidal volumes.

As a general rule it may be said that the dead space is increased during anaesthesia, although the changes are very variable. Cooper (1967) has suggested that the physiological dead space during anaesthesia with passive ventilation can be roughly estimated from the formula:

$$V_D/V_T = 33 + \frac{Age}{3} \text{ per cent}$$

Measurement of physiological dead space.—This is usually done by using Enghoff's modification of the Bohr equation which may be derived as follows:

$$(V_T - V_D)Pa_{CO_2} = V_T \times P\bar{E}_{CO_2}$$

This merely states that the volume of CO_2 in gas which has partaken in gas exchange (tidal volume V_T – physiological dead space V_D) is the same as the volume of CO_2 in mixed expired gas, although it is now diluted to a larger volume, the tidal volume V_T.

Rearranging this equation:

$$\text{physiological dead space } V_D = V_T \frac{(Pa_{CO_2} - P\bar{E}_{CO_2})}{Pa_{CO_2}}$$

The apparatus dead space should be subtracted from this amount. The assumption is made that Pa_{CO_2} is equal to alveolar P_{CO_2}.

Measurement of physiological dead space requires the collection of a sample of mixed expired air into a Douglas bag over a known number of breaths, and measurement of its carbon dioxide content and total volume. The arterial P_{CO_2} must also be measured in a blood sample taken during the period of gas collection. The values obtained for Pa_{CO_2}, $P\bar{E}_{CO_2}$ and V_T are then substituted in the equation, and V_D phys calculated. Allowance is then made for apparatus dead space.

3. **Apparatus dead space** consists of the volume of gas contained in any anaesthetic apparatus between the patient and that point in the system where rebreathing of exhaled carbon dioxide ceases to occur (e.g. the expiratory valve in a Magill system, or the side-arm in an Ayre's T-piece). The importance of apparatus dead space is so well known as hardly to need further emphasis, especially when anaesthetising small children. The interior volume of an adult face-piece and the connections up to the point of the expiratory valve in a Magill system may add as much as 125 ml of dead space to the patient. This problem is further discussed below.

Alveolar Ventilation

Alveolar ventilation is defined as that proportion of the tidal or minute volume which takes part in gas exchange. The normal value for alveolar ventilations is $2 \cdot 0$ to $2 \cdot 4$ l/min/square metre BSA*, or about $3 \cdot 5$ to $4 \cdot 5$ l/min in adults. Its importance lies in the fact that it is the pulmonary factor controlling the excretion of carbon dioxide by the lungs, and it is directly related to the tidal volume, physiological dead space and respiratory rate.

Alveolar Ventilation/Min = (Tidal Volume − Physiological Dead Space) × Respiratory Rate.

$$\text{or } \dot{V}_A = (V_T - V_D \text{ phys}) \times f$$

From this relationship it can be seen that a rise in physiological dead space or a fall in the respiratory rate will lead to a reduction in the alveolar ventilation provided the other factors remain fairly constant. So too will a fall in the tidal volume, although in normal man the physiological dead space also decreases, so that the effect on the alveolar ventilation is lessened.

For example, if we calculate the alveolar ventilation under various circumstances we find the following figures are obtained:

1. *Normal*
$$(V_T - V_D \text{ phys}) \times f = \dot{V}_A$$
$$(450 - 150) \quad \times 13 = 3 \cdot 9 \text{ l/min } (P_{CO_2} \text{ normal})$$

2. *Tidal Volume Reduced*
$$(300 - 100) \quad \times 13 = 2 \cdot 6 \text{ l/min } (P_{CO_2} \text{ raised})$$

* Body surface area.

3. *Physiological Dead Space Increased by Anaesthetic Apparatus*

$$(450 - 225) \times 13 = 2 \cdot 7 \text{ l/min (P}_{CO_2} \text{ raised)}$$

4. *Respiratory Rate Decreased*

$$(450 - 150) \times 8 = 2 \cdot 4 \text{ l/min (P}_{CO_2} \text{ raised)}$$

These simple calculations, although useful as a guide, do not always represent the true state of affairs. For instance, the addition of apparatus dead space of 100 ml (measured by filling the relevant volume with water) may represent a rather smaller addition when in clinical use. This is due to patterns of gas flow and channelling of gases within the apparatus. For example, the central core of the gas stream moves rapidly whilst gas in the periphery moves relatively slowly. Thus the central element represents the major portion of the ventilation, so reducing the role of the dead space. It should also be noted that in practice physiological mechanisms react to any of these changes and tend to return the P_{CO_2} towards normal values, so that the alterations in alveolar ventilation are not as great as those indicated above. However, under the influence of sedative or anaesthetic drugs these physiological responses may be depressed, so that any alteration in alveolar ventilation due to the addition of apparatus dead space may not be compensated fully. Deep anaesthesia, respiratory depressant drugs and the muscle relaxants all tend to depress alveolar ventilation. The resulting rise in alveolar carbon dioxide tension will produce a fall in alveolar oxygen tension unless extra oxygen is added to the inspired air. The explanation of this phenomenon is as follows: in very general terms, and provided that no great exchange of inert gases is occurring in the lungs, the alveolar oxygen tension can be calculated from the following equation, which is a simplification of the Alveolar Air Equation (Comroe *et al.*, 1962):

Alveolar oxygen tension =

$$\text{Inspired oxygen tension} - \frac{\text{Alveolar carbon dioxide tension}}{\text{Respiratory quotient}}$$

or $P_{A O_2} = P_{I O_2} - P_{a CO_2}/R$

Substituting normal figures into this equation:

$$P_{I O_2} - P_{a CO_2}/R = P_{A O_2}$$

$$150 - \frac{40}{0 \cdot 8} = 100 \text{ mm Hg} \quad (20 \cdot 0 - \frac{5 \cdot 3}{0 \cdot 8} = 13 \cdot 3 \text{ kPa})$$

If a rise in alveolar carbon dioxide tension to 60 mm Hg now occurs the equation will become:

$$P_{I O_2} - P_{a CO_2}/R = P_{A O_2}$$

$$150 - \frac{60}{0 \cdot 8} = 75 \text{ mm Hg} \quad (20 \cdot 0 - \frac{8 \cdot 0}{0 \cdot 8} = 10 \cdot 0 \text{ kPa})$$

Thus, if the alveolar carbon dioxide tension rises to 60 mm Hg ($8 \cdot 0$ kPa) the alveolar oxygen tension, and therefore the arterial oxygen tension, will fall to 75 mm Hg (10 kPa), and a rise in $P_{a CO_2}$ has resulted in arterial hypoxaemia. Because alveolar ventilation is almost invariably reduced by anaesthesia with spontaneous ventilation, and because other changes leading to arterial hypoxaemia occur in the lungs, it is always advisable to administer at least 33 per cent oxygen in all anaesthetic gas mixtures. This manoeuvre compensates for any rise in Pco_2, and also for the other pulmonary changes which occur. For example, if 30 per cent oxygen is administered, then the equation becomes:

$$PI_{O_2} - Paco_2/R = PA_{O_2}$$

$$230 - \frac{60}{0 \cdot 8} = 155 \text{ mm Hg} \quad (30 \cdot 7 - \frac{8 \cdot 0}{0 \cdot 8} = 20 \cdot 7 \text{ kPa})$$

and adequate oxygenation is therefore assured.

The clinical assessment of alveolar ventilation is one of the most important decisions that the anaesthetist has to make. When respiratory exchange is adequate the Po_2 and Pco_2 in the arterial blood are 100 mm Hg (13·3 kPa) and 40 mm Hg (5·3 kPa) respectively, yet at present it is impractical to measure these routinely in clinical work. Observation of the reservoir bag, the movements of the chest and abdomen, the rate of respiration, measurement of the minute volume using a respirometer, and the colour of the blood in the patient's capillary bed are all used in this assessment. Of these, the use of a respirometer is the only reliable method of assessing the patient's ventilation. The dangers of hypoventilation during anaesthesia cannot be overstressed. Equally, it is not sufficient merely to oxygenate a patient by raising the inspired oxygen percentage if adequate steps are not being taken at the same time to remove the carbon dioxide. Many beginners fall into the trap of believing that all must be well if the patient has a good colour during anaesthesia.

Vital Capacity

At the end of a normal expiration, a patient lying at rest and breathing quietly is capable of forcibly expiring a large quantity of air from his lungs—this is called the *expiratory reserve volume*. Similarly at the end of a normal inspiration, he is equally capable of taking in an even larger quantity of air—the *inspiratory reserve volume*. If the tidal volume is added to the sum of these two measurements, the patient's vital capacity will be known.

			Approximate Figure
	Tidal volume		500 ml
Vital capacity =	Inspiratory reserve volume		2500 ml
	Expiratory reserve volume		1000 ml
			4000 ml

The vital capacity can be simply measured with a spirometer. The patient is requested to take a maximum inspiration and then to expire completely into the spirometer. This test is not wholly reliable, as with a judicious use of the tongue some patients can give completely false readings. Modifications of it will be considered under the tests of lung function.

The vital capacity does not remain constant even in healthy adults, and is altered by such factors as age, physical training, changes in weight and an increase in height. For this reason it is often expressed in relation to the surface area of the body. Repeated examinations may lead, for no obvious reasons, to a steady improvement.

2/TABLE 4

NORMAL VALUES OF VITAL CAPACITY

	Athlete	Male	Female
Average vital capacity in ml/m² of body surface area	2800	2600	2100
Average vital capacity in ml/m² of height ..	2900	2500	2000

In view of the marked differences in values for normal people, a measurement of vital capacity cannot be considered abnormal unless it varies by more than 20 per cent from the above figures. A single reading is of little value, but repeated readings may be useful when undertaken on a comparative basis to study the progress of a patient's treatment.

The vital capacity may be reduced by many disease processes. Some of these are of particular interest to the anaesthetist.

1. **Alterations in muscle power.**—Clearly, any drug which depresses the activity of the ventilatory mechanisms, whether it be in the brain, nerve, or muscle fibre, must reduce the vital capacity. Similarly, lesions in the brain such as cerebral tumours, a raised intracranial pressure, lesions affecting the nerves, such as poliomyelitis and polyneuritis, or lesions of the neuromuscular mechanism such as occur in myasthenia gravis, will lead to a reduced vital capacity.

2. **Pulmonary disease.**—The commonest disease in this country in which a reduction in vital capacity is found is chronic bronchitis. Some other lung diseases which reduce the vital capacity are pulmonary fibrosis, lobar collapse, pneumonia, and asthma.

3. **Space-occupying lesion in the chest.**—Neurofibromata and other extrapleural tumours, kyphoscoliosis, pericardial and pleural effusions, pneumothorax, and some diseases—such as carcinoma of the lung with infiltration or consolidation—will reduce the vital capacity.

4. **Abdominal tumours which impede the descent of the diaphragm.**—The addition of 1 litre of water to the stomach brings about no significant change in the vital capacity, but if another litre is added a slight fall occurs, which returns to normal again on emptying the stomach (Mills, 1949). Although the gravid uterus displaces the diaphragm upwards, the vital capacity of a pregnant woman is not decreased. On the contrary, it is increased on average 10 per cent over the normal, since the thoracic cage is enlarged transversely and antero-posteriorly and there is marked splaying of the subcostal angle.

5. **Abdominal pain.**—The pain experienced after an operation involving the abdominal musculature leads to a reduction in vital capacity of 70–75 per cent in upper abdominal and 50 per cent in lower abdominal operations.

These figures have been confirmed by Simpson and his associates (1961), who advocated the use of a continuous thoracic epidural technique for the relief of post-operative pain. Using this method, they were able to produce not only complete freedom from pain, but also a very substantial improvement in the vital capacity (see Table 5). It is interesting to note, however, that in very few patients in their series was the vital capacity restored to the pre-operative level. It might be argued, therefore, that the epidural itself was responsible for limiting some respiratory activity, but Moir (1963) in a similar study, concluded that no important degree of respiratory paresis was produced by epidural blockade.

2/TABLE 5

VITAL CAPACITY READINGS EXPRESSED AS A % OF THE PRE-OPERATIVE VALUE

	Before epidural (In pain)			1 hour after epidural (Pain-free)			24 hours after epidural (Pain-free)		
	Range %	Mean %	No. of Cases	Range %	Mean %	No. of Cases	Range %	Mean %	No. of Cases
Upper Abdominal	20–56	35·2	54	44–139	69·0	54	61–139	83·2	50
Lower Abdominal	37–69	55·5	6	80–91	84·8	6	92–96	94·7	3

Vital capacity readings in 60 patients undergoing abdominal surgery (Simpson *et al.*, 1961).

There seems to be little doubt that a continuous epidural technique provides the most effective form of pain relief in combination with the maximum ventilatory function. Nevertheless, such techniques are time-consuming and require a high degree of technical skill if the thoracic level is used (in order to reduce the incidence of hypotensive complications). For these reasons this technique is best reserved for the special case.

6. **Abdominal splinting.**—Tight abdominal binders, strapping, or bandaging limit the range of respiratory movement. Elastic strapping applied in the vertical plane allows the greatest freedom of respiration in the post-operative period.

7. **Alterations in posture.**—Changes in posture in the conscious subject lead to considerable alterations in the vital capacity, and these are mainly related to positions which are calculated to alter the volume of blood in the lungs. Thus the capacity is greater when standing than when sitting or lying. It increases by as much as $\frac{1}{4}$–$\frac{1}{2}$ litre if there is an accumulation of blood in the legs. The inhalation of amyl nitrite causes an increase of about $\frac{1}{4}$ litre. The latter is probably mainly due to increased depth of inspiration.

The various positions in which an anaesthetised patient may be placed on the operating table have been shown to have a considerable effect on the vital capacity of the unanaesthetised subject. For example:

	Loss of Vital Capacity
Trendelenburg position (20°)	.. 14·5 per cent
Lithotomy	.. 18·0 per cent
Left lateral	.. 10·0 per cent
Right lateral	.. 12·0 per cent
Bridge in dorsal position ..	.. 12·5 per cent
Prone position, unsupported	.. 10·0 per cent

(Case and Stiles, 1946)

Significance during anaesthesia.—Alterations in the vital capacity are of little significance during anaesthesia unless extremely pronounced. During spontaneous ventilation the patient can nearly always maintain a satisfactory Pa_{CO_2} and during artificial ventilation the only noticeable consequence is that the lungs feel "stiff". It is only when the vital capacity begins to fall below the required tidal volume that respiratory difficulties arise during anaesthesia. Examples of conditions in which this may occur are tension pneumothorax, a large haemothorax, diaphragmatic hernia, exomphalos in the newborn, neuromuscular diseases and upper respiratory obstruction. Reductions in vital capacity do, however, become important in the post-operative period when the expulsion of secretions may be seriously impeded. If the vital capacity falls below about three times the tidal volume artificial help may be needed to maintain the airways clear of excessive secretions. Following the use of relaxants the patient may not be able to breath adequately for a short time and will therefore need artificial help until the relaxant has been completely eliminated.

Residual Volume

Residual volume is the amount of air that still remains in the lungs after the patient has made a maximal expiration. Normal average values range from 2,100 ml for males to 1,570 for females. Functional residual capacity is the amount of air remaining in the lungs after a normal expiration. Normal average values range from 3,300 ml for males to 2,300 ml for females.

Unfortunately neither of these two measurements can be made directly. There are, however, two indirect methods which use a known concentration of a relatively insoluble gas, i.e. one that does not readily traverse the alveolar membrane and become dissolved in the plasma.

Nitrogen technique.—The principle is to collect all the nitrogen that can be washed out of the patient's lungs. Following a maximal expiration (if residual volume is required) or a normal expiration (if functional residual capacity is required) the patient inspires oxygen from a special source and then expires into a spirometer which is known to be free of nitrogen. Over some minutes almost all the alveolar nitrogen is washed out of the lungs. In healthy adults this may be achieved after only two minutes, but in patients with severe emphysema at least 7–20 minutes may be needed. At the beginning of the test all the nitrogen is in the lungs and at the end it has all passed to the spirometer. The concentration of nitrogen in the spirometer can now be measured. The total volume of gases in the spirometer is known so that the total volume of nitrogen in the mixture can be calculated. As air contains 80 per cent nitrogen a suitable correction will reveal the total alveolar gas volume at the moment the test began.

Helium technique.—In this case a spirometer with carbon dioxide absorption is used. This is filled with a mixture of 10 per cent helium and 90 per cent oxygen and the patient then breathes in and out of it. At first, there is no helium in the patient's lungs, but gradually mixing takes place until after a few minutes the concentration of helium in the patient's lungs and in the spirometer is the same. Again, the volume of gas in the alveoli can then be calculated.

Significance.—As the residual volume represents the amount of air remaining in the lungs at the end of a maximal expiration, any increase in it signifies that the lung is larger than usual and cannot empty adequately. Increases in residual volume are usually associated with air-trapping in the lungs, but may occur temporarily without any actual structural change. For example, obstruction to the airway, as in asthma or over-inflation of the lungs after a thoracic operation, may cause an increase. If there is a marked increase in residual air the act of respiration may be difficult, since by implication the patient is unable to reduce the volume even by forced expiration, and it is likely that respiration is carried out with the mechanical disadvantage of a thorax already larger than normal.

In severe emphysema some air is "trapped" completely in the alveoli and never comes in contact with the respired gases. In emphysematous patients it is impossible to obtain a true reading of the residual volume by either of the methods mentioned above. This can only be obtained in a highly specialised respiratory unit where a body plethysmograph is available. Such an instrument measures the thoracic gas volume whether it is in free communication with the airway or not.

Functional Residual Capacity

The functional residual capacity is the volume of gas held in the lungs at the normal relaxed end-expiratory point. It is increased in certain diseases (such as asthma and chronic bronchitis) and as a result of the application of a positive end-expiratory pressure (Fig. 13a). It is decreased as a result of the induction of anaesthesia (Fig. 13b) and post-operatively, especially following abdominal surgery. The FRC is especially important in relation to the Closing Volume (see below) since if the latter rises above the FRC arterial hypoxaemia may occur.

Closing Volume (CV)

As the lungs become reduced in volume during expiration there comes a point at which some small airways begin to close and therefore prevent any further expulsion of gas from related alveoli, so that air-trapping occurs. The lung volume at which this phenomenon can first be detected is called the Closing Volume (CV). Measurements of this volume are made using a single breath

2/FIG. 13(a).—Spirometer tracing showing the effect of positive end-expiratory pressure (PEEP) on functional residual capacity (100 ml divisions).

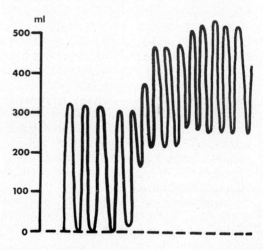

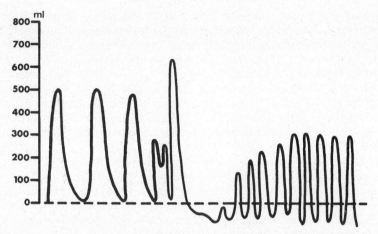

2/Fig. 13(b).—Spirometer tracing showing decrease in functional residual capacity at onset of anaesthesia—thiopentone (100 ml divisions).

nitrogen-washout technique. Whilst breathing air the subject slowly expires to residual volume, and then slowly takes a single breath of oxygen to maximum inhalation. The breath is held for a few seconds and then slowly and evenly expired. During this phase the instantaneous nitrogen concentration and volume of the expirate are recorded, and a characteristic curve is obtained (Fig. 14). This curve has four phases: (I) Dead space gas; (II) Mixed dead space and alveolar gas; (III) Mixed alveolar gas from all alveoli; and (IV) A phase in which there is a sudden rising concentration of nitrogen. The CV is the volume at which phase IV begins. The reasoning behind this is as follows. During inhalation the oxygen is preferentially distributed to the smaller alveoli in the dependent parts of the lung due to the shape in the alveolar compliance curve

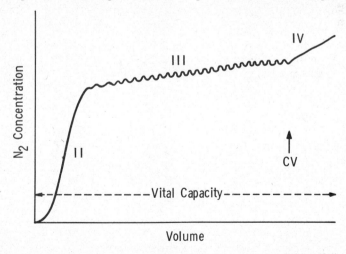

2/Fig. 14.—Measurement of closing volume by nitrogen wash-out technique (full explanation in text).

which assures a larger change in volume in smaller alveoli than in larger ones. Therefore the nitrogen is more diluted in the smaller alveoli. During expiration the mixed alveolar nitrogen concentration from all alveoli is measured (Phase III) until the point at which airway closure begins. At this moment the nitrogen concentration increases because the expulsion of gases from the smaller airways ceases and exhalation continues from those areas of the lung where the nitrogen concentration is higher. Other tracer gases such as helium, argon and [133]Xenon can be used in a similar fashion. The CV is usually presented as a fraction of the vital capacity, but may also be presented in relation to the FRC (e.g., CV—FRC, or FRC/CV).

In subjects with normal lungs the normal value for CV is intimately related to the age and position of the subject. Normal regression lines for CV in supine subjects with respect to age are shown in Fig. 15. From this figure it can be seen that the lowest values for closing volumes are to be found in the late teens, and that below (down to the age of about 5 years) and above this age it is progressively increased.

The important point to note is the relationship of the CV to the FRC. If the CV rises above the FRC some airways will be closed during part, or later perhaps the whole, of the range of normal ventilation with the result that blood passing through the closed areas of lung will not be fully oxygenated, and the arterial Po_2 will fall. In subjects with normal lungs CV becomes equal to FRC in the 60's and in the 40's in supine subjects. After this the CV continues to rise as age increases, and the arterial Po_2 begins to fall. A rise in CV is seen in smokers, obesity, rapid intravenous transfusion, early chronic bronchitis, left ventricular failure and following myocardial infarction. It is almost certainly increased after surgery, and may be an important factor in the genesis of post-operative hypoxaemia (Alexander et al., 1973; Fibuch et al., 1975). Although it is known that the FRC falls during anaesthesia, and therefore may encroach upon the CV, especially in the elderly, it is not known whether the CV itself is altered. This is because the manoeuvres required to measure the CV are difficult

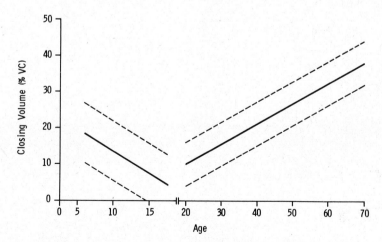

2/Fig. 15.—Relationship of age to closing volume in normal subjects.

to perform during anaesthesia. Air-trapping probably does occur in the anaes-thetised state (Don *et al.*, 1972; Rehder *et al.*, 1977) but the exact sequence of events is not clear. The use of a positive end-expiratory pressure probably raises the arterial Po_2 by increasing the FRC above the CV.

Thoracic Gas Volume

The principle of measuring the total volume of air contained in the thorax is based on a change of the air pressures inside and outside the thorax when the patient's airway is suddenly obstructed. First, the patient is enclosed in a body plethysmograph in a special chamber, and permitted to breathe the air within the chamber. The airway pressure and the plethysmograph pressure are noted. At the desired moment (usually at the end of a normal expiration) the airway is suddenly occluded by an electrical shutter. The patient will then attempt to inspire against a total obstruction. The chest expands, the intrathoracic pres-sure falls whilst the pressure in the plethysmograph rises. Alveolar pressure is as-sumed to equal mouth pressure under these circumstances, so that the pressure differences now enable the original thoracic gas volume to be calculated.

This method is rapid and relatively simple. It is often used in combination with the dilution methods of nitrogen and helium for in this manner it is easy to determine the amount of "non-ventilated" areas of lung in a particular patient. In a patient with severe emphysema these tests may reveal that as much as 1–3 litres of air are trapped within the alveoli.

Discussion.—All these tests must be interpreted with caution because there is a wide margin for normal values even in the healthy adult. Nevertheless, an increase in functional residual capacity is usually assumed to denote structural emphysematous changes in the lung. In reality it represents hyperinflation of the lung during quiet breathing and though this is commonly caused by emphysema and partial obstruction of the airway, it could in rare cases be due to a deformity of the thorax.

Minimal Air

Even after the pleural cavities have been opened and the lungs have collapsed, there still remains a very small, but nevertheless important, quantity of air entrapped in the lungs—the minimal air. In medico-legal circles the presence of air in the lungs of a newborn child suggests that it has breathed after birth, but this deduction does not hold if the lungs have been positively inflated during resuscitation. A piece of aerated lung when placed in water will float, whereas a piece of atelectatic lung (i.e. one which has not been aerated) will sink to the bottom.

Dynamic Tests of Ventilation

The tests of ventilatory function so far discussed are more or less static in nature. However, ventilation is essentially a dynamic process, and other function tests have been devised which attempt to quantitate ventilatory function in terms of the *rate* at which ventilation can take place, rather than in terms of volumes.

1. **Maximum breathing capacity (MBC).**—This test is designed to measure the speed and efficiency of filling and emptying the lungs during increased

respiratory effort, and is defined as the maximum volume of air that can be breathed per minute. It is. usually measured for 15 seconds and the result expressed in litres per minute. It is therefore a dynamic test, as opposed to the static measurement of vital capacity. As age increases there is a large reduction in the maximum breathing capacity, but it is in patients with pulmonary emphysema that it shows the most impairment. It also falls in the presence of bronchospasm and bronchiolar obstruction and the test has been used, therefore, to judge the effectiveness of bronchodilators in the treatment of bronchoconstriction. Cournand and Richards (1941) reported that the maximum breathing capacity is reduced by 15 per cent after a five-rib thoracoplasty but that this functional loss is considerably greater if a pronounced scoliosis develops.

A disadvantage of the maximum breathing capacity test is that results are apt to differ in the hands of separate workers; this is largely due to variations in technique, and to the different types of apparatus used for measurement. The instrument may introduce errors in certain circumstances, such as by adding resistance to respiration or influencing the rate of breathing. Furthermore the test is a tiring procedure and not without risk in severely disabled subjects, and the results can be fairly accurately predicted from the timed vital capacity (forced expiratory volume) (Needham et al., 1954). For these reasons it has fallen into disrepute at the present time. Average values for normal subjects range from 100–200 litres per minute depending upon the mode of measurement, but there is a big difference between these figures and those for abnormal subjects.

2. **Forced expiratory volume (FEV).**—The patient makes a maximal inspiration, expires as forcefully and rapidly as he can into a spirometer, and the total amount of air expelled over a given time is measured. The time intervals at which the total amount of air expelled is measured are 0·5, 1, 2 and 3 seconds. However, as there seems to be little advantage between the results taken at each of these intervals, it is customary to take only the volume expired at 1 second, called the FEV_1. This volume is expressed as a percentage of the forced vital capacity. In normal young subjects 83 per cent of the vital capacity should be expired during the first second. The lower limit of normal is usually taken as 70 per cent. In a patient with chronic bronchitis the FEV_1 may be only 50 per cent or less.

Recently the dry spirometer has come into common use to measure the vital capacity and FEV_1. One such instrument is the Vitalograph (Fig. 16). Expiring into it causes a bellows to expand and results in the vertical deflection of a pen writing on a calibrated chart. The initial act of expiration activates a pressure switch, and the whole chart is then moved sideways at a constant speed by an electric motor. A graph is drawn out on the chart, in which the vertical axis is expressed in litres, and the horizontal axis as time in seconds (see Fig. 17). The result is a graphical analysis of the rate and volume of the patient's forced vital capacity, from which the FEV_1 can be calculated. One of the main advantages of this type of instrument is that the records are produced on a small flat sheet of paper which can be filed away for reference, and subsequent tests can then be compared with previous records. A rough estimate of the peak expiratory flow rate can be obtained by measuring the slope of the steepest part of the curve.

3. **Peak expiratory flow rate (PEFR).**—After a maximal inspiration, the

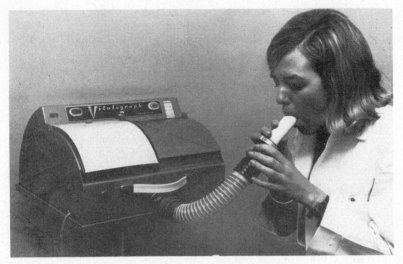

2/Fig. 16.—The "Vitalograph".

patient expires as forcefully as he can, and the maximum flow rate of air is measured. The measurement can be made either into a pneumotachograph, or by a specially designed instrument, such as the Wright Peak Flow Meter. The normal limits for the PEFR are taken as 450–700 l/minute in men, and 300–500 l/minute in women, although like all tests of ventilatory function the normal value varies with the age and build of the subject.

Discussion.—The results from measurement of both the FEV_1 and the PEFR can be improved with a little practice on the patient's part. For this reason

2/Fig. 17.—Examples of the time course of forced expiration taken with a "Vitalograph". Curve (i): normal male aged 40. FEV_1 = 3·7/5·0 = 74 per cent. Curve (ii): a patient with chronic bronchitis, showing both a restrictive and an obstructive lesion (see text). Curve (iii): the same patient after the inhalation of an isoprenaline aerosol, showing some improvement.

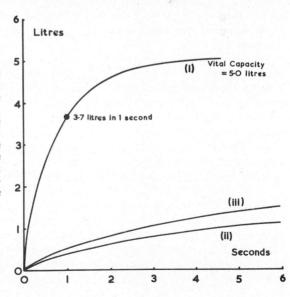

it is customary to perform the test five times, and then to take the average of the last three readings as the final result. Alternatively, the best of the five readings can be taken. It is of great importance to use apparatus with a low resistance to high gas flow rates.

Low values for the FEV_1 and PEFR usually indicate a higher than normal resistance to gas flow within the conducting airways (i.e. a diffuse airways obstruction). This type of abnormality is termed "obstructive" and is found in such conditions as asthma, chronic bronchitis, bronchitis and bronchospasm. The response to the inhalation of a bronchodilator aerosol can readily be tested. If reversible bronchoconstriction is present, then both the PEFR and FEV_1 improve after aerosol inhalation (see Fig. 17). This gives a guide as to whether bronchodilator drugs will or will not be an effective form of treatment, for example in combination with physiotherapy during the pre-operative preparation of such a patient. Some patients are found to have a reduced vital capacity, although their PEFR and FEV_1 values are within normal limits. This type of ventilatory defect is described as "restrictive". Although this distinction between obstructive and restrictive abnormalities of ventilation has been made, it is usual to find that both the vital capacity and the tests of flow rate are reduced so that both types of abnormality are present. Such is the case in chronic bronchitis where, apart from diffuse airway obstruction, air trapping also contributes to abnormally low PEFR and FEV_1 values.

If no apparatus is available for estimating the severity of an obstructive lesion, this can be judged by a simple bedside test. The patient is asked to take a deep breath, and then to exhale as forcibly as possible through his mouth. Normally this forced expiration is virtually complete after three seconds. Prolongation beyond this time is abnormal, and the severity of the obstructive lesion can be roughly judged from the time it takes to complete the expiration.

4. **Broncho-spirometry.**—The function of each lung can be studied separately by broncho-spirometry. This test has an advantage over most others in that it measures both ventilation and oxygen uptake at the same time. The introduction of the Carlens catheter (Carlens, 1949) has overcome some of the difficulties of the technique (Fig. 18a).

Under topical analgesia the special catheter is placed in the trachea so that the end rests in the left main bronchus with the hook over the carina (Fig. 18b). Inflation of the terminal balloon isolates the left lung and inflation of the proximal balloon the right. Each lung can then be connected separately to a spirometer fitted with carbon dioxide absorption, and a simultaneous record obtained from both lungs. In a normal subject one would expect 55 per cent of both the ventilation and the oxygen consumption to be carried out by the right lung and 45 per cent by the left. Figure 18c illustrates how disease in one lung may be suggested by a considerable alteration in this ratio.

This test is most useful when used to estimate the function of one lung when pneumonectomy or lobectomy on the opposite side is being considered.

5. **Uneven ventilation.**—The way in which inspired air is distributed to the alveoli may be influenced by local changes in airways resistance or pulmonary elasticity. The simplest method for detecting abnormal distribution of pulmonary ventilation involves studying the elimination of nitrogen from the alveoli when breathing 100 per cent oxygen. The subject inhales pure oxygen for a

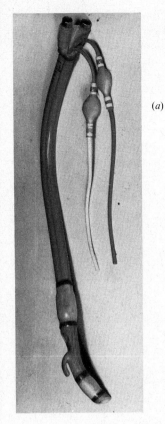

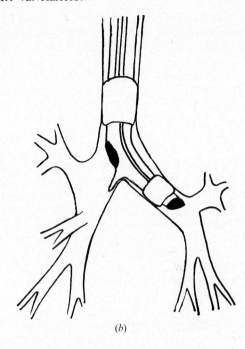

(a)

(b)

2/Fig. 18.—(a) Carlens catheter. (b) Carlens catheter *in situ* (diagrammatic).

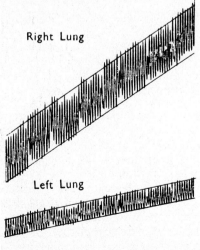

Right Lung

Left Lung

TIME IN MINUTES

2/Fig. 18(c).—Broncho-Spirometry

Spirometer tracings of individual lungs during broncho-spirometry (31-year-old woman with diseased left lung).

		Right lung
O$_2$ uptake ..	..	210 ml/min (77 per cent)
Ventilation ..	..	6·0 l/min (73 per cent)

		Left lung
O$_2$ uptake ..	..	63 ml/min (23 per cent)
Ventilation ..	..	2·16 l/min (27 per cent)

period of seven minutes, and at the end of this time the nitrogen concentration in a sample of alveolar air is measured using a nitrogen meter (see Chapter 3). If the concentration is above 2 per cent, it is considered to be an indication of abnormal distribution of ventilation, as washout of nitrogen has not been achieved in those alveoli which are being poorly ventilated. It should be remembered that the rate of nitrogen washout can also be affected by (1) the tidal and minute volumes and (2) the functional residual capacity.

THE PLEURAL CAVITY

Each lung is invested with a thin serous covering on its outer surface (visceral pleura) and this is reflected on to the inner aspect of the chest wall and the upper surface of the diaphragm (parietal pleura). The potential space between these two layers is the pleural cavity and under normal conditions the two surfaces are in apposition save for a small quantity of lymph which acts as a lubricant. In disease, adhesions may form between the two surfaces, but if the underlying lung is not involved there is no appreciable change in respiratory function.

At the apex of the pleural cavity the outer surface is surrounded by loose areolar tissue (extrapleural or Sibson's fascia) in which small fibrous bands can sometimes be demonstrated coursing over the dome of the lung (bands of Sebalot).

Intrapleural Pressure

Owing to the continual retractive force exerted by the elastic recoil of the lung, the intrapleural pressure under normal conditions is always negative. When the pleural cavity is opened the negative pressure returns to atmospheric, the lung collapses, and the mediastinum moves over towards the unaffected side.

The elastic recoil of the lung is made up of three factors:

1. The elastic tissue in the bronchial wall and also that coursing throughout the interstitial tissue of the lungs.
2. The arrangement of the muscle fibres of the bronchi and bronchioles in a "geodesic" network so that on contraction the bronchial tree not only becomes reduced in diameter but also shortened in length.
3. The surface tension of the fluid lining the alveolar walls.

In man the intrapleural pressure ranges from $-5 \cdot 6$ mm Hg ($-0 \cdot 7$ kPa) on inspiration to $-2 \cdot 6$ mm Hg ($-0 \cdot 3$ kPa) on expiration. It is less negative at the bottom than at the top of the lung. In normal circumstances the force required to separate the two pleural surfaces is prodigious unless air or fluid enters the pleural cavity. During a strong inspiratory effort with the glottis closed, pressures of -40 mm Hg ($-5 \cdot 3$ kPa) have been recorded, whereas forced expiration under similar conditions may lead to pressures as high as $+50$ mm Hg ($6 \cdot 7$ kPa). These variations in pressure have little bearing on the thoracic cage, but are reflected on the thin-walled surrounding structures, namely the heart and great vessels. A rise of intrathoracic pressure impedes the venous return and expels blood from the intrathoracic veins into the neck and abdomen.

Intrapleural Pressure Changes in Pulmonary Collapse

With the pleura intact, collapse of lung can take place only if the surrounding soft tissue structures such as those at the apex of the lung, the diaphragm, and the mediastinum move inwards to fill the vacant space. In practice, as the lung collapses, so the pressure in the intrapleural space falls. This is then reflected on the entire thoracic cavity but only the soft tissues can yield. When they do so, the intrapleural pressure rises and the lung can then collapse a little further. This cycle is repeated over and over again. The diaphragm is the principal tissue to be affected and, in cases with a large area of pulmonary collapse, it will be found to be raised.

In cases of severe post-operative pulmonary collapse, negative intrapleural pressures four times greater than normal have been recorded.

Pneumothorax

Air can enter the pleural cavity in a number of ways. If there is a free communication with the atmosphere, whether through a broncho-pleural fistula or a wound of the chest wall, the pneumothorax is described as *open*, whereas if there is no communication it is *closed*. A particularly dangerous type of pneumothorax is that in which air can enter but cannot escape (ball-valve), leading to a *tension* pneumothorax. Thus in an anaesthetised patient a pneumothorax may be found to be open, closed, or under tension.

It is important to remember in any discussion of the physiological changes occurring under these conditions that the pleural cavity in the experimental animal often differs profoundly from that in man. For example, the commonest animal to be used for such investigations is probably the dog, and in this animal the parietal and visceral pleura are of almost diaphanous texture, the mediastinum extremely mobile, and the two pleural cavities are often in direct communication. The extremely thin and lax pleural membranes permit pressure changes in one cavity to be rapidly transmitted to the other. In man, however, the pleural membrane is thicker and the mediastinum represents a fairly solid mass separating the two cavities, which have no communication. Thus a change of pressure in one cavity is only partially reflected in the other cavity.

Norris and his colleagues (1968) have shown a correlation between the extent of a pneumothorax as judged from a radiograph and the size of the anatomical shunt producing arterial oxygen desaturation. When the ratio of lung to intrapleural space is greater than 75 per cent the shunt does not exceed the normal value of 2 per cent of the cardiac output. Below 65 per cent the shunt increases as the size of the lung decreases. When the air is removed from the pleural space a delay of several hours occurs before the ventilation-perfusion upset in the lung improves, and this despite an early increase in the size of the lung. This delay is probably due to the relatively greater pressure required to open a ventilatory unit which is completely closed, than that needed for one that has remained at least partially open.

Open pneumothorax.—In the presence of a pneumothorax the size of the opening in relation to the diameter of the trachea will determine how much air enters the lungs. But patients breathing quietly under local analgesia can tolerate large openings in their chest wall although there is no negative intrapleural pressure and the lung is partially collapsed. The reason for this is that in the resting state only a small volume of air—the tidal air—is required, and this is a small fraction of the vital capacity. If, however, the patient becomes alarmed and attempts deep respirations, more air is sucked into the pleural space, the lung collapses further, and dyspnoea and cyanosis result. It must be clear, therefore, that those patients with a reduced vital capacity tolerate a pneumothorax badly. Under anaesthesia the detrimental effects of a pneumothorax are countered by intermittent positive-pressure respiration when the opening is between the pleura and the chest wall. If the opening is via a broncho-pleural fistula this treatment may lead to a tension pneumothorax unless special precautions are taken.

The degree of collapse of lung with the chest open depends on a number of factors which are altered in both health and disease:

1. Size of opening in the pleura.
2. The elastic recoil of the lung.
3. Airways resistance and bronchiolar patency.

Closed pneumothorax.—This may be accidentally acquired or result during the closure of a thoracotomy wound, or be induced for therapeutic reasons. An accidental pneumothorax may arise when an emphysematous bulla ruptures and partially fills the pleural space with air. As a thoracotomy wound is closed, a certain amount of air will remain entrapped in the pleural cavity. This volume can be considerably reduced if the anaesthetist ensures that the lung is fully distended just prior to complete closure of the wound. After such operations as lobectomy and pneumonectomy, a potential space is created which it is often impossible to fill with the surrounding soft tissues. In order to allow the remaining lung tissue to function adequately a negative intrapleural pressure must be re-established. Gases may be removed from this space in the following ways:

1. *Absorption.*—Any gas—including air—when introduced into the pleural cavity, is absorbed by the blood stream, because the visceral pleura is permeable to these gases. The rate of absorption of the contained gases depends largely on their respective partial pressures. Thus, air will be absorbed slowly, for the partial pressure of nitrogen is high in both the pleural space and the blood stream. Oxygen, however, is rapidly removed, and according to Dalton's Law this then raises the partial pressure of nitrogen so that it is now higher than that in the circulation; thus some nitrogen is absorbed. This process continues until all the air has been removed but, depending on the amount entrapped, may take up to three or four days to be completed.

2. *Aspiration.*—A pneumothorax apparatus may be used to take off small amounts of air in the operating theatre so that the patient returns to the ward with a normal negative intrapleural pressure.

3. *Water seal.*—This has two main functions—one to act as a drainage tube for any blood that may collect in the pleural cavity; the other to allow air to leave the cavity and to prevent its return. It is an efficient and simple type of unidirectional valve. A litre of sterile water is placed in a large glass bottle and the height of the water level is noted. A glass column starting just below the

surface of the water is connected by a length of rubber tubing directly with the intrapleural space via a leakproof circuit. On inspiration water is sucked up the glass column and falls again on expiration. If the patient coughs, or the lung is distended on expiration by increasing the respiratory resistance, then air is driven out of the chest and bubbles out into the bottle, which is in direct communication with the atmosphere. Using this method, provided there are no leaks either from the lung surface or bronchus, it is possible to re-establish a negative intrapleural pressure almost immediately after closure of the thoracic wound.

4. *Suction through a water seal.*—In order to be certain that all the air is removed from the pleural space suction may be applied to the air in the glass bottle. This will be transmitted via the drainage tube to the pleural cavity and thus rapidly establish a negative intrapleural pressure. It is an extremely useful method of treatment after segmental resection of lung, particularly where the remaining portion of lung continues to leak air into the pleural space. It must be remembered, however, that the indiscriminate use of suction may continue to keep open channels which might otherwise seal off.

Tension Pneumothorax

When air enters the intrapleural space but cannot leave it, a tension pneumothorax results. It may arise spontaneously or during anaesthesia, especially when intermittent positive pressure ventilation is used. In the earlier instance a bulla may rupture or a broncho-pleural fistula may be present. A quite normal lung may rupture if unduly high inflation pressures are allowed during anaesthesia.

A simple valve-system usually causes the pressure in the enclosed space to rise sometimes as high as $+20$ mm Hg ($2 \cdot 7$ kPa)—thus displacing the mediastinum and compressing the great veins and auricles.

Tension pneumothorax should be suspected during anaesthesia if inflation becomes increasingly difficult and the patient's condition steadily deteriorates. An unanaesthetised patient presents with cyanosis, hypotension and dyspnoea. Whether anaesthetised or not, tachycardia or bradycardia, depending on how far the condition has progressed, may be present. Pneumomediastinum and subcutaneous emphysema may or may not be present. In two recorded cases (Vance, 1968; Rastogi and Wright, 1969) the onset of marked respiratory wheezing led to the mistaken diagnosis of severe bronchospasm, and consequent ineffective treatment with bronchodilator drugs. Rarely a tension pneumothorax may occur due to the rupture of a bulla during an asthmatic attack when bronchospasm will also be present. Once a tension pneumothorax is suspected percussion of the chest wall will usually reveal the side which is affected. A wide-bore needle should be passed into the pleural space on that side and this should be connected to an underwater seal as soon as one is available. The rapid insertion of a wide-bore intravenous cannula over the most resonant area can be life-saving on such an occasion; once the stilette has been withdrawn and in combination with positive-pressure ventilation the entrapped air can readily pass to the atmosphere. Very occasionally, a tension pneumothorax may be bilateral (Rastogi and Wright, 1969) so that this possibility must always be borne in mind and the situation confirmed with a chest X-ray as soon as possible.

ABNORMAL CHEST AND LUNG MOVEMENTS

When the stability of the thoracic cage is destroyed either by trauma or surgical intervention, then abnormal movements of both chest wall and the underlying lung may occur. There are three principal conditions that must be considered, paradoxical respiration, pendelluft and mediastinal flap.

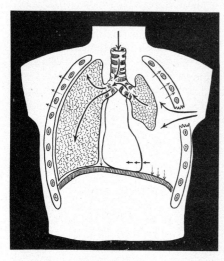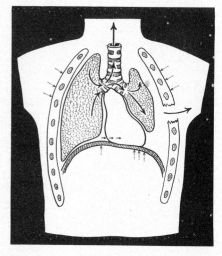

(*a*) Inspiration.   (*b*) Expiration.

2/FIG. 19.—PENDELLUFT

Paradoxical Respiration

In the presence of a crush injury of the chest wall or the deliberate surgical removal of part of the rib cage (as in a thoracoplasty), the affected part of the chest wall collapses inwards. On inspiration the unaffected side will expand in the normal fashion but the injured side will be sucked in. On expiration, the reverse takes place. This type of respiration—paradoxical respiration—is only seen in patients breathing spontaneously and is abolished by controlled ventilation. The presence of paradoxical respiration is an indication to apply external pressure (in the form of a pad) over the wound site to prevent this abnormal movement of the chest wall, or for artificial ventilation in the more severe cases.

Pendelluft

This signifies the pendulum-like movement of air that occurs from one lung to the other in the presence of an open pneumothorax in a patient breathing spontaneously. Thus, when the chest is opened the underlying lung partially deflates as the negative intrapleural pressure is lost. On inspiration, the lung on the normal side fills with air partly from the trachea and partly from the partially deflated lung on the affected side. On expiration, the converse takes place and some expired air from the normal lung passes over into the other side (Fig. 19). The physiological result of this pendulum-like flow of air is that the alveolar carbon dioxide tension rises.

Previously, this condition was always believed to occur in the presence of paradoxical respiration, but Maloney and his associates (1961) have shown that this concept is untrue. In a study of dogs using a bronchospirometric technique together with gas analysis they were able to prove that pendelluft does not occur in the presence of paradoxical respiration provided the pleural cavity is not open to the atmosphere.

In the presence of an open pneumothorax, pendelluft does not necessarily occur; much will depend on the size of the opening in the chest wall and the volume of the ventilation. If the size of the hole in the chest wall is less than the diameter of the trachea, then it is easier for air to enter via the trachea, so very little air will be sucked into the affected side and both lungs will expand on inspiration. Similarly, a patient breathing spontaneously can often tolerate a large opening in his pleural cavity provided he is breathing quietly. The moment ventilation increases both paradoxical respiration and pendelluft may result.

Mediastinal Flap

In man the mediastinum can move freely with the different phases of respiration. It remains, however, approximately in the middle of the thorax because the negative pressure in the pleural cavities balance each other. When the pleural cavity is opened, so that the lung collapses and the pressure around it becomes atmospheric, the negative intrapleural pressure on the other side will pull the heart and great vessels in the mediastinum towards the sound lung. This negative pull reaches its maximum during inspiration and, therefore, the mediastinum comes furthest over at this time (Fig. 20a). On expiration the intrapleural pressure becomes less negative and the mediastinum passes back to its original position.

During quiet breathing, even in the presence of a large hole in the chest wall, the mediastinum merely moves with a slight to and fro' motion. As the volume of ventilation increases so the flapping movement becomes more obvious. Its presence tends to embarrass respiration because it impairs the filling of the lung on the normal side. The actual range of movement is greatest when the patient is in the supine position but it is more dangerous in the lateral position because, then, the whole weight of the mediastinal contents is compressing the dependent normal lung. In addition, mediastinal flap interferes with the filling of the great veins, leading to a fall in cardiac output.

Treatment.—Paradoxical respiration, pendelluft, mediastinal flap and the disturbances caused by the weight of the mediastinal viscera, can all be prevented during anaesthesia by assisted or controlled respiration (Fig. 20b).

ASSISTED AND CONTROLLED RESPIRATION

In a normal conscious subject breathing spontaneously, the carbon dioxide tension of the blood varies between 36 and 44 mm Hg (4·8–5·9 kPa), and only rarely can values outside this range be recorded. Under the conditions of anaesthesia, when spontaneous respiration is maintained, the effective tidal exchange can be impaired by anaesthetic, analgesic and relaxant drugs, so that the level of carbon dioxide in the body will consequently rise. Moreover the patient's efforts may be further impeded by the resistance of the anaesthetic system. As oxygen is usually added to anaesthetic mixtures the tidal volume may well be sufficient to ensure oxygenation of the patient, yet inadequate to carry away all this carbon dioxide. There is no simple method available for measuring the carbon dioxide tension of blood or alveolar air and, as a result, the anaesthetist must estimate the balance and effectiveness of the tidal exchange on a purely empirical basis. When there is any doubt about this, respiration must be assisted, and arterial blood gases analysed.

Assisted Respiration

With this, the patient spontaneously commences inspiration and the anaesthetist then assists with positive-pressure down the trachea until the lungs are fully expanded. Expiration is then allowed to take place passively. Assisted respiration is useful when respiratory activity is temporarily depressed or hampered by such things as a small dose of central depressant like pethidine or a peripherally acting drug of the muscle relaxant type. It is, however, not easy to match spontaneous activity satisfactorily in this way, especially for long periods,

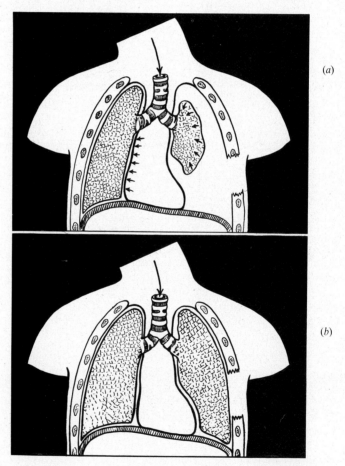

(a)

(b)

2/Fig. 20.—Effect of Pneumothorax on Mediastinum (Inspiration)

(a) Mediastinal flap + weight of heart and great vessels (spontaneous respiration).
(b) These factors corrected by positive-pressure ventilation.

and when it is possible to carry it out efficiently, apnoea tends to result as the carbon dioxide tension in the blood falls. Respiration is now said to be controlled. In other words efficient assisted respiration soon becomes controlled respiration.

Controlled Respiration

Controlled respiration can be initiated in three different ways:
1. Paralysis of the muscles of respiration.
2. Depression of the respiratory centre.
3. Removal of the carbon dioxide stimulus to the respiratory centre.

In practice a combination of all three methods is often used. A reduction of arterial P_{CO_2} (hyperventilation) and a reduced activity of the respiratory centre (analgesics) can enable the total dose of relaxant to be reduced. Provided the respiratory centre has not been heavily depressed by analgesic drugs then spontaneous respiratory activity can be resumed at will, even though the carbon dioxide tension of the blood has been reduced to a very low level.

The dangers of a high carbon dioxide tension are far greater than those of a low one, and during controlled respiration the anaesthetist should err, if at all, on the side of hyperventilation. This is particularly important during thoracotomy when a partially collapsed lung may cause gross defects of gas distribution and elimination.

Apart from its value to ensure adequate ventilation of the lungs in certain circumstances, controlled respiration can be made to provide ideal conditions for the surgeon, working either in the chest or abdominal cavity. The smooth, rhythmical inflation of the lungs and the movement of the diaphragm with controlled respiration is preferable to the jerky movements previously seen during spontaneous respiration under anaesthesia for abdominal and thoracic operations. The anaesthetist can also help the surgeon by momentarily preventing movement of the lungs and diaphragm during some critical manoeuvre.

The principal disadvantage of controlled respiration is the risk of persistent apnoea, which has become prominent since the introduction of muscle relaxant drugs.

DIFFUSION RESPIRATION

In a normal person the interchange of gases at the alveolar capillary membrane depends upon physical diffusion, while at tidal volumes smaller than 1 litre the movement of gas molecules from the alveolar ducts to the alveoli is almost entirely by diffusion. Some movement is caused by the contraction of the heart and by the ejection of blood from it leading to a pulsatile flow in the pulmonary vessels. If the nitrogen in the lungs is replaced by oxygen then these factors are sufficient to maintain an adequate uptake of oxygen in the blood in the absence of respiratory muscle activity. This process is known as diffusion respiration, but during it carbon dioxide is not removed from the blood. In fact the tension of carbon dioxide in the alveoli rises rapidly to equal that of the mixed venous blood (46 mm Hg—6·1 kPa) but thereafter more slowly.

Diffusion respiration can be produced in an anaesthetised patient following the use of a muscle relaxant and the endotracheal administration of oxygen, and is often deliberately practised during bronchoscopy (see Chapter 12).

RESPIRATORY MOVEMENTS IN ANAESTHESIA

During the induction of anaesthesia the respiratory pattern undergoes a whole series of changes. When ether is used, increasing concentrations of the drug in the body are only gradually achieved, so that the consequent effects on respiration are produced as a relatively slow and orderly process, and provide classical signs of progressively increasing depth of anaesthesia. These have been well-described by Guedel (1951) and are briefly reviewed here.

The movement of the thoracic cage on inspiration passes steadily from one of expansion during light anaesthesia to one of retraction in the late stages of ether anaesthesia. This transition occurs gradually and must be related to the paralysis of the various muscle groups. Thus, in light anaesthesia the abdominal muscles probably act as synergists and exert a steady isometric pull on the lower costal margin. The chest and abdominal wall rise and fall in unison (Stage III, Planes I and II). As the depth of anaesthesia increases so the synergistic muscles of respiration drop out one by one. In the second plane (Stage III, Plane II) respiratory rate, rhythm, and depth are similar to those found in the first plane, but when the third plane (Stage III, Plane III) is reached a characteristic expiratory pause may occur together with an absence of movement in the upper part of the thoracic cage. At the same time, the abdominal element of respiration becomes more marked and the abdomen begins to protrude just before the lower part of the thoracic cage moves outwards. Chest movements are in fact starting to lag behind those of the abdomen.

When the anaesthesia is deepened to the fourth plane (Stage III, Plane IV) the inspiratory phase is marked by a quick jerky protrusion of the abdominal wall as the diaphragm descends, followed immediately by a similar jerky retraction of the chest wall. This is often called diaphragmatic respiration and is characterised by paradoxical movements of the abdomen and thoracic cage. At this point, almost all the muscles of respiration, except the diaphragm, have ceased to function; thus, as the diaphragm descends, the intra-abdominal pressure is raised, and the abdominal wall is thrust out in a forceful manner. At the same time the descent of the diaphragm creates a relatively negative intrathoracic pressure and the intercostal muscles and ribs are sucked inwards. Expiration, by comparison, is a slow, prolonged movement during which the muscles return to their former positions. It is followed by a slight pause.

In the fourth stage of anaesthesia (Stage IV) this expiratory pause grows longer, inspiration becomes more jerky and irregular, until finally respiratory activity ceases altogether.

Tracheal Tug

In deep anaesthesia (Stage III, Plane III or IV) inspiration is associated with a tracheal tug. This is a sharp downward movement of the trachea on inspiration. The exact mechanism is obscure but there are two theories which deserve serious attention. Harris (1951) believes it is associated with the dual origin of the muscle fibres of the diaphragm. In deep anaesthesia there is a general loss of muscle tone so that the sternocostal fibres of the diaphragm are no longer supported by a rigid costal margin when they contract on inspiration. In consequence, these costal fibres contract ineffectively leaving the crural fibres alone to appear to be functioning. The result is that a sharp contraction of the central part of the diaphragm on inspiration is transmitted to the whole mediastinum. The root of the lung and trachea is then pulled downwards with each inspiration. This explanation, however, does not account for the occurrence of this condition in respiratory failure.

Another approach has been made on the basis of the part played by the elevating muscles of the larynx. In rats, the sternothyroid and sternohyoid muscles contract during inspiration and are directly controlled by the respiratory centre. In man, these muscles may help to raise the sternum as accessory muscles of respiration but their size and mobility make it unlikely they play an important role. In normal breathing the larynx remains stationary in both phases of respiration. This is due to the pull of its stabilising muscles (mylohyoid, stylohyoid, styloglossus and the posterior belly of the digastric), all of which are elevators of the larynx. It has been suggested that tracheal tug is due to a failure of these stabilising muscles to stand up to the forceful traction of the diaphragm (Campbell, 1958).

Apart from deep anaesthesia, tracheal tug may be noticed in partially curarised patients and in the presence of respiratory obstruction. In most cases it can be cured by returning full power to the muscles of respiration or removing the cause of the respiratory obstruction. Tracheal tug at the end of anaesthesia—in the absence of muscular paralysis—may be an indication for endotracheal suction or bronchoscopy, as the cause is not infrequently inadequate ventilation of one lung due to an accumulation of mucus.

Respiratory Patterns

The different wave forms of respiration can be visualised from tracings made either by a spirometer (tidal flow) or by a pneumograph (chest expansion and deflation). These offer a useful method for teaching the various patterns that may occur during anaesthesia.

Expiratory phase.—During quiet breathing in a conscious subject the duration of expiration is usually 1·3–1·4 times longer than that of inspiration. A pause at the end of expiration is present as a constant feature in both conscious and anaesthetised subjects, provided the rate of respiration is slow enough and the tidal volume sufficiently large (Morton, 1950). An increase in the rate and a diminution in the tidal volume lead to an abolition of this pause (Fig. 21). The presence of the pause in the third plane (Stage III, Plane III) of ether anaesthesia is largely related to the use of premedication. It may not occur, even in fourth-plane anaesthesia, if no central respiratory depressant has been used, yet is a marked feature in all patients who have previously received morphine. It is interesting to recall that this expiratory pause was not included by Guedel in his original description of respiratory activity under ether anaesthesia.

Inspiratory pause.—A pause at the peak of inspiration is seen during diaphragmatic respiration due to the use of muscle relaxants. This type of respiration has been described as "truncated" (Morton, 1950) because of the turret-shaped manner in which inspiration is suddenly interrupted by the prolonged pause (Fig. 22). Just as with the expiratory pause, an increase in the rate of respiration tends to diminish it. In deep anaesthesia or in the presence of good muscle relaxation, a small superadded inspiratory effort may also sometimes be seen, giving a sort of step-ladder effect. The cause of "truncated" respiration still remains unknown. The respiratory pattern is almost identical with normal respiration in which the "peaks" have been neatly sliced off. The reason for this plateau is more difficult to understand. Morton (1950) suggests that it may be due to partial paralysis of the muscles of respiration. There is no reason to believe that impulses do not continue to flow down the phrenic nerves when muscle relaxants are used. If only half of the usual number of muscle fibres in the motor unit responded to this stimulus, then inspiration would commence in

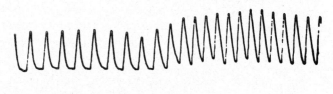

2/Fig. 21.—Respiratory tracing. Expiratory pause. Increasing the rate and volume of respiration abolishes this pause in both conscious and anaesthetised subjects.

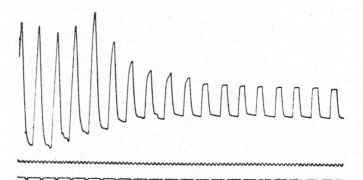

2/Fig. 22.—Respiratory tracing. Spirometer: Time in 1 and 4 seconds. Truncated respiration.

the normal manner but might be only half completed. Nevertheless, these fibres would remain in a state of contraction until the impulses from the phrenic nerve ceased. A step-ladder pattern is most commonly observed in the presence of a high carbon dioxide tension and when decamethonium is used as the relaxant. Again, its cause is obscure.

Sigh.—A deep sigh (Fig. 23) is occasionally seen in both conscious and anaesthetised subjects. In the latter it is commonly associated with deep anaesthesia, particularly when open ether is administered. Its occurrence may be misinterpreted by the surgeon as denoting too light anaesthesia, but in practice it is unrelated to surgical stimuli, nor is its cause known. It must be distinguished from the inspiratory gasp or breath-holding which is clearly related to surgical stimulation in the presence of inadequate suppression of reflex activity (Fig. 24).

Sighing in a conscious person is thought to be a mechanism by which during quiet respiration an occasional deep breath prevents underventilated alveoli from collapsing. However, Fletcher and Barber (1966) investigated conscious subjects breathing spontaneously and found that sighing was not followed by any change in lung mechanisms or in lung compliance. They were also unable to demonstrate any changes when sighing was almost completely abolished by intravenous morphine.

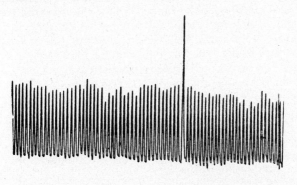

2/Fig. 23.—Sigh. Respiratory tracing to show typical sigh during anaesthesia.

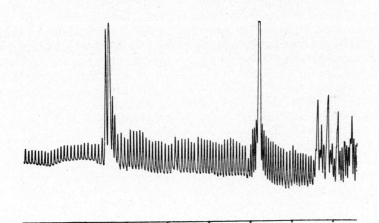

2/Fig. 24.—Inspiratory gasp. Result of surgical stimulation under too light anaesthesia.

Diaphragmatic Respiration

This type of respiration generally occurs under three conditions, and all should be readily distinguishable:

1. Deep ether anaesthesia (Stage III, Plane IV).
2. Curarisation (used in its widest sense) just short of total paralysis.
3. Respiratory obstruction.

A combination of any of these may occur in the same patient. Nevertheless, squeezing the rebreathing bag will quickly differentiate between the deeply anaesthetised or paralysed and the obstructed patient. In all these conditions respiratory activity may appear to take on an "inverted" pattern in which the abdomen contracts and moves in whilst the chest moves out. Attempts to measure an actual increase in the diameter of the chest reveal no change because a reduction in the antero-posterior measurement is exactly compensated for by an equal increase in the lateral one. Nevertheless this "see-saw" type of respiration is very characteristic. The mechanism in the paralysed patient has already been discussed (see "truncated" respiratory pattern).

The movements of the abdomen and chest wall in respiratory obstruction are more complex and there is little experimental evidence available. For descriptive purposes there would appear to be two distinct types of respiratory obstruction. One is *mechanical,* in which, for example, the tongue falls back and partially obstructs the glottis. The other is *reflex,* occurring in conjunction with laryngeal or bronchial spasm when the level of anaesthesia is insufficient to combat the stimulation of surgery.

In mechanical respiratory obstruction the patient continues to breathe in an entirely normal manner, but the expiratory pause disappears the moment the obstruction starts. In fact this is such a constant finding that it could be used as a method of diagnosing its presence. The explanation may well be that the restriction of the airway causes a prolongation of the duration of both expiration and inspiration, thus abolishing the expiratory pause.

Reflex obstruction is more complicated, since the effects of surgical or anaesthetic stimulation in the presence of inadequate reflex suppression may not only lead to laryngeal spasm (when the trachea is not intubated) but also to breath-holding and contraction of the abdominal muscles. The patient behaves as though impulses fan out from the spinal cord causing numerous muscle groups to contract. The carbon dioxide tension rises until, depending upon the threshold of the respiratory centre, an inspiratory effort occurs as the glottis partially or completely opens. At the same time the abdominal muscles momentarily relax. Thus in cases of partial reflex obstruction, the vocal cords open and the abdominal muscles relax on inspiration, only to contract again in the expiratory phase. The jerky movements of the abdominal musculature in this type of case give the impression of "see-saw" respiration, but in actual practice the movement is almost entirely abdominal and the chest wall remains relatively steady.

Hiccup

Hiccup is an intermittent clonic spasm of the diaphragm, of reflex origin. With each contraction the bronchial lumen is constricted and, in unintubated patients, the glottis closed. Fitzgerald (1967) has questioned the commonly accepted sequence of events. From a consideration of the anatomy of the central nervous system connections that are involved, he argues that the reverse is more likely, glottic closure preceding phrenic nerve stimulation through the respiratory centre. In mild cases, unassociated with anaesthesia, the spasm is usually a unilateral contraction of the diaphragm which, if the condition persists, gradually spreads across the whole muscle (Samuels, 1952). The left side is more often affected than the right.

Afferents can arise from almost any part of the body, including the central nervous system, but during anaesthesia are most frequently associated with visceral stimulation, usually in the upper abdomen, and probably transmitted through the vagus. Hiccup may also be caused by inflation of the stomach with anaesthetic gases, or from irritation below the diaphragm due to extraneous fluids, such as blood, pus or gastric juice.

Hiccup is not a common complication of deep anaesthesia but rather a product of modern methods when relaxation is produced by motor paralysis, and sensory reflex activity is by comparison relatively undepressed. It can be regarded as a reflex response of the partially anaesthetised respiratory centres and incompletely paralysed peripheral musculature to vagal stimulation.

Treatment.—Careful appraisal of the surgeon's technique will usually enable the anaesthetist to suppress reflex activity in advance of stimulation so that hiccup is prevented. A deeper level of anaesthesia than that previously maintained, or the addition of a further dose of relaxant just before a procedure which is known to be particularly stimulating, are often successful. Such preventive measures may be necessary even when the surgical conditions, in terms of relaxation, are satisfactory. Hiccup is often associated with the slow return of diaphragmatic activity as the degree of relaxation wears off, when it is no more than attempted forceful respiratory movement and should be treated as such. It also often occurs "out of the blue" in the presence of very adequate relaxation of the abdominal muscles.

Total paralysis will always prevent or stop hiccup, but the very large dose of muscle relaxant that this may entail in some patients is not always advisable, and may complicate the situation at the end of the operation. A large number of individual drugs, ranging from the administration of amyl nitrite to the addition of a sudden blast of ether vapour to the anaesthetic mixture, have been tried at one time or another. Salem *et al.* (1967) found that stimulation of the mid-pharynx behind the uvula, and opposite the second cervical vertebra, by gentle movement with the end of a catheter inserted through the nose stopped hiccups in 84 out of 85 patients. Such methods presumably act by reflex inhibition, and even though many of them stop the disturbance, they are usually only temporarily effective.

The best and most rational treatment for hiccup during anaesthesia is to block the reflex pathways concerned by a deeper level of anaesthesia (further supplementation with analgesic, hypnotic or more potent inhalational anaesthetic) or by incremental doses of a muscle relaxant.

In the post-operative period a cause for hiccup must be sought before special treatment is advised. Uraemia, subphrenic abscess and grossly distended bowels are some of the conditions which must be excluded, but in many patients no specific factor can be incriminated. Then, adequate sedation together with large doses of chlorpromazine and similar phenothiazine compounds should be tried. A method of treatment which often proves successful is initiation of the swallowing reflex with both nose and ears blocked. The patient sips repeatedly from a glass of water while his external auditory meatae and nose are obstructed. The success of this manoeuvre presumably depends on the afferent stimulus in the middle ear (from fluctuating pressure waves) being stronger than that which initiates the hiccup.

An oesophageal tube and suction are helpful to relieve distension. Carbon dioxide inhalation occasionally inhibits an attack. For prolonged and severe cases, after screening the patient to decide which side is affected, infiltration with local analgesic of a phrenic nerve in the neck should be considered. Chlorpromazine has been found useful in some cases.

The Work of Breathing

As the term suggests, the work of breathing comprises all the energy required to ventilate the lungs. Unfortunately the task of the respiratory muscles is not simply the inflation of a passive balloon (the lungs). Certain forces which tend to prevent the lungs being inflated must be overcome. There are three essential components in this opposition: (a) the force needed to overcome the elastic resistance of the lung; (b) the force to move non-elastic tissues (structural resistance); and finally (c), the force to overcome resistance to the flow of air through the tracheo-bronchial tree.

The **elastic resistance** of the lung is defined as the force tending to return the lung to its original size after stretching. It should not be thought of as the force required to expand the lung, as this is also a measure of the rigidity of the lung which varies with pulmonary congestion. The *compliance of the lung* is a measure of its change in volume per unit of pressure change. In cardiac and pulmonary disease the congestion and fibrosis which are frequently present lead to a fall in the "compliance" of the lung.

The **structural resistance** is composed of the thoracic wall, the diaphragm and the abdominal contents. It is related to the speed of the flow of air so that when this is maximal so is the structural resistance.

The **air resistance** is important because it is dependent on the length and size of the lumen of the bronchial tree. The anaesthetist adds an extra air resistance when he inserts an endotracheal tube. This matter is of particular importance in the intubation of a young child for whom too small an endotracheal tube may increase the air resistance enormously.

The flow of air through the bronchial tree may be laminar (streamlined) or turbulent. In this latter condition the air pursues an erratic course with the creation of many eddy-currents. The air resistance in laminar flow can be lowered by reducing the *viscosity*, whereas in turbulent flow it is the *density* that must be lowered. Anaesthetists sometimes use a mixture of helium and oxygen (79 per cent: 21 per cent) in certain cases of upper respiratory obstruction with the object of improving the patient's oxygenation. As the viscosity of this mixture is slightly *greater* than air, the resistance to laminar flow will be increased. On the other hand, its density is less than that of air, so the resistance to turbulent flow is decreased. As partial upper respiratory obstruction sets up turbulent flows the rationale of this therapy appears to be soundly based.

Compliance

The lungs and thoracic wall function as a single unit, and provided the tidal volume is in the normal range there is a linear relationship between the volume change and the pressure that produces it. If it is measured when the flow of air has ceased, as during breath-holding or during apnoea in anaesthesia, it is known as *static compliance*.

$$\text{Static compliance} = \frac{\text{Volume change in litres}}{\text{Pressure change in cm of } H_2O \text{ (kilopascals)}}$$

The compliance of the lungs and of the thoracic wall in a normal person are approximately the same, namely 0·2 litres/cm H_2O ($2·0 \times 10^{-2}$ l/kPa). Thus a volume change of 0·2 litres in the thorax is obtained by a pressure of 1 cm of H_2O ($9·8 \times 10^{-2}$ kPa) exerted against the lungs in conjunction with a pressure of 1 cm of H_2O ($9·8 \times 10^{-2}$ kPa) against the thoracic wall, giving a total thoracic compliance of 0·1 litre/cm H_2O ($1·0 \times 10^{-2}$ l/kPa) (Comroe et al., 1962).

When the volume change of the thorax in relation to pressure changes is measured during respiration it is known as *dynamic compliance*.

Measurement of total thoracic compliance.—The pressure gradient to be measured is that between the airway and the atmosphere, but it is difficult to obtain a reliable result unless the patient is able to relax completely. Thus the measurement of total thoracic compliance is best made in a patient who is relaxed and ventilated, either with the aid of a tank ventilator (conscious patient) or an endotracheal tube (unconscious patient).

(a) *Tank ventilator.*—The conscious patient is placed in the ventilator so that the transthoracic pressure can be measured. The volume of air inspired at each level of subatmospheric pressure within the tank reveals the data for a pressure-volume curve.

(b) *Endotracheal method.*—In the anaesthetised patient an endotracheal tube is inserted. This tube is then occluded and the pressure within the system during a period of apnoea is measured. After this the tube is unclamped and the volume of air or gas expired is collected in a spirometer. Again, a pressure-volume curve is plotted.

Measurement of lung compliance.—The pressure gradient to be measured is that between the airway and the pleural space. Direct measurements by placing the tip of a sampling needle (connected to a manometer) within the pleural space are dangerous. This disadvantage has been overcome by the method of Dornhorst and Leathart (1952) who have shown that the intrapleural pressure is transmitted directly through the thin-walled oesophagus to its lumen. Thus changes in oesophageal pressure represent alterations in intrapleural pressure. Since this measurement is a static one, it is made with the patient holding his breath after having inspired a known volume of air from a spirometer. The procedure is then repeated many times with different volumes so that a pressure-volume curve can be constructed. This is usually linear provided large volumes are not used, and will give an average value for lung compliance.

Measurement of thoracic wall compliance.—This is obtained by subtraction of lung compliance from total thoracic compliance.

Measurement of dynamic compliance.—This requires a very sensitive technique for the measurement of the pressure, volume and air flow.

Discussion

Values for compliance should always be related to the predicted normal value for a person of the same sex, age, height, weight and lung volume, and are preferably related to the functional residual capacity (FRC). For example, a simple change in posture can alter the FRC and thus produce a change in compliance.

One of the principal factors causing the elastic recoil of the lungs is the presence of elastic fibres within the pulmonary tissue. The important role of the surface tension of the fluid lining the alveolar walls has also been emphasised (see p. 33). This tends to draw the opposing walls closer together and so collapse the alveoli. If this fluid were pure water it would exert the very considerable pull of about 70 dynes/cm (70×10^{-3} Nm^{-1}), but fortunately it contains a "detergent-like" agent (surfactant) which reduces the surface tension to as little as 2–8 dynes/cm ($2\text{–}8 \times 10^{-3}$ Nm^{-1}).

Von Neergaard (1929) was the first to observe this effect. He demonstrated that much less pressure was required to inflate lungs filled with saline than those filled with air, the difference being due to abolition of the elastic pull of the surface tension exerted by the alveolar lining membrane. The detergent-like agent is believed to be absent in hyaline membrane disease of the newborn, and therefore to account for the very high inflationary pressures that are needed to expand the lungs in this condition.

Pulmonary oedema (altered surface tension with fluid in the alveoli), emphysema (destruction of elastic fibres) and mitral stenosis (increased pulmonary vascular congestion) are but some of the conditions that decrease the compliance of the lungs.

Under the conditions of anaesthesia so many factors are operating at the same time, and the situation changes so often, that it is frequently impossible to relate any change in compliance to a single agent or procedure. For example, a drug may affect the muscles of the thorax, the secretions in the respiratory tract, alter the cardiac output, constrict the bronchioles or dilate the pulmonary vessels.

However, very many investigations have been carried out and nearly all agree with Mead and Collier (1959) that there is a progressive fall in compliance during anaesthesia. This is almost entirely accounted for by changes in lung compliance, which decreases with time and with any action which tends to deflate the lungs. This has been accounted for by the absence of the periodic deep sighs that a conscious person takes unknowingly. Thus Gliedman et al. (1958) found that lung compliance fell more during ventilation with an automatic ventilator, which provides regular, even tidal volumes, than in those ventilated by hand. Particularly with a pressure preset ventilator, a reduction in compliance will lead to a reduction in tidal volume which will tend to cause a further reduction in compliance.

Egbert and his colleagues (1963) showed that occasional deep breaths during anaesthesia with intermittent positive pressure ventilation will prevent or lessen the occurrence of falls in compliance, and Sykes et al. (1965) have produced similar results by the use of large tidal volumes. Norlander et al. (1968), however, using the Engstrom ventilator at normal tidal volumes throughout, found no decrease in compliance and they believe this is due to the special flow-pressure pattern of that ventilator which—with an accelerating gas flow and a variable end-inspiratory pressure plateau—offers breath-to-breath mini-sighs.

Breathing and Oxygen Consumption

In a normal resting subject the work of breathing uses up approximately 0·5 ml oxygen for every litre of ventilation. Thus at average minute volume of 8 litres about 4 ml of oxygen are required, or about 1·5 per cent of the total oxygen consumption each minute. Increasing respiratory activity leads to a disproportionately high rate of oxygen consumption.

Respiratory Work and Disease

Just as in health, so it has been found in *heart disease* (e.g. mitral stenosis) that the metabolic needs of the body are met with the minimal amount of respiratory work (Marshall *et al.*, 1954). In patients with mitral stenosis the severity of the dyspnoea is directly proportional to the degree of pulmonary rigidity, which presumably is due to vascular congestion. Thus more work is required to inflate the lungs. It is this increase in respiratory work that makes the patient short of breath. The exact increase necessary to make the patient actually conscious of the respiratory effort varies from individual to individual.

Anaesthetists who commonly come in contact with cases of heart disease have often commented on the general improvement in the circulatory condition that frequently follows the induction of anaesthesia. This is particularly true when assisted or controlled respiration is used. The explanation may lie in the removal of this extra respiratory work by the mode of anaesthesia and the improved ventilation of the lungs.

In chest diseases, especially chronic ones, there is always an upset in respiratory mechanics with an increased work load. In pulmonary fibrosis the lung compliance is decreased, but to a small extent this is offset by a reduction in airway resistance which may occur because the traction exerted by the parenchymal tissue on the lung airways is increased. In diseases affecting the thoracic cage, such as ankylosing spondylitis or kyphoscoliosis, the chest wall compliance may be much reduced.

In obstructive lung conditions, such as severe asthma, chronic bronchitis, and emphysema there is an increased airway resistance and a reduced dynamic compliance. In emphysema marked changes take place in the structure of the lungs, associated with an increase in tissue rigidity leading to a complete loss of elasticity. This lack of elasticity markedly reduces the radial support of the peripheral airways and, combined with a possible intrinsic narrowing as well, means that during expiration the small bronchioles collapse before the alveoli distal to them have emptied completely, and air-trapping ensues. The lung-volume is increased, the intrathoracic pressure becomes less negative, and there is no lung-recoil when a pneumothorax is induced. The chest wall gradually becomes fixed in a position of inspiration.

All these changes make the emphysematous patient work harder to ventilate his lungs, and, owing to the fixed chest wall, put the respiratory muscles at a mechanical disadvantage. This increase in respiratory work leads to the onset of dyspnoea and the limitation of the maximal breathing capacity (McIlroy and Christie, 1954).

In the conscious state, the emphysematous patient can partially compensate for the loss of elastic tissue in the lung by actively contracting the abdominal muscles on expiration. It has already been pointed out that these muscles are the principal muscles of expiration. Anaesthesia, however, is frequently designed to relax them, so that while providing the surgeon with ideal conditions to explore the abdomen it deprives the emphysematous patient of his principal means for emptying the alveoli. In such circumstances, if spontaneous respiration is allowed, the level of carbon dioxide in the blood must necessarily rise. Therefore, on both theoretical and practical grounds, when marked abdominal relaxation is produced during general anaesthesia for an emphysematous patient, respiration should be controlled or assisted. Although intermittent positive-pressure respiration permits the anaesthetist to allow an adequate time for expiration to take place in these patients, it does not otherwise help to empty the alveoli. In crush injuries of the chest the use of intermittent positive-pressure ventilation ensures that both or all segments of the thoracic cage move uniformly without the varying pull of the external muscles. This eliminates the work of breathing and the possibility of paradoxical respiration, corrects the pathological changes consequent on the abnormal mechanics of breathing, and is the most efficient way of obtaining a normal gas exchange. It also reduces pain, and by splinting the damaged chest wall permits speedier healing of the fractures.

RESISTANCE TO VENTILATION

Under normal conditions of breathing the respiratory resistance comprises the force required to drive air to and fro' along the bronchial tree from the mouth to the alveoli. The resistance to the flow of air in a tube is the pressure difference between the two ends at a given flow rate. If a subject breathes through an anaesthetic apparatus then the resistance of the extra breathing pathway must be taken into account, because the respiratory muscles will have to do more work. A simple test can be made by asking a conscious subject to breathe through a small endotracheal tube (Magill No. 4 or 6) held between his lips, when the extra effort required soon becomes apparent. Expiration is affected most, because there is a rise in intrapulmonary pressure with inadequate emptying of the alveoli. This leads to an increase in carbon dioxide and, therefore, an increase in the depth of respiration in an attempt to wash out more carbon dioxide. The abdominal muscles soon come into action during expiration in an endeavour to drive air out of the lungs.

Nearly every piece of anaesthetic apparatus increases in varying degree the respiratory resistance. One of the most important factors is the type of flow of the gases. This largely depends upon the diameter and shape of the breathing tubes and connection pieces, the number, style and setting of valves in the system, and the size and packing of the soda-lime canister.

Gas flows.—When the flow of gas along a tube is smooth and regular it is called laminar, but as the rate of flow increases a critical velocity is reached at which the flow becomes turbulent (Fig. 25). The flow of air in the respiratory tract of a normal patient is laminar, and the flow of gases during inspiration in anaesthetic practice does not reach sufficiently high rates to produce turbulent flow. The internal diameter of the tubes along which the gases flow and the presence of obstruction in them may, however, affect the critical velocity and hence produce turbulent flow. It is important, therefore, that the anaesthetist should use the largest sized tube that will pass easily through the glottic aperture, since in the adult this is the narrowest portion of the respiratory tract between the lips and the carina. In children the cricoid is the limiting factor. Furthermore, the endotracheal connections should be of a wide bore, and curved rather than sharply angled (Fig. 26). Macintosh and Mushin (1946) have

described and illustrated the different effects of a No. 10 and No. 6 endotracheal tube on intrapleural pressure (Fig. 27).

Valves.—The number and the types of unidirectional valve used in the
different pieces of anaesthetic apparatus vary, but the majority are of the disc
type which is lifted by the flow of gases either against its own weight (simple
disc type) or against the resistance of a spring (spring-loaded type). Hunt (1955)
has described the optimum design of disc valves. They should be made to have
approximately equal cross-sectional flow areas for air at all the constricted
portions and these areas should be approximately equal to that of the main
duct. The disc should be as light as practicable and should have a lift approaching one quarter of the diameter of the duct. If a disc becomes wet from the
moisture of the expired gases a slight increase in respiratory resistance will
occur, not only from the greater weight of the disc but from the surface tension
of the water between the disc edges and its seating. For paediatric anaesthesia
not only is resistance of great importance but also the quantity of air contained
in the valve, since this may markedly increase dead space in a small infant (see
p. 1435 *et seq.*) The effects of various pieces of anaesthetic apparatus in the

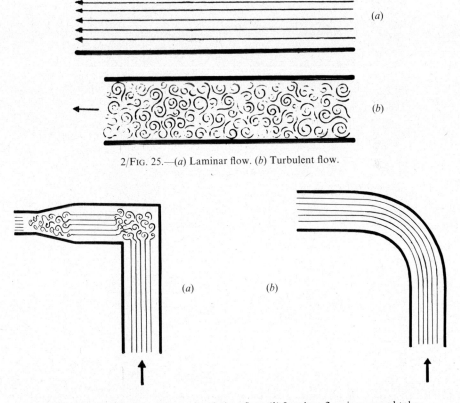

2/Fig. 25.—(*a*) Laminar flow. (*b*) Turbulent flow.

2/Fig. 26.—(*a*) Mixed laminar and turbulent flow. (*b*) Laminar flow in a curved tube.

external resistance to respiration in infants has been extensively reviewed by Smith (1961).

Soda-lime canister.—The insertion of a soda-lime canister into a respiratory system is, in the mechanical sense, an obstruction. The difference between breathing in and out of a spirometer with or without a soda-lime container can be easily demonstrated. The resistance or obstruction to the flow of gases of a conventional soda-lime canister is very much larger than that of the average valve, except when using very small flow rates. The manner in which the granules are packed into the canister plays an important part, for vigorous compaction will increase the resistance for any given flow rate. It is clearly best, therefore, to select as large a granule as possible which is compatible with adequate

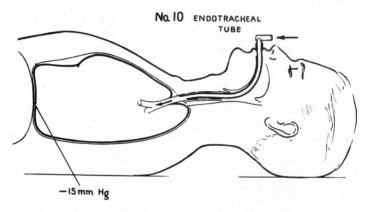

(*a*) Large-bore endotracheal tube means less resistance to respiration and therefore a lower intra-pleural pressure (− 15 mm Hg is − 2·0 kPa).

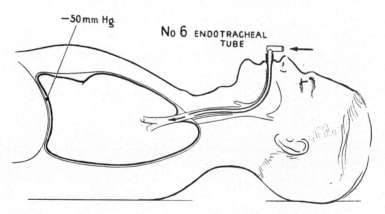

(*b*) Small-bore endotracheal tube means a greater resistance to respiration and therefore a high intrapleural pressure (− 50 mm Hg is − 6·7 kPa).

2/Fig. 27.—Diagrams to Show the Effect of Endotracheal Tube Size on Intrapleural Pressure, and therefore on Inspiratory Effort

absorption. For inhalational anaesthesia a blend of 4–8 mesh granules (see p. 115) has been found to offer optimum absorption efficiency with the minimum of resistance. In certain machines for measuring metabolic rate the efficiency of absorption is increased by using a range of 20–40 mesh granules; the resulting increase in resistance is offset by using mechanical blowers to circulate the gases. A wide, short canister (as used in circle absorbers) offers less resistance than the long narrow (Waters) canister, because the gases travel at a lower velocity between the granules and also have a shorter over-all passage through the canister.

Respiratory Effects of Resistance to Breathing

The diameter of the endotracheal tube, the pattern of the flow of gases along the flexible tubing, the valves, and the soda-lime canister are all capable of increasing resistance to respiration.

In a conscious patient even a moderate rise in respiratory resistance is followed by a fall in ventilation and in the slope of the CO_2 response curve. In turn, the muscles of respiration make a compensatory effort so that ventilation remains unchanged. Nunn and Ezi-Ashi (1961) found that this temporary reduction in ventilation was no greater in the anaesthetised patient. Furthermore, there was a wide range of compensatory response to the resistance but some patients were capable of overcoming it even when this resistance was relatively high.

Another finding of interest was the difference in the effect of a 5-kilogram weight placed first on the chest and then on the epigastrium. The anaesthetised patient showed almost no change in ventilation following pressure on the chest, whereas there was a 20 per cent reduction in ventilation if the same weight was placed on the upper abdomen (Table 6).

2/Table 6

EFFECT OF EXTERNAL INTERFERENCE WITH RESPIRATION ON VENTILATION

	Change in Lung volume (ml)	Change in tidal volume (%)	Change in respiratory rate (%)	Change in minute volume (%)
5 kg on sternum	−70	−4·1	+2·8	−1·7
5 kg on epigastrium	−45	−19·2	+2·0	−17·8

The reason for this discrepancy is that the diaphragm is the principle muscle of respiration and any pressure in the epigastric region will seriously impede its function. These figures help to emphasise the importance of intermittent positive-pressure respiration in patients undergoing upper abdominal surgery, particularly where firm retraction on liver or bowel is used to gain exposure.

The endotracheal tube is always considered an important source of resistance to respiration. It is known that the resistance presented by a tube is proportional to the flow of gases and the diameter of the tube. Munson and his colleagues (1963) have shown in a group of patients that whereas the mean peak flow rate in the conscious state was 21 litres/min, it rose to 28–43 litres/min when anaesthesia was induced. A glance at Fig. 28 shows how the peak flow rate is high

2/Fig. 28.—Peak inspiratory flow rate with various types of inhalational anaesthetic with and without narcotic premedication.

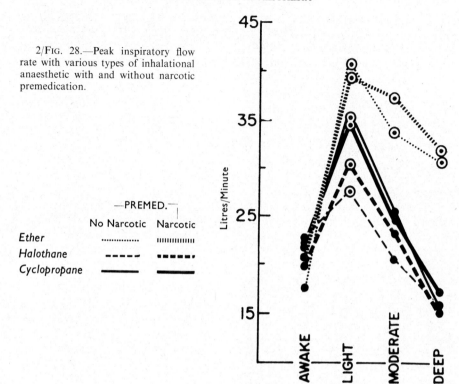

2/Fig. 29.—Resistance through endotracheal tubes. The Magill tube size is quoted.

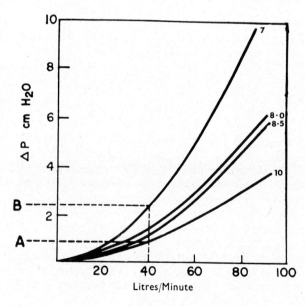

during light anaesthesia with most anaesthetic agents but drops down again when moderate or deep levels of anaesthesia are reached. With ether anaesthesia high peak flow rates are maintained at most levels of anaesthesia.

Interpretation of these flows in relation to the various sizes of endotracheal tube available reveals some interesting data. In adults, the difference in pressure gradients across a No. 10 and No. 7 Magill tube with a flow rate of 40 l/min is only 1 cm H_2O (0·1 kPa) (Fig. 29). Thus at this flow rate there is a very small increase in resistance over a wide range of adult endotracheal tube sizes. This discrepancy may in part be due to the large bore of the trachea being required for fight or flight rather than the more tranquil event of anaesthesia where only relatively low flow rates are present.

By contrast, in children the size of the endotracheal tube is of paramount importance. Here the difference in pressure gradients across a No. 0 and a No. 3 Magill tube at a flow rate of 40 l/min is now over 80 cm H_2O (8 kPa) (Fig. 30). However, it should be pointed out that this is an exaggeration of the real situation, as a child small enough to need a Magill 0 or 3 will not have a peak flow of anything like 40 l/min.

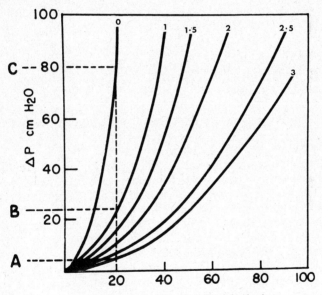

2/FIG. 30.—Resistance through endotracheal tubes.

Conclusion.—These various studies of resistance suggest that the anaesthetised patient can compensate for a temporary increase of respiratory resistance provided it is not too severe and it is not impeded by disease, depressant drugs or muscle relaxants. Nevertheless, any increase in resistance will be reflected in the circulation which is not considered here. In children the size of the endotracheal tube is of supreme importance and every effort should be made to pass the largest endotracheal tube that will easily traverse the narrow opening at the cricoid ring. In adults, however, sizes larger than No. 8 Magill have correspondingly little advantage to offer.

ANAESTHETIC BREATHING SYSTEMS

A badly designed or improperly used anaesthetic breathing system adversely affects the respiratory function of the patient. At the extremes of age, and in ill patients, such a disturbance may have serious consequences. The principles of good practice must be recognised when selecting and administering anaesthesia with any particular system, and the advantages and disadvantages peculiar to it appreciated. No one of the schemes to be described is perfect in itself, but some are of greater value for special types of case or anaesthesia than for routine use whatever the condition. When making a final choice, and after consideration of all the basic facts, the preference and experience of the anaesthetist concerned must be decisive.

The desirable features to be found in a good anaesthetic breathing system are:

1. Efficient elimination of exhaled CO_2.
2. The supply of an adequate inspired O_2 concentration.
3. Efficient exchange of anaesthetic gases.
4. A low apparatus dead-space.
5. A low resistance to gas flow except in certain well-defined circumstances, such as the application of a positive end-expiratory pressure.
6. Safety.
7. Convenience in use.

Circuits in common current use can be classified as follows:
(a) Open-mask methods.
(b) Circuits relying on an adequate fresh gas flow for efficient performance.
(c) Circuits relying on soda-lime for the elimination of carbon dioxide.

(a) Open-mask Methods

Volatile anaesthetic agents such as diethyl ether can be administered by a drop technique onto an open mask. Though not much used today in developed countries, the method is most suitable for use in children because of the practical difficulties of obtaining surgical anaesthesia in adults; although the technique requires much practical judgement in its use it is simple and safe, and particularly useful when more sophisticated apparatus is unavailable. An example of such apparatus is the Schimmelbusch mask, in which a simple metal frame is covered with layers of gauze. The patient's respirations pass through the gauze and vaporise the volatile agent which is dropped onto the gauze from a dropper bottle. He therefore inhales an air-anaesthetic mixture which is at a low temperature and the respiratory tree is called upon to raise the temperature to 37° C and also to saturate it with water vapour. It has been estimated that there is a heat loss from the patient of about 300 calories per minute using diethyl ether as the anaesthetic agent. Oxygen can be added to the inspired gas mixture by delivering it through a narrow tube inserted under the edge of the mask. Examples of agents which have been administered by this method are diethyl ether, divinyl ether, ethyl chloride and halothane.

(b) Circuits Requiring High Gas Flows

In this type of system CO_2 elimination is obtained by venting into the

atmosphere; the volume of exhaled gas thus discarded depending on the amount
of the fresh gas flow into the circuit. An expiratory valve or opening in the
system allows the exhaled gases to pass into the atmosphere, and the position of
the bag, the total flow of fresh gas and its site of entry into the circuit, and the
position of the expiratory port, are all important to the efficiency of the circuit.
Provided the apparatus dead space is low and that a sufficient fresh gas flow is
available to ensure satisfactory CO_2 elimination, then an inspired concentration
of oxygen equal to that in the fresh gas mixture and efficient exchange of anaesthetic gases are also assured. The total performance of these circuits can therefore be judged by examining the efficiency of CO_2 elimination. Various types of
systems were classified and analysed by Mapleson (1954), and are depicted in
Fig. 31. The fresh gas flows required to ensure CO_2 elimination are also shown
and these flows are related to the minute volume of the patient, itself related to
the CO_2 output and therefore the size and age of the patient.

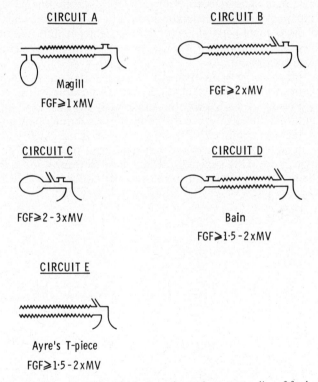

2/Fig. 31.—Classification of circuits which depend on adequate supplies of fresh gases to ensure
efficient operation (from Mapleson, 1954).

The Magill circuit (Mapleson "A").—During anaesthesia with spontaneous
ventilation the Magill attachment is still the best for an adult for economy in
total gas flow with virtual elimination of rebreathing. The fresh gas flow into
the Magill attachment has been investigated by Kain and Nunn (1967). These
workers, measuring minute volume and end-tidal CO_2 while reducing the

fresh gas flow in steps, found that significant rebreathing (as indicated by a rise in minute volume and end-tidal CO_2) did not occur until the gas inflow was reduced to between 2 and 4 litres/minutes, or about equal to the patient's alveolar ventilation (Fig. 32). Previously it had been considered that a gas inflow equal to the patient's minute volume was necessary to prevent rebreathing. This state of affairs only holds when the patient is breathing spontaneously, but not if such a system is used for intermittent positive-pressure respiration. Then a far greater flow of gases must be used to prevent carbon dioxide accumulation.

Ayre's T Piece (Mapleson "E")

With a "T" piece the dead-space gases pass down the open end of the tube first, while the alveolar gases, leaving last, may be reinspired. A high flow of gases (one and a half to twice the respiratory minute volume of the patient) is needed to prevent rebreathing with a "T" piece if the capacity of the expiratory limb of the system is to be ignored. Rebreathing can be eliminated with a small expiratory limb provided that the volume of the gases that can be held in it is no greater than the volume of fresh gases that can enter it during an expiratory pause (Mapleson, 1954). With a small expiratory limb some mixing with the atmospheric air may occur.

In paediatric anaesthesia an open-ended bag is usually attached to the open end of the expiratory limb converting the system to a Mapleson "D" type of circuit. With spontaneous ventilation the same fresh gas flow is required (1·5–2 times the minute volume) to prevent significant rebreathing depending on the length of the expiratory pause. With a short or absent pause twice the minute volume should be delivered, but if there is a significant pause then 1·5 times the minute volume is probably sufficient. When used to control the ventilation in adult patients the arterial P_{CO_2} can be maintained at low or just below normal levels by a fresh gas flow of 70–100 ml/min/kg body weight.

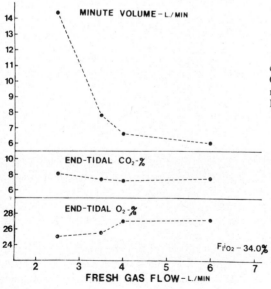

2/FIG. 32.—Diagram showing the changes in minute volume, end-tidal CO_2 and end-tidal O_2 with step-wise reductions in fresh gas flow into a Magill anaesthetic circuit.

Bain Circuit

This is a modification of the Mapleson "D" type of circuit in which the fresh gas flow is introduced through a narrow bore tube running inside a larger bore outer tube. For spontaneous ventilation a fresh gas flow of 1·5–2 times the minute volume is necessary to prevent significant rebreathing depending on the length of the expiratory pause. The characteristics of the circuit during controlled ventilation have recently been described by Henville and Adams (1976).

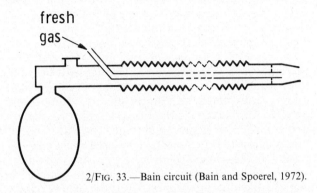

fresh gas

2/Fig. 33.—Bain circuit (Bain and Spoerel, 1972).

Using a tidal volume of 10 ml/kg and a respiratory rate of 10–15 breaths per minute the arterial Pco_2 can be controlled by the supply of fresh gas. They found that at a fresh gas flow of 70 ml/kg the mean arterial Pco_2 was 40·8 mm Hg, S.D. = ± 4·3 (5·4 ± 0·6 kPa) and with a flow of 100 ml/kg the mean arterial Pco_2 was 34·3 mm Hg, S.D. = ± 4·5 (4·6 ± 0·6 kPa). The arterial Pco_2 can therefore be fairly accurately controlled during anaesthesia. In patients weighing less than 40 kg the fresh gas flow should not be reduced below 3 l/min or higher Pco_2 values than predicted will result. This is a reflection of the higher metabolic rate of children and infants, and thus of a higher CO_2 output.

Circle Systems *Without* Absorber

The desire for greater control of the arterial Pco_2 during controlled ventilation whilst using large tidal volumes to maintain alveolar patency has lead to the investigation of circle systems *without* CO_2 *absorption* for this purpose (Suwa and Yamamura, 1970; Scholfield and Williams, 1974). The theory behind this system is that provided large tidal volumes are used, in the order of 10–15 ml/kg body weight, then equilibration of gases in the lungs and in the circle system will be approached. If a fresh gas supply about equal to the alveolar ventilation is then introduced into the circuit with the spill-valve open then the arterial Pco_2 will be maintained near normal values. It is however important that the point at which the fresh gas is introduced into the circuit and the point at which the spill-valve is situated are separated by a volume of at least 500–1000 ml. If the two are placed closer together then the fresh gas may be lost directly to the atmosphere and CO_2 elimination jeopardised. Different methods of estimating the fresh gas flow required in relation to the estimated CO_2 output of the patient have been tried. In practice the provision of a fresh gas flow of $4\frac{1}{2}$ l/min to adult females and 6 l/min to adult males will result in an arterial Pco_2 in the low normal range—mean 33 mm Hg (4·4 kPa), range 30–36 mm Hg (4·0–4·8 kPa) (Kerr, J. H., 1976, personal communication).

Non-rebreathing Valves

The non-rebreathing valve may be considered as a modification of the semi-closed system. Designed primarily to prevent rebreathing by ensuring unidirectional flow of all expired gases, such valves have therefore the additional advantage of enabling the patient to inspire a constant proportion of gases from the anaesthetic machine, since there is no mixing of these with those which are expired. At any one moment the anaesthetist can tell the exact proportion of gases that the patient is inspiring. Non-rebreathing valves are also useful for intermittent positive-pressure ventilation, but unless specially designed, the exhalation part of the valve may need to be held closed when the pressure is applied. A further advantage is that the patient cannot be hyperventilated if the total flow of gases is set to match the required minute volume of the patient.

An excellent valve of this type is the Frumin, which can be used for both spontaneous and controlled respiration (Frumin, Lee and Papper, 1959). It is so designed that a sudden rise in pressure (as produced by the anaesthetist's hand squeezing the reservoir bag) closes the expiratory leak so that all the gases pass to the patient. On release of the pressure at the end of inspiration the gases can then escape quietly again to the atmosphere. This valve can be used either with a face-mask or in a modified form to provide an "in-line" gas flow for use with an endotracheal tube. The resistance and dead space are minimal. The resistance to gas flow in the valve at either inspiration or expiration is 1·5 mm Hg at 60 litres/minute (0·2 kPa l^{-1} sec) flow rates.

Another valve of this type has been designed by Ruben (1955), the exhalation part of which automatically closes during controlled or assisted respiration. One of its principal advantages is the small dead space—only 9 ml. Similarly, the resistance is low. It can, however, only be described as "noisy" in practice.

(c) Circuits Requiring Low Gas Flows (Carbon Dioxide Absorption Techniques)

John Snow in 1850 was one of the first to realise the potentialities of carbon dioxide absorption, but it was not until the work of Dennis Jackson on animals (1915) and Waters' application of this work to man (Waters, 1924) that the method came to be widely adopted. The principle is that if sufficient oxygen is added to the anaesthetic system to supply the patient's basic metabolic requirements and the carbon dioxide is removed from the exhalation, then the same mixture of gases or vapours can be breathed over and over again.

The primary justification for absorption techniques in anaesthesia is economy. Heat preservation and moistening of the inspired gases are secondary and minor advantages. It must, however, be borne in mind that the ability of the anaesthetist to reduce the level of carbon dioxide to below normal levels in a patient by means of such a system was, and still is, one of the basic factors in inducing controlled respiration. The risk of an explosion with an inflammable anaesthetic can be minimised by using it in a closed system.

Soda-lime.—This is a mixture of about 94 per cent calcium hydroxide and 5 per cent sodium hydroxide, and 1 per cent potassium hydroxide is added to some preparations to enhance absorption. Small amounts of silica are sometimes added as this reacts with calcium and sodium hydroxide to form calcium and sodium silicate. The silicate of calcium is extremely hard and brittle, whereas sodium silicate is gelatinous. The more silica that is added, the harder the soda-lime becomes, and therefore the less dust that is formed. As a general rule, however, the efficiency of absorption of soda-lime varies inversely with its hardness: for this reason silicates are omitted altogether in many present-day preparations of soda-lime.

Sodium hydroxide, present in a 5 per cent proportion, plays the role of catalyst. Increasing this amount will improve absorption but unfortunately leads to excessive heating and "caking". Calcium hydroxide, on the other hand, represents the main bulk of soda-lime and absorbs well, but it forms dust easily and is hygroscopic. The optimum moisture content of the mixture is from 14–19 per cent and such soda-lime is described as "non-hygroscopic" because it does not readily absorb moisture from the surrounding atmosphere.

In preparation, the whole mass is fused into sheets and then allowed to harden. After this it is fragmented and then graded according to the size of the granules. For this purpose a wire mesh screen is used as a sieve. A 4-mesh screen means that there are four quarter-inch square openings per inch (approximately four 6·2 mm square openings per 25 mm); an 8-mesh screen signifies eight eighth-inch openings per inch (approximately eight 3·1 mm openings per 25 mm), and so on. In general anaesthesia the granules should be in the 4–8 mesh range, as this size represents the optimum surface area of absorption with the minimum resistance.

Hardness is measured by placing the granules in a standard steel pan together with 15 steel balls of fixed diameter. The whole is then shaken for thirty minutes, after which the granules are placed on a 40-mesh sieve and again shaken for a further three minutes. The amount retained on the screen should be not less than 75 per cent of the original and is described as the hardness number.

2/TABLE 7
SPECIFICATIONS FOR SODA-LIME
(*Based on B.P. and U.S.P. standards*)

Colour:	White
Content:	Calcium hydroxide 94 per cent
	Sodium hydroxide 5 per cent
	Potassium hydroxide 1 per cent
Moisture content:	Not less than 14 per cent
	Not more than 19 per cent
Granule size:	4–8 mesh
Hardness number:	75 or more

Baralyme.—This comprises 80 per cent calcium hydroxide and 20 per cent barium hydroxide. This mixture is sufficiently hard not to require the addition of silica. Barium hydroxide (like sodium hydroxide in soda-lime) plays the role of activator so that barium carbonate, calcium carbonate and water are formed. Heat is produced in a similar manner, but as both barium and calcium carbonate are insoluble, no interaction can take place. For this reason baralyme has no powers of regeneration like soda-lime, where any sodium carbonate (soluble) formed can combine with any unneutralised calcium hydroxide available. Studies by Adriani (1963) suggest that modern soda-lime is nearly 50 per cent more efficient than baralyme.

Indicators in soda-lime.—Many dyes will change colour as hydroxides are neutralised and converted to carbonates.

Ethyl violet is an example of a colourless base indicator which can be impregnated into soda-lime. The base of the indicator reacts with carbonic acid to form a soluble carbonate which is purple in colour. When all the sodium hydroxide is converted to sodium and calcium carbonate, a purple colour develops. Examples of other dyes are given in Table 8.

Too much reliance should never be placed on any indicator for soda-lime as hypercarbia can always develop before signs of soda-lime exhaustion are evident. Furthermore, complete reliance on a colour change may lead to a dangerous situation if a soda-lime without any indicator is suddenly used. Such findings as the presence of channelling along the sides of a canister may prove misleading in judging the time of exhaustion of soda-lime. Nevertheless, the presence of an indicator in soda-lime is a useful guide, particularly if a double canister system is being used, in that it allows one chamber to be replaced. The final proof of the efficacy of a particular soda-lime canister's contents can only lie in the periodic testing of the gases flowing through it for the possible presence of carbon dioxide. This can be achieved by using a simple analyser.

2/TABLE 8

Indicators	Soda-lime	
	Fresh	Exhausted
Methyl orange	Orange	Yellow
Phenolphthalein	Colourless	Pink
Ethyl violet	Colourless	Purple
Clayton yellow	Pink	Yellow

Mechanism of absorption.—When the patient's exhalations are passed through the canister containing the soda-lime granules the carbon dioxide combines with the hydroxides to form carbonates and water. This chemical change requires the presence of some moisture, which is provided by the patient's expiration, and at the same time it produces heat. There is also an overall increase in the weight of the canister contents which amounts to about 33 per cent when they are worn out.

(1) $CO_2 + 2NaOH \rightarrow H_2O + Na_2CO_3 + heat.$
(2) $Na_2CO_3 + Ca(OH)_2 \rightarrow 2NaOH + CaCO_3.$

A small quantity is also absorbed thus:

$$CO_2 + Ca(OH)_2 \rightarrow H_2O + CaCO_3 + heat.$$

The heat produced is known as the *heat of neutralisation*. Temperatures up to 60° C have been recorded inside canisters. The production of some heat is a sign that the soda-lime is functioning efficiently.

Regeneration of soda-lime.—The surface of the soda-lime granule rapidly becomes exhausted. There are pores, however, which penetrate into the interior and allow carbon dioxide to diffuse inwards to find a fresh hydroxide surface. Clinically it has been observed in the past that if soda-lime was taken out of the system and rested when apparently exhausted, then after a few hours it was again able to absorb carbon dioxide efficiently. This observation led to the suggestion of having two canisters and interchanging them every hour to allow one to have a rest period.

The explanation of this regeneration is complex but is clearly concerned with the pores in the granule. The sodium hydroxide in the moisture on the surface of the granule is more soluble than calcium hydroxide, so it combines with the carbon dioxide in the usual manner to form sodium carbonate. Now this substance is very soluble, so it passes into the interior of the granule through one of the pores to react with the less soluble calcium hydroxide lying in the inner sanctum. Here calcium carbonate, which is insoluble, is formed along with sodium hydroxide. The sodium hydroxide then diffuses out to the surface and the process is repeated.

Due to improved soda-lime, regeneration is rarely seen today. There are three main reasons (Adriani, 1963). First, less silica is now used. The granule is not so hard but is capable of better absorption. Second, the moisture content is better controlled and more uniform. Third, small quantities (1 per cent) of potassium hydroxide have been added to improve absorption. Furthermore, experiments using a tidal volume of 500 ml containing 200 ml of carbon dioxide have shown that the modern circle absorber will remove virtually all the carbon dioxide for the first three hours, but after that the content of carbon dioxide escaping from the canister rises rapidly to reach about 0·5 per cent after five hours. There was no evidence of regeneration.

The to and fro'.—The canister is placed between the breathing bag and face-piece or endotracheal tube. Fresh gases are introduced near the face-piece so that any alteration in the gas concentration is immediately transmitted to the patient. The presence of a warm canister so close to the patient's respiratory tract ensures that the heat and humidity loss is negligible, but the system has largely fallen into disfavour because of the inadequacy of the carbon dioxide absorption, the awkwardness of the apparatus so close to the patient's head, and the possibility of inhalation of dust particles.

A standard adult to and fro' canister is cylindrical and measures 8 by 13 cm. Ideally the air space should equal the patient's tidal volume. When filled with soda-lime the air capacity lies between 375 and 425 ml. As the patient breathes in and out of the canister, so the soda-lime nearest the mouth becomes exhausted. The respirations usually travel along the sides of the canister because in this region the flow of gases apparently encounters least resistance. With this system, as the soda-lime becomes exhausted, so the entrapped air around it becomes dead space because this air can now be rebreathed without first having the carbon dioxide removed. For the first $1\frac{1}{2}$ hours the standard canister appears to be capable of absorbing almost all the carbon dioxide but after that there is a progressive rise up to 0·5 per cent after $5\frac{1}{2}$ hours (Adriani, 1963).

A neat and simple method of obtaining a well-packed canister is to place a nylon pot scourer between the soda-lime and the cap (Robson and Pask, 1954). This also helps to prevent channelling of gases in the canister.

The circle.—In this system the gases have to pass great distances along flexible tubing so that the resistance to flow is higher than in a to and fro' apparatus. The presence of unidirectional valves also offers an increase in resistance, though if these are properly constructed with a wide surface area this is reduced to a minimum.

The canister itself requires a number of comments. First, it is immaterial whether it is placed vertically or horizontally though, in the latter case, there is a greater tendency to leave a gap along the upper surface in the packing or settling of the granules. The gases may enter from the top or the bottom of the canister. The capacity of the absorber should be at least equal to the patient's tidal volume; if the tidal volume is greater then some of the expired gases will pass directly through the canister without coming to rest in the interior, thus impeding efficient absorption. The total air space normally available in an absorber lies between 40–60 per cent of the total volume of the unit, but this volume can be varied by changing the size of the granules and also the firmness of the packing.

In recent years large canisters have become more popular because they ensure better absorption, in that their capacity far exceeds any predictable tidal volume and all expired gases are in contact with a large number of granules during their passage through the absorber. The ideal capacity has not yet been determined, but the greater this is the longer becomes the period of uninterrupted use before renewal is required. These units are often constructed of transparent plastic material so that a change in the colour of the indicator in the soda-lime can be seen. Nevertheless, the heat and alkali needed in absorption techniques tend to destroy rubber and plastic materials.

In some cases these large absorbers are made in two interchangeable sections so that one half can be replaced when exhausted. An alternative method to having one large canister in the circuit is to use two absorbers mounted in series. However, these large-size canisters should be used solely for the purpose of more efficient absorption rather than as an economy measure, for it is known that inadequate absorption commences before the indicator has changed completely.

Although soda-lime is believed to act as a bactericidal filter and the heat and presence of alkali possibly do have a germicidal effect, for a known infected patient it is advisable to use a "to and fro'" system since the soda-lime can be discarded and the apparatus can be thoroughly and efficiently sterilised at the end of the anaesthetic. If economy of anaesthetic gases or vapour is the primary consideration then very low flows can be used with the closed circle system provided the concentration of oxygen and anaesthetic agent in the inspired mixture is carefully monitored.

REFERENCES

ADRIAN, E. D. (1933). Afferent impulses in the vagus and their effect on respiration. *J. Physiol.* (*Lond.*), **79**, 332.

ADRIANI, J. (1963). *Chemistry and Physics of Anesthesia*. Springfield, Ill.: Charles C. Thomas.

ALEXANDER, J. I., SPENCE, A. A., PARIKH, R. K., and STUART, B. (1973). The role of airway closure in postoperative hypoxaemia. *Brit. J. Anaesth.*, **45**, 34.

ASKROG, V. F., PENDER, J. W., and ECKENHOFF, J. E. (1964). Changes in physiological deadspace during deliberate hypotension. *Anesthesiology*, **25**, 744.

BAIN, J. A., and SPOEREL, W. E. (1972). A streamlined anesthetic system. *Canad. Anaesth. Soc. J.*, **20**, 426.

BELLVILLE, J. W., and SEED, J. C. (1960). The effect of drugs on the respiratory response to carbon dioxide. *Anesthesiology*, **21**, 727.

BRADLEY, R. D., and SEMPLE, S. J. G. (1962). A comparison of certain acid-base characteristics of arterial blood, jugular venous blood and cerebrospinal fluid in man, and the effect on them of some acute and chronic acid-base disturbances. *J. Physiol. (Lond.)*, **169**, 381.

BRADLEY, R. D., SPENCER, G. T., and SEMPLE, S. J. G. (1965). In *Cerebrospinal Fluid and the Regulation of Ventilation*. Eds. Brooks, C. McC., Kao, F. F., and Lloyd, B. B. Oxford: Blackwell.

BURNS, B. D. (1963). The central control of respiratory movements. *Brit. med. Bull.*, **19**, 7.

BURNS, B. D., and SALMOIRAGHI, G. C. (1960). Repetitive firing of respiratory neurones during their burst activity. *J. Neurophysiol.*, **23**, 27.

CAMPBELL, E. J. M. (1954). The muscular control of breathing in man. (Ph.D. Thesis) Univ. London.

CAMPBELL, E. J. M. (1955). An electromyographic examination of the role of the intercostal muscles in breathing in man. *J. Physiol. (Lond.)*, **129**, 12.

CAMPBELL, E. J. M. (1958). *The Respiratory Muscles and the Mechanics of Breathing*. London: Lloyd-Luke (Medical Books).

CAMPBELL, E. J. M., and GREEN, J. H. (1953). The variations in intra-abdominal pressure and the activity of the abdominal muscles during breathing: a study in man. *J. Physiol. (Lond.)*, **122**, 282.

CAMPBELL, E. J. M., and HOWELL, J. B. L. (1963). Sensation of breathlessness. *Brit. med. Bull.*, **19**, 36.

CARLENS, E. (1949). A new flexible double-lumen catheter for broncho-spirometry. *J. thorac. Surg.*, **18**, 742.

CASE, E. H., and STILES, J. A. (1946). The effect of various surgical positions on vital capacity. *Anesthesiology*, **7**, 29.

COMROE, J. H., FORSTER, R. E., DUBOIS, A. B., BRISCOE, W. A., and CARLSEN, E. (1962). *The Lung. Clinical Physiology and Pulmonary Function Tests*, 2nd edit. Chicago: Year Book Medical Publishers.

COOPER, E. A. (1967). Physiological deadspace in passive ventilation. *Anaesthesia*, **22**, 199.

COURNAND, A., and RICHARDS, D. W., Jr. (1941). Pulmonary insufficiency: discussion of physiological classification and presentation of clinical tests. *Amer. Rev. Tuberc.*, **44**, 26.

DAVIE, I., SCOTT, D. B., and STEPHEN, G. W. (1970). Respiratory effects of pentazocine and pethidine in patients anaesthetised with halothane and oxygen. *Brit. J. Anaesth.*, **42**, 113.

DON, H. F., WAHBA, W. M., and CRAIG, D. B. (1972). Airway closure, gas trapping, and the functional residual capacity during anesthesia. *Anesthesiology*, **36**, 533.

DORNHORST, A. C., and LEATHART, G. L. (1952). A method of assessing the mechanical properties of lungs and air passages. *Lancet*, **2**, 109.

DUNBAR, B. S., OVASSAPIAN, A., and SMITH, T. C. (1967). The effects of methoxyflurane on ventilation in man. *Anesthesiology*, **28**, 1020.

EGBERT, L. D., LAVER, M. B., and BENDIXEN, H. H. (1963). Intermittent deep breaths and compliance during anaesthesia in man. *Anesthesiology*, **24**, 57.

FENCL, V., VALE, J. R., and BROCH, J. A. (1969). Respiration and cerebral blood flow in metabolic acidosis and alkalosis in humans. *J. appl. Physiol.*, **27**, 67.

FIBUCH, E. E., REHDER, K., and SESSLER, A. D. (1975). Preoperative CC/FRC ratio and postoperative hypoxemia. *Anesthesiology*, **43**, 481.

FINK, B. R. (1961*a*). Influence of cerebral activity in wakefulness on regulation of breathing. *J. appl. Physiol.*, **16**, 15.

FINK, B. R. (1961*b*). Electromyography in general anaesthesia. *Brit. J. Anaesth.*, **33**, 555.

FINK, B. R., HANKS, E. C., HOLADAY, D. A., and NGAI, S. H. (1960). Monitoring of ventilation by integrated diaphragmatic electromyogram: determination of carbon dioxide (CO_2) threshold in anesthetized man. *J. Amer. med. Ass.*, **172**, 1367.

FITZGERALD, P. (1967). The anatomy of hiccough. *Irish J. med. Sci.*, **6**, 529.

FLETCHER, G., and BARBER, J. L. (1966). Lung mechanics and physiologic shunt during spontaneous breathing in normal subjects. *Anesthesiology*, **27**, 638.

FREEMAN, J., and NUNN, J. P. (1963). Ventilation-perfusion relationships after haemorrhage. *Clin. Sci.*, **24**, 135.

FRUMIN, M. J., LEE, A. S., and PAPPER, E. M. (1959). New valve for non-rebreathing systems. *Anesthesiology*, **20**, 383.

GLIEDMAN, M. L., SIEBENS, A. A., VESTAL, B. L., TIMMES, J. J., GRANT, R. N., MURPHY, J. L., and KARLSON, K. E. (1958). Effect of manual versus automatic ventilation on the elastic recoil of the lung. *Ann. Surg.*, **148**, 899.

GORDH, T., and SILFERKIOLD, B. P. (1943). Body plethysmograph in infants. *Acta med. scand.*, **113**, 183.

GREEN, J. H., and HOWELL, J. B. C. (1955). Correlation of respiratory airflow with intercostal muscle activity. *J. Physiol. (Lond.)*, **130**, 33P.

GUEDEL, A. E. (1951). *Inhalation Anesthesia*, 2nd edit. New York: The Macmillan Co.

GUZ, A., NOBLE, M. I. M., TRENCHARD, D., COCHRANE, H. L., and MAKEY, A. R. (1964). Studies on the vagus nerves in man: their role in respiratory and circulatory control. *Clin. Sci.*, **27**, 293.

HANKS, E. C., NGAI, S. H., and FINK, B. R. (1961). The respiratory threshold for carbon dioxide in anesthetized man. Determination of carbon dioxide threshold during halothane anesthesia. *Anesthesiology*, **22**, 393.

HARRIS, T. A. B. (1951). *The Mode of Action of Anaesthetics* Edinburgh: E. & S. Livingstone.

HENVILLE, J. D., and ADAMS, A. P. (1976). The Bain Anaesthetic System. An assessment during controlled ventilation. *Anaesthesia*, **31**, 247.

HERING, E. (1868). Die Selbststeuerung der Athmung den Nervus vagus. *S.B. Akad. Wiss. Wien.*, *II. Abth.*, **57**, 672.

HUNT, K. H. (1955). Resistance in respiratory valves and canisters. *Anesthesiology*, **16**, 190.

JACKSON, D. E. (1915). A new method for the production of general analgesia and anaesthesia, with a description of the apparatus used. *J. Lab. clin. Med.*, **1**, 1.

KAIN, M. L., and NUNN, J. F. (1967). Fresh gas flow and rebreathing in the Magill Circuit with spontaneous respiration. *Proc. roy. Soc. Med.*, **60**, 749.

KAIN, M. L., PANDAY, J., and NUNN, J. F. (1969). The effect of intubation on the deadspace during halothane anaesthesia. *Brit. J. Anaesth.*, **41**, 94.

KARCZEWSKI, W. A. (1974). *International Review of Science: Respiratory Physiology*, pp. 197–219. London: Butterworth & Co.

KATZ, R. L., and NGAI, S. H. (1962). Respiratory effects of diethyl ether in the cat. *J. Pharmacol. exp. Ther.*, **138**, 329.

LANE, D. J. (1970). D. M. Thesis, University of Oxford.

LARSON, C. P., JR., EGER, E. I., II, MUALLEM, M., BUECHEL, D. R., MUNSON, E. S., and EISELE, J. H. (1969). Effects of diethylether and methoxyflurane on ventilation, II. A comparative study in man. *Anesthesiology*, **30**, 174.

LEUSEN, I. R. (1954a). Chemosensitivity of the respiratory centre. Influence of CO_2 in the cerebral ventricles on respiration. *Amer. J. Physiol.*, **176**, 39.

LEUSEN, I. R. (1954b). Chemosensitivity of the respiratory centre. Influence of changes on the H^+ and total buffer concentrations in the cerebral ventricles on respiration. *Amer. J. Physiol.*, **176**, 45.

LLOYD, B. B., JUKES, M. G. M., and CUNNINGHAM, D. J. C. (1958). The relation between alveolar oxygen pressure and the respiratory response to carbon dioxide in man. *Quart. J. exp. Physiol.*, **43**, 214.

McDOWALL, D. G., and HARPER, A. M. (1970). Cerebral blood flow and CSF pH during hyperventilation. In *Progress in Anaesthesiology. Proceedings of the Fourth World Congress of Anaesthesiologists*, p. 542. Amsterdam: Excerpta Medica Foundation.

McILROY, M. B., and CHRISTIE, R. V. (1954). The work of breathing in emphysema. *Clin. Sci.*, **13**, 147.

MACINTOSH, R. R., and MUSHIN, W. W. (1946). *Physics for the Anaesthetist*. Oxford: Blackwell Scientific Publications.

MALONEY, J. V., Jr., SCHMUTZER, K. J., and RASCHKE, E. (1961). Paradoxical respiration and "pendelluft". *J. thorac. cardiovasc. Surg.*, **41**, 291.

MAPLESON, W. W. (1954). The elimination of rebreathing in various semi-closed anaesthetic systems. *Brit. J. Anaesth.*, **26**, 323.

MARSHALL, R., McILROY, M. B., and CHRISTIE, R. V. (1954). The work of breathing in mitral stenosis. *Clin. Sci.*, **13**, 137.

MEAD, J., and COLLIER, C. (1959). Relation of volume history of lungs to respiratory mechanics in anaesthetized dogs. *J. appl. Physiol.*, **14**, 669.

MILLS, J. N. (1949). Variability of the vital capacity of the normal human subject. *J. Physiol. (Lond.)*, **110**, 76.

MITCHELL, R. A. (1965). In *Cerebrospinal Fluid and the Regulation of Ventilation*, p. 109. Eds. Brooks, C. McC., Kao, F. F., and Lloyd, B. B. Oxford: Blackwell.

MITCHELL, R. A. (1966). In *Advances in Respiratory Physiology*. p. 1. Ed. Caro, C. G. London: Edward Arnold.

MITCHELL, R. A., LOESCHCKE, H. H., MASSION, W. H., and SEVERINGHAUS, J. W. (1963). Respiratory responses mediated through superficial chemosensitive areas on the medulla. *J. appl. Physiol.*, **18**, 523.

MOIR, D. D. (1963). Ventilatory function during epidural analgesia. *Brit. J. Anaesth.*, **35**, 3.

MORTON, H. J. V. (1950). Respiratory patterns during surgical anaesthesia. *Anaesthesia*, **5**, 112.

MUALLEM, M., LARSON, C. P., JR., and EGER, E. I., II (1969). The effects of diethyl ether on Pa_{CO_2} in dogs with and without vagal, somatic and sympathetic block. *Anesthesiology*, **30**, 185.

MUNSON, E. S., FARNHAM, M., and HAMILTON, W. H. (1963). Studies of respiratory gas flows: a comparison using different anesthetic agents. *Anesthesiology*, **24**, 61.

MUNSON, E. S., LARSON, C. P., JR., BABAD, A. A., REGAN, M. J., BUECHEL, D. R. and EGER, E. I., II (1966). The effects of halothane, fluroxene and cyclopropane on ventilation: a comparative study in man. *Anesthesiology*, **27**, 716.

NEEDHAM, C. D., ROGAN, M. C., and McDONALD, I. (1954). Normal standards for lung volumes, intrapulmonary gas mixing, and maximum breathing capacity. *Thorax*, **9**, 313.

NGAI, S. H., FARHIE, S. E., and BRODY, D. C. (1961). Effects of trichloroethylene, halopropane and methoxyflurane on respiratory regulatory mechanisms. *J. Pharmacol. exp. Ther.*, **131**, 91.

NORLANDER, O. P., HERZOG, P., NORDEN, I., HOSSLI, G., SCHAER, H., and GATTIKER, R. (1968). Compliance and airway resistance during anaesthesia with controlled ventilation. *Acta anaesth. scand.*, **12**, 135.

NORRIS, R. M., JONES, J. G., and BISHOP, J. M. (1968). Respiratory gas exchange in patients with spontaneous pneumothorax. *Thorax*, **23**, 427.

NUNN, J. F., CAMPBELL, E. J. M., and PECKETT, B. W. (1959). Anatomical subdivisions of the volume of respiratory dead space and effect of position of the jaw. *J. appl. Physiol.*, **14**, 174.

NUNN, J. F., and EZI-ASHI, T. I. (1961). The respiratory effects of resistance to breathing in anesthetized man. *Anesthesiology*, **22**, 174.

NUNN, J. F., and EZI-ASHI, T. I. (1962). The accuracy of the respirometer and ventigrator. *Brit. J. Anaesth.*, **34**, 422.

PAPPENHEIMER, J. (1950). Standardisation of definitions and symbols in respiratory physiology. *Fed. Proc.*, **9**, 602.

PAPPENHEIMER, J. R., FENCL, V., HEISEY, S. R., and HELD, D. (1965). Role of cerebral fluids in control of respiration as studied in unanesthetized goats. *Amer. J. Physiol.*, **208**, 436.

PASKIN, S., SKOVSTED, P., and SMITH, T. C. (1968). Failure of the Hering-Breuer reflex to account for tachypnoea in anesthetized man. *Anesthesiology*, **29**, 550.

PITTS, R. F. (1946). Organisation of the respiratory center. *Physiol. Rev.*, **26**, 609.

PRIMROSE, W. B. (1952). Chest movements and the intercostal muscles. *Brit. J. Anaesth.*, **24**, 3.

RASTOGI, P. N., and WRIGHT, J. E. (1969). Bilateral tension pneumothorax under anaesthesia. *Anaesthesia*, **24**, 249.

READ, D. J. (1967). A clinical method for assessing the ventilatory response to carbon dioxide. *Aust. Ann. Med.*, **16**, 20.

REHDER, K., MARSH, H. M., RODARTE, J. R., and HYATT, R. E. (1977). Airway closure. *Anesthesiology*, **47**, 40.

RIGG, J. R. A., ENGEL, L. A., and RITCHIE, B. C. (1970). The ventilatory response to carbon dioxide during partial paralysis with tubocurarine. *Brit. J. Anaesth.*, **42**, 105.

ROBSON, J. G., and PASK, E. A. (1954). Some data on the performance of Waters' canister. *Brit. J. Anaesth.*, **26**, 333.

RUBEN, H. (1955). A new non-rebreathing valve. *Anesthesiology*, **16**, 643.

SALEM, M. R. (1967). An effective method for the treatment of hiccups during anesthesia. *Anesthesiology*, **28**, 463.

SAMUELS, L. (1952). Hiccup. A ten year review of anatomy, etiology and treatment. *Canad. med. Ass. J.*, **67**, 315.

SCHOLFIELD, E. J., and WILLIAMS, N. E. (1974). Prediction of arterial carbon dioxide tension using a circle system without carbon dioxide absorption. *Brit. J. Anaesth.*, **46**, 442.

SEVERINGHAUS, J. W., and LARSEN, C. P. (1965). Respiration in Anesthesia. In *Handbook of Physiology—Respiration II*, Chap. 49, p. 1223. Washington, D.C.: American Physiological Society.

SEVERINGHAUS, J. W., MITCHELL, R. A., RICHARDSON, B. W., and SINGER, M. M. (1963). Respiratory control at high altitude suggesting active transport regulation of CSF pH. *J. appl. Physiol.*, **18**, 1155.

SIMPSON, B. R., PARKHOUSE, J., MARSHALL, R., and LAMBRECHTS, W. (1961). Extradural analgesia and the prevention of post-operative respiratory complications. *Brit. J. Anaesth.*, **33**, 628.

SMITH, W. D. A. (1961). The effects of external resistance on respiration. Part I. General review. *Brit. J. Anaesth.*, **33**, 549.

SUWA, K., and YAMAMURA, H. (1970). The effect of gas inflow on the regulation of CO_2 levels with hyperventilation during anesthesia. *Anesthesiology*, **33**, 440.

SYKES, M. K., YOUNG, W. E., and ROBINSON, B. E. (1965). Oxygenation during anaesthesia with controlled ventilation. *Brit. J. Anaesth.*, **37**, 314.

VANCE, J. P. (1968). Tension pneumothorax in labour. *Anaesthesia*, **23**, 94.

VON NEERGAARD, K. (1929). Neue Auffassungen ueber einen Grundbegriff der Atem-mechanik, abhaengig von der Oberglaichen Spannung in der Alveolen. *Z. ges. exp. Med.*, **66**, 373.

WADE, O. L. (1954). Movements of the thoracic cage and diaphragm in respiration. *J. Physiol. (Lond.)*, **124**, 193.

WANG, S. C., NGAI, S. H., and FRUMIN, M. J. (1957). Organization of central respiratory mechanisms in the brain stem of the cat: genesis of normal respiratory rhythmicity. *Amer. J. Physiol.*, **190**, 333.

WATERS, R. M. (1924). Clinical scope and utility of carbon dioxide filtration in inhalation anesthesia. *Curr. Res. Anesth.*, **3**, 20.

WHITTERIDGE, D., and BÜLBRING, E. (1946). Changes in activity of pulmonary receptors in anaesthesia and their influence on respiratory behaviour. *Brit. med. Bull.*, **4**, 85.

WIDDICOMBE, J. G. (1961). Respiratory reflexes in man and other mammalian species. *Clin. Sci.*, **21**, 163.

YOUNG, I. M. (1957). Adrenaline Hyperpnoea. (Ph.D. Thesis) Univ. London.

FURTHER READING

BROOKS, C. McC., KAO, F. F., and LLOYD, B. B. (Eds.) (1965). *Cerebrospinal Fluid and the Regulation of Ventilation.* Oxford: Blackwell.

COMROE, J. H. (1965). *Physiology of Respiration. An Introductory Text.* Chicago: Year Book Medical Publishers.

COTES, J. E. (1968). *Lung Function.* Oxford: Blackwell Scientific Publications.

Chapter 3

PULMONARY GAS EXCHANGE AND ACID-BASE STATUS

THE function of the respiratory system is to provide an adequate supply of oxygen to the tissues and to regulate the excretion of carbon dioxide so as to help maintain a normal acid-base state. The lungs are one link in a complex chain of systems, and provide the mechanisms which allow the transfer of oxygen and carbon dioxide between blood and air. Three principal factors are concerned in their function, namely: ventilation, diffusion, and pulmonary blood flow. Ventilation must not only be sufficient to move an adequate volume of air, but its distribution throughout the lungs must be related to the distribution and quantity of pulmonary blood flow. Finally, each gas must be able to diffuse across the alveolar membrane with ease.

VENTILATION

The subject of the overall ventilation of the lungs is dealt with in Chapter 2, and distribution of ventilation later in this Chapter (p. 132).

ALVEOLAR GAS TRANSFER

The exchange of gases within the lung occurs through a process of passive diffusion across the alveolar-capillary membrane. This membrane consists of the alveolar membrane, interstitial fluid, and the capillary endothelium. In the case of oxygen, the plasma, red cell membrane and intracellular fluid must also be considered, as the rate of reaction of oxygen with haemoglobin plays an important part in determining the rate of diffusion. The rate of transfer of a gas is directly proportional to the area of the membrane, the solubility of the gas in liquid, and the partial pressure gradient across the membrane; and is inversely proportional to the molecular weight of the gas* and the distance across which diffusion has to occur. Carbon dioxide diffuses some twenty times more rapidly than does oxygen.

The most important variable in considering the diffusion of oxygen is the partial pressure gradient across the capillary wall. At the arterial end of the pulmonary capillary the partial pressure of oxygen (Po_2) in the blood is about 40 mm Hg (5·3 kPa) so that a gradient of about 65 mm Hg (8·6 kPa) is present between alveolus and blood. As oxygen passes across the membrane, the Po_2 of the blood rises, the rate of rise being determined by the rate of gas transfer and its rate of combination with haemoglobin, so that the pressure gradient driving the gas across the membrane falls. This process is shown in Fig. 1. From this diagram it can be seen that an average red blood corpuscle takes about 0·75 seconds to traverse a capillary, that the majority of the gas exchange occurs within the first third of this time, and that virtually complete equilibrium be-

---

* Graham's Law states that the rate of diffusion of gases through certain membranes is

$$\propto \frac{1}{\sqrt{\text{Mol. Wt}}}.$$

tween blood and alveolus has been established at the venous end of the capillary. From this data it is evident that there is a great reserve capacity in the diffusion process. For example during exercise almost complete equilibration still occurs even though the time available for gas transfer may be reduced by two-thirds. A similar but opposite and much more rapid process occurs during diffusion of carbon dioxide, although the driving pressures are much lower (maximum of 6 mm Hg (0·8 kPa) at the arterial end of the capillary).

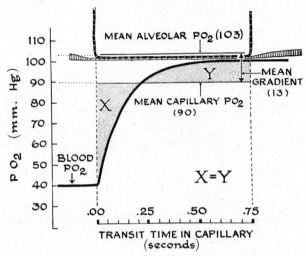

3/FIG. 1.—The change in oxygen tension of blood during its passage through a pulmonary capillary.

The alveolar-capillary membrane can be seen to be thickened in certain diseases, such as sarcoidosis, asbestosis, pulmonary fibrosis, and infiltrating carcinoma, and this thickening can produce defects in the diffusion process. This state of affairs has been given the name "alveolar-capillary block", and is characterised clinically by dyspnoea and profound cyanosis, especially on exercise, associated with a low arterial P_{CO_2}. However, it has been shown that the diffusion defect in these conditions is not nearly so severe as was once supposed, and that most of the hypoxia is due to ventilation/perfusion abnormalities (see below). At present it is considered that impairment of diffusion does not play nearly such an important role in clinical practice as was at one time suspected, except perhaps in acute severe pulmonary oedema.

Transfer Factor for Carbon Monoxide

An estimate of the efficiency of gas transfer from gas to blood can be made by measuring the Transfer Factor for carbon monoxide. This is usually done by a single breath technique using a test gas mixture containing CO 0·03 per cent, helium 14 per cent and air. The subject exhales to residual volume, takes a single breath of the prepared gas mixture, holds it for 10 seconds and then exhales slowly and fully to residual volume. During exhalation a mid-expired sample is collected and analysed for CO and helium concentrations. The time for which the breath was held and the inspired volume are also noted. From these data the transfer factor can be calculated (Cotes, 1968).

The transfer of CO from inspired gas to blood depends on three factors.

(1) *Ventilation.* This is because the concentration of CO in the alveoli depends on the depth and the distribution of ventilation when inhaling the test gas, and is therefore influenced by airways obstruction. This distribution factor can to some extent be compensated for by an estimate of the volume of lung into which the test gas was distributed, hence the helium which is contained in the mixture.

(2) *Pulmonary capillary blood volume,* especially the volume of red cells which are available to take up the CO. Thus anaemic patients tend to have a low transfer factor and polycythaemic patients a high one.

(3) *Diffusion.* CO is so diffusible that it only leads to a reduction in gas transfer factor when a major diffusion defect is present, such as in severe pulmonary oedema.

Other factors affecting the transfer factor are less important. It increases during growth and is higher in men than in women and is low in the presence of a low cardiac output. During exercise it may be doubled. However, the most important single factor which lowers the transfer factor is ventilation-perfusion maldistribution.

Low values for transfer factor are found in bronchitis, emphysema, diffuse pulmonary infiltrations and loss of functioning lung tissue (e.g. pulmonary collapse, pulmonary embolus).

THE PULMONARY CIRCULATION

The pulmonary circulation consists of the pulmonary artery and its branches, the precapillary vessels (which unlike those in the systemic circulation are thin-walled and easily distended), the pulmonary capillaries, the pulmonary venous system and the left atrium. It is a low-pressure system, easily distensible, with a low resistance to blood flow, and accepts all the blood that leaves the right side of the heart. The normal pulmonary artery pressure curve is similar in shape to the aortic pressure curve, but with a systolic pressure of 20–30 mm Hg (2·7–4·0 kPa), a diastolic pressure of 8–12 mm Hg (1·1–1·6 kPa), and a mean pressure of 12–15 mm Hg (1·6–2·0 kPa) at rest. The normal mean left atrial pressure is about 8 mm Hg (1·1 kPa), with an upper limit of 15 mm Hg (2·0 kPa). The system is very flexible in adapting itself to changes in blood flow and blood volume, its adaptability being almost entirely passive in nature. Thus, immediately after blocking the pulmonary artery to one lung, the pressure in the other only rises by about 5 mm Hg (0·7 kPa). Also, the low pulse pressure in the pulmonary artery, when compared with that in the aorta, is due to the high distensibility and low resistance of the system. The compliance of the entire pulmonary vascular tree resembles that of a large systemic vein in nature.

The pulmonary circulation normally contains about 10 per cent of the total blood volume, but this amount is easily altered by as much as 50 per cent. A rise in pulmonary blood volume is seen in negative-pressure breathing, the supine position when compared with the upright position, systemic vasoconstriction from any cause, over-transfusion, and left ventricular failure. A fall in pulmonary blood volume occurs during positive-pressure breathing, on assuming the upright posture, during Valsalva's manoeuvre, after haemorrhage, or as a result of systemic vasodilatation from any cause. Thus it is a simple matter to shift blood from the pulmonary circulation to the systemic circulation, and vice versa.

Although on histological examination the pulmonary blood vessels can be seen to contain smooth muscle, control of the distribution of the blood flow within the vessels, and of the resistance offered to flow, appears to be largely passive. Although more than a dozen active reflexes have been described, none of them is as yet generally accepted. The one exception to this is the response of the pulmonary circulation to alveolar hypoxia. If alveolar hypoxia occurs for any reason, either generally or locally within the lung, the result is *vaso-constriction* and a reduction in blood flow in those vessels supplying the hypoxic area, so that the blood is diverted to oxygenated parts of the lung. This response to hypoxia is the opposite to that which occurs in the systemic circulation. In man 50 per cent of the final shift in blood flow has occurred within 2 minutes of the onset of alveolar hypoxia, and it is complete after 7 minutes. The reflex is accentuated by a local rise in H^+ ion concentration. The mechanism of this reflex is as yet undecided although its purpose is more readily apparent. For example, if pulmonary collapse occurs in a portion of the lung, ventilation will be reduced in the collapsed area, and oxygenation of the venous blood flowing to that area will be less effective. The blood is therefore diverted to parts of the lung where it can become adequately oxygenated, thus tending to maintain a normal arterial oxygen saturation.

Pulmonary Hypertension

Pulmonary hypertension is said to be present when the systolic pressure rises above 30 mm Hg (4·0 kPa). It can be due either to an increase in flow, in pulmonary vascular resistance, or in left atrial pressure. An increase in pulmonary blood flow occurs when a left-to-right shunt is present, such as is found in atrial or ventricular defects or in the presence of a patent ductus arteriosus. In these conditions the blood flow through the lungs may be as much as three times the systemic cardiac output. If this state of affairs is allowed to persist, after some years the pulmonary vascular resistance begins to rise due to structural changes in the vessels and the pulmonary artery pressure rises even further. Eventually the pressure on the right side of the heart may exceed that in the left side, and a right-to-left shunt with central cyanosis then appears. The combination of a ventricular septal defect, pulmonary hypertension and a reversed shunt is called Eisenmenger's complex*.

A rise in left atrial and pulmonary venous pressures causes pulmonary arterial hypertension by back-pressure, and may be secondary to aortic or mitral valve disease, or to left ventricular failure from any cause. A rise in pulmonary vascular resistance occurs in such conditions as massive or multiple pulmonary emboli and in some lung diseases, notably advanced chronic bronchitis. Pulmonary hypertension in the latter condition is thought to be due to a combina-

---

* *Eisenmenger complex* is the condition which he originally described and comprises ventricular septal defect, a pulmonary resistance which is equal to or exceeds systemic vascular resistance, and right-to-left shunt.

Eisenmenger syndrome is any vascular connection between the left and right sides of the circulation at the atrial, ventricular or aortopulmonary level in which the pulmonary vascular resistance is equal to or exceeds systemic vascular resistance, causing a right-to-left shunt.

tion of chronic hypoxia and obliteration of the pulmonary vascular bed by the disease process.

Pulmonary Oedema

Normally the pressure in the pulmonary capillaries is low and is exceeded by the colloidal osmotic pressure of the plasma which tends to retain fluid within the circulation. If for any reason the pulmonary capillary pressure rises above the osmotic pressure, fluid passes across the alveolar-capillary membrane and pulmonary oedema results. This can occur in any disease in which the pulmonary venous pressure is high, such as those listed above, or as a result of over-transfusion, of brain damage, or following chemical or other damage to the pulmonary capillaries when their ability to retain protein is impaired.

Measurement of Pulmonary Blood Flow

There are four principal methods. First, use of radio-active gases. Second, the direct Fick method requiring the measurement of the oxygen uptake per minute in the pulmonary circulation. Third, the dye-dilution method; and fourth, the body plethysmograph. The last method has the advantage that it measures blood flow instantaneously. The patient, enclosed in the body plethysmograph, sits in an air-tight chamber, the interior pressure of which can be sensitively monitored. At the desired moment he inhales deeply from a bag inside the chamber containing a mixture of 80 per cent nitrous oxide and 20 per cent oxygen. The nitrous oxide rapidly leaves the bag and becomes dissolved in the pulmonary circulation. The bag empties and the interior pressure of the chamber decreases. The rate of pulmonary blood flow can then be calculated from a knowledge of the pressure of nitrous oxide in the patient's alveoli, the solubility of nitrous oxide in blood, and the volume of the alveoli.

Pulmonary Haemodynamics during General Anaesthesia

The haemodynamics of the pulmonary circulation in fit young volunteers during general anaesthesia have been described by Price and his colleagues (1969). They found that cyclopropane caused a rise in mean pulmonary artery pressure and wedge pressure, and that pulmonary vascular resistance was doubled. About 40 per cent of the rise in pulmonary artery pressure was estimated to be secondary to the increased vascular resistance, and about 60 per cent due to actions distal to the pulmonary capillaries. No significant change in these measurements was found during halothane anaesthesia, with or without nitrous oxide. A nitrous oxide/oxygen/d-tubocurarine sequence has no effect on the pulmonary artery pressure or vascular resistance, although both are elevated during ether anaesthesia (Wyant et al., 1962).

One important property of many anaesthetic agents has recently come to light, which is that they inhibit the pulmonary vascular vasoconstrictor response to alveolar hypoxia (Sykes et al., 1973). Thus the normal compensatory response to alveolar hypoxia which tends to limit the consequent fall in arterial Po_2 is reduced or absent. This effect may be an important aetiological factor in the arterial hypoxaemia which occurs in the anaesthetised patient (see p. 143).

Hypoxic Pulmonary Vasoconstrictor Reflex

The main cause of hypoxaemia during anaesthesia is now believed to be due

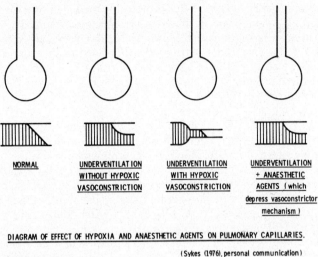

NORMAL | UNDERVENTILATION WITHOUT HYPOXIC VASOCONSTRICTION | UNDERVENTILATION WITH HYPOXIC VASOCONSTRICTION | UNDERVENTILATION + ANAESTHETIC AGENTS (which depress vasoconstrictor mechanism)

DIAGRAM OF EFFECT OF HYPOXIA AND ANAESTHETIC AGENTS ON PULMONARY CAPILLARIES.

(Sykes (1976), personal communication)

☐ = Oxygenated blood
▥ = De-oxygenated blood

3/Fig. 2.

to a reduction in functional residual capacity; in turn, this increases airway closure in dependent areas of the lung and so increases venous admixture.

In the normal conscious subject the lung possesses an intricate mechanism whereby hypoxaemia in a particular area of the lung is accompanied by a vasoconstriction of the pulmonary vessels supplying that area. This mechanism plays an important part in controlling and matching perfusion to ventilation. Inhalational anaesthetic agents (with the possible exception of halothane) are known to suppress this reflex pulmonary vasoconstriction thereby increasing the hypoxia (see Fig. 2 and Table 1). Intravenous anaesthetic drugs do not affect this reflex response.

3/Table 1

Effect of Various Anaesthetic Agents on the Hypoxic Pulmonary Vasoconstrictor Reflex in Animal and Man

Cat		Dog	Man
Isolated lung	Intact lung	Intact lung	Intact lung
Ether ↓ Halothane ↓ Trichloroethylene ↓ Methoxyflurane ↓ Nitrous oxide ↓ Cyclopropane 0	Ether ↓ Halothane 0	Ether ↓ Halothane 0 T.C.E. ↓ N₂O ↓	Ether ↓ Halothane 0

↓ = Reflex suppression.
0 = Nil or minimal suppression.

(Sykes, personal communication, 1976)

Mechanism.—The hypoxic reflex is probably mediated by a receptor (? mast cells) on the alveolar side of the alveolar capillary membrane. The most acceptable explanation is that these receptors release a vasoconstrictor substance. Nearly all inhalational anaesthetic agents (but not the intravenous ones), with the possible exception of halothane and cyclopropane, appear to depress the activity of these receptors (Sykes *et al.*, 1973; Sykes, personal communication, 1976).

DISTRIBUTION OF PULMONARY BLOOD FLOW

Many years ago it was suggested that in the erect posture the simple factor of the weight of a column of blood in the lung would cause the upper part of the lung to receive less blood than the lower part. Great advances have been made in the study of the amount and distribution of both air and blood in the lungs with the aid of radio-active techniques. Radio-active oxygen with a half-life of two minutes (West, 1963 *a* and *b*) or radio-active xenon with a half-life of 5·3 days are available (Ball *et al.*, 1962). So also is oxygen-15-labelled carbon dioxide. The principle of the method of measurement is simple. The patient's chest is surrounded with multiple counters which can detect radio-activity in a particular area of the lung. The subject then takes a single breath of radio-active gas. The distribution of this gas in the lung will reveal the regional ventilation per unit of lung volume. Alternatively, if the value of the pulmonary blood flow is required, then the technique differs according to which gas is used. In the case of oxygen (or oxygen-labelled carbon dioxide) the patient takes a breath and then holds it: the rate of the removal of this gas from the different areas of the lung signifies the pulmonary blood flow. In contrast, xenon is a relatively insoluble gas and is injected into an arm vein as a solution in saline: the xenon passes to the pulmonary capillaries and out into the alveoli. The precise areas in which this takes place are revealed by the counters.

In the normal conscious subject West (1962) found that, in the upright position, there was a nine-fold difference in the pulmonary blood flow between the first and fifth intercostal spaces, with almost no blood flow at the apex of the lung. From Fig. 3*a* it will be observed that in passing from the apex to the base of the lung, the volume of the organ only increases from 7 to 13 per cent, yet the blood flow alters from 0·07 l/min at the apex, to 1·29 l/min at the base. In the *supine* position the blood flow at the apex increases considerably, so that its distribution becomes uniform from apex to base, although now perfusion anteriorly is less than that posteriorly. It appears, therefore, that gravity plays a dominating role in determining the distribution of blood flow within the lungs. The mechanisms through which gravity controls the distribution of blood in the upright lung are shown in Fig. 3*c*. The lung has been divided into three zones by considering the relationships between the alveolar pressure (P_A), the pulmonary artery pressure (P_a) and the pulmonary venous pressure (P_v), and the effects these pressures have upon the collapsible pulmonary vessels. In zone 1, at the top of the lung, the alveolar pressure exceeds both the pulmonary artery and pulmonary venous pressures. The result is collapse of the local pulmonary vessels, and little or no blood flow. In zone 2 the pulmonary artery pressure exceeds the alveolar and pulmonary venous pressures. The pulmonary vessels are now held partly open, and blood flow begins to occur at the top of the zone, increasing rather rapidly down its length. In zone 3 the pulmonary artery pressure exceeds the pulmonary venous pressure, which itself is greater than the alveolar pressure. Blood flow continues to increase as we pass down zone 3, but at a slower rate than in zone 2. There is another important difference between zone 2 and zone 3. In zone 2, the blood flow depends mainly on the difference between the *alveolar* and *pulmonary artery* pressures, whereas in zone 3, it is the difference between the *pulmonary arterial* and *pulmonary venous* pressures which is important, the alveolar pressure having little influence.

The scheme outlined above satisfactorily explains most of the observed findings (e.g. the effect of lying supine). For instance, during exercise the perfusion of the lung becomes more evenly distributed, and this is probably due to the increase in pulmonary artery pressure which is observed under these conditions so that zone 1 becomes much smaller or disappears altogether.

mm Hg	kPa
132	17·6
28	3·7
89	11·9
42	5·6

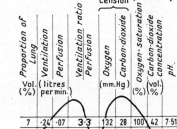
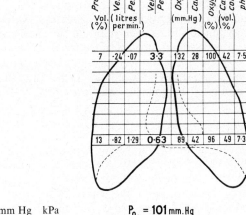
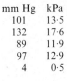

Proportion of Lung	Ventilation	Perfusion	Ventilation ratio Perfusion	Oxygen	Carbon-dioxide	Oxygen-saturation	Carbon-dioxide concentration	pH.
Vol. (%)	(litres per min.)			\ Alveolar tension \ (mm.Hg)		\ Capillary blood \ (%)	(vol. %)	
7	·24	·07	3·3	132	28	100	42	7·51
13	·82	1·29	0·63	89	42	96	49	7·39

3/Fig. 3(*a*).—Differences in ventilation, blood flow and gas exchange in the normal upright lung.

mm Hg	kPa
101	13·5
132	17·6
89	11·9
97	12·9
4	0·5

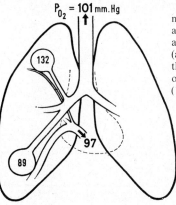

$P_{O_2} = 101$ mm. Hg

3/Fig. 3(*b*).—Diagram showing how normal alveolar-arterial oxygen difference arises. The P_{O_2} values in alveoli at the top and bottom of the lungs, in alveolar air (average value) and in mixed blood leaving the lungs are shown. Alveolar-arterial oxygen difference = 101 − 97 = 4 mm Hg (13·5 − 12·9 = 0·5 kPa).

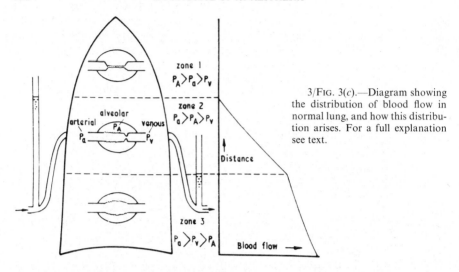

3/Fig. 3(c).—Diagram showing the distribution of blood flow in normal lung, and how this distribution arises. For a full explanation see text.

In the normal lung at lung volumes below total lung capacity, the interstitial pressure at the lung base is raised because the lung parenchyma is less well expanded than at the lung apex. Perivascular oedema isolates the vessel from the normal expanding action of the lung parenchyma, with the result that the vessel closes by virtue of the inherent tension in its wall. A modification of the three zone model to take account of the reduction of blood flow in the most dependent regions of the lung has been proposed by Hughes and his colleagues (1968). Under pathological conditions, interstitial oedema may further raise the interstitial pressure, thus further reducing the basal blood flow (West *et al.*, 1965).

DISTRIBUTION OF VENTILATION

In the normal upright lung the ventilation per unit lung volume is greater at the base than it is at the apex. The change in ventilation decreases approximately linearly with the distance up the lung, being about twice as great at the base than at the apex. These differences disappear in the supine position, the ventilation becoming almost even from apex to base. Also, the differences in regional ventilation become less during exercise, and are reversed in the inverted position. The mechanism by which ventilation is distributed within the normal lung has become clearer. In the upright position the lung tends to sag towards its most dependant part under the influence of gravity so that the alveoli are smaller at the base than they are at the apex. Small alveoli are more compliant than larger ones so that during inspiration a greater volume change occurs in the former and hence ventilation is preferentially distributed to the dependant parts of the lung, provided that the basal areas are not so compressed that airway closure has occurred. The local tension of carbon dioxide may also play a part. Severinghaus *et al.* (1961) found that a fall in alveolar CO_2 in one lung after occlusion of its pulmonary artery was accompanied by a fall in its ventilation of about 25 per cent.

In diseased lung the two main factors controlling the distribution of ventilation are the patency of the airways, and local changes in compliance within the lungs. Any factor which reduces the airway calibre, and therefore raises the resistance to airflow, will result in a fall in ventilation to the affected region. Similarly, any area in which the local compliance has decreased will be less well ventilated than the surrounding more expandable normal lung tissue.

THE RELATIONSHIPS BETWEEN VENTILATION AND PERFUSION IN NORMAL AND ABNORMAL LUNGS

The normal alveolar ventilation ($\dot{V}_A$) in an adult is approximately 4 l/min, and the total perfusion ($\dot{Q}$) about 5 l/min. Therefore the proportion of ventilation to perfusion is $\frac{4}{5} = 0.8$. This ratio is known as the VENTILATION/PERFUSION RATIO ($\dot{V}_A/\dot{Q}$). The ventilation/perfusion ratio for a whole lung is a composite of the ratios for each individual alveolus, and in an "ideal" lung the ratio for each alveolus should be the same as that for the whole lung (namely 0·8), so that ventilation and blood flow are distributed absolutely evenly to each individual alveolus. As is apparent from the foregoing discussions on the distribution of blood flow and ventilation within the normal lung, this is far from the case.

The differences in ventilation and perfusion at the top and bottom of the upright lung, together with their effects on gas exchange, are shown in Fig. 3a. At the bottom of the lung ventilation is exceeded by blood flow, so that $\dot{V}_A/\dot{Q}$ is low, namely 0·63. Because ventilation is proportionally low, the rate of supply of oxygen to these alveoli is less than the maximum rate at which it could be removed by the blood flow. This results in a low P_{O_2} in these over-perfused alveoli (i.e. 89 mm Hg, 11·8 kPa), and therefore, a low P_{O_2} in the blood leaving this portion of the lung. However, owing to the shape of the oxygen dissociation curve, a P_{O_2} of 89 mm Hg (11·8 kPa), only results in a small fall in oxygen saturation (to 96 per cent), as the curve is nearly horizontal at this level of P_{O_2}. Similarly, the excretion of carbon dioxide is impaired, because the ventilation is not sufficient to wash out all the carbon dioxide passing into the alveoli from venous blood without a small rise in its alveolar concentration ($P_{A\ CO_2} = 42$ mm Hg, 5·6 kPa). The result is that blood leaving the base of the lungs is slightly hypoxic and hypercapnic.

Passing up the lungs, both ventilation and perfusion decrease, but perfusion decreases at about three times the rate at which ventilation does. By the time the top of the lung is reached, perfusion is almost nil, so that ventilation at the apices is proportionally far greater than perfusion, and the ratio of the two becomes very high ($\dot{V}_A/\dot{Q} = 3.3$). Therefore oxygen is supplied to the upper alveoli at a greater rate than it is removed, with the result that a new equilibrium is established, and the alveolar P_{O_2} is high ($P_{A\ O_2} = 132$ mm Hg, 17·6 kPa). The blood leaving these areas has a similar P_{O_2} and the saturation rises to nearly 100 per cent. The alveolar carbon dioxide pressure is lower than at the bases ($P_{A\ CO_2} = 38$ mm Hg, 5 kPa) owing to excessive washout. Thus blood leaving the apices is almost 100 per cent saturated with a slightly low carbon dioxide content. It is clear that at the top of the lung much of the ventilation is "wasted", as it does not have the opportunity to partake in gas exchange owing to the very low blood flow. This wasted ventilation, therefore, becomes part of the physiological dead space by definition. Any further increase in the proportion of alveoli which are over-ventilated (i.e. with a *high* $\dot{V}_A/\dot{Q}$ ratio) will result in an increase in physiological dead space. This may be secondary to either an increase in relative ventilation in parts of the lung, or to a reduction in relative perfusion, because in both instances a rise in $\dot{V}_A/\dot{Q}$ will occur.

The term $\dot{V}_A/\dot{Q}$ *mismatch* refers to the situation where alveoli are either over- or underperfused relative to their ventilation. Some degree of $\dot{V}_A/\dot{Q}$ mismatch is normal, as explained above, but this may be increased.

$\dot{V}_A/\dot{Q}$ Mismatch and Carbon Dioxide Excretion

Variations in the relationship between ventilation and perfusion have a smaller effect on the excretion of carbon dioxide than on the uptake of oxygen. Because of the shape of the CO_2 dissociation curve (p. 156) blood passing through zones of lung with a high $\dot{V}_A/\dot{Q}$ ratio loses more CO_2 than normal and so can compensate for blood passing through zones of lungs with a low $\dot{V}_A/\dot{Q}$ ratio which will lose less CO_2 than normal. The same is not true for oxygen. Because of the shape of the haemoglobin-oxygen dissociation curve, blood passing through zones of lung with a high $\dot{V}_A/\dot{Q}$ ratio cannot pick up enough extra oxygen to compensate for blood passing through zones with a low $\dot{V}_A/\dot{Q}$ ratio. If blood from zones of high and low $\dot{V}_A/\dot{Q}$ ratios is mixed (Table 2) the CO_2 content and P_{CO_2} of the blood are close to normal whereas the oxygen content and P_{O_2} are reduced.

3/Table 2

	O_2 Content	CO_2 Content
(1) $V_{A/Q}$ ratio low	Low	High
(2) $V_{A/Q}$ ratio high	Increase not great enough to compensate for (1)	Low
(1) & (2) arterial blood	Low	Normal

Blood leaving those parts of the lung with different $\dot{V}_A/\dot{Q}$ ratios will become mixed in the left atrium and left ventricle, so that the arterial tensions of oxygen and carbon dioxide will be somewhere in between the extreme values found at the top and bottom on the lungs.

Alveolar-Arterial P_{O_2} Difference ($P_{A_{O_2}} - Pa_{O_2}$)

In normal young people the arterial P_{O_2} is about 97 mm Hg (12·9 kPa) and the P_{CO_2} about 40 mm Hg (5·3 kPa). As the normal average alveolar P_{O_2} is about 101 mm Hg (13·4 kPa) there is therefore a difference of about 4 mm Hg (0·5 kPa) between the alveolar and arterial P_{O_2} values. This difference is known as the *Alveolar-Arterial PO_2 Difference* ($P_{A_{O_2}} - Pa_{O_2}$) (see Fig. 3*b*).

The normal value for $P_{A_{O_2}} - Pa_{O_2}$ when breathing air ranges from 5–25 mm Hg (0·7–3·3 kPa), increasing with age (Raine and Bishop, 1963). The main factors responsible for an increase in this difference are shown below:—

1. Increased partial pressure of oxygen in inspired gas ($P_{I_{O_2}}\uparrow$)

2. Venous Admixture $\begin{cases} \text{LOW } \dot{V}_A/\dot{Q} \\ \text{TRUE SHUNT} \end{cases}$

3. Reduced partial pressure of oxygen in mixed venous blood ($P\bar{v}O_2\downarrow$).

Increased partial pressure of oxygen in inspired gas (PIO_2).—The higher the alveolar PO_2 the greater is the alveolar-arterial PO_2 difference. This is due to the shape of the haemoglobin-oxygen dissociation curve: a small difference in the oxygen content of blood at high levels of PO_2 is reflected by a large change in PO_2, whereas the same difference in the oxygen content of blood at low levels of PO_2 is reflected by a much smaller change in PO_2.

Venous admixture.—As a gross simplification, the blood returning to the left side of the heart can be considered to be made up of two fractions:

(a) Blood which has passed through "ideal" alveoli, that is alveoli with perfect ventilation and perfusion (i.e. no $\dot{V}A/\dot{Q}$ mismatch).

(b) Mixed venous blood. The oxygen and carbon dioxide contents of venous blood vary according to which organ or part of the body the blood has come from. By the time the venous blood has reached the pulmonary artery mixing has occurred, so that a blood sample taken from the pulmonary artery consists of *mixed venous blood*.

The blood from "ideal" alveoli obviously has a PO_2 equal to "ideal" alveolar PO_2. In order to produce the observed alveolar-arterial PO_2 difference a certain quantity of mixed venous blood would have to be added. This quantity is termed *venous admixture* and can be defined as the *CALCULATED* amount of mixed venous blood which would be required to mix with blood draining "ideal" alveoli to produce the observed difference between "ideal" alveolar and arterial PO_2. This is an entirely theoretical concept since some of the blood contributing to the venous admixture effect has a PO_2 lower than $P\bar{v}O_2$, e.g. Thebesian venous blood from the myocardium; and some have a higher PO_2 than PvO_2, e.g. blood which has passed through zones of relatively overventilated or underperfused lung. This less than fully oxygenated blood which is responsible for the venous admixture effect can be divided into

(a) blood which has passed from the right to the left side of the circulation and picked up *no* oxygen in the lungs—TRUE SHUNT;

(b) blood which has picked up *some* oxygen in the lungs but is still less than fully oxygenated, having passed through relatively overperfused or underventilated zones of lung—LOW $\dot{V}A/\dot{Q}$ RATIO.

The causes of true shunt are summarised in Table 3. Other terms sometimes encountered are:

(i) *Anatomical shunt*. This is the same as "true shunt".

(ii) *Pathological shunt*. Those forms of anatomical shunt which are not present in the normal subject, e.g. congenital heart disease with right-to-left shunting.

(iii) *Physiological shunt*. This refers to the normal degree of venous admixture and comprises admixture due to normal true shunt (Table 3) and admixture due to blood which has passed through relatively over-perfused or underventilated (low $\dot{V}A/\dot{Q}$) zones of lung.

(iv) *Atelectatic shunt*. Blood which has passed through collapsed (un-ventilated) zones of lung.

Venous admixture causes an increase in arterial CO_2 *content* which is similar in magnitude to the reduction in arterial O_2 *content*. In the normal subject both quantities are very small, about 0·3 vols per cent. Because of the shapes of the

CO_2 and O_2 dissociation curves this small increase in CO_2 content is reflected by only a small increase in $PaCO_2$ (less than 1 mm Hg, 0·1 kPa), whereas the small reduction in O_2 content is reflected by a large reduction in PaO_2 (15 mm

3/TABLE 3
CLASSIFICATION OF CAUSES OF "TRUE SHUNT"
(after Nunn, 1969)

	Normal	*Abnormal*
Extrapulmonary	Thebesian veins	Congenital disease of the heart or great vessels with right-to-left shunting.
Intrapulmonary	Bronchial veins Possibly some slight degree of atelectasis	Atelectasis Pulmonary infection Pulmonary arteriovenous shunts Pulmonary neoplasm including haemangioma Circulation through contused, damaged or oedematous lung.

Hg, 2·0 kPa). The arterial Po_2 is therefore the best indicator of venous admixture. Whether this is due to true shunt or to ventilation/perfusion mismatch can be determined by giving the subject 100 per cent O_2 to breathe. If there is only a relatively small increase in arterial Po_2, the hypoxaemia is likely to be due to true shunt. In the presence of a 50 per cent shunt, changes in inspired oxygen concentration have virtually no effect on arterial Po_2.

Venous admixture, which is normally up to 5 per cent of the cardiac output, may be calculated using the shunt equation and the alveolar air equation.

SHUNT EQUATION AND ALVEOLAR AIR EQUATION

The "shunt" equation can be derived as follows:—
Pulmonary capillary blood flow ($\dot{Q}c$) + blood flow through shunt ($\dot{Q}s$) = cardiac output ($\dot{Q}T$).

$$\dot{Q}c + \dot{Q}s = \dot{Q}T$$

This equation can be rewritten in terms of oxygen content:

$$(Cc'O_2 \times \dot{Q}c) + (C\bar{v}O_2 \times \dot{Q}s) = (CaO_2 \times \dot{Q}T)$$

($Cc'O_2$ is the oxygen content of pulmonary end-capillary blood; $C\bar{v}O_2$ is the oxygen content of mixed venous or pulmonary arterial blood; CaO_2 is the oxygen content of arterial blood).

Since $\dot{Q}c = \dot{Q}T - \dot{Q}s$,

$$(Cc'O_2 \times \dot{Q}T) - (Cc'O_2 \times \dot{Q}S) + (C\bar{v}O_2 \times \dot{Q}s) = (CaO_2 \times \dot{Q}T)$$

Dividing both sides by $\dot{Q}T$,

$$Cc'O_2 - \left(Cc'O_2 \times \frac{\dot{Q}s}{\dot{Q}_T}\right) + \left(C\bar{v}O_2 \times \frac{\dot{Q}s}{\dot{Q}_T}\right) = CaO_2$$

$$Cc'O_2 - CaO_2 = (Cc'O_2 - C\bar{v}O_2)\frac{\dot{Q}s}{\dot{Q}_T}$$

Therefore $\dfrac{\dot{Q}s}{\dot{Q}_T} = \dfrac{Cc'O_2 - CaO_2}{Cc'O_2 - C\bar{v}O_2}$

Of the quantities on the right-hand side of the equation, CaO_2 and $C\bar{v}O_2$ can be obtained by analysis of arterial and pulmonary arterial blood samples respectively. $Cc'O_2$ refers to the oxygen content of blood in equilibrium with "ideal" alveolar gas, which cannot be sampled since it becomes contaminated with alveolar dead-space gas. "Ideal" alveolar Po_2 can be derived using the alveolar air equation.

Nunn (1969) discusses different forms of the alveolar air equation, of which the following is the most satisfactory:

$$\text{ideal alveolar } Po_2 = Pio_2 - PaCo_2, \frac{Pio_2 - P\bar{E}o_2}{P\bar{E}Co_2}$$

For the derivation of this equation the reader is referred to West (1970) and Leigh and Tyrell (1968).

If the patient is breathing 100 per cent oxygen, then since alveolar gas contains only oxygen and carbon dioxide,

$$\text{ideal alveolar } Po_2 = Pio_2 - PaCo_2$$

The error involved in assuming that $PaCo_2$ (which can be measured) is the same as the ideal alveolar Pco_2 (which cannot be measured) is small.

Reduced partial pressure of oxygen in mixed venous blood ($P\bar{v}O_2$).—The lower the $P\bar{v}O_2$ the greater will be the effect of a given amount of venous admixture on the $Pao_2 - Pao_2$ difference. The commonest cause of a reduced $P\bar{v}O_2$, apart from arterial hypoxia, is a low cardiac output.

Considering the magnitude of the variations in ventilation/perfusion relationships within the normal upright lung, it is remarkable how efficient the lungs are at oxygenating venous blood when compared to the "ideal" lung. As mentioned above, the normal alveolar-arterial oxygen difference is only about 4 mm Hg (0·5 kPa), with a venous admixture of less than 5 per cent of the cardiac output. This is due to the shape of the oxygen dissociation curve since, for blood leaving the over- or underventilated regions of normal lungs, only the flat upper portion of the curve is involved. In blood leaving the lung bases, therefore, a Po_2 of 89 mm Hg (11·8 kPa) corresponds to a saturation of 96 per cent, not far below full saturation. Because the upper portion of the oxygen dissociation curve is almost a straight line, this small fall in saturation can be compensated for by blood leaving the overventilated regions of the lung. In these regions at the top of the lung the Po_2 in the blood is 132 mm Hg (17·6 kPa), corresponding to a saturation of nearly 100 per cent. The result is that when the two are mixed together the final Po_2 is 97 mm Hg (12·9 kPa) with a saturation of 97 per cent. However, arterial oxygenation is much less satisfactory when, for blood leaving the underventilated regions, the point of equilibration lies well down on the

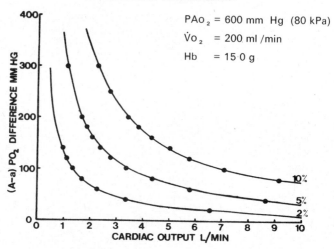

3/Fig. 4.—Graph showing the effect of venous admixture and cardiac output on the alveolar-arterial oxygen difference while breathing oxygen. As can be seen, for a given venous admixture, the alveolar-arterial oxygen difference rises steeply at low cardiac outputs. Also, a change in venous admixture causes a greater change in alveolar-arterial oxygen difference when the cardiac output is low.

steep part of the dissociation curve. Under these circumstances the slightly higher oxygen content found in the overventilated regions is now unable to compensate for the rather lower saturations in blood leaving the underventilated areas. Significant desaturation therefore occurs in the final blood mixture leaving the left ventricle. This situation occurs frequently in pathological states. For instance, if a region of atelectasis is present, in which no ventilation occurs, the blood leaving this part of the lung has an oxygen saturation equal to that in venous blood arriving at the lungs (i.e. $Po_2 = 40$ mm Hg (5·3 kPa); saturation $= 75$ per cent), as no oxygen has been added to the blood. Here we have a saturation which is considerably lower than that found in the under-ventilated areas of normal lung. The small rise in saturation in the overventilated regions is now unable to compensate for the low saturation in the blood which has passed through the atelectatic lung, and arterial desaturation inevitably follows. Clearly, compensation becomes even more difficult in the presence of a low cardiac output, when systemic venous saturation may fall to 50 per cent or less. The relation between cardiac output, venous admixture and arterial oxygenation is shown in Fig. 4. As can be seen, for a given venous admixture arterial oxygenation falls considerably at low cardiac outputs. This accounts for the very low arterial Po_2 values found in patients with cardiorespiratory failure.

SOME FACTORS AFFECTING PULMONARY FUNCTION
with special reference to anaesthesia

Advancing Age

The results obtained from almost any lung function test must be interpreted with the subject's age in mind. For the tests of ventilation increasing age is associated with a fall in maximum breathing capacity, forced expiratory volume, peak expiratory flow rate, vital capacity and total lung capacity. A progressive rise is seen in the ratios functional residual capacity/total lung volume and residual volume/total lung capacity. The physiological dead space rises, but the arterial P_{CO_2} remains constant. The alveolar-arterial oxygen difference rises, and may be as high as 25 mm Hg (3·3 kPa) in old age. The arterial P_{O_2} therefore falls progressively, and in an old person with clinically normal lungs may be as low as 75 mm Hg (10 kPa). A falling arterial P_{O_2} with advancing age is almost certainly related to a rise in the closing volume of the lungs (see p. 79). Once the closing volume becomes greater than the functional residual capacity airway closure occurs and the arterial P_{O_2} begins to fall.

Posture

Compared with the upright position, in a subject lying supine the distribution of both blood flow and ventilation becomes even from top to bottom of the lung. However, an anterior to posterior gradient now appears. In the inverted position ventilation is greater at the apex than at the base, the reverse of that found in the normal upright position.

When an anaesthetised patient, breathing spontaneously, is turned on his side, perfusion of the lowermost lung is encouraged at the expense of the upper. The proportion of the ventilation going to the lower lung is also increased because the diaphragm is able to contract more efficiently. This is due to the weight of the abdominal contents pushing the muscle higher up into the thorax and so permitting a greater range of movement on contraction. Thus, during spontaneous respiration both perfusion and ventilation of the lower lung are increased. Once the patient is paralysed and artificially ventilated, the upper lung now becomes preferentially ventilated, as its compliance is greater due partly to there being less pressure from the abdominal contents and diaphragm to be overcome, and partly because its vascular bed is less distended. If thoracotomy is now performed the amount of lung tissue which is ventilated but not perfused rises, and the fraction which is perfused but not ventilated (atelectatic shunt) also increases, but to a lesser extent (Virtue et al., 1966).

Effect of Artificial Ventilation

It is now widely accepted that anaesthesia with artificial ventilation results in an increased physiological dead space, sometimes up to 50 per cent or more of the tidal volume. This means that parts of the lungs have become relatively overventilated. The precise effects of artificial ventilation on the regional distribution of ventilation are at present uncertain although Bergman (1963) has suggested that there is no alteration from that found during spontaneous ventilation. The essential change is that the alveolar pressure is increased. It is, therefore, possible to predict some of the effects of positive pressure ventilation on the distribution of blood flow. An increase in alveolar pressure will result in an enlargement of zone 1, with the other two zones dropping down the lung. The amount of lung with a high $\dot{V}_A/\dot{Q}$ ratio is therefore greater, and an increased physiological dead space results. This effect was found by Campbell et al. (1958) who reported a rise in physiological dead space following a change from spontaneous to controlled ventilation, with no change in alveolar-arterial oxygen difference. For a further discussion of the effects of ventilation on the arterial oxygenation see the section on Anaesthesia (p. 143).

Effect of Duration of Inspiration

During intermittent positive-pressure ventilation in a normal subject the duration of inspiration is usually set at 1·0–1·5 seconds. A long inspiratory time increases mean intrathoracic pressure so reducing venous return and cardiac output. A short inspiratory time causes poor distribution of the inspired gas due to the characteristics of "fast" and "slow" alveoli (see below). The following Table summarises the advantages and disadvantages of an inspiratory time which is longer or shorter than this.

		Venous Return Cardiac Output	Distribution of Inspired Gas
Inspiratory Time	More than 1·5 sec	Bad	Good
	Less than 1·0 sec	Good	Bad

"Fast" and "Slow" Alveoli

Consider a balloon with a tube leading to it: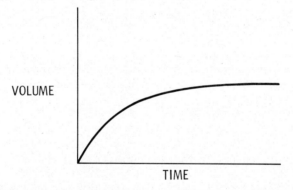

3/Fig. 5.

The inflation of the balloon in response to a given inflationary pressure is described by the exponential "wash-in" curve.

VOLUME

TIME　　　　3/Fig. 6.

If the tube leading to the balloon is narrowed the balloon will still reach the same final volume when inflated at the same pressure, but it will take longer to do so.

The compliance of the balloon wall is also of importance. If the wall has a low compliance (stiff) the balloon will reach a smaller final volume, when subjected to the same inflation pressure, and this volume will be reached after a shorter time.

The exponential curve can be described in terms of its time constant (γ) which is the time it would take for the balloon to reach its final volume if the initial gas flow rate was maintained throughout inflation ($\gamma = 1.44 \times$ the half-life). As we have seen, the time constant depends on the resistance and compliance of the system.

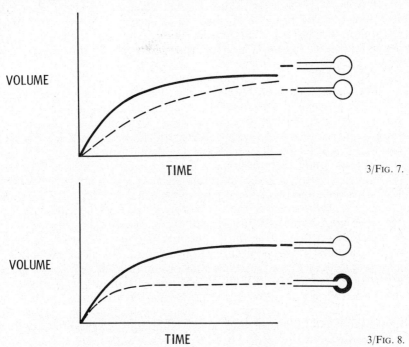

3/Fig. 7.

3/Fig. 8.

What has been said about the balloon can be applied to the lungs. Typical values for resistance (pulmonary and apparatus) and compliance for an anaesthetised patient are 1.0 kPa 1^{-1} sec (10 cm H_2O L^{-1} sec) and 0.5 l/kPa (50 ml/cmH$_2$O) respectively; the two multiplied together give the time constant:

$$\begin{array}{ccccc} \text{RESISTANCE} & \times & \text{COMPLIANCE} & = & \text{TIME CONSTANT} \\ 1.0 & \times & 0.5 & = & 0.5 \\ \text{kPa } 1^{-1} \text{ sec} & & \text{l/kPa} & & \text{sec} \end{array}$$

An increase in resistance or compliance gives rise to a longer time constant. Different parts of the lungs may have different time constants and this scatter of time constants is exaggerated in some forms of respiratory disease such as asthma and emphysema. A short inspiratory time will result in poor ventilation of those zones of lung having a long time constant and there will be a resulting increase in $\dot{V}A/\dot{Q}$ mismatch.

Effect of Total Blood Volume and its Distribution

Freeman and Nunn (1963) working with anaesthetised dogs, found an increase in physiological dead space in the presence of haemorrhage. In fact under these conditions it could be increased to nearly 80 per cent of the tidal volume. Askrog et al. (1964) found similar changes during controlled hypotension in man, especially if the patient was tipped head up. Both experimental findings can be explained by a fall in pulmonary arterial and venous pressures, in one case secondary to a fall in total blood volume, in the other because of a shift of blood from the pulmonary to the systemic circulation. From Fig. 3c it can be seen that this will result in an increase in zone 1, with the other two zones dropping down the lung. Therefore, an increase in dead space results, the amount depending on the fall in pulmonary arterial and venous pressures.

Premedication

It has been suggested (Tomlin *et al.*, 1964) that when arterial hypoxaemia is observed during and after general anaesthesia it may in part be due to the pulmonary effects of subcutaneous atropine. They found that the mean oxygen saturation in a group of patients premedicated with atropine (93·4 per cent) was significantly lower than in a second unpremedicated group (96·0 per cent). In a second study they observed a significant fall in arterial Po_2 following atropine given subcutaneously (from a mean of 95·4 mm Hg to 86·4 mm Hg, 12·7–11·5 kPa), and that post-operative hypoxaemia occurred in those patients premedicated with atropine but not in a group of unpremedicated patients. On the other hand, Nunn and Bergman (1964), in a study on conscious volunteers, observed that arterial oxygenation was unchanged in conscious subjects even after the administration of up to 2 mg of atropine intravenously. Conway (1964) has produced evidence that the route of administration may be important, hypoxaemia being most likely to appear after subcutaneous administration of the drug. Although the effect of atropine, if any, on arterial oxygenation has not yet finally been settled, there is general agreement that it increases both anatomical and physiological dead space. Nunn and Bergman (1964) found an increase in V_D/V_T ratio of 26·5 to 34·3 per cent. A similar increase in anatomical dead space has been reported by Smith *et al.* (1967) after both atropine (+ 22 per cent) and hyoscine (+ 25 per cent). The precise mechanism of this effect is not known, but it is probably related either to an action on the bronchial musculature or to an action on the lining membrane.

In 1965, Pierce and Garofalo found that arterial Po_2 was significantly lower in a group of patients awaiting open heart surgery after being given a mixture of pethidine, promethazine and pentobarbitone, although no change occurred in a second group given pentobarbitone alone. Arterial Pco_2, was unchanged in both groups. Egbert and Bendixen (1964) noted an alteration in the pattern of breathing after the administration of morphine, the main change being a large decrease in the frequency of spontaneous "sighing". They suggested that this might result in alveolar collapse, and therefore in arterial hypoxaemia. Fletcher and Barber (1966) agreed with this finding, but could detect no change in arterial Po_2, $Pa_{O_2} - Pao_2$, or in lung compliance, in spite of the absence of "sighing" after morphine for up to one and a half hours. A transient increase in compliance followed a voluntary maximum inspiration, but did not occur after spontaneous sighing. Martinez *et al.* (1967) have investigated the pulmonary effects of various premedications in patients with pulmonary or cardiovascular disease, but who were well compensated at the time. They studied the effects of intramuscular morphine (1·3 mg/10 kg), pentobarbitone (15 mg/10 kg) and atropine (0·07 mg/10 kg), morphine and hyoscine (0·07 mg/10 kg), hyoscine alone and a placebo.

Both arterial Po_2 and Pco_2 were unchanged in all groups after the drugs had been given, except for a small rise in Pao_2 after morphine alone and after pentobarbitone and atropine. The most significant finding was a fall in alveolar ventilation, ranging between 5·4 per cent and 12·7 per cent of control values, following each drug combination except the placebo. They considered that the arterial Pco_2 remained constant despite a fall in ventilation because this was accompanied by a reduction in CO_2 production. The study is remarkable for the lack of effects demonstrated. Gardiner and Palmer (1964), investigating healthy patients awaiting surgery, also found no change in arterial Po_2 or Pco_2 thirty minutes after premedication with either atropine alone or with papaveretum and hyoscine.

In spite of these studies it is well known that opiates, given in sufficient dosage, cause a reduction in alveolar ventilation and a rise in arterial Pco_2, and depress the ventilatory response to carbon dioxide (Smith *et al.*, 1967). They also cause systemic venodilatation, with a small shift of blood out of the pulmonary circulation (the likely mechanism through which they are effective in pulmonary oedema).

Anaesthesia

Although it had been suggested previously, the possibility that clinically unrecognised arterial hypoxaemia might occur during routine anaesthesia in healthy patients was first seriously considered following the publication of a paper by Bendixen and his colleagues in 1963. They reported that during anaesthesia with controlled respiration a progressive fall occurred in arterial Po_2 and total compliance, both of which could be reversed by passive hyperinflation. Pao_2 fell most rapidly in those patients who were ventilated at the lowest tidal volumes. In 1964 Bendixen *et al.* published similar findings during spontaneous respiration with ether/oxygen anaesthesia, and Egbert *et al.* (1963), measuring total compliance under a variety of anaesthetics, found that in the absence of deep breaths a fall in compliance could be demonstrated after 5 to 10 minutes, and that passive hyperinflation returned compliance to control levels. Gold and Helrich (1965) also found a decrease in lung compliance to below pre-anaesthetic levels during nitrous oxide/oxygen/halothane anaesthesia with spontaneous respiration, and noted that the decrease was related to the magnitude of the decrease in tidal volume. At this time Nunn (1964) also published a study showing abnormally high alveolar-arterial oxygen differences during anaesthesia with spontaneous respirations, and recommended an inspired oxygen concentration of at least 35 per cent to maintain normal oxygenation during surgery. In a second study, this time during controlled ventilation, Nunn *et al.* (1965) again found abnormally low arterial Po_2 values and noted that they fell progressively in their older patients. Passive hyperinflation was not always successful in reversing these changes. Slater *et al.* (1965), in a study of nitrous oxide/oxygen/curare anaesthesia, suggested that a minimum oxygen concentration of 33 per cent was necessary to maintain a Pao_2 of 80 mm Hg (10·7 kPa) or more in the majority of patients, and Sykes *et al.* (1965) found that high alveolar-arterial oxygen differences could be reduced by ventilating paralysed patients at high tidal volumes. At this time, therefore, it appeared that atelectasis, as shown by high alveolar-arterial oxygen differences and low compliance, was an

inevitable accompaniment of general anaesthesia. The atelectasis appeared to
be progressive, although Askrog and his colleagues (1964) could find no evidence
of this during either halothane, cyclopropane or nitrous oxide anaesthesia,
and in some cases it could be substantially reversed by passive hyperinflations.
However up to this time few workers had measured arterial oxygen tensions
immediately preceding the induction of anaesthesia, although many had
examined changes in Pao_2 during its course. In an investigation into the effects
of halothane and oxygen on functional residual capacity, compliance and
alveolar-arterial oxygen differences, Colgan and Whang (1968) were unable to
find any alteration from pre-operative values either during or after anaesthesia,
and stated that "progressive atelectasis was not a predictable consequence of
unassisted ventilation during anaesthesia in healthy dogs and man". However
it is evident from their figures in man that some alveolar collapse may have been
present in their patients after premedication but before the induction of anaesthesia, as they found abnormally high alveolar-arterial oxygen differences at
this time (mean $Pa_{O_2} - Pao_2 = 164$ mm Hg (21·9 kPa); mean $Pao_2 = 414$
mm Hg (55·2 kPa), breathing 100 per cent oxygen). An excellent investigation
has been reported by Marshall et al. (1969) covering the periods before, during

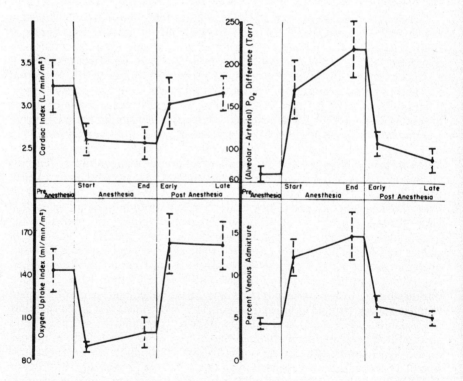

3/Fig. 9.—Changes in cardiac index, oxygen uptake, alveolar-arterial oxygen difference and
venous admixture during and after halothane/oxygen anaesthesia with spontaneous respiration.
The post-anaesthetic measurements were made 30 minutes ("early") and 3 hours ("late") after
discontinuing the halothane. Mean data from 10 patients, ± S.E.

and after halothane and oxygen anaesthesia in man. Before the induction of anaesthesia they found the following data; breathing 100 per cent oxygen, mean Pao_2 = 572 mm Hg (76·2 kPa); mean $PAo_2 - Pao_2$ = 70 mm Hg (9·3 kPa); mean shunt = 4·4 per cent of the cardiac output. Soon after induction evidence of an increase in intrapulmonary shunting had appeared (mean Pao_2 = 466 mm Hg (62·1 kPa); mean $PAo_2 - Pao_2$ = 170 mm Hg (22·7 kPa); mean shunt = 12·1 per cent) which had increased at the end of operation (mean Pao_2 = 427 mm Hg (56·9 kPa); mean $PAo_2 - Pao_2$ = 218 mm Hg (29·1 kPa); mean shunt = 14·8 per cent). These changes had all returned to pre-operative levels three hours after operation (Fig. 9).

There is no doubt that general anaesthesia is associated with the development of an intrapulmonary shunt. The actual value of this shunt is remarkably constant at about 10–15 per cent of the cardiac output with a large variety of anaesthetic agents and from investigator to investigator. It seems likely that the appearance of intrapulmonary shunting is related to the state of anaesthesia rather than to the actions of individual agents. Some workers have found little difference in venous admixture measurements made when breathing inspired oxygen concentrations of 21 per cent and 100 per cent, suggesting that ventilation/perfusion maldistribution plays little part in its aetiology (Bergman, 1967), and no changes have been reported in the distribution of either ventilation or perfusion following the induction of anaesthesia with or without controlled ventilation (Hulands et al., 1969). Low tidal volumes appear to predispose to greater shunting effects than high tidal volumes, although the ratio of inspiratory to expiratory time is not important (Lumley et al., 1969). Many workers have not found the changes to be progressive with time (Askrog et al., 1964; Sykes et al., 1965; Panday and Nunn, 1968; Lumley et al., 1969). However the volume history of the lungs immediately before taking blood for analysis is probably of great importance in determining the values found, and it is possible that during controlled ventilation small differences in techniques could explain the contradictory results of different workers.

Recent work has suggested that the reduced oxygen transfer during anaesthesia is related to changes in the functional residual capacity (FRC). There is no doubt that the FRC falls immediately after the induction of anaesthesia. This has been demonstrated by many workers, although the amount of the fall has been variously measured at between about 15 and 30 per cent of the control FRC. The fall occurs with both spontaneous (Hewlett et al., 1974a) and controlled ventilation (Hewlett et al., 1974b). It appears to be a constant accompaniment to anaesthesia although the exact mechanism of the change has not yet been worked out. The extent of the fall can be correlated with a drop in arterial Po_2 and rise in alveolar-arterial oxygen difference (Hickey et al., 1973), and provides a ready explanation for the changes discussed above. As the FRC falls so airway closure may occur resulting in the appearance of an area of relatively underventilated lung in its most dependant parts. The alveolar-arterial oxygen difference will then rise. The severity of the extent of alveolar underventilation will depend on the closing volume, the amount of fall in the FRC, the position of the patient and the mixed venous oxygen content. Another important contributary factor may be that, due to the effects of anaesthesia, pulmonary vasoconstriction in those vessels supplying the affected portions of lung does not occur, and the natural compensation for alveolar hypoxia is reduced or abolished (see p. 128). A sequence of events can thus be suggested:

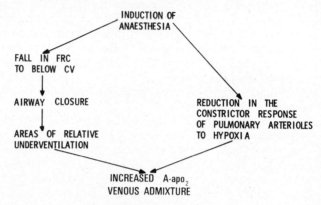

One incontrovertible fact arises out of these experiments, namely that during general anaesthesia the transport of oxygen through the lungs is often impaired, and that to ensure adequate arterial oxygenation during an anaesthetic at least 33 per cent oxygen should be administered in the inspired gas mixture.

The Ventilation/Perfusion Ratio and Carbon Dioxide Excretion

As well as affecting oxygen transfer within the lungs, anaesthesia also impairs the efficiency of carbon dioxide excretion. The most important adverse effect is due to a reduction in alveolar ventilation, brought about by (1) direct depression of the respiratory centres; (2) decreased ventilatory response to a rise in arterial Pco_2; (3) the addition of apparatus dead space; and (4) an increase in physiological dead space. Another factor which has to be taken into account is that the alveolar-arterial CO_2 difference (normal = less than 1 mm Hg, 0·1 kPa) rises during anaesthesia. Nunn and Hill (1960) found an average value of 4·5 mm Hg (0·6 kPa) during spontaneous respiration, and 4·7 mm Hg (0·6 kPa) during controlled ventilation. It has been suggested that these findings might be secondary to a fall in pulmonary artery pressure.

Post-operative Hypoxaemia

Although it has been known for many years that arterial hypoxaemia occurs after major thoracic and abdominal surgery, it has also been shown to be present after much simpler procedures. Nunn and Payne (1962) have reported a fall in arterial oxygen tension for as long as 12–24 hours following operation. The hypoxaemia is readily correctible by administering a modest concentration of oxygen (Conway and Payne, 1963).

The mechanism of post-operative hypoxaemia may be the same as that during general anaesthesia, namely that the FRC falls below the closing volume of the lungs.

Discussion

When an anaesthetised patient breathes 20 per cent oxygen and 80 per cent nitrous oxide the effects of maldistribution are sufficient to reduce the oxygen tension of the arterial blood. Fortunately, the shape of the oxygen dissociation curve for blood is so arranged that despite a significant drop in tension the saturation level is minimally affected. However, the tension may fall to a level where a further small reduction would lead to a dangerous drop in saturation.

These facts can best be emphasised by referring to the analogy of the child playing on a cliff top (Fig. 10). The sea, the cliff face and the grass field on top represent the oxygen dissociation curve. The conscious subject breathing air (21 per cent oxygen) is represented by the child at point A. It will be observed

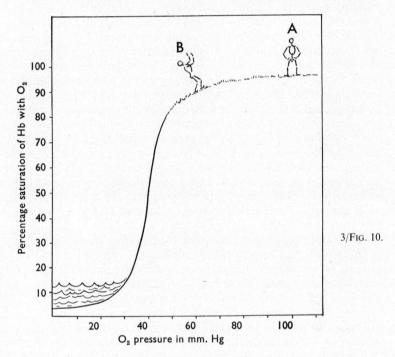

3/Fig. 10.

that fairly wide movements to the right or left will lead to only a very small change in oxygen saturation. The anaesthetised patient, or those in the immediate post-operative period under analgesic drugs, are quite different. Now the child has moved to point B. Any movement to the left (as, for example, with atelectasis or mild respiratory obstruction) can lead to a perilous descent towards desaturation. If, however, such patients are given extra oxygen, they are rapidly transported to the safety zone (point A) enjoyed by the conscious subject.

It is recommended, therefore, that at least *33 per cent* oxygen should be the *minimum* inspired concentration for the anaesthetised patient breathing spontaneously and also that a periodic hyperinflation should be used to simulate the "sigh" of the conscious subject. This work also underlines the value of oxygen therapy in the post-operative period, although in most instances good physiotherapy with encouragement of deep breathing is sufficient.

A simple assessment of respiratory function must always be made before operation and anaesthesia. Observation of the patient at rest and at light exercise, such as walking in the ward, together with a clinical examination, are likely to prove just as satisfactory as more complicated tests in the majority of cases. The breath-holding test of Sebrasez is a useful but rough method for estimating cardiorespiratory reserve. It consists of taking a maximum inspiration while at rest and then holding the breath for as long as possible. Failure to hold the breath for more than 25 seconds is abnormal.

Properly chosen and adequately given anaesthesia need not necessarily hamper respiratory function during the time of its administration if a mixture containing at least 33 per cent oxygen is breathed. Assisted or controlled respiration will compensate for most types of decreased ventilatory capacity, though there are occasions when even intermittent positive-pressure may be better avoided, e.g. cases of obstructive emphysema. The general reduction of metabolism and rest associated with a carefully chosen anaesthetic is a therapeutic factor of importance. In the immediate post-operative period and for some time after, however, unaided respiratory function must be sufficient to maintain a normal oxygen and carbon dioxide tension in the blood. Pain, the central respiratory effects of depressant doses of opiates and post-operative lung complications all tend in differing ways to reduce respiratory function; furthermore, the results of surgery on the lungs, and of post-operative complications in them, may be decisive factors leading to decompensation. It is the ability of the patient to withstand the immediate post-anaesthetic period as well as the period of operation that anaesthetists ought to try to assess pre-operatively.

Dyspnoea is the most obvious clinical symptom and sign of this incapacity; it is an index of the relation between ventilatory capacity and ventilatory volume. Subjects with a normal capacity may show dyspnoea on heavy exercise. In the presence of lung disease, however, the capacity is limited and a slight increase in ventilatory volume leads to difficulty in breathing. It is because so many thoracic operations are considered against a background of disease in the lungs that specialised tests may have to be carried out to determine the function of that portion which will remain.

The value of these tests to the anaesthetist is very limited, and it is doubtful whether, at the moment, they offer much more information in cases of disease than can be obtained by simple observation of the patient's dyspnoea and cyanosis. In so far as the special tests substantiate clinical investigation they may be helpful in the choice of practical anaesthesia. Thus emphysema or bronchial spasm may necessitate special techniques or special treatment. One of the difficulties in assessing the results of the tests is the differentiation between normal and abnormal, and in deciding from the results of respiratory function tests what the chances are of post-operative complications. Nevertheless, they do enable an objective assessment to be made of the severity of dyspnoea, and hence of true impairment of ventilatory function. This may be of value not only in evaluating the results of surgical treatment, but also in preparing patients for operation when the results of treatment could with advantage be measured and compared with previous figures. Broncho-spirometry, despite its many disadvantages, may occasionally give valuable information concerning the adequacy of the lung which is to be left after pneumonectomy.

The geriatric patient who is physically handicapped by pulmonary disease is increasingly frequently submitted to surgery and therefore to anaesthesia.

Although gross in its practical implications, the basic advantages of properly chosen and administered anaesthesia, and the relative tolerance to it of even diseased patients, enables most operations to be performed with a limited mortality and morbidity. If, however, any improvement is to be made on the present best, and the occasional patient is to be saved from a major complication, objective measurements of the pulmonary state of patients of this type before, during and after operation and anaesthetic, and following pre-operative treatment, must be carried out. Only by such means can progress eventually be made towards a reasoned pre-operative assessment of what a patient can be expected to tolerate during and after an operation.

Pre-operative Assessment and Lung Function

Milledge and Nunn (1975) studied the criteria of fitness for anaesthesia in patients with chronic lung disease. They concluded that the forced expiratory volume in one second (FEV_1) was a useful pre-operative screening test. If the values of FEV_1 fell below 1 litre then it was advisable to supplement this information with blood gas studies. The combination of these results enabled an anaesthetist to predict the post-anaesthetic course. Thus:—

Group I FEV_1 less than 1 litre
               + Normal $PaCO_2$ and PaO_2
                . . . . . normal post-operative course
Group II FEV_1 less than 1 litre
               + Normal $PaCO_2$ and low PaO_2
                . . . . . require prolonged use of oxygen therapy
Group III FEV_1 less than 1 litre
               + *high* $PaCO_2$ and *low* PaO_2
                . . . . . require ventilatory support

THE TRANSPORT OF GASES IN THE BLOOD

OXYGEN

In alveolar air the tension of oxygen is 100 mm Hg (13·3 kPa), whereas it is only 40 mm Hg (5·3 kPa) in the venous blood entering the pulmonary capillaries. This pressure gradient is sufficient to induce oxygen to pass rapidly across the alveolar membrane. On reaching the blood stream the oxygen becomes dissolved in the plasma before finally uniting with haemoglobin for its carriage to the tissues.

Simple solution of oxygen in the plasma.—Only a very small proportion of the total oxygen carried in the arterial blood—namely, 0·3 ml per 100 ml of blood (0·3 volumes per cent)—is physically dissolved in the plasma. Nevertheless this small quantity is of vital importance for it alone reflects the tension of oxygen in the blood (Po_2) and also acts as a pathway for the supply of oxygen to haemoglobin. When the blood reaches the tissues it is this small quantity that is first transferred to the cells, while its place is rapidly taken by more oxygen liberated from haemoglobin.

Haemoglobin.—Haemoglobin consists of the protein "globin" joined with the pigment "haem", which is an iron-containing porphyrin. The porphyrin nucleus consists of four pyrrol rings joined together by four methine bridges. The iron is in the ferrous (Fe^{++}) form and is attached to the N of each pyrrol ring and to the N of the imidazol group in the globin, thus creating a loose "bond" available for union with oxygen to form oxyhaemoglobin. The globin is made up of 4 amino acid chains. There are 2 α chains each containing 141 amino acids and 2 β chains each containing 146 amino acids. Other chains having different amino acid sequences also occur.

HbA	2α	2β	—	adult haemoglobin
HbF	2α	2γ	—	fetal haemoglobin
HbA$_2$	2α	2γ	—	accounts for 2 per cent of total haemoglobin in normal adults.

In sickle-cell anaemia (p. 718) the β chains are abnormal whereas in thalassaemia there is deficient production of either α or β chains.

Methaemoglobin consists of haemoglobin in which the iron is present in the ferric (Fe^{+++}) rather than ferrous (Fe^{++}) form, and is unable to combine with oxygen. Methaemoglobinaemia may occur

(a) because of inadequate conversion of methaemoglobin (which is normally present in small amounts) to haemoglobin—hereditary methaemoglobinaemia, or

(b) because of excessive production of methaemoglobin as occurs in poisoning by higher oxides of nitrogen—toxic or acquired methaemoglobinaemia. Conversion of methaemoglobin to haemoglobin can be hastened by reducing agents such as ascorbic acid or methylene blue.

Oxyhaemoglobin

The reaction of haemoglobin with oxygen occurs in four stages; the rate at which the final stage takes place is much higher than the rate of the other stages and so counteracts the slowing down of the rate of reaction of haemoglobin with oxygen which would be expected, on the basis of the law of mass action, as saturation nears completion (Staub *et al.*, 1961).

$$Hb + O_2 \qquad\qquad HbO_2$$
$$\text{Reduced Haemoglobin} \quad \rightleftharpoons \quad \text{Oxyhaemoglobin}$$

The union of oxygen and haemoglobin is broken as easily as it is formed. In arterial blood the Po_2 is 100 mm Hg (13·3 kPa) and consequently haemoglobin is almost completely in its oxygenated form. In the tissues, the blood Po_2 drops to 40 mm Hg (5·3 kPa) and the haemoglobin is now forced to give up some of the oxygen it is holding.

In males the average haemoglobin content of blood is 15·8 g per 100 ml of blood; in females it is 13·7 g. The average for both sexes is 14·5 g. One gram of haemoglobin when fully saturated can combine with 1·39 ml of oxygen; thus theoretically 100 ml of blood should carry about 20 ml of oxygen. Complete equilibration between the alveolar and arterial tension is never reached, so that arterial blood under normal conditions is seldom more than 95 per cent saturated, with an oxygen tension of 100 mm Hg (13·3 kPa). Thus the 15 g of haemoglobin present in 100 ml of blood can carry approximately 19 ml of oxygen. It will be seen, therefore, that every 100 ml of blood passing through the lungs takes up 5 ml of oxygen [19 ml (arterial) − 14 ml (venous) = 5 ml].

Equally, the tissues remove 5 ml per cent or about one-third to one-quarter of the available total (Table 4).

3/TABLE 4

Oxygen	Mixed Venous	Arterial
1. Amount in solution in plasma	0·13 ml per cent	0·3 ml per cent
2. Tension	40 mm Hg (5·3 kPa)	100 mm Hg (13·3 kPa)
3. Amount combined with haemo-globin (oxyhaemoglobin)	14 ml per cent	19 ml per cent
4. Saturation	75 per cent	98 per cent

Oxygen Flux

The amount of oxygen leaving the left ventricle per minute in the arterial blood has been termed the "oxygen flux" (Nunn, 1969). Ignoring the very small amount of oxygen in physical solution,

$$\frac{\text{Oxygen}}{\text{flux}} = \frac{\text{cardiac}}{\text{output}} \times \frac{\text{arterial}}{\text{oxygen}} \times \frac{\text{haemoglobin}}{\text{concentration}} \times 1\cdot39$$
$$\text{saturation}$$
$$= 5000 \text{ ml/min} \times \frac{98}{100} \times \frac{14\cdot7}{100} \text{ g/ml} \times 1\cdot31 \text{ ml/g}$$
$$= 1000 \text{ ml/min} \hspace{2cm} \text{(Gregory, 1974)}$$

where 1·39 is the volume of oxygen (ml) which combines with 1 g of haemoglobin. Normally about 250 ml of this oxygen is used up in cellular metabolism and the rest returns to the lungs in the mixed venous blood which is therefore about 75 per cent saturated with oxygen. Because the three variables in the equation (cardiac output, arterial oxygen saturation and haemoglobin concentration) are multiplied together, a relatively trivial reduction of each may result in a catastrophic reduction in oxygen flux; in addition the oxygen consumption may be increased above 250 ml/min for example in the post-operative patient suffering from "halothane shakes".

Oxygen Dissociation Curve

The amount of any gas which is taken up by plasma or blood varies according to the tension of the gas to which it is exposed. Taking oxygen as an example, the amount that is dissolved in plasma is directly proportional to the partial pressure even though this may be greater than that of the atmosphere i.e. there is a linear relationship. On the other hand, the iron in the haemoglobin molecule has a remarkable property of combining with oxygen to form oxyhaemoglobin. Whole blood (at body temperature and with a normal carbon dioxide content) has the familiar S-shaped dissociation curve (Fig. 11).

This type of curve is beautifully designed for the uptake of oxygen in the lungs and its release in the tissues. During oxygen loading of haemoglobin in the

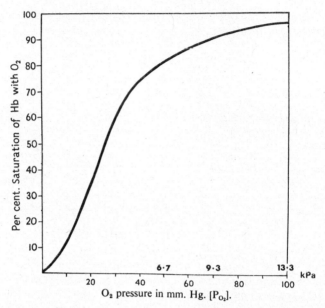

3/Fig. 11.—Oxygen dissociation curve of human blood (50 mm Hg = 6·7 kPa; 70 mm Hg = 9·3 kPa; 100 mm Hg = 13·3 kPa).

lungs variations in the Po_2 of blood leaving different portions of the lung have little effect on the oxygen content of the arterial blood because it is the flat upper part of the curve which is involved. For example, blood leaving alveoli with a Po_2 of 100 mm Hg (13·3 kPa) will be 98 per cent saturated, whereas blood leaving alveoli at a Po_2 of 70 mm Hg (9·3 kPa) will still be 91 per cent saturated, a drop of only 7 per cent. For unloading of oxygen, when the Po_2 falls below about 50 mm Hg (6·7 kPa) there is rapid release of oxygen from the haemoglobin so that at capillary Po_2 tensions oxygen is very readily available.

Other molecules as well as oxygen are carried by haemoglobin and these influence the exact position of the dissociation curve. The most important of these are carbon dioxide, hydrogen ions and 2,3 diphosphoglycerate (2,3 DPG), all associated with globin, and carbon monoxide which takes the place of oxygen on the haem radical. These molecules influence the position of the dissociation curve as follows.

(a) *Hydrogen ion* (Bohr effect).—Acidaemia shifts the curve to the right and alkalaemia to the left.

(b) *Carbon dioxide tension.*—A rise in carbon dioxide tension tends to shift the curve to the right, and vice versa. In the tissues the carbon dioxide tension is high, so that the haemoglobin can more readily give up its oxygen, whereas in the pulmonary capillary blood the carbon dioxide tension falls and therefore the oxygen dissociation curve is shifted to the left and the uptake of oxygen is aided. Carbon dioxide acts both by altering the H^+ ion concentration of the solution and also by the formation of carbaminohaemoglobin.

(c) *2,3 Diphosphoglycerate (2,3 DPG).*—Recently the importance of 2,3 DPG on oxygen uptake and release by haemoglobin has been highlighted

(Thomas *et al.*, 1974). The position of the dissociation curve is related to the concentration of 2,3 DPG within the red cell. This substance combines with globin and modifies oxygen access to the haem chain, a rise in 2,3 DPG being associated with a reduction in the affinity of haemoglobin for oxygen. Therefore a high concentration of 2,3 DPG shifts the curve to the right, and a low concentration shifts it to the left. Examples of factors influencing the 2,3 DPG level in the red cell are all types of chronic hypoxia, which raises the level, and storage of blood which lowers it. (See also p. 709.)

(*d*) *Temperature.*—A fall in temperature shifts the curve to the left. There is no evidence, however, that the tissues suffer hypoxia because there is a co-incidental fall in oxygen demand.

(*e*) *Anaesthetic drugs.*—There is evidence which suggests that halothane, and some other agents, may shift the curve to the right by a small amount.

(*f*) *Storage of blood.*—In ACD blood there is a rapid fall-off in the concentration of 2,3 DPG in the red cells and the dissociation curve shifts to the left so that recently transfused blood is reluctant to give up oxygen to the tissues. This change becomes significant almost immediately the blood is taken and may take 2–3 days to recover after infusion. The use of citrate-phosphate-dextrose (CPD) as the anticoagulant in stored blood delays the fall in 2,3 DPG for about ten days, at which time the 2,3 DPG level is still near to normal in CPD blood, but in ACD blood has been reduced to about 30 per cent of normal. After two weeks of storage the 2,3 DPG level is virtually zero in ACD blood, and even in CPD blood falls off rapidly during the following week.

Significance of Shifts in the Oxygen Dissociation Curve

Shifts in the dissociation curve of haemoglobin are usually presented as changes in the P_{50} value, defined as the Po_2 at which haemoglobin is 50 per cent saturated. The normal value for the P_{50} is 27·5 mm Hg (3·7 kPa). A shift to the left lowers the P_{50} and a shift to the right raises it. Changes in P_{50} have only a modest effect on the uptake of oxygen in the lungs, the main consequence of alterations being on the release of oxygen to the tissues. A low P_{50} decreases oxygen availability to the tissues and may therefore lead to cellular hypoxia. The importance of these changes in clinical practice have yet to be determined, but they may be crucial to survival of the patient following massive blood transfusion.

CARBON DIOXIDE

The tissues produce carbon dioxide and this is then given up to the blood circulating through the capillaries. It rapidly enters the plasma and then passes into the red cells. On reaching the pulmonary capillaries the tension of carbon dioxide (Pco_2) in the venous blood is 46 mm Hg (6·1 kPa); in the alveoli the tension is 40 mm Hg (5·5 kPa). There is, therefore, a pressure gradient of 6 mm Hg (0·8 kPa) driving carbon dioxide across the alveolar membrane. In normal circumstances each 100 ml of arterial blood carries 50 ml of carbon dioxide.

Carbon dioxide is distributed in the blood in the following manner:

(*a*) *In solution in the plasma.*—Only a small yet very important proportion of the total carbon dioxide (i.e 6 per cent) is carried in this manner. As with oxygen, this quantity is responsible for determining the tension of the gas in blood and also acts as the intermediary between the air in the alveoli and the inside of the red cell. The majority of the carbon dioxide is present in physical solution in the plasma, but a small proportion is combined with water to form carbonic acid—H_2CO_3.

(b) *As bicarbonate* (70 per cent).—Except for the small proportion that is physically dissolved in the plasma, most of the carbon dioxide passes to the red cells where the enzyme *carbonic anhydrase* aids its rapid union with water to form carbonic acid (H_2CO_3) (Fig. 12). This enzyme is not found in the plasma, and is destroyed both by heat and cyanide.

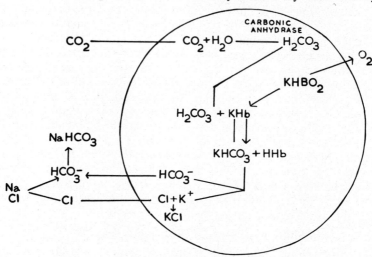

3/Fig. 12.—Chloride shift.

Normally carbon dioxide combines with water very slowly, but in the presence of carbonic anhydrase the whole process is greatly speeded up. Similarly, this enzyme has the remarkable property of accelerating the same process in the reverse direction when the pulmonary capillaries are reached. Recent studies have revealed that premature babies, neonates and young infants have a very low level of carbonic anhydrase enzyme activity. They, therefore, are particularly dependent on adequate ventilation for the elimination of carbon dioxide (Boutros and Woodford, 1963).

The role of carbonic anhydrase and haemoglobin is depicted in Fig. 12. The key to the whole process is the liberation of oxygen, thus:

$$Hb\,O_2 \longrightarrow Hb + O_2$$

Carbon dioxide diffuses into the red cell where in the presence of carbonic anhydrase it combines with water to form carbonic acid which dissociates into hydrogen ions and bicarbonate ions:

$$\text{carbonic anhydrase}$$
$$CO_2 + H_2O \rightleftharpoons H_2CO_3 \rightleftharpoons H^+ + HCO_3^-$$

This formation of bicarbonate cannot take place to such an extent in the plasma due to the absence of carbonic anhydrase. Deoxygenated haemoglobin combines with the hydrogen ions

$$Hb + H^+ \longrightarrow HHb$$

so favouring the formation of HCO_3^- by displacing the equilibrium of the bicarbonate-forming equation (above) to the right according to the law of mass action. The bicarbonate diffuses out of the red cell into the plasma, and, so that ionic equilibrium is maintained, chloride ions (Cl^-) diffuse in the opposite direction from plasma into the red cells. This is called the chloride shift or Hamburger phenomenon (Fig. 12).

When the blood reaches the capillaries of the lung there is a pressure difference of $46 - 40 = 6$ mm Hg ($6 \cdot 1 - 5 \cdot 3 = 0 \cdot 8$ kPa) of carbon dioxide on either side of the alveolar membrane, and as it diffuses across this barrier very rapidly this is quite sufficient to ensure an adequate interchange of gases. The process is the reverse of that already described for the uptake of carbon dioxide. First the small percentage physically dissolved in the plasma falls, then as the pressure gradient of dissolved carbon dioxide between the red cell and the plasma widens, so the carbon dioxide leaves the red cell and allows bicarbonate ions to enter. Thus the sodium bicarbonate in the plasma splits again so that the bicarbonate can pass back into the red cell and chloride ions move out into the plasma again. Following the formation of carbonic acid the enzyme carbonic anhydrase aids the breakdown to carbon dioxide and water so that finally carbon dioxide passes out into the plasma and from thence across the alveolar membrane.

Plasma bicarbonate, therefore, plays a very important role as the principal storehouse and carrier of carbon dioxide in the blood.

(c) *As a carbamino compound* (24 per cent).—Carbon dioxide can combine with the amino groupings of the haemoglobin to form carbamino-haemoglobin:

$$Hb.NH_2 + CO_2 \leftrightarrows Hb.NH.COOH$$

A smaller amount combines in a similar manner with the plasma proteins. The combination takes place directly between the carbon dioxide and the haemoglobin or plasma protein, as no enzyme—such as carbonic anhydrase—is required. The amount formed is influenced mainly by the degree of oxygen saturation of the blood and not by the carbon dioxide tension.

Christian and Greene (1962) have demonstrated that both ether and thiopentone-nitrous oxide-oxygen anaesthesia decrease the activity of carbonic anhydrase in blood, whereas cyclopropane is without effect.

Carbon Dioxide Dissociation Curve

The carbon dioxide dissociation curve relates the carbon dioxide content of blood to the P_{CO_2} to which it is exposed (Fig. 13). The position of this curve depends upon the degree of oxygenation of the blood. The more deoxygenated the blood becomes the more carbon dioxide it carries at a given P_{CO_2}: this is called the *Haldane effect*. In Fig. 13 curve B is the CO_2 content/P_{CO_2} curve for

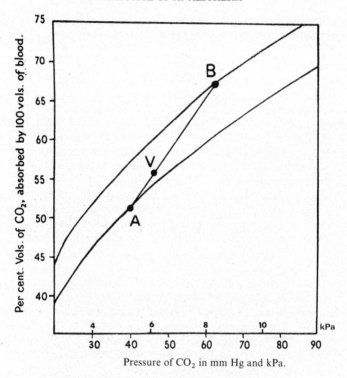

3/Fig. 13.—Carbon Dioxide Dissociation Curve.
Upper line = Fully reduced human blood.
Lower line = Fully oxygenated human blood.
A = volume and tension of CO_2 in arterial blood.
V = volume and tension of CO_2 in venous blood.
B = Conditions in fully reduced blood.

Line AV is the dissociation of CO_2 in human blood. A rise in the respiratory quotient moves it to the right. A fall in the respiratory quotient moves it to the left.

fully deoxygenated blood and curve A is for fully oxygenated or arterial blood. Note that the arterial and venous points, point B, and that part of the curve for fully oxygenated blood below A, approximate to a straight line. It is for this reason that blood from zones of lung with high $\dot{V}A/\dot{Q}$ ratios can compensate for blood from zones with low $\dot{V}A/\dot{Q}$ ratios (p. 134). The major component of the Haldane effect is the increased carriage of CO_2 by reduced haemoglobin as carbamino haemoglobin. In addition, CO_2 carriage as bicarbonate is increased.

$$CO_2 + H_2O \rightleftharpoons H_2CO_3 \rightleftharpoons HCO_3^- + H^+$$

Reduced haemoglobin buffers the hydrogen ions, so displacing the equilibrium of this equation to the right and increasing the concentration of bicarbonate (HCO_3^-).

Due to the Haldane effect, the uptake of CO_2 by capillary blood is facilitated. When this blood reaches the lungs and becomes oxygenated elimination of CO_2 is facilitated.

THE ACID-BASE STATUS OF THE BLOOD

Life is an acidogenic process and from birth until death the body is under a constant obligation to balance hydrogen ion output against hydrogen ion intake; the diet normally contains hydrogen ions, mostly in the form of sulphur-containing amino acids of proteins, and the urine is the sole channel of hydrogen ion excretion. The average intake is 50–80 mEq/day (mmol/day)—much the same as sodium and potassium: the important difference, which has tended to obscure the precisely adjusted external balance of hydrogen ions, is that intermediate metabolism can give rise to relatively enormous hydrogen ion loads. Such release of hydrogen ions is normally followed by rapid neutralisation before excretion and therefore has no net effect on hydrogen ion balance. Certain circumstances, of which tissue hypoxia is the commonest, give rise to acidosis because the stage of hydrogen ion production outstrips the stage of hydrogen ion neutralisation and the various buffer systems in the cells and extracellular fluid are the body's only means of defence against such accumulations. The acute buffer storage capacity is capable of absorbing up to 10 mEq (mmol) of hydrogen ions per kg body weight, i.e. 500–700 in an adult, or nearly ten times the average daily intake. If hydrogen ion intake ceases, hydrogen ion production continues as is made evident by the gradually progressive acidosis which develops in anuric patients. It is of practical importance that hydrogen ion concentration does not reach lethal levels for 7–10 days or even longer. During this time the hydrogen ions produced by metabolism are absorbed by the various buffer systems in the cells and extracellular fluid. Renal control of hydrogen ion output is slow to develop and several days are needed for urinary excretion of hydrogen ions to increase from average to maximal amounts: the kidneys make no significant contribution to the control of sudden fluxes in hydrogen ion concentration. Tissue hypoxia, starvation and diminished ventilatory reserve are accompaniments of many surgical operations: all will tend to strain the buffer capacity of the body and it is therefore important that patients are brought to surgery with the least possible encroachment of their capacity to deal with acute rises in hydrogen ion concentration. For this among other reasons diabetes, heart failure and uraemia should all be brought under control as far as is practicable before operation. The contribution of haemoglobin to the buffer capacity of blood is considerable and tends to be overlooked on account of its more obvious importance to oxygen carriage.

Terminology

The relationship between acids and bases can be described by the following equation:

$$\text{Acid} \rightleftarrows H^+ + \text{Base}^-$$

An acid is a hydrogen ion donor. A strong acid is almost completely dissociated when in an aqueous solution. A weak acid is less completely dissociated. *A base* is a hydrogen ion acceptor. A strong base is one for which the above equilibrium is displaced almost completely to the left, and a weak base is one for which it is displaced only partly to the left. *Buffers* are substances which by their presence in solution increase the amount of acid or alkali which must be added to cause a unit shift in pH. The combination in solution of a weak acid and its strong base (as a salt) is called a *buffer pair*. The weak acid is the *buffer acid* and the strong base is the *buffer base*. A buffer system obeys the Law of Mass Action, so that

$$K [Acid] = [H^+] \times [Base^-]$$

where K is a constant. Rearranging this formula

$$[H^+] = K \frac{[Acid]}{[Base^-]}$$

and converting to negative logarithms to the base 10, this equation becomes:

$$pH = pK' + \log \frac{[Base^-]}{[Acid]}$$

For the bicarbonate buffer system the equation becomes:

$$pH = pK' + \log \frac{[HCO_3^-]}{[H_2CO_3]}$$

This is the Henderson-Hasselbalch equation. $[HCO_3^-]$ represents the plasma bicarbonate, and $[H_2CO_3]$ represents the sum of the dissolved carbon dioxide and carbonic acid, according to the equation

$$CO_2 + H_2O \rightleftharpoons H_2CO_3$$

For plasma at 38° C, $pK' = 6 \cdot 1$ (the dissociation constant). Numerous graphic representations of the Henderson-Hasselbalch equation have been suggested, the best known being the pH-bicarbonate plot (Davenport, 1958), and the pH-log P_{CO_2} plot (Siggaard-Andersen, 1966).

The acidity of a solution depends on the concentration of hydrogen ions contained in it, and is most often expressed in pH units. pH is the negative logarithm of the molar hydrogen ion concentration (or, more correctly, the hydrogen ion activity). The normal pH of whole blood is 7·4 units, equivalent to a hydrogen ion concentration of 40 nano-equivalents/litre (nmol/l). A nano-equivalent is an equivalent $\times 10^{-9}$, or one millionth of a milli-equivalent. The relationship between pH and the hydrogen ion concentration is shown in Table 5.

3/TABLE 5
EQUIVALENT VALUES OF PH AND
HYDROGEN ION CONCENTRATION

$[H^+]$ nano Eq/l (nmol/l)	pH
100	7·0
63	7·2
40	7·4
25	7·6
16	7·8
10	8·0

The Pco_2 of a gas mixture saturated with water vapour at $37°$ C is given by the equation:

$$Pco_2 = Fco_2 \times (PB - 47) \text{ mm Hg } [Fco_2 \times (PB - 6.3) \text{ kPa}]$$

where Fco_2 is the fractional concentration of carbon dioxide in the mixture, PB is the barometric pressure (760 mm Hg, 101 kPa), and 47 mm Hg (6.3 kPa) is the saturated vapour pressure of water at $37°$ C. The Pco_2 of a solution of carbon dioxide in a liquid such as plasma is best understood by considering a gas-liquid system in equilibrium. The carbon dioxide tension of the liquid phase is equal to that in the gas phase when no net exchange of CO_2 occurs between the two phases. At any given equilibrium the carbon dioxide content of the liquid is a reflection of the Pco_2 of the gas phase, and therefore the CO_2 content of the liquid can be described by stating the Pco_2 of the gas phase. The Pco_2 of blood is thus defined as that Pco_2 in a gas mixture which, when in contact with the blood, results in no net exchange of CO_2 between the two phases.

An *acidosis* is said to be present when the hydrogen ion concentration in blood is higher than normal (low pH), or would be if no compensation had occurred. An *alkalosis* is present when the hydrogen ion concentration is lower than normal (high pH), or would be if compensation had not occurred. These definitions enable combinations of changes to be described, e.g. a respiratory acidosis and a metabolic alkalosis present at the same time, although the pH may lie within the normal range. A *respiratory acidosis* or *alkalosis* is a change, or potential change, in pH resulting from alterations in the Pco_2. A *metabolic acidosis* or *alkalosis* is a change, or potential change, in pH resulting from alterations in the non-volatile acids in the blood, e.g. lactic acid.

Buffer base is the sum of the buffer anions in the blood. It includes bicarbonate, haemoglobin, proteins and phosphates, and therefore alters with changes in the haemoglobin. The *total* buffer base does not alter with respiratory changes in the blood, but does alter as a result of non-respiratory (metabolic) changes. The total buffer base can therefore be used to quantitate a metabolic acidosis or alkalosis. Instead of measuring total buffer base, which is difficult, metabolic factors can be described in terms of the change in buffer base from its normal value. This change is termed the *base excess*, and is defined as the amount of titratable base on titration to normal pH at normal Pco_2 and temperature (i.e. to pH = 7.4, at Pco_2 = 40 mm Hg, [5.3 kPa,] and $38°$ C). A positive value for the base excess indicates a metabolic alkalosis, and a negative value a metabolic acidosis (sometimes termed a *base deficit*). The base excess as read from Astrup charts is independent of the haemoglobin level. *Standard bicarbonate* is the plasma bicarbonate concentration of fully oxygenated blood at $38°$ C when the Pco_2 has been adjusted to 40 mm Hg (5.3 kPa). By adjusting the Pco_2 to 40 mm Hg (5.3 kPa), alterations in the plasma bicarbonate in whole blood secondary to changes in Pco_2 disappear, and the standard bicarbonate, like base excess, therefore describes metabolic acid-base changes.

The normal values and changes found in the blood resulting from uncompensated alterations in acid-base status are shown in Table 6.

Buffering Systems in the Body
About three-quarters of the chemical buffering power in the body lies within

3/TABLE 6

THE NORMAL VALUES AND CHANGES FOUND IN THE BLOOD RESULTING FROM UNCOMPENSATED CHANGES IN ACID-BASE STATUS

	pH	P_{CO_2}	Plasma bicarbonate	Total buffer base	Base excess	Standard bicarbonate
Normal values	7·35–7·44	36–46 mm Hg (4·8–6·1 kPa)	23–28 mEq/litre (m mol/l)	44–48 mEq/litre (m mol/l)	0 ± 3 mEq/litre (m mol/l)	22–26 mEq/litre (m mol/l)
Respiratory acidosis	Low	High	High	Normal	Normal	Normal
Respiratory alkalosis	High	Low	Low	Normal	Normal	Normal
Metabolic acidosis	Low	Normal	Low	Low	Negative	Low
Metabolic alkalosis	High	Normal	High	High	Positive	High

the cells, and is due to the high concentration of intracellular proteins, phosphate and other inorganic compounds. The remainder is due to the buffering power of the extracellular fluids. The buffering power of a system depends on the pH at which it is working and on the concentrations of the buffer elements.

The bicarbonate buffer system.—As previously explained this system consists of a mixture of H_2CO_3 (the weak acid) and $NaHCO_3$ (the strong base). The relationship between their concentrations and the pH is described by the Henderson-Hasselbalch equation:

$$pH = pK' + \log \frac{[HCO_3{}^-]}{[H_2CO_3]}$$

so that the pH is determined by the ratio $\frac{[HCO_3{}^-]}{[H_2CO_3]}$. In Fig. 14 the relation between the relative concentrations of the two and the pH is shown. This S-shaped curve is typical of many buffers. The following points should be noted: (1) The buffering power of the system is greatest when the slope of the curve is steepest so that, for the addition of a given amount of acid or base the smallest change in pH occurs around this part of the curve. (2) The buffer system is most efficient when the concentrations of $HCO_3{}^-$ and H_2CO_3 are equal, or when

$pH = pK$ (under these conditions $\log \frac{[HCO_3{}^-]}{[H_2CO_3]} = O$). Once the relative con-

centrations of bicarbonate and carbonic acid exceed about 8:1 in either direction the buffering power of the system falls off rapidly. Normally the system functions at a pH of around 7·4, when the ratio of bicarbonate to carbonic acid is 20:1, well outside its optimal working range, but is very well placed to combat acidosis.

From these considerations it is evident that the *chemical* buffering power of the bicarbonate system in the body is poor. However, its efficiency is vastly improved by the fact that both the carbonic acid and bicarbonate concentrations can be regulated by the body, the former by the lungs and the latter by the kidneys. Herein lies the importance of the bicarbonate buffer in the regulation of the acid-base state of the body. It is the only buffer which can be physiologically adjusted to maintain a normal pH. For instance, if a strong acid is added to the blood the following reactions occur:

$$HCl + NaHCO_3 = H_2CO_3 + NaCl$$

$$H_2CO_3 \rightleftarrows H_2O + \boxed{CO_2} \rightarrow \text{Excreted by the lungs}$$

In the first instance the strong acid is "swapped" for a weak acid (chemical buffering). The carbonic acid dissociates into water and CO_2, and the latter is excreted by the lungs (physiological buffering).

The phosphate buffering system.—This works in exactly the same way as the bicarbonate system, except that the NaH_2PO_4 (sodium dihydrogen phosphate) is the weak acid and Na_2HPO_4 (disodium hydrogen phosphate) is the strong base. The system is a chemical buffer. The pK of the system is 6·8, so that it is working fairly close to its optimal pH.

Proteins as buffers.—Proteins are quantitatively the most important buffers in the body. They contain acidic and basic groups, which make up "buffer pairs". An example of an acidic group is $-COOH$, which can dissociate into $-COO^- + H^+$, and an example of a basic group is $-NH_2$, which can accept a hydrogen ion to form $-NH_3^+$. The pK's of the different protein buffer systems vary, but many are around 7·4, so that in blood and extracellular fluid they are working at or near their most efficient ranges.

Haemoglobin as a buffer.—Haemoglobin is responsible for half the buffering power of the blood. It acts as a buffer both because it is a protein and, more

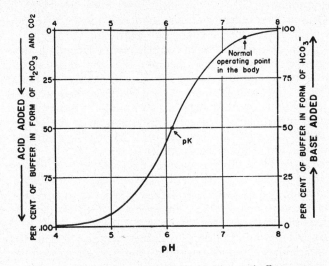

3/Fig. 14.—The reaction curve for the bicarbonate buffer system.

important, because of the ability of the imidazole groups within the molecule to accept H^+ ions. The acidity of these groups is influenced by the oxygenation and reduction of haemoglobin, the point to remember being that haemoglobin is a weaker acid in the reduced form than when it is oxygenated (Fig. 15). When oxygenated haemoglobin gives up oxygen to the tissues it becomes reduced and is therefore more able to accept H^+ ions and CO_2. In the lungs the reverse effect occurs.

The buffers in the blood, in order of importance, are haemoglobin, bicarbonate and plasma proteins, and phosphate. In interstitial fluid the main buffers are bicarbonate, phosphate, and interstitial proteins. In the cells the main buffers are proteins, phosphate, and other inorganic substances.

3/Fig. 15.—The effect of the oxygen saturation of haemoglobin upon the buffering power of the imidazole group.

Carbon Dioxide Stores

A large amount of CO_2 is contained in the body, about 120 litres in all. Because of this great volume the total amount can only be altered rather slowly as a result of an inappropriate change in ventilation. The CO_2 stores can be considered to be contained in three compartments depending on the possible rate of exchange of the gas—fast, medium and slow. The fast compartment consists of the blood and high blood-flow organs such as the brain, heart and kidneys in which the tissue P_{CO_2} levels tend to follow the alveolar P_{CO_2} rather closely. The medium compartment consists mainly of resting skeletal muscle, and the slow compartment of bone and fatty tissue. The size of the three compartments is different, the slow compartment having the greatest capacity for storing CO_2, and the fast one the smallest.

From the above facts it follows that the final arterial P_{CO_2} changes resulting from a stepwise change in ventilation will be delayed, and it will take time for a new equilibrium to be attained. This time is faster for a stepwise increase in ventilation than it is for a decrease. Thus following a sudden increase in ventilation a new equilibrium is reached after about 20 minutes, the half-time for the change being 3–4 minutes. Following a sudden decrease in ventilation the half-time is 15–20 minutes and a new equilibrium may not have been reached after as long as one hour.

Respiratory Acidosis (Hypercapnia, hypercarbia)

In a healthy conscious subject a reduction in the alveolar ventilation immediately leads to a rise in the arterial Pco_2. This in turn results in an attempt to increase the ventilation again and to return the Pco_2 to normal. For a discussion of the carriage of CO_2 in the blood see page 153. If for any reason the patient is unable to increase his ventilation, a respiratory acidosis develops. The Pco_2 rises, plasma bicarbonate rises and the pH falls. The kidney compensates for these changes by excreting H^+ ions and retaining bicarbonate. This secondary response is slow to develop, and it may take many days for full compensation to occur. The response to a chronic respiratory acidosis is therefore a metabolic alkalosis which tends to, and often succeeds in, returning the pH to normal. A fully compensated respiratory acidosis is then said to be present. In the presence of acute hypercarbia, such as happens during general anaesthesia, there is no time for any appreciable renal compensation to occur. During apnoea the arterial Pco_2 rises about 3–6 mm Hg (0·4–0·8 kPa) per minute and H^+ ions accumulate at a rate of 10 mEq/min (mmol/l). This is some 20 times faster than the kidney can excrete them.

The systemic effects of hypercapnia are widespread. The central nervous effects include impairment of mental activity and loss of consciousness, a rise in cerebral blood flow and CSF pressure and the stimulation of respiration, followed by depression if the Pco_2 rises further. General sympathetic overactivity occurs. If a high inspired oxygen tension is not delivered to the patient hypoxaemia follows hypercapnia (see p. 73). Profound effects are seen in the circulation. The heart muscle is depressed, although this effect is offset by the increased sympathetic activity, and a rise in cardiac output follows, accompanied by peripheral dilatation. Increased bleeding is seen in surgical wounds. The blood pressure rises, and the patient presents with a warm skin, dilated veins and a bounding pulse. Dysrhythmias occur, and are especially likely to happen during cyclopropane or halothane anaesthesia. For further discussion on the effects of hypercarbia see Chapter 4. It is important to remember that under anaesthesia many of the above signs are masked, and the only indications of hypercapnia may be an increase in the depth of respiration, or difficulty in controlling the ventilation.

Under anaesthesia hypercapnia may be caused by: (a) Badly chosen or malfunctioning apparatus, e.g. using adult apparatus on a child, incorrectly assembled apparatus or worn out soda-lime. (b) The accidental administration of carbon dioxide. (c) Hypoventilation due to such factors as central respiratory depression or the misuse of relaxants.

The treatment of hypercarbia due to apparatus faults or the accidental administration of carbon dioxide is self-evident. But a word of warning: the Pco_2 should be returned to normal values slowly or serious cardiac dysrhythmias and/or hypotension may be precipitated. Hypoventilation should be treated by assisting or controlling the respirations until the patient is himself once more able to maintain adequate ventilation. If hypercapnia is suspected a generous concentration of oxygen should be given in the inspired gas mixture.

Hypoventilation during anaesthesia.—Under anaesthesia the function of the lungs is often impeded. For example, most sedative and anaesthetic agents depress the activity of the respiratory centres. Thus, many patients breathing spontaneously through any anaesthetic system show a rise in the carbon dioxide tension of the blood. In some cases the degree of hypoventilation may be greater than realised and the P_{CO_2}, then rapidly reaches very high levels. It is, therefore, important to emphasise that during anaesthesia the anaesthetist (not the patient) is largely responsible for controlling the carbon dioxide tension at about the normal level. The principal difficulty for the anaesthetist is to recognise minor degrees of hypoventilation; the time-honoured custom of looking at the reservoir bag and thinking that ventilation is "adequate" is often grossly erroneous. Fluctuations in arterial P_{CO_2} from 40–60 mm Hg (5·3–8·0 kPa) are probably of little consequence in the normal, healthy patient but values in excess of 80 mm Hg (6·6 kPa) denote severe and dangerous hypoventilation. When the level rises to 110 mm Hg (14·6 kPa), carbon dioxide narcosis occurs and the patient will not recover consciousness when the anaesthetic drugs are withdrawn. If, at this moment, the patient is allowed to breathe room air simply because the operation is finished, he will not only have to contend with the disadvantages of alveoli filled with anaesthetic gases escaping from the circulation (Diffusion hypoxia, see p. 322) and the uneven ventilation-perfusion ratio which normally follows anaesthesia (see p. 143), but also with a reduced quantity of available oxygen from the lungs due to the high carbon dioxide tension. Hypoxia will occur, as shown in Table 7.

Fluctuations—both up and down—in the carbon dioxide content of the plasma are not always due to respiratory complications but may equally be the result of changes in tissue metabolism. Both respiratory acidosis and metabolic acidosis sometimes occur in a patient at the same time under conditions of

3/TABLE 7

PARTIAL PRESSURE OF GASES IN ALVEOLI, BREATHING AIR

	Normal ventilation (arterial P_{CO_2} = 40 mm Hg or 5·3 kPA)	Hypoventilation (arterial P_{CO_2} = 100 mm Hg or 13·3 kPa)
Oxygen	95 mm Hg (12·7 kPa)	35 mm Hg (4·7 kPa)
Nitrogen	578 mm Hg (77·0 kPa)	578 mm Hg (77·0 kPa)
Carbon dioxide	40 mm Hg (5·3 kPa)	100 mm Hg (13·3 kPa)
Water vapour	47 mm Hg (6·3 kPa)	47 mm Hg (6·3 kPa)
Total	760 mm Hg (101 kPa)	760 mm Hg (101 kPa)

anaesthesia. The reasons for this are not yet clear but may be related to pre-operative starvation, the reaction of the body to surgical trauma and to the effects of the various anaesthetic agents.

During controlled respiration in the presence of severe chronic bronchitis the ventilation required to maintain a normal or low P_{CO_2} may have to be much greater than in a patient with normal lungs. Tidal volumes of up to one litre may be necessary to produce a large enough alveolar ventilation to keep the P_{CO_2} from rising. Unless this point is borne in mind the patient may suffer from the effects of hypercapnia while the anaesthetist is happy in the mistaken belief that ventilation is adequate.

Respiratory Alkalosis (Hypocapnia, hypocarbia)

This state of affairs commonly occurs during controlled respiration. Excessive ventilation leads to a reduction in the P_{CO_2}. The kidney compensates for a rise in pH by excreting more HCO_3^- ions and reabsorbing more H^+ ions, thus producing an alkaline urine. The secondary response to a respiratory alkalosis is therefore a metabolic acidosis, but in an anaesthetised patient this secondary response is reduced by the fall in renal blood flow caused by the anaesthetic agents. However, it is not uncommon to find a mild metabolic acidosis in the anaesthetised and hyperventilated patient. An uncompensated respiratory alkalosis leads to the following changes in the blood: a low P_{CO_2}, a low plasma bicarbonate, a high pH and a normal base excess and standard bicarbonate.

Other features of alkalosis are hypokalaemia, increased neuromuscular excitability sometimes producing tetany, and a shift to the left of the haemo-globin-oxygen dissociation curve.

The principal theoretical danger of a respiratory alkalosis under anaesthesia is cerebral vasoconstriction, as it is known that the P_{CO_2} of the blood reaching the brain largely controls the diameter of these vessels. Thus, a severe alkalosis may produce intense cerebral vasoconstriction. Cerebral effects of hyper-ventilation, such as euphoria and analgesia, have been demonstrated but whether they are due to cerebral vasoconstriction or to a direct action of a low CO_2 tension on the cells is not definitely known, although the latter seems to be much more likely. Satisfactory evidence that long periods of even severe respiratory alkalosis lead to cerebral damage is still lacking and most clinicians believe that a mild respiratory alkalosis is more beneficial for the patient than a mild respiratory acidosis. Furthermore, severe vasoconstriction is probably prevented by the reaction of the cerebral vessels to the change of oxygen tension, because a reduced oxygen tension leads to cerebral vasodilatation.

During anaesthesia with controlled ventilation a low P_{CO_2} causes the cardiac output to fall. In fact one of the main determinants of the cardiac output during anaesthesia is the P_{CO_2} level (Prys-Roberts, 1968). As the P_{CO_2} rises from low, through normal to high values the cardiac output increases, at first due only to increases in the stroke volume, and then to increases in both stroke volume and in heart rate. These changes are accompanied by a rise in mean arterial pressure and in left ventricular stroke work, and by a fall in peripheral resistance.

Geddes and Gray (1959) have stressed the value of hyperventilation in association with complete muscular paralysis for providing ideal conditions for surgery. Using a mixture of nitrous oxide/oxygen (70:30 per cent) for ventilation together with electro-encephalographic recordings they found a state indistinguishable from that obtained with anaesthetic agents such as ether or halothane. On the other hand Bridge and Eger (1966) found that, during halothane anaesthesia, hyperventilation *per se* had no effect on the depth of anaesthesia.

The precise role of carbon dioxide in brain function is not yet clear but Bonvallet *et al.* (1956) found a low P_{CO_2} reduced activity in the reticular formation; Morrice (1956) suggested an adequate carbon dioxide tension was essential for the Krebs tricarboxylic acid cycle.

In the past it was often believed that when patients were hyperventilated the carbon dioxide level had to rise back to normal again before spontaneous respiration was resumed. Utting and Gray (1962) have emphasised the fallacy of this conception. In a study of twelve patients they found that spontaneous breathing recommenced even when a severe degree of respiratory alkalosis was present (Fig. 16). They concluded that provided the respiratory centre was not depressed by an anaesthetic or analgesic agent then respiration could be resumed with a peripheral stimulus.

Metabolic Acidosis

A metabolic acidosis follows the accumulation in the body of non-volatile acids, e.g. lactic acid, or aceto-acetic and α-keto-glutaric acids in uncontrolled diabetes mellitus. Uncompensated, the changes seen in blood are as follows: a low pH, low plasma bicarbonate, normal P_{CO_2}, a negative base excess and a low standard bicarbonate. These changes are usually followed by a secondary hyperventilation with a fall in the P_{CO_2}, so that the pH tends to return towards normal.

The effects of a metabolic acidosis may be severe. The heart muscle is depressed and the cardiac output falls. Intense peripheral vasoconstriction may occur. These changes tend to perpetuate the acidosis so that a vicious circle is set up. The hydrogen ions will tend to displace potassium ions from the intracellular fluid with the result that hyperkalaemia can be produced, especially if renal function is poor. The cardiovascular responses to sympathetic activity and sympathomimetic drugs are reduced so that the natural protective mechanisms are interfered with. Metabolic acidosis stimulates the peripheral chemoreceptors. If these are inactive and provided the acidosis is sufficiently intense, then H^+ ions may leak into the brain and stimulate the respiratory centre directly. There is no evidence available to support the clinical suggestion that metabolic acidosis is capable of depressing the activity of the respiratory centre.

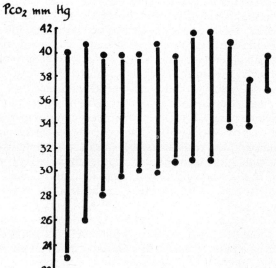

3/FIG. 16.—The results of P_{CO_2} estimations in twelve patients. The top dot represents the value of P_{CO_2} pre-operatively and the bottom dot signifies the level of P_{CO_2} as respiration recommenced after a period of hyperventilation.

It must also be remembered that the haemoglobin-oxygen dissociation curve is moved to the right.

A mild metabolic acidosis sometimes occurs in patients undergoing general anaesthesia (see below). It is commonly observed after a period of extracorporeal perfusion, after circulatory arrest and hypothermia, and immediately following the temporary occlusion of a major vessel such as the aorta. Other causes are massive blood transfusion, respiratory distress of the newborn, renal failure, diabetic coma and salicylate poisoning.

Treatment should be directed towards immediate correction of the acidosis with sodium bicarbonate or THAM, and treatment of the precipitating cause. The dose of bicarbonate can be calculated from the base excess, assuming that equilibration throughout the extracellular fluid will occur (about 20 per cent of the body weight).

$$\text{Dose (mEq) (mmol)} = \frac{\text{Base excess} \times \text{Body weight (kg)}}{3}$$

This dose should be given intravenously over about twenty minutes. The results of administering the dose of bicarbonate as suggested above are not always predictable due to the possible development of further acidosis since the original blood sample was taken, and because of altered equilibrium with the extracellular fluid in a deranged circulation. For these reasons it is essential to reassess the acid-base status of the arterial blood after the bicarbonate has been given, and to correct further if necessary. Sodium bicarbonate is a poor buffer in its own right, as explained previously, and acts mainly by combining with H^+ ions to form CO_2 and water:

$$H^+ + HCO_3^- \rightleftharpoons H_2CO_3 \rightleftharpoons CO_2 + H_2O$$

The administration of bicarbonate to correct a metabolic acidosis therefore presents a carbon dioxide load for the lungs to excrete, and efficient buffering of a metabolic acidosis depends on adequate pulmonary ventilation. One disadvantage of using bicarbonate as a buffer is that its use necessitates loading with sodium a circulation that may already be in failure. If this is considered to be undesirable then THAM may be used instead, as it is virtually sodium free.

Metabolic acidosis and anaesthesia.—During uncomplicated anaesthesia in normal man metabolic acidosis is rarely encountered (Bunker, 1962). In dogs, however, it is commonly observed during ether anaesthesia and this perhaps has tempted some authors to assume the same is true in man. The reason for this discrepancy is that ether anaesthesia causes equal amounts of adrenaline and noradrenaline to be liberated in the dog but principally noradrenaline in man. Noradrenaline is largely free of metabolic effects, whereas adrenaline stimulates the release of lactic acid from the tissues in dogs.

There are, however, a few exceptions to this rule. Small children who possess increased sympathetic nervous activity tend to produce a moderate metabolic acidosis during ether anaesthesia. Furthermore, adult patients who are suffering from metabolic diseases in which lactic acid utilisation is impaired (i.e. Cushing's disease, cirrhosis of the liver) also tend to develop severe metabolic acidosis during ether anaesthesia. This state of affairs is peculiar to ether anaesthesia and it is not observed after cyclopropane or thiopentone-nitrous oxide-oxygen anaesthesia.

3/TABLE 8

THE MECHANISMS BY WHICH PRIMARY ACID-BASE CHANGES ARE COMPENSATED. If the pH has been fully returned to normal the primary change is said to be FULLY COMPENSATED. If the pH has not been completely returned to normal the primary change is said to be PARTIALLY COMPENSATED.

Original acid-base change	Compensatory Mechanism	Compensating Organ
Respiratory Acidosis	Metabolic alkalosis, with a further rise in plasma $[HCO_3{}^-]$	Kidney
Respiratory Alkalosis	Metabolic acidosis, with a further fall in plasma $[HCO_3{}^-]$	Kidney
Metabolic Acidosis	Respiratory alkalosis, with a further fall in plasma $[HCO_3{}^-]$	Lungs
Metabolic Alkalosis	Respiratory acidosis, with a further rise in plasma $[HCO_3{}^-]$	Lungs

Metabolic Alkalosis

Under normal circumstances this is rarely observed in the anaesthetised patient. Two uncommon situations in which an alkalosis may be seen are (1) excessive administration of base to correct a metabolic acidosis, and (2) in the presence of severe pyloric stenosis. In the latter situation hyperventilation may be dangerous, as the combination of both a respiratory and a metabolic alkalosis will lead to a very high pH. A mild metabolic alkalosis is often observed post-operatively, especially in association with potassium depletion.

MEASUREMENT OF ACID-BASE STATUS

(1) Respiratory Acidosis and Alkalosis

Such measurements are in effect an assessment of the efficiency of ventilation. There are three principal methods:

1. *Tidal volume measurement.*—This is the simplest, yet least accurate, method available. The amount of air or gases expired with each breath by the patient can easily be measured by a suitable respirometer (e.g. Wright, Dräger or Monaghan). Most of these instruments add a small amount of resistance to respiration and are least accurate over low flow rates—the circumstances where they are most needed. Once the tidal volume and the number of respirations per minute have been assessed the minute volume can easily be calculated. This figure must then be related to the patient's metabolic requirements. The latter will depend on the age, body-weight, surface area and metabolic state of the patient. The correct requirements for each individual subject can best be calculated either with the aid of the Radford nomogram or the Nunn slide rule.

2. *Measurement of alveolar carbon dioxide tension.*—There are two principal ways in which this can be achieved—an end-tidal sampling method or a rebreathing technique. The *end-tidal sample* is taken at the close of expiration and provided there is a sufficient volume of ventilation it represents the contents of the alveolar air. The sample is then analysed for carbon dioxide content. One of the principal disadvantages of this technique is uneven ventilation, as is found in some patients with emphysema, for air-trapping will lead to consistently low readings. However, even in normal subjects the end-tidal CO_2 differs from arterial blood during anaesthesia by as much as 10 mm Hg (1·3 kPa) for reasons which are not yet explained. *The rebreathing technique* (Campbell and Howell, 1960; Collier, 1956) is based on the principle of equilibrating the air in the patient's lungs with oxygen in a rebreathing bag. First the patient breathes oxygen (spontaneously or by controlled respiration) for two minutes in and out of the bag, which is attached by a mask to the face or directly on to the end of an endotracheal tube. During this period the carbon dioxide content within the rebreathing bag gradually rises until it approximates the mixed venous carbon dioxide concentration. At this stage the method aims at obtaining a rough equilibration between the carbon dioxide tension in the bag and the mixed venous blood in the pulmonary artery. The contents of the bag are then temporarily sealed whilst the patient breathes room air or anaesthetic gases again for a few minutes. At the end of this period the mask is again applied and the patient rebreathes the contents in the bag for a further 45 seconds, which represents approximately the time taken for blood leaving the lungs at the beginning to recirculate. If the patient is unconscious or hypoventilating, then gentle assistance can be given to the bag to ensure that a true alveolar sample is obtained. At the end of the period the carbon dioxide content of the bag is analysed in a modified Haldane apparatus (Fig. 17). Now the CO_2 per cent is converted to partial pressure, multiply by $\dfrac{P_B - 47}{100}$ mm Hg $\left(\dfrac{P_B - 6·3}{100}\ \text{kPA}\right)^*$, and the figure obtained represents the P_{CO_2} of mixed venous blood. The arterial P_{CO_2} is obtained by subtracting 8 mm Hg (1·1 kPa). The main technical error arises from having leaks around the face-piece during rebreathing. The method is not affected by the presence of nitrous oxide or halothane provided 70 per cent potassium hydroxide is used for the absorption of the carbon dioxide. The principal advantage of this technique lies in its simplicity, the relative cheapness of the apparatus, and the rapidity with which successive estimations can be made. However, in cases with a very high alveolar carbon dioxide tension [i.e. 80 mm Hg (11·0 kPa) or above] the values obtained are consistently lower than those measured by a direct arterial technique. The reason for this anomaly is that in the rebreathing technique originally the bag contents are without CO_2 and insufficient time is available for equilibration. If one were to start with a higher value of CO_2 in the bag the correct answer could be obtained.

3. *Measurement of arterial carbon dioxide tension* (P_{CO_2}).—The most commonly used methods are the interpolation micro-method (Astrup, 1959) or the carbon dioxide electrode (Severinghaus, 1959).

  (*a*) *The interpolation micro-method* has the advantage that a sample of capil-

* P_B Barometric Pressure = 760 mm Hg (101 kPa). Water vapour pressure at 37° C = 47 mm Hg (6·3 kPa).

lary blood is sufficient for each measurement.* The method is based on the principle that the relation between the logarithm of P_{CO_2} and pH is always a straight line. If this line can be constructed for a particular sample of blood then merely knowing the pH will enable the P_{CO_2} to be predicted. The interpolation method, therefore, measures only the pH. Thus, a sample of blood is first taken from the patient and the pH measured; it is then exposed to a known high level of P_{CO_2} (e.g. 60 mm Hg, 8·0 kPa = Point A on Fig. 18) and a known low level of P_{CO_2} (e.g. 30 mm Hg, 4·0 kPa = Point B on Fig. 18) and the pH measured on each occasion. A straight line can now be drawn connecting points A and B. The actual pH of the sample is then located on this line. The pH of the blood sample is found to be 7·1 and this corresponds with a P_{CO_2} of 50 mm Hg (6·6 kPa).

(b) *The principle of the carbon dioxide electrode* (Smith and Hahn, 1969) is that it produces an electrical signal directly proportional to the logarithm of the

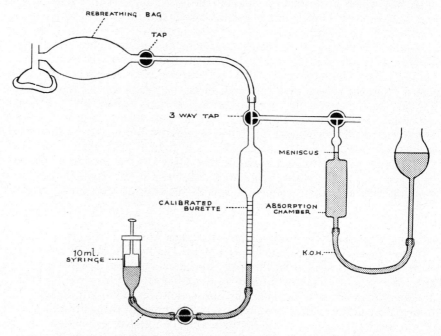

3/Fig. 17.—Modified Haldane Apparatus.

The calibrated burette is filled with mercury from the 10 ml syringe and after levelling the potassium hydroxide solution to the meniscus the tap above the meniscus is turned to position ⊥. The rebreathed sample is blown through and this tap is then closed. The sample is drawn into the burette. The tap above the calibrated burette is turned to position T and the first tap to position ⊣. The sample is then pushed into the absorption chamber fifteen times. The meniscus is levelled and the volume change due to carbon dioxide absorption is read from the burette.

* *Note on collection of blood for P_{CO_2} estimations.*

The best sample is one taken anaerobically into a sealed heparinised glass syringe from a large artery, stored in an ice-cold container for transport and then analysed without contact with the atmosphere. If venous or capillary blood is used, in addition to the foregoing precaution an attempt should be made to stimulate the peripheral circulation by warmth so that the errors associated with stagnation are minimised.

P_{CO_2} of a sample of either a liquid or a gas. It consists of a pH electrode separated from the sample by a teflon membrane which is permeable to CO_2 but not to ions in the sample. CO_2 diffuses through the membrane into a thin layer of dilute sodium bicarbonate solution controlling the pH of this solution. The electrode has the advantage that the partial pressure of CO_2 may be read directly from a meter in one to two minutes.

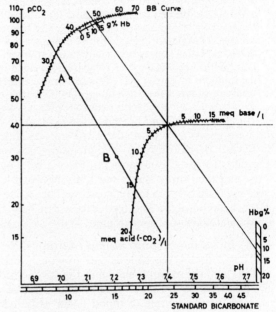

3/Fig. 18.—Graph showing calculations of $\varDelta$ acid-base or buffer base of a blood sample.

(2) Metabolic Acidosis and Alkalosis

The best way to quantitate the metabolic component of acid-base equilibrium has long been a matter for debate. However at present the most convenient and practical methods are to measure either the base excess/deficit or the standard bicarbonate. There are two principal ways of estimating the base excess:

(a) *By measuring the pH, P_{CO_2} and haemoglobin*

Measurement of pH.—The glass electrode.

This instrument is based on the characteristics of special glass which is selectively permeable to H^+ ions. This glass has the property that if each side of the glass is bathed in a solution of different pH, an e.m.f. is generated across it. This e.m.f. is directly and linearly proportional to the difference between the pH of the two solutions. If the pH on one side of the glass is stabilised, and a solution of unknown pH is introduced onto the other side of the glass, the e.m.f. thus generated gives an indication of the unknown pH. The e.m.f. across the pH sensitive glass can be measured by placing metal electrodes in the solutions on either side of it. But a problem arises here, because at any metal-electrolyte interface an e.m.f. is developed and this can obscure that across the glass. For this reason the electrodes on either side must be electrically very stable, so that little or no variation in potential occurs at their surfaces. If variations do occur it is impossible to separate these from alterations across the pH glass, which is what we are trying to measure. Suitably stable electrodes are (1) silver, coated with a layer of silver chloride, and immersed in a solution containing chloride ions; and (2) calomel coated mercury, in contact with saturated KCl. The general arrangement of a pH electrode is shown in Fig. 19. On one side of the glass is a solution of 0·1 M HCl (stable pH) into which is dipped a silver: silver chloride electrode. On the other side of the glass is the test solution. This is connected electrically via a liquid bridge to a saturated solution of KCl, which is itself in contact with a mercury: calomel electrode. A porous plug is inserted in the KCl to prevent contamination of the calomel electrode by the test solution. The e.m.f. across the whole assembly can now be measured by connecting the silver and calomel electrodes through a sensitive high resistance voltmeter. The instrument is calibrated by setting it up against solutions of known pH, and the pH of an unknown solution can then be measured by comparing the e.m.f. it generates with that produced by the solutions of known pH. Although for each measurement the potential across the whole apparatus is read, the stability of the system is such that changes in e.m.f. across the whole are due to changes across the pH sensitive glass.

If the pH, Pco_2 and haemoglobin content of a sample of blood are known, the base excess can be read from a special slide rule, such as that designed by Severinghaus, or from a nomogram such as that of Siggaard-Andersen (Fig. 20). To use this nomogram, place a ruler against the value for the blood Pco_2, and then bring it into line with the value for the pH. The ruler will now cross the large column for base excess. The lattice-work is due to various values of the haemoglobin. The base excess can now be read off directly from the appropriate haemoglobin column.

(b) By the interpolation method (Astrup, 1959)

This method is the same as that previously described for measuring the Pco_2 (p. 169), and the example shown in Fig. 18 can be used again. The lower curved line gives values for base excess. The point at which the straight line constructed for the sample of blood under examination cuts this curve gives the base excess value. In the example the line AB cuts the base excess line at the point marked − 15 mEq/litre (mmol/l), indicating a severe metabolic acidosis.

The standard bicarbonate can also be measured by dropping a perpendicular from the point at which the line AB cuts the $Pco_2 = 40$ mm Hg (5·3 kPa) line, and reading off its value from the point at which the perpendicular meets the

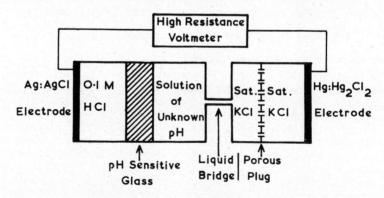

3/Fig. 19.—Schematic diagram of a pH electrode. See text for full details.

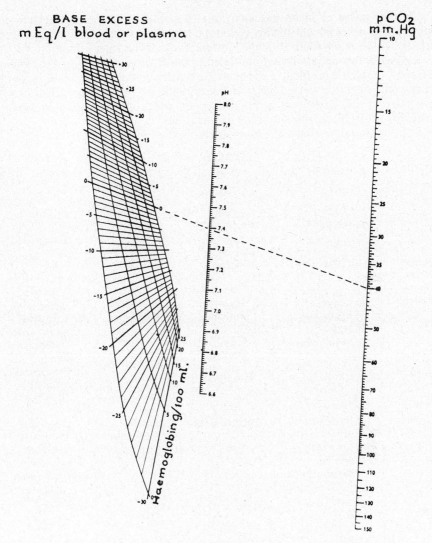

3/Fig. 20.—Nomogram for blood acid-base calculation (Siggaard-Andersen, 1963).

standard bicarbonate scale. In this example the standard bicarbonate is equal to 14 mEq/litre, a very low value (normal = 22–26 mEq/litre, mmol/l).

If we now had to decide how much bicarbonate would be required to correct such a metabolic acidosis, the dose can be calculated from the equation on page 167. Assuming that the patient weighs 60 kg, the dose of bicarbonate works out at $\dfrac{15 \times 60}{3}$ = 300 mEq (mmol). After this dose has been administered, another sample of arterial blood must be analysed, and a further dose given if necessary.

Interpretation of blood gas analysis.—The impact of the glass electrode system and development of this technique has made sweeping changes in the anaesthetist's requirements for the interpretation of laboratory data. Now that it is possible for the relatively uninitiated to make measurements of Po_2, Pco_2, and pH, the whole problem of the control of patients undergoing anaesthesia or in the post-operative period has been greatly simplified. If suitable apparatus is available, then a knowledge of Po_2, Pco_2, and pH is sufficient to diagnose the majority of problems of ventilation and acid-base balance.

The value of these measurements is emphasised in Table 9.

3/TABLE 9

CAUSES OF VARIATIONS IN Po_2, Pco_2 AND pH AND THEIR EFFECT ON ACID-BASE BALANCE

	Po_2 mm Hg (kPa)	Pco_2 mm Hg (kPa)	pH	Base excess or deficit (in mEq/litre) (mmol/l)
Normal values	100 (13·3)	40 (5·3)	7·4	0
Raised	(a) Oxygen inhalation (b) Hyper-ventilation	(a) Hypo-ventilation (b) Carbon dioxide inhalation	Alkalosis (a) Respiratory (b) Metabolic	+3 or more (a) Excessive bicarbonate administra-tion (b) Pre-existing metabolic alkalosis
Lowered	(a) Intrapulmon-ary factors (b) Lowered alveolar concentration 1. Low inspired conc. 2. Hypo-ventilation (c) R–L shunts (d) Low cardiac output states	Hyperventilation	Acidosis (a) Respiratory (b) Metabolic	−3 or less (a) Tissue ischaemia or hypoxia (b) Pre-existing metabolic acidosis

A few simple examples will illustrate the value of this table, e.g.

(a) *The patient's blood (whilst breathing air) reveals the following data:*

Po_2 60 mm Hg (8·0 kPa)
Pco_2 42 mm Hg (5·6 kPa)
pH   7·4
Base excess/deficit = 0 mEq/litre (mmol/l)

Interpretation.—The Po_2 is low yet the Pco_2, pH and base excess/deficit are normal. The normal P_{CO_2} signifies that ventilation is adequate whereas the low P_{O_2} indicates that there is some interference with the transfer of oxygen from the alveoli to the pulmonary circulation. The commonest cause of this situation is an alteration of the ventilation-perfusion ratio.

Diagnosis.—This situation is observed in patients with scattered areas of pulmonary collapse. It could also be present if the patient was inspiring a mixture with a low percentage of oxygen: however, the normal P_{CO_2} rules out the possibility of hypoventilation.

Treatment.—In the past it was often assumed that all areas of pulmonary collapse were secondary to blockage of the bronchiole by mucous secretions or "plugs". A number of investigators have found that under anaesthesia and in the post-operative period under sedation the normal control of the ventilation-perfusion ratio is altered (see p. 143). The patient should be given oxygen to breath, and re-expansion of the lungs should be encouraged with coughing and deep breathing. Conway and Payne (1963) have shown that this type of hypoxaemia occurring in the early post-operative period can readily be corrected by giving oxygen. An oxygen flow of 2 litres/minute into a plastic oxygen mask is perfectly satisfactory.

(b) *The patient's blood (whilst breathing air) reveals the following data:*

P_{O_2} 45 mm Hg (6·0 kPa)
P_{CO_2} 80 mm Hg (10·7 kPa)
pH   7·2
Base excess/deficit $= 0$

Interpretation.—The raised P_{CO_2} suggests under-ventilation and this could also account for the lowered P_{O_2}. A pH on the acid side without any change in the base excess confirms a respiratory rather than a metabolic problem.

Diagnosis.—Hypoventilation is the cause of the respiratory acidosis. Measuring the minute volume with a Wright respirometer will confirm this finding. If the patient was breathing 100 per cent oxygen rather than air when the test samples were taken then the P_{O_2}, would rise to 550 mm Hg (73·1 kPa) (if no increased shunt were present), yet the other figures would remain the same.

Treatment.—Improved ventilation. This can be achieved by applying intermittent positive-pressure ventilation, but careful monitoring of the P_{CO_2} level will be required before normal spontaneous respiration can be allowed to resume.

(c) *The patient's blood (whilst breathing air) reveals the following data:*

P_{O_2} 100 mm Hg (13·3 kPa)
P_{CO_2} 40 mm Hg (5·3 kPa)
pH   7·1
Base excess $= -17·5$ mEq/litre (mmol/l)

Interpretation.—Normal values for P_{O_2} and P_{CO_2} suggest that ventilation and oxygen transfer within the lungs are normal. A pH on the acid side with a large base deficit indicates a metabolic acidosis probably due to poor peripheral blood flow.

Diagnosis.—Metabolic acidosis due to poor peripheral perfusion.

Treatment.—Sodium bicarbonate, in the requisite amount, should be given on the basis of the patient's extracellular fluid volume to correct the metabolic acidosis. For example, if the patient has a weight of 70 kg and a base excess of -17.5 mEq/litre (mmol/l) then he requires an intravenous injection of $\dfrac{70 \times 77.5}{3} = 408$ mEq (mmol) to correct the metabolic acidosis.

REFERENCES

ASKROG, V. F., PENDER, J. W., and ECKENHOFF, J. E. (1964). Changes in physiological deadspace during deliberate hypotension. *Anesthesiology*, **25**, 744.

ASKROG, V. F., PENDER, J. W., SMITH, T. C., and ECKENHOFF, J. E. (1964). Changes in respiratory deadspace during halothane, cyclopropane and nitrous oxide anesthesia. *Anesthesiology*, **25**, 342.

ASTRUP, P. (1959). Ultra-micro methods for determining pH, pCO_2 and standard bicarbonate in capillary blood. In: *A Symposium on pH and Blood Gas Measurement*, pp. 81–92. Ed. R. F. Woolmer. London: J. & A. Churchill.

BALL, W. C., STEWART, P. B., NEWSHAM, L. G. S., and BATES, D. V. (1962). Regional pulmonary function studied with Xenon[133]. *J. clin. Invest.*, **41**, 519.

BENDIXEN, H. H., BULLWINKEL, B., HEDLEY-WHITE, J., and LAVER, M. B. (1964). Atelectasis and shunting during spontaneous ventilation in anesthetised patients. *Anesthesiology*, **25**, 297.

BENDIXEN, H. H., HEDLEY-WHITE, J., and LAVER, M. B. (1963). Impaired oxygenation in surgical patients during general anesthesia with controlled ventilation. A concept of atelectasis. *New Engl. J. Med.*, **269**, 991.

BERGMAN, N. A. (1963). Distribution of inspired gas during anesthesia and artificial ventilation. *J. appl. Physiol.*, **18**, 1085.

BERGMAN, N. A. (1967). Components of alveolar-arterial oxygen tension difference in anesthetised man. *Anesthesiology*, **28**, 517.

BONVALLET, M., HUGELIN, A., and DELL, P. (1956). Milieu intérieur et activité automatique des cellules réticulaires mésencéphaliques. *J. Physiol. (Paris)*, **48**, 403.

BOUTROS, A. R., and WOODFORD, V. R. (1963). Blood carbonic anhydrase activity. A possible role in the production of acid-base imbalance in children and infants. *Canad. Anaesth. Soc. J.*, **10**, 428.

BRIDGE, B. E., Jr., and EGER, E. I., II (1966). The effect of hypocapnia on the level of halothane anesthesia in man. *Anesthesiology*, **27**, 634.

BUNKER, J. P. (1962). Metabolic acidosis during anesthesia and surgery. *Anesthesiology*, **23**, 107.

CAMPBELL, E. J. M., and HOWELL, J. B. L. (1960). Simple rapid methods of estimating arterial and mixed venous P_{CO_2}. *Brit. med. J.*, **1**, 458.

CAMPBELL, E. J. M., NUNN, J. F., and PECKETT, B. W. (1958). A comparison of artificial ventilation and spontaneous respiration with particular reference to ventilation-blood flow relationships. *Brit. J. Anaesth.*, **30**, 166.

CHRISTIAN, G., and GREENE, N. M. (1962). Blood carbonic anhydrase activity in anesthetized man. *Anesthesiology*, **23**, 179.

COLE, R. B., and BISHOP, J. M. (1963). Effect of varying inspired oxygen tension on alveolar-arterial oxygen tension difference in man. *J. appl. Physiol.*, **18**, 1043.

COLGAN, F. J., and WHANG, T. B. (1968). Anesthesia and atelectasis. *Anesthesiology*, **29**, 917.

COLLIER, C. R. (1956). Determination of mixed venous carbon dioxide tension by rebreathing. *J. appl. Physiol.*, **9**, 25.

COMROE, J. H., FORSTER, R. E., DUBOIS, A. B., BRISCOE, W. A., and CARLSEN, E. (1962).
  The Lung. Clinical Physiology and Pulmonary Function Tests, p. 103, 2nd edit. Chicago:
  Year Book Medical Publishers.
CONWAY, C. M. (1964). Arterial oxygen tensions in surgical patients. In: *Oxygen Measure-
  ments in Blood and Tissue and their Significance*, p. 173. Eds. J. P. Payne & D. W. Hill.
  London: J. & A. Churchill.
CONWAY, C. M., and PAYNE, J. P. (1963). Post-operative hypoxaemia and oxygen therapy.
  Brit. med. J., **1**, 844.
EGBERT, L. D., and BENDIXEN, H. H. (1964). Effect of morphine on the breathing pattern.
  J. Amer. med. Ass., **188**, 485.
EGBERT, L. D., LAVER, M. B., and BENDIXEN, H. H. (1963). Intermittent deep breaths and
  compliance during anesthesia in man. *Anesthesiology*, **24**, 57.
FLETCHER, F. and BARBER, L. (1966). Lung mechanics and physiological shunt during
  spontaneous breathing in normal subjects. *Anesthesiology*, **27**, 638.
FREEMAN, J., and NUNN, J. P. (1963). Ventilation-perfusion relationships after haemorrhage.
  Clin. Sci., **24**, 135.
GARDINER, A. J. S., and PALMER, K. N. V. (1964). Effect of premedication and general
  anaesthesia on arterial blood gases. *Brit. med. J.*, **2**, 1433.
GEDDES, I. C., and GRAY, T. C. (1959). Hyperventilation for the maintenance of anaesthesia.
  Lancet, **2**, 4.
GOLD, M. I., and HELRICH, M. (1965). Pulmonary compliance during anesthesia. *Anesthe-
  siology*, **26**, 281.
GREGORY, I. C. (1974). The oxygen and carbon monoxide capacities of fetal and adult
  blood. *J. Physiol. (Lond.)*, **236**, 625.
HEWLETT, A. M., HULANDS, G. H., NUNN, J. F., and HEATH, J. R. (1974a). Functional
  residual capacity during anaesthesia II: spontaneous ventilation. *Brit. J. Anaesth.*,
  46, 486.
HEWLETT, A. M., HULANDS, G. H., NUNN, J. F., and MILLEDGE, J. S. (1974b). Functional
  residual capacity during anaesthesia III: artificial ventilation. *Brit. J. Anaesth.*, **46**,
  495.
HICKEY, R. F., VISICK, W., FAIRLEY, H. B., and FOURCADE, H. E. (1973). Effects of halothane anaesthesia on functional residual capacity and alveolar-arterial oxygen difference. *Anesthesiology*, **38**, 20.
HUGHES, J. M. B., GLAZIER, J. B., MALONEY, J. E., and WEST, J. B. (1968). Effect of lung
  volume on the distribution of pulmonary blood flow in man. *Resp. Physiol.*, **4**, 58.
HULANDS, G. H., GREENE, R., ILIFE, L. D., and NUNN, J. F. (1969). Influence of anaesthesia
  on the regional distribution of perfusion and ventilation in the lung. *Brit. J. Anaesth.*,
  41, 789.
LEIGH, J. M., and TYRRELL, M. F. (1968). Respiratory gas equations: a geometric approach.
  Brit. J. Anaesth., **40**, 430.
LUMLEY, J., MORGAN, M., and SYKES, M. K. (1969). Changes in arterial oxygenation and
  physiological deadspace under anaesthesia. *Brit. J. Anaesth.*, **41**, 279.
MARSHALL, B. E., COHEN, P. J., KLINGENMAIER, C. H., and AUKBERG, S. (1969). Pulmonary
  venous admixture before, during and after halothane: oxygen anesthesia in man.
  J. appl. Physiol., **27**, 653.
MARSHALL, B. E., and GRANGE, R. A. (1966). Changes in respiratory physiology during
  ether/air anaesthesia. *Brit. J. Anaesth.*, **38**, 329.
MARTINEZ, L. R., VON EULER, C., and NORLANDER, O. P. (1967). Ventilatory exchange and
  acid-base balance before and after preoperative medication. *Acta anaesth. scand.*,
  11, 139.
MILLEDGE, J. S., and NUNN, J. F. (1975). Criteria for fitness for anaesthesia in patients
  with chronic obstructive lung disease. *Brit. med. J.*, **3**, 670.

MORRICE, J. K. W., (1956). Slow wave production in E.E.G., with reference to hyperpnoea, carbon dioxide and autonomic balance. *Electroenceph. clin. Neurophysiol.*, **8,** 49.

NUNN, J. F. (1964*a*). Factors influencing the arterial oxygen tension during halothane anaesthesia with spontaneous respiration. *Brit. J. Anaesth.*, **36,** 327.

NUNN, J. F. (1964*b*). Personal communication.

NUNN, J. F. (1969). *Applied Respiratory Physiology.* London: Butterworth & Co.

NUNN, J. F., and BERGMAN, N. A. (1964). The effect of atropine on pulmonary gas exchange. *Brit. J. Anaesth.*, **36,** 68.

NUNN, J. F., BERGMAN, N. A., and COLEMAN, A. J. (1965). Factors influencing the arterial oxygen tension during anaesthesia with artificial ventilation. *Brit. J. Anaesth.*, **37,** 898.

NUNN, J. F., and HILL, D. W. (1960). Respiratory deadspace and arterial to end-tidal CO_2 tension difference in anesthetized man. *J. appl. Physiol.*, **15,** 383.

NUNN, J. F., and PAYNE, J. P. (1962). Hypoxaemia after general anaesthesia. *Lancet*, **2,** 631.

PANDAY, J., and NUNN, J. F. (1968). Failure to demonstrate progressive falls of arterial Po_2 during anaesthesia. *Anaesthesia*, **23,** 38.

PIERCE, J. A., and GAROFALO, M. L. (1965). Preoperative medication and its effect on blood gases. *J. Amer. med. Ass.*, **194,** 487.

PRICE, H. L., COOPERMAN, L. H., WARDEN, J. C., MORRIS, J. J., and SMITH, T. C. (1969). Pulmonary haemodynamics during general anesthesia in man. *Anesthesiology*, **30,** 629.

PRYS-ROBERTS, C. (1968). Ph.D. Thesis, Univ. of Leeds.

RAINE, J. M., and BISHOP, J. M. (1963). A—a difference in O_2 tension and physiological deadspace in normal man. *J. appl. Physiol.*, **18,** 284.

SEVERINGHAUS, J. W..(1959). Recent developments in blood O_2 and CO_2 electrodes: In: *A Symposium on pH and Blood Gas Measurement*, pp. 126–142. Ed. R. F. Woolmer, London: J. & A. Churchill.

SEVERINGHAUS, J. W., SWENSON, E. W., FINLEY, T. N., LATEGOLA, M. T., and WILLIAMS, J. (1961). Unilateral hypoventilation produced in dogs by occluding one pulmonary artery. *J. appl. Physiol.*, **16,** 53.

SLATER, E. M., NILSSON, S. E., LEAKE, D. L., PARRY, W. L., LAVER, M. B., HEDLEY-WHITE, J., and BENDIXEN, H. H. (1965). Arterial oxygen tension measurements during nitrous oxide/oxygen anesthesia. *Anesthesiology*, **26,** 642.

SMITH, A. C., and HAHN, C. E. W. (1969). Electrodes for the measurement of oxygen and carbon dioxide tensions. *Brit. J. Anaesth.*, **41,** 731.

SMITH, C. A. (1950). In Mitchell-Nelson's *Textbook of Pediatrics*, 5th edit. Philadelphia: W. B. Saunders.

SMITH, T. C., STEPHEN, G. W., ZEIGER, L., and WOLLMAN, H. (1967). Effects of pre-medicant drugs on respiration and gas exchange in man. *Anesthesiology*, **28,** 883.

STAUB, N. C., BISHOP, J. M., and FORSTER, R. E. (1961). Velocity of O_2 uptake by human red blood cells. *J. appl. Physiol.*, **16,** 511.

SYKES, M. K., DAVIES, D. M., CHAKRABATI, M. K., and LOH, L. (1973). The effect of halothane, trichloroethylene, and ether on the hypoxic pressor response and pulmonary vascular resistance in the isolated perfused cat lung. *Brit. J. Anaesth.*, **45,** 655.

SYKES, M. K., YOUNG, W. E., and ROBINSON, B. E. (1965). Oxygenation during anaesthesia with controlled ventilation. *Brit. J. Anaesth.*, **37,** 314.

THOMAS, H. M. (III), LEFRAK, S. S. *et al.*, (1974). The oxyhaemoglobin dissociation curve in health and disease. Role of 2,3-diphosphoglycerate. *Amer. J. Med.*, **57,** 331.

TOMLIN, P. J., CONWAY, C. M., and PAYNE, J. P. (1964). Hypoxaemia due to atropine. *Lancet*, **1,** 14.

UTTING, J. E., and GRAY, T. C. (1962). The initiation of respiration after anaesthesia accompanied by passive pulmonary hyperventilation. *Brit. J. Anaesth.*, **34,** 785.

VIRTUE, R. W., PERMUTT, S., TANAKA, R., PEARCY, C., BANE, H., BROMBERGER-BARNEA, B. (1966). Ventilation-perfusion and changes during thoracotomy. *Anesthesiology*, **27**, 132.

WEST, J. B. (1962). Regional differences in gas exchange in the lung of erect man. *J. appl. Physiol.*, **17**, 893.

WEST, J. B. (1963a). Blood-flow, ventilation and gas exchange in the lung. *Lancet*, **2**, 1055.

WEST, J. B. (1963b). Distribution of gas and blood in normal lungs. *Brit. med. Bull.*, **19**, 53.

WEST, J. B. (1970). *Ventilation/Blood Flow and Gas Exchange*. Oxford: Blackwell Scientific Publications.

WEST, J. B., DOLLERY, C. T., and HEARD, B. E. (1965). Increased pulmonary vascular resistance in the dependant zone of the isolated dog lung caused by perivascular oedema. *Circulat. Res.*, **12**, 301.

WYANT, G. M., CHANG, Chung Ai, and MERRIMAN, J. E. (1962). The effect of anesthesia upon pulmonary circulation. *Anesth. Analg. Curr. Res.*, **41**, 338.

FURTHER READING

CHERNIACK, R. M., and CHERNIACK, L. (1961). *Respiration in Health and Disease*. Philadelphia: W. B. Saunders Co.

COMROE, J. H., FORSTER, R. E., DUBOIS, A. B., BRISCOE, W. A., and CARLSEN, E., (1962). *The Lung*, 2nd edit. Chicago: Year Book Medical Publishers.

COTES, J. E. (1968). *Lung Function*. Oxford: Blackwell Scientific Publications.

DAVENPORT, H. W. (1958). *The ABC of Acid-Base Chemistry*. Chicago: Univ. of Chicago Press.

NUNN, J. F. (1969). *Applied Respiratory Physiology*. London: Butterworth & Co.

SIGGAARD-ANDERSEN, O. (1966). *The Acid-Base Status of the Blood*. Copenhagen: Munksgaard.

WEST. J. B. (1970). *Ventilation/Blood Flow and Gas Exchange*. Oxford: Blackwell Scientific Publications.

Chapter 4

OXYGEN AND ASSOCIATED GASES

OXYGEN (O_2)

History

Although Stephen Hale prepared oxygen along with many other gases in 1727, the full credit for its discovery and the realisation of the importance of this gas as a normal constituent of air must go to Priestley (1777). Following upon this discovery Lavoisier and his colleagues (1780 and 1789) demonstrated that it was absorbed by the lungs and, after metabolism in the body, eliminated as carbon dioxide and water. Since that time its value as a therapeutic agent has gradually increased with improved methods of administration.

Commercial Preparation

Fractional distillation of liquid air is the method now almost universally adopted. Before liquefaction of the air carbon dioxide is removed, and afterwards the nitrogen and oxygen are separated by making use of the difference in their boiling points (oxygen = $-182\cdot5°$ C: nitrogen = $-195\cdot8°$ C). The gaseous oxygen is then collected and stored in cylinders, coloured black with white shoulders, at a pressure of approximately 120 atmospheres, or roughly 1800 lb/sq inch (12·4 MPa).

Presentation

Cylinders up to 48 cu ft capacity for anaesthetic use are supplied with pin index valves. Cylinders larger than 48 cu ft are supplied with bull-nosed threads.

Large volume users may consider piped oxygen supplies to be justified. The oxygen may be supplied to piped systems in large compressed gas cylinders attached to a manifold in banks of two or more cylinders. Various devices are employed to ensure a continuity of gas supply, one bank of cylinders "running" whilst the other is held in reserve, with facilities for automatic opening of the reserve when the "running" bank nears exhaustion and with the simultaneous activation of a warning device.

Another form of oxygen supply is from liquid oxygen. In general, users in excess of 5,000 cubic feet of oxygen per week will find the liquid oxygen source economical. In one type of installation the liquid oxygen is boiled in a vacuum insulated evaporator (VIE) and supplied to the pipeline at 60 lb per sq inch (4·14 kPa). No compressor is necessary with such an installation.

Physical Properties

Oxygen is a tasteless, colourless and odourless gas; with a specific gravity of 1·105 (air = 1) and a molecular weight of 32. At normal atmospheric pressure it liquefies at $-183°$ C, but on increasing the pressure to 50 atmospheres, the temperature at which liquefaction occurs rises to $-119°$ C. The liquid may be cooled to a solid which melts at $-218°$ C. The solubility in water is 2·4 volumes per cent at 37° C and 4·9 volumes per cent at 0° C.

Inflammability

Oxygen cannot be ignited, but its presence aids combustion. Fires which occur during oxygen therapy are due to the rapid conflagration favoured by the high concentration of oxygen, though oxidisable substances such as cloth, wool or rubber must be present. With oil or grease, oxygen under pressure may cause an explosion, and this type of fire was particularly liable to happen when the old type of Endurance reducing valve was used. As the cylinder was turned on, a sudden jet of gas through this valve might come in contact with extraneous grease and result in an explosion. Combustion was favoured by the rubber diaphragm in the valve and enhanced by the continual flow of oxygen. The present-day Adams valve is less susceptible to this risk, but nevertheless grease should always be avoided in the presence of oxygen.

Pharmacological Actions

Oxygen is a normal constituent of air, and in order to appreciate the importance of an oxygen-rich atmosphere it is necessary to recall a few fundamental facts concerning respiration. About one-fifth 20·9 per cent) of the air we inhale at each breath consists of oxygen. Thus, in the inspired air, oxygen has a partial pressure of one-fifth of the atmospheric pressure, i.e. 20·9 per cent of 760 mm Hg = 159 mm Hg (20·9 per cent of 101·3 kPa = 21·2 kPa). As the air passes down the bronchial tree it becomes mixed with expired gases which are partially depleted of their oxygen so that the partial pressure of oxygen in the alveoli is about 100 mm Hg (13·3 kPa). This is the force that drives the oxygen across the pulmonary membrane, because the tension of oxygen in the venous blood is only 40 mm Hg (5·3 kPa).

1. *Oxygen Content*

The oxygen content of the blood is the amount of oxygen that can be extracted from 100 ml of blood. It is expressed in ml of dry gas at standard temperature and pressure (STPD).

2. *Oxygen Capacity*

The oxygen capacity is the volume of oxygen at STPD carried by 100 volumes of blood after saturation with room air.

The oxygen capacity of blood includes oxygen in combination with haemoglobin (1·39 ml O_2 per gram Hb) and oxygen in solution in the plasma (0·3 ml O_2 per 100 ml blood).

3. *Oxygen Saturation*

Oxygen saturation is the oxygen content of a sample compared with the oxygen capacity of that sample expressed as a percentage.

More exactly, it is the

$$\frac{O_2 \text{ combined with Hb}}{O_2 \text{ combined with Hb after equilibration with air}} \times 100$$

$$= \frac{O_2 \text{ content} - \text{dissolved } O_2}{O_2 \text{ capacity} - \text{dissolved } O_2} \times 100$$

The oxygen saturation may be obtained by spectrophotometric methods but

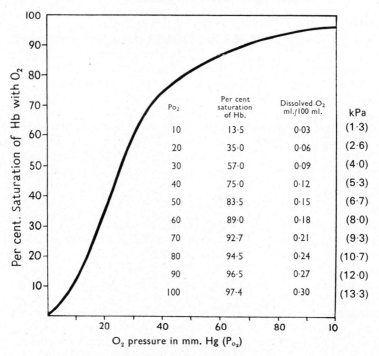

P_{O_2}	Per cent saturation of Hb.	Dissolved O_2 ml./100 ml.	kPa
10	13·5	0·03	(1·3)
20	35·0	0·06	(2·6)
30	57·0	0·09	(4·0)
40	75·0	0·12	(5·3)
50	83·5	0·15	(6·7)
60	89·0	0·18	(8·0)
70	92·7	0·21	(9·3)
80	94·5	0·24	(10·7)
90	96·5	0·27	(12·0)
100	97·4	0·30	(13·3)

4/FIG. 1.—The oxygen dissociation curve. The oxygen pressures in kilopascals are given in the margin in parenthesis.

it should be noted that actual oxygen content may not be obtained in this manner.

Oxygen content is traditionally measured by the manometric method of Peters and Van Slyke which was first described in 1924, but the modern micro-manometric technique of Natelson (1951) is presently favoured. More recently an excellent correlation with such techniques has been obtained by Davies (1970) using a gas chromatograph.

In the arterial circulation, 100 ml of blood carries about 19·8 ml of oxygen combined with haemoglobin, while a small amount (0·3 ml) of oxygen is also carried in solution in the plasma. Although this latter quantity is not large its importance is great, because it is via this pathway that the oxygen passes to and from the haemoglobin and so reaches the tissues.

The percentage saturation of haemoglobin with oxygen depends largely on the tension of oxygen in the blood. An increase in oxygen tension results in a rise in the amount of oxygen carried by the haemoglobin, but the relationship is not linear as it is with the oxygen in solution in the plasma. The graph obtained is expressed as the *oxygen dissociation curve* (Fig. 1). This dissociation curve of haemoglobin is of particular importance to anaesthetists because it is possible to vary the percentage of oxygen in the inspired mixtures of gases (thus altering the tension of oxygen, i.e. P_{O_2}) and so determine the oxygen saturation of the patient's blood. The peculiar S-shape of the curve has certain advantages for the patient. First, the tension of oxygen (P_{O_2}) in the arterial blood can fall from 95 mm Hg (12·7 kPa) to 80 mm Hg (10·7 kPa), as may happen with slight respiratory obstruction yet the haemoglobin of arterial blood remains virtually fully saturated (i.e. 97·0 per cent). In fact, the Po_2 has to fall to about 60 mm Hg (8·0 kPa) before cyanosis is visible and even then the arterial oxygen saturation is around 85 per cent. Secondly, at the beginning of the curve when the Po_2 is low in the tissues the haemoglobin readily gives up its oxygen content.

The small, but vital amount of oxygen (0·3 ml/100 ml blood) which is dissolved in the plasma does not have any such dissociation curve, for the oxygen content of plasma bears a direct linear relationship to the tension to which it is exposed. Thus, a patient breathing air will have an alveolar partial pressure of oxygen of 100 mm Hg (13·3 kPa), and this will give a 95–97 per cent saturation of the haemoglobin. The total oxygen content of 100 ml of blood is about 20·1 ml of which only 0·3 ml is carried by the plasma (Table 1).

4/TABLE 1
MEAN VALUES FOR OXYGEN IN BLOOD

	Arterial	Venous
Oxygen tension (Po_2) in mm Hg (kPa)	95 (12·7 kPa)	40 (5·3 kPa)
Oxygen dissolved in plasma (ml/100 ml blood)	0·3	0·12
Total oxygen content (ml/100 ml blood)	20·3	15·5
Total oxygen carried by haemoglobin (ml/100 ml blood)	20	15·4
Per cent saturation of haemoglobin	97	75

(Adapted from Comroe et al., 1962)

Increasing the arterial tension of oxygen to 300 mm Hg (40 kPa) will raise the haemoglobin saturation to virtually complete saturation (i.e. 100 per cent). Such a tension, though leading to an almost negligible increase in the amount actually carried by the haemoglobin, causes a threefold rise in the quantity dissolved in the plasma. This amount is directly proportional to the partial pressure no matter how high the Po_2 rises, i.e. an increase of 0·003 ml O_2 100 ml blood for each mm Hg rise in partial pressure.

The exact degree of saturation achieved with a given tension of oxygen can be influenced by various factors. An increase in carbon dioxide tension shifts the curve to the right and a decrease, as in hyperventilation, to the left. Similarly, variations in temperature and pH can influence the oxygen dissociation curve (see p. 151). Oxygen saturation can be measured by means of an oximeter.

At normal rates of metabolism the body tissues remove about 5 ml of oxygen from every 100 ml of blood. When a subject is exposed to 2·3 atmospheres of oxygen, sufficient oxygen is dissolved in the plasma to supply all the tissue requirements without the presence of haemoglobin being necessary.

OXYGEN LACK

The failure of the tissues to receive adequate quantities of oxygen is variously described as anoxia, hypoxia, or oxygen lack, but strictly interpreted anoxia means *total* lack of oxygen. The lack of oxygen represents a severe hazard to the tissues and has been aptly described by Haldane as causing "not only stoppage of the machine, but also total ruin of the supposed machinery." Under ordinary conditions the body has certain regulatory mechanisms which prevent the tissues from suffering oxygen deprivation, but during the course of anaesthesia oxygen lack may become a factor of prime importance. There are four main types of hypoxia that may occur, viz. (1) Anoxic, (2) Anaemic, (3) Stagnant, (4) Histotoxic.

1. Anoxic Hypoxia

The haemoglobin is insufficiently oxygenated in the lungs. During anaesthesia the simplest cause of anoxic hypoxia is a failure to administer a sufficient percentage of oxygen in the inspired air. Usually it is inadvisable to use less than 30 per cent oxygen from the anaesthetic machine, since the actual concentration inspired by the patient after mixing with expired gases may be much less. Hypoxia is frequently caused by mechanical factors, such as laryngeal spasm, simple obstruction to the airway by the tongue, or the presence of foreign material like blood, vomit, mucus and sputum, and partial respiratory paralysis. Shallow breathing or periods of apnoea also influence the oxygen saturation of blood. Moreover, collapse of part of a lung may lead to oxygen lack. In all these instances prevention is the best form of cure, and no amount of oxygen therapy is likely to cure the hypoxia until the primary cause has been removed.

Another common cause of anoxic hypoxia is the administration of a "gas", or nitrous oxide anaesthesia. Opinion is sharply divided as to how much of the unconsciousness produced is simply due to hypoxia and how much to the anaesthetic properties of nitrous oxide. During a rapid induction in an unpremedicated patient it would seem highly probable that the speed at which unconsciousness is reached is closely related to the degree of oxygen deprivation (see Nitrous Oxide).

During thoracic anaesthesia it is often necessary to place a "blocker" or balloon in one of the main bronchi to prevent secretions leaking out and flowing over to the other side. It should be remembered that whilst the balloon is in position, and until the affected lung has been allowed to collapse fully by opening the pleural cavity, about half the cardiac output is passing through that lung. A period of half to one hour may pass during which it is found to be increasingly difficult to keep the patient well oxygenated unless the percentage inspired is increased. On opening the pleural cavity the lung collapses readily on handling and a rapid improvement in the patient's oxygenation is often noted. The exact mechanism of the transfer of gases in a lung shut off from the atmosphere by a blocker is not sufficiently understood, but this cause of hypoxia can be largely offset by filling the patient's lungs with a high percentage of oxygen before the blocker is placed in position (see Chapter 12).

Diffusion hypoxia.—Fink (1955) has drawn attention to a mild condition of anoxic hypoxia that may occur in the immediate period following a long anaesthesia with nitrous oxide and oxygen and which is due to the outward diffusion of nitrous oxide from the pulmonary blood lowering the alveolar partial pressure of oxygen in the inhaled air. He has measured the arterial oxygen saturation on such occasions and finds that it may fall 5 to 10 per cent, often reaching values below 90 per cent. Although this type of hypoxia is rarely severe and can be simply prevented by administering oxygen to a patient for five to ten minutes from the time that anaesthesia ceases, its clinical significance may well be important, since it could account for occasional mishaps in ill patients.

2. Anaemic Hypoxia

When there is a reduction in the oxygen-carrying power of the blood, then anaemic hypoxia may result. It occurs either because there is insufficient haemoglobin in the blood or because some of the haemoglobin has been modified so that it can no longer transport oxygen. Lack of haemoglobin occurs in many chronic disease states, and particularly in the presence of infections, haemorrhage, and carcinomata, but during surgery the primary cause is blood loss. Anaemic hypoxia is characterised by a fall in the oxygen capacity of arterial blood.

Methaemoglobinaemia and Sulphaemoglobinaemia

Characteristically the cyanosis (due to the presence of either methaemoglobin or sulphaemoglobin in the blood) is unaccompanied by evidence of cardiac or respiratory abnormalities. In severe cases there may be symptoms and signs of hypoxaemia such as headache, tiredness, dizziness, dyspnoea, tachycardia and in chronic cases of polycythaemia. The condition can prove fatal.

Methaemoglobinaemia is the commonest of the two conditions and may be either *inherited* or *acquired*. The latter can be caused by a number of drugs and chemicals such as nitrites, nitrates (which are converted to nitrites in the gut) phenacetin, acetanilide, sulphanilamide and prilocaine (Citanest). Sulphaemoglobinaemia may be produced by most of the compounds that cause methaemoglobinaemia and the two conditions frequently coexist.

Methaemoglobin (Hb Fe^{+++} OH) is produced in small quantities by oxidation of the ferrous porphyrin complex, but, under normal circumstances, this ferric form is promptly reduced, thereby keeping the level of methaemoglobin in the blood at a low level. Coal-tar derivatives and other substances (mentioned above) interfere with this process and allow methaemoglobin to accumulate.

Methaemoglobinaemia gives a chocolate-brown appearance whereas sulphaemoglobinaemia produces a cyanotic tinge which is sometimes described as leaden-blue or mauve-lavender. The principal reason for attempting to distinguish between these two conditions (i.e. different wavelengths of their respective absorption spectra) is that methaemoglobinaemia can be treated whereas sulphaemoglobinaemia cannot. There are no known measures which will convert sulphaemoglobin to haemoglobin, though concentrations of sulphaemoglobin sufficient to endanger life do not seem to occur.

Treatment of methaemoglobinaemia.—The *inherited* form of methaemoglobinaemia can be successfully retarded by taking large doses of vitamin C (500 mg/diem) or oral methylene blue. The *acquired* form requires removal of the causative agent and, if necessary, the intravenous administration of 1 per cent methylene blue solution (1–2 mg/kg body weight) over a period of 5 minutes (Mahomedy *et al.*, 1975).

Carbon monoxide.—A further possible cause of anaemic hypoxia is the great affinity of haemoglobin for carbon monoxide, resulting in the formation of carboxyhaemoglobin. Although it is unlikely that a patient would require surgical intervention whilst suffering from acute carbon monoxide poisoning, it should be remembered that haemoglobin has about 300 times greater affinity for carbon monoxide than for oxygen and significant levels are found in cigarette smokers (see also Methaemoglobinaemia and Sulphaemoglobinaemia).

3. Stagnant Hypoxia

When both the cardiac output and the peripheral blood flow fall to a low level, the circulation through the tissues becomes too slow to meet the requirements of the cells for oxygen: the result is stagnant or ischaemic hypoxia. This type of hypoxia is most commonly seen in states of shock, trauma, and haemorrhage. It may be local or generalised. For example, during anaesthesia the lobe of an ear or the bed of the finger nail may be seen to look dusky or cyanosed, yet if they are squeezed and rubbed briskly, fresh oxygenated blood enters, giving a bright tinge to the colour of the skin. This local phenomenon is particularly well seen in cases with poor peripheral vasomotor control, and is also seen as a more generalised state in association with intense vasoconstriction at the end of a long and perhaps haemorrhagic operation, or as a compensatory measure in cases with a low cardiac output due to heart disease. The state of the peripheral circulation may be used as an index of the onset or degree of "shock".

In hypotensive anaesthesia combined with posture there is widespread vasodilatation with pooling of the blood in the most dependent parts. The large veins become distended with blood and these parts usually show some signs of stagnant hypoxia due to local pooling of the blood. In itself, this is not necessarily detrimental to the patient, but when the venous return is handicapped, the cardiac output falls.

4. Histotoxic Hypoxia

It is commonly believed that the production of unconsciousness by most anaesthetic drugs is due to depression of tissue oxidation by interference with the dehydrogenase systems (see Central Nervous System section). This has been considered as a form of histotoxic hypoxia, which is classically and most grossly typified by the effect of cyanide on the body. It also occurs in alcohol poisoning. In histotoxic hypoxia the blood does not unload oxygen during its passage through the tissues, since the cells are unable to utilise it. This condition, therefore, is characterised by a venous oxygen saturation higher than normal.

Cyanosis

The term indicates a bluish colour of the skin or mucous membranes which becomes evident when the absolute amount of reduced haemoglobin present in the blood is greater than 5 g per cent. In almost every case its onset is closely associated with that of hypoxia and in considering the possible causes the two conditions are best taken together (see Table 2). Cyanosis and hypoxia are not necessarily synonymous, however, and either condition can occur independently of the other, particularly during anaesthesia.

In polycythaemia, there may be a great increase in the number of red cells and consequently also in the total amount of reduced haemoglobin. When the level rises above 5 g per cent, cyanosis is present yet there is no hypoxia. Alternatively, in severe anaemia, hypoxia may be present without any cyanosis, because there is less than a total of 5·0 g per cent of reduced haemoglobin in the circulation. In patients with Fallot's tetralogy the chronic hypoxia leads to a compensatory polycythaemia, so that hypoxia and cyanosis are both present.

4/TABLE 2

HYPOXIA AND CYANOSIS

Possible Causes likely to be met by the Anaesthetist

---

1. Factors present before operation:
   (a) Lesions involving the respiratory tract
       Oedema of the glottis, e.g. Ludwig's angina, bilateral quinsy.
       Carcinoma of the larynx.
       Tracheal compression and stenosis.
       Foreign bodies in bronchus.
       Neoplasms in bronchial tree.
       Asthma and severe bronchitis.
       Pulmonary disease, e.g. tuberculosis, emphysema, fibrosis, etc.
       Space-occupying lesions of the chest wall.
       Air or fluid in the pleural space.
       Paresis of the muscles of respiration, e.g. poliomyelitis, myasthenia gravis, etc.
   (b) Lesions involving the circulation
       Cyanotic heart disease.
       Pulmonary oedema (e.g. mitral stenosis).
       Congestive cardiac failure.
       "Shock" states (e.g. blood loss; coronary thrombosis).
       Polycythaemia.

N.B. Methaemoglobin, sulphaemoglobin, and the injection of blue dyes give the appearance of cyanosis.

---

2. Factors developing during operation:
   (a) Lesions of the respiratory tract
       Inhalation of blood or vomit.
       Mucus or sputum.
       Laryngeal spasm.
       Insufficient oxygen in respired mixture.
       Inadequate ventilation due to paresis of respiratory muscles.
       Central respiratory depression.
       Collapse of trachea and bronchial bronchiolar spasm.
       Insertion of bronchial blocker.
   (b) Lesions of the circulation
       Stagnation of the peripheral circulation.
       Cardiac failure and pulmonary oedema.
       Injection of blue dye.

---

3. Factors developing after operation:
   (a) Lesions of the respiratory tract
       Tongue falling back and obstructing glottis.
       Inhalation of blood or vomit.
       Mucus or sputum.
       Laryngeal spasm.

Inadequate ventilation.
Pulmonary collapse.
Tracheal collapse.

(b) Lesions of the circulation
Cardiac failure and pulmonary oedema.
Peripheral circulatory failure.
Excessive transfusion therapy.

Comment

The preceding description is based on the old terminology outlined by Haldane (1926). Alternatively, Van Liere and Stickney (1963) have suggested that hypoxia should be considered in three parts, that is

Anoxic Hypoxia	= Gas Phase Hypoxia
Anaemic Hypoxia	= Fluid Phase (Constituents)
Stagnant Hypoxia	= Fluid Phase (Flow)
Histotoxic Hypoxia	= Tissue Phase Hypoxia

Hypoxia

The basis of this classification is that hypoxia caused by an alteration of the oxygen content in inspired gases is termed the *Gas* phase, that due to a factor concerning the blood is named the *Fluid* phase, and finally a cause arising in the tissues is labelled *Tissue* phase (for classification see Table 3).

4/TABLE 3
REVISED CLASSIFICATION OF HYPOXIA

Type		Principal lesion	Examples

GAS PHASE		Low F_IO_2	Altitude:
			    Hypoxic gas mixture
			    Diffusion (Fink)

		Low P_AO_2	Hypoventilation:
			    Polio
			    Polyneuritis
			    Muscle relaxant
			Consolidation:
			    Collapse

		Diffusion defect	R.D.S. Fibrosis
FLUID PHASE	Constituents	Anaemia Carboxyhaemoglobinaemia Methaemoglobinaemia	Various anaemias Carbon monoxide poisoning: car exhaust, smoking Prilocaine
	Flow	Low cardiac output R–L shunts	Cardiac failure Fallot's: V.S.D.
TISSUE PHASE		Inhibition of oxidative enzymes	Cyanide poisoning

Effect of Oxygen Lack

The physiological response to hypoxia.—The catalogue of responses to hypoxia is large and depends on the speed of occurrence and the severity. However, the response may be considered as *Direct* or *Indirect*.

The direct effects are principally upon the cardiorespiratory system, whilst the secondary effects are those due to failure within organs such as the brain, liver, kidney when the oxygen tension falls below a critical level.

Cardiac Response

The heart is an organ with a high oxygen consumption $(8-10 \text{ ml } O_2/100 \text{ g}^{-1}/\text{min})$ even at rest and is thus relatively hypoxic. To enable this organ to cope with increased oxygen demands in exercise, it is able to metabolise lactate. This is also a property which enables the heart to withstand hypoxia.

The normal response to hypoxia is a tachycardia, which will tend to obviate the peripheral effects of hypoxia by an increased cardiac output and oxygen carrying capacity.

The effect of hypoxia on the systemic vessels in the periphery is to dilate them, but this vasodilatation is partly offset by (1) increased catecholamine excretion and (2) carotid body stimulation. Kravec and his co-workers (1972) measured the systemic vascular response to hypoxia and found:—

	Control	Breathing 12–14 per cent O_2
Mean B.P. (mm Hg)	77 ± 10 (SD)	78 ± 8 *not significant*
Cardiac Output (l/min)	$5 \cdot 2 \pm 0 \cdot 8$	$6 \cdot 6 \pm 1 \cdot 6$ *significantly increased*
Systemic Resistance (dynes/cm^{-5})	1165 ± 211	996 ± 360 *significantly reduced*

Thus, in the early stages of hypoxia the increased cardiac output partly compensates for the reduced peripheral resistance, but as the hypoxia advances towards anoxia so the myocardial output fails and bradycardia and hypotension supervene.

The Respiratory Response

The most obvious response to hypoxia is hyperventilation due to peripheral chemoreceptor stimulation. Hyperventilation leads to a fall in $PaCO_2$, and

$$\text{Since } PAO_2 = P_1O_2 - \frac{PaCO_2}{R} \text{ (Simplified alveolar gas equation)}$$

a fall in the $PaCO_2$ will allow the alveolar oxygen tension (PAO_2) to rise. A higher alveolar oxygen tension will increase the saturation of pulmonary capillary blood.

Pulmonary Vascular Response

The changes which take place in the pulmonary vasculature in response to hypoxia are the least obvious. Pulmonary arterioles vasoconstrict in response to hypoxia. If the increase in cardiac output and hyperventilation are considered protective mechanisms, the action of the pulmonary vasculature seems paradoxical. It is thought that the response is an attempt to balance pulmonary blood flow from underventilated alveoli to those with adequate ventilation (see

Chapter 3, p. 128). However, in patients with intracardiac shunts, e.g. ventricular septal defects, hypoxia will cause a raised right ventricular pressure (due to pulmonary vasoconstriction) and possibly a right-to-left shunt with consequent arterial desaturation.

Secondary Effects on Other Organs

Cerebral function is a most sensitive indication of oxygen lack. Changes of mood occur and performance gradually deteriorates, culminating in loss of consciousness. In the EEG, slow waves of large amplitude are typical.

Hepatic cells, arranged in lobules with centrilobular (portal blood supply) and peripheral (systemic blood supply) show a characteristic pattern of disorder in hypoxic conditions. The centrilobular cells exhibit the first changes, being most remote from the systemic blood supply. In acute hypoxia, centrilobular necrosis is seen whilst in more chronic hypoxic states, a fibrosis develops.

The effect of hypoxia on the kidney is largely due to vascular reactions and intra-renal redistribution of blood flow. The kidney is the source of erythro-poietin which stimulates marrow formation of erythrocytes.

Acute Hypoxia in Man and Primates

The effects of brief, intense hypoxia have been studied in man by Billings and Ernsting (1974). Their subjects, breathing air, were rapidly decompressed from a simulated altitude of 2438 m (8000 ft) to between 10,000 and 12,000 m (40,000 ft). In 16 out of 72 decompressions the subjects lost consciousness. A plot of end-tidal PO_2 (approximating to alveolar PAO_2) of each subject against time produced a curve, and the area of the portion of that curve below 30 mm Hg (4 kPa) Po_2 was proportional to the severity of the period of hypoxia. It was also found that the area so described was proportional to the impairment of psychomotor performance (Ernsting, 1969).

If the area of severe hypoxia was in excess of 140 mm Hg (18·7 kPa) seconds (end-tidal PO_2 × time in seconds), then loss of consciousness could be expected (Fig. 2).

Ernsting (1975) describing experiments where baboons were exposed to square wave decompression, concluded that permanent brain damage was unlikely to be produced if exposure was to altitudes between 9144 m (30,000 ft) and 11,278 m (37,000 ft). (The PO_2 at these altitudes correspond to 45 mm Hg (6·0 kPa) and 32 mm Hg (4·3 kPa) respectively).

The duration of exposure was terminated when the respiratory rate of the baboons fell to 4/min, which occurred after 10–16 minutes.

Post-operative Hypoxia

Since Nunn and Payne (1962) showed that post-operative hypoxaemia was an inevitable consequence of any form of anaesthesia, the precise cause of this defect has been sought. Whilst no single cause has been shown, many features have been demonstrated.

In nearly all instances of observed post-operative hypoxaemia, the $PaCO_2$ level has been within normal limits, eliminating hypoventilation as a cause. The possibility of atelectasis in the absence of an inert gas was excluded by Webb and Nunn (1967).

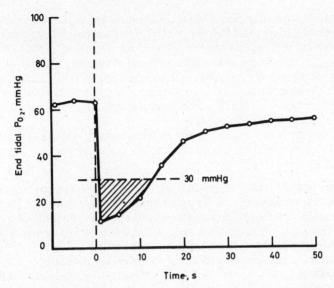

4/FIG. 2.—Method of quantifying intensity of hypoxia induced by rapid decompression. The hatched area represents the conditions where consciousness may be lost according to duration of exposure and depth of hypoxia, i.e. 1 second at Po_2 of 16 mm Hg (2·1 kPa) or 10 seconds at Po_2 of 21 mm Hg (2·8 kPa).

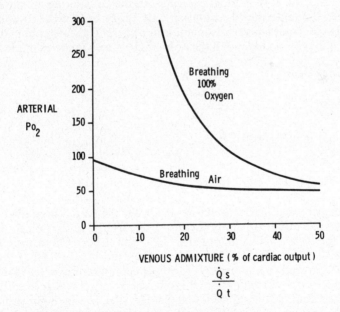

4/FIG. 3.—The effect of venous admixture due to anatomical (true) shunt (as opposed to $\dot{V}/\dot{Q}$ mismatch) on arterial Po_2 during air and oxygen breathing.

The site of operation has a marked effect on the degree of post-operative hypoxaemia (Diament and Palmer, 1967), upper abdominal surgery producing the greatest fall in oxygen tension. Spence and Alexander (1972) also showed hypoxaemia to be marked after upper abdominal surgery, but that this could be ameliorated by efficient pain relief with thoracic epidural blockade (Spence and Smith, 1971). They postulated a reduction of the functional residual capacity (FRC). Kitamura *et al.* (1972) considered the main defect to be an increase in the maldistribution of ventilation.

Whatever the cause of post-operative hypoxaemia, it is usually corrected by enrichment of the inspired oxygen concentration to 30 per cent (Conway and Payne, 1963).

Chronic oxygen lack.—A gradual decline in the oxygen tension of inspired air occurs most commonly on flying to high altitudes; this matter therefore is more naturally concerned with aviation medicine. As the altitude increases so the total atmospheric pressure is reduced and the partial pressure of oxygen declines proportionately. Thus:

At sea level—partial pressure of O_2 in air = 159 mm Hg (21·2 kPa)
At 10,000 ft   ,,   ,,   ,,   ,, = 110 mm Hg (14·7 kPa)
At 20,000 ft   ,,   ,,   ,,   ,, = 73 mm Hg (9·7 kPa)
At 50,000 ft   ,,   ,,   ,,   ,, = 18 mm Hg (2·4 kPa)

The tension of oxygen in arterial blood (P_{O_2}) is nearly identical with that in the alveoli. Unfortunately, the concentration of oxygen in the alveoli is not the same as that in air. The reasons for this are simple: oxygen is removed from the alveolar gases and carbon dioxide enters. All the air entering is fully saturated with water and under quiet ventilation only 14 per cent of the composition of the alveolar air comes directly from the atmosphere. The difference in the partial pressure of oxygen in air and in the alveoli is best seen in the example below:

Partial pressure of:

Air	*Alveolar air*
	O_2 = 103 mm Hg (13·7 kPa)
O_2 = 159 mm Hg (21·2 kPa)	CO_2 = 40 mm Hg (5·3 kPa)
N_2 = 601 mm Hg (80·1 kPa)	N_2 = 570 mm Hg (76·0 kPa)
	Water = 47 mm Hg (6·3 kPa)
Total = 760 mm Hg (101·3 kPa)	Total = 760 mm Hg (101·3 kPa)

The higher the altitude, therefore, the lower the partial pressure of oxygen in the alveoli and consequently the lower the arterial saturation of blood. At sea level the $P_{A\,O_2}$ is 100 mm Hg (13·3 kPa) and the arterial saturation 95 per cent: on rising to 10,000 feet (3048 metres) the $P_{A\,O_2}$ is 67 mm Hg (8·9 kPa) and the arterial saturation has dropped to 90 per cent, whereas at 30,000 feet (9144 metres) the $P_{A\,O_2}$ is 21 mm Hg (2·8 kPa) and the arterial oxygen saturation is only 20 per cent. Mountaineers and people who live at high altitudes can partially compensate for this lower arterial oxygen saturation by increasing the number of red blood cells in the circulation (compensatory polycythaemia).

A normal person loses consciousness when the arterial oxygen saturation falls to 50 per cent or below. Breathing air, this gives an upper ceiling of 23,000 feet (7010 metres), but if oxygen is substituted for air a height of 47,000 feet (14,326 metres) may be reached before unconsciousness ensues.

The various physiological changes that can be noted in a patient suffering from chronic hypoxia are:

(a) Decreased mental efficiency.

(b) Sleepiness, headache, lassitude and fatigue.

(c) Euphoria.

(d) Increased ventilation. Above 8000 feet (2438 metres) the arterial saturation falls to 93 per cent or less and this is sufficient to stimulate the chemoreceptors into activity leading to increased ventilation.

The persistent increase in pulmonary ventilation results in a reduction in the alveolar carbon dioxide tension. This respiratory alkalosis is partly compensated for by the kidneys which excrete more bicarbonate, so producing a metabolic acidosis.

The most significant instances of chronic oxygen lack are to be found in patients with severe lung or heart disease when there is interference with the oxygen transport mechanism.

Oxygen Excess (see also Chapter 5)

"Oxygen remains a fascinating paradox. Essential to mammalian life within a narrow spectrum of partial pressures, it is lethal at pressures outside that range" (Smith, 1975).

A considerable weight of evidence is accumulating to substantiate this statement. It has long been known that fit adults breathing pure oxygen can suffer toxic effects (Donald, 1947). Most of the effects described initially concerned the central nervous system. Then Nash et al. (1967) reported pulmonary lesions in patients undergoing IPPV with oxygen.

Clark et al. (1973) demonstrated the lethal nature of oxygen at 2 atm in dogs and Shields et al. (1975) showed this to be due to acute pulmonary oedema with cellular damage. Whilst Nash and his co-workers (1967) suggested that the pulmonary lesions were primarily due to a raised PaO_2, Penrod (1958) in an experiment on cats found otherwise. He cannulated each bronchus independently and ventilated one lung with oxygen and the other with an inert gas. Only the oxygen-ventilated lung showed pathological changes. Clearly, it is not the concentration of oxygen in the inspired mixture that is toxic, as spacemen have lived for prolonged periods in environments of pure oxygen, though being at a reduced pressure (Herlocher et al., 1964).

The cause of pulmonary oxygen toxicity is not yet elucidated but there is electron microscopic evidence of mitochondrial damage suggestive of enzyme malfunction (Clark and Lambertson, 1971a). Certainly surfactant production is impaired (Motlagh et al., 1969). The histological changes are not specific but are characterised by atelectasis, pulmonary capillary congestion, interstitial and alveolar oedema, capillary degeneration and haemorrhage.

Winter and Smith (1972) have summarised the cycle of events in lung damage following exposure to excessive oxygen fractions (see Chapter 5, Fig. 9). In normal human subjects, the onset of pulmonary changes may be inferred by estimation of changes in vital capacity after lengthening periods of exposure to oxygen at increased concentrations and pressures (Clark and Lambertson, 1971b).

When venous admixture exceeds about 30 per cent of the cardiac output, an increase in the inspired oxygen concentration has relatively little effect on the arterial Po_2, and a very high inspired oxygen concentration may make matters worse by producing toxic changes in the lungs.

Circulatory system.—In studies in volunteers breathing pure oxygen (Eggers et al., 1962) it has been shown that there is a slight fall in both heart rate and cardiac output during the inhalation. The most striking feature was the generalised increase in peripheral resistance and systemic pressure. The effects of oxygen inhalation on the general circulation have been likened to the effects of administering a peripheral vasoconstrictor, for the blood pressure goes up and the heart rate goes down. On this basis it is suggested that the slowing of the heart rate may be a reflex action following upon stimulation of the baroreceptors rather than any direct action on the chemoreceptors.

Blood.—Inhalation of 100 per cent oxygen for as long as three days has not been found to affect significantly the number of red or white cells, or the amount of haemoglobin (Comroe et al., 1945). Nevertheless, using the shorter life span of the red blood cell in sickle-cell anaemia and chronic haemolytic anaemia, Reinhard et al. (1944) and Tinsley et al. (1949) have clearly demonstrated that inhalations of a high concentration of oxygen will, within the safe period of administration, lower the red blood cell count in the peripheral blood. A decline in reticulocytes (young red cells) appears about the fourth or fifth day of oxygen therapy and is followed on the sixth or seventh day by the start of a fall in the number of red cells. In these patients a rise in the red cell count began about 48 hours after the cessation of oxygen therapy.

Elimination of nitrogen.—The inhalation of 100 per cent oxygen leads to a rapid fall in the nitrogen content of the arterial circulation so that the blood is almost completely cleared in a few minutes, but the loss from other tissues is more gradual. The brain takes 15–20 minutes before it is largely free of nitrogen. The cerebrospinal fluid clears relatively slowly, only 50 per cent leaving in the first hour, while fat tissues—with their poor blood supply—may take many hours before denitrogenation is complete. Oxygen inhalation may also be used to remove air from body cavities such as the gastro-intestinal tract and cerebral ventricles.

Other Effects of Oxygen Excess

Retrolental fibroplasia (see page 225 and Chapter 45, p. 1418 in Treatment of Respiratory Distress Syndrome).

Indications for Oxygen Therapy

Oxygen therapy is clearly indicated in the presence of acute cyanosis, yet it is well-known that the oxygen tension of arterial blood can fall to dangerously low levels without there being obvious changes in the colour of the skin. Nevertheless, during surgery observation of the shade of red exhibited by arterial blood will usually give a rough but valuable guide to the state of oxygenation of the patient.

It is often falsely assumed that the anaesthetised patient requires only the same percentage of oxygen as is present in air to maintain a normal arterial oxygen saturation. Recent work has shown that for a variety of reasons the anaesthetised patient requires *more* oxygen than the conscious patient breathing air (see Chapter 3).

Anaesthesia appears to increase the difficulty of maintaining the tissue oxygen tension for a number of reasons. First, the shunt in the pulmonary vessels is increased, so that a larger quantity than usual of the blood passing down the pulmonary arteries by-passes the alveoli and thus passes directly to the left side of the heart. Secondly, variations in the ventilation-perfusion ratio lead to an increasing degree of maldistribution of the blood and gas in the lungs so that they become less efficient as an oxygenator (see Chapter 3, p. 133). It seems that anaesthesia in some way interferes with the careful mechanism which normally ensures that the pulmonary blood flow passes to alveoli that are functioning, and vice versa. Thus, whereas in the normal conscious state only about 1–5 per cent of the blood entering the pulmonary arteries fails to be exposed to the alveolar gases, in the anaesthetised patient this figure may rise to as much as 10–15 per cent. To these two must be added the effect of hypoventilation due to respiratory depressant drugs. In these circumstances, the tissue oxygen tension can fall to very low levels.

Anaesthesia, however, does offer the patient some advantages as far as oxygen requirements are concerned. On the credit side the induction of unconsciousness depresses metabolism and this may lower the total body oxygen consumption by as much as 15–20 per cent. Hypothermia can increase this figure. Furthermore, if the patient breathes a mixture of nitrous oxide and oxygen the "diffusion effect" (see p. 322) *increases* the oxygen saturation of the blood during the period of *uptake* of the gas. Finally, if hyperventilation is used this can raise the alveolar oxygen tension just as hypoventilation can lower it.

The various factors influencing the tissue oxygen tension of the anaesthetised patient breathing an inhalational anaesthetic with 21 per cent oxygen (same as air) are summarised below (Table 4).

4/TABLE 4

SUMMARY OF FACTORS INFLUENCING OXYGEN TENSION OF TISSUES IN
ANAESTHETISED PATIENT

(a) Factors lowering oxygen tension.
   1. Pulmonary shunt.
   2. Maldistribution, i.e. alteration in the ventilation-perfusion ratio.
   3. Hypoventilation (if present).
   4. Reduction of cardiac output.

(b) Factors raising oxygen tension.
   1. Depression of metabolism.
   2. Diffusion effect.
   3. Hyperventilation.

The practical significance of all these various factors is best exemplified by referring to studies of the arterial oxygen saturation of a patient *spontaneously* breathing anaesthetic concentrations of halothane and air. It is found that the oxygen saturation in the arterial blood often falls below normal. For this reason the optimum concentration of oxygen in the inspired mixture for a patient under general anaesthesia is nearer 30 per cent than 20 per cent. A concentration of 33 per cent oxygen in the inspired gases will compensate for the detrimental effects of anaesthesia except in the presence of hypoventilation, severe anaemia, or a reduced cardiac output (see also Chapter 3).

So far only the anaesthetised patient has been considered, but it must be remembered that many of these factors persist for a number of hours after the anaesthetic has been withdrawn. During anaesthesia suboxygenation is unlikely to occur in skilled hands, but it can commonly be observed in the post-operative period. Several workers have demonstrated that nearly all patients undergoing general anaesthesia have a period of reduced oxygen saturation lasting for many hours after operation. In this period, hypoventilation is liable to play a much more important role and for the first quarter of an hour or so diffusion hypoxia (see pp. 146 and 322) will also work to the patient's disadvantage if nitrous oxide has been used.

Just how important changes in oxygen saturation of the blood are in the post-operative patient is not yet clear. Fortunately, owing to the shape of the oxygen dissociation curve, a large fall in the oxygen saturation of the blood is only reflected in a relatively small reduction in tissue oxygen tension (see Chapter 3, Fig. 10). Nevertheless, this dissociation curve has been likened to a precipice and once over the cliff edge it will be seen that both saturation and tension fall fast. In practice, once on the descent of the curve, for a given fall in tension there is now a very large fall in saturation (relative to what happens on the horizontal part of the curve). Clearly it is better for the patient to be kept on the plateau, well away from the dangerous cliff edge.

The importance of the oxygen saturation of the blood can be emphasised with a few simple examples. Assuming a cardiac output of 5 litres per minute, then with an arterial oxygen saturation of 100 per cent there is 1,000 ml of oxygen available to the tissues (100 ml of blood at 100 per cent saturation carries about 20 ml of oxygen). Thus, the tissues' oxygen requirements are covered fourfold. Even under conditions of hypoxia, when the arterial saturation may drop to 40 per cent, there will still be enough oxygen available for the tissues (e.g. 400 ml), but the gradient between the tension of oxygen in the plasma and that in the tissues may now be insufficient for the transfer process. For example, when the arterial saturation falls to 40 per cent the Pao_2 will be about 23 mm Hg (3·1 kPa); although the blood still contains adequate quantities of oxygen it is known that consciousness is lost when the Po_2 in the internal jugular vein falls below about 20 mm Hg (2·7 kPa). Nevertheless, even in these adverse circumstances the inhalation of 100 per cent oxygen will immediately raise the amount of oxygen available to the tissues above the danger level.

Effects of Oxygen Therapy

1. **Oxygen saturation of the blood.**—With the inhalation of air in a normal subject at sea level the tension of oxygen in the alveoli is about 104 mm Hg (13·8 kPa) and 100 mm Hg (13·3 kPa) in the arterial blood, giving a saturation of 95–97 per cent. If 100 per cent pure oxygen is now breathed the alveolar oxygen tension rises to 673 and the arterial tension to 640 with a saturation of 100 per cent.

Thus, breathing:

	Air	100 per cent oxygen
Alveolar Po_2 (mm Hg)	104	673
Arterial Po_2 (mm Hg)	100	640
Arterial O_2 per cent saturation	97	100

A study of these figures reveals a point of importance. Oxygen tension gives a far wider range and therefore a better indication of the state of oxygenation of the patient's blood than oxygen saturation.

2. **Carbon dioxide tension of the blood.**—Theoretically, breathing pure oxygen can interfere with the transport of carbon dioxide because reduced haemoglobin is a stronger base than oxyhaemoglobin, and therefore carries more carbon dioxide. This only becomes of practical importance when oxygen is breathed at high pressures. Nevertheless, in patients with diseased lung tissue in whom chronic hypoxia and a raised Pco_2 are present, the sudden inhalation of oxygen may lead to hypoventilation and a rise in carbon dioxide tension of the blood, due to removal of the hypoxic stimulus to the peripheral chemo-receptors.

3. **Ventilation.**—The clinical effects of breathing excess of oxygen have already been considered (p. 193). The immediate result of the inhalation of oxygen in normal man is a slight decrease in minute volume, lasting for a few minutes only. This is presumably due to the temporary reduction of stimuli reaching the respiratory centre from the carotid and aortic bodies. Following this slight reduction in ventilation there is an increase of approximately 10 per cent minute volume during the period of inhalation. The cause of this increase is unknown but it may be due either to oxygen acting as an irritant to the lower respiratory tract or to a local increase in the Pco_2 of cells in the respiratory centre, due either to vasoconstriction from the raised Po_2 or to the diminished amount of reduced haemoglobin available for the removal of carbon dioxide (Comroe et al., 1962).

In any consideration of oxygen therapy it is important to stress that occasionally it is possible to do more harm than good. This is most likely to occur in two principal situations. First, the patient with severe chronic bronchitis and emphysema who is admitted to hospital with cyanosis and respiratory failure. Secondly, the post-operative patient who has received large doses of respiratory depressant drugs. In both these instances respiration is probably largely maintained by the "anoxic drive" of the chemoreceptors of the carotid and aortic bodies. The sudden inhalation of a high concentration of oxygen leads to diminished ventilation with an increase in Pco_2 and a fall in Po_2. However, if a careful watch is undertaken to prevent underventilation, oxygen therapy can do no harm and may certainly do a lot of good, provided the concentration does not exceed 50 per cent.

4. **Blood volume and haemorrhage.**—The role of oxygen in the treatment of haemorrhage has been controversial (Wood et al., 1940; Frank and Fine, 1943). Freeman and Nunn (1963) demonstrated that oxygen has an important part

to play in patients with acute haemorrhage or a reduced blood volume. In such instances, the fall in cardiac output leads to a drop in peripheral blood flow. In turn, this leads to stagnant anoxia in the tissues and a metabolic acidosis develops. The increased acidity of the blood stimulates the respiratory centre and hyperventilation or "air hunger" develops.

Studies on dogs undergoing haemorrhage have revealed that raising the inspired oxygen from 21 per cent (air) to 30 per cent nearly halves the mortality (Freeman, 1962). One of the most remarkable features is that the physiological dead space in the haemorrhagic animal rises from a normal value of 30 per cent of the tidal volume to nearly 80 per cent. This must, of course, seriously reduce the effective alveolar ventilation.

The explanation of this reduction in effective alveolar ventilation probably lies in a fall in cardiac output and therefore of pulmonary blood flow. Under these conditions, it is possible to visualise that "only a thin trickle of blood passes through certain favoured alveoli leaving the rest ventilated but unperfused—a state which accords closely with the necropsy appearances" (Freeman and Nunn, 1963).

Anaesthesia or heavy sedation in the post-operative period may not only depress the activity of the respiratory centre and thus reduce the compensatory hyperventilation, but it may also lead to an increase in peripheral vasodilatation and a further reduction in cardiac output. For these reasons, there now seems to be good evidence for the administration of an increased percentage of oxygen to the patient with a reduced blood volume, though clearly adequate blood transfusion is most important.

(For details of Oxygen Toxicity see Chapter 5, p. 225).

Methods of Oxygen Therapy

Selection of equipment.—There are three principal types of apparatus available for oxygen therapy: face-masks, nasal catheters including spectacles, and oxygen tents. The selection of a particular piece of apparatus will depend on several factors. First, the concentration of oxygen required for the patient. In an emergency in an unconscious patient the only satisfactory way to give 100 per cent oxygen is to use intermittent positive-pressure ventilation with a mask, valve and a bag. Secondly, the equipment must be reliable. Many of the earlier models of plastic disposable masks did not mould accurately to the contours of the patient's face so that the concentration of oxygen varied greatly. Finally, comfort is an important factor in the conscious or semi-conscious patient. Humidity and flow rate influence the comfort of a particular mask.

General considerations.—During recent years great strides have been made in the design of equipment for oxygen therapy. The need for accuracy arose from the treatment of patients with chronic respiratory failure (e.g. severe bronchitis and emphysema). The sudden administration of a high inspired oxygen concentration removes the respiratory drive created largely by the low oxygen tension, ventilation becomes reduced and acute acidosis and carbon dioxide narcosis may follow. A small increase in inspired oxygen tension may have little in the way of a depressant effect on ventilation but at the same time produce a relatively large increase in arterial oxygen saturation due to the steepness of the oxygen dissociation curve at these levels of Po_2.

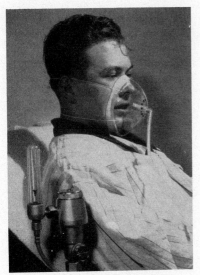

4/Fig. 4.—The "MC" mask.

Oxygen masks.—There are a great many available but only two of those in use are listed here.

"*MC*" *mask* (Fig. 4).—This is a disposable mask that is very suitable for patients in recovery areas. At gas flows of 4 litres/min an inspired concentration of approximately 45 per cent oxygen can be obtained.

"*Ventimask*" (Fig. 5).—This mask uses the venturi principle so that a low flow of oxygen can be used to draw in large quantities of air. The advantage of this principle is that it is not only economical with oxygen but it also permits accuracy in the concentration of oxygen delivered to the patient, even in the presence of a poorly fitting mask.

The mask is disposable and contains a single inlet tube. There are three types designed to give an under-mask concentration of either 24, 28, or 35 per cent oxygen in air.

Nasal catheters.—A size 9 rubber Jacques catheter, with two or three side holes cut in the terminal part to prevent all the flow of oxygen impinging on the same area of pharyngeal mucosa, is satisfactory for adults. It should be well-lubricated before use and inserted so that the tip lies in the oropharynx. Too deep insertion leads to gastric dilatation. Flows up to 3 litres/minute are well tolerated and give an inspired oxygen concentration of 27 per cent. Higher flows of 4–6 litres are often possible and give a concentration of between 30–40 per cent inspired oxygen (Miller, 1962).

4/Fig. 5.—The "Ventimask".

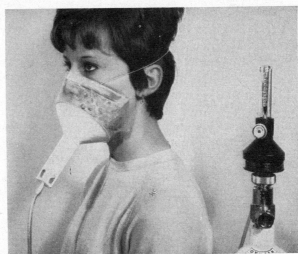

Comment

The performance of these devices for oxygen therapy has been assessed on "patient-model" devices (Bethune and Collis, 1967) and on patients (Leigh, 1970). The results emphasise the irregular performance of high-flow devices with regard to carbon dioxide accumulation, whilst the low-flow venturi devices provide inspired oxygen tensions close to the specification.

Oxygen tents.—A tent must be used when other methods of oxygen administration are impracticable. Such occasions arise when the patient is very young or incapable of tolerating a mask or catheter.

Hewer and Less (1957) have listed the essential components of a modern oxygen tent:

1. Positive ventilation of the atmosphere in the tent must be secured.
2. The temperature and humidity of the atmosphere in the tent must be amenable to regulation.
3. Carbon dioxide must not be allowed to accumulate within the tent.
4. Adequate provision must be made for nursing, flushing the tent, and sampling the internal atmosphere.
5. The materials from which the tent is made must be non-inflammable.
6. It must be possible to sterilise the interior of the tent.

The established design of an oxygen tent was re-examined by Wayne and Chamney (1967) who described an economical, efficient model which enables an oxygen concentration of 47 per cent to be achieved within the tent.

CARBON DIOXIDE (CO₂)

History

Carbon dioxide was first isolated by Black in 1757. Henry Hill Hickman (1800–1830) carried out experiments on animals with carbon dioxide, and he wrote a letter in 1824 on "Suspended Animation". A medal is awarded in commemoration of his work by the Royal Society of Medicine of London. The physiological significance of this gas was not fully appreciated until the work of Yandell Henderson in the United States (1925) and J. S. Haldane in England (1926). It soon gained widespread popularity amongst anaesthetists as a stimulus to respiration, but in more recent years the emphasis has been on its elimination rather than its addition in view of the high figures for carbon dioxide tensions in the blood that have been recorded with certain anaesthetic systems and techniques.

Preparation

In the laboratory.—The addition of any strong mineral acid to a carbonate or bicarbonate frees carbonic acid, which is an unstable, volatile substance. Thus it liberates its anhydride—carbon dioxide.

$$NaHCO_3 + HCl \rightarrow NaCl + H_2O + CO_2$$

| Sodium bicarbonate | Hydrochloric acid | Sodium chloride | Water | Carbon dioxide |

Commercially.—Carbon dioxide is a common by-product in the preparation of the alkaline earth oxides, notably calcium and magnesium, from their respective carbonates, and is also collected from fermentation vats in breweries:

$$\text{CaCO}_3 \quad \xrightarrow{\text{Heat}} \quad \text{CaO} \quad +\text{CO}_2$$

Calcium	Calcium	Carbon
carbonate	oxide	dioxide

Physical Properties

Carbon dioxide is a very stable substance, representing a minute proportion of the atmosphere—namely 0·03 per cent. It combines readily with water to form carbonic acid, the solubility diminishing as the temperature increases. The gas has a pungent odour which in high concentrations may be irritating to mucous membranes. The molecular weight is 44. On compression by a pressure of 50 atmospheres (5065 kPa) at 20° C it forms a colourless liquid and as such is stored in cylinders for medical use. The cylinders are coloured grey.

Inflammability

Carbon dioxide—in a concentration of 5 per cent—is very effective in reducing the range of inflammability of any mixtures of gases, because it possesses a high molar heat capacity. Charges of static electricity are more easily dissipated when the concentration of carbon dioxide in the atmosphere is 0·5 per cent or greater.

Pharmacological Actions

Carbon dioxide is a waste product of tissue metabolism. It is carried in the blood in three forms, namely in physical solution, combined with the protein in the red cell and plasma as carbamino-protein, and as bicarbonate in the plasma (see transport of carbon dioxide, p. 153).

Carbon Dioxide Excess

A high concentration of carbon dioxide can produce unconsciousness. After a few breaths of 40 per cent carbon dioxide with oxygen a patient will show many of the signs of anaesthesia. In psychiatric practice, a mixture of 50 per cent carbon dioxide with oxygen was sometimes used to produce a convulsion, as an alternative to electric shock treatment. It may well be that a high carbon dioxide tension in the blood is the reason why some patients with a "prolonged apnoea" do not recover consciousness during a period of inadequate artificial respiration without an anaesthetic mixture.

Respiratory effects.—When the concentration of carbon dioxide in the body is allowed to rise slowly (as in partial respiratory obstruction) the depth, and later the rate, of respiration is increased. The respiratory centre is stimulated both by a direct action of the gas and by changes in the pH of the blood. This latter mechanism can also activate the centre reflexly through the medium of the chemoreceptors in the carotid and aortic bodies and the central chemoreceptor on the ventrolateral surface of the medulla (see Chapter 3). High concentrations of carbon dioxide depress respiration.

The carbon dioxide tension of arterial blood is normally controlled within narrow limits even in the face of large increases in metabolic CO_2 production, for example during exercise. The mechanism whereby the control system achieves this remarkable stability of arterial P_{CO_2} remains a controversial subject.

Circulatory effects.—A rise in carbon dioxide tension leads to a rise in the systolic blood pressure with a complementary bradycardia, and an increase in the cardiac output and the blood flow through the brain and skin capillaries. The mechanism of the pressor response is believed to be both direct and reflex (chemoreceptor) stimulation of the vasomotor centre. High concentrations of carbon dioxide depress nervous conduction in the heart, particularly in the bundle of His, so that heart block and a slow ventricular rhythm are commonly observed with an increased myocardial irritability. A rise in the carbon dioxide level of the blood increases the excretion of catecholamines (principally noradrenaline) from the sympathetic nerve-endings within the myocardium. Thus, with most anaesthetic agents—principally cyclopropane and halothane—the higher the carbon dioxide level of the blood the greater is the chance of dysrhythmias. As both these agents are respiratory depressants hypoventilation bears a close correlation with the onset of ventricular arrhythmia. Furthermore, both these agents "sensitise" the myocardium to this increased catecholamine excretion so that clinically both improving ventilation and reducing the depth of anaesthesia will help to restore normal rhythm.

In dogs, dramatic changes in cardiac rhythm can be produced by a sudden termination of a period of hypercarbia. Severe dysrhythmias are observed if a vigorous attempt to lower the Pco_2 is made. Under the conditions of clinical anaesthesia in man there is no satisfactory evidence to support the view that a similar situation arises. In fact, it appears to be quite the contrary (Price, 1960) and it would appear to be both safe and advisable to remove the excess CO_2 from the body at a rapid rate, though care must be taken to monitor serum potassium (raised in acute hypercapnia and reduced in acute hypocapnia). Capillary dilatation in the tissues, together with hypertension, is the cause of increased oozing from excess carbon dioxide during an operation.

In a patient who is slowly recovering consciousness after an anaesthetic, the presence of partial respiratory obstruction or inadequate ventilation, with a consequent rise in the tension of carbon dioxide in the blood, may cause many of the signs just mentioned. To the untrained observer, the circulatory state of such a patient will seem satisfactory, as exemplified by a normal blood pressure and pulse rate. As time passes, however, the effects of the anaesthetic finally wear off and ventilation improves. The excess carbon dioxide is now rapidly removed and this stimulus to the vasomotor centre is no longer present. At this moment the patient may well pass into a state of apparent circulatory collapse, as the blood pressure falls to a low level. The heart rate may reflexly increase. Before the dangers of inadequate ventilation were fully appreciated, this form of post-operative circulatory collapse occurred relatively frequently. It was also sometimes associated with deep cyclopropane anaesthesia, when it certainly accounted for many cases of "cyclopropane shock" (see p. 253).

Use of Carbon Dioxide in Anaesthesia

For anaesthetic purposes a concentration of 5 per cent is usually sufficient to produce a temporary increase in the depth of respiration during induction with an irritant volatile agent such as ether. The mechanisms regulating the concentration of carbon dioxide in the blood are extremely sensitive, however, and the administration of anaesthetic and analgesic drugs can so depress the respiratory centre that it may no longer respond to even gross changes in the tension of the gas, and only be reflexly stimulated by the chemoreceptors. Morphine, pethidine and the barbiturates are most commonly responsible.

In the presence of respiratory depression, concentrations of carbon dioxide which are themselves depressant to the respiratory centre may accumulate. The opportunity for such an occurrence is very much increased in anaesthetic practice when patients are inadequately ventilated after the use of muscle relaxants or anaesthetised with unphysiological techniques. Pask (1955) has drawn attention to the potential danger of this combination of circumstances, and the culminating effect during the early post-operative period of slight respiratory obstruction—due perhaps to loss of tone in the muscles of the jaw and tongue—with a further rise in carbon dioxide. Tensions as high as 160 mm Hg (21·3 kPa) have been reported in partially paralysed patients during anaesthesia. On the other hand, with excessive hyperventilation and the use of carbon dioxide absorption techniques the tension of carbon dioxide may fall as low as 15–20 mm Hg (2·0–2·7 kPa).

Clinical Use

The most reasonable indication for the use of carbon dioxide occurs at the end of operation when it is desired to restart spontaneous respiration after a period of properly controlled respiration, which is normally maintained in part by moderate hyperventilation with temporary hypocapnia. Some patients with chronic bronchitis are especially likely to need carbon dioxide at this stage, as their respiratory centres are normally accustomed to a high tension of the gas.

The intermittent inhalation of carbon dioxide may be beneficial in the treatment of post-operative hiccup.

The inhalation of 5 per cent carbon dioxide has been used to produce cerebral vasodilatation during anaesthesia for carotid artery surgery.

HELIUM (He)

History

Helium was first noted by Lockyer and Eden in 1867 when examining the spectrum of the sun. It was isolated by Ramsay and Lockyer in 1895.

Preparation

The main source is from the abundant supplies of natural gas found in the United States, chiefly in Texas and Kansas. The other gases present are removed by absorption, liquefaction or scrubbing with water and sodium hydroxide. Helium is difficult to liquefy, so that when the temperature is lowered to $-195°$ C the other gases can easily be removed and helium remains as a gaseous residue.

Physical Properties

Helium is an inert, colourless, odourless gas. It is one of the "rare gases" present in air, the others being radon, argon, xenon and krypton. Apart from hydrogen, helium is the lightest known gas, with a molecular weight of 4 and specific gravity of 0·178 (air = 1). The oil/water solubility ratio is 0·187 at 37° C. It diffuses through skin and rubber.

Clinical Use

The therapeutic value of helium lies in its capacity to lower the specific gravity of any mixture of gases of which it forms a part. Thus in the presence of respiratory obstruction a helium-oxygen mixture may be of greater benefit than oxygen alone. Dean and Visscher (1941) have shown that factors other than density must be taken into account, such as the type of gas flow in the respiratory tract. In normal circumstances this is streamlined but if the speed of flow is increased, as is the case with any incomplete obstruction in the upper respiratory tract, a velocity is reached at which the flow becomes turbulent. The pressure required to move a streamlined gas flow is proportional to the rate of flow and the *viscosity* of the mixture. The viscosity of air is 1·00 compared with 1·11 for a mixture of 80 per cent helium and 20 per cent oxygen, so that air is best under such conditions. The pressure required to move a turbulent flow is proportional to the square of the rate of flow and to the *density* of the mixture. A mixture of 80 per cent helium and 20 per cent oxygen with a density of 0·33 is under these conditions better than air with a density of 1·00. Doll (1946) reviewing the therapeutic value of helium in the light of these facts, recommends this gas when respiratory obstruction exists in the larger air passages but presents evidence to show that in asthma—a disease of the smallest passages where air flow is not turbulent—it is unlikely to be of value.

The inhalation of a helium-oxygen mixture for a short period prior to the induction of anaesthesia in cases with upper respiratory obstruction, will considerably improve the arterial oxygen saturation and may enable a rapid intubation to be performed with safety. For such a purpose cylinders are available containing 79 per cent helium and 21 per cent oxygen. Alternatively, helium can with advantage be added to a mixture of inhalational gases to decrease the specific gravity of the anaesthetic mixture and increase the speed of induction for the patient when there is some obstruction in the upper respiratory tract. A mixture of 25 per cent oxygen, 15 per cent cyclopropane and 60 per cent helium has a specific gravity of 0·50, or half that of air.

PRINCIPLES OF GAS ANALYSIS

In anaesthetic practice a knowledge of the concentration of a gas such as oxygen, carbon dioxide, or nitrous oxide is often required for the satisfactory management of the patient. This information can be obtained in a variety of ways depending on the apparatus available. In general the methods available can be classified in three groups—first, those based on *chemical* analysis; second, those requiring *physical* measurement; and third, the use of a *specific electrode*.

Chemical Analysis

The principal methods require the absorption of a gas by a particular reagent. After the gas has been removed from the sample the volume change is measured. Under these conditions both the temperature and the pressure must be kept constant. Examples of this type of apparatus are the Haldane, Orsat-Henderson and Van Slyke (see Rebreathing Technique, p. 169). The Scholander micropipette analyser is based on the same principle but has the advantage that very small quantities of gas are required, yet accurate determinations of oxygen and carbon dioxide can be obtained.

A variation of this system is the manometric technique, where both the volume and the temperature are kept constant and variations in pressure can be measured by an apparatus such as that of Van Slyke and Niell. This type has the advantage of great accuracy and permits the determination of the pressure of gases in blood. Oxygen, for example, is absorbed by sodium hydrosulphite and carbon dioxide by sodium hydroxide. Nitrous oxide interferes with the estimation but allowance can be made for its presence. A micro-manometric modification of the Van Slyke method of analysis has been described by Natelson (1951).

Physical Analysis

In recent years such techniques have become more popular because of the introduction of electronics in medicine and also because the very small quantities required permit continuous gas analysis.

The principal methods employed are:

Magnetic.—Oxygen is a paramagnetic gas and will thus alter the magnetic flux existing between the poles of a permanent magnet. A small dumb-bell-shaped vessel containing nitrogen—a weakly diamagnetic gas—is suspended between the poles of the magnet. This dumb-bell will rotate in the presence of a paramagnetic gas such as oxygen to a degree proportional to the concentration of oxygen present. A mirror attached to the dumb-bell reflects a light beam which is displayed on a calibrated ground-glass screen.

A high degree of accuracy is obtainable.

Infra-red analyser.—A sample gas is compared continuously with a reference gas—usually carbon dioxide—for absorption of infra-red radiation. An infra-red radiator is "shone" through the sample and the reference cell alternately by means of a rotating shutter which "chops" the infra-red beam. The difference in the signal obtained from the detector when the beam is transmitted through the sample and the reference is a measure of the concentration of gas in the sample. The speed of rotation of the "chopper" determines the response time of the system. The response of the analyser should be sufficiently rapid to enable end-tidal analysis of each expiration to be seen. It should be noted that an infra-red analyser will not measure oxygen.

Gas chromatography.—The measurement of gases and vapours by the gas chromatograph has advanced considerably, but the basic technique remains the same in principle. Measurement of blood oxygen and carbon dioxide content may now be performed rapidly using this technique (Davies, 1970).

A column consisting of crushed firebrick or Celite (or Kieselguhr, a diatomaceous earth) is usually heated to $70°–100°$ C. A carrier gas, being hydrogen, nitrogen, helium, argon or carbon dioxide, is used to carry the constituents to be distinguished. Each constituent then separates in the column and arrives at the detector as a separate entity and is revealed as an individual response. The various substances are distinguished by the time taken following injection for the response to appear. The record is usually displayed on a pen recorder and the amount of each constituent represented as a peak height. More exactly, it is proportional to the area under the peak, and the output of the detector may be fed directly to an integrating amplifier and the result obtained as a digital print out.

The detectors in gas chromatographs are of three main types:

1. Hot wire (katharometer) which detects changes in the thermal conductivity of the carrier gas.

2. Gas density.

3. Ionisation

(i) Micro-argon using Sr^{90} as a radioactive source of β rays.

(ii) Electron capture, using Ni_{63} as a source of free electrons.

(iii) Flame ionisation. A hydrogen flame is the means whereby ions are formed. This type of detector is extremely sensitive to organic compounds.

Specific Electrodes

During recent years great progress has been made in the development of gas electrode systems so that these are now commercially available for oxygen, carbon dioxide and pH. For blood gas analysis several manufacturers now produce complete electrode systems. The analysis can be carried out on capillary tube blood samples, and some systems are self-calibrating.

1. **Oxygen electrode.**—The principle is that a platinum electrode is polarised from a mercury cell battery to about 650 mV. Oxygen molecules in the vicinity of the electrode (cathode) become polarised thus:

$$O_2 + 4e \rightarrow 2\,O^{--}$$

The ionised molecules may thus carry a current to a silver/silver chloride electrode of the opposite polarity (anode), the resulting current being proportional to the concentration of oxygen in the solution. The electrodes are separated from the blood sample by a semi-permeable membrane of polypropylene, and immersed in a solution of potassium chloride and phosphate buffer to minimise the effect of gases other than oxygen. Basically, the present-day model is a development of the original Clark electrode.

2. **Carbon dioxide electrode.**—The design and principle of this electrode has already been described (see Chapter 3, p. 169).

3. **pH electrode.**—Developments in this type of electrode have included the return to the use of capillary glass electrodes, with the sample inside the capillary to ensure anaerobic measurement.

Mass Spectrograph

This device is able to analyse the concentrations of respirable gases. There are two types:

1. *The Magnetic Mass Spectrograph*

This analyser ionises the gas mixture as it is introduced into a high-vacuum chamber where it is subjected to a high magnetic field. The arc of ionic deflection is specific for each ion. Detectors distinguish the concentration of different ionised gases.

2. *Quadropole Mass Spectrograph*

The gas particles are again ionised in a vacuum chamber but subjected to an electrical field within 4 rods. The precise nature of this field may be altered, but at any given frequency only ions of a single mass will move along the axis. It, in effect, acts as an ion filter.

The Fuel Cell

The fuel cell can be used to measure the concentration of oxygen by record-ing the electrical energy produced when oxygen is exposed to a fuel cell. One commercially available consists of a lead anode and gold cathode in caesium hydroxide. A teflon membrane allows oxygen to permeate into the cell where it is reduced to hydroxyl ions which, in turn, react with the lead anode. The potential thus produced is proportional to the oxygen tension.

LAPAROSCOPY

Laparoscopy is an increasingly used technique for examination of abdominal and pelvic viscera under direct vision. The abdomen is distended with gas, usually carbon dioxide, and the patient postured so that the free viscera fall from the field of view. In pelvic laparoscopy, the peritoneal cavity is filled with gas and the patient placed in a steep head-down position.

Clearly, spontaneous respiration by the patient is embarrassed to a con-siderable extent. The distending gas will tend to prevent descent of the dia-phragm and, in addition, the weight of viscera in the head-down position will lie against the diaphragm. It is these two aspects of the technique which have led workers to advocate controlled or assisted respiration (Desmond and Gordon, 1970).

The chief danger of filling the peritoneal cavity with gas is that this gas may inadvertently be introduced into the circulation. The effects of such a gas embolism will be less if the gas used is highly soluble in blood. In addition, since diathermy is often used during laparoscopy (e.g. laparoscopic sterilisation) the gas should not support combustion or make explosive mixtures with enteric gas (hydrogen and methane—Robinson et al., 1975). Carbon dioxide satisfies these requirements but can have dangerous effects upon the cardiovascular system (Arthure, 1970). Nitrous oxide has also been advocated (Corall et al., 1975), but because of its lower solubility and the theoretical ability to support combustion in the presence of diathermy, it will probably not find wide support (see Chapter 43).

REFERENCES

ARTHURE, H. (1970). Laparoscopy hazard. Brit. med. J., 4, 492.

BETHUNE, D. W., and COLLIS, J. M. (1967). The evaluation of oxygen masks: a mechanical method. Anaesthesia, 22, 43.

BILLINGS, C. E., and ERNSTING, J. (1974). Protection afforded by phased dilution oxygen equipment following rapid decompression—performance aspects. Aerospace Med., 45, 132.

CLARK, J. M., and LAMBERTSON, C. J. (1971a). Pulmonary oxygen toxicity. A review. Pharmacol. Rev., 23, 37.

CLARK, J. M., and LAMBERTSON, C. J. (1971b). Rate of development of pulmonary oxygen toxicity in man during oxygen breathing at 2·0 Atm. J. appl. Physiol., 30, 739.

CLARKE, G. M., SMITH, G., SANDISON, A. T., and LEDINGHAM, I. McA. (1973). Acute pulmonary oxygen toxicity in spontaneously breathing anaesthetized dogs. Amer. J. Physiol., 30, 739.

COMROE, J. H., Jr., and DRIPPS, R. D. (1950). Physiological Basis for Oxygen Therapy. Springfield, Ill.: Charles C. Thomas.

COMROE, J. H., Jr., DRIPPS, R. D., DUMKE, P. R., and DEMING, M. (1945). Oxygen toxicity. *J. Amer. med. Ass.*, **128**, 710.

COMROE, J. H., FORSTER, R. E., DUBOIS, A. B., BRISCOE, W. A., and CARLSEN, E. (1962). *The Lung. Clinical Physiology and Pulmonary Function Tests,* 2nd edit. Chicago: Year Book Medical Publishers.

CONWAY, C. M., and PAYNE, J. P. (1963). Post-operative hypoxaemia and oxygen therapy. *Brit. med. J.*, **1**, 844.

CONWAY, C. M., PAYNE, J. P., and TOMLIN, P. J. (1965). Arterial oxygen tensions of patients awaiting surgery. *Brit. J. Anaesth.*, **37**, 405.

CORALL, I. M., ELIAS, J. A., and STRUNIN, L. (1975). Laparoscopy explosion hazards with nitrous oxide. *Brit. med. J.*, **4**, 288.

COURNAND, A., RILEY, R. L., BRADLEY, S. E., BREED, E. S., NOBLE, R. P., LAWSON, M. D., GREGERSON, M. I., and RICHARDS, D. W. (1943). Studies of the circulation in clinical shock. *Surgery*, **13**, 964.

DAVIES, D. D. (1970). A method of gas chromatography for quantitative analysis of blood gases. *Brit. J. Anaesth.*, **42**, 19.

DEAN, R. B., and VISSCHER, M. B. (1941). The kinetics of lung ventilation. An evaluation of the viscous and elastic resistance to lung ventilation with particular reference to the effects of turbulence and the therapeutic use of helium. *Amer. J. Physiol.*, **134**, 450.

DESMOND, J., and GORDON, R. A. (1970). Ventilation in patients anaesthetised for laparoscopy. *Canad. Anaesth. Soc. J.*, **17**, 378.

DIAMENT, M. L., and PALMER, K. N. V. (1967). Venous-arterial pulmonary shunting as the principal cause of post-operative hypoxaemia. *Lancet*, **1**, 15.

DOLL, R. (1946). Helium in the treatment of asthma. *Thorax*, **1**, 30.

DONALD, K. W. (1947). Oxygen poisoning in man. *Brit. med. J.*, **1**, 667.

EGGERS, G. W. N., Jr., PALEY, H. W., LEONARD, J. J., and WARREN, J. V. (1962). Haemodynamic responses to oxygen breathing in man. *J. appl. Physiol.*, **17**, 75.

ERNSTING, J. (1965). The influence of alveolar nitrogen and environmental pressure on rate of gas absorption from non-ventilated lung. *Aerospace Med.*, **36**, 948.

ERNSTING, J. (1969). The prevention of hypoxia on rapid decompression to altitudes between 40,000 and 50,000 ft. in transport aircraft. *Proc. 41st Annual Meeting of Aerospace Med. Assn.*

ERNSTING, J. (1975). In: *Oxygen Measurements in Biology and Medicine*, p. 231. London: Butterworth & Co.

FINK, R. B. (1955). Diffusion anoxia. *Anesthesiology*, **16**, 511.

FRANK, H. A., and FINE, J. (1943). Traumatic shock, V. A study of the effects of oxygen on haemorrhagic shock. *J. clin. Invest.*, **22**, 305.

FREEMAN, J. (1962). Survival of bled dogs after halothane and ether anaesthesia. *Brit. J. Anaesth.*, **34**, 832.

FREEMAN, J. (1966). *Oxygen Measurements in Shock. Symposium on Oxygen Measurement in Blood and Tissues*, pp. 221–243. London: Churchill.

FREEMAN, J., and NUNN, J. F. (1963). Ventilation-perfusion relationships after haemorrhage. *Clin. Sci.*, **24**, 135.

GUESS, W. L., and STETSON, J. B. (1968). Tissue reactions to organotin-stabilized polyvinyl chloride catheters. *J. Amer. med. Ass.*, **204**, 580.

HALDANE, J. S. (1926). Some bearings of the physiology of respiration on the administration of anaesthetics. *Proc. roy. Soc. Med.*, **19**, Sect. of Anaesth., p. 33.

HENDERSON, Y. (1925). Physiological regulation of the acid-base balance of the blood and some related functions. *Physiol Rev.*, **5**, 131.

HERLOCHER, J. E., QUIGLEY, D. G., and BEHAR, V. S. (1964). Physiologic response to increased oxygen partial pressure. I. Clinical observations. *Aerospace Med.*, **35**, 613.

HEWER, C. L., and LEE, J. A. (1957). *Recent Advances in Anaesthesia and Analgesia*, 8th edit. London: J. & A. Churchill.

KITAMURA, H., SAWA, T., and IKEZONO, E. (1972). Postoperative hypoxaemia. *Anesthesiology*, **36**, 244.

KRAVEC, T. F., EGGERS, G. W. N. Jr., and KETTEL, L. J. (1972). Influence of patient age on forearm and systemic vascular response to hypoxaemia. *Clin. Sci.* **42**, 555.

LAVOISIER, A. L., and DE LA PLACE, P. S. (1780). Mémoire sur la chaleur. *Mém. prés Acad. Sci. (Paris)*, **94**, 355.

LEIGH, J. M. (1970). Variation in performance of oxygen therapy devices. *Anaesthesia*, **25**, 210.

MAHOMEDY, M. C., MAHOMEDY, Y. H., CANHAM, P. A. S., DOWNING, J. W., and JEAL, D. E. (1975). Methaemoglobinaemia following treatment dispensed by witch doctors. *Anaesthesia*, **30**, 190.

MICHAEL, E. L. (1960). Exposure to oxygen tension of 418 mm Hg for 168 hours. *Aerospace Med.*, **31**, 138.

MILLER, W. F. (1962). Oxygen therapy catheter, mask, hood and tent. *Anesthesiology*, **23**, 445.

MILLIKAN, G. A. (1942). Oximeter, instrument for measuring continuously oxygen saturation of arterial blood in man. *Rev. sci. Instrum.*, **13**, 434.

MOTLAGH, F. A., KAUFMAN, S. Z., and GUSTI, R. (1969). Electron microscopic appearance and surface tensions properties of the lungs ventilated with dry or humid air or oxygen. *Surg. Forum*, **20**, 219.

MOTLEY, H. L., COURNAND, A., WERKO, L., HIMMELSTEIN, A., and DRESDALE, D. (1947). The influence of short periods of induced acute anoxia upon pulmonary artery pressures in man. *Amer. J. Physiol.*, **150**, 315.

NASH, G., BLENNERHASSETT, J. B., and PONTOPPIDAN, H. (1967). Pulmonary lesions associated with oxygen therapy and artificial ventilation. *New Engl. J. Med.*, **276**, 368.

NATELSON, S. (1951). Routine use of ultra micro methods in the clinical laboratory. *Amer. J. clin. Path.*, **21**, 1153.

NUNN, J. F. (1965). Influence of age and other factors on hypoxaemia in the post-operative period. *Lancet*, **2**, 466.

NUNN, J. F., and PAYNE, J. P. (1962). Hypoxaemia after general anaesthesia. *Lancet*, **2**, 631.

PASK, E. A. (1955). Committee on deaths associated with anaesthesia. Review of cases where post-operative care was inadequate to meet the circumstances which arose. *Anaesthesia*, **10**, 4.

PENROD, K. E. (1958). Lung damage by oxygen using differential catheterisation. *Fed. Proc.*, **17**, 123.

PRICE, H. L. (1960). Effects of carbon dioxide on the cardiovascular system. *Anesthesiology*, **21**, 652.

PRIESTLEY, J. (1777). *Experiments and Observations on Different Kinds of Air*. London.

RAINE, J., and BISHOP, J. M. (1963). Alveolar-arterial differences in oxygen tension and physiological dead space in normal man. *J. appl. Physiol.*, **18**, 284.

RAMSAY, —., and LOCKYER, J. N. (1895). L'hélium, élément terrestre. (Abstr.) *Rev. sci.*, **3**, 654.

REINHARD, E. H., MOORE, C. V., DUBACH, R., and WADE, L. J. (1944). Depressant effects of high concentrations of inspired oxygen in erythrocytogenesis. *J. clin. Invest.*, **23**, 682.

ROBINSON, J. S., THOMPSON, J. M., and WOOD, A. W. (1975). Laparoscopy explosion hazards with nitrous oxide. *Brit. med. J.*, **3**, 764.

ROSS, J. M., FAIRCHILD, H. M., WELDY, J., and GUYTON, A. C. (1962). Autoregulation of blood flow by oxygen lack. *Amer. J. Physiol.*, **202**, 21.

SÉGUIN, A., and LAVOISIER, A. L. (1789). Premier mémoire sur la respiration des animaux. *Mém. prés. Acad. Sci. (Paris)*, **103**, 566.

SHIELDS, T. G., SMITH, G., and LEDINGHAM, I. McA. (1975). Mechanisms of oxygen toxicity. *Brit. J. Anaesth.*, **47**, 904.

SMITH, G. (1975). (Editorial) Oxygen and the lung. *Brit. J. Anaesth.*, **47**, 645.

SPENCE, A. A., and ALEXANDER, J. (1972). Mechanisms of post-operative hypoxaemia. *Proc. roy. Soc. med.*, **65**, 12.

SPENCE, A. A., and SMITH, G. (1971). Post-operative analgesia and lung function: A comparison of morphine with extradural blockade. *Brit. J. Anaesth.*, **43**, 144.

STORSTEIN, O. (1952). Effect of pure oxygen breathing on circulation in anoxaemia in patients with lung and heart diseases and normal individuals subjected to experimental anoxaemia. *Acta med. scand.*, **142**, Suppl. 1, p. 269.

TINSLEY, J. C., Jr., MOORE, C. V., DUBACK, R., MINNICH, V., and GRINSTEIN, M. (1949). The role of oxygen in the regulation of erythropoiesis. Depression of the rate of delivery of new red cells to the blood by high concentrations of inspired oxygen. *J. clin. Invest.*, **28**, 1544.

VAN LIERE, E. J., and STICKNEY, J. C. (1963). *Hypoxia*. Chicago: Univ. of Chicago Press.

VON EULER, U. S., and LILJESTRAND, G. (1946). Observations on the pulmonary arterial blood pressure in the cat. *Acta physiol. scand.*, **12**, 301.

WAYNE, D. J. and CHAMNEY, A. R. (1967). A new oxygen tent. *Lancet*, **2**, 344.

WEBB, S. J. S., and NUNN, J. F. (1967). A comparison between the effects of nitrous oxide and nitrogen on arterial Po_2. *Anaesthesia*, **22**, 69.

WHITBY, L. E. H., and BRITTON, C. J. C. (1957). *Disorders of the Blood*, 8th edit. London: J. & A. Churchill.

WINTER, P. M., and SMITH, G. (1972). The toxicity of oxygen. *Anesthesiology*, **37**, 210.

WOOD, G. O., MASON, M. F., and BLALOCK, A. (1940). Studies on effects of inhalation of high concentrations of oxygen in experimental shock. *Surgery*, **8**, 247.

Chapter 5

HYPERBARIC PHYSIOLOGY AND MEDICINE

INTEREST in hyperbaric techniques stems from use in four areas of medical practice. It can be used to overcome or prevent certain types of hypoxia when conventional treatment has failed. Secondly, hyperbaric oxygen appears to augment the efficacy of radiotherapy in the management of certain tumours. Also, hyperbaric oxygen appears to have a place in the management of some infections. In addition there is currently considerable interest in the effects of high environmental pressures as in tunnel construction or deep water exploration.

In this chapter the fundamental principles of hyperbaric medicine will be discussed, the various dangers and complications due to exposure to a hyperbaric environment will be described and the indications for hyperbaric oxygenation enumerated.

Definition.—The scope of hyperbaric medicine embraces all those circumstances in which, either total environmental pressure is increased above that which obtains at sea level, or in which the partial pressure of inspired gases are increased by change in composition of the components of air breathed at sea level. This therefore includes oxygen inhalation using a mask at sea level, the use of a pressure chamber at sea level, and immersion in deep water. Oxygen therapy has been covered elsewhere in this book and will not be mentioned further here.

Physics and physiology.—At sea level the atmosphere exerts a pressure of 760 mm Hg (1 Atmosphere or 101·3 kPa). This pressure is referred to as one atmosphere absolute (1 AT.A). However, confusion arises because engineers insist on ignoring the 760 mm Hg (101·3 kPa) pressure of our own atmosphere and set their gauges to read zero. Thus, when working with a hyperbaric chamber, if the gauge reads 760 mm Hg (101·3 kPa) the pressure in reality is 1 Atmosphere at sea level + 1 Atmosphere (chamber pressure) i.e. 2 Atmospheres Absolute. As this terminology is so confusing only mm Hg and kPa pressures and Atmospheres Absolute will be used throughout this chapter.

In physical terms, compression or decompression of a given amount of gas basically does three things: it changes volume, it changes density, and it changes the partial pressures of constituent gases. Physiological responses and problems due to exposure to a hyperbaric environment stem directly from these physical changes and may be categorised and differentiated into complications due to the direct *physical effects* of pressure, and *secondary complications* due to abnormally high volumes of respiratory gases dissolved in the blood and tissues. The first of these physical effects is due to hydrostatic pressure, which, when associated with injury will be considered later under the broad heading of *Barotrauma*. The more elusive secondary reactions may be grouped together: a high inspired partial pressure of nitrogen is responsible for *Nitrogen Narcosis*, and *Decompression Sickness*; a high inspired partial pressure of oxygen has therapeutic applications and can in certain circumstances result in various forms of *Oxygen Toxicity*.

What happens then when man is placed in a compressed air environment? Both the soft tissues and the air cavities of the body must be considered. Soft tissues of the body behave as liquid and as such, are incompressible. The laws which apply to liquids can be applied to the tissues of the human body when subjected to an increase in environmental pressure as in a pressure chamber or with immersion in water. Gases in the cavities of the body obey the "gas laws", and of these Boyle's law is of fundamental importance. This law states that for a given quantity of gas whose temperature remains constant, the pressure varies inversely with volume. Put more simply this means that if the pressure of a given amount of gas is doubled, then it must be compressed to half its volume. These points are illustrated in Fig. 1 which represents the changes taking place

BOYLE'S LAW AND DIVING
PV = K

Depth	Diving Bell	Volume	Pressure		Gas	mm.Hg	kPa
AIR SEA	Diving Bell	1 vol	101 kPa	= 1 AT.A	O_2	150	20
					N_2	600	80
10 m		$\frac{1}{2}$ vol	203 kPa	= 2 AT.A	O_2	300	40
					N_2	1200	160
20 m		$\frac{1}{3}$ vol	304 kPa	= 3 AT.A	O_2	450	60
					N_2	1800	240
30 m		$\frac{1}{4}$ vol	405 kPa	= 4 AT.A	O_2	600	80
					N_2	2400	320
40 m		$\frac{1}{5}$ vol	507 kPa	= 5 AT.A	O_2	750	100
					N_2	3000	400
50 m		$\frac{1}{6}$ vol	608 kPa	= 6 AT.A	O_2	900	120
					N_2	3600	480

5/Fig. 1.—As the diving bell submerges ambient pressure increases and water rises within the bell reducing the volume of trapped air (Boyle's law) and increasing the partial pressures of oxygen and nitrogen (Dalton's law). Thus as pressure increases from 1 to 6 atmospheres absolute, air within the bell is compressed to 1/6th of its original volume, and partial pressures of oxygen and nitrogen are increased sixfold.

in an inverted bucket or diving bell pushed under water. At sea level the bucket contains a given mass of air which occupies the volume of the bell and exerts a pressure equal to the environment of 1 AT.A (101 kPa). If the bucket is now pushed down in water to a depth of 10 metres, the pressure inside the bucket is equal to that of the surrounding water which is 2 AT.A (202 kPa). The pressure has now been doubled and therefore the air within it must contract to half its volume. This is achieved by the water level rising halfway up inside the bucket. Similarly if the bucket is lowered to 30 metres, where the pressure is 4 AT.A (405 kPa), the air would be compressed to one-quarter of its original volume.

The air cavities of the body including respiratory passages, lungs, sinuses, middle ear and viscera are all subjected to changes in pressure as environmental pressure changes. As pressure increases either within the pressure chamber, or when submersed in water, the incompressible tissues take up the pressure of the environment but do not change their shape and are undistorted. This state, however, can only be upheld if the pressure within the air cavities of the body are also increased and equal to that of enclosing tissues. Within the pressure chamber, equalisation of pressure between gas cavities and surrounding tissue does not usually present difficulty; under water however, air must be supplied artificially by delivering compressed gas at a pressure equivalent to the water pressure at that depth. If this is not done two things may happen. If the surrounding tissues will allow it, the enclosing air may contract to meet the increasing pressure. Failing this, if the volume cannot be reduced the pressure will be unchanged and a pressure difference will build up between the air and the surrounding tissues. Barotrauma is the term used to describe tissue damage which may occur whenever pressure gradients exist between tissues.

Study of partial pressures of the gases within the inverted bucket will also serve to explain some of the *secondary complications* of increase in environmental pressure referred to above. These are also shown in Fig. 1. For example, in the inverted bucket at a depth of 30 metres, the partial pressure of oxygen has risen from 150 mm Hg (20 kPa) at sea level to 600 mm Hg (80 kPa). Pressure of nitrogen has increased from 600 mm Hg (80 kPa) at the surface to 2400 mm Hg (320 kPa) at 30 metres. Obviously, as a consequence of these greatly increased values of partial pressure, the amount of gas dissolved in body liquids will be proportionately increased.

Pulmonary Barotrauma

This condition is due to distortion of lung tissue which may occur during decompression either within a pressure chamber or during ascent in water. If during pressure reduction, there is any restriction or resistance to the release of air from the lungs, then as surrounding pressure falls, so the trapped air being unable to expand, will remain at a pressure above that of surrounding tissues. This excessive air-over-tissue pressure may expand the lungs and chest until the alveoli rupture and air escapes into the interstitial tissues, the pleural cavity, or into the circulation. Air may be trapped in this way in lung cysts, or by airway obstruction, bronchospasm, laryngospasm, or by breath holding. Sometimes air entering the pulmonary circulation through tears in lung tissue may pass to the left side of the heart to be distributed as arterial emboli.

Three clinical syndromes of pulmonary barotrauma, namely *pneumothorax*, *interstitial emphysema*, and *air embolism* can be recognised. Of these air embolism is by far the most serious. The clinical picture of air embolus depends on the final resting place of the offending bubble. The most serious sign is that of loss of consciousness immediately following decompression or soon after. Convulsions have occurred, and muscle paralysis and visual changes are also fairly common following air embolism. Any form of air embolism should respond to rapid recompression of the patient; the object being to reduce the volume of the embolism until it passes the point of obstruction or better, to redissolve the gas in the blood. Following resolution of symptoms, slow decompression is undertaken so that the bubbles will not form again. Schedules of treatment for these accidents have been published and are available in various forms as "Therapeutic Decompression Tables".

Pneumothorax or interstitial emphysema must be managed symptomatically. In the case of pneumothorax the air may be released by introducing a catheter into the pleural cavity and connecting it to some form of one-way valve, such as an underwater drain.

Interstitial emphysema is more difficult to manage by virtue of its position. Recompression will reduce the size of the trapped air but absorption of the gas from these sites is slow and sometimes other means for removal must be adopted. This may necessitate surgical intervention by direct cannulation of the air pockets.

Aural Barotrauma

Normally the Eustachian tube serves to equalise pressures between nasopharynx and middle ear. In healthy individuals the Eustachian tube opens during swallowing and this is quite sufficient to maintain the necessary pressure adjustments without conscious awareness. When the Eustachian tube fails to open freely a pressure gradient develops across the tympanic membrane when environmental pressure increases; this results in inward bulging of the membrane with stretching, pain, haemorrhage and ultimately perforation. It is recommended that unconscious or anaesthetised patients should have a preliminary myringotomy to obviate this problem before being subjected to changes in environmental pressure. Sometimes underwater swimmers wear tight-fitting rubber hoods or caps which trap air in the external auditory meatus. As the water pressure rises so the hood is pressed firmly against the ear until the contained air volume can shrink no further. Meanwhile, as environmental pressure increases, the pressure in the respiratory tract also increases. If the Eustachian tube opens this pressure may be passed to the middle ear resulting in the air pressure in the outer ear becoming relatively lower than the pressure in the middle ear. This results in outward bulging of the drum and the appearance of oedematous swelling of the linings of the external auditory meatue with blebs and large haemorrhagic blisters—a condition known as "reversed ear".

Respiratory Sinuses

The air-filled sinuses of the skull are normally connected by foramina to the nasopharynx. This allows pressure equilibrium to be maintained between them and the rest of the respiratory system. When one of these channels becomes blocked, for example by catarrhal swelling, polypi, or deviated septa, air cannot pass freely in or out. Should environmental pressure be increased in these circumstances then the pressure of the surrounding tissue will exceed that within the sinus, its lining will swell and the space may fill with transudate and blood.

Dental Problems

Small pockets of gas sometimes exist around the roots of teeth and are the result of fermentation. These being isolated, would, during compression, shrink and the space they occupy possibly fill with blood and transudate. On surfacing the bubble would expand resulting in an increase in pressure. The result is a severe toothache.

Gas in the Intestinal Tract

Usually gas in abdominal viscera does not present any problems with changes in environmental pressure. However, on occasions fermentation continues in the gut and this can produce abdominal distension, discomfort and painful flatulence. Some people are air swallowers, particularly when anxious, and on occasions this can produce difficulties when swallowed air expands producing extreme discomfort and inconvenience.

Pressure and Clothing

Pockets of compressed air trapped within clothing close to the skin of a patient or diver may produce a deep impression on the skin during exposure to high environmental pressure.

Consequences of High Inspired Partial Pressure

Nitrogen and Inert Gas Narcosis

It is now widely recognised that men and animals exposed to a hyperbaric environment of air will exhibit signs and symptoms of intoxication and narcosis. The occurrence of narcosis was first reported by Junod in 1835. He noted that when breathing compressed air "the function of the brain was activated, imagination was lively, thoughts had a peculiar charm, and, in some persons, symptoms of intoxication". Since that time many workers have confirmed these observations. In recent years, Cousteau in 1964, referred to it in an apt and descriptive way as "l'ivresse des grands profondeurs", ("the raptures of the deep"). In Britain divers refer to it less romantically as "The Narks".

The narcosis observed when breathing compressed air is not an isolated phenomenon. The noble so called "rare gases" cause the same signs and symptoms but vary in the narcotic effect. The cause of inert gas narcosis is complex and cannot be related to any one factor. Many attempts have been made to correlate the narcotic effects of the inert gases: helium, neon, argon, krypton and xenon, to their various physical properties such as lipid solubility, partition coefficients, molecular weight, absorption coefficients, thermodynamic activity, and the formation of clathrates. However, the best correlation is afforded by lipid solubility (Table 1). Thus xenon is an anaesthetic at atmospheric pressure, and krypton causes dizziness. Helium is a very weak narcotic and it is mainly for this reason that it is used for deep diving or deep pressure chamber work beyond 10 AT.A.

The narcosis observed when breathing compressed air is of particular relevance. Obviously medical personnel working in a hyperbaric chamber, compressed with air, would have their efficiency impaired if faced with some unusual or complicated clinical event. Also in deep-sea diving nitrogen narcosis is of considerable importance because it reduces the efficiency of the diver and can result in behaviour which is detrimental to safety. Sufficient is known about the responses of an average man to increasing inspired partial pressures of nitrogen, and it is possible to tabulate the sequence of events as follows: at a depth of 30–45 metres the atmospheric pressure is 4–5 AT.A and the inspired pressure of nitrogen will amount to 2500 mm Hg (333 kPa) with the result that euphoria, increasing self-confidence, and lightheadedness are noted. When depths of 60 to 75 metres are reached the atmospheric pressure is 8–9 AT.A, corresponding to an inspired nitrogen of about 5000 mm Hg (665 kPa). In this instance the power of concentration is considerably reduced and many mistakes are made in the performance of even simple tasks. There may be peripheral

5/TABLE 1

Correlation of narcotic potency of the inert gases with lipid solubility and other physical characteristics

Gas	Molecular weight	Sol. in lipid	Temp. °C	Oil–water sol. ratio	Relative narcotic potency
					(least narcotic)
He	4	0·015	37°	1·7	4·26
Ne	20	0·019	37·6°	2·07	3·58
H_2	2	0·036	37°	2·1	1·83
N_2	28	0·067	37°	5·2	1
A	40	0·14	37°	5·3	0·43
Kr	83·7	0·43	37°	9·6	0·14
Xe	131·3	1·7	37°	20·0	0·039
					(most narcotic)

numbness and tingling. Personal safety tends to be disregarded. At even greater depths of 90–115 metres with an atmospheric pressure of 12–13 AT.A— corresponding to an inspired nitrogen pressure of 10,000 mm Hg (1330 kPa)— many individuals may be approaching unconsciousness, although it is possible that some of the signs and symptoms are due to oxygen poisoning. The first quantitative evidence of nitrogen narcosis reported by Shilling and Willgrube (1937) perhaps serves to stress the dangers of compressed air narcosis in so far as operating room personnel and deep-sea divers are concerned.

Decompression Sickness ("Bends", "Chokes", "Diver's Palsy" or "Caisson Disease")

At sea level body tissues are normally in equilibrium or saturated with the nitrogen in atmospheric air at atmospheric pressure. When ambient pressure is raised, as in a pressure chamber or during deep-sea diving, greater amounts of gas dissolve in the tissues until, after some time, tissue saturation is attained at the higher inspired pressures. When pressure is reduced gas dissolved in the tissues must be carried by the blood to the lungs to be eliminated. Should decompression be too rapid, bubble formation may occur with relatively in-soluble nitrogen being the main constituent of the bubbles. The physiological basis of decompression sickness is the local release of nitrogen bubbles in the tissues and blood. The signs and symptoms will vary according to the extent and location of the bubbles. The term decompression sickness in practice refers only to those conditions which are the result of an excessively rapid reduction of environmental pressure and are caused by liberation of bubbles of gas from tissues and blood which have been supersaturated. This definition does not usually include those conditions which are caused mainly by the physical effect of gas expanding within a body cavity such as the lungs, and not actually dissolved in any tissue (barotrauma).

The early signs and symptoms of decompression sickness, the result of bubble formation, can be conveniently divided into two types.

Type 1.—This includes cases where pain is the only symptom, together with those showing cutaneous or lymphatic involvement either alone or with joint pain. Skin manifestations are usually preceded by intense itching localised in one or perhaps a number of areas asymmetrically distributed. Lymphatic occlusion may produce distal oedema for example in a painful limb. The skin distal to the obstruction may have the typical peau d'orange or pigskin appearance.

Type 2.—This category includes all cases of a more serious nature with central nervous and cardiopulmonary system involvement. The symptomatology may be multifocal and often unpredictable. The pulmonary manifestations sometimes known as the "Chokes" in traditional diving parlance, are probably the result of bubbles in pulmonary capillaries, and are usually evident at an early stage. Neurological upsets of many forms occur. Disturbances of cerebral function may account for almost any bizarre symptom or pattern of behaviour. Psychotic conditions have been simulated, but visual blurring, diplopia, scotomata, hemianopia, and migrainous headaches are commonly seen. Sometimes the clinical appearance suggests local involvement of the spinal cord with paralysis. Almost every possibility has been described. The effect on the legs, and consequently the gait, which may occur as a result of this condition, is referred to by divers as "The Staggers", and may be a disturbance of labyrinthine function with vertigo, nystagmus, nausea and vomiting.

Delayed Decompression Sickness

Aseptic necrosis of bone is considered to be a form of decompression sickness which does not occur in the acute stages, but only after a delay of many months. It is suggested that this condition, like the other lesions of decompression sickness, is the result of bubbles of nitrogen producing infarcts in bones. This may, in time, cause joint deformity and arthritic changes. Common sites of aseptic necrosis are the head of the femur, proximal or distal ends of the humerus, and proximal end of the tibia.

Prevention of Decompression Sickness

Decompression sickness can be almost completely avoided by the strict adherence to the rules which have been laid down to guide individuals working in a high pressure environment. The following factors are of importance:

1. **Limitation of pressure in the chamber.**—Since tissues can be moderately saturated with an inert gas without the formation of bubbles, it is possible to spend unlimited time in a chamber at 2 AT.A (200 kPa) without the need for slow decompression.

2. **Limitation of time.**—Experience with deep-sea diving has suggested that

when the time spent at a given atmospheric pressure is limited, then no decompression is necessary. The longer the period spent in a compressed environment the greater the problems of decompression.

3. **Limitation of rate of decompression.**—It is apparently safe to be decompressed rapidly to half the original working pressure, but a suitable pause must be made at this new pressure before further decompression is undertaken.

4. **Use of helium and oxygen mixtures.**—Substitution of helium for nitrogen as the inert gas eliminates the dangers of narcosis and also reduces the problems of decompression sickness. Helium also reduces the time required for decompression because it is only about one-half as soluble as nitrogen in the body, and in addition it diffuses out much more rapidly. Thus the amount of helium absorbed at a given time will be considerably less than nitrogen under the same conditions, and the rate of elimination will be faster.

5. **Oxygen decompression.**—It has already been stated that rapid decompression to half the original pressure can be achieved with safety. On reaching this stage, the time required at this new level can be shortened if the subject breathes oxygen. This ensures the maximum possible gradient between the nitrogen in the tissues and the zero level of nitrogen in the alveoli. This will speed the elimination of nitrogen and the decompression time will be shortened. In civil engineering practice involving tunnel work, workers may be frequently exposed to pressures in excess of 3 AT.A (300 kPa) for shift periods of up to 8 hours each. Here rigid adherence to decompression schedules is clearly of great importance.

HYPERBARIC OXYGEN

Physiology.—Much of the recent interest and the benefits of hyperbaric therapy follow from its effects on the absorption and transport of oxygen. The higher the PO_2 of the inspired gas, the higher the arterial PO_2 in an almost linear relationship. The higher the arterial PO_2, the higher the actual amount of oxygen carried in physical solution in arterial blood. However it should be noted that a high arterial oxygen level does not necessarily mean that tissue levels will be elevated; these depend on a number of other factors including the properties of haemoglobin, the cardiac output, regional tissue perfusion, and upon the diffusion of oxygen from capillaries into tissues.

Fresh air contains 20·93 per cent oxygen, the remainder being mainly nitrogen. At the sea-level barometric pressure of 760 mm Hg (101·3 kPa) the partial pressure of oxygen in inspired air is thus 158 mm Hg (21 kPa), which is 20·93 per cent of 760 mm Hg (101·3 kPa). When air is inspired it rapidly becomes saturated with water vapour at body temperature, and on entering the lungs mixes with alveolar gas which contains carbon dioxide; the water vapour and the carbon dioxide accounts for 47 mm Hg (6·3 kPa) and about 40 mm Hg (5·3 kPa) respectively of the total alveolar pressure, leaving 673 mm Hg (90 kPa) for the combined pressures of nitrogen and oxygen. When oxygen alone is inspired, nitrogen is displaced from the alveoli, leaving only the oxygen, water vapour and the carbon dioxide. The alveolar PO_2 then equals the total alveolar pressure minus the sum of the saturated water vapour pressure and the alveolar PCO_2. The alveolar oxygen pressures obtained when breathing oxygen at various ambient pressures can be readily calculated from the following formula:

$PAO_2 = PIO_2 - PH_2O - PACO_2$ where $PIO_2 = $ inspired partial pressure of oxygen and $PACO_2 = $ Alveolar partial pressure of CO_2 (usually 40 mm Hg or 5·3 kPa), $PH_2O = $ Alveolar pressure of water vapour (47 mm Hg or 6·3 kPa at 37° C).

Table 2 shows alveolar oxygen pressures calculated in this way for atmospheric pressures ranging from 1 to 6 atmospheres (100–600 kPa).

The alveolar PO_2 is the principal determinant of arterial PO_2, normally the difference between the two is small and is mainly due to venous admixture (see page 134).

5/TABLE 2

ALVEOLAR OXYGEN PRESSURES OBTAINABLE WITH OXYGEN ADMINISTRATION AT AMBIENT PRESSURES RANGING FROM 1–6 ATMOSPHERES (101·3–607·8 kPa)
(assuming body temperature 37° C and PA CO_2 40 mm Hg–5·3 kPa)

Ambient pressure		Alveolar PO_2	
AT.A	kPa	mm Hg	kPa
1	101·3	673	90
2	202·6	1433	191
3	303·9	2193	292
4	405·2	2953	393
5	506·5	3713	494
6	607·8	4473	595

Oxygen is carried in blood by chemical combination with haemoglobin, and in physical solution with plasma as dissolved oxygen (see page 182). One gram of haemoglobin combines with 1·34 ml of oxygen. Assuming a haemoglobin concentration of 14·6 grams per 100 ml of blood, the amount of oxygen which can be carried in the chemical combination with haemoglobin will be 19·6 ml per 100 ml of blood. When breathing air at atmospheric pressure, haemoglobin is only 97 per cent saturated with oxygen so only 19 ml of oxygen are carried per 100 ml of blood. In a healthy individual when 100 per cent oxygen is breathed at atmospheric pressure the haemoglobin becomes fully saturated.

The amount of physically dissolved oxygen is proportional to the partial pressure of oxygen in equilibrium with the blood no matter how high the oxygen pressure (Henry's Law) (i.e. 0·003 ml O_2/100 ml blood/mm Hg PO_2). When breathing room air at an alveolar PO_2 of 100 mm Hg (13·3 kPa) oxygen in physical solution mounts to 0·3 ml O_2 per 100 ml blood. If the PO_2 rose to 600 (80 kPa) (because the patient breathed a high oxygen mixture) the dissolved oxygen would be 1·8 ml; if a subject breathed O_2 at 3 AT.A (300 kPa), and the arterial PO_2 was 2000 mm Hg (266 kPa), the dissolved oxygen would be 6 ml O_2/100 ml blood (Table 3 and Fig. 2). In the latter case dissolved oxygen would be sufficient to supply all the oxygen required by a resting man and venous blood would return to the lungs with the haemoglobin still fully saturated.

Thus at normal atmospheric pressure the oxygen content of arterial blood is largely dependent on the haemoglobin content. When hyperbaric oxygen is inhaled the haemoglobin cannot increase its oxygen load because it is already

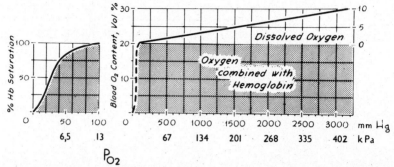

5/FIG. 2.—The oxygen content of blood when equilibrated with oxygen. From the standard oxygen dissociation curve on the left it can be seen that haemoglobin is almost fully saturated with oxygen when the Po_2 is 100 mm Hg (13 kPa). When the partial pressure is increased (right-hand graph) additional oxygen is carried in physical solution. At 3 atmospheres (304 kPa) oxygen, the pressure usually used in clinical hyperbaric chambers, an additional 6 ml oxygen/100 ml blood can be carried. From the graph it will be apparent that the amount of oxygen dissolved in plasma is very much less than that combined with haemoglobin, and that only a minor decrease in physically dissolved oxygen will reduce the Po_2 much more than a similar decrease in oxyhaemoglobin.

fully saturated, and, as the Po_2 rises, the oxygen content increases only by the carriage of additional oxygen as a simple solution in the plasma.

When an individual is breathing room air his oxygen stores are extremely limited and confined mainly to oxygen carried by haemoglobin and the small amount within the functional residual volume of the lungs. However oxygen stores are considerably increased when hyperbaric oxygen is given. At 3 AT.A (300 kPa) oxygen will be physically dissolved in body water to the extent of about 6 ml/100 ml. In a 70 kg adult with 50 litres body water this would create a potential oxygen reservoir of 6 × 500 = 3000 ml of oxygen. Such increases will theoretically allow tissues to survive temporary anoxia for much longer periods than are possible without hyperbaric oxygen.

It was stressed above that tissue oxygen levels depend not only on the arterial oxygen tension but also upon other factors which are responsible for oxygen delivery; these include haemoglobin, cardiac output and its distribution, and transfer factors. Hyperbaric oxygen may result in physiological adjustments which tend to offset increases in tissue oxygen levels. Cerebral blood vessels may constrict, for example, in response to changes in carbon dioxide transport thus limiting the increase in cerebral tissue oxygen tension.

Indications for Hyperbaric Oxygen

The indications and current status of hyperbaric oxygen are difficult to define, and it would be perhaps prudent to regard it for the present, as experimental. On theoretical grounds hyperbaric oxygen has much to offer in certain disease processes; however the nub of the matter and the therapeutic objective, is the restoration or elevation of the tension of the gas in the probable area of maximum cellular activity—that is in the mitochondria. It should not be presumed that tissue oxygen is commensurate with the inhaled or arterial oxygen levels. A variety of haemodynamic adjustments are possible which may limit increases in the tissue oxygen levels.

5/TABLE 3

OXYGEN LEVELS IN PLASMA OBTAINABLE WITH OXYGEN ADMINISTRATION AT AMBIENT
PRESSURES RANGING FROM 1–6 ATMOSPHERES (101·3–607·8 kPa)
(Assuming body temperature of 37° C, a PA CO_2 40 mm Hg [5·3 kPa] and a physiological
shunt of about 5 per cent cardiac output).

Ambient pressure			Approximate Arterial PO_2		Oxygen in simple solution
AT.A	kPa	%O_2	mm Hg	kPa	ml/100 plasma
1	101·3	20·93	100	20	0·3
1	101·3	100	600	80	1·8
2	202·6	100	1400	186	4·2
3	303·9	100	2000	268	6·0
4	405·2	100	2850	372	8·5
5	506·5	100	3650	485	11·0
6	607·8	100	4350	579	13·1

Clinical applications of hyperbaric oxygen today are confined to relatively unusual disease processes and include: carbon monoxide poisoning, gas gangrene, congenital cardiac anomalies, peripheral vascular insufficiencies and cancer therapy. Such limited application makes comparative scientific evaluation of hyperbaric oxygen difficult, and a great deal of work needs to be done to establish the benefits of the technique in relation to the conventional therapeutic regimes. A significant advance in hyperbaric oxygen would be the demonstration of its efficiency in the treatment of common diseases. Well controlled clinical trials of myocardial infarction or in the shock syndrome are currently being conducted in various centres throughout the world; their conclusions are awaited with interest.

The indications for hyperbaric oxygen may be classified in two groups according to their clinical application: current and possible.

CURRENT APPLICATIONS OF HYPERBARIC OXYGEN

Carbon Monoxide Poisoning

Carbon monoxide has considerably greater affinity for haemoglobin than oxygen; consequently exposure to even low concentrations of carbon monoxide rapidly leads to "anaemic hypoxaemia" because the gas interferes with the ability of haemoglobin to transport oxygen. Prompt institution of hyperbaric oxygen therapy has an important part to play in this condition. Oxygen at between 2 to 3 AT.A (200–300 kPa) alleviates the situation in three ways: first, it provides enough dissolved oxygen in the plasma to keep the patient alive. Secondly it moves the oxygen-haemoglobin dissociation curve to the right, thus enabling the remaining oxyhaemoglobin to give up more oxygen. Thirdly, it accelerates the rate of dissociation of carboxyhaemoglobin to twice that achieved by conventional treatment with 5 per cent CO_2 in O_2. Treatment should be continued until carboxyhaemoglobin is no longer detectable in the blood, by which time consciousness will return provided there has been no brain damage. Clearance time seems to be related to the period of exposure to carbon monoxide rather than to the blood level of carboxyhaemoglobin or the clinical condition of the patient. Although few people doubt the efficacy of hyperbaric oxygen treatment in CO poisoning, there is little evidence to support the fact that such therapy saves many lives.

Infections

It would seem reasonable to suspect that organisms such as *Clostridium welchii* and *Clostridium tetani*, which thrive under conditions of low oxygen level, might be adversely affected by hyperbaric oxygenation. In Clostridial gas gangrene hyperbaric oxygen therapy appears to have an established place. Hyperbaric oxygen appears to inhibit the growth of the causative organisms, thus allowing normal body responses to deal with the bacteria, and stops the production of the Clostridial alpha toxins. Van Zyl (1967) analysed results from world-wide reports of other workers on the use of hyperbaric oxygen in the management of 170 patients with histotoxic Clostridial infections. He compared these results with those obtained by conventional or traditional forms of therapy, including antibiotics, and concluded that high pressure oxygen eliminated the conventional requirements for urgent radical excision of infected tissue, and that after high pressure oxygen therapy subsequent tissue preservation was much greater than one would anticipate in patients who had been treated conservatively.

Although hyperbaric oxygen would seem to be logical in the treatment of tetanus, results have not been convincing. The total number of tetanus cases treated in which benefit has been claimed has been small, and in most the therapeutic effect of hyperbaric oxygen was masked by conventional therapy. Although hyperbaric oxygen therapy is unlikely to play a part in the treatment of established tetanus, it is possible it may find an adjunctive use in the early stages of the disease.

Certain aerobic organisms are known to be sensitive to hyperbaric oxygen; experimentally it is known to be effective against coagulase-positive staphlococci and *Pseudomonas pyocyaneus*. Clinically, the main benefit has been obtained in surface involvement, as in infected burns, leg ulcers, and areas of infected devitalised tissues such as pressure sores or amputation stumps.

Cancer Therapy

Hyperbaric oxygen appears to have a useful part to play in potentiation of radiation therapy for inoperable cancer. The rationale for the use of hyperbaric oxygen in radiotherapy depends upon the fact that the radiosensitivity of a normal cell rendered hypoxic declines to about one-third of its original levels. On the other hand hyperoxygenation of a normal cell produces only a relatively small increase in sensitivity. Tumor cells are frequently hypoxic and treatment with hyperbaric oxygen raises their oxygen tension, restoring their sensitivity to radiation. Churchill-Davidson et al. (1955) have reported good results with this therapy, and Siegel and Morton (1967) have commented favourably on its use with cytotoxic drugs.

Arterial Insufficiency

Tissues deprived of their blood supply either by trauma, embolism or thrombosis can be supported during the critical period in an attempt to diminish the area of anoxaemia and permit the improvement of collateral flow. Hyperbaric oxygen has been used in plastic surgery for the treatment of ischaemic pedical grafts (Perrins, 1966, 1967).

Decompression Sickness and Air Embolism

It is customary to treat decompression sickness by recompression in air and the details of recompression procedures are well documented (Lanphier, 1966). The purpose of recompression is to provide prompt and lasting relief of symptoms and signs in decompression sickness and air embolism. The recompression procedure is intended to reduce the size of the gas bubble rapidly and to ensure that no symptom-producing bubbles form upon subsequent decompression. The increase in pressure during recompression causes compression of bubbles according to Boyle's law. However, decrease in diameter of nitrogen bubbles with increasing pressure is disappointingly small (Fig. 3). Under normal

GAS VOLUME vs DIMENSION CHANGE WITH BOYLE'S LAW

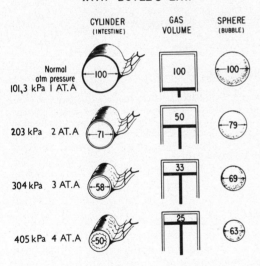

5/Fig. 3.—Change in diameter of gas bubbles of three different shapes with compression. The volume of each is progressively reduced as ambient pressure increases; however, reduction in diameter of cylindrical and spherical bubbles is disappointingly small, even negligible at higher pressures, and proportionately much less than the reduction in length of cylindrical bubbles.

conditions, any bubble containing normal atmospheric components tend to disappear by outward diffusion of gas. When tissues are super-saturated with gas this may no longer be true; the bubble may then grow by increasing diffusion of gas into it from surrounding tissues. To prevent this, the ambient pressure during treatment must at least equal the pressure of dissolved gas in the surroundings of the bubbles. The process of gas diffusion from bubbles may be slow and methods of speeding it up are desirable. Most effective is the administration of oxygen at increased pressure, preferably at about 3 AT.A.

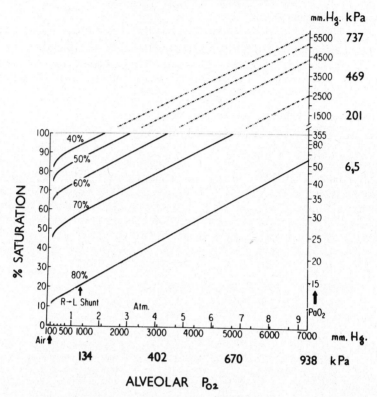

5/Fig. 4.—As physiological shunt increases (Q_s/Q_t) (diagonal lines), the effect of increasing the inspired oxygen tension (horizontal scale) upon the arterial oxygen tension or saturation (vertical scales) becomes less and less. At shunt fractions above 40 per cent the risk of oxygen toxicity must be carefully weighed against the small increase in Pao_2 as inspired oxygen is increased beyond 350 mm Hg (47 kPa). At a shunt of 80 per cent it is impossible to get a Pao_2 above 60 mm Hg (8 kPa) even with an alveolar Po_2 of 7000 mm Hg (930 kPa).

(This graph was computed assuming a blood pH of 7·4; a body temperature of 37° C, and an A–V O_2 difference of 6 volumes per cent.)

Possible Clinical Applications

The beneficial effect of hyperbaric oxygen therapy in hypoxia secondary to severe cardiac disease is obvious. During cardiac surgery hyperbaric oxygen will theoretically permit lower flows during cardiopulmonary bypass, will allow longer periods of circulatory arrest, and in addition will obviate the need for using red blood cells in the priming fluid of cardiopulmonary bypass pumps. Despite these theoretical benefits however, hyperbaric oxygen has not been adopted in current practice for this purpose.

The use of oxygen to correct arterial hypoxaemia due to increase in physiological shunt is well established. However it is important to realise that the increase in arterial oxygen tension for a given increase in alveolar oxygen tension decreases markedly as the shunt increases (Fig. 4). For high shunt fractions there is little increase in systemic oxygen as the fractional concentration of oxygen in inspired gas (FIO_2) increases; on the other hand even a small reduction in shunt fraction is associated with a considerable increase in systemic oxygen.

METHODS OF ADMINISTRATION OF HYPERBARIC OXYGEN

Two types of hyperbaric chamber are in use for hyperbaric oxygen administration. One is a single-person chamber in which only the patient is subjected to compression, and the staff remain outside (Figs. 5 and 6). Here the patient alone is exposed to oxygen.

The other is a large operating room pressure chamber enclosing both the patient and medical attendants. Large pressure chambers can be used for surgery (Fig. 7). The chamber is compressed with air which is breathed by the medical attendants, while the patient breathes 100 per cent oxygen at the same ambient pressure either from a mask or cuffed endotracheal tube according to the state of consciousness. In the conscious patient, the efficacy of oxygen administration is dependent on the efficiency of the oxygen supply system; here the fit of the mask to the patient's face is of prime importance. Any leakage around the mask will lead to a fall in inspired oxygen tension. Best results are obtained by administering oxygen using a close-fitting pilot's type face mask connected to a low-pressure demand regulator.

Basic Design Requirements of a Pressure Chamber

Five design features are important.

1. *Compressed air pump*.—Usually there are two. One pump is used for rapid compression, the other is used to maintain ventilation of the chamber once the requisite pressure has been reached. It is desirable that the compressors produce a steady rise of pressure within the chamber because this tends to reduce the incidence of painful effect of pressure changes on the middle ear and the skull sinuses. To avoid risk of explosion with high concentrations of oxygen the compressor pump must be oil-free.

2. *Climate control*.—There must be provision for heating, cooling and humidifying the air in the chamber.

3. *Electric equipment*.—All electric equipment within the chamber must be spark proof.

4. *Anaesthetic gases* and *oxygen* are best administered from cylinders stored within the chamber with facilities for spent gases to be vented.

5. *Sterile instruments*.—There must be some provision such as an air-lock for allowing instruments to be passed to and from the chamber.

OXYGEN TOXICITY

Oxygen toxicity is a complex phenomenon which, in spite of much investigation over many years, remains an enigma. Although it is possible that high oxygen tensions could affect many, if not all, organ systems, it would appear that certain systems are more susceptible than others. These are:

1. *Pulmonary toxicity*, which is the most prominent manifestation of oxygen overdosage seen in clinical practice (Lorrain-Smith Effect, Smith, 1899).

2. *Retrolental fibroplasia* in neonates.

3. *Hypoventilation*, seen in patients with chronic hypoxaemia and hypercarbia.

4. *Central nervous system oxygen toxicity* (Paul Bert Effect, Bert, 1878).

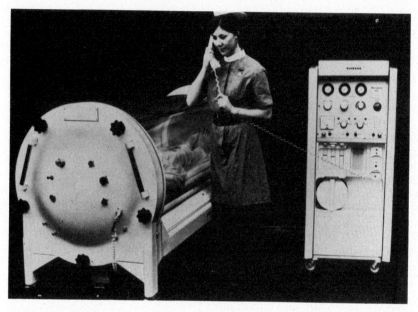

5/Fig. 5.—Single person transparent hyperbaric oxygen chamber (Vickers Ltd.). This general purpose model is designed to work at 3 atmospheres (304 kPa) pressure using recirculation with carbon dioxide absorption.

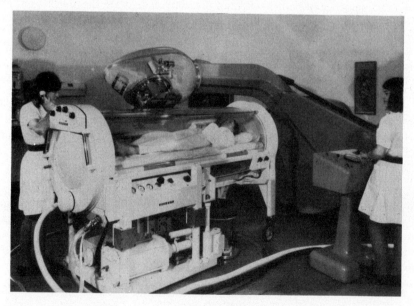

5/Fig. 6.—Hyperbaric system with cantilevered radiotherapy unit. Designed to work at 4 atmospheres pressure (405 kPa).

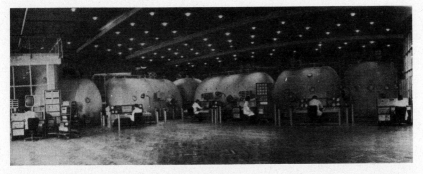

5/Fig. 7.—Hyperbaric facility at Research Institute of Clinical and Experimental Surgery in Moscow. This system consists of a series of interconnected hyperbaric chambers including entry locks, decompression chamber, group therapy chamber, operating theatre and experimental laboratory. Pressures range from 6–9 ats (608–912 kPa).

PULMONARY OXYGEN TOXICITY

The current clinical concept of oxygen toxicity has evolved from numerous observations in man and animals. With regard to pulmonary oxygen toxicity three clinically important generalisations may be justified from the many studies which have been done.

(a) There is at present no evidence that pulmonary oxygen toxicity develops in man at an inspired tension below about 0·5 atmospheres (51 kPa) even with prolonged exposure.

(b) There is no reliable data to support the contention that measurable toxicity can develop in man breathing oxygen for 24 hours or less.

(c) There is no evidence that patients with pre-existing pulmonary disease are more sensitive to oxygen than normal volunteers.

A pathologist, Lorrain-Smith (1899), was the first to carry out extensive investigations into the effects of increased oxygen tensions on the lungs of animals. He showed that oxygen was a lung irritant producing inflammation and congestion and that these effects occurred at a partial pressure of oxygen less than that required for the onset of convulsions. These findings, often referred to as the "Lorrain-Smith Effect", have been amplified by various workers in studies carried out usually within the range of 0·7 to 3·0 AT.A (70–304 kPa) oxygen; it is within this range that lung damage is the predominant sign of oxygen poisoning. At pressures less than 0·5 AT.A (51 kPa) oxygen, the damage occurs very slowly if at all, as mentioned above, and at pressures greater than 3·0 AT.A (304 kPa) oxygen, the problem is overshadowed by the signs of central nervous system toxicity.

In man, despite the ethical difficulty in organising detailed studies, there is now sufficient data to demonstrate unequivocally that pulmonary oxygen toxicity is a real entity. The rate of development and degree of damage to the lungs appears to be proportional both to the dose of oxygen and to the duration of exposure. Because it is impossible to do detailed examinations of the lungs of normal volunteers to determine the rate of onset and course of toxicity, indirect measures have been adopted. Many have used "onset of symptoms" to describe tolerance curves. The earliest symptom is often described as substernal distress which begins as a mild irritation in the area of the carina and may be accompanied by occasional coughing. If exposure continues, pain becomes more intense, and is exacerbated by coughing or deep breathing. Time to onset of symptoms varies inversely with the partial pressure of oxygen (Fig. 8). Because of wide variability in the onset of symptoms, more objective criteria have been sought as indicators of the onset of oxygen toxicity. Among these, reduction in vital capacity is perhaps the most sensitive. It has been shown that vital capacity is progressively reduced during inhalation of between 0·5–1·0 AT.A (51–100 kPa) oxygen by Comroe *et al.* (1945), and at 2·0 AT.A (200 kPa) by Clark and Lambertsen (1966). As toxicity progresses, other changes become measureable. Minute ventilation, respiratory rate, compliance, and blood/ gases all significantly deviate from normal as time passes.

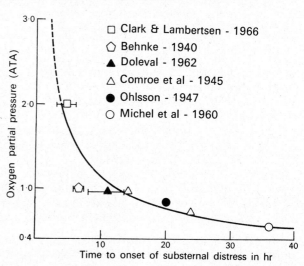

5/Fig. 8.—Time to onset of symptoms in normal volunteers.

Our understanding of the pathological changes of oxygen-poisoned lungs has been advanced considerably recently by application of histological techniques which enable quantification of lung damage, and in addition increasing application of electronmicroscopy has played a role. Although many of the changes described in detail refer to animal experiments, there is good reason to believe that the human lung behaves in a similar fashion when exposed to high oxygen tensions for sufficient periods of time. When monkeys are exposed to concentrations of between 90 to 100 per cent oxygen at 1 AT.A (100 kPa), the first change after a few days was slight swelling of endothelial cells, together with a small amount of interstitial oedema fluid. Following four days exposure, there was considerable destruction of alveolar cells, mainly of Type 1 (membranous pneumocytes). There was an increase in the thickness of the air-blood barrier, largely due to a 35 per cent increase in endothelial thickness and also an increase in the interstitial fluid volume (40 per cent of which was represented by an increase in oedematous tissues). After seven days, hyperplasia of Type 2 alveolar epithelial cells (granular pneumocytes) had led to a marked increase in alveolar thickness with almost complete destruction of Type 1 cells. The endo-thelium differed from region to region, with gross variations in thickness. At the end of twelve days, the proliferative changes seen in the granular pneumocytes were accentuated, which resulted in a further reduction in the alveolar spaces. The air-blood tissue barrier at the time was increased in thickness by approxi-mately 370 per cent. During these experiments half of the animals died of acute toxicity within 7 days of commencing the experiment, some survived beyond that time apparently having become adapted. Two animals were weaned back to ambient air and then sacrificed 56 and 84 days after completion of the experi-ment. In both, considerable chronic change in lung structure had occurred. Al-though there are differences in the pathological changes seen in the lung of various species of animals exposed to high oxygen tensions, certain changes appeared consistently and are summarised in Fig. 9.

Proposed Mechanisms of Oxygen Toxicity

Despite detailed documentation of the pathological effects induced by inhalation of oxygen, comparatively little progress has been made towards precise delineation of the mechanisms involved. A number of speculative hypotheses have been advanced regarding possible mechanisms, but supporting evidence is far from conclusive. These will be briefly discussed in turn.

Absorption Collapse

It has been suggested that a major cause of oxygen-induced pulmonary damage is simple atelectasis resulting from a blockage of the small airways, with resultant absorption of gases trapped peripheral to the obstruction. However, this hypothesis has been challenged on the grounds that histologically the sequence of events in the course of the development of lung damage was capillary congestion progressing later to alveolar exudation and damage, and finally to secondary changes such as atelectasis.

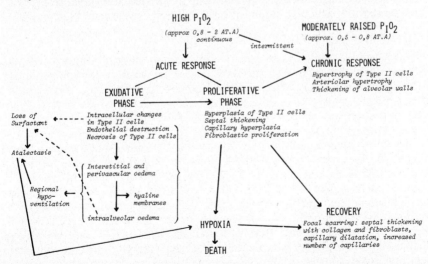

5/FIG. 9.—Diagrammatic representation of pathological responses of mammalian lung to oxygen.

While there is no doubt that collapse of lung is an important part of the clinical syndrome and sequelae of oxygen toxicity, it is not currently regarded as an initiating event. In clinical practice manoeuvres which ensure patency of the airways, such as physiotherapy of the chest, use of high tidal volumes, and techniques which increase the FRC by the use of positive end-expired pressures (PEEP) should receive particular attention.

Lung Surfactant

Alveoli have a natural tendency to collapse because of mechanical properties of lung tissue; this collapse is prevented by a lining of lipoprotein material about 50 Å thick (surfactant), which lowers the surface tension of the lungs, thereby stabilising the alveoli (Pattle, 1955, 1961 a and b, 1965). The low surface tension also prevents transudation from capillaries which would otherwise occur. Surface-active properties of the lipoprotein material is believed to be due to phospholipid dipalmityl lecithin (Brown, 1964). It follows from the above that if for any reason the amount of lung surfactant is decreased, the resultant rise in alveolar surface tension might be expected to bring about alveolar collapse and transudation. There have been many studies of the effect of oxygen at hyperbaric and atmospheric pressure on lung surfactant, some showing reduced surfactant activity, and others showing no effect. However, it is technically extremely difficult to obtain samples of lung extracts which give a true representation of the state of the surface tension of the fluid lining the alveoli. Although it seems certain that there are measurable changes in surface tension in the late stages of acute pulmonary oxygen toxicity, it is not clear whether these are the result of direct effects or indirect effects consequent upon mechanical changes induced by oxygen. Type 2 alveolar epithelial cells are thought to be the source of the surfactant.

In summary, the results obtained on the effects of oxygen on lung surfactant are inconclusive but sufficiently encouraging to warrant additional research on this subject with particular emphasis on improving experimental techniques.

Metabolic Upset

The possibility that oxygen toxicity is brought about by inhibition of enzyme systems vital to the metabolism has received ever increasing attention. Although there is great variability in enzymatic resistance to high levels of oxygen, many reactions are very sensitive and easily inactivated. Those which have received much attention are those containing SH groups, the sulphydryl enzymes. Several mechanisms for the oxidation of SH groups have been proposed, and it is not known which pathways are involved. It is possible that the inactivation of sulphydryl groups is brought about either by oxidation or by the formation of free radicals produced under hyperbaric conditions. Inactivation of SH enzymes can have profound effects at many sites of action. Several such enzymes are involved in the tricarboxylic acid cycle. An enzyme essential to glycolysis—glyceraldehyde phosphate dehydrogenase—is susceptible to oxygenation. In cellular respiration several flavo-proteins are particularly vulnerable, and Chance et al. (1965, 1966) have demonstrated that oxygen interferes with chain electron transportation systems (Fig. 10). Other investigations have demonstrated altered metabolism of glutamate and *GABA*, which may be fundamental

PATHWAYS OF FORWARD AND REVERSED ELECTRON TRANSFER

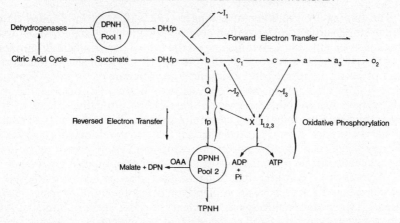

5/Fig. 10.—Schematic diagram of respiratory chain including reversed and forward pathways of electron transfer, with special emphasis on the possible site of action of hyperbaric oxygen (Chance *et al.*, 1966).

to the central nervous system effects of high-pressure oxygen (Fig. 11.)

Myocardial Failure

Experiments *in vivo* have revealed that myocardial metabolism may be depressed by oxygen. This prompts the question that heart failure may be responsible for the pulmonary oedema of pulmonary oxygen toxicity. However, although evidence for this hypothesis is conflicting, it would appear to be unlikely that myocardial failure *per se* makes an important contribution to acute pulmonary oxygen toxicity.

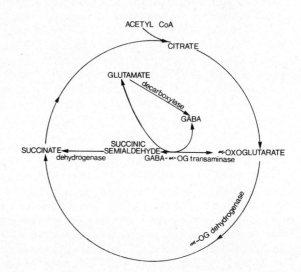

5/Fig. 11.—Metabolic reactions involving GABA and their relationship to the tricarboxylic acid cycle. Only the cycle intermediates relevant to the present discussion are shown.

Role of the Endocrine System

The finding by Faulkner and Binger (1927) that warm-blooded animals were more sensitive to oxygen than cold-blooded animals suggests that overall metabolic rate may exert an influence on the rate of development of pulmonary oxygen toxicity. Thus thyroxin or thyroid extract has been shown to hasten the onset of both convulsions and pulmonary oxygen damage in cats. Conversely, depression of metabolism by anaesthesia or hypothermia is associated with a reduction in susceptibility to oxygen. Part of the protective effects of hypo-physectomy against pulmonary oxygen toxicity may be related to a reduction in TSH secretions. Also it has been shown that the development of pulmonary damage is retarded by adrenalectomy, while conversely cortisone or similar adrenal corticoids increase the rate of development of pulmonary damage.

There is also considerable evidence that change in sympatho-adrenal medullary activity may exert an influence on development of oxygen toxicity in animals; sympathomimetic agents augment the onset of the pulmonary oxygen damage, whilst sympatholytic agents delay development.

CENTRAL NERVOUS SYSTEM TOXICITY

Paul Bert (1878) noted convulsions in animals exposed to oxygen pressures in excess of 3 AT.A (300 kPa), which he was able to demonstrate were due to the partial pressure of oxygen and not the total environmental pressure. Man also is subject to the convulsive effects of hyperbaric oxygen. Bornstein and Stroink (1912) reported muscle spasms in the legs with exercise after exposure for 50 minutes to oxygen at 3 AT.A (300 kPa).

These early findings have been amply confirmed and extended by others (Behnke *et al.* 1934–36), and our current understanding of the progressive nature of the clinical picture of oxygen poisoning is most aptly expressed by Lambertsen (1953) as follows:

"The convulsions are usually but not always preceded by the occurrence of localised muscular twitchings, especially about the eyes, mouth and forehead. Small muscles of the hand may be involved and inco-ordination of diaphragm activity in respiration may occur. These phenomena increase in severity over a period which may vary from a few minutes to nearly an hour with essentially clear consciousness being retained. Eventually an abrupt spread of excitation occurs and the rigid tonic phase of the convulsion begins. The tonic phase lasts for about 30 seconds and is accompanied by an abrupt loss of consciousness. Vigorous clonic contractions of the muscular groups of head and neck, trunk and limbs then occur becoming progressively less violent over about one minute."

Our current knowledge on the toxic neurological effects of hyberbaric oxygen is derived from the extensive study of Donald (1947). In Donald's studies, the time to onset of symptoms was used as a quantitative measure of susceptibility. The symptom usually noted was lip twitching, but in a few instances it was nausea, vertigo or convulsions. In these studies an extremely large variation in susceptibility, not only between individuals, but also in any one person from day to day was noted. Also onset of symptoms occurred consistently sooner when studies were done during exercise, and in studies done under water rather than in a dry chamber. In view of this work and studies done at the U.S. Navy Experimental Diving Unit it is now current practice to limit the depth at which oxygen diving is done to about 10 metres; and Lanphier (1955) has constructed an oxygen limit curve showing the underwater working limits (Fig. 12).

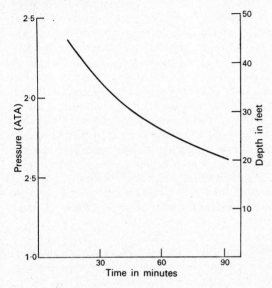

5/Fig. 12.—Oxygen limit curve for man (Lanphier, 1955).

In dry conditions when no exercise is being undertaken, and when medical personnel are in attendance, a more lenient attitude can be tolerated. During radiotherapy for cancer Foster and Churchill-Davidson (1976 personal communications) reported only six cases of convulsions in 2965 exposures to 3 AT.A (300 kPa) oxygen for periods lasting 20 to 66 minutes.

Diagnosis

The suddenness of onset of convulsions make the detection of the pre-convulsive state difficult. However, the pattern of the electro-encephalogram will reveal hyper-irritability prior to their onset and an electromyogram of the lip muscles has been used to detect the earliest signs of muscle twitching.

Treatment

Provided the high pressure of oxygen is immediately withdrawn and the patient allowed to breathe air (either at atmospheric pressure or above) the convulsions will cease and no permanent cerebral damage will result. The danger of oxygen convulsions *per se* lies in the possible injury to the individual during a spasm in a small chamber.

However, if the patient is lying in a small single chamber then rapid decompression is not always advisable because in the conscious state laryngeal spasm may develop during the convulsions and close the glottis. In this case, a sudden drop of environmental pressure would lead to a dangerously high pressure trapped within the lungs thus increasing the possible risk of rupture. If the patient continues to breathe spontaneously (denoting an open glottis) or there is an endotracheal tube *in situ* (as in the anaesthetised subject), then the dangers of rapid decompression under hyperbaric oxygen are minimal.

ANAESTHESIA IN A HYPERBARIC CHAMBER

Time is the factor which limits the period for which temporary occlusion of circulation to the vital organs is undertaken in certain cardiovascular and neurosurgical procedures. Extension of the time factor by hyperoxygenation prior to occlusion of circulation is one of the outstanding theoretical contributions of hyperbaric oxygen to surgery. These benefits may be augmented by hypothermia which favours oxygen solubility, and simultaneously reduces metabolic requirements. However, although early clinical experience with this technique in the surgery of congenital heart disease in infants was encouraging, development of satisfactory pump oxygenators specifically designed for infants have largely supplanted hyperbaric oxygen in cardiac surgery. Today there are probably few indications for anaesthesia under hyperbaric conditions, with a possible exception of deep-sea emergencies and radiotherapy; and even with regard to the latter, most patients tolerate the hyperbaric conditions required without need for anaesthesia. To cover the few remaining indications for providing anaesthesia under hyperbaric conditions, there is need to rehearse some of the problems involved.

Selection of Anaesthetic Agents

Where the main object of the hyperbaric chamber is to secure high tissue oxygen level, then obviously the anaesthetic technique must allow for an inspired oxygen level which is as high as possible. Nitrous oxide therefore has little place as an anaesthetic under these circumstances. Some form of intravenous anaesthesia with tracheal intubation and spontaneous breathing is suitable for those patients who need anaesthesia during radiotherapy in a single-subject chamber. For major surgery the use of a volatile agent such as halothane, vaporised by 100 per cent oxygen in association with controlled ventilation using non-rebreathing circuits, is probably the best. Expired gases should be led to the exhaust port of the chamber. The actual level of controlled ventilation is important; the aim is to ensure that arterial carbon dioxide tensions are maintained at about normal levels; in this way cerebral blood flow is maintained and hence cerebral oxygenation. Ether and cyclopropane are not used because of their inflammability. Halothane can under certain circumstances be inflammable, it is however safe when vaporised in 100 per cent oxygen below 4 atmospheres pressure (400 kPa).

Anaesthetic Equipment

In the pressure chamber.—Cylinders containing the gases used in anaesthesia are usually at a pressure high enough to function normally in a hyperbaric environment. Reducing valves, similarly, work normally provided the supply pressure is sufficiently high; this means that any gas piped to them from outside the chamber must have a higher pressure than usual pipeline pressure of 60 lb per sq inch (4·3 kPa).

Rotameters become inaccurate in the pressure chamber because of the gas density. At 2 AT.A (200 kPa) rotameters read about 30 per cent higher compared with readings from the same flows at 1 atmosphere (100 kPa). Because of these discrepancies, flow meters should be individually calibrated using a spirometer at the pressure at which the flow meter is used. Vaporisers of the "Fluotec" type should deliver the set concentration because the partial pressure of vapour in equilibrium with its liquid is proportional to the absolute temperature, and is not affected by total ambient pressure. In practice, however, it has been shown that individual vaporisers exhibit variation in the partial pressure of halothane delivered, probably due to change in the ratio of gas passing through the bypass and vaporising chambers. They tend to be accurate when the concentration setting is 2 per cent or above, but below this values tend to be high. Vaporisers, when not in use, should have their filler plug open during change in ambient pressure so as to avoid the danger of explosion. In some types of vaporiser liquid anaesthetic could be forced back up the inlet pipe during compression if appropriate precautions are not taken.

Changes in gas volume on compression or decompression necessitate a number of commonsense precautions. Cuffs on endotracheal tubes and intravenous and bladder catheters should be filled with water or saline to prevent large volume changes which would apply if they were filled with air. Similarly thoracotomy drainage tubes should be left open during decompression to avoid development of tension pneumothorax. Intragastric tubes should be left open. Intravenous transfusion may present problems because of expansion of air in the bottle; however, this may be prevented by the use of plastic infusion bottles. Multidose containers should have needles introduced through their tops to prevent pressure change of contents.

Electrically operated ventilators should not be used because of the potential fire hazard from sparking. Pressure operated ventilators are satisfactory, but those powered by compressed air from outside the chamber will require an increase of pipeline pressure for efficient operation. Oil and grease must be excluded absolutely from those parts of the respirator exposed to high-pressure oxygen because of the fire hazard.

Suction apparatus taken from a direct suction pipeline outside the chamber tends to operate excessively when the chamber is operating at high pressure because of the pressure differential. The recommended procedure is to have a pressure reducing suction regulator within the chamber, thus making negative pressure of the sucker independent of the chamber pressure.

Patient Monitoring Within the Pressure Chamber

Because of the fire risk from electrical apparatus electro-encephalographic, electro-cardiographic, and gas analysers should be left outside the chamber but connected to the interior via leads. Oscilloscopes and panelmeters of the monitoring apparatus may be visualised from the interior of the chamber utilising the chamber portholes.

Respiratory monitoring using pneumotachographs or a Wright's respirometer will need recalibration at the pressure at which they are to be used.

Temperature recording may be done using battery-operated thermistor probes, although care must be taken to avoid the possibility of electrical sparking within the apparatus.

Blood gas and acid-base analysis may be done within the chamber but this necessitates having the necessary equipment actually within the chamber complete with required calibrating gases. Only equipment which is safe can be used under these circumstances.

End-expired carbon dioxide levels may be monitored by passing a fine tube from the region of the endotracheal tube to an appropriate carbon dioxide analyser outside the chamber.

REFERENCES

BEHNKE, A. R., FORBES, H. S. & MOTLEY, E. P. (1935–6). Circulatory and visual effects of oxygen at 3 atmospheres pressure. *Amer. J. Physiol.* **114**, 436–442.

BEHNKE, A. R., JOHNSON, F. S., POPPEN, J. R. & MOTLEY, E. P. (1934–5). The effect of oxygen on man at pressures from 1 to 4 atmospheres. *Amer. J. Physiol.* **110**, 565–572.

BEHNKE, A. R., SHAW, L. A., SHILLING, C. W., THOMSON, R. M. & MESSER, A. C. (1934). Studies on the effects of high oxygen pressure. 1. Effect of high oxygen pressure upon the carbon dioxide and oxygen content, the acidity, and the carbon dioxide combining power of the blood. *Amer. J. Physiol.*, **107**, 13–28.

BERT, P. (1878). *La Pression Barometrique.* Eng. Trans. by Hitchcock. M. A. & Hitchcock, F. A., 1943. Columbus, Ohio: College Book Company.

BORNSTEIN, A., and STROINK, M. (1912). Ueber Sauerstoffvergiftung. *Dtsch. med. Wschr.*, **38**, 1495–1497.

BROWN, E. S. (1964). Isolation and assay of dipalmityl lecithin in lung extracts. *Amer. J. Physiol.*, **207**, 402–406.

CHANCE, B., JAMIESON, D., and COLES, H. (1965). Energy-linked pyridine nucleotide reduction: Inhibitory effects of hyperbaric oxygen *in vitro* and *in vivo*. *Nature (Lond.)*, **206**, 257–263.

CHANCE, B., JAMIESON, D., and WILLIAMSON, J. R. (1966). Control of the oxidation-reduction state of reduced pyridine nucleotides *in vivo* and *in vitro* by hyperbaric oxygen. In *Proc. 3rd. Intern. Conference on Hyperbaric Medicine.* Ed. Brown, I. W., and Cox, B. G., pp. 15–41. Washington, D.C.: Nat. Acad. Sci., Nat. Res. Council.

CHURCHILL-DAVIDSON, I., SANGER, C., and THOMLINSON, R. H. (1955). High pressure oxygen and radiotherapy. *Lancet*, **1**, 1091.

CLARK, J. M., and LAMBERTSEN, C. J. (1966). Rate of development of pulmonary O_2 toxicity in normal men at 2 ATA ambient. *Fed. Proc.*, **25**, 566.

COLLIER, C. R. (1963). Pulmonary surface activity in O_2 poisoning. *Fed. Proc.*, **22**, 339.

COMROE, J. H., DRIPPS, R. D., DUMKE, P. R., and DEMING, M. (1945). Oxygen toxicity. The effect of inhalation of high concentrations of oxygen for twenty-four hours on normal men at sea level and at a simulated altitude of 18,000 feet. *J. Amer. med. Ass.*, **128**, 710.

COUSTEAU, J., (1964), At home under the sea. *Nat. Geograph.*, **125**, 465.

DONALD, K. W. (1947). Oxygen poisoning in man. *Brit. med. J.* **1**, 667–672.

FAULKNER, J. M., BINGER, C. A. L. (1927). Oxygen poisoning in cold blooded animals. *J. Exp. Med.*, **45**, 865–871.

JUNOD, T. (1835). Recherches sur les effets physiologique et therapeutiques de la compression et des rarefaction de l'air taut sur le corps que les membres isoles. *Ann. gen. Med.*, **9**, 157.

LAMBERTSEN, C. J., KOUGH, R. H., COOPER, D. Y., EMMEL, G. L., LOESCHCKE, H. H., and SCHMIDT, C. F. (1953). Comparison of relationship of respiratory minute volume to Pco_2 and pH of arterial and internal jugular blood in normal man during hyperventilation produced by low concentrations of CO_2 at 1 atmosphere and by O_2 at 3·0 atmospheres. *J. appl. Physiol.*, **5**, 803–813.

LANPHIER, E. H. (1955). Use of nitrogen oxygen mixtures in diving. From *Proceedings of the Underwater Physiology Symposium*, edited by L. G. Goff. Washington, D.C.: Nat. Acad. Sci., Nat. Res. Council.

LANPHIER, E. H., and BROWN, I. W., Jr. (1966). The physiological basis of hyperbaric therapy. From *Fundamentals of Hyperbaric Medicine*. Publication No. 1298, p. 33. Washington, D.C.: Nat. Acad. Sci., Nat. Res. Council.

PATTLE, R. E. (1955). Properties, function and origin of the alveolar lining layer. *Nature (Lond.)*, **175**, 1125–1126.

PATTLE, R. E. (1965). Surface lining of lung alveoli. *Physiol. Rev.*, **45**, 48–79.

PATTLE, R. E., and BURGESS, F., (1961). The lung lining film in some pathological conditions. *J. Path. Bact.*, **82**, 315–331.

PATTLE, R. E., and THOMAS, L. C. (1961). Lipoprotein composition of the film lining of the lung. *Nature (Lond.)*, **189**, 844.

PERRINS, D. J. D. (1966). Hyperbaric oxygenation of ischaemic skin flaps and pedicles. *Proc. Third Internat. Conf. on Hyperbaric Medicine*. Ed. I. W. Brown, Jr. Washington, D.C.: Nat. Acad. Sci. Publication No. 1404, p. 613.

PERRINS, D. J. D. (1967). Influence of hyperbaric oxygen on the survival of split skin grafts. *Lancet*, **1**, 868.

SHILLING, C. W., and WILLGRUBE, W. W. (1937). Quantitative study of mental and neuro-muscular reactions as influenced by increased air pressure. *U.S. nav. med. Bull.*, **35**, 373–380.

SIEGEL, B. V., and MORTON, Jane I. (1967). Potentiation of the immunosuppressive effect of cytoxan by hyperbaric oxygen. *Experientia (Basel)*, **23**, 758.

SMITH, J. Lorrain (1899). The pathological effects due to increase of oxygen tension in the air breathed. *J. Physiol.*, **24**, 19.

VAN, ZYL, JAKOBUS J. W. (1967). Hyperbaric oxygenation in bacterial infections; with emphasis on those caused by the histotoxic clostridial organisms. From *Hyperbaric Oxygenation, a general review*. M.D. Thesis, University of Stellenbosch.

FURTHER READING

CHEW, H. E. R., HANSON, G. C., and SLACK, W. K. (1969). Hyperbaric oxygenation. *Brit. J. Dis. Chest.*, **63**, 113.

ELIOT, D. H., and BENNETT, P. B. (1975). *The Physiology and Medicine of Diving*. London: Baillière Tindall.

Chapter 6

INHALATIONAL ANAESTHETIC AGENTS

THE continued dominance of inhalation methods of anaesthesia, over regional and intravenous techniques, is attributed to many factors but particularly to their inherent safety and almost universal applicability. Because of this, and the fact that new inhalational agents are in the process of development and introduction, it is proposed to rehearse briefly the properties we should anticipate of the ideal inhalational agent; later certain aspects such as metabolism and potency standards which are common to all drugs in this group will be discussed. Finally each individual inhalational agent in current clinical use will be described in detail.

New inhalational agents should allow a pleasant rapid induction, and rapid emergence. They should be chemically stable in storage, and in contact with all materials used in construction of anaesthetic circuits, also they should not be inflammable. They should be biochemically stable and non-toxic to parenchymatous organs even with prolonged or repeated use; it would be a considerable advantage if the drug was excreted as given with virtually no biotransformation. The agent should be capable of inducing unconsciousness or sufficiently deep hypnosis to ensure amnesia, and sufficiently potent as an analgesic to prevent pain perception due to surgical stimuli; in addition it should produce some degree of skeletal muscle relaxation. Potency of the agent should be sufficient to allow high inspired oxygen levels which are occasionally required to compensate for increases in venous admixture during anaesthesia. It should have a high oil solubility which is usually indicative of anaesthetic potency, and rather low water solubility to ensure mobility. The ideal agent will have no deleterious effect upon the heart and will not be subject to serious interactions with drugs such as adrenaline or monoamine oxidase inhibitors.

METABOLISM OF VOLATILE ANAESTHETIC AGENTS

Volatile anaesthetic agents were originally assumed to be unaffected by passage through the body and to be eliminated unchanged from the lungs. However, even though it was known that they may be liable to undergo biotransformation, in the case of chloroform since Zeller's report in 1883, and in the case of trichloroethylene since the 1930s, these observations were considered to be esoteric unique features of the two drugs and not applicable to other inhalational agents. These views had to be revised however in the early 1960s when Van Dyke and others (1964) demonstrated in animals biodegradation of halothane, ether, chloroform, and methoxyflurane—observations which were soon to be amply confirmed by numerous investigators in man. Now it is known that all volatile agents are biotransformed, and in a number it has been measured quantitatively: up to 10–20 per cent halothane (Rehder et al. 1967), or fluroxene (Blake and Cascorbi, 1970), and about 50 per cent methoxyflurane (Holaday et al., 1970) taken up in man may be biodegraded rather than eliminated unchanged. Over the last 15 years anaesthetic metabolism has been the subject of many investigations which have in the main followed two general trends.

Firstly, a number of studies have been biochemically orientated and have sought to demonstrate the chemical reactions involved, factors governing rate and extent of the reactions, and the fate of the resulting metabolites themselves. The second approach has had a clinical bias; of special interest has been the possibility that a relationship might exist between metabolism of anaesthetic agents and their toxicity. The three main aspects of toxicity which have received attention include: histotoxicity, abortifacient activity, and teratogenicity. Recently also a further clinical implication of anaesthetic metabolism emerges from the reports of Tinker *et al.* (1976) of plasma bromide levels after halothane, which clearly indicate a potential for prolonged sedation particularly after a long exposure to halothane. The close relationship between anaesthetic metabolism and histotoxicity can be demonstrated for both chloroform and methoxyflurane. Nephrotoxicity can readily be shown to be related to certain methoxyflurane metabolites, and hepatotoxicity is clearly directly and immediately related to chloroform metabolites. However, convincing evidence for hepatotoxicity following halothane has not been forthcoming despite considerable research, and the same may be said regarding the possibility that these metabolites might indirectly provoke damage by forming antigens capable of initiating sensitisation reactions involving the liver. Indeed, there is even doubt that the syndrome "halothane hepatitis" really exists (see Chapter 38).

The two other aspects of toxicity mentioned above: abortifacient activity and teratogenicity, mainly concern personnel and their associates working in or near operating units which are contaminated or polluted with anaesthetic gases and vapours. There appears to be some evidence that chronic exposure to traces of anaesthetic in the environment can be hazardous. A number of studies suggest that there is an increased incidence in operating-room workers of spontaneous abortion, congenital abnormalities in their offspring, cancer in female anaesthetists, liver disease, and renal disease in nurses (Ad Hoc Committee, American Society of Anesthesiologists, 1974). However, although a cause-effect relationship has not yet been established (and may indeed be impossible to prove conclusively) it would seem to be prudent to take all reasonable steps to monitor, and where feasible to reduce, ambient levels of anaesthetic vapour within operating rooms, particularly as this may be effectively accomplished by relatively simple measures (See Chapter 8).

Minimum Alveolar Anaesthetic Concentration (MAC)

MAC is the minimum alveolar concentration of anaesthetic at 1 atmosphere that produces immobility in 50 per cent of those patients or animals exposed to a noxious stimulus. The term was first suggested in 1963 when Merkel and Eger described a technique for the determination in dogs of the minimum alveolar concentration of anaesthetic (MAC) required to prevent gross muscular movement in response to a painful stimulus. Since then sufficient evidence has accumulated to lead us to accept MAC as a measure or index of anaesthetic potency (potency equals the reciprocal of the partial pressure of an agent to achieve a given anaesthetic effect), which would allow, for example, comparison of circulatory or respiratory effects of equipotent doses of two or more inhalational agents. The term MAC was chosen, and has gained wide acceptance, as an index of potency for three main reasons. Firstly MAC is perhaps the most readily measured index of partial pressure of drug at the anaesthetic site of action—the brain. Secondly MAC appears to be equally applicable to all inhalational agents; and does not rely on fickle physical signs or side-effects which vary from drug to drug. Finally MAC provides a useful number for the clinician in describing the dose of drug required to achieve the essential end point of anaesthesia: analgesia and amnesia.

NITROUS OXIDE (N_2O)

Nitrous oxide was first prepared by Priestley in 1772, and its anaesthetic properties were first demonstrated by Sir Humphrey Davy in 1800. It was not until 1844, however, that it came to be used in clinical practice. In that year Gardner Quincy Colton, a lecturer in chemistry, gave a demonstration of the effects of inhaling nitrous oxide at Hartford, Connecticut. Amongst his audience was Horace Wells, a local dentist, who was so impressed that he persuaded Colton to give him some nitrous oxide the following day for extraction of a tooth. The procedure was completely painless. Later that year Wells gave a demonstration of the technique at Harvard Medical School, but the patient complained of pain and Wells was dubbed a fraud. The introduction of ether soon afterwards delayed a full appreciation of nitrous oxide until nearly twenty years later, when Colton reintroduced it for use in dental practice.

Preparation

In the laboratory.—Small amounts may be prepared by reacting iron with nitric acid. Nitric oxide (NO) is first produced, but this is reduced to nitrous oxide since an excess of iron is present:

$$2NO + Fe \rightarrow FeO + N_2O$$

Commercially.—Nitrous oxide is produced by heating ammonium nitrate to between 245 and 270° C.

$$NH_4NO_3 \xrightarrow[245-270° C]{Heat} N_2O + 2H_2O$$

The processes involved in drying and purifying the gas may vary but that used by the British Oxygen Company in the United Kingdom is briefly as follows (British Oxygen Co., 1967). A strong solution of ammonium nitrate when heated produces nitrous oxide with ammonia, nitric acid, nitrogen and traces of nitric oxide (NO) and nitrogen dioxide (NO_2). Cooling of the emerging gases results in reconstitution of the ammonia and nitric acid to ammonium nitrate and this is returned to the reactor. The gases are now passed through water scrubbers which remove any residual ammonia and nitric acid, and then through caustic permanganate scrubbers which remove the higher oxides of nitrogen to leave a residuum of 1 Vpm (volume per million) of nitric acid and nitrogen dioxide with the purified nitrous oxide and some nitrogen. Acid scrubbers now remove any final traces of ammonia and the gases are then compressed and dried in an aluminium drier. As the gases leave the drier continuous sampling takes place by passing a small stream of them through a visual bubbler. This consists of two solutions in series, the first containing acid potassium permanganate which

6/Table 1. Physical and Chemical Constants of Some Inhalational Agents

Agents	Molecular Weight	Flammability	Vapour Pressure at 20°C	Solubilities			MAC	Maximum Safe Concentration (per cent)
				Oil/Gas	Blood/Gas	H_2O/Gas		
Nitrous Oxide N_2O	44	no	800 psi (5515 kPa)	1·4	0·47	0·44	105	80
Cyclopropane C_3H_6	42	yes	90 psi (620 kPa)	11·2	0·42	0·20	9·2	30
Xenon Xe	131	no		1·9	0·20	0·10	71	80
Diethyl Ether C_2H_5—O—C_2H_5	74	yes	440 mm Hg (59 kPa)	65	12·1	13·1	1·92	8
Chloroform $CHCl_3$	119	no	170 mm Hg (23 kPa)	265	8·4	3·8	0·7	1·0
Trichloroethylene CCl_2=$CHCl$	131	no	60 mm Hg (8 kPa)	960	9·2	1·55		1·5
Halothane $CF_3CHClBr$	197·4	7·0 Air 5·4 O_2	243 mm Hg (32 kPa)	224	2·3	0·74	0·75	3
Methoxyflurane CH_3—O—CF_2CHCl_2	165·0	no	22·5 mm Hg (3 kPa)	825	13·0	4·5	0·16	1·5
Enflurane CHF_2—O—CF_2CHFCl	184·5	no	184 mm Hg (24 kPa)	98·5	1·8	0·82	1·68	5
Isoflurane CHF_2—O—$CHClCF_3$	184·5	no	250 mm Hg (33 kPa)	99	1·4	0·61	1·2	5

converts any nitric oxide to nitrogen dioxide. The second consists of a colourless solution of Saltzman reagent in which any nitrogen dioxide present dissolves causing a chemical reaction which produces a magenta colour. The compressed and dried gases are now expanded into a liquefier with resultant liquefaction of the nitrous oxide and escape of the gaseous nitrogen. The pure nitrous oxide is now evaporated, compressed to a liquid, and passed through a second aluminium drier to the cylinder filling line. At this stage visual and electronic checks are carried out on samples leaving the drier to ensure that the nitrogen dioxide content does not exceed 1 Vpm.

About nine tenths of the contents of a full nitrous oxide cylinder are in liquid form. Great care is taken during manufacture to prevent moisture being included in the cylinder contents, since water vapour tends to freeze as it passes through a reducing valve and leads to a drop in the flow of gas.

When a nitrous oxide cylinder is turned on, the gaseous tension within it is first reduced and then immediately built up again as some of the liquid vaporises. In a discussion on the value of the use of pressure gauges on nitrous oxide cylinders Jones (1974) has pointed out that it is a misconception to believe that the pressure of the gas in the cylinder is maintained whilst liquid nitrous oxide is present. In fact, when flow rates of 10 litres/minute are used there is a sharp linear fall in pressure whereas only a small but nevertheless progressive fall occurs with a flow rate of 2 litres/minute. However, he points out that even a short interruption in flow will rapidly allow the gas pressure to build up again as more liquid vaporises until finally no liquid remains. Then a pressure gauge would act in a similar manner to other gas cylinders. It is true, therefore, that pressure gauges on nitrous oxide cylinders will not indicate total contents until all the liquid is exhausted. Nevertheless they do warn against failure of flow. Most of the recent models of anaesthetic machines now incorporate them in their design.

Latent heat is required for the vaporisation of liquid nitrous oxide and this is obtained from the casing of the metal cylinder, which, as a result, rapidly cools. This in turn leads to freezing of the water vapour in the air immediately surrounding the cylinder, and to the formation of a layer of ice on the cylinder.

Nitrous oxide cylinders are marketed in various sizes, and coloured blue. In the United Kingdom 100 and 200 gallon cylinders are the most commonly used.*

Physical Properties

Nitrous oxide is non-irritating, sweet-smelling and colourless, and is the only inorganic gas used to produce anaesthesia in man. The molecular weight is 44·01 and the specific gravity is 1·527 (air = 1). It is readily compressible under 50 atmospheres pressure at 28° C. to a clear and colourless fluid with a boiling point of − 89° C. It is stable in the presence of soda-lime. The oil/water solubility ratio is 3·2. The blood/gas solubility coefficient is 0·47.

Impurities

The main impurities which may occur have already been mentioned, and to them carbon monoxide should be added. This may be produced from burning

*100 gallons of nitrous oxide weigh 30 oz: US gallon is 5/6th Imperial gallon.

particles of the sacks in which ammonium nitrate is delivered. The consequences of inhaling higher oxides of nitrogen, especially nitrogen dioxide, in concentrations over 50 Vpm are reflex inhibition of breathing with laryngospasm, and the rapid onset of intense cyanosis (Prys-Roberts, 1967). The last is due to both the formation of methaemoglobin and to altered pulmonary gas exchange. Pulmonary oedema may occur in the acute phase, but with concentrations lower than 50 Vpm it may not appear for some hours. If the patient does not die quickly, chronic chemical pneumonitis may follow, with resultant pulmonary fibrosis. Respiratory acidosis, from associated ventilatory failure, and metabolic acidosis, from production of nitric and nitrous oxide formed from solution of the gases in the body fluids, may occur. Hypotension may be marked and results from the effect of nitrate and nitrite ions on vascular smooth muscle. The cases of poisoning described by Clutton-Brock (1967) illustrate vividly the clinical consequences.

The detection of higher oxides of nitrogen has been reviewed by Kain *et al.* (1967). In clinical practice the best method involves the use of a starch iodide paper. The moistened paper is placed in a 20 ml syringe and 15 ml of oxygen are drawn up, followed, by 5 ml of the sample gas. Any nitric oxide will be oxidised by the oxygen to nitrogen dioxide, and the latter by oxidising iodide to iodine will turn the starch from a faint purple to a bright blue, depending on the amount of iodine present. The sensitivity of this test is 300 Vpm.

The principles of treatment of poisoning by the higher oxides of nitrogen have been discussed by Prys-Roberts (1967). He stresses that the advice he gives, although based on current concepts for the correction of the physiological disturbances that occur, is only a conjectural suggestion for those faced with the problem. Oxygen, either by spontaneous or assisted ventilation, and methylene blue, 2 mg/kg of body weight intravenously, will be required initially to overcome the intense cyanosis resulting from methaemoglobinaemia. Further increments of methylene blue may be required, but excessive amounts can result in the production of methaemoglobin and also haemolytic anaemia.

Bronchial lavage and suction, together with endobronchial and parenteral steroids, have been suggested for the treatment of the chemical pneumonitis. The use of fibre-optic endoscopic equipment will allow bronchial toilet to be done in a far more efficient and safe manner than has been hitherto possible using the standard bronchoscope. The acid-base and blood gas status of the patient should be regularly checked and appropriate measures taken to correct acidaemia, hypoxia, or hypercarbia. The cardiovascular status of the patient should be monitored at least by electrocardiograph, and occasionally measurement of central venous, pulmonary artery and pulmonary wedge pressures may be useful. The severe systemic hypotension from vasodilation can be improved by intravenous fluid and minimal doses of a vasopressor. The use of dimercaprol is suggested for severe cases since it has a protective action against the higher oxides of nitrogen.

Inflammability

It is neither inflammable nor explosive but will support combustion of other agents, even in the absence of oxygen, because at temperatures above 450° C it does decompose to nitrogen and oxygen.

Pharmacological Actions

Nitrous oxide is rapidly absorbed from the alveoli and 100 ml of blood will carry 45 ml of nitrous oxide in its plasma. It does not combine with haemoglobin nor does it undergo any chemical combination within the body, so that elimination is as speedy as absorption.

Anaesthetic action.—Nitrous oxide is a weak anaesthetic. At one time it was thought that any anaesthetic action that followed its use was produced solely by the exclusion of oxygen from the brain cells, since it is 15 times more soluble in plasma than nitrogen, and 100 times more so than oxygen.

Some patients can be rendered unconscious by the inhalation of mixtures containing at least 20 per cent oxygen—indeed a few subjects lose consciousness with mixtures containing equal parts of nitrous oxide and oxygen. If nitrogen is substituted for nitrous oxide in such a mixture anaesthesia rapidly ceases, and even if the oxygen is reduced to 10 per cent—with 90 per cent nitrogen—no anaesthesia occurs (Goodman and Gilman, 1955). Faulconer and Pender (1949) showed that a 50:50 mixture of nitrous oxide and oxygen at 2 atmospheres pressure rapidly produces surgical anaesthesia with complete oxygen saturation of the arterial blood, whereas the same concentration at atmospheric pressure in their patients did not produce loss of consciousness.

There is nowadays, therefore, no doubt that nitrous oxide is a weak anaesthetic agent, but the problem still remains as to how much of the anaesthesia produced (when it is used without supplement) is due to the potency of the gas and how much to the hypoxia which so frequently accompanies its use in these circumstances. The fact that these two features are intimately connected is emphasised by the following statement of Clement (1951): ". . . control of anaesthesia is synonymous with control of oxygen". In the past a case of anoxic damage to the brain, or even of death, has been reported following the use of nitrous oxide for a short period. Faulconer *et al.* (1949) showed that to produce in man surgical anaesthesia (stage III) with nitrous oxide a partial pressure of 760 mm Hg (101·3 kPa) is required if full oxygenation is maintained. Since an 80 per cent mixture of nitrous oxide in oxygen at normal atmospheric pressure results in a partial pressure of nitrous oxide of only about 600 mm Hg (80 kPa), surgical anaesthesia cannot be achieved without some hypoxia. The use of a mixture of nitrous oxide and oxygen in the proportion 85:15 for induction causes a marked fall in arterial saturation in approximately two minutes, even when previous preoxygenation is carried out for three minutes. When pure nitrous oxide is used to induce anaesthesia, loss of consciousness is rapid enough —about 60 seconds—to suggest that this is primarily caused by displacement of oxygen from the brain rather than by saturation with nitrous oxide to a degree sufficient to cause anaesthesia without hypoxia (Bourne, 1954). In modern anaesthetic practice, nitrous oxide (even at sea level) is no longer used as an induction agent save in exceptional circumstances because of the danger of the accompanying hypoxia. However, because it is a weak anaesthetic agent and when accompanied by at least $33\frac{1}{3}$ per cent oxygen it has proved an immensely valuable agent for volatilising other liquid anaesthetics.

Haemodynamic Effects of Nitrous Oxide

Nitrous oxide has been long regarded as devoid of cardiovascular side-effects, a viewpoint supported both by considerable clinical experience extending over a period of more than a hundred years, and by a number of well-controlled haemodynamic trials. However the observations by Price and Helrich (1955) that the drug possessed myocardial depressant properties was followed by isolated clinical reports in which it was blamed for the profound hypotension that occurred when the agent was given to patients anaesthetised with oxygen and halothane (Johnstone, 1959; Bloch, 1963). Interpretation of these observations is difficult because nitrous oxide was given against a background of other drugs with the possibility of complex interactions. In an attempt to resolve these difficulties two groups gave the drug on its own. Eisele and Smith (1972) demonstrated that substitution of 40 per cent nitrogen by 40 per cent nitrous oxide in oxygen in trained healthy volunteers was associated with significant reductions in heart rate (6 to 9 per cent); there was no change in blood pressure and consequently derived peripheral vascular resistance increased significantly. Thornton et al. (1973) confirmed these observations in a study on ten patients with heart disease during cardiac catheterisation.

In view of the widespread and expanding indications for nitrous oxide in the fields of post-operative, obstetric and coronary care analgesia, further studies were undertaken to determine the level at which nitrous oxide inhalation was associated with haemodynamic effects. Nitrous oxide was given in incremental steps of 10 per cent up to 50 per cent; 21 per cent oxygen and nitrogen formed the balance of the inspired mixtures. No change in heart rate, blood pressure or cardiac output was noted, suggesting that the high inspired oxygen level utilised in other studies was in some way responsible for the cardiovascular depression noted (Kaul and Coleman, 1975).

In clinical practice therefore it would appear to be reasonable to ignore the possibility that nitrous oxide may be associated with cardiovascular depression.

Nitrous oxide does not sensitise the heart to adrenaline; the latter may therefore be infiltrated to produce ischaemia of the surgical field provided the concentration does not exceed about 1 in 200,000, the total dose 1 mg and the patient is moderately overventilated with arterial Po_2 of more than 100 mm Hg (13·3 kPa) and Pco_2 less than 35 mm Hg (4·6 kPa). Alternatively ornithine-8-vasopressin (POR 8) may be used (Coleman and Baker, 1973).

Contra-indications to nitrous oxide anaesthesia.—There are no contra-indications to the use of nitrous oxide in combination with an adequate percentage of oxygen. But present practice suggests that there are no occasions when this combination alone is justified. It is always preferable either to precede the inhalation by an intravenous induction of anaesthesia or to supplement it with a more potent inhalational agent, thereby ensuring a satisfactory level of oxygenation in the inspired mixture at all times. Indeed, a minimum concentration of 30 per cent oxygen is recommended when nitrous oxide is used for anaesthetic purposes.

Methods of Administration

Nitrous oxide can be administered by intermittent or continuous flow machines.

Intermittent flow.—This is an economical method as gas only flows during inspiration, and it is based upon two different techniques.

The first technique depends upon nitrous oxide and oxygen flowing into a mixing bag from which the patient inspires via corrugated tubing and a mask. As the bag empties, so it is refilled from the cylinders, and when it is full the flow of gases is automatically cut off until the next inspiratory effort starts the process once more (see Chapters 42 and 9). This type of apparatus is used almost entirely in midwifery and dental practice. The percentage of gas and oxygen in the mixture breathed can be readily adjusted by setting the dial to the required figure, and a simple device enables the intermittent flow to be replaced by continuous flow at various pressures—a factor which may be particularly useful in dental anaesthesia. Many machines incorporate a small trichloroethylene or halothane inhaler and a reservoir bag between the patient and the machine.

The second technique makes use of a premixed cylinder of nitrous oxide and oxygen under pressure with a demand valve to allow a high flow of gas to the patient on inspiration. The premixing of these two gases in the same cylinder was first suggested by Barach and Rovenstine (1945). At room temperature and at a pressure of 2000 pounds per square inch certain proportions of nitrous oxide in oxygen exist as a single phase gas, due to the solvent action (Poynting effect) of the oxygen at this pressure. Tunstall (1961) described this pheno- menon, making the point that up to 75 per cent nitrous oxide-oxygen remains in the gas phase under these conditions. He also reported the clinical use of a mixture of 50 per cent nitrous oxide and 50 per cent oxygen contained in one cylinder for the relief of pain in childbirth. Cooling such a mixture produces liquid nitrous oxide at the bottom of the cylinder, and this remains even when the cylinder is rewarmed (Cole, 1964). In these circumstances, if the cylinder is used it will first deliver a mixture with an oxygen content that is higher than intended, and then one that is lower. Delivery of a constant mixture from the cylinder can be assured either by preventing cooling or, should cooling occur, by briskly inverting the cylinder several times after rewarming (Tunstall, 1963; Cole, 1964). The use of premixed nitrous oxide and oxygen (Entonox) for the relief of pain in labour is described in Chapter 42.

Continuous flow.—A continuous flow of gases is supplied from the anaes- thetic machine, and a semi-closed system is most frequently used, with almost all the expired mixtures passing into the atmosphere through the expiratory valve. A completely closed system with absorption of carbon dioxide is not indicated when nitrous oxide is used, since it is extremely difficult to adjust the patient's oxygen requirements accurately and to maintain anaesthesia with this weak agent in such circumstances. Semi-closed anaesthesia is, however, fre- quently practised with a carbon dioxide absorber in place so that a more econo- mical flow of gases can be used (see below).

CLINICAL USES OF NITROUS OXIDE

For the reasons already stated, there is no place for the use of nitrous oxide as the sole anaesthetic.

Nitrous Oxide Analgesia

The introduction of premixed cylinders of 50:50 nitrous oxide and oxygen has revolutionised the use of nitrous oxide for analgesia. Parbrook (1968) has reviewed the possible indications, which include obstetric analgesia, the relief of pain in acute trauma and for cardiac ischaemia—particularly when a high oxygen content of the inspired gases is required—and other more traditional situations such as burns and painful dressings. Parbrook (1967) has also outlined four zones of analgesia, which are essentially subdivisions of Stage I of anaesthesia, and he believes that the first of these is the most useful, because in it the patient remains in full contact with his surroundings. This zone is generally achieved with concentrations of 6–25 per cent of nitrous oxide.

Nitrous Oxide for Dental Anaesthesia (see Chapter 9)

Nitrous Oxide with Supplements

Though lacking in potency nitrous oxide is the least toxic of all the various anaesthetic agents available and has come to occupy an important role in anaesthetic technique. It is often used in conjunction with oxygen as the vehicle for delivering an anaesthetic vapour such as halothane or ether to the patient. In this respect as a weak anaesthetic agent it reduces the amount of the inhalational agent required for the same level of anaesthesia. It is also used extensively, sometimes with supplements of thiopentone, pethidine or other narcotic analgesics in conjunction with the muscle relaxants in major surgery.

It is frequently administred in a ratio of $66\frac{2}{3} : 33\frac{1}{3}$ per cent nitrous oxide and oxygen. The $33\frac{1}{3}$ per cent oxygen in the normal patient is sufficient to maintain adequate saturation of arterial blood; the increased inspired oxygen concentration is necessary to compensate for any alteration in the ventilation/perfusion ratio caused by anaesthesia as described in Chapter 3. In seriously ill patients requiring a high oxygen intake then nitrous oxide is not the most suitable agent.

Significance of uptake.—The high cost of some inhalational anaesthetic agents has increased the interest in using a low-flow technique. As nitrous oxide is the principal carrier gas it is important to emphasise a few points in relation to its uptake by the blood. Nitrous oxide is relatively insoluble in blood, therefore the tension rises rapidly on induction and falls equally fast at the end of anaesthesia. The brain, an organ with a rich blood supply, has a similar solubility to that of blood so the brain tension also rises fast. Equilibrium between alveolar blood and brain concentrations is achieved in a few minutes, but this must not be interpreted as meaning that a state of complete saturation has been achieved. Other tissues such as muscle and fat with a relatively low blood supply will gradually extract nitrous oxide from the blood, so that even after many hours some gas is still leaving the circulation. For example, with a patient breathing 75:25 per cent nitrous oxide/oxygen the uptake by the body (mostly muscle and fat) is about 175 ml/minute at the end of one hour, and at two hours it is still around 100 ml/minute. After about thirty hours complete saturation could theoretically be achieved but this is thwarted by the constant loss of 5–10 ml/minute of nitrous oxide through the skin.

Low-flow technique.—The flow rate of nitrous oxide is important for two reasons. First, if it is the sole induction agent (in combination with oxygen) and it is used in a circle system (i.e. rebreathing allowed but carbon dioxide absorbed), then a 1 litre flow of 75:25 N_2O/O_2 will not render the patient unconscious even after 10 minutes of breathing this mixture. The reason for this is that the capacity of air in the lungs and in the anaesthetic apparatus is so great that they dilute the nitrous oxide to a level below which unconsciousness can be produced. On the other hand, if an 8 litre flow of the same mixture is used then unconsciousness is lost within two minutes because the apparatus is rapidly flushed out (Eger, 1960). Therefore, if a low-flow nitrous oxide technique is to be used it should always start with a high flow for a few minutes before reducing to smaller flows.

Once on a low-flow technique it must not be assumed that because the inspired concentration of oxygen is 25 per cent the alveolar concentration is at this level. Assuming for a moment that the input flow is 1·0 litre per minute and the oxygen consumption is 250 ml/minute and also that "complete saturation" with nitrous oxide has been achieved, then after one breath all the oxygen in the alveoli (i.e. 25 per cent of 1 litre = 250 ml) will be taken up by the blood and the alveoli will then contain pure nitrous oxide. This will remain to dilute the next breath containing the inspired concentration of 75:25 N_2O/O_2. Consequently the oxygen content in the alveoli is considerably below the 25 per cent in the inspired concentration. This example emphasises the paramount importance of using an oxygen analyser in the circle system when low flows of nitrous oxide are being administered. Provided the concentration of oxygen in the inspired mixture does not fall below 25 per cent and total minute volume is adequate then this technique can safely be used, but for reasons described in Chapter 2 et seq., it is best not to use an inspired mixture of less than 33 per cent oxygen.

Finally, it is interesting to consider the question of what happens to the patient with abdominal distension or a closed pneumothorax who also breathes a mixture of N_2O/O_2. Nitrous oxide, though relatively insoluble in blood, is still much more soluble than nitrogen. Therefore more molecules will present themselves at the cavity site and for every one molecule of nitrogen leaving, at least ten molecules of nitrous oxide will be available. On this basis the induction of nitrous oxide and oxygen anaesthesia might be predicted to increase distension of the gas bubble. (See also Chapter 7, p. 321).

ETHYLENE (C_2H_4)

There is a wide discrepancy in the anaesthetic literature as to the origin of the hydrocarbon, ethylene. In 1779 Priestley gave the credit to Ingenhousz, but the exact date of preparation remains obscure. Other authorities claim that Becher, in 1669, was the first person to prepare the gas. In 1923 Brown, whilst working in the Henderson Laboratory at Toronto, published some observations on the anaesthetic properties of this gas in animals. That same year Luckhardt and Carter of Chicago reported their findings on the use of this drug in human subjects. The evidence available suggests that the credit for its introduction as an anaesthetic should go to Luckhardt, since he had observed its anaesthetic and analgesic properties in animals years before.

Preparation

In the laboratory: Ethyl bromide is reacted with alcoholic potassium hydroxide to form ethylene, potassium bromide, and water.

$$C_2H_5Br + KOH \rightarrow C_2H_4 + KBr + H_2O$$

Ethyl bromide + potassium hydroxide → Ethylene + potassium + water
(alcoholic)   bromide

Commercially: by dehydration of ethyl alcohol with either sulphuric (H_2SO_4) or phosphoric (H_2PO_4) acid.

$$150° C +$$

$$C_2H_5OH + H_2SO_4 \rightarrow C_2H_4 + H_2O$$
Ethyl alcohol + Sulphuric acid   Ethylene + Water

At temperatures below 150° C ethyl ether may be formed when sulphuric acid is used.

Natural gas can be used to produce ethylene by a process of breakdown or "cracking" with heat. Propane is formed as an intermediate process.

Physical Properties

Ethylene is a colourless, non-irritating gas with a slightly sweetish and unpleasant odour. It is lighter than air, having a specific gravity of 0·97 (air = 1). Molecular weight is 28·03. It liquefies at 10° C under 60 atmospheres pressure and the boiling point of this liquid is —104° C. It is the least soluble in blood of the commonly used anaesthetic agents having an Ostwald blood-gas solubility coefficient of 0·140 (*cf.* nitrous oxide = 0·468). The oil/gas coefficient is 1·28 and the solubility in blood and tissue (e.g. heart and brain) is about equal, i.e. 1·0 and 1·2 respectively (Marshall and Grollman, 1928; Meyer and Hopff, 1923; Kety, 1951). It is not altered by soda-lime but diffuses through rubber.

Impurities

These are either contaminants from the manufacturing process or from decomposition. Alcohol, aldehydes, ether, oxides of sulphur or phosphorus, carbon dioxide, carbon monoxide, olefins or acetylenes may be present.

Inflammability

Ethylene is highly combustible, when mixed with oxygen or air, and exposed to sparks or flames. Thus in air 3·1–32·0 per cent ethylene is explosive, while in oxygen the range is from 3·0–80·0 per cent. The risk of explosion is increased on account of its low density which allows it to rise in the atmosphere.

The addition of nitrous oxide (40 per cent) to a mixture of ethylene (50 per cent) and oxygen (10 per cent) does not prevent an explosion, but helium and nitrogen, when used as diluents, reduce the explosive range.

Pharmacological Actions

Ethylene is rapidly absorbed from the alveoli and, when given in a concentration of 100 per cent, it brings about unconsciousness slightly more rapidly than nitrous oxide. Ethylene in mixtures of 20–40 per cent with oxygen is said to produce analgesia, but 80–90 per cent is required for anaesthesia. The main advantages over nitrous oxide are a more rapid induction, greater muscular relaxation, and the ability to use a slightly higher percentage of oxygen. Against these must be set the disadvantage of a highly explosive agent with an unpleasant odour.

In a report from the United States of nearly 200,000 cases of ethylene-oxygen anaesthesia, there were five deaths in the operating room and three in the post-operative period attributed to this agent. There were three non-fatal explosions in this series.

Ethylene is rapidly eliminated through the lungs, although a very small percentage may be excreted through the skin. The incidence of post-operative nausea and vomiting is greater than that with nitrous oxide.

Method of Administration

This is similar to that already described for nitrous oxide.

CYCLOPROPANE (C_3H_6)

Cyclopropane, or trimethylene, was first prepared by the chemist Freund in 1882. Nearly fifty years later, in 1929, Lucas and Henderson of Toronto noted that it possessed better anaesthetic properties than propylene, in which they were primarily interested. In 1933 Waters and his colleagues, at Madison, Wisconsin, introduced cyclopropane into clinical anaesthesia.

Preparation

Cyclopropane can be prepared from the natural gas found in the United States, or from trimethylene glycol. This substance is produced during the fermentation of molasses to obtain glycol. In the first stage trimethylene glycol is reacted with hydrobromic acid to form trimethylene dibromide, and in the second stage this latter substance is treated with zinc which brings about the production of cyclopropane and zinc dibromide.

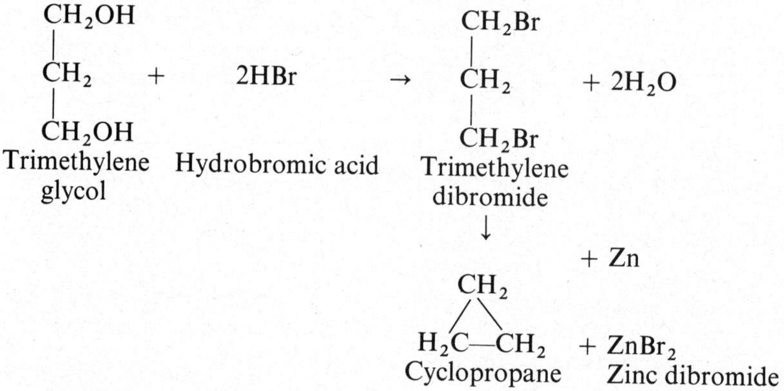

$$
\begin{array}{ccccc}
CH_2OH & & & CH_2Br & \\
| & & & | & \\
CH_2 & + & 2HBr & \rightarrow & CH_2 & + 2H_2O \\
| & & & | & \\
CH_2OH & & & CH_2Br & \\
\text{Trimethylene} & \text{Hydrobromic acid} & & \text{Trimethylene} \\
\text{glycol} & & & \text{dibromide}
\end{array}
$$

$$
\begin{array}{c}
\downarrow \\
+ \; Zn \\
CH_2 \\
/ \backslash \\
H_2C\!-\!CH_2 \quad + \; ZnBr_2 \\
\text{Cyclopropane} \quad \text{Zinc dibromide}
\end{array}
$$

Physical Properties

Cyclopropane is a pleasant, sweet-smelling gas, which is irritating to the respiratory tract when inhaled in concentrations over 40 per cent. The molecular weight is 42·08 and the vapour density 1·42 (air = 1), and because it is heavier than air it tends to gravitate towards the floor. When subjected to pressures of five atmospheres or more, it liquefies. It is stored as a liquid at a pressure of 75 lb per square inch in light metal cylinders which are coloured orange. Because of this relatively low pressure no reducing valves are required, the flow being regulated through a simple fine-adjustment pin. One ounce of the liquid gives 3·5 U.K. gallons or 4·29 U.S. gallons of gas. The boiling point is −33° C and freezing point −127° C. It has a solubility coefficient in blood of 0·415 (*cf.* nitrous oxide 0·468) and therefore it is relatively insoluble in blood. This accounts for the rapid induction and recovery that can be achieved with this agent. The solubility coefficient in human fat is 6·8 and the solubility in the tissues is about the same as in blood. Cyclopropane is not altered or decomposed by alkalis, and so undergoes no change in the presence of soda-lime, but diffuses through rubber.

Impurities

Propylene, allene, cyclohexane, carbon dioxide, various halides such as brom- or chlor-propane and, finally, nitrogen, are possible impurities. Concentrations of propylene above 3 per cent may prove dangerous.

Inflammability

Cyclopropane, when mixed with air, oxygen or nitrous oxide, becomes explosive over a variable range. In air 2·4–10·4 per cent cyclopropane is explosive, in oxygen 2·5–60·0 per cent, and in nitrous oxide 3–30 per cent.

Pharmacological Actions

Uptake.—Cyclopropane, when inhaled, is absorbed from the alveoli and carried in the circulation attached principally to the red cells by virtue of their high protein and lipoprotein content. Some is attached to the serum protein but as the water solubility of cyclopropane is relatively low (0·204 as opposed to 15·61 for ether) only a small portion is physically dissolved in the plasma.

Elimination.—Cyclopropane is excreted almost entirely by the lungs, although a small quantity is lost through the skin. Approximately 50 per cent of cyclopropane in the body is removed within ten minutes of discontinuing its administration.

Concentration for anaesthesia.—The amount of cyclopropane required for induction must necessarily be higher than that used for maintenance because of the dilution caused by the contents of the lungs and the anaesthetic apparatus. For a rapid induction of anaesthesia the reservoir bag of the apparatus should be filled with 50:50 cyclopropane and oxygen. The patient is asked to take five or six deep breaths of this mixture. Unconsciousness sets in within thirty seconds and this is rapidly followed by a period of apnoea in most cases. Sometimes un-co-ordinated twitching movements may be observed throughout the body lasting for about half a minute.

Inhalation of a concentration of 4 per cent cyclopropane in oxygen produces analgesia, 6 per cent abolishes consciousness, 8 per cent light anaesthesia and 20–30 per cent deep anaesthesia. These figures, however, are of limited value since the concentration of cyclopropane inhaled and its effect vary widely, depending on the response of the patient and the duration of the inhalation.

Action on the respiratory system.—Cyclopropane given with oxygen to the unpremedicated patient produces a progressive decrease in alveolar ventilation as the depth of anaesthesia increases (Jones *et al.*, 1960). The depression of ventilation is due to a fall in tidal volume, for the respiratory rate increases as anaesthesia deepens. This increase in rate was at one time thought to result from a sensitisation by cyclopropane of the pulmonary stretch receptors in the respiratory tract, but there is strong evidence that anaesthetics abolish this reflex (Paskin, 1968). If morphine or pethidine are used as part of the premedication then there is a progressive decrease in tidal volume without any change in respiratory rate. This leads to profound hypoventilation at a much lighter level of anaesthesia than would be experienced in the unpremedicated patient. From a clinical standpoint heavy premedication with analgesics before cyclopropane anaesthesia invariably leads to apnoea long before a sufficient concentration is given for adequate muscular relaxation. Munson and his colleagues (1966) suggest that at equipotent anaesthetic concentrations cyclopropane is less depressant to respiration than halothane.

In the experimental animal cyclopropane produces bronchial constriction and though such a response is not commonly seen in clinical practice, it should be remembered when considering this agent for anaesthesia for a patient liable to bronchospasm.

Action on the circulatory system.—*General response.* Much work has been done on the study of the effects of cyclopropane on the circulation (Price, 1961). In the past, most of the data concerning the effects of this anaesthetic have been based on studies involving premedication of the patient, intermittent positive-pressure ventilation, endotracheal intubation and the trauma of surgery. All of these are believed to influence the action of cyclopropane on the circulation and therefore the actions quoted below are those reported as being due solely to cyclopropane anaesthesia.

Effect on the heart.—Cyclopropane when administered to the heart-lung preparation causes a depression of cardiac contractility which is directly related to the concentration used. In direct contrast, in anaesthetised man cyclopropane brings about an increase in cardiac output with a rise in right ventricular stroke volume, stroke work and end-diastolic pressure. This increase in cardiac output is only seen under light anaesthesia, for the output falls to normal or below as depth is increased. These findings in intact man suggest that the increase in cardiac output under light anaesthesia is related to the stimulation of the sympathetic nerves supplying the heart. It is known that the noradrenaline concentration in the myocardium increases proportionately with the concentration of cyclopropane. The adrenaline concentration is not affected. Thus, the increase in cardiac output in light anaesthesia may be due to increased noradrenaline production and as anaesthesia deepens so the direct depressant effect of cyclopropane on the myocardium becomes manifest. If, however, cyclopropane is administered to a patient with sympathetic blockade then only the depressant action on the myocardium could be anticipated.

Effect on the heart rate.—It is widely believed by all users of cyclopropane that this anaesthetic agent produces a slowing of the pulse rate. Yet, if the patient is not premedicated with a narcotic, the effect of cyclopropane on the heart rate is negligible. As the anaesthetic depth is increased no obvious change in pulse rate is observed. If, however, some premedication is given in the form of morphine, then a bradycardia may be observed with cyclopropane anaesthesia (Li and Etsten, 1957).

In the absence of any premedicant drugs concentrations of cyclopropane as high as 14–18 vols. per cent can be inspired without any observable change in pulse rate (Price, 1961). Furthermore, if a large dose of atropine (1·0–2·0 mg) is then given, a very dramatic increase in pulse rate takes place (i.e. an average increase of 70 beats/minute). This increase is far greater than that produced by the same dose of atropine without cyclopropane anaesthesia. The inference is made, therefore, that cyclopropane may increase vagal activity and this effects cardiac impulse generation, conduction and improved atrial contractility. At the time it increases vagal activity it also stimulates sympathetic activity within the heart. In the unpremedicated patient these two forces balance each other out and there is little change of pulse rate. When atropine is given not only is vagal activity blocked but sympathetic activity is allowed to proceed unheeded. Hence the dramatic tachycardia. However, atropine administration during cyclopropane anaesthesia leads to a high incidence of dysrhythmias, and might lead to ventricular fibrillation (Eger, 1962).

Dysrhythmias.—An increase in the alveolar carbon dioxide tension precipitated the onset of dysrhythmias in every one of a series of twenty-eight patients anaesthetised with cyclopropane (Price *et al.*, 1958). It is known that both hypercapnia and cyclopropane increase the rate of noradrenaline liberation from sympathetic nerves terminating in the myocardium. Catecholamines liberated from other areas of the body are relatively ineffective. It would appear, therefore, that the combination of a raised carbon dioxide tension of the blood and cyclopropane lead to an excessive noradrenaline excretion in the myocardium. Nevertheless, Price *et al.* (1968) demonstrated that cyclopropane itself has a direct effect on the myocardium. Thus, during sympathetic nerve stimulation there is an increased chronotropic response and this is not directly related to the amount of transmitter substance released. Clinically, therefore dysrhythmias under cyclopropane anaesthesia can largely be prevented if particular attention is paid to the prevention of hypoventilation. In fact Price and his colleagues (1960) concluded that "in persons anaesthetised with cyclopropane the most reliable circulatory indication of hypercarbia was the presence of cardiac dysrhythmias."

"Cyclopropane shock".—This term became popular during the era of cyclopropane to explain the sudden cardiovascular collapse that was sometimes observed at the end of a long anaesthetic under deep cyclopropane. At first it was believed to be solely due to the accumulation of carbon dioxide brought about by the respiratory depression of the deep cyclopropane. Now it would seem that it is a combination of both cyclopropane and carbon dioxide causing a period of intense sympathetic nervous activity. The hypotension and collapse that occurs at the end of the anaesthesia is believed to be due to the sudden withdrawal of this activity.

Action on various organs.—*The kidney.* Cyclopropane produces a reduction of renal blood flow in direct proportion to the concentration. Thus under light anaesthesia there is about a 30 per cent fall in renal blood flow, whereas under deep anaesthesia it may fall to as low as 80 per cent of normal. This fall in renal blood flow with increasing concentrations of cyclopropane signifies that the agent produces a constriction of the renal vessels (Miles *et al.*, 1952). Deutsch and his co-workers (1967), studying normal unpremedicated human subjects, found that cyclopropane anaesthesia produced a dramatic reduction in both glomerular filtration and renal plasma flow (about 40 per cent). They concluded that their findings could be explained on the basis of increased sympathetic nervous system activity during cyclopropane anaesthesia. At the same time they observed that cyclopropane anaesthesia was associated with an antidiuresis which was probably brought about by increased production of antidiuretic hormone (ADH), and they also noted an increase in plasma renin levels. The latter finding is particularly interesting as the renin-angiotensin system has been considered to be responsible for the autoregulation of renal blood flow, so it is theoretically possible that cyclopropane may act on the renal blood flow through the mechanism of this system.

The liver.—Cyclopropane reduces liver blood flow in direct relation with the depth of anaesthesia (Shackman *et al.*, 1953). This finding has been corroborated by the work of Price and his colleagues (1965) who found that cyclopropane reduced splanchnic blood flow to both the gut and the liver. They concluded that this effect was brought about not only by increased sympathetic activity in the vasoconstrictor fibres to the liver and intestine but also by sensitisation of the vascular smooth muscle to the action of noradrenaline.

The uterus.—Cyclopropane depresses the contractions of the gravid uterus again in direct relation to the concentration used. It passes quickly through the placental barrier and equilibrium between maternal and fetal blood is rapidly established. For this reason high concentrations of cyclopropane are rarely used for Caesarean section or forceps delivery in obstetrical anaesthesia, though if cyclopropane is used as an induction agent only, the respiratory depression of the fetus is eliminated within a few minutes of the withdrawal of the agent.

The lungs.—Cyclopropane increases central venous pressure. This may be due to stimulating vagal activity but it results in the right heart and great veins becoming firmer with increased tone. Thus, when the lungs are inflated with positive pressure the veins (and indirectly the cardiac output) are less susceptible to this compression. This may explain why the blood pressure does not usually fall under cyclopropane anaesthesia even in the seriously ill patient. Nevertheless, hypotension and diminished cardiac output do sometimes occur on induction with cyclopropane anaesthesia, particularly if a narcotic agent has been used. As time progresses this depression is usually offset and the blood pressure returns to normal, suggesting that some homeostatic mechanism is at work. This may be due to stimulation of baroreceptor reflex activity. Price and Widdicombe (1962) have demonstrated in dogs and cats that cyclopropane anaesthesia acts by a direct stimulant effect on the baroreceptors in the carotid sinus. Another possible explanation, supported by some evidence in animal experiments, is that cyclopropane diminishes the sensitivity of the medullary vasomotor centre to afferent inhibitory impulses, causing an increase in the centre's efferent discharge and consequent vasoconstriction.

Central nervous system.—Price and his colleagues (1969), working with cats, have confirmed that cyclopropane increases sympathetic nervous activity and they conclude that this effect is brought about by a selective depression of certain neurones in the medulla oblongata. Thus, cyclopropane inhibited the "depressor" neurones whilst stimulating the "pressor" ones. An additional excitatory action on the spinal cord neurones could not be excluded but appeared relatively unimportant.

Cyclopropane and adrenaline.—Price and his co-workers (1958) studied the different blood levels of adrenaline required to produce ventricular dysrhythmias with either a simple infusion technique or that produced by a raised carbon dioxide level of the blood. They found that hypercapnia was far more effective in producing dysrhythmias than adrenaline infusion. In fact, the catecholamine level under hypercapnia was only one-tenth as high as in the infusion series yet the incidence of dysrhythmias was high, suggesting that endogenous adrenaline is far more effective than the exogenous material.

Matteo and his associates (1963), however, found that the subcutaneous injection of a 1:60,000 solution of adrenaline during cyclopropane anaesthesia with adequate ventilation (i.e. normal CO_2 level) led to a 30 per cent incidence of ventricular dysrhythmias. From data available it would seem that the use of a subcutaneous infiltration with even a weak solution of adrenaline (i.e. 1:200,000) is contra-indicated during cyclopropane anaesthesia in man.

Clinical Use

Owing to the risk of an explosion, the popularity of cyclopropane as an anaesthetic has gradually faded with the introduction of newer and non-inflammable anaesthetics. Cyclopropane may, however, be the agent of choice for the induction of anaesthesia when a rapid loss of consciousness is necessary, coupled with a high concentration of oxygen and maintenance of the systemic blood pressure. This type of induction is most commonly required in obstetric practice, but is also useful for those patients in whom any cardiovascular depression is dangerous. In such circumstances cyclopropane is best administered as a 50:50 mixture with oxygen (Bourne, 1954). The patient breathes from a six-litre bag filled with the mixture. Five to six breaths are sufficient to produce loss of consciousness. Some motor excitement (tonic or clonic contractions) may be observed at this point, and its onset is usually associated with a momentary period of breath-holding which lasts for a few seconds.

Summary

Cyclopropane anaesthesia is particularly suitable as an anaesthetic agent for the seriously-ill patient because it is accompanied by a high oxygen concentration and a rise of cardiac output (under light anaesthesia only), peripheral vasoconstriction, and virtually no change in heart rate. The result is that the blood pressure is well maintained even when intermittent positive-pressure respiration is introduced. The latter procedure is often necessary because cyclopropane diminishes tidal volume. Most of the beneficial effects of cyclopropane on the myocardium are abolished if a narcotic is given as part of the premedication. Barbiturates, phenothiazine derivatives and atropine do not have this adverse effect. Morphine and pethidine also reduce ventilation in their own right so that when combined with cyclopropane there is a serious risk of hypoventilation; both the increased carbon dioxide level of the blood and cyclopropane combine to raise the amount of noradrenaline excreted in the myocardium so that the risk of dysrhythmias is increased. The presence of these dysrhythmias under cyclopropane anaesthesia should suggest inadequate ventilation or too deep anaesthesia; in either case it has often been observed that the inhalation of a low concentration of ether vapour will bring about a return of normal rhythm.

Disease, trauma and narcotic agents appear to influence both the sympathetic and the parasympathetic responses to cyclopropane. Atropine tends to remove the effect of increased vagal stimulation whereas ganglion-blocking drugs will remove the sympathetic response and may cause cyclopropane to produce a profound hypotension through direct myocardial depression.

DIETHYL ETHER $(C_2H_5)_2O$

Ether was first described by Valerius Cordus in 1540. In 1841, Crawford Long used ether in his own home in Jefferson, Georgia, and, in the following year, he used it during three surgical operations. Unfortunately these events were not published until after William Morton's famous demonstration of the potentialities of ether as an anaesthetic at the Massachusetts General Hospital in 1846 (Morton, 1847). After this, ether became widely publicised and the news spread to London, where Drs. Boott and Squire soon used it on surgical cases at University College Hospital.

Preparation.—Dehydration of alcohol by sulphuric acid at a temperature below 140° C.

$$C_2H_5OH + H_2SO_4 \rightarrow C_2H_5HSO_4 + H_2O$$
$$\text{Ethyl alcohol} \quad \text{Sulphuric acid}$$

$$C_2H_5HSO_4 + C_2H_5OH \rightarrow H_2SO_4 + C_2H_5OC_2H_5$$
$$\text{Ethyl alcohol} \qquad\qquad \text{Diethyl ether}$$

Physical properties.—Ether is a colourless, volatile liquid (boiling point 36·5° C) with a characteristic pungent smell. At room temperature (20° C) it has a vapour pressure of approximately 425 mm Hg (57 kPa).

Significance of vapour pressure.—A knowledge of the vapour pressure of a volatile anaesthetic agent enables the anaesthetist quickly to calculate the inspired concentration being delivered to the patient by a "bubble-through" type of vaporiser e.g. copper kettle or "Vernitrol". It is of very little value if only a portion of the stream of gases are exposed to the liquid as in a "blow-over" type of vaporiser e.g. Boyle's bottle. Even when the latter type of vaporiser is converted to "bubbling" then the constantly changing temperature of the liquid make a calculation difficult unless this temperature is known.

The principle of the copper kettle (Fig. 1) is that the vaporiser is constructed of a highly conductive metal and when attached directly to an anaesthetic table-top of similar material it has a large heat reservoir available which will prevent the temperature in the vaporiser from falling. A known flow of oxygen is then bubbled through the liquid anaesthetic agent at room temperature.

Taking ether as an example, at a room temperature of 20° C the vapour pressure is 425 mm Hg (57 kPa). With flow rates of up to 500 ml of oxygen per minute passed through this instrument the temperature does not alter appreciably. Above this figure it falls in proportion to the flow rate. However, if the temperature of the liquid is known then the concentration of the ether vapour emitted can still be accurately predicted. For example, at a room temperature of 20° C the vapour pressure is 425 mm Hg (57 kPa) (Fig. 2) and the ether concentration is 52 vols per cent; if the temperature of the liquid dropped to −10° C (Fig. 2) the same inflow would only meet ether at a vapour pressure of 120 mm Hg (16 kPa) giving a concentration of ether vapour of about 14 vols per cent.

The important part played by a changing temperature in vaporisation is well illustrated by studying the glass Boyle's bottle type of vaporiser during ether anaesthesia. When a liquid becomes a vapour, heat is required for the process so the liquid cools (i.e. latent heat of vaporisation). A point is soon reached when the liquid is so cool that it freezes the moisture on the outside of the glass vapor-

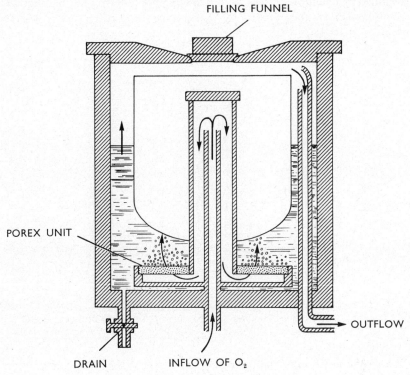

FILLING FUNNEL

POREX UNIT

OUTFLOW

DRAIN   INFLOW OF O₂

6/FIG. 1.—Diagram of flow of gases through a copper kettle. (After Morris.)

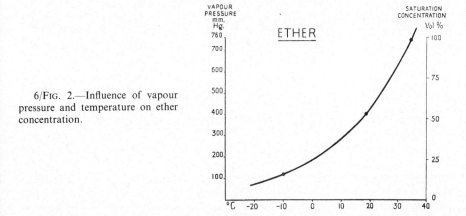

6/FIG. 2.—Influence of vapour pressure and temperature on ether concentration.

VAPOUR PRESSURE mm. Hg.

SATURATION CONCENTRATION Vol %

ETHER

iser and frost appears. This can be prevented by placing a jacket of warm water around the glass bottle. Alternatively, the ether can be kept constantly above its boiling point (36·5), so that it is under pressure trying to escape. This principle is used in the construction of the Oxford Vaporiser Mark II where the ether is surrounded by chemical crystals with a melting point above that of ether. Once these crystals have been melted by warm water then ether vapour will issue spontaneously (Fig. 3).

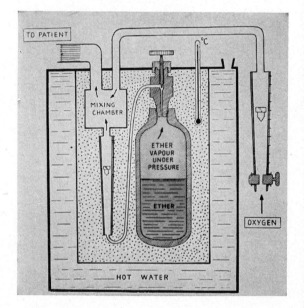

6/FIG 3.—Oxford Vaporiser Mark II.

If a "bubble-through" vaporiser (copper kettle) is used at a room temperature of 20° C then a flow of 500 ml of oxygen through this instrument will give an output of 1000 ml of 50 per cent ether vapour. Except for the total volume involved it is easier to think of this as 500 ml of pure ether vapour. When this total is added to 4 litres of nitrous oxide and oxygen the patient will then receive a 10 per cent ether concentration, viz.

$$\left.\begin{array}{c} \text{4 litres of } N_2O/O_2 \\ + \\ \text{1 litre of 50 per cent ether vapour} \end{array}\right\} \begin{array}{c} \text{5 litres total gas flow including 500 ml} \\ \text{of ether vapour.} \end{array}$$

= 5 litres of 10 per cent ether vapour in nitrous oxide/oxygen.

Inflammability.—Ether is a highly inflammable liquid which ignites at a temperature of 154° C (the presence of peroxides may lower the ignition point to 100° C). Provided sufficient oxygen is present, low concentrations of ether burn with a clear blue flame, whereas high concentrations explode. In air, the range of inflammability of ether is 1·9–48·0 per cent, but with the addition of more oxygen this is increased to 2·0–82·0 per cent. Since ether vapour is two-and-a-half times heavier than air, the vapour collects like an invisible blanket over the floor. A spark from an electric motor or a switch can ignite this, causing a characteristic "cold blue" flame to spread slowly across the floor. In daylight this flame may be invisible. The chief danger is that it may reach a richer source of oxygen than the air, thus causing an explosion of devastating consequences.

Stability.—The two important impurities caused by decomposition of ether are acetic aldehyde and ether peroxide, the former can be detected by Nessler's solution (complex mercuric iodide solution), and the latter by potassium iodide solution—both of which are turned yellow. Decomposition is favoured by air, light and heat but prevented by copper and hydroquinone. Ether should, therefore, be kept in sealed, dark bottles in a cool cupboard.

Other impurities are alcohol, sulphuric acid, sulphur dioxide, mercaptans, and ethyl esters.

Some doubt has been expressed about the toxicity of these impurities of ether in man. An investigation in animals revealed that aldehyde (0·5 per cent) was without significant effect, whereas mercaptans (1·0 per cent) and peroxide (0·5 per cent) could cause gastric irritation but had no other obvious deleterious action. During anaesthesia the presence of mercaptans in the ether should be suspected if the patient's expirations have a peculiar "fishy" odour; in such cases tachycardia and an unexplained hypotension may also occur.

Pharmacological Actions

Uptake and distribution.—Ether has a blood/gas solubility coefficient of 12·1 (Eger *et al.*, 1963). This signifies that blood has a tremendous capacity for absorbing ether so that it is constantly being removed from the alveoli. Consequently it takes a long time for the alveolar tension to rise to the same height as the inspired tension. As alveolar tension is virtually synonymous with brain tension then induction of anaesthesia will be slow and equally recovery will be affected in the reverse manner. This combined with the fact that it is irritant to the respiratory tract means that it will take 15–25 minutes to achieve deep anaesthesia.

The solubility of ether in the various tissues is similar to that of blood (Table 2).

6/TABLE 2

THE TISSUE/BLOOD COEFFICIENT FOR ETHER

1·14 in Brain tissue
1·2 in Lung tissue
3·3 in Fat tissue
(Eger *et al.*, 1963).

Significance of oil/gas solubility.—The value for ether is 65; this signifies a relatively low lipoid solubility when compared with other agents, e.g. 224 for halothane and 960 for trichloroethylene. The oil/gas solubility coefficient is another way of indicating anaesthetic potency. For example, to produce the 1st plane of surgical anaesthesia with ether an alveolar concentration of 2·5 vols per cent is required, whereas with trichloroethylene only 0·17 vols per cent is needed (Eger, personal communication).

Estimation of ether concentration.—In the past the concentration of ether in the blood was measured by complex chemical analysis of the level in blood

(Andrews *et al.*, 1940). Newer methods such as gas chromatography or infra-red analysis are now available and these indicate the alveolar concentration of ether in vols per cent (Table 3).

6/TABLE 3
APPROXIMATE BLOOD AND ALVEOLAR LEVELS OF ETHER IN RELATION TO
DEPTH OF ANAESTHESIA

	Blood level in mg per cent	Alveolar concentration in vols per cent
Stage I	10– 40	0·284–1·14
Stage II	40– 80	1·14 –2·27
Stage III, Plane I	80–110	2·27 –3·12
Plane II	110–120	3·12 –3·41
Plane III	120–130	3·41 –3·69
Plane IV	130–140	3·69 –3·98
Stage IV	140–180	3·98 –5·11

Excretion.—Only a small quantity of ether undergoes biodegradation. The majority (85–90 per cent) is excreted unchanged through the lungs and the remainder is metabolised or eliminated via the skin, body secretions and urine.

Action on the respiratory system.—Ether, in anaesthetic concentrations, is an irritant to the mucosa of the respiratory tract. It increases the amount of bronchial secretions but at the same time it also increases the internal diameter of the bronchi and bronchioles. For this reason, it is an extremely useful anaesthetic agent for patients with asthma or bronchiolar spasm. Ether does not affect the action of surfactant in reducing surface tension in the alveoli (Miller and Thomas, 1967).

Ether is believed to stimulate the nerve endings in the bronchial tree and thus reflexly excite the respiratory centre. It may also sensitise the baroreceptors. The ultimate effect is to increase the *rate* of respiration. At a later stage, as the paralysant action of ether manifests itself in deep anaesthesia, the minute volume steadily declines until apnoea finally supervenes. Larson and his colleagues (1969) have shown that in healthy unpremedicated patients, the resting preinduction arterial carbon dioxide tension does not rise until deep levels of ether anaesthesia (alveolar ether concentrations of 6 per cent) are reached. They doubt the need for controlled or assisted ventilation to maintain a satisfactory arterial carbon dioxide tension during anaesthesia.

Action on the cardiovascular system.—There is still a wide margin of discrepancy in the reported findings of the action of ether on the cardiovascular system in man. This is because countless studies have been made but each has varied the technique or the quantity or quality of premedicant and other drugs used. As most patients undergoing ether anaesthesia require premedication, it has been argued that studies made on patients without premedication are only academic, yet it is only through such studies that it is possible to determine the precise effect of ether anaesthesia in man.

If ether vapour is added to the circulation in a heart-lung preparation there is a dramatic depression of myocardial activity. Brewster and his colleagues

(1953) working with adrenalectomised dogs have convincingly shown that ether can depress the myocardium. Jones and his co-workers (1962) have demonstrated that ether produces increased sympathetic nervous activity, mainly in the form of liberation of noradrenaline. The plasma level of noradrenaline rises with increasing depth of ether anaesthesia (Black *et al.*, 1969) (Fig. 4).

Ether anaesthesia produces remarkably small alterations in blood pressure and pulse rate. It rarely leads to cardiac irregularities and does not sensitise the myocardium (like cyclopropane) to the action of noradrenaline and adrenaline. In fact, in the past, small concentrations of ether were often given to stop irregularities produced by cyclopropane anaesthesia. The evidence of tachycardia when ether is given without atropine premedication is taken as an indication of the parasympathetic blocking action of ether. To summarise, ether appears to increase sympathetic nervous activity and block parasympathetic activity in normal man (Price, 1961). The increase in noradrenaline liberation under ether anaesthesia partially offsets the direct myocardial depressant action of ether seen in the isolated heart preparation. Deep ether anaesthesia, therefore, should be used with caution in those patients with reduced catecholamine secretion or in the presence of ganglion blockade. β-blocking agents, such as propranolol, may be dangerous during ether anaesthesia (Jorfeldt *et al.*, 1967).

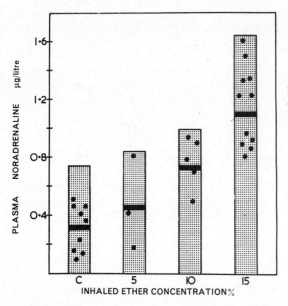

6/Fig. 4.—Plasma noradrenaline levels in relation to increasing concentration of inhaled ether. The horizontal black lines indicate mean values (Black *et al.*, 1969).

Action on the peripheral circulation.—McArdle and his colleagues (1968) have measured the effects on forearm blood flow and conclude that increasing the concentration leads to a reduction in flow. There is no change in flow with inspired concentrations of 5 per cent ether, a slight fall with 10 per cent and a significant reduction with 15 per cent. When the sympathetic nerve supply to one forearm is blocked by local analgesia, the reduction in blood flow to that side still equals the fall on the unblocked side as increasing concentrations of ether are inspired, thus suggesting that the vasoconstriction is not nervously mediated. Black *et al.* (1969) suggest that there is a close relationship between the increase in vascular resistance and a rising plasma noradrenaline concentration.

Action on skeletal muscle.—Ether causes skeletal muscle relaxation by depressing the central nervous system (Ngai *et al.*, 1965), and by affecting the nerve, the motor end-plate and the muscle itself. Concentrations used in clinical practice cause a block at the motor end-plate (Secher, 1951*a*), and there is some evidence that the post-junctional membrane is affected (Karis *et al.*, 1966). The mode of action is probably similar (but not identical) to that of *d*-tubocurarine (Secher, 1951*b*), so that when these two drugs are used in the same patient an additive effect results from their synergism. The effect of ether at the motor end-plate can be reversed by neostigmine (Gross and Cullen, 1943).

Action on other organs.—Ether provokes sickness in two ways. First, it is absorbed in saliva and passed to the stomach where it irritates the mucosa. Secondly, it stimulates the vomiting centre in the medulla.

The smooth muscle of the intestines is depressed by ether in direct relation to the concentration of the anaesthetic in the blood.

Prolonged administration of ether, particularly in the presence of hypoxia, may lead to damage of liver cells. Since ether stimulates the autonomic nervous system and leads to the release of adrenaline, glycogen is mobilised from both the liver and muscle tissue and a marked rise in blood sugar follows.

Renal blood flow is depressed, and albuminuria from tubular irritation, occurs in a proportion of patients.

Ether reduces the tone of the gravid uterus even in slight concentrations. High concentrations lead to complete relaxation. It rapidly passes from the maternal placental circulation into that of the fetus, so that equilibrium between the two is soon achieved.

Clinical Use

The objective in the administration of any anaesthetic is not only to produce unconsciousness but also to suppress the reflex activity of the patient to just a sufficient degree to enable the surgeon to perform a particular operation. Modern anaesthetic techniques often go far beyond this maxim, but ether still remains the safest and most effective means of gradually producing reflex suppression.

In the conscious state, if the skin of a patient's hand is incised with a knife, the hand is rapidly withdrawn unless the patient deliberately brings other muscles into force which overcome this withdrawal reflex. The moment unconsciousness is produced, the central controlling force is removed, and the patient responds to stimuli in a reflex manner. Now, if the skin is cut, not only is the limb withdrawn but, owing to "facilitation" produced by the reflex, there is a spread to many other pathways, so that the larynx may close, the abdominal muscles may contract, and the other limbs move across in an unco-ordinated effort to ward off the stimulus. As the depth of anaesthesia increases so, one by one, the reflex pathways become blocked, until finally all are suppressed. The exact position in which the reflex arc is broken differs with the various anaesthetic agents. Ether not only has a direct suppressant action on the central nervous system but also raises the excitation threshold of the motor end-plate, in a similar manner to d-tubocurarine chloride, thus producing a neuro-muscular block.

Even in minimal concentrations ether irritates the bronchial tree, stimulating the vagal afferent fibres leading to an increase in depth and rate of respiration together with an outpouring of mucous secretions. The latter reflex is success-fully depressed by adequate doses of atropine or hyoscine. As the depth of anaesthesia increases the respiratory pattern changes, more reflexes become suppressed, and characteristic changes in the size of the pupil can be seen. This slow progression of change has made it possible to divide up the various altera-tions in reflex activity into stages of ether anaesthesia. First described by Guedel after an exhaustive study of open ether anaesthetics, these stages remain today amongst the basic requirements for the student of anaesthesia. They are given in Table 4.

The pre-operative use of even small doses of the opiates prevents the correct interpretation of the pupil signs. The changes are best seen in children pre-medicated with barbiturates. During rapid lightening of ether anaesthesia the changes in pupillary diameter (together with all the other reflexes) tend to lag behind the more accurate respiratory-pattern changes. Sometimes even the respiratory patterns of deep anaesthesia may persist until the patient is practically awake.

Guedel's classification refashioned.—Many authors have attempted to re-fashion Guedel's classification to embrace the changes seen with such anaes-thetic drugs as halothane or the muscle relaxants. With ether, a relatively slow process of events underlines the stages and enhances the intrinsic safety of the drug. Newer agents do not respect such an orderly sequence; amongst others, the capacity of the intravenous thiobarbiturates to depress respiration in light anaesthesia, and of muscle relaxants to simulate most of the signs of anaesthesia yet produce no anaesthesia at all, are well known. The idea of anaesthetic depth is outmoded when combinations of drugs are used, but the need for a guide to the assessment of anaesthesia remains. Mushin (1948) and Laycock (1953) have restated the orthodox stages in modern terms. Analgesia, characterised by consciousness and disorientation, is an essential feature of the first stage, and merges into the second, when unconsciousness supervenes, often with marked reflex activity. Both these stages may be lost, however, when the induction of anaesthesia is rapid. It is in the third stage that surgery is performed when the reflexes are depressed. The fourth stage represents overdosage.

Each or all of these stages of general anaesthesia can usually be assessed from the specific and objective signs that surgical stimuli produce. Thus modern polypharmacy in anaesthesia is devised to select a combination of drugs, each with a more or less distinct action, and to avoid the unnecessary depression of other parts of the body that must occur occasionally when a single agent is used. Gray (1957) has summarised this type of technique in the single word "control". Others have termed it "balanced anaesthesia", but this idea of utilising more than one agent to offset the disadvantages of a single one, was suggested long before anaesthesia reached its present state (Lundy, 1926).

The anaesthetist chooses a drug or mixture of drugs that best fits the antici-pated needs of the operation, and as Laycock (1953) has written, reflexes are his

6/TABLE 4. THE STAGES AND SIGNS OF ETHER ANAESTHESIA

	Respiration			Pupils		Reflex Depression
	Rhythm	Volume	Pattern	Size	Position	
Stage I (Analgesia) Analgesia to loss of consciousness	Irregular	Small		Small	Divergent	Nil
Stage II (Excitement) Loss of consciousness to rhythmical respiration	Irregular	Large		Large	Divergent	Eyelash Eyelid
Stage III (Surgical anaesthesia) Plane I Rhythmical respiration to cessation of eye movement	Regular	Large		Small	Divergent	Skin Vomiting Conjunctival Pharyngeal Stretch from limb-muscles
Plane II Cessation of eye movement to start of respiratory muscle paresis (excl. diaphragm)	Regular	Medium	*	½ dilated	Fixed centrally	Corneal
Plane III Respiratory muscle paresis to paralysis	Regular Pause after expiration	Small		¾ dilated	Fixed centrally	Laryngeal Peritoneal
Plane IV Diaphragmatic paresis to paralysis	Jerky Irregular Quick inspiration Prolonged expiration, i.e. "see-saw"	Small		Fully dilated	Fixed centrally	Anal sphincter Carinal
Stage IV Apnoea						

* If the respiration rate is slow, an expiratory pause may be seen in Plane II.

essential guides in this matter. He must understand them, look out for them, nurse them, leave them alone, depress or abolish them.

Methods of Administration

A patient can be anaesthetised with ether by any one of the three standard methods, namely open, semi-closed and closed with carbon dioxide absorption.

For an open technique the Schimmelbusch mask is commonly used. This consists of a wire frame covered with a layer or two of gauze or a single layer of lint. The ether is dropped on to it from a suitable bottle, the aim being to supply the maximum concentration that the patient will tolerate without coughing or breath-holding. The mask should be kept moist over its whole surface since this will provide the maximum vapour concentration, bearing in mind that the liquid vaporises very rapidly. It is helpful during open ether administration to allow a slow trickle of oxygen under the margin of the mask, and during the induction of anaesthesia to add a little carbon dioxide to increase the depth of respiration. An alternative to the addition of carbon dioxide is to allow some of this gas to accumulate from the patient's exhalations by covering the mask with gamgee gauze so that the system becomes semi-open. Such an arrangement also helps to contain the ether vapour.

The chief disadvantage of these techniques is the unpleasant induction, but this can be mitigated by the use of ethyl chloride prior to ether. Very high vapour concentrations are seldom achieved—indeed the concentration may be insufficient for some adults. Under experimental conditions, using an external method of warming, concentrations of 40 per cent or more have been obtained, but in clinical practice the rapid evaporation of ether results in a corresponding fall in temperature and therefore in the volume concentration of the inspired vapour.

In the semi-closed method the ether is vaporised in a glass container by a flow of anaesthetic gases and oxygen. One of the factors adding to the safety of ether as an anaesthetic agent, when used in this way, is that as vaporisation increases, so the temperature of the liquid ether falls which in turn slows the rate of vaporisation. If, therefore, the control is set to deliver a strong concentration of ether vapour, the depth of anaesthesia increases, but after a time, with the control still in the same position, there is a reduction in the vapour concentration. It is inadvisable to warm the outside of the glass container unless a strong concentration is required during the induction of anaesthesia. Even then this practice is generally considered too dangerous and it is safer to surround the bottle with cold water to prevent icing.

The vaporisation of ether in a closed system depends upon the particular type of apparatus. When it is to and fro', vaporisation is exactly as in a semi-closed system, but owing to the small basal flow of gases, only slight concentrations of ether can be obtained. In a circular system the whole volume of ventilation can be passed through an ether bottle, so that high concentrations of ether can be relatively quickly built up. Moreover, vaporisation is assisted both by heat from the patient and by heat produced in the canister.

The E.M.O. inhaler.—This "draw-over" inhaler was designed by Epstein and Macintosh (1956) to deliver a required concentration of anaesthetic vapour irrespective of variations in the temperature of the liquid anaesthetic throughout the range likely to be met in clinical practice. The apparatus incorporates a water bath which surrounds the vaporising chamber and, by acting as a heat buffer, prevents sudden, marked changes in the temperature of the liquid anaesthetic. A bellows type thermostat automatically ensures that a constant vapour concentration of anaesthetic leaves the inhaler. The E.M.O. inhaler must be calibrated to suit the particular volatile anaesthetic used in it.

Convulsions occurring during ether anaesthesia (see Chapter 31).

DIVINYL ETHER $(C_2H_3)_2O$

In 1887 Semmler described a substance which he believed to be divinyl ether. The anaesthetic properties of divinyl ether were first described by Leake and Chen in 1930, and three years later Gelfan and Bell (1933) published the first report on its use in clinical anaesthesia.

Preparation.—This is a complicated and costly process. Ether is first chlorinated to prepare $\beta\beta$-dichlor-ether which is then fused with molten potassium hydroxide to produce divinyl ether, potassium chloride and water.

$$(C_2H_4Cl)_2O + 2KOH \rightarrow (C_2H_3)_2O + 2KCl + 2H_2O$$

| $\beta\beta$-dichlor-ether | + Potassium hydroxide | → Divinyl ether | + Potassium chloride | + Water |

Physical properties.—Divinyl ether is a colourless, non-irritating liquid with a sweet odour. The molecular weight is 70, the specific gravity of the liquid is 0·77 and of the vapour 2·2 (air = 1). The boiling point is 28·3° C. Divinyl ether is believed to be less soluble in water than ethyl ether, but the oil/water solubility ratio is a matter of disagreement. Adriani (1952) claims it is 41·3, whereas Kochmann (1936) states it is similar to that of diethyl ether, or 3·2. The very rapid recovery from anaesthesia with this agent favours Adriani's figure.

Stability.—Divinyl ether has a relatively low stability, which is made worse by acids and improved by alkalis. When it is chemically pure it is so volatile that moisture tends to freeze on the anaesthetic face-piece. For this reason 3·5 per cent absolute alcohol is added to diminish volatility. A non-volatile organic base—phenyl-alpha-naphthylamine—in a concentration of 0·01 per cent is also added to improve the stability. The commercial product is known as "Vinesthene" in the United Kingdom. The liquid decomposes on exposure to air, light and heat to form formaldehyde, acetaldehyde, formic and acetic acid. It is, therefore, best kept in dark, well-stoppered bottles in a cool place. The manufacturers do not recommend use two years after production and it is inadvisable to use the contents of a bottle that has been opened for more than two weeks. It is not affected by soda-lime even when the heat in the canister reaches temperatures as high as 70° C.

Inflammability.—Divinyl ether is explosive when mixed with air in concentrations between 1·7 and 27·0 per cent, and with oxygen between 1·8 and 85·0 per cent.

Pharmacological Actions

Divinyl ether is absorbed and eliminated almost entirely through the lungs, but a small percentage is excreted through the skin. A vapour, with a concentration of 4 per cent, will give a light plane of anaesthesia with a blood concentration of 20–30 mg per cent, whereas a vapour with 10 per cent divinyl ether may lead to a blood level of 70 mg per cent and respiratory arrest. Induction is more rapid and pleasant than with ether owing to the increased potency and the absence of irritation of the bronchial tree. Recovery is also more rapid than after ether.

Action on the cardiovascular system.—Divinyl ether has similar effects to diethyl ether. The pacemaker may be displaced, leading to auricular extrasystoles, but the adrenergic stimulation leads to improvement in myocardial contraction.

Action on the respiratory system.—Bronchial dilatation is produced, and in light anaesthesia respiration is increased in rate. An overdose leads to failure of the respiratory centre before the heart finally stops beating.

Action on the alimentary system.—Divinyl ether can cause toxic damage to the liver if used in high concentration for prolonged periods. Central lobular necrosis is produced, and though this complication is rare it is inadvisable to use the agent for more than 30 minutes at one administration. As with chloroform, the incidence of this complication can be greatly reduced by pre-operative treatment with glucose, protein and amino acids in order to protect the liver, and also by a high percentage of oxygen with a low carbon dioxide tension during anaesthesia.

Other actions.—Salivation is apt to be produced by divinyl ether, particularly if premedication has been omitted. It has few side-effects and causes little or no nausea and vomiting after short administrations. It depresses uterine tone in labour and quickly crosses the placenta into the fetus.

Clinical Use

Divinyl ether is both volatile and expensive, so that its clinical use is restricted; although it has some value for the induction of anaesthesia, divinyl ether alone is generally used in a special closed inhaler as a single dose method. A quantity of the agent is evaporated in the bag of an inhaler which has previously been filled with oxygen. About 3–5 ml of divinyl ether will produce anaesthesia in about six breaths and give approximately 2–3 minutes of unconsciousness, depending upon the size of the patient. The method is particularly suitable for guillotine tonsillectomy, and sometimes for dental extractions, in children.

A mixture of 75 per cent diethyl ether and 25 per cent divinyl ether marketed under the trade name of "Vinesthene Anaesthetic Mixture" (V.A.M.) has a wider application, however, since it gives a rapid induction of anaesthesia with less irritation of the bronchial tract than does diethyl ether alone. V.A.M. may be vaporised by any of the methods described for ether.

ETHYL CHLORIDE (C_2H_5Cl)

Ethyl chloride was first prepared by Basil Valentine during the early part of the seventeenth century. Flourens in 1847 (Flourens 1847 *a* and *b*) and Heyfelder in 1848 described its general anaesthetic properties, but it continued to be used solely for local refrigeration analgesia until in 1894 Carlson inadvertently produced unconsciousness in a patient whilst spraying the gum for a dental extraction. In the past it has been used extensively in anaesthesia.

Preparation.—There are two common methods of preparation:
(a) By reacting ethylene with hydrochloric acid:

$$C_2H_4 + HCl \rightarrow C_2H_5Cl.$$

(b) By treating ethyl alcohol with hydrochloric acid:

$$C_2H_5OH + HCl \rightarrow C_2H_5Cl + H_2O.$$

Physical properties.—Ethyl chloride is a clear fluid with an ethereal odour which is not irritating to the respiratory tract. Frequently this is masked by the addition of eau-de-Cologne. The molecular weight is 64·5. The specific gravity of the liquid is 0·921 at 20° C and of the vapour 2·28 (air = 1). The boiling point is 12·5° C, so that at ordinary room temperatures it is a vapour. Nevertheless, it is easily compressed to form a highly volatile liquid which can be stored in glass or metal tubes. It has a high lipoid solubility, for at 38° C five volumes of vapour dissolves in one volume of blood.

Impurities.—It may contain traces of alcohol, aldehydes, chlorides or poly-halogenated ethanes.

Inflammability.—The vapour is heavier than air and is capable of explosion when mixed with air in concentrations between 3·8–15·4 per cent and with oxygen between 4·0 and 67·0 per cent.

Pharmacological Actions

Ethyl chloride is non-irritant to the respiratory mucosa. Concentrations of 3–4·5 per cent in the inspired air produce anaesthesia and a blood concentration of 20–30 mg per cent leads to the signs of surgical anaesthesia. Forty mg per cent leads to respiratory arrest.

Action on the cardiovascular system.—There is very little evidence that ethyl chloride produces an irritable myocardium, and dysrhythmias are rare during induction. The pulse rate may be slowed from stimulation of the vagal centre and there is widespread vasodilatation due to vasomotor depression. As anaesthesia progresses the heart dilates slightly, owing to the effect on the myocardium. Although both the cardiac output and peripheral vascular tone are depressed in deep anaesthesia, there is no evidence that myocardial failure will occur before respiratory arrest—most cases of sudden circulatory failure during the induction of anaesthesia can be traced to relative overdosage at the time rather than to peculiar side-effects. Overdosage easily and quickly results on account of the physical properties of the drug.

Other actions.—Ethyl chloride anaesthesia is frequently followed by headache, nausea and vomiting. It depresses uterine tone in labour and quickly crosses the placenta into the fetus.

Clinical Use

Local analgesia.—A fine spray is allowed to fall on the operation area. The liquid vaporises and the skin cools to −20° C, and the surrounding water vapour freezes and deposits fine snowy crystals over the wound. The incision is painless but as the thaw sets in the pain may become excruciating.

General anaesthesia.—Ethyl chloride is an extremely potent and simple anaesthetic to administer—so much so that the greatest possible care should be exercised in its use. It is particularly suitable for induction in children, but once a rhythmical respiratory exchange has commenced it should be abandoned: if necessary, the anaesthesia can be maintained by the much safer agent—diethyl ether.

It is inadvisable to spray more than 5 ml of the ethyl chloride on to an open mask for the induction of anaesthesia; subsequent doses should be much smaller. Great care should be taken to prevent a child holding its breath for a prolonged period and then taking a large inspiration of a highly-concentrated vapour, which can lead to circulatory collapse.

Ethyl chloride may be used with oxygen in a closed inhaler in a manner similar to that described for divinyl ether. A dose of 3–5 ml is sufficient for a single administration.

TRICHLOROETHYLENE (CCl_2CHCl)

Originally described by E. Fischer, a German chemist, in 1864, it was first used as an anaesthetic agent in animals by Lehmann in 1911 whilst working at Wurzburg University.

The finding that trichloroethylene was a powerful grease solvent led to its wide application in industry for the removal of grease from metal and machinery. This led to toxic symptoms in some of the factory workers, however, and in 1915 Plessner described the syndrome of acute trichloroethylene poisoning— one of the main features of which is sensory paralysis of the fifth cranial nerve. Such symptoms were almost certainly due to the impurities associated with trichloroethylene. In the same year Oppenheim described twelve cases of trigeminal neuralgia that were successfully treated by inhalations of trichloroethylene vapour.

In 1934, Dennis Jackson of Cincinnati University redescribed its anaesthetic properties and one year later, at the same University, Striker and his colleagues published the first report of the successful administration of trichloroethylene to 304 patients for dental extractions or minor operative procedures. Hewer and Hadfield (1941) popularised it in the United Kingdom.

Preparation.—Acetylene when treated with chlorine forms tetrachlorethane; this is reacted with calcium hydroxide in a "lime slurry" to form trichloroethylene, which is purified by distillation.

$$C_2H_2 \quad + \quad 2Cl_2 \quad \rightarrow \quad C_2H_2Cl_4$$
Acetylene   Chlorine   Tetrachlorethane

$$2C_2H_2Cl_4 \quad + Ca(OH)_2 \rightarrow \quad 2C_2HCl_3 \quad + \quad CaCl_2 \quad + 2H_2O$$
Tetrachlorethane   Calcium   Trichloroethylene   Calcium   Water
hydroxide   chloride

Physical properties.—Trichloroethylene is a heavy colourless liquid with a low volatility (boiling point 87·5° C) and has a smell similar to that of chloroform but not so sweet. The vapour pressure at 20° C is about 57 mm Hg (7·6 kPa). Thus with a high boiling point and low vapour pressure it is relatively difficult to vaporise high concentrations.

However, it has an oil/gas solubility coefficient of 960; on this basis it is the most potent of all known anaesthetic agents and it is calculated that a concentration as low as 0·17 vols per cent will achieve the 1st plane of surgical anaesthesia (or minimal anaesthetic concentration).

Trilene, the trade name for the preparation which is used in anaesthesia in Great Britain, consists of purified trichloroethylene, thymol (stabilising agent) 1:10,000 and waxoline blue (dye) 1:200,000. The dye is added to distinguish it from chloroform.

In the United States the trade name is Trimar. It consists of 99–99·5 per cent purified trichloroethylene with the remainder alcohol. Ammonium carbonate is added as a preservative.

Stability.—Trichloroethylene is decomposed by strong light or by contact with hot surfaces into phosgene and hydrochloric acid. It is, therefore, best kept in metal containers.

It is contra-indicated in the presence of soda-lime for two reasons—first, it decomposes to phosgene and hydrochloric acid when in contact with a hot surface. Secondly, in the presence of an alkali and heat it may be broken down to hydrochloric acid and dichloracetylene, a substance which is both inflammable and toxic. Dichloracetylene may itself decompose to phosgene and carbon monoxide. Thus:

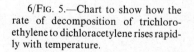

1. $\underset{\text{CCl}_2}{\overset{\text{CHCl}}{\|}}$ $\xrightarrow{\text{NaOH}}$ $\underset{\text{CCl}}{\overset{\text{CCl}}{\mbox{\(\mkern1mu\|\|\|\)}}}$ + HCl (absorbed by NaOH)

     Trichloroethylene + Heat → Dichloracetylene + Hydrochloric acid

2. $\underset{\text{CCl}}{\overset{\text{CCl}}{\mbox{\(\|\|\|\)}}}$ $+ O_2 \xrightarrow{}$ $COCl_2$ +   CO

     Dichloracetylene + Oxygen → Phosgene + Carbon monoxide

The rate of decomposition of trichloroethylene in the presence of soda-lime depends largely on the temperature. At 15° C it is slow, but over 60° C the rate rises sharply (Fig. 5). It has been suggested that decomposition can be inhibited by the addition of 10 per cent silica.

Some of the early cases of cranial nerve palsy following the use of trichloro-

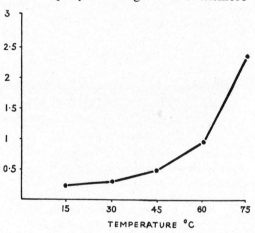

6/Fig. 5.—Chart to show how the rate of decomposition of trichloroethylene to dichloracetylene rises rapidly with temperature.

TEMPERATURE °C

ethylene in the presence of soda-lime are believed to have been due to the high percentage of sodium hydroxide present in the absorbents used. Soda-lime of this type was five times more hygroscopic and also generated more heat than that available today. It has also been shown that the temperature of modern soda-lime rarely rises above 40° C during clinical anaesthesia, nevertheless at this temperature small amounts of dichloracetylene can be formed.

It is inadvisable to use cautery or diathermy in the immediate presence of trichloroethylene vapour, such as during an oral operation, because at temperatures above 125° C phosgene and hydrochloric acid may be rapidly formed, particularly if a high percentage of oxygen is present (Carney and Gillespie, 1945; Firth and Stuckey, 1945).

Toxicity.—Cranial nerve lesions are amongst the commonest toxic manifestations of impure trichloroethylene or its degradation products, such as dichloracetylene. The fifth nerve is the most commonly involved but lesions of all the nerves except the first, ninth and eleventh have been reported.

The onset of toxic symptoms and signs is usually characterised by a complaint of numbness or coldness around the lips starting about twenty-four to forty-eight hours after the anaesthetic ceased. During the next few days the area of sensory loss spreads to involve the whole field supplied by the trigeminal nerve. There is no motor involvement. Recovery usually begins between the fifth and tenth days and may be complete in a fortnight.

Inflammability.—Trichloroethylene vapour is non-inflammable and non-explosive in the concentrations used in anaesthesia (see also Chapter 8).

Pharmacological Actions

Uptake and distribution.—Trichloroethylene has a blood/gas solubility coefficient of 9·15, which indicates that it is relatively soluble in blood. In other words blood has a great capacity for taking up trichloroethylene. A long time will elapse, therefore, before alveolar tension reaches equilibrium with the inspired concentration. Clayton and Parkhouse (1962) found that the administration of a 1 per cent v/v trichloroethylene concentration resulted in an arterial concentration in the blood of 12·17 mg/100 ml. Furthermore, in slim subjects the concentration in venous blood approximated to that of arterial blood after about 30 minutes, whereas in fat subjects it took twice as long. This is because trichloroethylene is extremely soluble in human fat due to its high oil/gas solubility; in fact, it is probably 100 times more soluble in fat than in muscle.

To summarise, this agent has a low volatility and a high blood solubility. The slow induction is partially offset by the high degree of potency due to the remarkable oil/gas solubility. Recovery, however, is prolonged.

Trichloroethylene is partly excreted unchanged by the lungs and partly metabolised. Depending upon the duration of time for which the vapour is inhaled, the percentage recovery of trichloroethylene in expired gases varies from 67 to 83 per cent (Malchy and Parkhouse, 1969). Metabolic degradation is slow, and the metabolic products are found in the urine from 10 to 18 days following a single period of trichloroethylene administration. Assuming that approximately 20 per cent of inspired trichloroethylene is metabolised, then 10 per cent of trichloroethanol and 10 per cent of trichloracetic acid will result (Greene, 1968).

Action on the cardiovascular system.—Almost every known form of cardiac dysrhythmia has been reported during trichloroethylene anaesthesia, but always in association with high concentrations of the inhaled vapour. Sinus tachycardia and bradycardia, nodal rhythm and partial heart block are usually associated with light anaesthesia, whereas ventricular extrasystoles may occur in deep anaesthesia.

The incidence of cardiac dysrhythmias is likely to be increased if adrenaline is used during anaesthesia. Opinion is divided on the incidence of primary cardiac failure due to trichloroethylene, though it appears that this condition may very rarely occur (Edwards *et al.*, 1956).

Trichloroethylene produces no significant alteration in forearm blood flow, heart rate or mean arterial blood pressure (McArdle *et al.*, 1968).

Action on the respiratory system.—Trichloroethylene in moderate concentrations (1–3 per cent) is non-irritant to the respiratory tract; in high concentrations, however, it may cause tachypnoea. The increased respiratory rate leads to a diminished tidal volume and in severe cases this may be so reduced that hypoxia occurs.

Other actions.—Post-operative vomiting and headache occasionally follow trichloroethylene anaesthesia, while circumoral herpes has been reported.

Trichloroethylene causes a rise in intracranial pressure. Jennett and his associates (1969) report that such an increase occurs even when the arterial carbon dioxide is low, and that it is associated with cerebral vasodilation and an increased cerebral blood flow.

Trichloroethylene will depress the contractions of the uterus during labour. Analgesic concentrations—0·5 per cent v./v. in air or less—have little effect on uterine muscle unless inhaled for periods approaching 4 hours, when accumulation of the drug in the body occurs. At this stage both the rate and tone of uterine contraction may be decreased. Trichloroethylene rapidly crosses the placenta into the fetal circulation, and animal experiments (sheep) show that within sixteen minutes the fetal concentration is higher than that in the maternal circulation (Helliwell and Hutton, 1950).

The effect of trichloroethylene on the liver has been studied by determining concentrations of glutamic acid, pyruvic acid, transaminase and lactic dehydrogenase in the blood of patients undergoing anaesthesia. Elevated values were not found in any case (Bløndal and Fagerlund, 1963).

Clinical Use

The fact that trichloroethylene is non-inflammable, relatively non-irritant and with minimal post-operative side-effects, has made it popular as a supplement to the sequence thiopentone, nitrous oxide and oxygen for the maintenance of light anaesthesia. The chief disadvantage in general surgery is that it is unsuitable for the production of muscular relaxation, since when this is attempted tachypnoea and cardiac dysrhythmias are quickly encountered. Nevertheless, within the safe limits of its application it is a useful agent. For the production of analgesia it is widely used in both obstetrics and dentistry. It is also useful for post-operative analgesia, particularly during physiotherapy (Ellis and Bryce-Smith, 1965; Hovell *et al.*, 1967).

Administration.—The low volatility makes trichloroethylene barely suitable for administration on an open mask, but as it is over four times as heavy as air this route can be used to produce analgesia if no apparatus is available. The drug is most commonly used in a semi-closed system using a Tritec vaporiser or, for analgesia, in a "draw-over" type of apparatus (see Chapter 42). It can also be given in an accurate concentration by volume in air from an E.M.O. inhaler after suitable calibration of the apparatus.

CHLOROFORM (CHCl₃)

Chloroform was independently discovered by Soubeiran, Liebig and Guthrie in 1831. Its chemical and physical properties were first described by Alexandre Dumas in 1835, and twelve years later, in 1847, Flourens reported on its anaesthetic properties (Flourens, 1847 *a* and *b*). That same year James Simpson, acting on a suggestion from a Liverpool chemist David Waldie, experimented upon himself and his colleagues, and finally gave it to patients with great success. Soon after its introduction into clinical practice chloroform largely replaced ether in popularity, but since then its popularity has gradually waned.

Preparation.—Chloroform may be prepared in a number of ways, but those most commonly encountered are:

In the laboratory: acetone or ethyl alcohol is heated with bleaching powder and the mixture is then submitted to steam distillation.

$$2CH_3.CO.CH_3 + Ca(OCl)_2 \rightarrow CH_3COCCl_3 + CHCl_3 + Ca(CH_3.COO)_2$$

| Acetone | Bleaching powder | Trichlor-acetone | Chloroform | Calcium acetate |

Commercially: carbon tetrachloride and hydrogen are allowed to react in the presence of iron.

$$\begin{array}{c} Cl \\ | \\ Cl-C\ \ Cl + 2H \\ | \\ Cl \end{array} \xrightarrow{\ \ Fe\ \ } \begin{array}{c} Cl \\ | \\ Cl-C-H + HCl \\ | \\ Cl \end{array}$$

| Carbon tetrachloride | Hydrogen | | Chloro-form | Hydrochloric acid |

Physical properties.—Chloroform is a colourless transparent fluid with a sweet smelling odour. The boiling point is 61° C and the vapour pressure at 20° C is 150 mm Hg (20 kPa).

The oil/gas solubility coefficient is 265 (*cf.* 960 for trichloroethylene and 11·2 for cyclopropane) denoting considerable solubility in lipoid tissues and also anaesthetic potency. In fact, an alveolar concentration of only 0·62 vols. per cent is required for 1st plane surgical anaesthesia.

Stability.—Prolonged exposure to light or heat results in the breakdown of chloroform, the most serious oxidation product being phosgene, which is highly irritant to the respiratory tract. For this reason it should be stored in dark bottles in a cool place. Stability is increased by the addition of 1 per cent ethyl alcohol, an agent which would also convert any phosgene present to diethyl carbonate.

Chloroform can be used with soda-lime without danger of undue decomposition. In theory several reactions may take place when chloroform comes into contact with an alkali (Bassett, 1949):

1. Decomposition of chloroform into sodium formate

$$CHCl_3 \quad + \quad 4NaOH \quad \rightarrow \quad 3NaCl \quad + \quad H.COONa \quad + \quad 2H_2O$$

| Chloroform | Sodium hydroxide | Sodium chloride | Sodium formate | Water |

2. Decomposition of chloroform into sodium chloride and carbon monoxide

$$CHCl_3 \quad + \quad 3NaOH \quad \rightarrow \quad 3NaCl \quad + \quad CO \quad + \quad 2H_2O$$

| Chloroform | Sodium hydroxide | Sodium chloride | Carbon monoxide | Water |

3. Decomposition of chloroform into sodium chloride and phosgene

$$CHCl_3 \quad + \quad NaOH \quad + \quad O \quad \rightarrow \quad NaCl \quad + \quad COCl_2 \quad + \quad H_2O$$

| Chloroform | Sodium hydroxide | Oxygen | Sodium chloride | Phosgene | Water |

There seems little doubt that under the conditions of anaesthesia little, if any, decomposition takes place, particularly if fresh soda-lime is used, and that the courses represented in equations 1 and 2 are the most likely, while the production of phosgene is extremely improbable. Bassett was able to show in soda-lime used clinically with chloroform that only very slight decomposition had taken place. Even if all the chloroform destroyed in his cases had been converted to carbon monoxide, only about 16 ml of the gas would have been produced throughout the anaesthetic. Other products which may be present are hydrochloric acid, acetone, free halogens, organic halides, ethyl chloride, aldehydes and peroxides.

Inflammability.—Chloroform is non-inflammable.

Pharmacological Actions

Uptake and distribution.—The blood/gas solubility coefficient of chloroform is 10·3 denoting that the blood is capable of taking up large quantities. Induction, therefore, is slow but this is partially offset by the high degree of anaesthetic potency of this agent. Recovery is slow.

The greater part of the chloroform inhaled is not altered in the body but is excreted unchanged by the lungs, nearly all of it leaving the circulation within sixty minutes of the end of anaesthesia. That which remains may not be eliminated for many hours and a small part is broken down in the body to hydrochloric acid and a residual hydrocarbon. Animal studies suggest that about 4 per cent of inhaled chloroform is metabolised (Cohen and Hood, 1969).

Chloroform has a direct depressant action on the myocardium, the respiratory centre, the vasomotor centre, and tissue cells in general, so that all of the four types of anoxia—anaemic, anoxic, stagnant and histotoxic—are possible in some degree when it is used.

Action on the cardiovascular system.—Chloroform depresses cardiac muscle and conducting tissue and also the smooth muscle of the peripheral vessels, with a resulting general depression of the circulation. These are direct effects, but both heart and circulation are also depressed reflexly from an action on the vagal and vasomotor centres. The situation is aggravated by anoxaemia resulting from respiratory depression and a reduction of the oxygen-carrying capacity of the blood.

Vagal inhibition of the heart may occur during induction. Since Levy's classical work in 1912 on ventricular fibrillation during chloroform anaesthesia (Levy, 1913) there has been a tendency to discountenance the view that irritant concentrations of chloroform reaching vagal receptors in the respiratory tract can induce cardiac arrest. Although this complication may be rare it seems very likely that it can occur, and not only with chloroform but with trichloroethylene and even agents such as ether, provided sufficiently irritant concentrations reach the vagal receptors in the lower air passages (Johnstone, 1955). It is particularly likely to happen when any one of these volatile agents is given to a patient who has had some muscle relaxant. During the period of paralysis abnormally high concentrations may be blown into the patient's lungs, creating a situation which would be impossible were the volatile anaesthetic agent alone used.

In spite of the possibility of vagal inhibition of the heart, death during the induction with chloroform in man is probably most commonly due to ventricular fibrillation. This was first suggested by Levy working with cats; he demonstrated that chloroform sensitises the myocardium to the stimulating effects of injected adrenaline. In man during chloroform induction the pulse rate is slowed, partly due to vagal stimulation in the medulla, and partly due to direct depression of conducting tissue in the heart. Moreover, the efficiency of the myocardium is decreased by a reduction in its refractory period. All in all, the heart is sensitised to the effects of sympathetic stimulation, which are frequently met during the induction of anaesthesia. It is believed, too, that chloroform may stimulate the afferent endings of the vagus nerve in the upper respiratory tract, causing a reflex excitation of the cardiac sympathetic nerves. Cardiac irregularities are also accentuated by carbon dioxide retention and hypoxia, both of which are likely concomitants of chloroform anaesthesia.

The pre-operative use of atropine, by reducing vagal tone, will decrease the incidence of cardiac irregularities, but not by any means prevent them all from occurring. Indeed electrocardiographic monitoring during chloroform anaesthesia has shown that irregularities of all types, but particularly multifocal ventricular extrasystoles—the precursors of ventricular fibrillation—occur more frequently than not (Hill, 1932). Waters (1951) studied fifty-two patients, and in this small series noted four cases of temporary cardiac arrest, and only seven cases in which no cardiac irregularities occurred. In all induction deaths with chloroform the heart stops before repiration ceases.

During the inhalation of moderate concentrations of chloroform (1·5–2 per cent) the cardiac output and peripheral resistance are progressively decreased, together with a continuous fall in blood pressure. It is incorrect to assume, however, that maintenance of light anaesthesia with low constant concentrations of chloroform leads to a steady fall in blood pressure. In fact perfectly reasonable pressures can be maintained.

Action on the respiratory system.—Chloroform depresses respiration both by a direct effect on the respiratory centre and by the production of progressive depression of the respiratory muscles.

Action on the liver.—It is generally accepted that central hepatic necrosis occurs in some degree after chloroform anaesthesia or analgesia irrespective of the concentration used or the length of administration. But Rollason (1964) using serum glutamic pyruvic transaminase (SGPT) activity in patients with good nutrition could find no evidence of liver damage following chloroform anaesthesia, provided the concentration did not exceed 2·25 per cent in an oxygen-rich mixture and there was no carbon dioxide retention. Repeated short administrations may sensitise the liver, and certainly increase the risk of a bad attack. In severe cases, leading to death, section of the liver will show necrosis with fatty degeneration of the cells surrounding the vein in the centre of the lobule. Signs and symptoms of poisoning are produced only by severe necrosis.

Delayed chloroform poisoning was originally described by Casper in 1850. The first symptoms may occur as early as six hours after the operation, although more commonly they present themselves twenty-four to forty-eight hours later. Nausea and vomiting start early and progressively increase in severity. The diagnosis becomes certain with the development of jaundice, and death, preceded by coma, may occur at any time during the first ten days. Delayed chloroform poisoning is not restricted in its symptomatology to the liver, the heart and kidneys also being affected. Fatty degeneration of the heart and necrosis of the tubular epithelium of the kidneys take place and result in incipient cardiac and renal failure.

A poor nutritional state increases the risk of this complication, whereas the pre-operative use of carbohydrates, proteins and amino acids helps to protect the liver. Moreover, the avoidance of hypoxia and carbon dioxide retention is of practical help. Waters (1951) has shown that if chloroform is given in the presence of a high percentage of oxygen, and if steps are taken to avoid carbon dioxide accumulation, hepatic and renal function tests in a group of patients show no significant difference from those of controls.

The treatment of delayed chloroform poisoning consists primarily of the administration of intravenous fluids, together with carbohydrates, protein and amino acids. Of the various amino acids methionine is the most useful because it plays an important part in building up the reserves of glycogen in the liver.

Action on the kidneys.—The toxic effects of chloroform are mainly on the renal tubules, which at microscopy can be seen to be swollen with the lumina filled with fat globules and coagulated serum. After chloroform anaesthesia transient albuminuria is a common occurrence, while prolonged administration often leads to glycosuria. In cases of delayed poisoning as described above ketonuria also occurs.

Other actions.—Toxic effects may be found in other organs. In severe cases fatty degeneration occurs in the pancreas and spleen, while nausea and vomiting in some degree usually follow all but the briefest anaesthetic. Chloroform depresses uterine contractions during labour and quickly crosses the placenta to reach the fetus.

Clinical Use

The main advantages of chloroform are a sweet-smelling, non-irritant vapour, portability, potency, and non-inflammability. It permits a rapid, smooth induction, while the decreased bleeding which results from circulatory depression was the forerunner of the "hypotensive" technique. Low volatility and a high potency make it particularly valuable in hot and humid countries, while the fact that an experienced administrator can produce such excellent conditions for surgery from a small bottle and simple mask has undoubtedly done much to recommend it in the past. It is interesting to recall in this respect that John Snow is believed to have given 4000 chloroform anaesthetics without any mortality.

Nevertheless, despite all these advantages, chloroform is not nowadays commonly used. As long ago as 1912 the Committee on Anesthesia of the American Medical Association went so far as to say that in their opinion the use of chloroform for major surgical operations was no longer justifiable. The reason for its elimination from major anaesthetic practice is to be found in the toxic effects it produces on the various parts of the body, and the fact that most, if not all, of its advantages can be obtained with a combination of other agents and with less risk to the patient. Only on an occasion where there is no suitable alternative, such as may occur for instance in certain circumstances in domiciliary midwifery, should chloroform now be used.

Administration

Chloroform may be dropped on to an open mask. One drop weighing 20 mg, if vaporised in 500 ml of air, forms a 1 per cent concentration of the vapour. At the start of induction 20 drops a minute is adequate, increasing later to 30 drops a minute. Great care should be taken to prevent the sudden inspiration of a high concentration, which is most likely with a struggling patient, and to avoid liquid chloroform reaching the skin, since it may cause a burn. Sometimes patients breathe shallowly during induction and then suddenly take a deep inspiration just before the second stage is reached. Nosworthy (1958) found that this could be avoided by adding a little carbon dioxide to the inspired mixture so that the depth of respiration could be regulated from the onset of unconsciousness. Once rhythmical and regular respiration has become established it is advisable to change over to ether or a chloroform-ether mixture (1 part chloroform to 4 parts diethyl ether). The safety of chloroform is at all times increased by the addition of oxygen to the inhaled mixture.

Administration in a semi-closed system has the advantage that it can be combined with an adequate oxygen flow and a more accurate increase in vapour concentration, but both in this type of system, and particularly in a closed system, the danger of accumulation cannot be over-emphasised.

THE FLUORINATED HYDROCARBONS

The introduction of halothane into clinical practice provides one of the great landmarks in the development of anaesthesia. In an attempt to find an agent that was basically as "safe" as ether yet non-inflammable, Suckling (1957) examined a number of fluorinated hydrocarbons. This group was known to be highly stable, volatile and non-inflammable (under clinical conditions).

In these compounds the fluorine atoms have a strong chemical bond with the carbon atoms. The result is that the fluorine atom is quite unreactive, particularly when the compound contains a CF_2 or CF_3 grouping. Such agents would be unlikely to interfere with body metabolism because of their high chemical stability, and therefore would tend to have a low toxicity (Sadove and Wallace, 1962).

Robbins (1946) in a study of many of the fluorinated hydrocarbons found that those with low boiling points produced convulsive movements; that the potency increased as the boiling point rose, yet recovery time became more prolonged, and that substitution of a bromine atom in the fluorohydrocarbon not only increased potency but also appeared to improve the safety margin.

The inclusion of several halogen atoms in a compound confers inflammability in the clinical range. If the halogen selected is a fluorine atom then there is no decrease in volatility, but the presence of at least one hydrogen atom is necessary for anaesthetic potency.

A large number of fluorinated hydrocarbons have been synthesised but only three have to date received extensive clinical trials. These are halothane, methoxyflurane and fluroxene:

$$
\begin{array}{ccc}
\underset{\underset{\displaystyle \text{F}}{|}}{\overset{\overset{\displaystyle \text{F}\quad\text{Br}}{|\quad|}}{\text{F}-\text{C}-\text{C}-\text{H}}}\underset{\displaystyle \text{Cl}}{} &
\underset{\underset{\displaystyle \text{Cl}}{|}}{\overset{\overset{\displaystyle \text{Cl}\quad\text{F}}{|\quad|}}{\text{H}-\text{C}-\text{C}-\text{O}-\text{C}-\text{H}}} &
\text{F}-\text{C}-\text{C}-\text{O}-\text{C}=\text{C}
\end{array}
$$

Halothane	Methoxyflurane	Fluroxene
(B.P. 50·2° C)	(B.P. 104·65° C)	(B.P. 43·2° C)

Of these three compounds halothane has received the widest clinical acclaim. One of the principal features of these fluorohydrocarbons is that they have relatively low boiling points (with the exception of methoxyflurane) when compared with similar agents containing only chlorine or bromine. For example, if all of the five halogens in halothane were chlorine then the boiling point would be 162° C. In fact, the boiling point of halothane is 50·2° C at atmospheric pressure.

A fourth compound that has had limited clinical trials during recent years is teflurane, or 1,1,1,2-tetrafluoro-bromethane, which is similar in structure to halothane. The incidence of cardiac dysrhythmias during light surgical anaesthesia with this agent is so high that it cannot be considered as a potentially useful addition to the existing fluorinated hydrocarbons of proven safety.

HALOTHANE (FLUOTHANE)

Halothane was prepared and examined by Raventós (1956). It was introduced into clinical anaesthesia by Johnstone (1956) and Bryce-Smith and O'Brien (1956).

Physical properties.—Halothane is a heavy, colourless liquid with a sweet smell somewhat resembling chloroform. It contains 0·01 per cent of thymol for stability. The formula is:

$$
\underset{\underset{\displaystyle \text{F}\quad\text{Cl}}{|\quad|}}{\overset{\overset{\displaystyle \text{F}\quad\text{Br}}{|\quad|}}{\text{F}-\text{C}-\text{C}-\text{H}}}
$$

Halothane

It has a molecular weight of 197·39 and a boiling point of 50·2° C (at 760 mm Hg, 101·1 kPa). It does not react with soda-lime. One of the contaminants is betene in a concentration of 0·001 per cent. When exposed to light for several days it will decompose to various halide acids such as HCl, HBr, free chlorine, bromine radicles and phosgene. The presence of thymol helps to prevent the liberation of free bromine.

The vapour pressure of halothane is 241 mm Hg (32 kPa) at 20° C. It is, therefore, very suitable for vaporisation in a bubble-through (e.g. copper kettle) or temperature and flow-controlled vaporiser (e.g. "Fluotec"). If a flow of 100 ml of oxygen is passed through the copper kettle (or "Vernitrol") vaporiser then as the vapour pressure is $\frac{240}{760}$ mm Hg or approximately $\frac{1}{3}$ of an atmosphere 100 ml of oxygen will pick up 50 ml of halothane (i.e. a total of 150 ml of $33\frac{1}{3}$ per cent halothane or 50 ml of pure halothane vapour). If this quantity (i.e. 50 ml of halothane vapour) is added to 5 litres of nitrous oxide and oxygen then the patient will receive an inspired concentration of 1 per cent halothane. Similarly, if 200 ml is put through the vaporiser and this is again added to 5 litres of nitrous oxide and oxygen the patient will receive a 2 per cent halothane vapour.

In the absence of water vapour halothane does not attack most metals. However, if water vapour is present it will attack aluminium, brass and lead. Copper and fault-free chromium are not attacked.

Halothane is readily soluble in rubber (coefficient 121·1 at 760 mm and 24° C) and less so in polyethylene (coefficient 26·3). This significant rubber solubility together with the large amount of this material used in an anaesthetic system means that the uptake of halothane by rubber could be significant if a low-flow circle absorption technique is used. High flows eliminate this problem (Eger et al., 1962).

Analysis.—Halothane can be estimated by gas chromatography (Dyjverman and Sjövall, 1962) or by infra-red (Robson et al., 1959) or ultra-violet light analysis.

Pharmacology

Uptake and distribution.—Halothane has a blood solubility coefficient of 2·3 (*cf.* nitrous oxide 0·46 and ether 12·1) and might be described as being in the medium range of solubility. Because it is relatively insoluble in blood it is not taken up very rapidly from the alveoli. This means that the alveolar concentration or tension can soon approach the inspired concentration. Now alveolar *tension* is virtually synonymous with brain *tension*, so a high tension is rapidly achieved in the brain. This means induction of anaesthesia is relatively rapid. On withdrawal of the anaesthetic the same process is reversed so that recovery is rapid.

Mapleson (1962) has shown that though the rate of uptake is high at the start, after twenty minutes, for every 1 per cent of halothane vapour in the inspired mixture, the patient has an uptake of 10 ml of halothane vapour per minute. This first goes to the organs with a rich blood supply such as the heart and brain. Resting muscle and fat have a much poorer blood supply so that they receive their quota of halothane long after the tension in the alveoli and brain have reached equilibrium. Thus, in the first few minutes of halothane anaesthesia most goes to the heart, brain, liver and kidneys. After ten or twenty minutes the muscles are tending to remove their quota from the circulation so that 10 ml of halothane vapour is removed from the lungs every minute. In time even the poorly perfused fat receives its share. In this manner the body continues almost indefinitely to keep removing halothane vapour from the lungs. If, therefore, a 1 per cent inspired concentration is given to a patient it is estimated that it will take 5 days or more for the concentration in the alveoli to rise to this level. In fact, equilibrium between inspired and alveolar concentrations is probably never reached because a small amount is lost through the skin.

One of the principal reasons for the prolonged uptake of halothane by the body is the remarkable capacity of human fat to absorb it. So great is this affinity—the solubility coefficient of halothane in fat is 60·0 (*cf*, nitrous oxide = 1·0)—that it is capable of removing almost all the halothane it receives in the circulation. Other tissues also show a slightly greater affinity for halothane than blood.

6/Table 5
Tissue/Blood Solubility Coefficient of Halothane
2·6 in Brain
2·6 in Lung
1·6 in Kidney
3·5 in Muscle
60 in Fat

Metabolism.—Isotope labelling techniques have now established that about 12 per cent of inspired halothane is metabolised by the liver microsomes and the resulting products are excreted in the urine (Van Dyke and Chenoweth, 1965). Halothane undergoes both oxidation and dehalogenation to form trifluoracetic acid, as well as bromide and chloride radicals (Rehder *et al.*, 1967). This metabolism may be stimulated by barbiturates and also by further doses of halothane itself (Cascorbi *et al.*, 1970).

Work with mice has shown that the metabolites of halothane may persist in the liver for as long as twelve days after administration (Cohen, 1969). Chronic exposure to halothane can impair liver cell function in small mammals and this may be due to the accumulation of metabolites. A matter of some concern to all anaesthetists, as well as those working in operating theatres, is whether such small concentrations of expired halothane from patients could have any harmful effects on the attendant staff.

Action on respiration.—Halothane is a respiratory depressant. This is more marked in the presence of narcotic premedication. Increasing the inspired concentration of halothane leads to a progressive diminution of volume rather than rate of respiration. In fact, surgical stimulation under light anaesthesia decreases basal metabolism in direct proportion to the depth of anaesthesia; in surgical anaesthesia the oxygen consumption is reduced about 20 per cent (Severinghaus and Cullen, 1958; Nunn and Matthews, 1959).

In view of the respiratory depressant action of halothane it is advisable occasionally to assist the ventilation whenever spontaneous respiration is present. At least 30 per cent oxygen should always be present in the inspired mixture.

The action of surfactant in the lungs is not affected by halothane anaesthesia (Miller and Thomas, 1967).

Halothane may be accidentally injected intravenously, in which case severe pulmonary lesions may occur, leading to death. Sandison and his colleagues (1970), in an experimental study of intravenous halothane in dogs, found that the predominant lesions produced in the lungs were generalised oedema and patchy alveolar haemorrhages, and that pathological changes occurred in other organs and in the blood. They note that in the dog, a dose equivalent to 3–5 ml for an adult human can cause severe lung damage.

Action on the heart.—One of the principal problems in the study of the action of halothane on the cardiovascular system is the wealth of contradictory evidence. This appears to be largely due to the multiplicity of premedicant and intravenous drugs used in the study. Price (1960), however, administered halothane and oxygen alone to a group of unpremedicated patients and observed the results. The cardiac contractile force was diminished; stroke volume and cardiac output were reduced despite an increased venous pressure. The heart rate and arterial pressure were also reduced, but the total systemic peripheral resistance was only slightly affected. Atropine reversed the bradycardia but failed to correct the arterial hypotension or to improve the cardiac output. Prys-Roberts and his colleagues (1967) found no significant change in calculated systemic peripheral resistance during oxygen-halothane anaesthesia with spontaneous respiration.

There appears to be unanimity of opinion amongst most authors that myocardial depression is directly related to the depth of halothane anaesthesia (Mahaffey et al., 1961; Morrow and Morrow, 1961; Severinghaus and Cullen, 1958; Wenthe et al., 1962), and animal experiments suggest that this is due to inhibition of enzyme activity in the muscle (Brodkin et al., 1967). Nevertheless, an overall picture of the action of halothane is more complex. For example, the ability of atropine to reverse the bradycardia suggests that halothane has a parasympathetic stimulant action as well as producing myocardial depression.

An interesting hypothesis that might explain most of the actions of halothane throughout the body is that in increasing concentration it gradually blocks the action of noradrenaline at the effector sites in the heart, central nervous system and peripheral tissues (Price, 1960). Two important findings support this suggestion. First, unlike most other anaesthetic agents, halothane does not produce an increase in the plasma catecholamine level of blood. Secondly, halothane partially blocks the constrictor action of noradrenaline on the skin vessels (Black and McArdle, 1962). On this basis the effect of halothane on the heart would be to reduce the secretion and activity of noradrenaline at the sympathetic nerve endings in the myocardium and at the same time to sensitise the parasympathetic nerve endings leading to bradycardia. There is experimental evidence from dogs to show that halothane can inhibit and, in adequate concentration, completely block stellate ganglion transmission (Price and Price, 1967).

Dysrhythmias occurring during halothane anaesthesia bear a direct relationship to hypercapnia from respiratory depression. Adrenaline can be safely used in the presence of halothane provided the concentration and total dose used are within acceptable limits and the patient is neither hypercapnic nor hypoxic. Katz and Katz (1966) suggest concentrations of 1 in 100,000 to 1 in 200,000 and a total dose of the former of not more than 10 ml in any one ten-minute period. Whenever an infiltration of adrenaline is used during anaesthesia it is important to remember that the adrenaline itself is the most dangerous factor, and that this danger is enhanced when the injection is made in a vascular part of the body. The prophylactic administration of propranolol intravenously before infiltrating with adrenaline has been recommended (Ikezon *et al.*, 1969), but there are inherent dangers in using propranolol during general anaesthesia, particularly with halothane, and these may well be greater than those of the controlled use of adrenaline.

Action on the peripheral circulation.—Despite a wealth of studies on the action of halothane on the myocardium, there are singularly few available on the action of this drug on the peripheral circulation. Black and McArdle (1962) investigated a group of unpremedicated patients inhaling 1–4 per cent halothane (with thiopentone induction and nitrous oxide/oxygen maintenance). They found a persistent vasodilatation of the skin and muscle vessels along with a fall in both the arterial pressure and the vascular resistance.

In an attempt to explain the mechanism of the vasodilatation produced by halothane they infused a solution of noradrenaline into the brachial artery of a series of patients. In the absence of halothane anaesthesia, noradrenaline promptly produced severe vasoconstriction, but when halothane was inhaled this constrictor action of noradrenaline was partially blocked.

In another study they found that if a nerve block was produced in one arm then halothane anaesthesia had no effect on the blood flow through this arm, yet it produced an increase in the normal arm.

These results suggest that halothane does not have a direct action on the vessel wall itself but acts rather by blocking the action of noradrenaline. This concept fits well with the possible action of halothane on the myocardium mentioned above.

Action on kidney and liver.—Halothane causes a decrease in renal flow probably related to a fall in glomerular filtration rate and a reduction in ADH release (Deutsch *et al.*, 1966). It also leads to a fall in hepatic blood flow (Epstein *et al.*, 1966). The possible association of halothane and liver damage is considered below.

Action on uterus.—Halothane anaesthesia relaxes uterine muscle in direct relation to the depth of anaesthesia and *in vitro* studies suggest that this may be due to stimulation of the adrenergic β-receptors in the uterus (Klide *et al.*, 1969). For this reason it has been expressly recommended in anaesthesia for external version, manual removal or contraction ring (Crawford, 1962). Vasicka and Kretchmer (1961), from experimental studies in women, found that uterine contractions recurred twice as quickly after halothane as compared with ether, when these anaesthetics were given in concentrations that produced comparable levels of clinical anaesthesia.

This last observation suggests that halothane may not be so liable to produce postpartum haemorrhage as has been stated. Some authors have stressed the possible dangers of increased bleeding from the uterus after the use of halothane. Like most other inhalational anaesthetic agents it readily crosses the placental barrier.

Action on gastro-intestinal tract.—In anaesthetic concentrations halothane depresses the motility of the jejunum, colon and stomach in dogs; activity promptly returns on withdrawal of the agent. It is also capable of antagonising the contractions produced by the parenteral administration of neostigmine (Marshall *et al.*, 1961).

Action on skeletal muscles.—Halothane has minimal neuromuscular blocking action but potentiates the action of the non-depolarising agents, whilst antagonising the effect of drugs which act by depolarisation (Graham, 1958; Hanquet, 1961; Katz and Gissen, 1967).

Action on the cerebral blood flow and intracranial contents.—Cerebral blood flow is increased and cerebral vascular resistance decreased during halothane anaesthesia. These changes occur when the arterial carbon dioxide tension is maintained within normal limits and provided there is not a considerable fall in mean arterial blood pressure (McDowall, 1967; Christensen *et al.*, 1967). At normal arterial carbon dioxide tension halothane causes a rise in cerebrospinal fluid pressure, but this can be prevented if the patient is hyperventilated before the addition of halothane to the anaesthetic gases (McDowall *et al.*, 1966). Intracranial pressure rises during halothane anaesthesia, especially so in those patients who have space-occupying intracranial lesions (Jennett *et al.*, 1969). Headache may follow halothane anaesthesia (Tyrell and Feldman, 1968).

Shivering.—Intense muscle spasms are occasionally observed in the early part of the post-operative period. These movements are sometimes jocularly referred to as the "halothane shakes". Moir and Doyle (1963) studied a large group of patients and found that the body temperature in those who "shivered" after operation was $0.5°$ C lower than those who did not shiver, and Jones and McLaren (1965) noted a close relationship between falls in central body temperature and shivering following halothane anaesthesia. Bay and his colleagues (1968) studied arterial oxygen and carbon dioxide tensions and cardiac output during post-operative shivering. They found that both ventilation and cardiac output were adequate for the increased demands imposed by shivering, but that there is a potential danger of hypoxaemia in patients who have ventilatory embarrassment or a fixed low cardiac output. The high incidence of shivering after halothane anaesthesia is probably related to the vasodilatory action of the drug and the environmental temperature.

Action on cells.—Experimental work by Nunn *et al.* (1969) has shown that halothane interferes with mitosis in cells.

Clinical Use

There is little doubt that halothane has proved one of the most useful agents in the whole history of clinical anaesthesia. It is non-inflammable, potent and non-irritating to the respiratory tract in anaesthetic concentrations. Furthermore, it has a low post-operative incidence of nausea and vomiting. In abdominal surgery it is often combined with a muscle relaxant in order to achieve good relaxation without resorting to high concentrations of halothane that would depress the systemic pressure. It is widely used in anaesthesia for all types of surgery including neurosurgery, ear, nose and throat, orthopaedic and paediatric cases. A reduction in blood pressure, which at one time was regarded as an undesirable side-effect, is now often used to advantage in major surgery to reduce the blood loss.

Methods of vaporisation.—Halothane can be vaporised in a number of ways but its high cost demands that reasonable economy be used. For this reason it is unsuitable for open-mask application. When placed in a bubble-through vaporiser (copper kettle, see Fig. 1) (Morris, 1952), a flow rate of 100 ml of oxygen through the apparatus (at room temperature) when added to 5 litres of nitrous oxide and oxygen will give an inspired concentration of 1 per cent. Similarly 200 ml of oxygen will give a concentration of 2 per cent.

On the other hand, the "Fluotec" vaporiser (Fig. 6a) receives all the inspired gas en route to the patient and adds a predicted amount of halothane to the mixture of gases. This apparatus is both temperature- and flow-controlled (Fig. 6b) and it is a satisfactory vaporiser for routine clinical use (Paterson *et al.*, 1969).

Vaporiser inside or outside circle system.—Various authorities have argued for and against the policy of whether the vaporiser should be always placed outside the circle system or whether it is safe to incorporate it inside the system to permit rebreathing and thereby exercise economy.

Halothane with a relatively high vapour pressure, low boiling point and low blood solubility can be regarded as a potent anaesthetic in which low concentrations (i.e. 0·4 per cent with nitrous oxide/oxygen) are capable of maintaining unconsciousness. The only justification, therefore, for using a vaporiser within the circle system is on the grounds of economy.

Vaporiser inside the circle system.—One of the principal fears of using a halothane vaporiser within the circle system has been the possibility that the concentration of halothane would rapidly rise to a fatal level; in fact this does not occur if the patient is breathing spontaneously because not only does the patient continue to remove halothane from the system but as soon as the anaesthetic concentration rises the respiratory minute volume becomes depressed. In this manner the patient will then vaporise less halothane and this acts to prevent a rapid build up of halothane within the system. The patient, at this point, will show all the clinical signs of deep halothane anaesthesia, i.e. depressed ventilation, slow pulse rate and hypotension. Provided the anaesthetist uses these signs and reduces (or turns off) the concentration delivered by the vaporiser then this method can be used. However, to achieve a satisfactory level of anaesthesia, in some cases it is necessary to depress ventilation below normal. If the anaesthetist then institutes assisted or controlled respiration without modifying the vaporiser setting a rapid and fatal concentration of halothane may develop. In short, the vaporiser should only be used within the circle system in the presence of spontaneous respiration. If assisted respiration is required then great care must be exercised to see that the concentration of halothane does not rise unexpectedly.

Vaporiser outside the circuit.—If the vaporiser is placed outside the circle system then the concentration within the system cannot rise above that entering it. In fact, due to the constant uptake of halothane by the body it takes many hours or even days for the alveolar concentration to reach equilibrium with the inspired concentration. A vaporiser outside the circle system, therefore, is relatively safe provided an excessive concentration is not used and the patient is carefully observed for the signs of increasing depth of anaesthesia.

It is often not fully realised that even though the vaporiser is placed outside

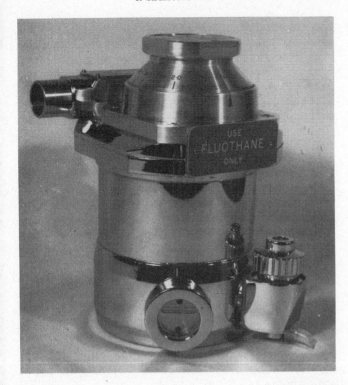

6/Fig. 6(a). — The "Fluotec" Mark III vaporiser.

6/Fig. 6(b).—Diagram to illustrate the interior of the "Fluotec" Mark III showing direction of flow of gases. The rotary valve controls the amount of the gas passing to the vaporising chamber. The remainder of the gas flows into the by-pass chamber and then to the outlet.

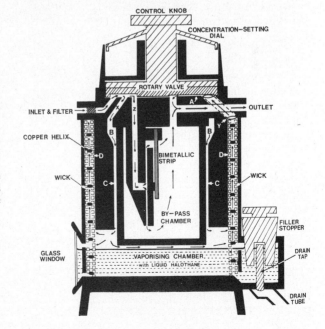

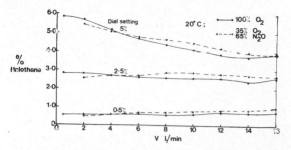

6/Fig. 7.—The effects of varying flow rates on halothane concentration ("Fluotec" Mark III).

the circle system, fluctuations in concentration can occur when assisted or controlled respiration is used (Hill and Lowe, 1962). On squeezing the bag the back-pressure in the anaesthetic apparatus rises to 15–20 cm of water. This forces more gases into the interior of the vaporiser and this increased volume of gases collects additional vapour. The exact increase in the vapour concentration delivered to the patient will depend on the flow of gases used. If a high flow of gases is used then the extra 50 ml or so that can be compressed into the vaporiser does not pick up enough vapour to seriously increase the concentration. On the other hand, if a low flow is used then it is possible the concentration received by the patient may actually be double that indicated by the vaporiser. For this reason a flow of gases of at least 4 litres/minute is recommended for use on the circle system even when the vaporiser is outside the circuit. Some vaporisers contain a special device to prevent this back-flow of anaesthetic gases during controlled respiration.

A small, convenient and inexpensive vaporiser that will only develop a maximum concentration of halothane of not more than 2·3 vols per cent is illustrated in Fig. 8.

The Fluorinated Hydrocarbons and Jaundice

In a review of the laboratory and clinical data available Sadove and Wallace (1962) reached certain tentative conclusions on the hepatotoxic effects of anaesthetic agents in general and halothane in particular. First, there appears to be a marked species variation in regard to the hepatotoxicity of various anaesthetic agents. Secondly, in man halothane is probably no more or less hepatotoxic than other commonly used anaesthetic agents, excluding chloroform. Thirdly, many other factors will accentuate the toxic potentiality of anaesthetic agents,

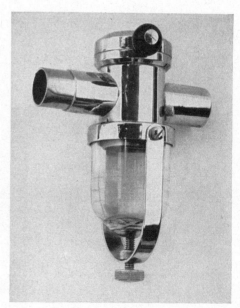

6/Fig. 8.—The Goldman vaporiser.

particularly the pre-operative nutritional state of the patient, blood transfusions, and the occurrence of hypoxia, hypercarbia or hypotension during or after anaesthesia (Morris and Feldman, 1963).

Since that time a number of reports have appeared in the literature linking both halothane and methoxyflurane with liver damage. Prior to 1963 there were only a handful of cases giving a possible link between halothane and toxic hepatitis (Burnap et al., 1958; Virtue and Payne, 1958; Barton, 1959; Vourc'h et al., 1960; Temple et al., 1962). In 1963 two reports appeared in the *New England Journal of Medicine* which attracted particular attention. The first entitled "Liver necrosis after halothane anaesthesia" (Bunker and Blumenfeld, 1963) reviewed two cases with a fatal outcome. One of these cases was a young girl (*aet.* 16) who had a lacerated wrist repaired under halothane anaesthesia lasting $4\frac{1}{2}$ hours. The anaesthesia and post-operative course were uneventful, but the patient developed signs of a hepato-renal syndrome on the 10th post-operative day and died three days later. Post-mortem examination showed profound central lobular necrosis of the liver.

In the second report (Lindenbaum and Leifer, 1963) the association between recurrent fever and hepatic dysfunction after repeated use of halothane anaesthesia was noted. A retrospective study revealed eight similar cases and these authors concluded that there was a relationship between halothane or methoxyflurane anaesthesia and hepatic dysfunction.

Since this time a number of reports attempting to link halothane anaesthesia and hepatic disturbance have appeared in the world literature (Tornetla and Tamaki, 1963; Gordon, 1963; Brody and Sweet, 1963; etc.).

Although no definite cause and effect relationship has yet been established it is important to consider every possibility, such as blood transfusion, viral hepatitis, antibiotics and other therapeutic agents (see also Chapter 38).

Laboratory studies.—Studies *in vitro* of the effects of halothane on cultures of human liver cells show little or no detectable alterations in cell morphology, unless the period of exposure is very prolonged (2 days) and the concentration of halothane equivalent to that which would be required to produce deep surgical anaesthesia. Even at these extremes, the cell vacuolation which is produced is partially reversible on withdrawal of the halothane (Corssen et al., 1966; Rees and Zuckerman, 1967).

A number of impurities are known to be present in halothane in minute quantities. One of these compounds—dichlorohexafluorobutene—has a higher boiling point than halothane and is said to increase twofold or more during the clinical use of halothane in a vaporiser (Cohen et al., 1963). Albin et al. (1964) cannot substantiate this finding, and state that the impurity is *not* increased when the copper kettle is used with halothane. Preliminary animal studies have suggested the possible toxicity of this compound in man.

The presence of copper appears to accelerate the formation of this butene compound and a possible pathway has been suggested (Cohen *et al.*, 1963) as follows:

$$
\begin{array}{ccc}
& F & Cl \\
& | & | \\
F\!-\!\!&C\!-\!\!&C\!-\!Br \xrightarrow{\;Cu\;} Cu \\
& | & | \\
& F & H
\end{array}
$$

Halothane

$$
Br + F\!-\!\underset{\underset{F}{|}}{\overset{\overset{F}{|}}{C}}\!-\!\underset{\underset{Cl}{|}}{\overset{\overset{H}{|}}{C}}\!-\!\underset{\underset{Cl}{|}}{\overset{\overset{H}{|}}{C}}\!-\!\underset{\underset{F}{|}}{\overset{\overset{F}{|}}{C}}\!-\!F \xrightarrow{\;O_2\;} F\!-\!\underset{\underset{F}{|}}{\overset{\overset{F}{|}}{C}}\!-\!\underset{\underset{Cl}{|}}{C}=\underset{\underset{Cl}{|}}{C}\!-\!\underset{\underset{F}{|}}{\overset{\overset{F}{|}}{C}}\!-\!F \; + H_2O
$$

Dichlorohexaflurobutene

The possible role of butene as a cause of liver damage following halothane anaesthesia has attracted much publicity. It has been suggested that the presence of copper accelerates the production of butene. On this basis, as the vaporisers in the United States are predominantly copper whilst those in Great Britain are either copper-nickel plate or glass, it was felt this discrepancy might be used to explain the higher incidence of post-operative jaundice in the United States. However, Nagel (1965) has studied the butene content in the residue of four commercially available vaporisers (one made of copper, the remainder of bronze or coated with copper-nickel plate). He failed to find an increasing concentration of butene from the vaporisation of halothane as the residue of the anaesthetic in the vaporiser approached zero. Furthermore, although each of the vaporisers was operated continuously for eight weeks, again there was no steady increase in the butene content of the residue. This evidence appears to suggest that the butene content of the residue in a vaporiser (including a copper one) does not rise to toxic levels under ordinary clinical conditions, even if the apparatus is not regularly drained.

Pharmacological studies.—This butene compound has been shown to be acutely toxic to various organs in dogs when concentrations present in the anaesthetic range are used. It is also highly toxic to rats (Lu *et al.*, 1953).

Clinical studies.—The typical clinical picture is composed of the onset of fever, leucocytosis with eosinophilia and later jaundice within 5–21 days after anaesthesia. The presence of liver dysfunction is confirmed by a positive cephalincholesterol flocculation test, positive thymol turbidity, raised serum alkaline phosphatase or raised serum glutamic oxaloacetic transaminase level.

Pathological studies.—In a review of the microscopy findings of 20 patients showing hepatic dysfunction after halothane anaesthesia, Klatskin (1964, personal communication) noted that the outstanding feature in all the cases was extensive hepatocellular necrosis, predominantly central and mid-zonal in location. In most cases the necrosis was sharply delineated, coagulative in type and accompanied by varying degrees of cytoplasmic vacuolation. Many of the pathological features resembled "those seen after the administration of a hepatotoxin or following massive haemorrhage especially when treated by a vaso-pressor drug."

Conclusion

The role of halothane in the production of post-operative jaundice, liver failure and death remains unsettled. Slater and his associates (1964) and Mushin and his colleagues (1964) were unable to discover any difference in the effect on the liver between halothane and other anaesthetics. The National Halothane Study (1966) carried out in the United States was retrospective but concluded that halothane-related hepatic necrosis, if indeed it occurred, was very rare. On the other hand, occasional cases are still reported in which there appears to be a clear relationship between post-operative jaundice and halothane anaesthesia. Moreover, there is some evidence that in certain very rare individuals, exposure to halothane may lead to sensitisation so that subsequent halothane anaesthesia may be followed by severe, and indeed fatal, jaundice (Belfrage *et al.*, 1966; Klatskin and Kimberg, 1969). Unexplained fever and leucocytosis with eosino-philia occurring in a patient during the first 24–72 hours after halothane anaes-thesia might reasonably be taken as a contra-indication to the use of halothane on a subsequent occasion in that patient. Some authorities recommend omitting halothane from the anaesthetic sequence if multiple administrations for the same patient are anticipated. Mushin *et al.* (1971) suggest that halothane should not be given to the same patient twice within a period of four weeks.

Methoxyflurane ($CHCl_2 CF_2OCH_3$)

Methoxyflurane (Penthrane) is 2·2 dichlorofluroethyl methyl ether. It was first studied by Van Poznak and Artusio (1960); the formula is as follows:

$$\begin{array}{ccccc} Cl & F & & H & \\ | & | & & | & \\ H-C-&C-&O-&C-&H \\ | & | & & | & \\ Cl & F & & H & \end{array}$$

Methoxyflurane

Physical properties.—It is a clear colourless liquid with a characteristic fruity odour. The boiling point is just greater than that of water i.e. 104·65° C at atmospheric pressure (760 mm Hg—101·3 kPa). The vapour pressure of methoxyflurane at room temperature (20° C) is approximately 23 mm Hg (3·1 kPa); in other words at this temperature the maximum concentration of vapour that can be obtained with a bubble-through vaporiser (e.g. copper kettle) is $\frac{23}{760} \times 100 = 3$ per cent.

Methoxyflurane is extremely soluble in rubber. This solubility is so great that 25–35 per cent of all the methoxyflurane introduced into the anaesthetic circuit can be absorbed by the rubber, and even after one hour as much as 20 per cent may still continue to be removed by the rubber (Eger and Brandstater, 1963).

Inflammability.—Methoxyflurane is not flammable except at abnormally high vapour concentrations and temperatures. Up to 4 per cent in concentration and below a temperature of 75° C it will not ignite. Thus, under conditions of clinical anaesthesia it can be considered as a non-inflammable agent unless some unusual method of vaporisation (involving heat) is used. Under hyperbaric conditions methoxyflurane shows evidence of becoming flammable though not explosive, in the presence of a sustained high voltage spark (Gottlieb *et al.*, 1966).

Pharmacology

Uptake and distribution.—The blood/gas solubility coefficient of methoxyflurane is 13·0 (*cf.* nitrous oxide 0·46). This signifies it is very soluble in blood. The high blood solubility together with the high solubility in rubber means that it takes a long time for the inspired concentration to equal alveolar concentration. Thus, about one-third of the output of the vaporiser is lost to rubber and that which reaches the alveoli is rapidly absorbed into the circulation. As tension of the vapour in the alveoli is virtually the same as brain tension, the build-up of tension in alveoli and brain is slow.

Methoxyflurane, however, has one very unusual physical attribute, namely a very high lipoid solubility; the oil/gas coefficient is 825 (*cf.* ether = 65). A high lipoid solubility signifies good anaesthetic potency, and this is borne out in practice. A steady alveolar concentration of only 0·30 vols per cent is required to maintain the 1st plane of surgical anaesthesia (Eger, 1964, personal communication). This high anaesthetic potency, together with the absence of irritation of the respiratory tract, helps to reduce the time taken for induction of anaesthesia.

With the exception of the fatty tissue, methoxyflurane is only a little more soluble in other tissues than it is in blood (Table 6).

6/TABLE 6
TISSUE/BLOOD SOLUBILITY COEFFICIENT OF METHOXYFLURANE

2·34	Brain tissue/White matter
1·70	Brain tissue/Grey matter
1·34	Muscle
38·5	Fat

Action on the respiratory system.—Methoxyflurane depresses respiration in direct relationship with the depth of anaesthesia. The tidal volume is affected more than the rate of respiration. This agent does not appear to stimulate salivation or bronchial secretions and is relatively free from irritant effects on the respiratory mucosa.

Action on the cardiovascular system.—Walker and his colleagues (1962) have measured the effects of methoxyflurane in unpremedicated patients. They observed a decrease in cardiac output, systemic vascular resistance and stroke volume. There was an increase in heart rate. The cardiovascular effects of methoxyflurane resembled halothane rather than ether, and they concluded that the hypotension produced by methoxyflurane was primarily due to a fall in cardiac output. Bagwell and Woods (1962) working with dogs found that methoxyflurane produced a progressive depression of ventricular contractile force, aortic pressure and total aortic flow with increasing concentration of the anaesthetic agent. Miller and Morris (1961) demonstrated that methoxyflurane does not increase the concentration of plasma catecholamines in the dog.

Action on skeletal muscle.—The basis for the profound muscular relaxation during methoxyflurane anaesthesia has been studied in man (Ngai *et al.*, 1962). It was found that even when anaesthesia was deepened to a stage where electromyographic activity in the diaphragm was abolished, the twitch response to ulnar nerve stimulation remained unaffected. This suggests that the principle cause of muscle paralysis in methoxyflurane anaesthesia is an action on the central nervous system (probably the spinal cord).

Action on the kidney.—Cousins and Mazze (1973) have conclusively demonstrated that there is a relationship between the total amount of methoxyflurane administered and the incidence of renal damage. High concentrations over a long period of time may lead to nephrotoxicity. A metabolite (an inorganic fluoride) is believed to be responsible. For this reason, methoxyflurane should only be used (if necessary) for short periods of time and in low concentrations. It is contra-indicated in the presence of nephrotoxic drugs or renal insufficiency.

Action on other organs.—As with all the halogenated hydrocarbon anaesthetic agents there is no positive evidence definitely proving that these drugs produce toxic reactions in the liver. Such damage, however, has been reported in patients who have received these agents, yet there is no evidence at present definitely connecting the two events. Moricca and his co-workers (1962) studied liver function in normal dogs and found a consistant modification of cellular function after methoxyflurane anaesthesia.

Clinical use

Methoxyflurane can be used as the principal anaesthetic agent for most surgical procedures (Boisvert and Hudon, 1962; Denton and Torda, 1963; McCaffrey and Mate, 1963). It has a relatively slow induction time (Thomason *et al.*, 1962) and some patients may complain about the unpleasant odour. In abdominal surgery the relaxation obtained is not as profound as that with a muscle relaxant (Jarman and Edghill, 1963). Deep anaesthesia leads to respiratory depression and hypotension. If high concentrations are used for a long period of time then recovery time is delayed and the patient may undergo a prolonged period of somnolence (Campbell *et al.*, 1962).

ENFLURANE (CHF_2—O—(F_2CHFCl)

History.—Enflurane (Ethrane) like its isomer isoflurane is a methyl ethyl ether. It was discovered by Terrell in 1963 and first introduced into anaesthesia by Virtue and his colleagues in 1966 and Dobkin *et al.* (1968). Enflurane is now second only to halothane in popularity in the United States and during 1975 was used in over 2 million administrations, and is now available in the U.K.

Physical properties.—Enflurane is a clear volatile liquid with a mild ethereal odour. It boils at $56 \cdot 5°$ C and has a vapour pressure of 184 mm Hg ($24 \cdot 5$ kPa) at room temperature ($20°$ C).

The formula is as follows:

$$\begin{array}{ccccccc}
 & F & F & & F & & \\
 & | & | & & | & & \\
H- & C- & C- & O- & C- & H \\
 & | & | & & | & & \\
 & Cl & F & & F & &
\end{array}$$

Enflurane

Enflurane is more stable than halothane and does not break down in the presence of strong light and requires no stabilisers. The greater stability of enflurane is reflected in lesser metabolism by body tissues; Chase *et al.* (1971) demonstrated much less metabolism for enflurane compared with published values for trichloroethylene, methoxyflurane, and halothane. These authors were able to recover more than 80 per cent of the enflurane administered.

Inflammability.—Enflurane is non-inflammable in all concentrations in air, nitrous oxide and oxygen.

Pharmacology

Uptake and distribution.—The blood/gas solubility coefficient of enflurane is 1·8 (*cf.* nitrous oxide 0·46). This signifies that it is relatively insoluble in blood. Under these circumstances a relatively rapid induction and recovery from anaesthesia could be anticipated. In clinical practice, induction does not appear to be as rapid as with halothane given in equipotent concentrations. Recovery, on the other hand, would appear to be more rapid than with halothane and this may be explained on the basis of the lower solubility of enflurane in blood and the demonstrably more rapid rate of elimination (Torri *et al.*, 1972). These authors also found a 25–35 per cent lower solubility in fatty tissues for enflurane as compared with halothane (see Table 7) but this poorly perfused area is hardly likely to influence recovery time.

6/Table 7
TISSUE/BLOOD SOLUBILITY COEFFICIENT OF ENFLURANE
1·45 Brain tissue
2·1   Liver
1·7   Muscle
36·2 Fat (Halothane 60)

The minimal anaesthetic concentration (MAC) for enflurane is 1·68 and the maximum safe concentration for inhalation is 5 per cent. The oil/gas solubility coefficient is 98·5.

Action on the respiratory system.—Enflurane is non-irritating to the respiratory tract with no excessive salivation, but in high concentrations it can cause coughing and even laryngospasm. Of particular importance is the finding that enflurane is a profound respiratory depressant so that even only twice the minimal anaesthetic concentration (MAC) cannot be reached without first producing apnoea (Eger—personal communication, 1976). In fact, enflurane would appear to have a greater respiratory depressant activity than any other volatile anaesthetic agent.

Action on the cardiovascular system.—Enflurane profoundly depresses cardiac contractility and output. With increasing concentrations, the blood pressure falls to the same or even greater extent than with halothane. Enflurane is probably the most depressant to the circulatory system of all the volatile anaesthetic agents (Eger—personal communication, 1976; Ascorve *et al.*, 1976). Nevertheless, topical or injected adrenaline is less likely to lead to cardiac irregularities in the presence of enflurane as compared with halothane.

Action on skeletal muscle.—Enflurane is compatible with the relaxant drugs in current clinical use although it considerably potentiates the action of the non-depolarising drugs. This potentiation is greater for enflurane than for halothane in equipotent doses.

Action on the central nervous system.—Change in the electro-encephalograph pattern is seen with increasing depth of anaesthesia characterised by high voltage, high frequency spike and dome activity alternating with periods of silence or frank "seizure" activity. These observations are aggravated by hypocapnia and may be terminated by decreasing inspired enflurane level. In a few instances abnormal neuromuscular activity is seen taking the form of twitching, clonus, or stiffness of extremities. No permanent adverse neurological sequelae attributable to enflurane have been described.

Action on the uterus.—Although there is no evidence that enflurane anaesthesia is associated with teratogenetic effects, its safety in pregnancy has not yet been established. The agent has been used with nitrous oxide and oxygen for Caesarian section (Coleman and Downing, 1975) and appeared to be well tolerated by both mother and fetus. Uterine bleeding was not excessive.

Pathological studies.—Enflurane or its metabolites have not been shown to produce toxic effects. Biotransformation results in low levels of serum fluoride ion averaging 15 mmol/l (mEq/l) but these levels are well below those known to produce renal damage [i.e. 50 mmol/l (mEq/l)]. However, it is possible that these levels could result in renal damage when function is impaired by pre-existing disease. No cases of significant hepatic or renal damage have been reported (Eger—personal communication, 1976).

ISOFLURANE ($CHF_2 OCHClCF_3$)

Isoflurane (Forane) is 1-chloro-2,2,2-trifluoroethyl difluoromethyl ether and an isomer of enflurane. It proved particularly difficult to isolate but was finally prepared by R. C. Terrell in 1965. The structural formula is below:

Isoflurane

Isoflurane was first introduced into anaesthesia by Stevens and his co-workers in 1971.

Physical properties.—Isoflurane is a clear colourless liquid with a boiling point of 48·5° C. Vapour pressure at 20° C is 250 mm Hg (33·3 kPa). It is non-inflammable in air, nitrous oxide and oxygen (Vitcha, 1971). The solubility coefficients are given below:

Oil/Gas	(at 37° C)	99
Blood/Gas	(at 37° C)	1·4
Water/Gas	(at 37° C)	0·61

It is a very stable compound and does not breakdown in the presence of warm soda-lime or strong light and requires no stabiliser (Eger—personal communication, 1976).

Pharmacology

The minimal anaesthetic concentration (MAC) is approximately 1·3. As the blood/gas solubility coefficient is as low as 1·4 (nitrous oxide 0·46) this indicates that induction and recovery from anaesthesia should be rapid. The outstanding pharmacological property of isoflurane is the finding that cardiac output is maintained (even with increasing depths of anaesthesia) despite the fact that there is a reduction in stroke volume. Cardiac output is maintained by an increase in heart rate. The pattern of circulatory changes could be accounted for by a combination of β-adrenergic stimulation and the effect of a raised Pa_{CO_2} due to depression of spontaneous respiration. Accompanying the maintained cardiac output there is a dose-related decrease in peripheral resistance (Stevens et al., 1971). This increase in peripheral flow is mainly due to dilatation of vessels in skin and muscle. The result of all these circulatory changes is that during isoflurane anaesthesia the cardiac output remains good but the blood pressure falls (along with peripheral resistance) to the same or an even greater extent than with halothane (Eger—personal communication, 1976).

Isoflurane, like enflurane is a profound respiratory depressant. However, surgical stimulation partially compensates for this depression thus preventing a large rise in the $PaCO_2$ (Eger et al., 1972 and Groves et al., 1974). As mentioned earlier the raised carbon dioxide tension may be partially responsible for the maintenance of the cardiac output.

Isoflurane, like enflurane but unlike halothane, does not sensitise the heart to dysrhythmic doses of adrenaline (Joas and Stevens, 1971). No abnormal motor activity has been observed. Like enflurane, isoflurane markedly potentiates the action of the non-depolarising muscle relaxants.

Metabolism.—Halsey and his co-workers (1971) working on hepatic extraction in swine were unable to measure any metabolites, but Hitt and his colleagues (1974) found some metabolism of isoflurane to ionic fluoride (trifluoracetic acid) but only at about one-fifth the rate established for methoxyflurane.

Pathological studies.—No significant cases of renal or hepatic failure have been reported. However, it has been suggested (but not substantiated) that isoflurane has carcinogenic properties (Brodeur, 1975).

REFERENCES

ADRIANI, J. (1952). The Pharmacology of Anesthetic Drugs, 3rd edit. Springfield, Ill.: Charles C. Thomas.

ALBIN, M. S., HORROCKS, L. A., and KRETCHMER, H. E. (1964). Halothane impurities and the copper kettle. Anesthesiology, 25, 672.

ANDREWS, E., POTTER, R. M., FRIEDMAN, J. E., and LIVINGSTONE, H. M. (1940). Determination of ethyl ether in blood. J. Lab. clin. Med., 25, 966.

ASCORVE, A., CRIADO, A., PERAL, P., AVELLO, F., and CONEJERO, P. (1976). A haemodynamic study of patients anesthetised with enflurane and halothane. Anesth. Intens. Care, 4, 151.

BAGWELL, E. E., and WOODS, E. F. (1962). Cardiovascular effects of methoxyflurane. Anesthesiology, 23, 51.

BARACH, A. L., and ROVENSTINE, E. A. (1945). The hazards of anoxia during nitrous oxide anesthesia. Anesthesiology, 6, 449.

BARTON, J. D. M. (1959). Jaundice and halothane. *Lancet*, **1**, 1097.

BASSETT, H. L. (1949). Action of soda-lime on chloroform. *Lancet*, **2**, 561.

BAY, J., NUNN, J. F., and PRYS-ROBERTS, C. (1968). Factors influencing arterial P_{O_2} during recovery from anaesthesia. *Brit. J. Anaesth.*, **40**, 398.

BELFRAGE, S., AHLGREN, I., and AXELSON, S. (1966). Halothane hepatitis in an anaesthetist. *Lancet*, **2**, 1466.

BLACK, G. W., and MCARDLE, L. (1962). The effects of halothane on the peripheral circulation in man. *Brit. J. Anaesth.*, **34**, 2.

BLACK, G. W., MCARDLE, L., MCCULLOUGH, H., and UNNI, V. K. N. (1969). Circulatory catecholamines and some cardiovascular, respiratory, metabolic and pupillary responses during diethyl ether anaesthesia. *Anaesthesia*, **24**, 168.

BLAKE, D. A., and CASCORBI, H. F., (1970). A note on the biotransformation of fluroxene in two volunteers. *Anesthesiology*, **32**, 560.

BLOCH, M. (1963). Some systemic effects of nitrous oxide. *Brit. J. Anaesth.*, **35**, 631.

BLØNDAL, B., and FAGERLUND, B. (1963). Trichloroethylene anaesthesia and hepatic function. *Acta anaesth. scand.*, **7**, 147.

BODLEY, P. O., MIRZA, V., SPEARS, J. R., and SPILSBURY, R. A. (1966). Obstetric analgesia with methoxyflurane. *Anaesthesia*, **21**, 457.

BOISVERT, M., and HUDON, F. (1962). Clinical evaluation of methoxyflurane in obstetrical anaesthesia: a report on 500 cases. *Canad. Anaesth. Soc. J.*, **9**, 325.

BOURNE, J. G. (1954). General anaesthesia for out-patients with special reference to dental extraction. *Proc. roy. Soc. Med.*, **47**, 416.

BOURNE, J. G. (1957). Fainting and cerebral damage. A danger in patients kept upright during dental gas anaesthesia and after surgical operations. *Lancet*, **2**, 499.

BRECHNER, V. L., WATANABE, R. S., and DORNETTE, W. H. L. (1958). Values for serum glutamic oxalacetic transaminase following anesthesia with Fluoromar. *Anesth. Analg. Curr. Res.*, **37**, 257.

BREWSTER, W. R., Jr., ISAACS, J. P., and WAINØ-ANDERSEN, T. (1953). Depressant effect of ether on myocardium of the dog and its modification by reflex release of epinephrine and nor-epinephrine. *Amer. J. Physiol.*, **75**, 399.

BRITISH OXYGEN CO. LTD. (1967). Current methods of commercial production of nitrous oxide. *Brit. J. Anaesth.*, **39**, 440.

BRODEUR, P. (1975). Annals of Chemistry. A compelling intuition. *The New Yorker*, 24th November, 122–149.

BRODKIN, W. E., GOLDBERG, A. H., and KAYNE, H. L. (1967). Depression of myofibrillar A.T.Pase activity of halothane. *Acta anaesth. scand.*, **11**, 97.

BRODY, G. L., and SWEET, R. B. (1963). Halothane anesthesia as a possible cause of massive hepatic necrosis. *Anesthesiology*, **24**, 29.

BROWN, W. E. (1923). Preliminary report on experiments with ethylene as a general anaesthetic. *Canad. med. Ass. J.*, **13**, 210.

BRYCE-SMITH, R., and O'BRIEN, H. D. (1956). Fluothane. A non-explosive anaesthetic agent. *Brit. med. J.*, **2**, 969.

BUNKER, J. P., and BLUMENFELD, C. M. (1963). Liver necrosis after halothane anesthesia. *New Engl. J. Med.*, **268**, 531.

BURNAP, T. K., GALLA, S. J., and VANDAM, L. D. (1958). Anesthetic circulatory and respiratory effects of Fluothane. *Anesthesiology*, **19**, 307.

CAMPBELL, M. W., HVOLBOLL, A. P., and BRECHNER, V. L. (1962). Penthrane. A clinical evaluation in fifty cases. *Anesth. Analg. Curr. Res.*, **41**, 134.

CARNEY, T. P., and GILLESPIE, N. A. (1945). (Letter) *Brit. J. Anaesth.*, **19**, 39.

CASCORBI, H. F., BLAKE, D. A., and HELRICH, M. (1970). Differences in the biotransformation of halothane in man. *Anesthesiology*, **32**, 119.

CHASE, R. E., HOLADAY, D. A., FISEROVA-BERGEROVA, V., SAIDMAN, L. J., and MACK, F. E. (1971). The biotransformation of ethrane in man. *Anesthesiology*, **35**, 262.

CHRISTENSEN, M.Stig., HØEDT-RASMUSSEN, K., and LASSEN, N. A. (1967). Cerebral vaso-dilatation by halothane anaesthesia in man and its potentiation by hypotension and hypercapnia. *Brit. J. Anaesth.*, **39**, 927.

CLAYTON, J. I., and PARKHOUSE, J. (1962). Blood trichloroethylene concentrations during anaesthesia under controlled conditions. *Brit. J. Anaesth.*, **34**, 141.

CLEMENT, F. W. (1951). *Nitrous Oxide-Oxygen Anesthesia*, 3rd edit. Philadelphia: Lea & Febiger.

CLUTTON-BROCK, J. (1967). Two cases of poisoning by contamination of nitrous oxide with higher oxides of nitrogen during anaesthesia. *Brit. J. Anaesth.*, **39**, 388.

COHEN, E. N. (1969). Halothane-$2^{14}C$ metabolism in the mouse. *Anesthesiology*, **31**, 560.

COHEN, E. N., BELLVILLE, J. W., BUDZIKIEWICZ, H., and WILLIAMS, D. H. (1963). Impurity in halothane anesthetic. *Science*, **141**, 899.

COHEN, E. N., and HOOD, N. (1969). Application of low-temperature autoradiography to studies of the uptake and metabolism of volatile anesthetics in the mouse. I. Chloroform. *Anesthesiology*, **30**, 306.

COHEN, E. N. (Chairman) *et al.* (1974). Occupational disease among operating-room personnel: a national study. (Report of an ad hoc Committee on the effect of trace anesthetics on the health of operating-room personnel, American Society of Anesthesiologists, 1974). *Anesthesiology*, **41**, 321.

COLE, P. V. (1964). Nitrous oxide and oxygen from a single cylinder. *Anaesthesia*, **19**, 3.

COLEMAN, A. J., and BAKER, L. W. (1973). Some cardiovascular effects of ornithine-8-vasopressin. *Brit. J. Anaesth.*, **45**, 511.

COLEMAN, A. J., and DOWNING, J. W. (1975). Enflurane anesthesia for cesarean section. *Anesthesiology*, **43**, 354.

CORSSEN, G., SWEET, R. B., and CHENOWETH, M. B. (1966). Effects of chloroform, halothane and methoxyflurane on human liver cells *in vitro. Anesthesiology*, **27**, 155.

COUSINS, M. J., and MAZZE, R. I. (1973). Methoxyflurane toxicity. A study of dose response in man. *J. Amer. med. Ass.*, **225**, 1611.

CRAWFORD, J. S. (1962). The place of halothane in obstetrics. *Brit. J. Anaesth.*, **34**, 386.

DAVY, H. (1800). *Researches, Chemical and Philosophical, chiefly concerning Nitrous Oxide.* London.

DENTON, M. V. H., and TORDA, T. A. G. (1963). Methoxyflurane: clinical experience in fifty orthopaedic cases. *Anaesthesia*, **18**, 279.

DEUTSCH, S., GOLDBERG, M., STEPHEN, G. W., and WEN-HSIEN, W. U. (1966). Effect of halothane on renal function in normal man. *Anesthesiology*, **27**, 793.

DEUTSCH, S., PIERCE, E. C., and VANDAM, L. D. (1967). Cyclopropane effects on renal function in normal man. *Anesthesiology*, **28**, 547.

DOBKIN, A. B., HEINRICH, R. G., ISRAEL, J. S., ASHLEY, A. L., NEVILLE, J. F., and OUNKASEM, K. (1968). Clinical and laboratory evaluation of a new inhalation agent, compound 347. *Anesthesiology*, **29**, 275.

DRAGON, A., and GOLDSTEIN, I. (1967). Methoxyflurane: preliminary report on analgesic and mood-modifying properties in dentistry. *J. Amer. dent. Ass.*, **75**, 1176.

DYJVERMAN, A., and SJÖVALL, J. (1962). Estimation of Fluothane by gas chromotography. *Acta anaesth. scand.*, **6**, 171.

EDWARDS, G., MORTON, H. J. V., PASK, E. A., and WYLIE, W. D. (1956). Deaths associated with anaesthesia. A report on 1,000 cases. *Anaesthesia*, **11**, 194.

EGER, E. I. (II) (1960). Factors affecting the rapidity of alteration of nitrous oxide concentration in a circle system. *Anesthesiology*, **21**, 348–358.

EGER, E. I. (II) (1962). Atropine, scopolamine, and related compounds. *Anesthesiology*, **23**, 365.

EGER, E. I. (II), and BRANDSTATER, B. (1963). Solubility of methoxyflurane in rubber. *Anesthesiology*, **24**, 679.

EGER, E. I. (II), DOLAN, W. D., STEVENS, W. C., MILLER, R. D., and WAY, W. L. (1972). Surgical stimulation antagonises the respiratory depression produced by Forane. *Anesthesiology*, **36**, 544.

EGER, E. I. (II), LARSON, P., and SEVERINGHAUS, J. (1962). The solubility of halothane in rubber, soda lime and various plastics. *Anesthesiology*, **23**, 356.

EGER, E. I. (II), SHARGEL, R., and MERKEL, G. (1963). Solubility of diethyl ether in water, blood and oil. *Anesthesiology*, **24**, 676.

EISELE, J. H., and SMITH, N. Ty. (1972). Cardiovascular effects of 40 per cent nitrous oxide in man. *Anesth. Analg. Curr. Res.*, **51**, 956.

ELLIS, M. W., and BRYCE-SMITH, R. (1965). Use of trichloroethylene inhalation during physiotherapy. *Brit. med. J.*, **2**, 1412.

EPSTEIN, H. G., and MACINTOSH, Sir R. (1956). An anaesthetic inhaler with automatic thermo-compensation. *Anaesthesia*, **11**, 83.

EPSTEIN, R. M., DEUTSCH, S., COOPERMAN, L. H., CLEMENT, A. J., and PRICE, H. L. (1966). Splanchnic circulation during halothane anaesthesia and hypercapnia in normal man. *Anesthesiology*, **27**, 654.

FAULCONER, A., PENDER, J. W., and BICKFORD, R. G. (1949). The influence of partial pressure of nitrous oxide on the depth of anesthesia and the electro-encephalogram in man. *Anesthesiology*, **10**, 601.

FIRTH, J. B., and STUCKEY, R. E. (1945). Decomposition of Trilene in closed circuit anaesthesia. *Lancet*, **1**, 814.

FISCHER, E. (1864). Ueber die Einwirkung von Wasserstoff aus Einfach-Chlorkohlenstoff. *Jena. Z. Med. Naturw.*, **1**, 123.

FLOURENS, M. J. P. (1847a). Note touchant l'action de l'éther sur les centres nerveux. *C. R. Acad. Sci. (Paris)*, **24**, 340.

FLOURENS, M. J. P. (1847b). Note touchant l'action de l'éther injecte dans les artères. *C. R. Acad. Sci. (Paris)*, **24**, 482.

FREUND, A. (1882). Über Trimethylene. *Mschr. Chemie.*, **3**, 625.

GELEAN, S., and BELL, I. R. (1933). The anesthetic action of divinyl oxide on humans. *J. Pharmacol. exp. Ther.*, **47**, 1.

GOODMAN, L. S., and GILMAN, A. (1955). *The Pharmacological Basis of Therapeutics*, 2nd edit. New York: The Macmillan Company.

GORDON, J. (1963). Jaundice associated with halothane anaesthesia. *Anaesthesia*, **18**, 299.

GOTTLIEB, S. F., FEGAN, F. J., and TIESLINK, J. (1966). Flammability of halothane, methoxyflurane and fluroxene under hyperbaric conditions. *Anesthesiology*, **27**, 195.

GRAHAM, J. D. P. (1958). The myoneural blocking action of anaesthetic drugs. *Brit. med. Bull.*, **14**, 15.

GRAY, T. C. (1957). Reflections on circulatory control. *Lancet*, **1**, 383.

GREENE, N. M. (1968). The metabolism of drugs employed in anesthesia. Part II. *Anesthesiology*, **29**, 327.

GROSS, E. G., and CULLEN, S. C. (1943). The effect of anesthetic agents on muscular contraction. *J. Pharmacol. exp. Ther.*, **78**, 358.

GROVES, C. L., MCDERMOTT, R. W., and BIDWAI, A. (1974). Cardiovascular effects of isoflurane in surgical patients. *Anesthesiology*, **41**, 486.

GUEDEL, A. E. (1951). *Inhalation Anesthesia*, 2nd edit. New York: The Macmillan Co.

HALSEY, M. J., SAWYER, D. C., EGER, E. I. (II), BAHLMAN, S. H., and IMPELMAN, D. J. K. (1971). Hepatic metabolism of halothane, methoxyflurane, cyclopropane, ethrane and forane in miniature swine. *Anesthesiology*, **35**, 43.

HANQUET, M. (1961). The action of halothane on inhibitors of neuromuscular transmission (observations carried out in humans). *Anesth. et Analg.*, **18**, 461.

HELLIWELL, P. J., and HUTTON, A. M. (1950). Trichlorethylene anaesthesia. *Anaesthesia*, **5**, 4.

HENDERSON, V. E., and LUCAS, G. H. W. (1930). Cyclopropane: a new anesthetic. *Curr. Res. Anesth.*, **9**, 1.

HEWER, C. L., and HADFIELD, C. F. (1941). Trichlorethylene as an inhalation anaesthetic. *Brit. med. J.*, **1**, 924.

HEYFELDER, F. (1848). *Die Versuche mit dem Schwefeläther, Salzäther und Chloroform, und die daraus gewonnenen Resultate in der chirurgischen Klinik zu Erlangen.* Erlangen.

HILL, D. W., and LOWE, H. J., (1962). Comparison of concentration of halothane in closed and semiclosed circuits during controlled ventilation. *Anesthesiology*, **23**, 291.

HILL, I. G. W. (1932). The human heart in anaesthesia. An electrocardiographic study. *Edinb. med. J.*, **39**, 533.

HITT, B. A., MAZZE, R. I., COUSINS, M. J., EDMUNDS, H. N., BARR, G. A., and TRUDELL, J. R. (1974). Metabolism of isoflurane in Fischer 344 rats and man. *Anesthesiology*, **40**, 62.

HOLADAY, D. A., RUDOFSKY, S. F., and TREUHAFT, P. S. (1970). The metabolic degradation of methoxyflurane in man. *Anesthesiology*, **33**, 579.

HOVELL, B. C., MASSON, A. H. B., and WILSON, J. (1967). Trichloroethylene for postoperative analgesia. *Anaesthesia*, **22**, 284.

IKEZONO, E., YASUDO, K., and HATTORI, Y. (1969). Effects of propanolol on epinephrine-induced arrhythmias during halothane anesthesia in man and cats. *Anesth. Analg. Curr. Res.*, **48**, 598.

JACKSON, D. E. (1934). A study of analgesia and anesthesia with special reference to such substances as trichlorethylene and vinesthene (divinyl ether), together with apparatus for their administration. *Curr. Res. Anesth.*, **13**, 198.

JARMAN, R., and EDGHILL, H. B. (1963). Methoxyflurane (Penthrane): a clinical investigation. *Anaesthesia*, **18**, 265.

JENNETT, W. B., BARKER, J., FITCH, W., and McDOWALL, D. G. (1969). Effect of anaesthesia on intracranial pressure in patients with space occupying lesions. *Lancet*, **1**, 61.

JOAS, T. A., and STEVENS, W. C. (1971). Comparison of the arrythmic doses of epinephrine during Forane, halothane and Fluroxene anaesthesia in dogs. *Anesthesiology*, **35**, 48.

JOHNSTONE, M. (1955). Some mechanisms of cardiac arrest during anaesthesia. *Brit. J. Anaesth.*, **27**, 566.

JOHNSTONE, M. (1956). The human cardiovascular response to Fluothane anaesthesia. *Brit. J. Anaesth.*, **28**, 392.

JOHNSTONE, M. (1959). Collapse after halothane. *Anaesthesia*, **14**, 410.

JONES, H. D., and McLAREN, A. B. (1965). Postoperative shivering and hypoxaemia after halothane, nitrous oxide, oxygen anaesthesia. *Brit. J. Anaesth.*, **37**, 35.

JONES, P. L. (1974). Some observations on nitrous oxide cylinders during emptying. *Brit. J. Anaesth.*, **46**, 534.

JONES, R. E., GULDMANN, N., LINDE, H. W., DRIPPS, R. D., and PRICE, H. L. (1960). Cyclopropane Anesthesia III. Effects of cyclopropane on respiration and circulation in normal man. *Anesthesiology*, **21**, 380.

JORFELDT, K., LÖFSTRÖM, B., MÖLLER, J. and ROSEN, A. (1967). Propranolol in ether anesthesia. Cardiovascular studies in man. *Acta anaesth. scand.*, **11**, 159.

KAIN, M. L., COMMINS, B. T., DIXON-LEWIS, G., and NUNN, J. F. (1967). Detection and determination of higher oxides of nitrogen. *Brit. J. Anaesth.*, **39**, 425.

KARIS, J. H., GISSEN, A. J. and NASTUK, W. L. (1966). Mode of action of diethyl ether in blocking neuromuscular transmission. *Anesthesiology*, **27**, 42.

KATZ, R. L., and GISSEN, A. J. (1967). Neuromuscular and electromyographic effects of halothane and its interaction with *d*-tubocurarine in man. *Anesthesiology*, **28**, 564.

KATZ, R. L., and KATZ, G. J. (1966). Surgical infiltration of pressor drugs and their interaction with volatile anaesthetics. *Brit. J. Anaesth.*, **38**, 712.

KAUL, S. U., and COLEMAN, A. J., (1975). Unpublished observations of the effects of nitrous oxide, oxygen, nitrogen mixtures.

KETY, S. S. (1951). Theory and application of exchange of inert gas at the lungs and tissues. *Pharmacol. Rev.*, **3**, 1.

KLATSKIN, G., and KIMBERG, D. V. (1969). Recurrent hepatitis attributable to halothane sensitization in an anesthetist. *New Engl. J. Med.*, **280**, 515.

KLIDE, A. M., PENNA, M., and AVIADO, D. M. (1969). Stimulation of adrenergic beta receptors by halothane and its antagonism by two new drugs. *Anesth. Analg. Curr. Res.*, **48**, 58.

KOCHMANN, M. (1936). Narkotica der Fettreihe. *In* Heffter's *Handbuch der experimentellen Pharmakologie*. Berlin: Ergünzungswerk, Vol. 2.

KRANTZ, J. C., CARR, C., LU, G., and BELL, F. K. (1953). The anesthetic action of trifluorethyl vinyl ether. *J. Pharmacol. exp. Ther.*, **108**, 488.

KUBOTA, Y., SCHWEIZER, H. J., and VANDAM, L. D. (1962). Haemodynamic effects of diethyl ether in man. *Anesthesiology*, **23**, 306.

LARSON, C. B., Jr., EGER, E. I. (II), MUALLEM, M., BUECHEL, D. R., MUNSON, E. S., and EISELE, J. H. (1969). The effects of diethyl ether and methoxyflurane on ventilation: II. A comparative study in man. *Anesthesiology*, **30**, 174.

LAYCOCK, J. D. (1953). Signs and stages of anaesthesia. A restatement. *Anaesthesia*, **8**, 15.

LEAKE, C. D., and CHEN, M. Y. (1930). Anesthetic properties of certain unsaturated ethers. *Proc. Soc. exp. Biol. (N.Y.)*, **28**, 151.

LEHMANN, K. B. (1911). Experimentelle Studien über den Einfluss technisch und hygienisch wichtiger Gase und Dämpfe auf den Organismus. Die gechlorten Kohlenwasserstoffe der Fettreihe nebst Betrachtungen über die einphasische und zweiphasische Giftigkeit ötherischer Körper. *Arch. Hyg. (Berl.)*, **74**, 1.

LEVY, A. G. (1913). The exciting causes of ventricular fibrillation in animals under chloroform anaesthesia. *Heart*, **4**, 319.

LI, T. H., and ETSTEN, B. (1957). Effect of cyclopropane anesthesia on cardiac output and related hemodynamics in man. *Anesthesiology*, **18**, 15.

LINDENBAUM, J., and LEIFER, E. (1963). Hepatic necrosis associated with halothane anesthesia. *New Engl. J. Med.*, **268**, 525.

LITTLE, D. M., BARBOUR, C. M., and GIVEN, J. B. (1958). The effects of fluothane, cyclopropane and ether anesthesias on liver function. *Surg. Gynec. Obstet.*, **107**, 712.

LU, G., JOHNSON, S. L., LING, M. S., and KRANTZ, J. C., Jr. (1953). Anesthesia XLI: The anesthetic properties of certain fluorinated hydrocarbons and ethers. *Anesthesiology*, **14**, 466.

LUCAS, G. H. W., and HENDERSON, V. E. (1929). A new anaesthetic gas: cyclopropane. A preliminary report. *Canad. med. Ass. J.*, **21**, 173.

LUCKHARDT, A. B., and CARTER, J. B. (1923). Ethylene as a gas anesthetic: preliminary communication. Clinical experience in 106 surgical operations. *J. Amer. med. Ass.*, **80**, 1440.

LUNDY, J. S. (1926). Balanced anesthesia. *Minn. Med.*, **9**, 399.

MCARDLE, L., BLACK, G. W., and UNNI, V. K. N. (1968). Peripheral vascular changes during diethyl ether anaesthesia. *Anaesthesia*, **23**, 203.

MCARDLE, L., UNNI, V. K. N., and BLACK, G. W. (1968). The effects of trichloroethylene on limb blood flow in man. *Brit. J. Anaesth.*, **40**, 767.

MCCAFFREY, F. W., and MATE, M. J. (1963). Methoxyflurane. A report of 1,200 cases. *Canad. Anaesth. Soc. J.*, **10**, 103.

MCDOWALL, D. G. (1967). Effects of clinical concentrations of halothane on the blood flow and oxygen uptake of the cerebral cortex. *Brit. J. Anaesth.*, **39**, 186.

MCDOWALL, D. G., BARKER, J., and JENNETT, W. B. (1966). Cerebrospinal fluid pressure measurements during anaesthesia. *Anaesthesia*, **21**, 189.

MACINTOSH, R. R., MUSHIN, W. W., and EPSTEIN, H. G. (1963). *Physics for the Anaesthetist*. 3rd Edit. Oxford: Blackwell Scientific Publications.

MAHAFFEY, J. E., ALDINGER, E. E., SPROUSE, J. H., DARBY, T. D., and THROWER, W. B. (1961). The cardiovascular effects of halothane. *Anesthesiology*, **22**, 982.

MAJOR, V., ROSEN, M., and MUSHIN, W. W. (1967). Concentration of methoxyflurane for obstetric analgesia by self-administered intermittent inhalation. *Brit. med. J.*, **4**, 767.

MALCHY, H., and PARKHOUSE, J. (1968). Respiratory studies with trichloroethylene. *Canad. Anaesth. Soc. J.*, **16**, 119.

MAPLESON, W. W. (1962). The rate of uptake of halothane vapour in man. *Brit. J. Anaesth.* **34**, 11.

MARSHALL, E. K., and GROLLMAN, A. (1928). Method for determination of the circulatory minute volume in man. *Amer. J. Physiol.*, **86**, 117.

MARSHALL, F. N., PITTINGER, C. B., and LONG, J. P. (1961). Effects of halothane on gastro-intestinal motility. *Anesthesiology*, **22**, 363.

MATTEO, R. S., KATZ, R. L., and PAPPER, E. M. (1963). The injection of epinephrine during general anesthesia with halogenated hydrocarbons and cyclopropane in man. *Anesthesiology*, **24**, 327.

MERKEL, G., and EGER, E. I., (II) (1963). A comparative study of halothane and halo-propane anesthesia—including a method for determining equipotency. *Anesthesiology*, **24**, 346.

MEYER, K. H., and HOPFF, H. (1923). Theorieder Narkose durch Inhalationoanesthetika. *Hoppe-Seylers Z. physiol. Chem.*, **126**, 281.

MILES, B. E., DE WARDENER, H. E., CHURCHILL-DAVIDSON, H. C., and WYLIE, W. D. (1952). The effect of the renal circulation of pentamethonium bromide during anaesthesia. *Clin. Sci.*, **11**, 73.

MILLER, R. A., and MORRIS, M. E. (1961). A study of methoxyflurane anaesthesia. *Canad. Anaesth. Soc. J.*, **8**, 210.

MILLER, R. N., and THOMAS, P. A. (1967). Determination from lung extracts of patients receiving diethyl ether or halothane. *Anesthesiology*, **28**, 1089.

MOIR, D. D., and DOYLE, P. M. (1963). Halothane and post-operative shivering. *Anesth. Analg. Curr. Res.*, **42**, 423.

MORRICA, G., CAVALIERE, R., MANNI, C., and MASSONI, P. (1962). Effects of methoxy-flurane on the liver. *Gazz. int. Med. Chir.*, **67**, 1293.

MORRIS, L. E. (1952). A new vaporiser for liquid anesthetics. *Anesthesiology*, **13**, 586.

MORRIS, L. E., and FELDMAN, S. A. (1963). Influence of hypercarbia and hypotension upon liver damage during halothane anaesthesia. *Anaesthesia*, **18**, 32.

MORROW, D. H., and MORROW, A. G. (1961). The effects of halothane on myocardial contractile force and vascular resistance. *Anesthesiology*, **22**, 537.

MORTON, W. T. G. (1847). *A memoir to the Academy of Sciences at Paris on a new use of sulphuric ether.* Reprinted by Henry Schuman, New York, 1946.

MUNSON, E. S., LARSON, C. P., Jr., BABAD, A. A., REGAN, M. J., BUECHEL, D. R., and EGER, E. I. (II) (1966). The effects of halothane, fluroxene and cyclopropane on ventilation. A comparative study in man. *Anesthesiology*, **27**, 716.

MUSHIN, W. W. (1948). The signs of anaesthesia. *Anaesthesia*, **3**, 154.

MUSHIN, W. W., ROSEN, M., BOWEN, D. J., and CAMPBELL, H. (1964). Halothane and liver dysfunction: a retrospective study. *Brit. med. J.*, **2**, 329.

MUSHIN, W. W., ROSEN, M., and JONES, F. V. (1971). Post-halothane jaundice in relation to previous administrations of halothane. *Brit. med. J.*, **2**, 18.

NGAI, S. H., HANKS, E. C., and BRODY, D. C. (1962). Effect of methoxyflurane on electro-myogram, neuromuscular transmission and spinal reflexes. *Anesthesiology*, **23**, 158.

NGAI, S. H., HANKS, E. C., and FARHIE, S. E. (1965). Effects of anesthetics on neuro-muscular transmission and somatic reflexes. *Anesthesiology*, **26**, 162.

NOSWORTHY, M. D. (1958). Personal communication.

NUNN, J. F., DIXON, K. L., and LOUIS, J. D. (1969). Effects of halothane on mitosis. *Anesthesiology*, **30**, 348.

NUNN, J. F., and MATTHEWS, R. L. (1959). Gaseous exchange during halothane anaesthesia: the steady respiratory state. *Brit. J. Anaesth.*, **31**, 330.

OPPENHEIM, H. (1915). Über Trigeminuserkrankung infolge von Trichloräthylenvergiftung (Discussion), *Neurol. Zbl.*, **34**, 918.

OSTLERE, G. (1953). *Trichlorethylene Anaesthesia.* Edinburgh: E. & S. Livingstone.

PACKER, K. J., and TITEL, J. H. (1969). Methoxyflurane analgesia for burns dressings: experience with the Analgizer. *Brit. J. Anaesth.*, **41**, 1080.

PARBROOK, G. D. (1967). The levels of nitrous oxide analgesia. *Brit. J. Anaesth.*, **39**, 974.

PARBROOK, G. D. (1968). Therapeutic uses of nitrous oxide. *Brit. J. Anaesth.*, **40**, 365.

PASKIN, S., SKOVSTED, P., and SMITH, T. C. (1968). Failure of the Hering-Breuer reflex to account for tachypnea in anesthetized man. *Anesthesiology*, **29**, 550.

PATERSON, G. M., HULANDS, G. H., and NUNN, J. F. (1969). Evaluation of a new halothane vaporiser. The Cyprane Fluotec Mark 3. *Brit. J. Anaesth.*, **41**, 109.

PITTINGER, C. B. (1966). *Hyperbaric Oxygenation,* p. 74. Springfield, Ill.: Charles C. Thomas.

PLESSNER, W. (1915). Über Trigeminuserkrankung infolge von Trichloräthylenvergiftung. *Neurol. Zbl.*, **34**, 916.

PRICE, H. L. (1960). General anaesthesia and circulatory homeostasis. *Physiol. Rev.*, **40**, 187.

PRICE, H. L. (1961). Circulatory actions of general anesthetic agents. *Clin. Pharmacol. Ther.*, **2**, 163.

PRICE, H. L., DEUTSCH, S., COOPERMAN, L. H., CLEMENT, A. J., and EPSTEIN, R. M. (1965). Splanchnic circulation during cyclopropane anesthesia in normal man. *Anesthesiology*, **26**, 312.

PRICE, H. L., and HELRICH, M. (1955). The effect of cyclopropane and diethyl ether, nitrous oxide, thiopentone and hydrogen ion concentration on myocardial function in the dog. *J. Pharmacol. exp. Ther.*, **115**, 206.

PRICE, H. L., LURIE, A. A., BLACK, G. W., SECHZER, P. H., LINDE, H. W., and PRICE, M. L. (1960). Modifications by general anesthetics (cyclopropane and halothane) of circulatory and sympathoadrenal responses to respiratory acidosis. *Ann. Surg.*, **152**, 1071.

PRICE, H. L., LURIE, A. A., JONES, F. E., PRICE, M. L., and LINDE, H. W. (1958). Cyclopropane anesthesia. *Anesthesiology*, **19**, 619.

PRICE, H. L., and PRICE, M. L. (1967). Relative ganglionic blocking potencies of cyclopropane, halothane, nitrous oxide and the interaction of nitrous oxide with halothane. *Anesthesiology*, **28**, 349.

PRICE, H. L., WARDEN, J. C., COOPERMAN, L. H., and MILLAR, R. A. (1969). Central sympathetic excitation caused by cyclopropane. *Anesthesiology*, **30**, 426.

PRICE, H. L., WARDEN, J. C., COOPERMAN, L. H., and PRICE, Mary L. (1968). Enhancement by cyclopropane and halothane of heart rate responses to sympathetic stimulation. *Anesthesiology*, **29**, 478.

PRICE, H. L., and WIDDICOMBE, J. (1962). Actions of cyclopropane on carotid sinus baroreceptors and carotid body chemoreceptors. *J. Pharmacol. exp. Ther.*, **135**, 233.

PRIESTLEY, J. (1774). *Experiments and observations on different kinds of Air.* London.

PRIESTLEY, J. (1779). *Experiments in Natural Philosophy, with continuation of the Observations on Air.* Vol. I.

PRYS-ROBERTS, C., KALMAN, G. R., KAIN, M. L., and GREENBAUM, R. (1967). Cardiac output—blood carbon dioxide levels during halothane anaesthesia in man. *Brit. J. Anaesth.*, **39**, 687.

RAVENTOS, J. (1956). The action of Fluothane—a new volatile anaesthetic. *Brit. J. Pharmacol.*, **11**, 394.

REES, K. R., and ZUCKERMAN, A. J. (1967). Lack of toxicity of halothane on differentiated liver cell cultures. *Brit. J. Anaesth.*, **39**, 851.

REHDER, K., FORBES, J., ALTER, H., HESSLER, O., and STIER, A. (1967). Biotransformation in man; a quantitive study. *Anesthesiology*, **31**, 560.

ROBBINS, B. H. (1946). Preliminary studies of the anaesthetic activity of fluorinated hydrocarbons. *J. Pharmacol. exp. Ther.*, **86**, 197.

ROBSON, G., GILLIES, D. M., CULLEN, W. G., and GRIFFITH, H. R. (1959). Fluothane (Halothane) in closed circuit anesthesia. *Anesthesiology*, **20**, 251.

ROLLASON, W. N. (1964). Chloroform, halothane and hepatotoxicity. *Proc. roy. Soc. Med.*, **57**, 307.

SADOVE, M. S., BALAGOT, R. C., and LINDE, H. W. (1957). The effect of Fluoromar on certain organ functions. *Anesth. Analg. Curr. Res.*, **36**, 47.

SADOVE, M. S., and WALLACE, V. E. (1962). *Halothane*. Philadelphia: F. A. Davis Co.

SAIDMAN, L. J., and EGER, E. I. (II) (1965). Effect of nitrous oxide and of narcotic premedication on the alveolar concentration of halothane required for anesthesia. *Anesthesiology*, **26**, 67.

SANDISON, J. W., SIVAPRAGASAM, S., HAYES, J. A., and WOO-MING, M. O. (1970). An experimental study of pulmonary damage associated with intravenous injection of halothane in dogs. *Brit. J. Anaesth.*, **42**, 419.

SECHER, O. (1951a). The peripheral action of ether estimated on isolated nerve-muscle preparation. (IV.) Measurement of action potentials in nerve. *Acta pharmacol. (Kbh.)*, **7**, 119.

SECHER, O. (1951b). The peripheral action of ether estimated on isolated nerve-muscle preparation. (III.) Antagonistic and synergistic action of ether and neostigmine. *Acta pharmacol. (Kbh.)*, **7**, 103.

SEVERINGHAUS, J., and CULLEN, S. C. (1958). Depression of myocardium and body oxygen consumption with Fluothane in man. *Anesthesiology*, **19**, 165.

SHACKMAN, R., GRABER, I. G., and MELROSE, D. G. (1953). Liver blood flow and general anaesthesia. *Clin. Sci.*, **12**, 307.

SIMPSON, J. Y. (1847). *Account of a new anaesthetic agent as a substitute for sulphuric ether in surgery and midwifery*. Edinburgh.

SLATER, E. M., GIBSON, J. M., DYKES, H. M. H., and WALZER, S. G. (1964). Post-operative hepatic necrosis. Its incidence and diagnostic value in association with the administration of halothane. *New Engl. J. Med.*, **270**, 983.

STEVENS, W. C., CROMWELL, T. H., HALSEY, M. J., EGER, E. I., SHAKESPEARE, T. F., and BAHLMAN, S. (1971). The cardiovascular effects of a new inhalation anaesthetic in human volunteers. *Anesthesiology*, **35**, 8.

STRIKER, C., GOLDBLATT, S., WARM, I. S., and JACKSON, D. E. (1935). Clinical experiences with the use of trichloroethylene in the production of over 300 analgesias and anesthesias. *Curr. Res. Anesth.*, **14**, 68.

SUCKLING, C. W. (1957). Some chemical and physical features in the development of Fluothane. *Brit. J. Anaesth.*, **29**, 466.

TEMPLE, R. L., COTE, R. A., and GORENS, S. W. (1962). Massive hepatic necrosis following general anesthesia. *Anesth. Analg. Curr. Res.*, **41**, 586.

THOMASON, R., LIGHT, G., and HOLADAY, D. A. (1962). Methoxyflurane anesthesia. *Anesth. Analg. Curr. Res.*, **41**, 225.

THORNTON, J. A., FLEMING, J. S., GOLDBERG, A. D., and BAIRD, D. (1973). Cardiovascular effects of 50% nitrous oxide and 50% oxygen mixture. *Anaesthesia*, **28**, 484.

TINKER, J. H., GANDOLFI, A. J., and VAN DYKE, R. A. (1976). Elevation of plasma bromide levels in patients following halothane anesthesia. Time correlation with total halothane dosage. *Anesthesiology*, **44**, 194.

TORNETLA, F. J., and TAMAKI, H. T. (1963). Halothane jaundice and hepatotoxicity. *J. Amer. med. Ass.*, **184**, 658.

TORRI, G., DAMIA, G., FABIANI, M. L., and FROVA, G. (1972). Uptake and elimination of enflurane in man. *Brit. J. Anaesth.*, **44**, 789.

TUNSTALL, M. E. (1961). Obstetric analgesia. The use of fixed nitrous oxide and oxygen mixture from one cylinder. *Lancet*, **2**, 964.

TUNSTALL, M. E. (1963). Effect of cooling on premixed gas mixtures for obstetric analgesia. *Brit. med. J.*, **2**, 915.

TYRELL, M. F., and FELDMAN, S. (1968). Headache following halothane anaesthesia. *Brit. J. Anaesth.*, **40**, 99.

VAN DYKE, R. A., and CHENOWETH, M. B. (1965). Metabolism of volatile anaesthetics II. *Biochem. Pharmacol.*, **14**, 603.

VAN DYKE, R. A., CHENOWETH, M. B., and VAN POZNAK, A. (1964). Metabolism of volatile anaesthetics. I. Conversion *in vivo* of several anaesthetics to 14CO-2 and chloride. *Biochem. Pharmacol.*, **13**, 1239.

VAN POZNAK, A., and ARTUSIO, J. F. (1960). Anaesthetic properties of a series of fluorinated compounds. *Toxicol. appl. Pharmacol.*, **2**, 374.

VASICKA, A., and KRETCHMER, H. (1961). Effect of conduction and inhalation anesthesia on uterine contraction. *Amer. J. Obstet. Gynec.*, **82**, 600.

VIRTUE, R. W., LUND, L. O., PHELPS, M., Jr., VOGEL, J. H. K., BECKWITT, H., and HERON, M. (1966). Difluoromethyl 1,1,2-trifluoro-2-chloroethyl ether as an anaesthetic agent: results with dogs and a preliminary note on observations with man. *Canad. Anaesth. Soc. J.*, **13**, 233.

VIRTUE, R. W., and PAYNE, K. W. (1958). Post-operative death after Fluothane. *Anesthesiology*, **19**, 562.

VITCHA, J. F. (1971). A history of Forane. *Anesthesiology*, **35**, 4.

VOURC'H, G., SCHNOEBELEN, E., BUCK, F., and FRUHLING, L. (1960). Hepatonéphrite aiguë mortelle après anesthésie comportant de l'halothane (Fluothane). *Anesth. et Analg.*, **17**, 466.

WALKER, J. A., EGGERS, G. W. N., and ALLEN, C. R. (1962). Cardiovascular effects of methoxyflurane anesthesia in man. *Anesthesiology*, **23**, 639.

WATERS, R. M. (1951). *Chloroform. A Study after 100 years.* Madison: Univ. Wisconsin Press.

WENTHE, F. M., PATRICK, R. T., and WOOD, E. H. (1962). Effects of anesthesia with halothane on the human circulation. *Anesth. Analg. Curr. Res.*, **41**, 381.

ZELLER, A. (1883). Ueber die schicksale des iodoforms und chlororms im organismus. *Z. Physiol. Chem.*, **8**, 70.

Chapter 7

UPTAKE AND DISTRIBUTION OF VOLATILE ANAESTHETIC AGENTS

SURGICAL anaesthesia continues to rely today mainly on drugs given by inhalation, but although the principles governing uptake and distribution of inhaled anaesthetics are often overlooked, an understanding of the fundamentals involved reveals valuable and diverse information on speed of induction, maintenance procedure, safety, and rate of recovery from a particular agent. It is possible to master techniques of inhalation anaesthesia by empiric methods, learning slowly by trial and error and adopting rules of thumb; but this approach is time consuming and potentially hazardous. The proper and rational way to learn is to base practical experience on a sound background knowledge of the principles involved. This chapter considers these principles in detail.

The goal in inhalational anaesthesia is the development of a critical tension of anaesthetic agent within the brain; depth of anaesthesia and its side-effects correlate closely with brain tension. The factors controlling brain levels are consequently of fundamental importance in applying techniques of inhalational anaesthesia. These can be considered in a logical sequence of four interrelated steps: firstly, the production and delivery of a suitable concentration of anaesthetic drug for inhalation; secondly, the factors influencing distribution of the agent to the lungs; thirdly, uptake therefrom, and finally, the delivery of anaesthetic agent from circulation to brain (Fig. 1).

FORM AND FUNCTIONS OF ANAESTHETIC SYSTEMS

An anaesthetic system is a device for presenting a suitable anaesthetic mixture to the patient. Many different systems are available, and although the performance of each may be scrutinised and judged according to the criteria itemised in Table 1, we need here to consider only the factors affecting the inspired level of anaesthetic agent. The anaesthetic circuit and the manner in which it is used exert considerable influence because it is difficult to give a well-controlled anaesthetic without accurate knowledge of the inspired level of anaesthetic agent, and there are often considerable differences between the level of anaesthetic agent set by the anaesthetist on the machine, and the level actually inspired by the patient (see also Chapter 2).

Open Systems

Circuits which have no reservoir and do not permit rebreathing such as an open-drop mask, the insufflation method, and the Ayre's T-piece may be described as open systems. These systems are inexpensive, and simple in construction, but make prediction of inspired anaesthetic gas and oxygen levels difficult. Dilution of anaesthetic with ambient air may occur with high patient inspiratory flow rates therefore it is difficult to maintain a steady level of inhalational anaesthetic agent.

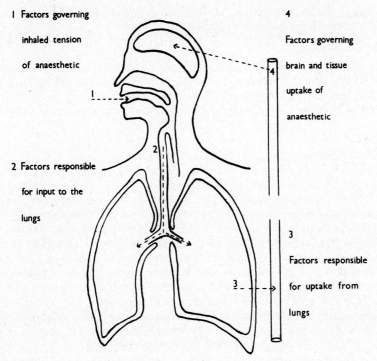

1 Factors governing inhaled tension of anaesthetic

2 Factors responsible for input to the lungs

4 Factors governing brain and tissue uptake of anaesthetic

3 Factors responsible for uptake from lungs

7/Fig. 1.—Diagrammatic illustration of the four factors influencing the brain tension of volatile anaesthetic agents and gases.

7/TABLE 1
FUNCTION OF ANAESTHETIC SYSTEM

Principal criteria
1. PREDICTABLE INSPIRED ANAESTHETIC CONCENTRATION.
2. ELIMINATION OF CARBON DIOXIDE.
3. PREDICTABLE INSPIRED OXYGEN LEVEL.
4. ABILITY TO MONITOR OR CONTROL VENTILATION OF LUNGS.

Secondary criteria
5. ECONOMY OF EQUIPMENT AND DRUGS.
6. EASE OF CLEANING AND STERILISATION.
7. SIMPLICITY IN CLINICAL USE.
8. POLLUTION OF THEATRE ENVIRONMENT. (Noise and gases).

Semi-open Systems

Semi-open circuits such as the Magill (Mapleson-A), the Magill with non-rebreathing valve, the Jackson Rees modification of the Ayre's T-piece (Mapleson-E) all have a reservoir, and when properly used prevent rebreathing. Prediction of the inspired level of anaesthetic with these circuits presents no difficulty, it is the same as that set by the anaesthetist. These circuits do not suffer the defects of the open system, an increase in minute ventilation cannot dilute inspired anaesthetic gas concentration.

Closed Systems

In addition to reducing theatre pollution, absorption of carbon dioxide gives a closed system great economic advantages over open and semi-open systems, but they are more cumbersome. If proper adjustments are made, they allow reduction of inspired anaesthetic gas levels to take any rebreathing into account.

Vaporisers

Some vaporisers are more efficient than others. The familiar glass Boyle's bottle will deliver varying concentrations depending on such factors as temperature of the liquid, the vapour pressure, and the surface area exposed to vaporisation. Other vaporisers such as "the copper kettle" and "Fluotec" are more accurate because they can compensate for changes in temperature due to latent heat of vaporisation. The output of most modern vaporisers is not affected by the flow rate of fresh gas passing through them; however it should be noted that the efficiency of certain of the older types of vaporiser is reduced by either very low or very high fresh gas flow rates. When a vaporiser is used in conjunction with a closed circuit, it may be either placed within the circle system (vaporiser in circle, V.I.C.), or outside (vaporiser outside circle V.O.C.). In these circumstances inspired concentrations of anaesthetic may differ substantially from that set on the vaporiser controls, and depend upon a number of facts including the minute ventilation, and the fresh carrier gas flow rate.

DELIVERY OF ANAESTHETIC AGENT TO THE LUNGS AND ALVEOLAR LEVELS

For an understanding of the many factors involved in the uptake and distribution of anaesthetic agents the author acknowledges with gratitude the contribution and help of Dr. Eger (1974) and the publishers Williams & Wilkins Co.

The tension of anaesthetic agent achieved within the lungs is of paramount importance because it is mirrored closely by levels within the brain; thus depth and some of the side-effects of anaesthesia correlate closely with the alveolar level. The alveolar level of an anaesthetic is the resultant of two entities: factors which promote delivery to the lungs on the one hand, and the factors which are responsible for uptake from the lungs on the other.

Delivery depends upon two factors: the inspired concentration, and the level of the alveolar ventilation.

Effect of Inspired Concentration

The inspired concentration is of obvious importance, the rate of rise of anaesthetic drug within the lungs must bear some direct relationship to the concentration inspired. The "concentration effect" rules that the higher the inspired concentration, the more rapid the rise in alveolar concentration. Two elements are responsible for this: the first is a *concentrating* effect which is illustrated as follows:

Consider a mythical lung filled with 100 per cent of an anaesthetic agent. Under these conditions no matter how much or how little gas is removed by the circulation, the concentration in the lungs must remain at 100 per cent even though the lung gets smaller. If, however, this lung is filled with only 80 per cent anaesthetic agent, and the remaining 20 per cent is an insoluble diluent gas, then as the anaesthetic agent is absorbed, so the proportion must be altered as the concentration of diluent gas remains the same. In other words, the diluent gas comes to represent a greater proportion of the whole and the concentration of anaesthetic gas must fall. Rate and degree of fall depends largely on the solubility of the particular anaesthetic agent in blood (Fig. 2).

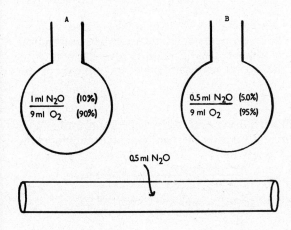

7/Fig. 2.—*The concentration effect*: the higher the inspired concentration of anaesthetic agent, the greater the rate of increase in alveolar concentration. When alveolus A is filled with a low concentration of N_2O (e.g. 10 per cent in oxygen), uptake of half reduces the alveolar concentration by half (alveolus B). However at a higher concentration of N_2O (e.g. 80 per cent in oxygen, alveolus C), uptake of half reduces the concentration by a smaller amount (alveolus D).

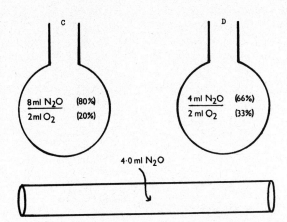

The second element of the concentration effect is an increase in the input or inspired ventilation. When appreciable volumes of anaesthetic are taken up rapidly, the lungs do not collapse; instead subatmospheric pressure created by anaesthetic uptake causes passive inspiration of an additional volume of gas to replace that lost by uptake.

The concentration effect modifies the influence of uptake from the lung on rate of rise of alveolar concentration towards the concentration inspired. At low inspired concentration, the alveolar concentration results from a balance between ventilatory input and circulatory uptake: if the latter removes half the anaesthetic introduced by ventilation, then the alveolar concentration is half that inspired. The influence of uptake diminishes as inspired concentration increases. At 100 per cent inspired concentration, uptake ceases to influence the alveolar concentration, and the relationship of ventilation to functional residual capacity alone determines the rate of rise in concentration of anaesthetic within the alveoli (Figs. 3 and 4).

Second Gas Effect

Passive increase in inspired ventilation, due to rapid uptake of large volumes of anaesthetic (e.g. N_2O), may have secondary consequences when a second gas is given concomitantly (e.g. halothane). This increase in alveolar ventilation accelerates the rate of rise of the second gas regardless of its inspired concentration (Fig. 5).

Effect of Ventilation

The second factor governing the delivery of anaesthetic agent to the lungs is the level of alveolar ventilation. The greater the ventilation the more rapid the

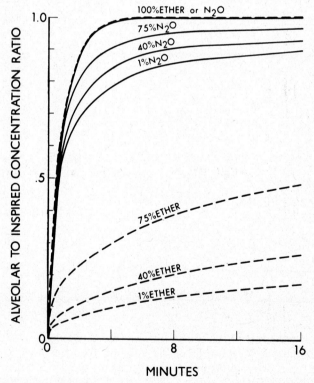

7/Fig. 3.—Increase in the inspired concentration of nitrous oxide and ether from 1 to 40 per cent and to 75 per cent increases the rate of increase of alveolar concentration. At 100 per cent inspired concentration, the rate of rise of nitrous oxide and ether is identical and depends on rate of wash-in.

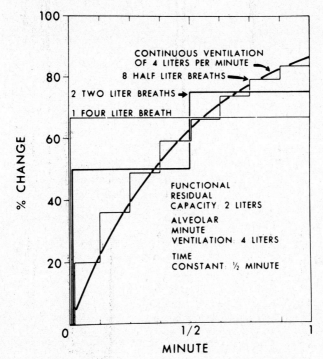

7/FIG. 4.—Rate of increase in alveolar concentration of an insoluble gas, expressed as a percentage of the inspired concentration, depends on the ratio of alveolar ventilation to functional residual volume. The larger the ratio, the greater the rate of rise of alveolar concentration. Size of tidal volume is relatively unimportant, two 2-litre breaths produce almost the same increase as 8 half-litre breaths.

approach of the alveolar gas level to that which is inspired. This effect is limited only by lung volume; the larger the functional residual volume (FRC), the slower the wash-in of new gas. If uptake is ignored for the present, ventilation in the early moments of induction of anaesthesia produces a rapid increase in alveolar level of anaesthetic. Imagine a hypothetical lung with an FRC of 2 litres during induction of anaesthesia with 100 per cent nitrous oxide. Allow each breath to amount to 500 ml and alveolar ventilation to be 4 litres per minute. At the end of the first breath the alveolar concentration of nitrous oxide would be 20 per cent (500 ml N_2O + 2000 ml FRC); at the end of the second breath 36 per cent (500 ml N_2O introduced by ventilation plus 400 ml N_2O already within FRC making 900 ml in a total of 2500 ml). By application of simple but tedious arithmetic, calculation of the concentration of N_2O at the end of the first minute would be approximately 86 per cent. A quicker way of determining the rate of wash-in of a new gas would be to determine the *time constant*: in this context, the time constant is the time required for the flow (ventilation) through a container to equal the capacity of the container (Lung volume FRC). It is also the time required for 63 per cent wash-in of a new gas into the lungs. The time constant in the example above is half a minute, because it took half a minute for a 4-litre flow (4 l/min alveolar ventilation) to equal the 2-litre capacity of the

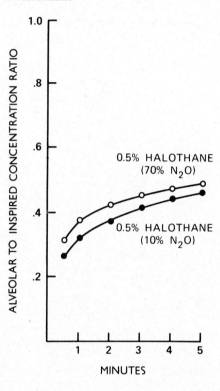

7/Fig. 5.—The second gas effect. The rate of increase in alveolar concentration of halothane is more rapid when it is administered together with 70 per cent compared with 10 per cent nitrous oxide.

0.5% HALOTHANE (70% N_2O)

0.5% HALOTHANE (10% N_2O)

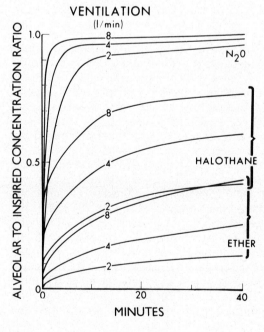

7/Fig. 6.—Influence of ventilation on alveolar level of anaesthetic agent. If uptake (cardiac output) is held constant, then rate of increase of alveolar concentration will be accelerated by increases in ventilation. This effect is greater with soluble anaesthetics.

container (FRC = 2 litres). In this example the concentration of N_2O in the lungs after half a minute was 63 per cent; doubling this period to one minute allows the N_2O concentration to increase to 86 per cent (63 per cent of difference between 63 per cent and 100 per cent), (Fig. 6).

UPTAKE OF ANAESTHETICS FROM THE LUNG

As mentioned above, alveolar levels of anaesthetic are the resultant of rate of delivery on the one hand, versus rate of uptake on the other. Uptake from the lungs is the product of three factors: solubility of anaesthetic in blood, the cardiac output, and the difference between the level of agent in venous blood and the level in the alveolar gas. An increase in any of these factors will increase anaesthetic uptake and consequently will slow the rate of rise of alveolar tension.

Solubility

There are a number of ways of expressing or describing the extent to which an anaesthetic will dissolve in blood and tissues. "Solubility" is the term used to describe how a gas or vapour is distributed between two media, for example between blood and gas or between tissue and blood. Figure 7 illustrates the derivation of the blood/gas partition coefficient. At equilibrium, that is when the partial pressure of anaesthetic in the two phases is equal, concentration of anaesthetic in the blood was two volumes per cent, and in the alveoli was one volume per cent. The blood/gas solubility coefficient is therefore 2. Partition coefficients of some inhalational anaesthetics in common use are illustrated in Table 2. If other things are equal, the greater the blood/gas partition coefficient, the greater the uptake of anaesthetic, and the slower the rate of increase in the alveolar concentration. Table 2 also lists the anaesthetics in order of increasing blood gas partition coefficients. Those at the top of the list achieve their effects rapidly compared with those at the bottom, or higher coefficients result in slow inductions. This impediment to rapid induction may be partly or completely overcome by raising the inspired concentrations to levels well in excess of that required for maintenance of anaesthesia (overpressure). The importance of solubility on the behaviour of the drug in clinical practice is illustrated in the following examples: if an anaesthetic is totally insoluble in blood (i.e. blood/gas partition coefficient = 0), then none of it will be taken into the circulation; consequently the alveolar concentration will rise at a rate determined solely by ventilation and the functional residual volume and will soon equal the inspired concentration (Fig. 8). On the other hand, if an anaesthetic has a low blood solubility, then only small quantities can be carried by the blood stream, and both alveolar concentration and tension will consequently rise rapidly. As concentration determines the tension of the anaesthetic in the arterial circulation, the tension in the blood will also rise rapidly even though only a very small amount is present in the circulation. As this blood passes round the various tissues in the body, it gives up some of the anaesthetic molecules, so venous blood returning to the lungs has a reduced tension. Nevertheless, the fact that the venous blood contains some of the anaesthetic agent means that the tension gradient between it and the alveoli is necessarily reduced. Nitrous oxide and cyclopropane are examples of inhalational anaesthetics with low blood solubilities. When fixed concentrations of such gases are given, diffusion across

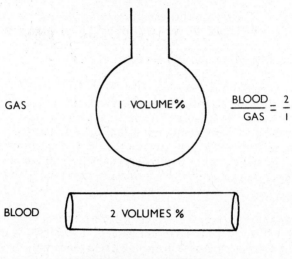

PARTITION COEFFICIENT = 2

7/FIG. 7.—Derivation of blood/gas partition coefficient. At partial pressure equilibrium, an alveolar concentration of 1 volume per cent resulted in a blood level of 2 volumes per cent; the blood/gas partition coefficient is therefore 2.

alveolar capillary membranes is rapid. Because of the low blood solubility only a small quantity is absorbed, the alveolar concentration therefore rises rapidly so that the tension of the gas is also rapidly increased (Fig. 9).

If the gas or vapour has a high solubility, then large amounts can be absorbed just as though the blood were like a piece of blotting paper, so that it is difficult for the alveolar concentration to rise rapidly (Fig. 10). As concentration in the alveolus remains low, the tension in the blood is also low, so that induction of anaesthesia is slow.

Figure 11 illustrates this point further; the approach of alveolar concentration to the concentration inspired varies inversely with solubility. It is slow with a very soluble agent such as ether, but quickly nears 100 per cent with insoluble agents like nitrous oxide or cyclopropane.

Cardiac Output

Because blood carries anaesthetic away from the lungs, the greater the cardiac output, the greater the uptake, and consequently the slower the rate of rise of alveolar level (Fig. 12). As with changes in ventilation, the magnitude of this effect is related to solubility: the most soluble agents are affected more than the least soluble. This effect is more readily visualised at extremes of solubility. There is no uptake of a totally insoluble agent, and therefore changes in cardiac output do not affect the alveolar concentration. If an agent is highly soluble, then most of the anaesthetic molecules that reach the alveoli are taken up by the blood. Doubling the cardiac output cannot appreciably increase the extraction of an agent from the lungs because most of the molecules will have been absorbed anyway. This is illustrated in Fig. 12. Thus induction of anaesthesia in a patient with a high cardiac output, as for example an extremely

7/TABLE 2
PARTITION COEFFICIENTS OF SOME INHALATIONAL ANAESTHETICS
AT $37°\ C \pm 0.5°\ C$

Agent	Blood/Gas	Tissue/Blood
Cyclopropane	0·42	1·34 (brain) 0·81 (muscle)
Nitrous oxide	0·47	1·0 (lung) 1·06 (brain) 1·13 (heart)
Fluroxene	1·37	1·44 (brain)
Isoflurane	1·41	2·6 (brain) 2·5 (liver) 4·0 (muscle) 45·0 (fat)
Enflurane	1·78	1·45 (brain) 2·1 (liver) 1·7 (muscle) 36·2 (fat)
Halothane	2·36	1·6 (kidney) 2·6 (brain) 2·6 (liver) 3·5 (muscle) 60·0 (fat)
Chloroform	10·3	1·0 (heart) 1·0 (brain)
Diethyl ether	12·1	1·2 (lung) 1·14 (brain)
Methoxyflurane	13·0	1·34 (muscle) 1·70 (brain—grey) 2·34 (brain—white)

(After Eger and Larsen, 1964)

nervous or thyrotoxic patient, will take longer than usual when a soluble agent such as ether is used. On the other hand if there is a low cardiac output (for example due to haemorrhage or heart disease) then the rate of induction of anaesthesia will be greatly increased.

Influence of Alveolar to Venous Anaesthetic Difference

The difference between the alveolar anaesthetic partial pressure and partial pressure in the returning venous blood is the third determinant of uptake. During induction the tissues remove nearly all the anaesthetic brought to them.

INSPIRED TENSION

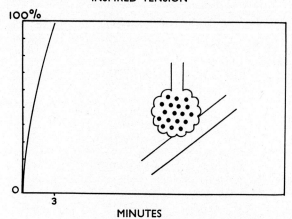

7/Fig. 8.—Rate of increase in alveolar tension of a gas which is totally insoluble in blood.

INSPIRED TENSION

7/Fig. 9.—Rate of increase in alveolar tension of a gas which is poorly soluble in blood (e.g. N_2O).

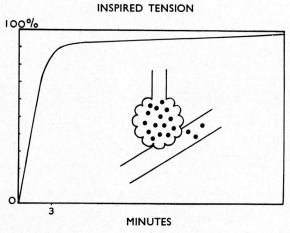

INSPIRED TENSION

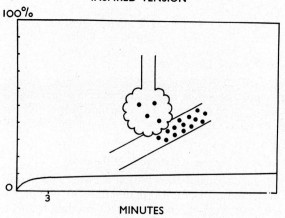

7/Fig. 10.—Rate of increase in alveolar tension of a gas which is highly soluble in blood (e.g. ether).

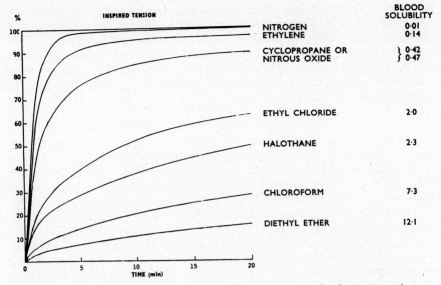

7/Fig. 11.—The influence of solubility of an anaesthetic agent on alveolar concentration.

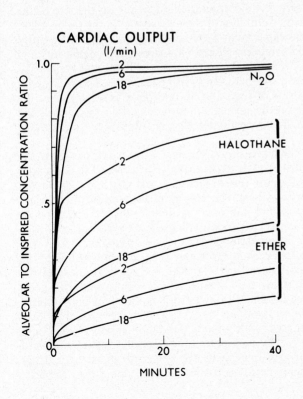

7/Fig. 12.—Influence of cardiac output on alveolar level of anaesthetic agent. If delivery (ventilation and inspired concentration) is held constant, then rate of increase of alveolar concentration will be retarded by increases in cardiac output. This effect is greater with soluble anaesthetics.

This lowers the venous anaesthetic partial pressure far below that of arterial blood. The result is a large alveolar to venous anaesthetic partial pressure difference which causes the maximum anaesthetic uptake. As time passes, the increasing tissue anaesthetic concentrations reduce the rate of uptake and the anaesthetic concentration in venous blood rises. The resulting rise in venous anaesthetic partial pressure narrows the alveolar to venous difference and thereby reduces uptake.

DELIVERY OF ANAESTHETIC TO TISSUES

The uptake of anaesthetic from the lungs is equal to the sum of uptakes by the individual tissues. If the tissues were not removing the anaesthetic, then the blood would return to the lungs with as much anaesthetic as it carried away. The alveolar to venous difference would be zero, there would be no uptake, and the alveolar concentration would quickly approach the concentration inspired.

The uptake by the tissues is governed by the same considerations that determined uptake from the lungs; firstly the solubility of anaesthetic drug in the tissues, secondly tissue blood flow, and finally the anaesthetic partial pressure difference between arterial blood and tissue. An increase in any of these factors will increase uptake and vice versa. Similarly these factors may limit uptake; if a factor approaches zero then uptake must approach zero regardless of the magnitude of the remaining factors. Thus as tissues become saturated uptake must approach zero.

The capacity of the tissues to hold anaesthetic depends on the size of the tissue and on the affinity or the solubility of the anaesthetic in the tissue under consideration. Therefore the capacity of a tissue to absorb anaesthetic drugs equals the product of tissue solubility (tissue-blood partition coefficient) and tissue volume. The greater the solubility or the tissue volume, the greater the capacity of that tissue for the anaesthetic. In a tissue which has a large capacity and a small blood flow, the rate of rise of anaesthetic level is slow, permitting the tissue to continue to extract the anaesthetic for a long time. Conversely the rate of rise usually is rapid in highly perfused tissue, and uptake by such a tissue soon ceases.

Tissue-blood partition coefficients vary far less than blood/gas partition coefficients (ignoring fat which is relatively avascular). The lowest tissue-blood/gas partition coefficient is about 1 (nitrous oxide), and the highest about 4 (halothane). This means that the rate at which tissue anaesthetic partial pressure approaches the arterial level is fairly uniform for all anaesthetics, and depends on the blood supply to the tissue. It is possible on the basis of blood flow to tissues, and their volume, to assign each body tissue to a group, and in this way to get an idea of the contribution each group makes to overall uptake and to the mixed venous anaesthetic partial pressure of anaesthetic agent. In this way the tissues may be divided into four groups. There are tissues with an extremely good blood supply—the vessel rich group (VRG); a group made up of body muscle and skin which has a moderately good blood supply (MG); a group comprising skeleton, ligaments and cartilages with a negligible blood supply (VPG); and finally body fat which has a relatively poor blood supply, but by virtue of high solubility, relatively far greater capacity for absorbing anaesthetic drugs (FG). The VRG includes highly perfused tissues such as brain, heart, kidneys, splanchnic bed (including liver) and endocrine glands. Although these tissues make up only about 10 per cent of the total body mass, they receive about three-quarters of the cardiac output. The high flow per unit volume of such tissue results in a small time constant, and rapid equilibration to the arterial anaesthetic partial pressure. These organs cease to remove appreciable volumes of anaesthetic from the lungs within 5 to 15 minutes of induction of anaesthesia. The relationship between tissue blood supply and organ size is illustrated in Table 3. The importance of blood supply may be illustrated by considering

7/TABLE 3

Group	Region	Mass in kg	Per cent Cardiac output
Vessel-rich	Brain	1·4	14
	Liver (splanchnic)	2·6	28
	Heart	0·3	5
	Kidney	0·3	23
Intermediate	Muscle	31·0	16
	Skin	3·6	8
Fat	Adipose tissue	12·5	6
Vessel-poor	Residual tissue	11·3	Nil
Total	—	63·0	100

(After Bard, 1961)

uptake of a relatively insoluble agent such as nitrous oxide (Fig. 13). The initial uptake of nitrous oxide is undertaken by those organs with a large blood supply (e.g. brain), and equilibrium is established in about ten minutes. After this period, the importance of the intermediate group (e.g. muscle) becomes obvious, and these structures are responsible for a large proportion of the total anaesthetic uptake in succeeding minutes. In time, even these organs achieve equilibrium with the alveolar concentration and the task of further uptake finally falls upon fatty tissues. Fat depots, having a large lipoid content with special affinity for anaesthetic agents, continue to remove the drugs from the circulation for many hours.

The effect of tissue uptake on rate of alveolar rise of ether, halothane, cyclopropane and nitrous oxide is illustrated in Fig. 14. Dissimilarities in uptake caused by differences in solubility determine the position of each curve; the greater the solubility, the lower the alveolar concentration. Although the curves vary in position they have a common shape; the alveolar concentration initially rises rapidly regardless of solubility. Even the start of the ether curve shows this rapid upswing. The reason for this is that at the start of anaesthesia, the alveolar concentration is zero and remains low during the first few breaths. The alveolar to mixed venous anaesthetic partial pressure difference at this time is too small, and there is little uptake of anaesthetic. Without uptake, alveolar ventilation

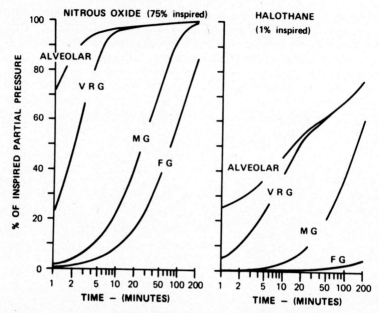

7/Fig. 13.—Influence of tissue uptake on alveolar level of anaesthetic agent. Tissue groups with relatively good blood supply (VRG) equilibrate to the alveolar tension more rapidly than the regions with relatively poor perfusion (MG and FG). Uptake into VRG tissues virtually ceases after 15 minutes for both nitrous oxide and halothane. Thereafter the muscle group dominates uptake.

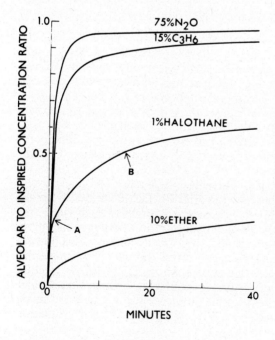

7/Fig. 14.—Influence of solubility of anaesthetic agent on shape and position of the alveolar concentration curves. The curves for nitrous oxide, cyclopropane, halothane and ether have different heights according to solubility, but are similar in shape. The rapid upswing to point A (halothane curve) is due to unopposed ventilation, whilst a slower continuing upswing to point B is due to uptake by VRG (vessel-rich group). The line continues with a slower uptake by MG (muscle) and FG (fat).

produces a rapid and unopposed increase in alveolar concentration. After a few minutes, however, a significant partial pressure difference develops and uptake increases in proportion with this difference. When uptake of anaesthetic from alveoli equals input by ventilation, a balance is achieved and the rapid rise in alveolar concentration slows considerably. This results in the first bend or knee in the curves corresponding to point A on Fig. 14. If uptake were to continue at the same rate as at induction of anaesthesia, then the alveolar curves would plateau. However, because of the progressive and rapid saturation of the VRG, initial uptake is not maintained. As the vessel-rich group reaches saturation, 75 per cent of the blood returning to the lungs contains anaesthetic at the same partial pressure as when it left. This reduction in the tension difference between alveolar and mixed venous blood thereby reduces uptake, and continued ventilation of the lungs permits the alveolar concentration to rise. Thus equilibration of the VRG to the arterial anaesthetic tension is nearly complete within 5 to 15 minutes. A second bend or knee is then seen corresponding to point B in Fig. 14. Uptake now is into the MG and FG. Were uptake to these groups to continue indefinitely, there would be no further rise in the curves. It should be noted however, that equilibration of muscle and fat has little influence on the alveolar partial pressure during the first hour of anaesthesia. The VRG saturation is of overwhelming importance during this time.

The Effect of Abnormalities of Cardiopulmonary Function on Uptake of Anaesthetic Agents

Thus far uptake of anaesthetic agents has been considered against a background of ventilation, cardiac output and regional perfusion within the normal range. When diseases or drugs adversely affect respiratory or circulatory function obviously there must be some change in anaesthetic uptake. The effect of certain changes in ventilation and cardiac output have been considered above. Here the effects of hyperventilation, ventilation-perfusion inequalities, reduced cardiac output, and changes in cerebral blood flow will be considered.

Hyperventilation and Cerebral Blood Flow

Although hyperventilation increases the rate at which an anaesthetic agent is delivered to the lungs, it also lowers the arterial carbon dioxide level which in turn reduces cerebral blood flow. Thus increasing ventilation twofold may halve both the arterial CO_2 and the cerebral blood flow. This reduction in cerebral perfusion delays the rate of rise of anaesthetic in the brain and thus opposes the tendency for the more rapid rise in alveolar anaesthetic concentration to hasten induction. The balance between these effects differs according to the solubilities of different anaesthetics. The effect of a modest increase in alveolar concentration of a poorly soluble agent such as cyclopropane or nitrous oxide produced by hyperventilation is more than offset by the reduction of cerebral blood flow, with the result that induction of anaesthesia is delayed. On the other hand the considerable rise in alveolar concentration induced by hyperventilation with a very soluble agent cannot be offset by reduced cerebral blood flow. Thus, induction of anaesthesia with methoxyflurane or ether is accelerated by hyperventilation. The intermediate solubility of halothane permits an almost perfect balancing of the increased alveolar anaesthetic rate of rise and reduced brain perfusion.

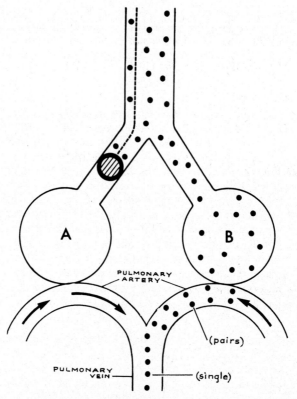

7/FIG. 15.—Effect of ventilation-perfusion inequality on uptake of anaesthetic agent. The dots represent molecules of anaesthetic agent.

Reduction of Cardiac Output and Cerebral Blood Flow

Uptake of anaesthetic from the lungs is reduced by low cardiac output thus increasing the rate of rise in alveolar partial pressure. However, when low cardiac output is associated with low cerebral blood flow, then the rate of transfer of anaesthetic agent from lung to brain is diminished. With soluble agents the increased rate of rise of anaesthetic agent within the lungs is sufficient to balance the effect of reduced cerebral perfusion. The initial rise in the brain, therefore, is normal; eventually however, the higher alveolar partial pressure resulting from a reduced cardiac output is associated with a higher brain level regardless of difference in solubility.

The Effect of Venous Admixture

Some degree of venous admixture (physiological shunt) is normal, and is due to venous blood entering the left ventricle both from pleural, bronchial and Thebesian veins, and from ventilation-perfusion mismatch, which together amounts to about 5 per cent of cardiac output. However, in many cardiopulmonary diseases and during anaesthesia venous admixture may be greatly increased (see Chapter 3). Referring to Fig. 15, all the anaesthetic agent is now being delivered to lung B. If the agent is soluble, the blood flow to that lung will take up an increased amount of the agent and so compensate to some extent for the blood flow from lung A which has taken up none of the agent. If the anaesthetic agent is insoluble, then partial pressure equilibration occurs rapidly between alveolar gas and alveolar capillary blood, limiting further uptake of the agent. The amount of the agent in the blood coming from lung B is therefore only slightly increased and cannot compensate for the absent uptake by blood passing through lung A.

THE EFFECT OF ANAESTHETIC AGENTS ON AIR AND GASES IN CLOSED BODY CAVITIES

Under normal circumstances, with the exception of the lungs, middle ear, sinuses, and intestines, there is no air in the various body cavities. However, during a pneumo-encephalogram, air is introduced into the ventricles of the brain, in a pneumothorax it is found in the pleural cavity, and in acute intestinal obstruction it accumulates in the lumen of the intestines. If such patients are anaesthetised with nitrous oxide and oxygen (70 per cent and 30 per cent), the anaesthetic gas will rapidly enter the enclosed space and the volume will increase. The reason for this is that nitrous oxide is 34 times more soluble than nitrogen in blood, but because of partial pressure difference between N_2O in the blood and the air in the body cavity, a larger quantity of nitrous oxide will enter the gas cavity than nitrogen will diffuse out. When the wall of the cavity is elastic, as in the case of intestines, distention occurs, but when it is rigid there is an increase in pressure. Eger and Saidman (1965), using 70–75 per cent nitrous oxide with oxygen for pneumo-encephalography in dogs, and in man, have shown that there is a dramatic rise in cerebral fluid pressure. Their finding suggested that this form of anaesthesia could cause a considerable increase in the cerebrospinal fluid pressure if used when air is present or injected into the ventricles; and that this rise in pressure might be clinically harmful in the presence of an already increased intracranial pressure. When the nitrous oxide is turned off, the cerebrospinal fluid pressure returns to its original value in about 10 minutes. Clinically, therefore, on the basis of this evidence, it would appear to be potentially harmful to use nitrous oxide/oxygen for pneumo-encephalogram if air is to be used as a filling medium. However, this risk would be removed if either nitrous oxide or oxygen were used to outline the ventricles. Similar problems occur when a pneumothorax, pneumoperitoneum, or pneumopericardium are present or when air is trapped either in the middle ear, intestine or respiratory tract (Fig. 16).

Recovery from Anaesthesia

When an inhalation anaesthetic is withdrawn at the end of surgery, the factors which affect elimination of the anaesthetic agent and recovery from anaesthesia are identical to those which were present during induction of anaesthesia. The effect of pulmonary ventilation to lower alveolar concentration is opposed by the same three factors which controlled uptake of drug from alveoli to blood. These are solubility of the anaesthetic agents in blood, cardiac output, and the venous to alveolar anaesthetic partial pressure difference. An increase in any one of these three factors will oppose the effect of ventilation, limit the fall in alveolar level, and thus prolong the time period for recovery from anaesthesia. The concentration effect which during uptake operated to increase uptake proportional to the inspired concentration has no effect on the output of the anaesthetic agent. However, there is a concentrating effect on non-anaesthetic gases, the outpouring of nitrous oxide at the end of anaesthesia may dilute the alveolar oxygen, thereby producing "diffusion hypoxia".

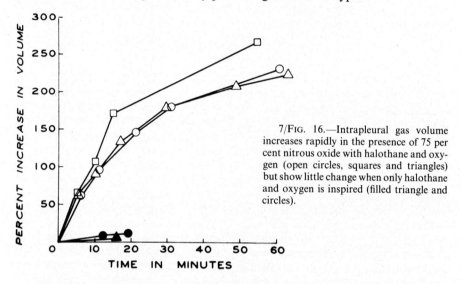

7/Fig. 16.—Intrapleural gas volume increases rapidly in the presence of 75 per cent nitrous oxide with halothane and oxygen (open circles, squares and triangles) but show little change when only halothane and oxygen is inspired (filled triangle and circles).

Diffusion Hypoxia

At the end of an anaesthetic when the mask is withdrawn the patient breathes room air. The alveoli will soon become filled with a mixture of nitrogen, oxygen, carbon dioxide and water vapour. Nevertheless, there is still an appreciable quantity of nitrous oxide dissolved in the circulation and tissues because although nitrous oxide is always referred to an insoluble anaesthetic agent it is some 34 times more soluble than nitrogen. This means that blood can carry that much more nitrous oxide than nitrogen. Thus during the first few minutes of breathing air large quantities of nitrous oxide leave the body. Following an anaesthetic with a 75:25 per cent mixture of nitrous oxide and oxygen, as much as 1500 ml of nitrous oxide may be expired in the first minute, 1200 ml in the second and 1000 ml during the third. The net result of this exodus is that temporarily the volume of expiration exceeds that of inspiration, so that an increased volume of carbon dioxide is removed from the alveoli. This lowers the arterial carbon dioxide tension and thus reduces ventilatory drive, even producing apnoea.

The other and even more important effect of this mass movement of nitrous oxide into the alveoli is the dilution of alveolar oxygen tension. Normally in the alveoli there is approximately 14 per cent oxygen, but under these conditions the concentration may drop to as low as 10 per cent. This results in a degree of hypoxia which may be extremely dangerous in the elderly and critically ill (Fig. 17).

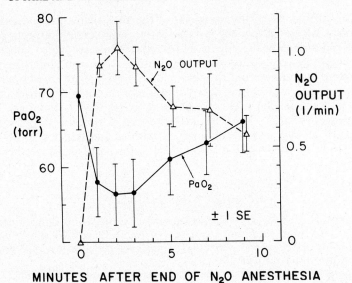

7/Fig. 17.—Diffusion hypoxia. A change in inspired gases from 21 per cent oxygen and 79 per cent N_2O to 21 per cent oxygen and 79 per cent nitrogen causes a fall in arterial oxygen tension which at its nadir coincides with the period of maximum nitrous oxide excretion.

Clinically, diffusion hypoxia is only significant when nitrous oxide oxygen technique is employed, because this is the only anaesthetic agent that is commonly used in high concentrations. The effect is only likely to persist in a rapidly diminishing manner, for about ten minutes at the end of a nitrous oxide anaesthetic. After anaesthesia, in the presence of normal ventilation, diffusion hypoxia is of little significance in healthy patients; however when ventilation is depressed it becomes increasingly important. The adverse effects of diffusion hypoxia can be prevented by giving the patient oxygen for about five minutes after discontinuation of nitrous oxide, and the concomitant drop in alveolar carbon dioxide may be prevented by judicious addition of 5 per cent carbon dioxide to the oxygen. This may be particularly important after controlled hyperventilation anaesthesia in which body stores of carbon dioxide are much depleted.

A reduced cardiac output or increased ventilation permits a more rapid fall in the alveolar anaesthetic concentrations. These changes may hasten recovery following anaesthesia with more soluble agents but the concomitant delay in tissue wash-out may retard recovery with poorly soluble agents. Concomitant increases in ventilation and circulation will accelerate recovery unless the increased perfusion is directed mainly to tissues of normally low perfusion, such as muscle or fat.

Finally, it should be noted that if a patient continues to breathe from an anaesthetic circuit at termination of anaesthesia, recovery may be delayed both by rebreathing and by the presence of anaesthetic vapour emerging from tubes and other components of the anaesthetic apparatus.

The point at which the patient is said to have recovered from anaesthesia is difficult to define. From the viewpoint of the anaesthetist the endpoint is that moment at which the patient is sufficiently awake. Safety aspects suggest a suitable endpoint to be the stage at which reflexes have recovered sufficiently for a patient to tolerate cardiopulmonary stresses. A patient cannot be regarded as recovered for example, unless he can maintain a safe airway in all eventualities, and can tolerate postural changes without clinical signs of a drop in cardiac output. The anaesthetic level corresponding to this stage is unknown, but Eger (1974) suggests that at "MAC awake" (the level at which a patient will obey a command), airways can be maintained without assistance. "MAC awake" appears to be about 0·6 of the MAC value of the particular anaesthetic.

FURTHER READING

CHENOWETH, M. B., Ed. (1972). *Modern Inhalation Anaesthetics*. Berlin: Springer-Verlag.
EGER, E. I. (II) (1974), *Anaesthetic Uptake and Action*. Baltimore: Williams & Wilkins Co.
PAPPER, E. M., and KITZ, R. J., Eds. (1962). *Uptake and Distribution of Anesthetic Agents*. New York: McGraw-Hill.
Symposium on Pharmacokinetics of Inhalation Anaesthetic Agents (1964). *Brit. J. Anaesth.* (No. 3), **36**.

Chapter 8

ENVIRONMENTAL HAZARDS AND SAFETY MEASURES IN THE OPERATING ROOM

RISKS are involved whenever an anaesthetic is administered, because anaesthesia requires the depression of many of a patient's protective reflexes, in order to allow access to a given part by a surgeon. Other chapters describe how this access may be achieved with minimal risk to the patient from drugs and apparatus used to administer them. This chapter is concerned with acute risks to the patient and operating room staff which anaesthetic techniques may produce, and chronic risks to staff from prolonged exposure to abnormal conditions.

FIRES AND EXPLOSIONS

The first of such acute risks to be described was the explosion which could occur because of the flammable nature of some anaesthetics. These anaesthetics as well as some other agents, such as fluids used for skin or instrument cleaning, could also be involved in fires.

There is no essential difference between a fire and an explosion. A *fire* becomes an *explosion* if the combustion is sufficiently rapid to cause pressure changes which result in the production of sound waves. For example, paraffin poured on to a red coal fire will increase the rate of combustion sufficiently to make it "roar". Ether vapour and oxygen, in certain proportions, will, if ignited in a confined space, cause an explosion. In certain circumstances, the speed of combustion may be so high that a pressure wave is produced which ignites adjacent gas mixtures by compression rather than by the speed of a flame. Such combustion is extremely violent and is known as "detonation". This phenomenon is similar to the compression ignition which occurs in diesel engines. Ether will detonate in certain circumstances in oxygen, but not in air.

The risk of an anaesthetic explosion in the United Kingdom has never been high. Even before the Report of the Working Party on Anaesthetic Explosions by the Ministry of Health (H.M.S.O., 1956) the risk of death from explosion of a flammable anaesthetic was less than one in three million. After the introduction of anti-static precautions which followed the publication of the Report of the Working Party and the introduction of halothane in the same year, the number of fires and explosions associated with anaesthesia fell to almost insignificant proportions in England and Wales. In 1966 and 1967 no explosion was reported. In 1968 there was one. The last time a death was reported following an anaesthetic explosion was in 1964.

In spite of this it is still necessary to discuss the risks, because ether and cyclopropane have their uses, and more detailed investigations into the flammability of newer compounds such as halothane and methoxyflurane have shown that these and other drugs are not "non-flammable" in an absolute sense. Indeed some workers (Schön and Steen, 1968) have been able to make even nitrous oxide burn, given an ignition source of enormous energy (200 watts/second for

0·5–1·0 second). Such freak conditions would never be encountered in clinical anaesthetic practice, but whenever a new technique or apparatus is introduced into the operating room its effects as an ignition source must be considered. Whenever a new volatile drug is introduced its pharmacological advantages must be weighed against any physical disadvantages such as flammability. For example, hexafluorobenzene (Burns *et al.*, 1961) is a drug with interesting anaesthetic properties. It has been shown to support blood pressure and respiration and to be safe when adrenaline is used (Garmer and Leigh, 1967). It has also been shown (Hall and Jackson, 1973) to double cardiac output in ponies in deep anaesthesia. Although it is non-flammable in air, six per cent can be made to burn in oxygen, and about four per cent is needed to produce anaesthesia. This might be an acceptable risk in some circumstances.

Flammable Anaesthetic Vapours

The essential conditions for an explosion are the presence, close enough together, of an *explosive mixture* and a spark of sufficient *energy*, or a surface hot enough to cause *ignition*. Whenever ether, cyclopropane, ethyl chloride or ethylene is used in anaesthetic concentrations, an *explosive mixture* is present, and even the low energy spark provided by static electricity is sufficient to cause *ignition*. Flammability limits of other drugs shown in Table 1 are either outside the anaesthetic concentrations or cannot be obtained in unheated vaporisers at room temperature (18–22° C). This table shows the flammability limits of inhalational anaesthetic drugs in air, oxygen and nitrous oxide. It is of interest that nitrous oxide lowers the *lower* limit of flammability for each drug. As oxygen is added to a mixture of an inhalational anaesthetic in nitrous oxide, a wider range of the concentrations used in anaesthesia becomes non-flammable.

It is interesting and not always recognised that all inhalational anaesthetics in use today are more flammable in nitrous oxide than in oxygen. This is illustrated graphically in Fig. 1 where the flammability of halothane in oxygen/ nitrous oxide mixtures at 20° C and atmospheric pressure is shown. The experimental data, supplied by the manufacturers of Fluothane only covered concentrations up to 20 per cent v/v. Extrapolation of this data to include all concentrations up to saturation at 20° C has been made. The concentrations of oxygen and nitrous oxide are given on the X-axis and increase from 0–100 per cent v/v from right to left and left to right respectively. The halothane concentration is given on the Y-axis and increases from 0–32 per cent v/v, the saturated vapour pressure concentration at 20° C. The horizontal lines give the greatest concentration of halothane possible at 1, 2 and 4 atmospheres pressure.

The figures were obtained using a cerium-magnesium fusehead ignition source. This is more powerful than any ignition source likely to be found in an operating theatre.

The addition of a non-combustible material, such as water vapour, to flammable mixtures of any kind, will reduce their flammability. This led Miller and Dornette (1961) to recommend the use of fluroxene in closed circuits even when the cautery is used. They claim that the water vapour present from the patient's expired gases raises the lower limit of flammability of fluroxene to 7·5 per cent.

8/TABLE 1

Drug	Limits in air per cent v/v		Limits in oxygen per cent v/v		Limits in 100% nitrous oxide per cent v/v	
	lower	higher	lower	higher	lower	higher
Diethyl ether	1·9	48·0	2·0	82·0	1·5	24·0
Divinyl ether	1·7	27·0	1·8	85·0	1·4	25·0
Cyclopropane	2·4	10·4	2·5	60·0	—	—
Ethyl chloride	3·8	15·4	4·0	67·0	2·0	33·0
Trifluoro-ethyl-vinyl-ether, fluroxene (Fluoromar)	3·0 (Krantz et al., 1953)	—	4·5 (Miller and Dornette, 1961)	80·0	—	—
Ethylene	3·1	32·0	3·0	80·0	1·9	40·0
Trichloroethylene (Trilene)	non-flammable		10·0	65·0	2·0/2·5*	

Halothane (Fluothane) F-C-C-Cl (with F, H, F, Br substituents)	non-flammable	non-flammable	4·0/5·0*
Methoxyflurane (Penthrane) H-C-C-O-C-H (with Cl, F, H, Cl, F, H substituents)	9·0* 28·0*	5·2* 28·0*	4·0* —
Teflurane F-C-C-F (with F, H, F, Br substituents)	"non-flammable" (Artusio, 1963)		
Enflurane (Ethrane) Cl-C-C-O-C-H (with F, F, F, H, F, F substituents)	"non-explosive in anaesthetic concentrations" (Krantz, 1964)		
Isoflurane (Forane) H-C-O-C-C-F (with F, F, H, Cl, F, F substituents)	"non-flammable" (Vitcha, 1971)		
Halopropane Br-C-C-C-H (with H, F, F, H, F, F substituents)	non-flammable (Fabian *et al.*, 1960)		

These values are taken from the U.S. Bureau of Mines Bulletin 503, Washington 1952, except for those marked (*) which are manufacturers' figures and those for the last four compounds, where other references are given. Although figures are given for lower limits of flammability in oxygen for trichloroethylene and in air and oxygen for methoxyflurane, it should be remembered that these concentrations cannot be obtained in unheated vaporisers at normal operating theatre temperatures (18–22° C).

Anaesthesia at hyperbaric pressures.—The manufacturers of halothane (Fluothane) give the following recommendation for this drug when it is used with oxygen in hyperbaric conditions up to 4 atmospheres pressure and at ordinary temperatures:—"In small volumes, such as closed circuit anaesthetic equipment, the concentration of Fluothane should not exceed 2 per cent v/v; in large volumes, any concentration up to that given by its saturated vapour pressure may be used." They do not recommend the use of oxygen/ nitrous oxide mixtures with halothane at hyperbaric pressures.

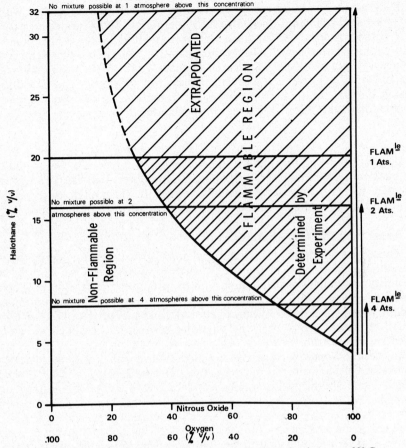

8/FIG. 1.—Flammability diagram for halothane in O_2/N_2O mixtures at 20° C.

In addition to flammable anaesthetic vapours in use on a patient, other combustible substances must be considered.

Residual gases.—Bracken and Wilton-Davies (1963) showed that 29 ml of cyclopropane gas could be dissolved in 1 ml of liquid trichloroethylene at 20° C. If cyclopropane is run through a trichloroethylene vaporiser, an explosive mixture could be delivered during subsequent use. The risk would last for about three minutes, if a gas flow of eight litres per minute were used.

No data is available for the cyclopropane solubility in halothane but it would be unwise to run cyclopropane through a halothene vaporiser. Cyclopropane and ether are adsorbed on to rubber, and a rubber hose recently used with these flammable gases will pass them into a subsequent gas mixture. It is wise to flush out rubber hoses and breathing bags with oxygen before use.

Persistence of flammable exhalation.—Vickers (1965) and Nicholson and Crehan (1967) have shown that even after long periods of cyclopropane or ether administration the exhaled flammable agent is present in the patient's breath at concentrations well below those which are flammable, once the patient has breathed a non-flammable mixture for five minutes.

Body gases.—Carroll (1964) describes an incident when a patient with a distended stomach had it opened with the diathermy. The gases which escaped were ignited, and burned for some ten seconds with an intense blue flame. A loud explosion was heard outside the operating room. Gases present in the alimentary tract include hydrogen and methane, both of which are flammable. Woodward (1961) proposed a scheme for clearing the bowel, and introducing carbon dioxide. In the absence of such precautions, some would question whether diathermy should be used for opening the large intestine.

PREVENTION

Fires in operating theatres may be prevented in three main ways—the use of non-flammable gas mixtures, the elimination of every sort of spark or flame of sufficient energy to ignite any flammable mixture which might be present, or the separation at a safe distance of flammable gases from ignition sources.

Non-Flammable Gas Mixtures

There is no doubt that from a physical point of view the soundest method of preventing explosions is to use drugs which cannot be made to burn in any circumstances in the operating room; but the prevention of explosions is by no means the only problem for the anaesthetist. Many regard ether or cyclopropane, or both, as indispensable to the production of good anaesthesia in certain cases, and there are occasions when the physiological risk to the patient of a non-explosive anaesthetic is greater than the risk of an explosion. Vapours with highly desirable pharmacological properties, but capable of ignition may be discovered. In such cases, if the diathermy can be dispensed with, or its spark kept at a safe distance, without increasing the risk to the patient, a flammable agent may be the drug of choice. In such a case, both the surgeon and anaesthetist must be prepared to understand the other's problems.

A non-flammable theatre.—It has been suggested that if a group of anaesthetists agreed to use only non-flammable drugs, their operating rooms need not be designed to eliminate sources of ignition. But such a suggestion is not without risk. A visiting anaesthetist, in the habit of using ether or cyclopropane, might well come to work in such theatres and not be in agreement with the view that flammable gases are unnecessary, or he might forget the limitations of the theatres. Furthermore, if a new drug were introduced, having extremely desirable pharmacological properties but ignitable in some extreme conditions, the existence of such theatres might stand in the way of progress in clinical anaesthesia.

Existing non-flammable drugs.—Although the introduction into clinical use of halothane and other fluorinated anaesthetics has greatly simplified the problem, it has not completely solved it. The pharmacological properties of drugs available are sometimes considered to be unsuitable for certain patients.

New drugs.—The most promising method of removing all flammable mixtures from the operating room is the discovery of new drugs. Shortly after the end of the Second World War, the introduction of curare into clinical use resulted in the development of "balanced anaesthesia" where several drugs were used to provide good operating conditions with analgesia and safety for the patient. The only gases used were nitrous oxide and oxygen, which are completely non-flammable in clinical use.

During the war, fluorinated hydrocarbons were studied in an effort to produce non-flammable lubricants and refrigerants. When it was realised that the substitution of fluorine for hydrogen did not significantly alter the properties of the compounds, apart from making them less "reactive", the possibility of producing a non-flammable ether was investigated. Go Lu et al. (1953) were among the first to demonstrate the anaesthetic properties of fluorinated hydrocarbons. The most promising of those he investigated was trifluoroethyl vinyl ether (fluroxene—Fluoromar) which contains three fluorine atoms in place of three hydrogen atoms. Its formula is given in Table 1. Presumably because of its five remaining hydrogen atoms, this drug is still flammable, but less so than diethyl ether. Its lower ignition limit in air is given as three per cent (Krantz et al., 1953), although Miller and Dornette (1961) give the lower limit as 7·5 per cent in the moist conditions of the closed circuit. Substitution of more hydrogen atoms by fluorine was found to reduce anaesthetic potency greatly.

Halothane was the first truly non-flammable fluorinated drug to be introduced into anaesthesia (Raventós, 1956) and has many useful properties besides that of non-flammability. It may be used with soda-lime in a closed system, is a potent anaesthetic and shares with ether the ability to minimise expiratory spasm in asthmatic patients. Unfortunately, it cannot be claimed to be the complete answer, because there are still occasions when some anaesthetists feel that ether or cyclopropane is the drug of choice.

More fluorinated compounds will probably be made and investigated, and possibly one or more of these will enable anaesthetists to dispense with the use of flammable drugs entirely, without prejudicing the safety of the patient or the convenience of the surgeon. In the meantime, care must be taken that new, non-flammable drugs are used on patients only if they offer a real clinical advantage and after most thorough pharmacological study. There are too many instances in medicine where drugs or techniques which appear attractive at first, prove to have totally unexpected side-effects either when used alone or in combination with some other drug. To justify its use on human patients, any new drug must claim to offer a *major* advantage over existing drugs. It is then for the anaesthetist to decide whether this advantage is sufficiently great in the case of a particular patient to outweigh the known risk of using any new compound.

Other fluorine compounds which have reached clinical practice since the introduction of halothane and fluroxene are Teflurane (Artusio et al., 1967), which may be regarded as halothane with the chlorine replaced by fluorine, Enflurane (Virtue et al., 1966) which is an ethyl methyl ether of similar structure to methoxyflurane, and Isoflurane (Pauca and Dripps, 1973) which is an isomer of Enflurane. No new compound has so far been discovered which has fewer side-effects than halothane and yet is equally non-flammable.

Inert diluents added to otherwise flammable drugs.—In theory, volatile drugs such as ether and cyclopropane could be made effectively non-flammable by the addition of an inert diluent. This could work either by (a) absorbing the thermal energy of an incipient explosion or (b) absorbing free radicals. These free radicals result from the absorption of thermal energy by a molecule of an explosive gas, and, if they are not deactivated, will combine with oxygen and initiate a chain reaction, which results in an explosion (Ubbelohde, 1935; Hinshelwood, 1940).

Any added substance has to satisfy certain requirements:

1. It must not be toxic to the patient.

2. It must have physical properties which enable the necessary vapour concentration to be obtained at room temperature.

3. It must not react with soda-lime.

4. The concentration of the substance required to prevent an explosion must be relatively low, so that it does not interfere with the amounts of anaesthetic and oxygen which have to reach the patient.

(a) Energy absorbing diluents.—Carbon tetrafluoride is an example of this type of diluent. Jones *et al.* (1950) have shown that a concentration of 68 per cent of this substance will completely inhibit the combustion of cyclopropane/oxygen mixtures.

A more practical member of this group is nitrogen. Figure 2 is a "triple graph", showing the flammability limits for trichloroethylene/oxygen/nitrogen mixtures (Jones and Scott, 1942). As the concentration of nitrogen is increased, the upper limit of flammability is lowered. Unfortunately, there is little effect

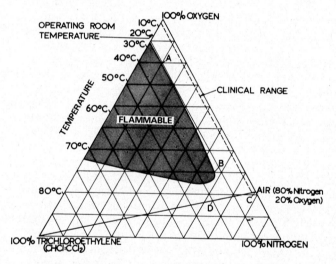

8/Fig. 2.—The flammability limits for trichloroethylene/oxygen/nitrogen mixtures.

on the lower limit, which remains at between ten and twelve per cent until the nitrogen reaches over 70 per cent. As it is the lower limit which is of most interest to anaesthetists, the use of nitrogen, or, for that matter, helium, as an inert diluent is not of much practical value.

Figure 2 shows "air" on the right side, near to "100 per cent nitrogen", and a long way from "100 per cent oxygen", since it is just over 20 per cent oxygen and just under 80 per cent nitrogen. The line joining "air" to "100 per cent trichloroethylene" shows that no mixture of trichloroethylene in air passes through the flammable area. It may also be seen from the parallel line next to and to the left of the line joining "100 per cent oxygen" and "100 per cent nitrogen" (the "ten per cent trichloroethylene line") that less than ten per cent trichloroethylene will never burn, in any mixtures of oxygen and nitrogen. The temperatures down the left side of the graph show that 10 per cent trichloroethylene cannot exist below 20° C, and so it is almost impossible to produce a flammable mixture of trichloroethylene in air or oxygen at room temperature. It is regarded as non-flammable in such mixtures, because the concentration needed for anaesthesia is only about 1 per cent. However, if nitrous oxide and oxygen are used, instead of air, flammable mixtures are produced with about 5 per cent trichloroethylene (see Table 1).

The lack of effect of increasing concentrations of nitrogen on the *lower limit* of flammability of a gas is a fairly constant phenomenon (Coward and Jones, 1952). The upper limit is affected to a much greater extent. Hence the range of flammability is always greater in oxygen than in air, although the *lower limit* is not significantly different.

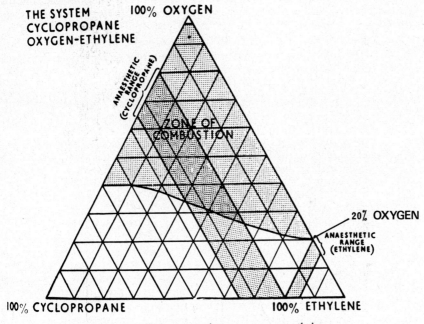

8/Fig. 3.—The system cyclopropane-oxygen-ethylene.

(b) "Free-radical" absorbers.—The value of a free radical absorbing diluent has been investigated by adding ethylene to mixtures of cyclopropane and oxygen (Jones *et al.*, 1943). This is depicted in Fig. 3 which shows that an explosion cannot occur so long as the oxygen concentration remains below 20 per cent. A non-explosive mixture containing 30 per cent oxygen can be produced provided the cyclopropane concentration is not reduced or the oxygen increased. Such a mixture has been tested clinically, but extremely careful control was necessary to keep it within the non-explosive limits (Horton, 1940). Coleman (1952) has shown that only about four per cent of some bromine containing fluorocarbons is necessary to inhibit the combustion of n-hexane in air. This is a readily ignitable substance, often used in the testing of fire extinguishers. It is thus possible that a chemical could be found which would render a flammable gas non-flammable and yet leave it clinically useful. It has been shown that 7 per cent halothane will prevent the ignition of cyclopropane/ oxygen mixtures (Bracken, personal communication) but as this is more than enough halothane to produce deep anaesthesia itself, the discovery is not of practical use.

The Elimination of Ignition Sources

The *energy* required to ignite gases varies according to the nature of the gases and how nearly their concentration approaches the stoichiometric, at which ignition is most easy. The stoichiometric mixture of any fuel is that at which, theoretically, combustion can be complete and all the fuel and oxygen molecules in the mixture react to form the products of combustion. The two main sources of ignition in the operating theatre are static electricity and diathermy.

The Report of the Working Party on Anaesthetic Explosions (H.M.S.O., 1956) lists the following probable *sources of ignition* in thirty-six explosions reported to the Ministry of Health from 1947 to 1954:

	Number	*Percentage*	
Static spark	22	61·1	
Static spark or open gas burner ..	1	}	} 69·4
Static spark or electric heater	1	8·3	
Static spark or smouldering towel ..	1		
Diathermy	5	14·0	
Spark in switch or cut-out	3	8·3	
Faulty valve in gas cylinder	1	}	
Foreign matter in valve	1	8·3	
Smoking (?)	1		

Static electricity.—It is almost impossible to ensure that a dangerous accumulation of static electricity will never occur in an operating room. Nevertheless most explosions due to static can be traced to a failure to observe fairly simple precautions. It is now believed that the danger from static is confined to a space even smaller than the area of 25 cm round the anaesthetic equipment outlined by Vickers (1970). The most important precaution for the anaesthetist to take against a dangerous accumulation of static electricity is to make sure that all breathing tubes and masks and apparatus locally associated with them are anti-static. In England and Wales equipment which is not anti-static is now allowed in parts of the operating room which are more than 25 cm from anaesthetic equipment. For the same reason, switches and electrical apparatus at a greater distance than 25 cm from anaesthetic apparatus need not be spark proof.

Anti-static precautions in operating rooms are aimed at removing all non-essential articles which readily acquire static charges and at providing a limited path to earth from all personnel and equipment close to anaesthetic circuits. In this way any static charges that develop are dissipated as quickly as possible, without significantly increasing the risk of electrocution. In general terms it involves ensuring that there is a resistance of not more than 100 megohms* and not less than 50,000 ohms between each such person or article, in the operating room and earth.

Static charges may be produced by *movement, friction* and *induction*. Trolleys when *moved* about the theatre can acquire dangerous static charges. This risk may be minimised by using wheels fitted with conducting rubber tyres.

Charges may be produced by *friction* in woollen blankets when these are quickly shaken or drawn across a trolley, and may be *induced* on equipment by the presence of certain types of electrical apparatus in the theatre. In such cases there is no contact between the source of the current and the article on which the charge is induced.

Materials.—Certain materials, such as Perspex and nylon, are inherently dangerous, since they readily acquire static charges. It is usually possible to find suitable alternative materials which are not so troublesome, but where this is not possible the offending materials can be treated with an anti-static wax.

Personnel.—Theatre staff should not wear clothing which readily acquires a static charge. Plastic aprons and woollen garments should therefore not be worn.

Conducting footwear should be worn by everyone in the operating room involved in anaesthesia. Anti-static shoes or boots are most satisfactory, but light canvas shoes with anti-static rubber soles can also be worn with safety. People who enter the operating room for only a short time are no longer required to wear anti-static footwear (in Great Britain) unless they are concerned with anaesthesia.

As far as personal clothing is concerned, the most important thing is to wear a close-fitting cotton or other anti-static outer garment. It should fit closely to reduce movement between the clothes and the wearer.

Woollen blankets should not be brought into the theatre. They should be replaced by cotton blankets, a towel, or some other anti-static fabric. Closely fitting woollen stockings worn by patients are not a serious static risk since they become moist, and provided they are not removed or roughly handled in the theatre, are not likely to acquire a charge of static electricity.

It is sometimes suggested that nurses and others should not wear nylon stockings in the theatre, as this material might insulate the wearers. Quinton (1953) has shown that this does not occur. No significant difference in resistance between the thigh and the outside of the sole of the shoe was found in a volunteer nurse who wore different types of stockings. Apparently the skin of the foot makes contact with the inside of the shoe through the mesh of the stocking.

Floors.—It is obviously essential that the floor in an operating theatre should have a conductivity of the same order as the items resting on it. The most satisfactory types of flooring in use at present are terrazzo or concrete with a resistance of from 0·1 to 10 megohms. To replace all unsatisfactory floors would be a most expensive undertaking, but it is now possible to lay conductive rubber or

*1 megohm = 1 million ohms.

plastic on top of an existing floor and so render it satisfactory. Where an anaesthetic is only occasionally given, and the floor is unsuitable, it is sufficient to stand the anaesthetic trolley on a moistened sheet large enough to prevent anyone from touching the trolley without himself also making contact with the sheet.

Relative humidity.—The generation of static electricity is more difficult in a damp atmosphere, while moisture on the surface of an article renders it more conductive. It is good practice, therefore, to wet rubber breathing tubes before use if their anti-static properties are in doubt. A 1 per cent solution of a wetting agent is more effective than plain water.

A high relative humidity reduces the risk of a static explosion, but cannot entirely remove the hazard. It must also be remembered that articles have to be exposed to a humid atmosphere for about ten minutes before any significant amount of moisture collects on their surfaces.

No exact figure can be given for an optimum relative humidity, and different authorities in this country recommend from 50–65 per cent. It is, however, very difficult to raise the humidity in a theatre; washing down the floor with hot water barely raises it by 8 per cent—and even if it were possible, there are few theatres in which the temperature could be kept low enough to make it comfortable to work in a high humidity. Where full air conditioning exists, a relative humidity of over 70 per cent is quite comfortable provided the temperature is not allowed to rise above 20–21° C (68–70° F).

Ideally, all operating theatres should be equipped with hygrometers of the paper or human hair type. When the humidity falls below 50 per cent the anaesthetist should be told, and he should take whatever steps he thinks necessary for the safety of the particular patient he is anaesthetising. These might involve the wetting of floor and walls, or the use of non-explosive anaesthetics.

Rubber equipment.—There is little doubt that non-conducting rubber is the main source of dangerous static electricity (H.M.S.O., 1956). Sometimes the charge is generated on the rubber, sometimes the rubber prevents the rapid discharge of static produced elsewhere. Only anti-static rubber should be used in association with anaesthetic equipment. This rubber is made by the addition of carbon to the rubber "mix". It owes its conductivity to the proximity of the carbon particles and it is thus possible for ordinary wear and tear to reduce its conducting properties. For complete safety, therefore, all anti-static rubber should be tested about once every year.

From the practical point of view, when there is any doubt about the anti-static properties of rubber equipment, it should be kept moist. If an anti-static article does not retain all the desirable properties of its non-conductive equivalent, an ordinary rubber one may be used, provided it is kept moist. The only anti-static item which is really markedly unsatisfactory in practice is the endotracheal tube. It is reasonable to use endotracheal tubes made of ordinary rubber, since they are kept moist when in position in the patient.

The instrument most commonly used for testing the conductivity of a material is a 500-volt D.C. insulation tester. The two leads of the apparatus are applied to different areas of the object to be tested, and the handle of the instrument is turned. A direct reading of the conductivity between the two test points is then given on a scale.

Ionisation.—Quinton (1953) has designed an apparatus which conducts away static charges by ionising the air in the neighbourhood of the anaesthetic trolley and the operating table. The ionised air is electrically conductive and serves to dissipate static charges. The apparatus is spark-proof, and the radio-active source is so arranged that theatre personnel cannot be exposed to radiation.

Diathermy.—If it is considered that a patient's best interests are served by the use of a flammable anaesthetic, the simplest solution to the problem of an explosion is to do without the diathermy. But this might seriously prejudice the success of the operation. It is then necessary to approach the problem in the third way—that of separating the ignition source from the flammable gas by a safe distance. This may be done by using a fully closed system for the administration of the anaesthetic, in a properly ventilated theatre.

Many anaesthetists have used ether or cyclopropane in a fully closed system with complete safety, provided the diathermy spark is some distance from any possible leak of flammable anaesthetic. In this connection, the lungs are not an effective barrier between explosive gases and diathermy sparks, and so such a technique cannot be used with safety if the chest is open. It must also be remembered that, however well the diathermy is separated from the explosive gases, the risk from static electricity with flammable gases remains, unless full-anti-static precautions are taken. It is also theoretically possible, if the lead from the diathermy plate attached to the patient is faulty, for the current from the diathermy to flow to earth via the patient and the anaesthetic apparatus, or via the anaesthetist. The current, unable to return to the diathermy apparatus along the plate lead, takes the shortest path to earth. This path may well be through the anaesthetist, should he be touching the patient, and can lead to the formation of a spark between the anaesthetist's fingers and the patient, if this contact is broken while the current is flowing. It is essential that the earth lead should be known to be functioning whenever the diathermy is used.

In connection with the leak of flammable gases from anaesthetic systems, Vickers (1970) has shown that as close as 10 cm from an expiratory valve delivering 15 per cent ether in eight litres of air/minute, the highest concentration of ether detectable was only 0·85 per cent of the lower limit of flammability. He concluded "that, as far as the mixtures escaping in clinical anaesthesia are concerned, there seems no likelihood of explosive concentrations occurring at a distance greater than 25 cm from the expiratory valve".

OTHER ELECTRICAL HAZARDS

The second group of hazards is concerned with the side-effects of electricity, other than the ignition of flammable gases and materials. According to Dobbie (1975) *surgical diathermy* is responsible for the greatest number of electrical accidents in hospitals. The commonest trouble is failure of the earth lead. If this is not intact, current will return to earth by the shortest possible route, and if this is via some other lead, such as that of an ECG, a burn may occur where the small electrode makes contact with the skin. If part of the patient's skin is touching a piece of metal which is connected to earth, current may take this course, and a burn occur at the point of contact.

To minimise these and other risks of damage from the diathermy, the following precautions may be taken:

1. Use an "earth-free" diathermy set.
2. Use two plate leads.
3. Use a monitored plate lead, which sounds an alarm if the lead breaks, or test the continuity of the plate lead before use.
4. Use a large area with good blood supply. Ischaemia makes tissues less conductive.
5. Ensure regular servicing of apparatus.
6. Train staff in the reasons for the precautions.
7. Put the plate as close as possible to the operation site, and avoid putting it below the knee, because the knee joint conducts electricity poorly.
8. Place ECG and other monitoring electrodes as far away as possible from the operation site. They should be at least one square centimetre in area. As far as possible fully isolated equipment should be used and *all ECG leads should have a* 10,000 *ohms resistor moulded into them.*
9. Encourage the operating surgeon to use the foot pedal himself. This should have an audible warning when current is flowing, and as little current as possible should be used.
10. Encourage the return of the active electrode to its quiver, whenever not in use and beware of pushing the foot pedal under the operating table.
11. The diathermy should be used with extra care in the neighbourhood of plastic drapes, if they are close to the outlet of anaesthetic gases. There is a risk that certain mixtures of nitrous oxide and oxygen could cause the ignition of such drapes by the diathermy (Cameron and Ingram, 1971).
12. Use of the diathermy presents real problems if the patient has an artificial cardiac pace-maker. In most cases the safest thing for such a patient is for diathermy to be avoided.

Mains electricity can be dangerous if the "live" lead becomes connected by external contacts to a person who is connected to earth. This can produce "gross shock", which can be prevented by the use of properly designed and maintained equipment. Mains operated instruments should be earthed and equipped with internal isolating transformers. They should be enclosed in earthed metal cases, which should be regularly checked. Some countries favour the use of non-earthed mains supplies for operating rooms. This system is expensive and requires complex isolation monitoring circuits.

Very much smaller currents can be dangerous if they flow to a contact in, or very close to, the myocardium. Such contacts can be provided by cardiac pace-makers or cardiac catheters which may be filled with conductive fluids. In order to prevent such *"microshock"* Hull (1972) recommends that all intra-cardiac leads and catheters should be *totally isolated* from earth, including circuitry and transducers which may be attached to them.

Although more and more monitoring devices are being used on anaesthetised patients to increase their safety, it must be remembered that even monitors carry risks, such as giving a false alarm, electrocution or a burn. An artificial monitoring device should only be connected to a patient if the anaesthetist in charge of the case believes that he will be able to give a better anaesthetic with it than without it. False alarms, such as those produced on an ECG by the diathermy, can distract an anaesthetist from clinical observation. A twenty-year-old patient undergoing minor surgery is reported to have been killed by electrocution because the anaesthetist wanted to try out a new ECG machine, which turned out to have an electrical fault. Burns continue to be reported at ECG plates when diathermy earth leads fail and the ECG leads have no built in resistor.

POLLUTION

Relatively recently it has become possible to measure volumes per million (vpm) of gases by portable and fairly simple physical methods such as gas chromatography and mass spectrometry. With the growing interest in general environmental conditions, such instruments have been used to measure small amounts of anaesthetic vapours present in operating rooms and other areas involved in anaesthesia. Whitcher *et al.* (1971) measured halothane concentrations within a three-foot radius of anaesthesia equipment, and found about nine vpm when a semi-open (10 l/min) circuit was used in an operating room with about ten air changes per hour without recirculation. The writer (1974) has measured halothane concentrations of 45 vpm in semi-open systems, 3 vpm in closed systems with a small leak and less than 1 vpm with fully closed systems at two feet from anaesthesia equipment in an operating room with twelve air changes per hour without recirculation. The figures for nitrous oxide in similar systems were semi-open 4400 vpm, semi-closed 200 vpm, and closed—nil.

Nothing is known about the effects on general health of breathing such concentrations of anaesthetic vapours for long periods intermittently over many years, but a retrospective national study of disease among operating room personnel was published in *Anesthesiology* (A.S.A. Committee, 1974). The authors believed that their results showed that female workers in the exposed group were subject to increased risk of spontaneous abortion, congenital abnormalities in their children, cancer and hepatic and renal disease, but their title was biased in that they described their report as being on "The effect of *trace anaesthetics* on the health of operating room personnel". The investigation could only be described fairly as being on the *effects of employment in a certain type of work*. Others (Walts *et al.* 1975) criticised the logic used by the authors of the national study. They believe that the data on spontaneous abortion, for example, would lead to the conclusion that "any increase in its rate amongst operating room personnel is LESS likely to be due to inhalation of trace anaesthetic vapours, than to result from other environmental factors". They show from the Study's figures that "the tendency towards spontaneous abortion is not dose related to anesthetic vapour", since the rate of spontaneous abortion was lower among physician anaesthesiologists and nurse anaesthetists than among operating room nurses and technicians. Levels of anaesthetic exposure are agreed to be higher for physician anesthesiologists and nurse anaesthetists than for operating room nurses and technicians.

It should also be remembered that, to such a retrospective study there are certain fundamental objections:

1. Only survivors and less than 50 per cent of them replied to the questionnaire.

2. It is difficult to avoid bias in the title. The questionnaire was headed "Effects of waste anesthetics on health".

3. Women are known to vary in what they consider to be abortions, between 8–25 per cent.

Bruce *et al.* (1974*b*) published a prospective study of anaesthesiologist mortality, which showed that "death rates, both overall and by categories, of anesthesiologists were lower than those for the control group, with the exception of suicide".

However, Bruce *et al.* (1974*a*) claimed that traces of anaesthetic gases can impair the performance of those working in operating rooms. In the present circumstances therefore, it would appear prudent to minimise the amount of anaesthetic vapours inhaled by those who work in such areas; but steps to do this must not be allowed to add a significant risk to the safety of the patient.

When considering pollution the following points appear to be worth stressing:

1. There is work which is believed by some to show that those who work in operating rooms are exposed to certain extra risks. There is no evidence to associate these risks with the inhalation of trace amounts of anaesthetic gases.

2. There is work which is believed by some to show that anaesthesiologists live longer than the average population.

3. There is work which is believed by some to show that mental ability is impaired by prolonged breathing of 1 vpm halothane in 50 vpm nitrous oxide (Bruce *et al.*, 1974*a*).

4. In modern operating rooms with 12 air changes an hour with no recirculation, a closed system of anaesthesia (4 l/min) with a leak will keep halothane levels below 3 vpm and nitrous oxide levels below 200 vpm.

5. The need for "scavenging" systems applies mainly where flow rates above 4 l/min are used. They may be active, involving a pump, or passive, where gases are carried to a disposal point by pressure existing at the patient's expiratory valve. An alternative to discharging gases to the outside is to pass them through a device such as the Cardiff adsorber, which removes many anaesthetic gases, but, unfortunately, has very little effect on nitrous oxide.

Scavenging systems (Fig. 4*a* and *b*) carry some obvious risks. In *passive* systems the patient is exposed to additional expiratory resistance. This will vary with the type of pipe (metal or corrugated rubber), the number and nature of bends, and the risk of obstruction. In *active* systems positive or negative pressure may become applied to the respiratory circuit. In *either system* the siting of the outlet may be critical. For example, there is a risk of back pressure from sources outside the operating room, and risk of an explosion if flammable gases have been used. The tubing may carry infection, and will need regular sterilisation. There is a risk that moist, inhaled anaesthetic gases may react with materials used in the system. The tubing may become misconnected. There have already been disasters where experienced anaesthetists have been involved in the misconnection of normal ventilators.

A totally closed system of anaesthesia removes the problem of pollution, and some anaesthetists believe it offers many other advantages and is more convenient than is generally realised, now that it is possible to monitor halothane concentrations by the use of a small meter. When such a totally closed system is used, the halothane concentration in the operating room remains below 1 vpm, and with no nitrous oxide in the system another source of pollution is eliminated. It appears logical to produce the minimum of vapours from volatile liquids if these are regarded as pollutants. Less than 10 ml of halothane are vaporised per hour in a closed system, and this results in considerable economy in running costs, as well as doing away with the need for piped gas systems. The absence of

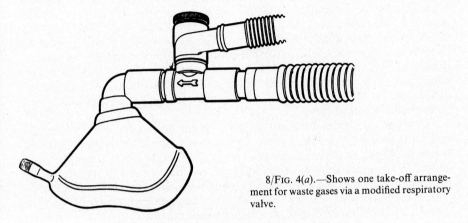

8/Fig. 4(a).—Shows one take-off arrangement for waste gases via a modified respiratory valve.

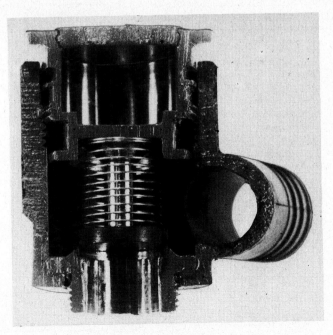

8/Fig. 4(b).—Shows a cross-section of the valve.

nitrous oxide minimises the risk of misconnected pipe lines. The use of *one carrier gas* is inherently safer than the use of two. The lack of nitrous oxide in the system also minimises the risk of oxygen failure. If the oxygen supply were to cease most ventilators would stop working, and with spontaneous respiration the patient's efforts at breathing from an empty bag would quickly attract attention. There is no risk that a patient's lungs would become filled with nitrous oxide.

Other interesting advantages of a totally closed system are that the patient's water vapour is conserved and fewer calories are lost. Oxygen is produced *physically* by the distillation of liquid air. It is therefore less liable to contain impurities than nitrous oxide, which is produced chemically. Nitrous oxide increases the flammability of all anaesthetic gases—even halothane can be made to burn in it. One final hazard worth mentioning is the effect which the presence of nitrous oxide has on cavities which do not normally contain it. The presence of nitrous oxide increases the risk associated with air embolism. It causes gut distension, produces gas bubbles in the middle ear, and over-distension of the cuffs of endotracheal tubes.

There is at present certainly some evidence to suggest that working in operating rooms carries extra risks. But there is no evidence to show that these risks are related to the inhalation of traces of anaesthetic gases. Indeed, those closest to the gases show the lowest morbidity. However, any steps to reduce the contamination of the working environment which do not add any risk for the patient should be encouraged. One method of doing this would appear to be the use of totally closed systems with adequate monitoring.

It would be tragic if a patient were to die through being misconnected to a scavenging device, or from infection carried by it, or from some other related cause, while the morbidity to staff remained unchanged.

REFERENCES

AMERICAN SOCIETY OF ANESTHESIOLOGISTS (1974). Report of an Ad Hoc Committee on the effect of Trace Anesthetics on the Health of Operating Room Personnel. *Anesthesiology*, **41**, 321.

ARTUSIO, J. F., Jr. (1963). *Halogenated Anesthetics*. Philadelphia: F. A. Davis Co.

ARTUSIO, J. F., VAN POZNAK, A., WEINGRAM, J., and SOHN, Y. J. (1967). Teflurane. A nonexplosive gas for clinical anesthesia. *Anesth. Analg. Curr. Res.*, **46**, 657.

BRACKEN, A., and WILTON-DAVIES, C. C., (1963). Explosion risk in a "non-flammable" system. *Anaesthesia*, **18**, 439.

BRUCE, D. L., BACH, M. J., and ARBIT, J. (1974a). Trace anaesthetic effects on perceptual, cognitive, and motor skills. *Anesthesiology*, **40**, 453.

BRUCE, D. L., EIDE, K. A., SMITH, N. J., SELTZER, F., and DYKES, M. H. M., (1974b). A prospective survey of anesthesiologist mortality, 1967–1971. *Anesthesiology*, **41**, 71.

BURNS, T. H. S., HALL, J. M., BRACKEN, A., and GOULDSTONE, G. (1961). An investigation of new fluorine compounds in anaesthesia. (3) The anaesthetic properties of hexafluorobenzene. *Anaesthesia*, **16**, 333.

CAMERON, B. G. D., and INGRAM, G. S. (1971). Flammability of drape materials in nitrous oxide and oxygen. *Anaesthesia*, **26**, 281.

CARROLL, K. J., (1964). Unusual explosion during electrosurgery. *Brit. med. J.*, **2**, 1178.

COLEMAN, E. H. (1952). Effect of fluorinated hydrocarbons on the inflammability limits of combustible vapours. *Fuel*, **31**, 445.

COWARD, H. F., and JONES, G. W. (1952). Limits of flammability of gases and vapours. Washington: U.S. Bureau of Mines, Bulletin 503.

DOBBIE, A. K., (1975). Paper at Symposium on Environmental Hazards. Faculty of Anaesthetists, London.

FABIAN, L. W., DEWITT, H., and CARNES, M. A. (1960). Laboratory and clinical investigation of some newly synthesized fluorocarbon anesthetics. *Anesth. Analg. Curr. Res.*, **39**, 456.

"Fluothane": A report to the Medical Research Council by the Committee on Non-explosive Anaesthetic Agents. *Brit. med. J.*, 1957, **2**, 479.

GARMER, N. L., and LEIGH, J. M. (1967). Some effects of hexafluorobenzene in cats. *Brit. J. Pharmacol.*, **31**, 345.

HALL, L. W., and JACKSON, S. R. K., (1973). Hexafluorobenzene. Further studies as an anaesthetic agent. *Anaesthesia*, **28**, 155.

HINSHELWOOD, C. N. (1940). *The Kinetics of Chemical Change*. London: Oxford Univ. Press.

H.M.S.O. (1956). *Report of a Working Party on Anaesthetic Explosions, including safety code for equipment and installations*. London: H. M. Staty. Office.

HORTON, J. S. (1940). *Bull. Amer. Assn. Nurse Anesthetists*, **8**, 285.

HULL, C. J. (1972). Symposium on Hazards in the operating theatre. Royal College of Surgeons at Newcastle upon Tyne.

JONES, C. S., FAULCONER, A., Jr., and BALDES, E. J. (1950). Preliminary investigations of carbon tetrafluoride as an inert diluent gas to prevent explosions of mixtures of cyclopropane and oxygen. *Anesthesiology*, **11**, 562.

JONES, G. W., KENNEDY, R. E., and THOMAS, G. J. (1943). U.S. Bureau of Mines, Technical Paper 653. Washington.

JONES, G. W., and SCOTT, G. S. (1942). U.S. Bureau of Mines, Report of Investigation 3666. Washington.

KRANTZ, J. C., Jr. (1964). Unpublished reports.

KRANTZ, J. C., Jr., CARR, C. J. C., LU, G., and BELL, F. K. (1953). Anesthesia XL. The anesthetic action of trifluoroethyl-vinyl ether. *J. Pharmacol. exp. Ther.*, **108**, 488.

LU, G., LING, J. S. L., and KRANTZ, J. C., Jr. (1953). Anesthesia XLI. The anesthetic properties of certain fluorinated hydrocarbons and ethers. *Anesthesiology*, **14**, 466.

MILLER, G. L., and DORNETTE, W. A. L. (1961). Flammability studies of Fluoromar-Oxygen mixtures used in anesthesia. *Anesth. Analg. Curr. Res.*, **40**, 232.

NICHOLSON, M. J., and CREHAN, J. P. (1967). Fire and explosion hazards in the operating room. *Anesth. Analg. Curr. Res.*, **46**, 412.

PAUCA, A. L., and DRIPPS, R. D. (1973). Clinical experience with isoflurane (Forane). *Brit. J. Anaesth.*, **45**, 697.

QUINTON, A. (1953). Safety measures in operating theatres and the use of a radioactive thallium source to dissipate static electricity. *Brit. J. appl. Phys.*, Suppl. No. 2, S 92.

RAVENTÓS, J. (1956). The action of Fluothane—a new volatile anaesthetic. *Brit. J. Pharmacol.*, **11**, 394.

SCHÖN, G., and STEEN, H. (1968). Explosion limits and ignition temperatures of some inhalation anaesthetics in mixtures with various oxygen carriers. *Anaesthesist*, **17**, 6.

UBBELOHDE, A. R. (1935). Investigations on the combustion of hydrocarbons. I. The influence of molecular structure on hydrocarbon combustion. II. Absorption spectra and chemical properties of intermediates. *Proc. roy. Soc. A*, **152**, 354 and 378.

VICKERS, M. D. (1965). The duration of the explosion hazard following induction with ether or cyclopropane. *Anaesthesia*, **20**, 315.

VICKERS, M. D. (1970). Explosion hazards in anaesthesia. *Anaesthesia*, **25**, 488.

VIRTUE, R. W., LUND, L. O., PHELPS, M., Jr., VOGEL, J. H. K., BECKWITT, H., and HERON, M. (1966). Difluoromethyl 1,1,2-trifluoro-2-chloroethyl ether as an anaesthetic agent: results with dogs, and a preliminary note on observations with man. *Canad. Anaesth. Soc. J.*, **13**, 233.

VITCHA, J. F. (1971). A history of Forane. *Anesthesiology*, **35**, 4.

WALTS, L. F., FORSYTHE, A. B., and MOORE, J. G. (1975). Occupational disease among operating room personnel. *Anesthesiology*, **42**, 608.

WHITCHER, C. D., COHEN, E. N., and TRUDELL, J. R. (1971). Chronic exposure to anesthetic gases in the operating room. *Anesthesiology*, **35**, 348.

WOODWARD, N. W. (1961). Prevention of explosion while fulgurating polyps of the colon. *Dis. Colon Rect.*, **4**, 32.

ANAESTHESIA FOR DENTAL SURGERY
AND FOR SURGERY OF THE EARS, NOSE AND THROAT

ANAESTHESIA FOR DENTAL SURGERY

History

Gardner Quincy Colton first administered nitrous oxide to Horace Wells for the extraction of a tooth in 1844. It is just over 100 years since anaesthesia for dental extractions was introduced into England by Thomas Evans, an American dental surgeon, in 1868. A brief period of unconsciousness was induced using nitrous oxide delivered via a face-mask, allowing enough time for the painless removal of one or two teeth. The method was not associated with fatalities nor, as far as is established, with cerebral complications (Goldman, 1968). The invention of the nosepiece about 1899 allowed a longer period of unconsciousness, and hence more surgical time. This greatly increased the dangers to the patient as it allowed protracted periods of hypoxia. The introduction of the demand-flow apparatus by McKesson in 1910 and the technique of secondary saturation in which nitrogen and oxygen were "washed out" of the lungs by nitrous oxide, further added to the hazards of dental surgery. Even though a very large number of anaesthetics were given safely, fatalities and cerebral complications were far from rare. This era of "anoxic unconsciousness" (Goldman, 1968) to provide pain-free dental extraction continued until recent years. Klock (1955) and Tom (1956) demonstrated that oxygen restriction at any stage was unnecessary, but even after the dangers of hypoxia were well-established, 31 patients died undergoing dental treatment under anaesthesia in the dental chair between the years 1961–1965 (Editorial *Brit. J. Anaesth.*, 1968). The dangers of hypoxia are stressed in a recent assessment of deaths occurring during dental out-patient treatment (Tomlin, 1974) and there is absolutely no place for hypoxic methods of induction to be used in current practice.

General anaesthesia in dentistry is, however, an expanding field. There are now about 2 million general anaesthetics given for dental patients each year in the United Kingdom, a number exceeding the sum total of anaesthetics given for all other branches of surgery. The vast majority of these are given to healthy individuals for the extraction of teeth or conservative dentistry as out-patients either in dental surgeries, clinics, or out-patient departments. A much smaller number are given to hospital in-patients for oral and maxillofacial surgery.

Problems in Dental Surgery

Dental operations are rarely life-saving. Most are elective and the mortality, or even morbidity, are as often attributed to anaesthesia as to the operation. The anaesthetist's concern is to provide with safety a quiet patient and an uncongested operating field and this demands a clear airway. The airway, however, is shared with the surgeon and as it lies in close proximity to the operation site, must be protected from inhalation of blood, saliva and operation debris. Further, dental burrs, when used for surgery of conservation, are irrigated with water. Careful packing of the oropharynx is therefore essential and facilities for adequate suction should always be available and in perfect working order. The surgeon requires a wide open unobstructed mouth, the anaesthetist a clear unobstructed airway.

For out-patient surgery there is a combination of problems not encountered in any other surgical field. Firstly, the average person regards dental treatment as a minor event, arriving in the dental surgery relatively unassessed and unprepared, and expecting to return to the normal routine of life shortly after the procedure is completed; secondly, many patients are still seated upright during the anaesthetic. The upright position is used in certain neurosurgical and neuro-radiological procedures, but both are carried out under careful anaesthetic control and monitoring. By comparison, the relatively unprepared and unassessed patient is also met for minor procedures in the Casualty Department, but these are performed with the patient in the supine position.

The combination of these two factors makes anaesthesia for out-patient dentistry unique. The safety of the individual must depend to a great extent not only on the brevity of surgery (most patients having only one or two teeth extracted) but also their youth and fitness. Dental extraction technique was originally developed to cope with quick removal of a tooth causing unbearable pain. The sitting position became so entrenched in the extraction technique that it was carried on into the age of multiple extractions undertaken to remove sepsis rather than alleviate severe pain (Love, 1963), and in recent years is still practised for conservative dentistry. The supine position for out-patient dental treatment under general anaesthesia has been advocated for many years (Scott, 1952; Bourne, 1957; Love, 1963; Bourne, 1973), the erect posture for such treatment being considered reckless as long ago as 1873 (Morrison). It requires a different surgical approach, to which most operators adapt easily, and its use appears to have become widespread in dental surgeries during the past five years.

Whatever position is adopted the dental surgeon requires certain things of his anaesthetist in order that a large number of cases can be treated with skill and safety (Moore, 1968). Induction of anaesthesia must be smooth and swift. During the operation the patient should be still and quiet, breathing spontaneously without obstruction, retching or coughing, especially if instruments such as dental drills and chisels are used in the mouth. There should be sufficient relaxation of jaw muscles to allow the mouth to be opened by gentle pressure of a gag and to allow insertion and changing of dental props and packs without difficulty. Recovery has been divided into waking time, walking time and the time it takes before the patient is able to leave the surgery or recovery room (Young and Whitwam, 1964). This period should be as short as possible. Control of blood or foreign material does not cease at the end of the operation, since the risk of aspiration and obstruction is considerable in the immediate post-operative period; indeed during the period 1963–1968 one-third of all deaths in dental chair cases happened during the recovery period (Tomlin, 1974). Straining or fighting which may encourage post-operative bleeding or cause damage to oral wounds or appliances must be avoided.

POSITION IN THE DENTAL CHAIR

Traditionally, out-patient dental treatment under general anaesthesia was performed with the patient seated upright in the dental chair. Although the safety of this position has been challenged for many years and the supine position championed as a safer alternative (Bourne, 1973) it should be remembered that over a six-year period (1963–1968), when the upright position still monopolised dental treatment, the crude death rate was only 1:300,000 despite a wide variation in anaesthetic techniques and the variable skills of the administrators. The circulatory effects of posture, and particularly their influence have been the centre of the arguments for or against either position. Other factors; airway control, airway protection from blood and debris and regurgitation of stomach contents may be of equal importance in patient safety (Green and Coplans, 1973).

Man spends most of his waking life in the upright position. If this position is chosen it is essential that those mechanisms which ensure adequate brain cell oxygenation in everyday life are not lost under general anaesthesia. Respiratory activity and ventilation-perfusion are better in the upright position than if the patient is lying flat, so long as the patient is allowed to breathe without the restriction of tight clothing. Blood drains by gravity to the lung bases where there is a much larger area for gas exchange than in other parts of the lung. The lung bases are also better ventilated by unimpeded diaphragmatic excursion. The better vital capacity found in the upright position (15 per cent more than if lying supine) may be of particular value in severe cardiorespiratory disorders and in the obese.

Whatever the patient's position the cerebral blood flow is adequately maintained over a wide range of mean arterial pressure. In the upright position the mean arterial pressure is kept higher due to overcompensation for the effect of gravity by the carotid sinus and aortic baroreceptors. Cerebrovascular resistance is minimal in the upright, increased in the supine and in a head-down position may be so high as to impede flow.

During anaesthesia in the dental chair cerebral blood flow may be altered by certain factors. Hypoxia is known to increase flow, a 35 per cent increase being produced when a mixture containing only 10 per cent oxygen is breathed (Keele and Neill, 1966). This was probably the safety factor which allowed millions of dental extractions to be performed under hypoxic conditions with remarkably few disasters. The baroreceptors are sensitised by halothane so that any fall in systemic pressure may be increased by the addition of this agent.

Diminished cerebral blood flow occurs if the arterial blood pressure is severely reduced (below 60 mm Hg—8 kPa). A marked fall in arterial pressure occurs in certain circumstances during dental treatment under local or general anaesthesia, including failure of venous return, central cardiac failure, loss of peripheral resistance and direct stimulation of the carotid sinus.

Failure of Venous Return

The venous return is dependent on the compression of veins by voluntary muscles, the thoracic pump mechanism, venous valves and the arteriovenous pressure gradient. Most of the capacitance of the circulatory system is in veins below the level of the heart. In the upright position under anaesthesia muscular action on the veins in this capacitance area ceases. In addition, anaesthetic agents such as halothane will produce vasomotor depression. Pooling in the venous system under direct i. fluence of gravity occurs especially in the legs. Reduction in venous return leads to a fall in cardiac output and hence a fall in mean arterial pressure.

It has been suggested (Green and Coplans, 1973) that venous pooling will be avoided by raising the legs to the horizontal position, whilst no further improvement is necessarily obtained by also lowering the head to the horizontal.

Central Cardiac Failure

Patients suffering from cardiovascular disease are more commonly seen in the dental surgery now that improved dental care has enabled more old people to keep their own teeth. Whilst frank cardiac failure is easily spotted and extra care taken, latent disease, early asymptomatic coronary occlusion, for example, may be missed and cardiac failure precipitated by or in association with dental anaesthesia.

In recent years there have been reports of a high incidence of cardiac dysrhythmias during general anaesthesia for minor oral surgery in patients with normal hearts. Although the exact mechanism for the production of these dysrhythmias is not certain it has been suggested that they are due to the beta effects of catecholamines acting on a myocardium sensitised by halothane (Plowman et al., 1974). Such dysrhythmias are uncommon if local anaesthesia is used alone or if purely intravenous techniques are used.

"Fainting"

Sudden profound hypotension associated with a fall in total peripheral resistance and bradycardia is known as a vasovagal attack or fainting.

Initially, impulses from the anterior hypothalamus, discharged in response to emotional stress or pain, lead to sympathetic overactivity shown by cutaneous vasoconstriction (pallor) and active vasodilatation in voluntary muscles. On this is superimposed massive parasympathetic discharge resulting in sweating and, via the vagus, extreme bradycardia. The bradycardia magnifies the effect of the fall in total peripheral resistance, the resultant reduction in cardiac output leading to profound hypotension. Muscle tone is reduced, consciousness lost and fainting occurs. Once the body is supine improved cerebral blood flow leads to a return of consciousness and the situation is reversed.

Fainting in the dental chair is common. Predisposing factors include anxiety and emotional stress, fatigue, fasting prior to the anaesthetic and poor health. Fear, pain and the upright position contribute. Two per cent of 3000 consecutive dental out-patients treated under local analgesia at a dental teaching hospital had fainting reactions, many losing consciousness (Hannington-Kiff, 1969). The young are more likely to faint than the old, but any person may suffer in this way, and it is impossible to predict who will faint in response to a given stimulus.

Fainting may occur with little warning. Restlessness, yawning, nausea and sweating occur. There is extreme pallor. It is important to observe carefully if the patient becomes detached from his surroundings or makes no response to direct questioning. It may happen at any stage in the dental surgery especially prior to induction of anaesthesia or during the recovery period. Careful monitoring of the pulse rate at all times is vital so that bradycardia is not missed. In the dental chair the upright patient may be actively prevented from falling into the horizontal position and if the faint is not recognised soon enough severe brain damage and even death will result.

Bourne (1960, 1966, 1970) has for many years considered that most catastrophies in the dental chair are due to the common fainting attack. Although such a view has been challenged (Tomlin, 1974) and it seems unlikely that fainting can occur once general anaesthesia has been induced, it will be more common until the traditional upright position of the patient is abandoned in favour of the supine position during dental treatment. Even then, safety is not guaranteed and faints in the horizontal position have been recorded (Weissler et al., 1959; Verrill and Aellig, 1970).

If a faint has occurred, after initial recovery of consciousness, the patient should be kept flat until complete recovery has taken place. The tendency to faint may persist for many hours after the initial episode and recurrence may occur if an attempt is made to stand up again too soon.

To summarise, fainting in the dental chair is not uncommon and has led to disaster. The dental anaesthetist must carefully watch for pallor and change in pulse rate at all stages of the procedure. Once recognised, simple treatment should be started as soon as possible.

Carotid Sinus Stimulation

During anaesthesia pressure by the anaesthetist on the soft tissues below the mandible may rarely lead to carotid sinus stimulation and a fall in blood pressure. Care should be taken to support the jaw correctly to avoid this complication.

OTHER ASPECTS OF POSTURE

Regurgitation of Stomach Contents

Silent regurgitation or active vomiting of stomach contents is a hazard during anaesthesia in any unprepared patient. Silent regurgitation is especially likely to occur in the presence of an undiagnosed hiatus hernia, a pharyngeal pouch or in late pregnancy. The upright position protects against this problem and the complication is rarely if ever encountered in the sitting position (Coplans, 1962). It is, however, often encountered in unprepared patients in the supine position. Active vomiting may occur during anaesthesia if the patient has a full stomach. Although this should not occur in adults requiring treatment, fear of dental treatment may keep undigested food in the stomach for many hours. It may also be a hazard in anaesthesia for children, who may have been given sweets to pacify them on the way to the dental surgery. The upright position gives no protection against active vomiting, indeed the position is ideal for overwhelming invasion of the trachea. This situation can only be avoided if the reason for pre-operative fasting is clearly explained; many patients and parents think it is only to avoid the unpleasantness of being sick. A careful smooth induction of anaesthesia is important. Premature insertion of the pack invariably leads to retching, and vomiting may follow. The supine position does not protect against either silent regurgitation or active vomiting, indeed regurgitation may become a commoner complication now that the horizontal position is becoming more universal. The supine position does, however, make immediate treatment such as turning the patient on the side much easier and is especially valuable if the head of the table or dental chair can quickly be tipped down.

Inhalation of Blood and Debris

Inhalation of blood and debris may occur as readily in the upright position as in the supine despite appearances to the contrary. Love (1963) states that the patient in the sitting position is safer from inhalation of material spilled in the mouth only when the floor of the mouth is horizontal or tilted forwards. In this position it is difficult to maintain a clear airway and surgical access is also difficult. In fact there is usually a change in the patient's position after induction of anaesthesia, either because the patient slips down in the chair or the dental surgeon actually tilts the chair backwards prior to surgery to gain better access to the upper teeth. The head will also tilt backwards if the anaesthetist does not apply adequate counter-pressure to the patient's head or if he is trying to maintain a good airway. Head retraction will occur if the patient is too lightly anaesthetised. These effects will produce a situation similar to that found with the supine position in which blood and debris will pool in the pharynx and are very liable to be inhaled. This is especially the case if back teeth are extracted. Correct placing of the pack therefore is just as vital in the upright position as in the supine to absorb blood as it gravitates to the back of the tongue. There should be adequate packing of the back of the mouth from one retromolar triangle to the other. The pack should be placed and maintained by the dental surgeon to guard the glottic area without encroaching on the airway. Positioning and maintenance of the pack without airway obstruction is technically easier in the upright than in the supine position. Careful watch should be kept on the area where the pack touches the buccal walls as there is often a space here through which blood and debris can pass (Love, 1963). Further points recommended by Love to avoid inhalation include tranquil anaesthesia, unhurried surgery, reliable suction and careful positioning of the patient in the immediate post-operative period. Respiratory obstruction, coughing, struggling, vomiting and heavy bleeding all make the likelihood of inhalation greater, whatever the position of the patient and these factors are mostly under the anaesthetist's control.

Airway Control

Once anaesthesia has been induced with the patient in the supine position, the relaxed tongue falls backwards by gravity against the posterior pharyngeal wall causing varying degrees of airway obstruction. The operator may aggravate the situation by displacing the mandible and the tongue backwards. In the upright position the tongue will fall into the floor of the mouth with less likelihood of obstruction so long as the head is held forward and surgical displacement is easier to counteract in the upright than in the supine position. Airway obstruction and resultant hypoxia is thus more of a danger in the supine than in the upright position. A nasopharyngeal airway may not improve the situation but intubation in the dental chair has been considered and may be essential in prolonged or difficult cases.

Conclusion

No posture guarantees absolute safety. The supine position eliminates certain cardiovascular hazards but may be associated with a higher degree of obstruction and hence hypoxia. Regurgitation may be a more common event in the supine position although it is easier to deal with stomach contents that have reached the pharynx than if the patient is upright. The reclining position with the feet horizontal may prove a safe compromise. Whatever position is adopted constant attention to vital signs is needed from the moment the patient is positioned in the chair prior to anaesthesia to the moment of full recovery.

OUT-PATIENT DENTAL SURGERY

Indications for General Anaesthesia

The majority of out-patient dental procedures, either extractions or conservation work, can be performed under local analgesia, and this will provide adequate operating conditions. There are, however, certain groups of patients in whom general anaesthesia is either definitely indicated or is of great value (Ministry of Health, 1967; Goldman, 1968).

1. Young children do not like local techniques.
2. Acute infective conditions, except where there is oedema of the floor of the mouth or Ludwig's angina, and in whom acute sepsis has not lead to trismus with limitations of the opening of the mouth. Due to the low pH of infected tissues local anaesthetics will not relieve pain. When severe infection is present treatment is best carried out as an in-patient.
3. Unco-operative patients, either those who are mentally subnormal or who have physical infirmity enough to become uncontrollable under local analgesia, e.g. spastics.
4. Multiple extractions, in more than one quadrant of the mouth.
5. Those individuals who are "sensitive" to local anaesthetics and the added vasoconstrictor drug.
6. A large number of people, often very intelligent, who are extremely nervous of all forms of dental treatment and to whom general anaesthesia for conservative dentistry as well as for extractions is a great benefit.

Preparation of the Patient

It is important to stress at the outset that in no other form of anaesthesia is the "psychological approach" more important than when giving an anaesthetic to a patient in the dental chair. The administrator is often required to assess the clinical state of an out-patient, whom he has never seen before, without causing any unnecessary alarm, and at the same time allay any apprehension. Commonsense and a few simple questions are what is needed. Indeed, even if there were time to do a full clinical examination (which is rarely the case), it is doubtful whether the information gained in most patients would be worth the apprehension produced.

Some simple instruction should be given to the patients before they come up for treatment. They should take no food or drink for at least four hours prior to the time of anaesthesia, and Young (1975) suggests 5 hours starvation to allow some latititude in the patient's interpretation of this request. Special precautions should be taken with children as they and/or their parents, may have differing ideas as to what is meant by food. The bladder should be emptied to avoid micturition during anaesthesia. Patients should be instructed to wear clothing which is not too tight around the neck or waist and have sleeves that are easily drawn up above the elbow in case intravenous agents are used. False teeth should be removed and shoes taken off.

In the limited time available clinical observation of the patient's general condition and features is much more important than detailed physical examination, indeed the latter may add little to the general assessment but merely increase the patient's anxiety. The age, muscular build and degree of mental apprehension can be assessed. As Thompson (1964) notes: Is the patient pale, panicky, panting, plethoric, porcine, pregnant or purple? The patient or parent should be questioned about any previous serious illness, recent illness or visits to the local doctor or hospital, and previous anaesthetic experiences; whether they have been taking any pills, capsules or other medicines and when they last had anything to eat or drink.

Whilst these questions are being asked a finger on the patient's pulse and careful observation will detect any obvious signs of disability. It may also be advisable to check the blood pressure in older patients. Absolute contra-indications to general anaesthesia as an out-patient include recent food or fluid, coronary disease, respiratory obstruction especially if there is oedema of the floor of the mouth or swelling of the neck, limited opening of the jaw from trismus, and cerebrovascular disease. There are many relative contra-indications to general anaesthesia. They include diabetes, pregnancy, congenital and acquired heart disease, obstructive respiratory disease and anaemia including sickle-cell anaemia (see p. 718). The urgency and importance of dental treatment may also be factors influencing the decision to give an anaesthetic in the dental surgery.

Drugs used in the treatment of disease may modify the patient's response to dental anaesthesia. Hypoglycaemic agents, antidepressants, tranquillisers, antihypertensives and anticoagulants are but a few examples of the multiplicity of drugs that may be met. It is important that the anaesthetist should know exactly the nature of the patient's treatment for concurrent disease. Whilst some drugs will have little effect on the patient's response to anaesthesia in the dental chair, others, for example the monoamine oxidase inhibitors, may have a profound effect. If necessary the patient should be referred to hospital for treatment and if thought advisable have his dental treatment as an in-patient.

Premedication is unnecessary for most patients and is a disadvantage for the ambulant as the recovery period may be increased and the time of departure delayed. Most patients can be calmed by a proper approach to their fears. The promise of an intravenous induction will allay the fears of the most nervous individuals.

Methods of Administration

Dental anaesthetic machines are designed to deliver accurate mixtures of nitrous oxide and oxygen either by intermittent or continuous flow. A suitable vaporiser, able to deliver accurate concentrations of an adjuvant should be included.

Intermittent flow.—The intermittent or demand flow method is theoretically

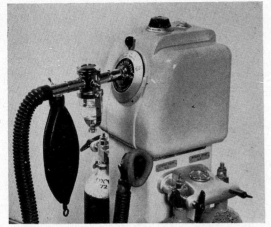

9/FIG. 1.—The "Walton Five" apparatus.

economical because gases flow only during inspiration into a mixing bag from which the patient inspires via corrugated tube and a mask. As the bag empties, so it is refilled from the cylinders, and when it is full of gases, automatically cuts off until the next inspiratory effort starts the process once more. In practice the resistance of the working parts is too great for comfortable spontaneous breathing if the pressure control is set at zero. A small positive flow of gases is therefore provided by adjusting the pressure control and thus gives a combination of continuous and intermittent flow. The "Walton Five" (Fig. 1), the A.E. machines and the McKesson Simplex are the most common demand flow machines still in use for dental anaesthesia in the United Kingdom. Apart from the pressure control, the percentage of gas and oxygen in the mixture breathed can be readily adjusted by setting the dial to the required figure. The mixture control is accurate in the machines mentioned, but accurate oxygen percentages are not possible with machines manufactured earlier than the "Walton Five". A vaporiser and the reservoir

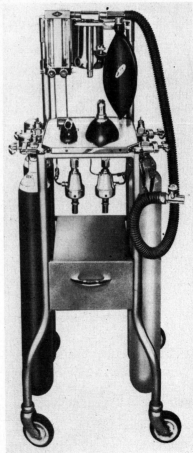

9/FIG. 2.—The "Salisbury" apparatus.

bag are incorporated between the patient and the machine. Although the reservoir bag is actually not necessary in a demand flow situation, as variations in the patient's tidal volume are compensated by the patient's own inspiratory effort, it may be life saving if manual inflation of the lungs should become necessary for example in respiratory obstruction or failure.

It would seem that the use of demand flow machines should now be abandoned in favour of the more accurate and simpler continuous flow anaesthetic machine. In fact, production of the "Walton Five" and the A.E. machines ceased in 1974.

Continuous flow.—A continuous flow of gases is supplied from the machine, almost all the expired gases passing into the atmosphere through the expiratory valve. A standard Boyle machine can be perfectly satisfactory for dental anaesthesia and simplified versions of the apparatus, such as the "Salisbury" machine (Fig. 2) have been introduced for this purpose. In the continuous flow method, a reservoir bag must be included in the system. A high flow is needed to ensure an adequate volume during induction when the mask or nose-piece is not applied to the face but is held some distance away (Goldman, 1968), a situation desirable especially when inducing anaesthesia in children.

Position in the Dental Chair

If the upright position is chosen the patient should sit comfortably with the seat of the dental chair tilted slightly backwards (Fig. 3). The occiput should rest on a head-rest which is adjusted to bring the head into a more upright position or that of "Sniffing the morning air". The hands rest across the abdomen without restriction and the knees are bent with the legs dependent. If the legs are supported in the horizontal position the chair should be tilted backwards further to place the patient in a more comfortable sloping position.

If the supine position is adopted a tilting trolley is ideal for the purpose especially in hospital out-patient practice, the patient recovering on the same trolley (Fig. 4). A pillow is placed under the shoulders to allow extension of the neck and the anaesthetist is able to rest his elbows on the trolley to facilitate correct support of the jaw during surgery. Children are easily managed in this position. In the upright position small children are more easily controlled in a special seat attached to the back of the dental chair.

Care should be taken to prevent lamps shining in the patient's face. A bib is placed round the neck to prevent any soiling of the clothes. A mouth prop is often inserted before induction in adults but can easily be inserted when the patient is asleep and should not be inserted in children until they are fully anaesthetised.

Anaesthesia for Dental Extractions

If an inhalational technique is chosen not less than 25 per cent oxygen should be delivered with the nitrous oxide from the commencement of induction if an adjuvant such as halothane is used. Latham and Parbrook (1966) suggest the use of pre-mixed 50:50 nitrous oxide and oxygen as this is a constantly accurate mixture and therefore safer and incidentally more economical than using separate cylinders of the two gases.

Adults and older children can be encouraged to breathe the gases through

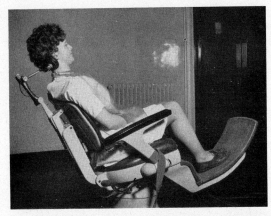

9/Fig. 3.—Posture for
dental anaesthesia.

a nose-piece. A high flow should be used but the gases should not be delivered at a pressure which is unpleasant for the patient. If the nose breathing is found difficult or impossible a mouth attachment or a pack held over the mouth may be of value. An alternative would be to use a standard face-mask which is gradually lowered to cover both nose and mouth during induction. The mask should initially be held away from the face especially in children. In small children a nose-piece may be used to cover both mouth and nose for induction, being reapplied to cover the nose only when surgical anaesthesia has been achieved.

Halothane is the commonest adjuvant to nitrous oxide in use in dental anaesthesia. It has many desirable features for out-patient dental treatment, as it is relatively non-irritant, provides a smooth quick induction, and adequate

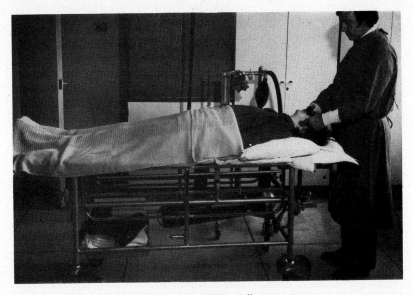

9/Fig. 4.—Tilting trolley.

muscle relaxation so that the mouth can be opened without force. Also, halothane is non-explosive and therefore safe to use in the presence of dental instruments which sometimes produce sparks from friction with the teeth. The patient recovers quickly and post-operative nausea and vomiting are uncommon. It can be vaporised from a Goldman vaporiser or some modification if a demand flow machine is used, or from a "Fluotec" or similar compensated vaporiser if a continuous flow machine is used.

Halothane can be added at the start of induction, 1 per cent halothane vapour being given initially and gradually increased to 2 per cent after a few breaths. Light surgical anaesthesia is quickly achieved so long as there is no breath holding or obstruction to breathing. Resistant cases require longer to achieve this state and nervous patients commonly mouth-breathe, prolonging induction time.

Light surgical anaesthesia can be recognised by the onset of regular rhythmical ventilation, expiration being about twice as long as inspiration. The eyelash reflex goes at the same time and adequate muscle relaxation will have been achieved to insert the dental prop and pharygeal pack at this stage. A mouth-gag may be introduced to allow the dental prop to be switched over to the other side if this is necessary. Once light surgical anaesthesia has been achieved, the halothane vaporiser can be turned down to deliver 0·5–1 per cent for simple extraction of one or more teeth and can be turned off altogether once the prop and pack have been inserted. Although the less halothane used the quicker the recovery time, this should not be an excuse for an inadequate depth of anaesthesia during surgery. Indeed too light a level of anaesthesia can only lead to danger of obstruction and inadequate dental treatment, and a correct level must be achieved even if this requires higher concentrations of halothane and in consequence a longer recovery period.

During the phase of returning consciousness the prop is removed and the pack either removed or replaced. At this stage the head should be held well forward with the jaw supported allowing any blood to drain forwards. The supine patient should be turned on his side for the recovery phase. Whatever the technique of anaesthesia employed, it is important that there are adequate facilities for recovery—a couch or trolley where those patients who take longer than a few seconds to wake up can be recovered on their sides, in good lighting conditions with adequate suction facilities. An additional safety factor is to allow recovery to take place without the patient being moved onto another surface.

Intravenous Induction

An intravenous induction may be preferable to inhalational methods and has indeed become much more popular. It is the method of choice for nervous or extremely robust individuals. Three agents, methohexitone, propanidid and althesin are in common use.

Methohexitone raises cardiac output and produces a more rapid return of consciousness compared with equipotent doses of thiopentone. Recovery time is quicker, methohexitone is broken down, mainly by the liver, at a rate of approximately 20 per cent per hour although a hypnotic effect with reduced mental alertness may persist for up to twenty-four hours after a single dose.

Propanidid has a significantly shorter duration of action. It is completely broken down in the body within 30 minutes. There are therefore no hangover effects as are found after methohexitone and there is complete mental awareness.

Both cause excitatory movements during induction with involuntary arm movements and hiccup if larger doses are given. Although both can produce cardiovascular depression this should be unusual following a single dose normally used for induction. Whereas methohexitone causes transitory respiratory depression if too large an induction dose is given, propanidid has a biphasic respiratory effect with initial hyperventilation leading to transient apnoea. *Propanidid* being produced in viscous solution is more difficult to inject but can be diluted satisfactorily with water or normal saline. Extravascular injection is not painful using propanidid. Methohexitone causes pain both on intra- and extravenous injection and venous thrombosis has been reported after use of either agent, though more commonly after multiple injection rather than after a single dose. Methohexitone is given as a one per cent solution in a minimum sleep dose of 1 mg/kg, propanidid in a 2·5 per cent solution, the initial minimum sleep dose being 5–10 mg/kg.

Althesin is the most recent induction agent to be tried. The rate of induction is slightly slower than with the others but smooth, the recovery time is only slightly longer than with propanidid and there is no hangover effect. There appears to be a greater incidence of involuntary movements however and emergence delirium is common (Warren, 1972; Rollason *et al.*, 1974).

Patients suffering from porphyria should not be given barbiturates and methohexitone is also best avoided in patients with a history of epilepsy. Allergic reactions are more common with both propanidid and althesin and hence methohexitone might be considered the drug of choice where a history of allergy is present. For most patients, however, the induction agent can be decided by personal preference although propanidid and althesin which cause no local tissue reaction and less hangover than methohexitone have marginal advantages.

Whatever intravenous agent is used for induction, as soon as the patient is asleep a nose-piece is placed directly on the face, the expiratory valve partially closed and anaesthesia continued using 50 per cent nitrous oxide and oxygen. If a long period of operating time is required or if it is found difficult to open the mouth it may be necessary to add 0·5–1·0 per cent halothane to the mixture.

Nausea and vomiting occur commonly after out-patient dental surgery. This is partially due to stimuli from the operative area and also as a result of swallowed blood in the stomach. Factors which are associated with a high incidence of sickness include a period of anaesthesia longer than five minutes and the use of halothane as the principal anaesthetic agent (Muir *et al.*, 1976; Smith and Young, 1976). Propanidid has also been incriminated and the technique associated with the lowest incidence of vomiting appears to be methohexitone either alone or followed by nitrous oxide and oxygen (Dundee 1965; Muir *et al.*, 1976).

Many patients expect to walk out of the dental chair and resume normal activities immediately after a general anaesthetic, although recent trends have shown that patients are now much more willing to take the whole day off for dental treatment than even five years ago.

Intubation in the Dental Chair

Intubation in the dental chair was suggested by Danziger (1962) and may be most valuable where the supine position is being used, especially when the dental surgery is likely to be prolonged or technically difficult. The recovery period is longer than normal and such patients may be best treated as day cases, arriving in the early morning and being escorted home in the late afternoon.

The best method of relaxation for insertion of the endotracheal tube is not firmly established. The incidence of muscle pains after suxamethonium in ambulatory patients is low when a small dose of non-depolarising relaxant such as gallamine 10–20 mg is given prior to suxamethonium. Where a relaxant is avoided and the tube inserted under deep halothane there appears to be a high incidence of post-operative headache (Smith and Young, 1976).

Anaesthesia for Conservative Dentistry

Traditionally, conservative dentistry or "fillings" (as opposed to "extractions") has been carried out under local analgesia, either by local infiltration or nerve block techniques. There is a great problem of fear of pain in dental treatment of this type, indeed fear of pain is probably the greatest deterrent to proper dental care (Monheim, 1957). Despite the improvement in local analgesic agents, the use of local sprays and analgesic jellies, and the use of sharp disposable needles, there has been little change in this inherent fear of the discomfort involved. Wide individual variation exists in the pain threshold and the degree of discomfort may to some extent depend on the patient's past experience. Conservative dental treatment means not only physical pain, but great mental stress. This is especially the case when a long period of time is necessary for treatment or when multiple nerve blocks are required. To deal with this problem local analgesia can be supplemented by sedation or dispensed with altogether, treatment being performed under intermittent intravenous general anaesthesia. These allow the dental surgeon to complete treatment, if necessary in more than one quadrant of the mouth, at a single sitting rather than subject the patient to the mental stress of several visits to the surgery. With all these methods the same care must be taken to assess the patient's general condition as if he were to undergo a full general anaesthetic. It should be stressed that whether supplements are added to the local block or intravenous anaesthesia is employed this is an additional hazard to the patient's welfare and should only be justified after careful consideration of all factors. It should not be given just because the patient demands the service.

Supplements to Local Analgesia (Sedation)

Although sedation helps minimise the discomfort of treatment, recovery time is undoubtedly prolonged. There must be facilities therefore to allow patients to recover slowly and in safety. Sedatives can be given orally. This route of administration, though comparatively safe, is unpredictable both in timing and effectiveness. Hypnotics, tranquillisers, analgesics and even alcohol have all been tried with variable results. They may be of value in helping the moderately anxious. For the very nervous patient, the intravenous route is more certain of producing the ideal tranquil situation as the dose can be finely adjusted to suit the individual requirements. At the same time, care ensures that a relative overdose, through individual variation, leading to respiratory or cardiovascular depression does not occur.

One of the best-known methods of intravenous sedation was introduced by Jorgensen and Leffingwell (1961) and was designed to make dentistry acceptable to the very nervous, and prolonged operations endurable to all. Consciousness is not abolished. Pentobarbitone, pethidine and hyoscine are used to provide sedation, amnesia and additional analgesia. Pentobarbitone is injected first, 5 mg being given intravenously as a test dose. Further doses of 10 mg are then given at half-minute intervals until the patient seems relaxed and at ease. Up to 100 mg can be given. At this stage a mixture of pethidine 25 mg and hyoscine 0·2 mg diluted in 5 ml of water is given slowly, 2–5 ml of the mixture being given. The patient is now in a state of "light sedation" and the local analgesic can be injected without much discomfort. Although good results will be achieved in expert hands it may be difficult to judge correct doses and there is always a marked "hangover". It is probably best to operate with the patient lying in the supine position.

Variations on the original Jorgensen technique have been tried using a wide range of hypnotic and analgesic drugs. When intermittent methohexitone is used as part of such a technique it is worth remembering that the potential convulsive properties of methohexitone may summate with those of intravenous lignocaine.

Diazepam (Valium) has been widely used as an intravenous tranquilliser prior to dental treatments. It provides a feeling of well-being, a shortening of the patient's time sense (even the most prolonged treatment appears to last only a few minutes) and amnesia for the event. The patient should be supine. 10–20 mg diazepam is given slowly intravenously over a period of two minutes. Care should be taken to retain consciousness to avoid the danger of respiratory obstruction. Injection should be made into a large vein because injections into small veins may be painful and also lead to venous thrombosis. The local block can be started immediately after the diazepam has been given. The technique gives satisfactory operating conditions for the dental surgeon even in the most anxious patient, and Healy *et al.* (1970*a*) consider it a real and practical advantage in the management of such patients. There is deep sedation and total amnesia for the first ten minutes after the injection and good tranquillisation lasting one hour in most individuals. Healy *et al.* (1970*b*) used an intravenous dose of up to 0·2 mg/kg and found no untoward physiological disturbance other than incompetence of largyngeal closure during the first few minutes after drug administration. Dixon *et al.* (1973) found that oxygen saturations and Po_2 did not fall following diazepam injection so long as the patient remained awake.

Recovery time is very slow but most patients are clinically safe to leave the surgery accompanied by a responsible adult within 90 minutes of administration of the drug. Delayed "hangover" effects have been observed though less commonly than after the "Jorgensen technique", but the patient should be told not to drive a vehicle for 24 hours (Dixon and Thornton, 1973).

Intermittent Intravenous Anaesthesia

For many years Drummond Jackson (1952) pioneered the use of an intravenous barbiturate, such as hexobarbitone or thiopentone, as the sole agent to provide pleasant yet relatively safe conditions for out-patient dental surgery, which he described (1962) as introducing "an era of pleasanter dentistry for both patient and dentist".

More recently methohexitone, propanidid and althesin have been widely used for this purpose. A patient's response to dental pain differs from the response to cutaneous pain. Cutaneous pain, for example cutting the skin with a knife, evokes brisk reflex defensive movement prohibiting surgery unless full surgical anaesthesia is established. Dental pain evokes much less response, allowing treatment to continue at a level of narcosis short of full surgical anaesthesia. A period of amnesia is especially common after methohexitone amnesia. During this "ultra-light" phase the patient appears to be awake but does not respond even to painful procedure so that additional increments of methohexitone may not be required. There are various ways of producing so-called "ultra-light" anaesthesia with intravenous agents. A common technique is described here. The patient should be settled comfortably with an arm fixed to a board. An indwelling needle is placed in a suitable vein. After a dental prop has been inserted into the mouth, the intravenous agent of choice is given, the size of the initial and subsequent doses being titrated against the patient's response to the stimulus of surgery. The aim—to provide a steady semi-narcotised state throughout the procedure—is difficult to achieve and requires high skill on the part of the administrator in judgement of size and timing of each dose. As doses are given intermittently an even plane of narcosis cannot be achieved, periods of full surgical anaesthesia alternating with periods of partial environment detachment (Howells, 1968). There is also wide individual variation in response to the drug used. Too light a plane of narcosis will evoke a marked response from the patient, but even if he cries out there appears to be amnesia of the event. Treatment is best carried out in the horizontal position.

Bourne (1967) recommends the following initial dosage scheme for methohexitone:

patients under 20 years of age	2·2 mg/kg body weight
patients between 20–40 years of age	1·5 mg/kg body weight
patients between 40–60 years of age	1·1 mg/kg body weight
patients over 60 years of age	0·75 mg/kg body weight.

Less should be given to the obese and those in poor health. With all patients it is best to err on the side of caution. Increments vary with individual requirements but up to 20 mg/min may be needed. Howells (1968) recommends the initial dose of propanidid to be 4–5 mg/kg whilst Cadle *et al.* (1968) suggest a higher initial dose especially in young females. Increments of 100–200 mg propanidid per minute may be necessary. Rollason and associates (1974), using althesin, found an initial dose of 4–12 ml satisfactory with increments of 1–2 ml when necessary. Whatever drug is used, an increment is given when the patient reacts to the surgical stimulus either by screwing up the eyes or by slight limb movement. Involuntary muscle movements occur during the use of all three drugs, Warren (1972) observing such movements in as many as 45 per cent of cases during dental conservation under althesin. Warren also noted a high level of post-althesin emergence delirium.

For periods of treatment lasting less than 20 minutes, propanidid or althesin would seem to be the drugs of choice, both being rapidly metabolised without the hangover effects seen after methohexitone. High doses of propanidid which would be required for longer periods of treatment, have occasionally led to stiffening of limbs suggestive of extra-pyramidal influences (Cadle *et al.*, 1968). Anaesthesia may have to be continued by this method for more than an hour. Great care must therefore be taken to ensure that a perfect airway is maintained and that neither respiratory depression nor hypotension occur. This requires even greater vigilance on the part of the anaesthetist than during an ordinary general anaesthetic. Cossham and Dixon (1973) have reported safe oxygen saturation figures during the use of propanidid, but Mann *et al.* (1971) and Wise *et al.* (1969) have been less happy about this aspect of patient safety using intermittent methohexitone.

The advantages of such a method appear great, both to the patient and surgeon. Induction is swift and certain and even in the most robust or nervous, management is less complicated than with inhalational methods and recovery more pleasant. It is certain that many more patients have attended for conservative dental treatment since the use of such intravenous agents became widespread. Perhaps it may be of special value to attract a patient back to regular dental care with a long initial treatment under intermittent intravenous anaesthesia followed by subsequent less unpleasant treatments performed under local analgesia only.

Faced with such facts the trend for the single-handed operator to give his own intravenous anaesthetic is to be deplored. The joint sub-committee of the Ministry of Health on dental anaesthesia (Ministry of Health, 1967) deprecated the practice and more recently it has been deemed inexcusable (*Brit. med. J.* Leader, 1975).

Anaesthesia for In-Patient Dental Surgery

When more extensive surgery is required than can be dealt with in the dental surgery, or when the patient's general condition contra-indicates out-patient treatment, he should be admitted to hospital. Although the majority of patients treated on an in-patient list are young healthy adults who require removal of impacted wisdom teeth, every list is likely to contain patients whose general condition demands a full general anaesthetic for their dental treatment. Amongst these are diabetics, patients with severe heart disease and chronic respiratory disease, mental defectives, spastics, mongols and those with some haemorrhagic disorder such as haemophilia or those with a history of post-extractional haemorrhage. Careful pre-operative assessment is therefore of the greatest importance. Local hazards should also be assessed. The patient may have loose teeth, prostheses, bridges and other dental work or a deviated nasal septum. Finally, it is valuable to know the extent to which the patient can open his mouth prior to surgery.

A nasal endotracheal tube is used except for certain procedures involving the maxilla. Nasal tubes are usually uncuffed, but special streamlined cuffed tubes can be used. A smaller diameter nasal tube has to be used than the equivalent oral tube and resistance to breathing is therefore greater. Damage can easily be done to the nasal mucosa resulting in haemorrhage and this can be severe on occasions. Infection present in the nose may also be carried to the bronchial tree. Because many patients for dental surgery, especially those who have had wisdom teeth extracted, will be ambulant within 12 hours, the incidence of muscle pains (suxamethonium) will be high unless it is preceded by a small dose of a non-depolarising agent, or intubation is performed without this relaxant drug (see Chapter 26).

Packing of the pharynx is essential. Common throat packs include gauze soaked in sterile saline, gauze soaked in "Vaseline" (autoclaved) and tampons soaked in sterile saline. Choice is by individual preference. A pack is not so efficient as a cuff, but in practice acts as a good seal to fluids since it tends to absorb them. The use of any pack increases post-operative pharyngitis, particularly if it becomes dry and remains in place for a long time. Towels are usually wrapped firmly around the face, hence the eyes must be protected and connections safely secured.

Although no method of anaesthesia is ideal, nitrous oxide-oxygen-halothane with spontaneous breathing is satisfactory. Bleeding is seldom severe. The intensity of monitoring will depend on the patient's condition. Young healthy adults having impacted wisdom teeth removed require only routine careful assessment throughout the operation with special care to note pulse irregularities (Plowman et al., 1974). Full dental clearance in an ill patient prior to cardiac surgery is a different matter, more intensive monitoring obviously being required in such cases. Unlike out-patient anaesthesia, both analgesics and anti-emetics can be used when necessary.

At the end of the procedure the pharyngeal pack must be removed as total laryngeal obstruction quickly results if the pack is left in the pharynx after removal of the endotracheal tube. Gauze packs are placed in the cheeks to stop oozing and an oral airway inserted. The nasal tube is best removed with the patient turned on to the side in the post-tonsillectomy position. At this stage, post-operative obstruction may easily occur. Post-halothane shivering, an annoying hazard, can be avoided by giving up to 10 mg of methyl phenidate just prior to extubation.

MAJOR ORAL AND MAXILLO-FACIAL SURGERY

Moore (1973) divided elective maxillo-facial operations into certain categories of which the following are relevant to this section:
1. Corrective operations of the jaws such as mandibular and maxillary osteotomies, and building-up procedures which may include the use of bone grafts.
2. Removal of tumours of the mandible and maxilla ranging from the enucleation of simple cysts to the removal of an extensive jaw carcinoma which may involve excision of adjacent soft tissues.
3. Operations on the tongue and floor of the mouth.

The problems involved during these procedures are similar to those described in the previous section, with the added knowledge that the establishment of an adequate airway during induction of anaesthesia and its maintenance in the post-operative period may cause complex problems. Blood loss may also be severe enough to require transfusion.

The choice between an oral and nasal tube depends on the site of surgical intervention and distortion of normal anatomy especially in cases of tumours which sometimes require blind introduction of a nasal tube. The position of the tube should not obstruct the surgical field and should be discussed with the surgeon beforehand. If extreme facial deformity is present and especially if the mandible is grossly underdeveloped (e.g. the Treacher Collins syndrome), intubation may be extremely difficult. Blind intubation may be necessary and is best performed with the patient breathing spontaneously. It should therefore be remembered that the use of intravenous agents for induction may be unsafe. The Huffman prism on the laryngoscope blade may be of help (Huffman and Elam, 1971). Cricothyroid puncture has been performed using a Tuohy epidural needle, the endotracheal tube being fed into the larynx using the epidural catheter as a guide. Finally, pre-operative tracheostomy under local anaesthesia may have to be considered in very severe cases.

Major maxillo-facial surgery is often prolonged. Although the nitrous oxide-halothane sequence with variations is satisfactory it may be preferable to use a cuffed endotracheal tube and employ a relaxant, controlled respiration and analgesic technique. This is especially valuable if the jaws are immobilised with either elastic bands or wire at the end of the operation as it allows rapid, smooth recovery. Controlled hypotension may be indicated (Davies and Scott, 1968). Swelling of the soft tissues after major jaw surgery often leads to marked post-operative'oedema and consequent respiratory obstruction.

If wiring is performed the pharyngeal pack is removed immediately prior to immobilisation. To help maintain the airway post-operatively, the nasal tube is partially removed and left in place as a nasopharyngeal airway. A safety-pin is inserted into the proximal end of the tube which is cut close to the nose. This pharyngeal airway is left in position at least until full recovery from the anaesthetic has taken place, but if tolerated it is best left until the following day. These patients are best nursed in an intensive care unit for the first 24 hours post-operatively. The nursing staff should know the position of wires or elastic bands. Wire cutters must be beside the patient for use in case of emergency such as severe respiratory obstruction which is not quickly relieved by simple measures. Post-operative vomiting must be avoided by using anti-emetics, although it is debatable whether swallowed blood should be allowed to remain in the gut. If vomiting occurs the patient should be placed in the post-tonsillectomy position allowing stomach contents to drain through the space between the molar teeth and cheek. Efficient suction must be immediately available throughout the period the jaws are wired.

Acute Trauma

Trauma may cause a wide variety of maxillo-facial injuries. These injuries range in severity from fracture of the nasal bones requiring simple reduction to complicated injuries involving facial bones, nose, maxilla and mandible. There may be considerable soft tissue damage. Concomitant injuries to the head with loss of consciousness, the chest and abdomen, and limb fractures may also be present. Many patients with maxillo-facial injuries sustain concussion. When the head injury is serious, treatment of the face may have to be delayed while an assessment of the head injury is made and priority of treatment given if it is considered the more dangerous to life (Ennis and Gilchrist, 1968). Maxillo-facial injuries seldom require immediate operation unless there is uncontrollable haemorrhage or an obstructed airway. Other injuries must be carefully assessed and hypovolaemia corrected.

An obstructed airway is frequently present as a result of blood, teeth and dentures (rarely radio-opaque) lying in the pharynx. There may be direct obstruction when a fractured maxilla has been displaced downwards and backwards on to the dorsum of the tongue, or by the tongue itself falling back when the anterior position of the mandible has been severely comminuted.

Atropine only should be given for premedication and opiate drugs avoided as there may be bleeding in the mouth and pharynx, and the stomach may contain swallowed blood. In addition, in an acute emergency the patient may have had a recent meal.

Intubation is the first important step. If the mouth can be opened sufficiently it may be simpler to pre-oxygenate and then go on to a thiopentone-suxamethonium with cricoid pressure and a rapid intubation sequence, especially as it may be difficult to induce anaesthesia by inhalation alone if a face mask cannot be properly applied. A cuffed tube is an added safety factor. If an inhalational induction is considered safer, this may be prolonged. A head-down position will allow blood to drain freely and be sucked out if necessary. If respiratory obstruction cannot be relieved, tracheostomy under local analgesia may be life-saving and induction can then take place via this route. The route of the endotracheal tube will depend on the extent and position of the injuries and the direction of the tube may have to be changed during the procedure. Once the respiratory tract is protected blood and debris can be removed from the pharynx and a large bore oesophageal tube passed to remove blood and other contents from the stomach. If cerebrospinal fluid is seen draining from the nose, a nasal tube should not be used because of the danger of infection. Any anaesthetic sequence allowing quick post-operative recovery is satisfactory for maintenance.

Post-operative management is similar to that described for other major jaw surgery and will depend on whether or not there is immobilisation of the jaws. Severe head injury and concomitant injuries to the chest may make tracheostomy essential. Intensive care facilities may be invaluable. Sedation should be avoided unless the patient actually complains of pain. Pain, in fact, is usually minimal post-operatively in these patients (Davies and Scott, 1968).

The treatment of facial injuries is rarely life-saving but the restoration of the normal contours of the facial skeleton and repair of soft tissues with minimal scarring are of the utmost importance to the patient. Correct management of such patients during the acute phase is therefore vital.

ANAESTHESIA FOR SURGERY OF THE EARS, NOSE AND THROAT

The problems of anaesthesia for surgery in this region of the body are similar to those already discussed in the sections on in-patient dental treatment and maxillo-facial surgery. Complete control of the airway is essential. Thus, an endotracheal method is usually indicated, although some procedures may be managed without a tube especially when operating time is short. Oral intubation is preferable to the nasal route when the site of operation permits. The tracheo-bronchial tract may require protection against inhalation of blood both during and after operations in the mouth and nasal cavities, and patients undergoing such procedures should recover in the semi-prone position, preferably over a pillow, so that the head and neck are at a lower level than the glottis—the "post-tonsillectomy position". Early return of reflex activity is also important in this respect.

The technique employed should provide an uncongested operating field. Both spontaneous breathing using halothane, and controlled ventilation using muscle relaxants are satisfactory and widely used. Attention to posture, the capillary vasoconstriction of controlled ventilation, and small doses of halothane can produce a satisfactory field for this type of surgery. However, inadequate ventilation, or coughing and straining with subsequent venous engorgement, will lead to excessive bleeding thus hampering the surgeons vision in what are often very confined spaces. General anaesthesia for many nasal and aural operations is often combined with the use of locally applied or injected vasoconstricting solutions.

Anaesthesia for Specific Operations

Dissection Tonsillectomy in Children

Tonsillectomy in children is still a very common procedure. The principles of speedy induction, control of the airway, protection of the trachea and bronchi from aspiration of blood are best achieved by use of an endotracheal tube. An oral tube can be accommodated via a modified Boyle Davis gag (Doughty, 1957) without obstructing the surgeon's operating field. Care should be taken that the endotracheal tube or its connections are not compressed by the blade of the gag or by the teeth. The operation is carried out with the patient supine and the shoulders raised on a sandbag or pillow, so that the head and neck lie at a lower level. Bleeding must be adequately controlled by the surgeon at all times. A nitrous oxide-oxygen-halothane sequence with spontaneous breathing is satisfactory. At the end of the operation the endotracheal tube should be removed only when the patient is in the post-tonsillar position.

The insufflation method of anaesthesia using a Boyle Davis gag without intubation is still used but cannot be recommended in view of the inherent dangers of obstruction and aspiration of blood. It is still used for guillotine tonsillectomy with ether or halothane as the principal anaesthetic agents.

Post-Tonsillectomy Bleeding

Post-operative haemorrhage after removal of tonsils and adenoids is not uncommon and is severe enough to require surgical ligation in about 1–2 per cent of cases (Gorham, 1964). It is the chief cause of death after the operation. Severe shock or even death, though rare, normally result from failure to judge the severity of blood loss. Assessment of this may be difficult. There may be continuous slow loss over many hours. Although bleeding from the tonsillar fossa can be seen by looking in the mouth, bleeding from the adenoid bed cannot be observed in this way. More blood may be in the stomach than on the pillow (Tate, 1963). Restlessness may be attributed to pain rather than blood loss and opiates wrongly given, the central depression masking the important signs and resulting in collapse. There is the additional hazard of vomiting or regurgitation, blood being aspirated into the lungs.

Such post-operative blood loss is especially dangerous in small children who may have lost a higher proportion of their blood volume at the time of operation (usually unmeasured). Wilson and associates (1973) found an average blood loss of 4·1–4·5 per cent of the blood volume of children during guillotine tonsillectomy and adenoidectomy. It is vital that haemostasis is secured under general anaesthesia as quickly as possible before the patient becomes dangerously shocked. If further surgery is necessary, the problem of the patient with a full stomach (i.e. blood) is paramount. Induction of anaesthesia is best carried out with the patient on his side and with a slight head-down position so that if regurgitation or vomiting occur, blood will not enter the larynx. Pre-operative sedation is unnecessary and should never be given. Induction of anaesthesia should be performed on a tipping table with a sucker in good working order close at hand. Any hypovolaemia should be corrected. Althesin may be used for induction but a gaseous induction using cyclopropane or halothane and oxygen may be considered safer. An endotracheal tube is passed via the mouth using either deep halothane or suxamethonium to provide relaxation. Once the airway is protected, the patient can be turned on to his back and the operation commenced using a nitrous oxide-oxygen-halothane sequence. Blood should be sucked out of the stomach using a wide bore tube. This will often produce an improvement in the patient's general condition and blood can be transfused whilst the source of bleeding is located. The recovery procedure is the same as after tonsillectomy with more careful observation of the general condition.

Aural Operations

Many aural operations are now performed under the microscope and the surgeon therefore requires an uncongested field with a quiescent patient. Endotracheal anaesthesia with the patient breathing spontaneously is satisfactory, but often better conditions for surgery can be produced with controlled ventilation. Although bleeding may be troublesome, hypotensive techniques are best reserved for cases in which the anatomy of the ear has been grossly distorted.

Saidman (1965) and Eger (1965) jointly, have shown that nitrous oxide anaesthesia influences the pressures and volumes in closed gas-filled cavities. Nitrous oxide is about thirty times more soluble than nitrogen in blood and therefore nitrous oxide molecules will collect in the air spaces more quickly than nitrogen molecules leave, causing a temporary increase in the size of the cavities. Both Thomsen (1965) and Matz et al., (1967) considered it possible that nitrous oxide inhalation, with its resultant rise in middle-ear pressure, might be responsible for tympanic perforation, otitis media, and other aural sequelae, particularly in patients with any interference of normal eustachian tube function. It is suggested, therefore, in such patients that a halothane-oxygen sequence is used avoiding nitrous oxide altogether, or that the nitrous oxide should be turned off about 10 minutes prior to final closure of the middle ear cavity.

Many aural operations are followed in the post-operative period by severe vestibular disturbances so that nausea is common with any head movement. This complication may be prevented by the use of an intramuscular phenothiazine given at the end of the operation and by giving oral prochlorperazine 25 mg b.d. for two to three days post-operatively.

Microlaryngeal Surgery

Microlaryngoscopy and microsurgery of the larynx require the combined use of a suspension laryngoscope and operating microscope. There should be total access to the mouth, the larynx should be immobile, relaxed and continuously under vision throughout. Controversy centres around whether or not an endotracheal tube should be employed. Advocates of non-intubation (Gordon and Sellars, 1971; Rajagopalan et al., 1972) make use of the venturi principle for intermittent positive-pressure breathing. Intermittent thiopentone and suxamethonium provide sleep and relaxation and oxygen is delivered to give adequate ventilation for prolonged periods. There is no interference with free access and visualisation of the larynx, but equally no airway protection from bleeding if biopsies are taken or tumours removed. The use of a small endotracheal tube provides such protection without seriously decreasing the easy access to most of the entrance of the larynx (Coplans, 1976). A 5 mm cuffed endotracheal tube which is kink-resistant is passed via the nose. Thiopentone, intermittent suxamethonium, nitrous oxide, oxygen and halothane provide excellent safe operating conditions. Other advocates of endotracheal tubes include Kleinsasser (1968) and Carden and Crutchfield, (1973) and the use of such tubes would seem to provide safer conditions for this type of surgery.

Laryngectomy

In this operation the anaesthetic sequence is largely conditioned by the surgical technique, and whether or not a tracheostomy has already been performed. If there is a tracheostomy, a suitable plastic tracheostomy tube should be inserted into which an adaptor can secure an airtight fit between tracheostomy tube and catheter mount.

In cases where there is no tracheostomy the anaesthetist is faced with problems of intubation and a change of tube at the stage during the operation when the lower end of the larynx is divided from the trachea. Pre-operative assessment of the degree of respiratory obstruction is essential. If the patient is slightly obstructed and stridor is present, respiratory depressant drugs should be omitted and atropine only given for premedication. Distortion of the normal anatomy by tumour or oedema may make intubation difficult and it may only be possible to insert a small size tube. This should be introduced with great care to avoid the risk of trauma to the neoplastic area with consequent haemorrhage. The anaesthetic method throughout the operation will depend on how easy the change over will be from the original endotracheal tube to the alternative cuffed tube system when the lower end of the larynx is divided before laryngectomy. If this can be easily accomplished it may be more satisfactory to employ muscle relaxation and intermittent positive-pressure ventilation throughout, for what is usually a poor-risk patient. If this is impractical, then spontaneous breathing using halothane may be better, the anaesthetic being deepened before the change over period to stop the patient wakening or coughing at this stage. Haemorrhage may be severe and if glands are to be excised, controlled hypotension should be considered. At the end, the second tube will have to be removed so that a permanent tracheostomy can be formed by sewing the skin to the edges of the trachea. The patient should be breathing spontaneously by this stage and adequate suction used to prevent aspiration.

Tracheostomy

Tracheostomy is performed either as an emergency procedure to relieve upper respiratory obstruction or as a planned manoeuvre to facilitate long-term ventilation. In both cases the operation is made safer and easier if an endotracheal tube is present in an anaesthetised patient. When the patient is completely obstructed and *in extremis*, intubation may prove to be impossible and the surgeon will have to perform the tracheostomy without anaesthesia as quickly as possible. Where upper respiratory obstruction is severe no premedication will be necessary and intravenous induction agents should never be used as they may add central respiratory depression to an already desperate situation. Such patients are usually sitting up in order to breathe more easily and should be brought to theatre and induced in the sitting position. An inhalational method with active respiration is the safest choice and cyclopropane and oxygen, or halothane and oxygen, are suitable combinations. A variety of tube sizes and introducers should be available.

Most planned tracheostomies for long-term ventilation have no such problems. An endotracheal tube may already be in place or easily inserted using a local anaesthetic spray, an intravenous induction agent and suxamethonium or a non-depolarising relaxant. The tube is left in the upper trachea and not withdrawn completely until the surgeon and anaesthetist are satisfied that the correct size of tracheostomy tube has been inserted and that it is firmly tied in position. Adequate suction will be necessary to remove retained secretions especially if these have accumulated in large quantities whilst the upper respiratory problem progressed.

REFERENCES

BOURNE, J. G. (1957). Fainting and cerebral damage. *Lancet*, **2**, 499.

BOURNE, J. G. (1960). *Nitrous Oxide in Dentistry: its Dangers and Alternatives*. London: Lloyd-Luke.

BOURNE, J. G. (1966). A dental anaesthetic death. *Lancet*, **1**, 879.

BOURNE, J. G. (1967). *Studies in Anaesthetics: including Intravenous Dental Anaesthesia*. pp. 56 and 103. London: Lloyd-Luke.

BOURNE, J. G. (1970). Deaths with dental anaesthetics. *Anaesthesia*, **25**, 473.

BOURNE, J. G. (1973). Deaths associated with general dental anaesthesia. *Brit. med. J.*, **1**, 293.

British Journal of Anaesthesia (1968). Editorial, **40**, 151.

British Medical Journal (1975). Leader, **2**, 408.

CADLE, D. R., BOULTON, T. B., and SPENCER SWAINE, M. (1968). Intermittent intravenous anaesthesia for out-patient dentistry. A study using propanadid. *Anaesthesia*, **23**, 65.

CARDEN, E., and CRUTCHFIELD, W. (1973). Anaesthesia for microsurgery of the larynx. *Canad. Anaesth. Soc. J.*, **20**, 378.

COPLANS, M. P. (1962). An assessment of the safety of the "sitting position" and hypoxia in dental anaesthesia. *Brit. dent. J.*, **113**, 15.

COPLANS, M. P. (1976). A cuffed nasotracheal tube for microlaryngeal surgery. *Anaesthesia*, **31**, 430.

COSSHAM, P. G., and DIXON, R. A. (1973). Subanaesthetic dosage of propanadid as a sedative for dentistry: a controlled clinical trial. *Brit. J. Anaesth.*, **45**, 369.

DANZIGER, A. M. (1962). Tracheal intubation for anaesthesia in the dental chair. *Brit. dent. J.*, **113**, 426.

DAVIES, R. M., and SCOTT, J. G. (1968). Anaesthesia for major oral and maxillo-facial surgery. *Brit. J. Anaesth.*, **40**, 202.

DIXON, R. A., DAY, C. D., ECCERSLEY, P. S., and THORNTON, J. A. (1973). Intravenous diazepam in dentistry: monitoring results from a controlled clinical trial. *Brit. J. Anaesth.*, **45**, 202.

DIXON, R. A., and THORNTON, J. A. (1973). Tests of recovery from anaesthesia and sedation: intravenous diazepam in dentistry. *Brit. J. Anaesth.*, **45**, 207.

DOUGHTY, A. G. (1957). A modification of the tongue-plate of the Boyle-Davis gag. *Lancet*, **1**, 1074.

DRUMMOND JACKSON, S. L. (1952). *Intravenous Anaesthesia in Dentistry*. London: Staples.

DRUMMOND JACKSON, S. L. (1962). A milestone in intravenous anaesthesia. *Brit. dent. J.*, **113**, 303.

DUNDEE, J. W. (1965). Comparison of side effects of methohexitone and thiopentone with propanadid. *Acta anaesth. scand.*, Suppl., **17**, 77.

EGER, E. I. (II), and SAIDMAN, L. J. (1965). Hazards of nitrous-oxide anesthesia in bowel obstruction and pneumothorax. *Anesthesiology*, **26**, 61.

ENNIS, G. E., and GILCHRIST, D. T. (1968). In: *Fractures of the Facial Skeleton*, p. 554. Eds. Rowe, N. L., and Killey, H. C. Edinburgh: E. and S. Livingstone.

GOLDMAN, V. (1968). Inhalational anaesthesia for dentistry in the chair. *Brit. J. Anaesth.*, **40**, 155.

GORDON, M., and SELLARS, S. L. (1971). Anaesthesia for microsurgery of the larynx. *Anaesthesia*, **26**, 199.

GORHAM, A. P. (1964). The role of the anaesthetist in the management of post-tonsillectomy haemorrhage in children. *Anaesthesia*, **19**, 565.

GREEN, R. A., and COPLANS, M. P. (1973). *Anaesthesia and Analgesia in Dentistry*. London: H. K. Lewis.

HANNINGTON-KIFF, J. G. (1969). Fainting and collapse in dental practice. *Dent. Practit. dent. Rec.*, **20**, 2.

HEALY, T. E. J., LAUTCH, H., HALL, N., TOMLIN, P. J., and VICKERS, M. D. (1970a). Inter-disciplinary study of diazepam sedation for outpatient dentistry. *Brit. med. J.*, **3**, 13.

HEALY, T. E. J., ROBINSON, J. S., and VICKERS, M. D. (1970b). Physiological responses to intravenous diazepam as a sedative for conservative dentistry. *Brit. med. J.*, **3**, 10.

HOWELLS, T. H. (1968). Intravenous anaesthetic agents in dental anaesthesia. *Brit. J. Anaesth.*, **40**, 182.

HUFFMAN, J. P., and ELAM, J. O. (1971). Prisms and fiberoptics for laryngoscopy. *Anesth. Analg. Curr. Res.*, **50**, 64.

JORGENSEN, N. B., and LEFFINGWELL, F. (1961). Premedication in dentistry. *Dent. Clin. N. Amer.*, July, 299.

KEELE, C. A., and NEIL, E. (1966). Sampson Wright's *Applied Physiology*, 11th edit., p. 141. London: Oxford University Press.

KLEINSASSER, O. (1968). *Mikrolaryngoskopie und Endolaryngeale Mikrochirurgie*, p. 12, Stuttgart: F. K. Schattauer.

KLOCK, J. H. (1955). New concepts of nitrous-oxide anesthetic. *Anesth. Analg. Curr. Res.*, **34**, 379.

LATHAM, J., and PARBROOK, G. D. (1966). The use of premixed nitrous-oxide and oxygen in dental anaesthesia. *Anaesthesia*, **21**, 472.

LOVE, S. H. S. (1963). The dangers of inhalation of debris during anaesthesia. *Brit. dent. J.*, **115**, 503.

MANN, P. E., HATT, S. D., DIXON, R. A., GRIFFIN, K. D., PERKS, E. R., and THORNTON, J. A. (1971). A minimal increment methohexitone technique in conservative dentistry. *Anaesthesia*, **26**, 3.

MATZ, G. J., RATTENBORG, C. G., and HOLADAY, D. A. (1967). Effects of nitrous oxide on middle ear pressure. *Anesthesiology*, **28**, 948.

MINISTRY OF HEALTH (1967). *Dental Anaesthesia.* (Report of a joint sub-committee of the Standing Medical and Dental Advisory Committee). London: H.M.S.O.

MONHEIM, L. M. (1957). *Local Anesthesia and Pain Control in Dental Practice.* St. Louis: C. V. Mosby.

MOORE, J. R. (1968). The surgeon's requirements for intra-oral surgery. *Brit. J. Anaesth.,* **40,** 152.

MOORE, P. (1973). In *Anaesthesia and Analgesia in Dentistry.* Eds. Green, R. A. and Coplans, M. P., London: H. K. Lewis.

MORRISON, E. M. (1873). *Brit. J. dent. Sci.,* **16,** 566.

MUIR, V. M. J., LEONARD, M., and HADDAWAY, E. (1976). Morbidity following dental extraction. *Anaesthesia,* **31,** 171.

PLOWMAN, P. E., THOMAS, W. J. W., and THURLOW, A. C. (1974). Cardiac dysrhythmias during anaesthesia for oral surgery: the effect of local blockades. *Anaesthesia,* **29,** 571.

RAJAGOPLAN, R., SMITH, F., and RAMACHANDRAN, P. R. (1972). Anaesthesia for microlaryngoscopy and definitive surgery. *Canad. Anaesth. Soc. J.,* **19,** 83.

ROLLASON, W. N., FIDLER, K., and HOUGH, J. M. (1974). Althesin in outpatient dental anaesthesia. *Brit. J. Anaesth.,* **46,** 881.

SAIDMAN, L. J., and EGER, E. I. (II) (1965). Change in cerebrospinal fluid pressure during pneumoencephalography under nitrous-oxide anesthesia. *Anesthesiology,* **26,** 67.

SCOTT, G. W. (1952). Inhalation and chest infection following dental extraction. *Guy's Hosp. Rep.,* **101,** 77.

SMITH, B. L., and YOUNG, P. N. (1976). Day stay anaesthesia. A follow-up of day patients undergoing dental operations under general anaesthesia with endotracheal anaesthesia. *Anaesthesia,* **31,** 181.

TATE, N. (1963). Deaths from tonsillectomy. *Lancet,* **2,** 1090.

THOMPSON, P. W. (1964). Dental anaesthesia. *Ann. roy. Coll. Surg. Engl.,* **35,** 362.

THOMSEN, K. A. (1965). Middle ear pressure during anaesthesia. *Arch. Otolaryng.,* **82,** 609.

TOM, A. (1956). An innovation in technique for dental gas. *Brit. med. J.,* **1,** 1085.

TOMLIN, P. J. (1974). Death in out-patient dental anaesthetic practice. *Anaesthesia,* **29,** 551.

VERRILL, P. J., and AELLIG, W. H. (1970). Vasovagal faint in the supine position. *Brit. med. J.,* **4,** 348.

WARREN, J. B. (1972). Althesin in the dental chair. *Postgrad. med. J.,* **48,** Suppl. 2, 130.

WEISSLER, A. M., WARREN, J. V., and DURHAM, N. C. (1959). Review: Vasodepressor syncope. *Amer. Heart. J.,* **57,** 786.

WILSON, S. M., OWEN, M., DUFF, T. B., and MALCOLM-SMITH, N. A. (1973). Operative blood loss in guillotine tonsillectomy and adenoidectomy in children: a comparison of 3 premedicant drugs. *Brit. J. Anaesth.,* **45,** 86.

WISE, C. C., ROBINSON, J. S., HEATH, M. J., and TOMLIN, P. J. (1969). Physiological response to intermittent methohexitone for conservative dentistry. *Brit. med. J.,* **2,** 540.

YOUNG, D. S., and WHITWAM, J. G. (1964). Observation on dental anaesthesia introduced with methohexitone. II: maintenance and recovery. *Brit. J. Anaesth.,* **36,** 94.

YOUNG, J. V. I. (1975). General anaesthesia for ambulant dental patients. *Brit. J. hosp. Med.,* **13,** 441.

Chapter 10

ARTIFICIAL RESPIRATION

DURING normal spontaneous respiration air is drawn into the lungs by expansion of the thoracic cavity and expelled during passive relaxation of the respiratory muscles, aided by the elasticity of the lungs themselves. Adequate gaseous exchange is thereby maintained. Failure of any of the structures involved in this process may lead to inadequate gaseous exchange which must then be maintained artificially until the failure has been corrected. Many methods of maintaining ventilation artificially have been described and Whittenberger (1955) has classified them under five headings:

1. Manual manipulation of the thoracic cage.
2. Gas pressure applied to the upper respiratory tract.
3. Pressure changes applied to the trunk but not the head.
4. Displacement of sub-diaphragmatic structures.
5. Electrical stimulation of the respiratory muscles.

HISTORY

Chapter Four of the Second Book of Kings in the Old Testament contains a remarkable account of the resuscitation of an apparently dead Shunammite child by the Prophet Elisha. Verses 34 and 35 read:

"And he went up, and lay upon the child, and put his mouth upon his mouth, and his eyes upon his eyes, and his hands upon his hands: and he stretched himself upon the child; and the flesh of the child waxed warm . . . and the child sneezed seven times, and the child opened his eyes".

We are not told where Elisha learnt the technique, but this possibly represents the first recorded account of resuscitation which may have been by artificial respiration.

The idea that drowned or collapsed people might be restored to life by artificial respiration recurs sporadically throughout recorded history, and has been entertainingly reviewed by Shackleton (1962). The first attempt to consider the problem constructively was made in Amsterdam in 1769, when the "Society for the Recovery of Drowned Persons" was formed. Interest in the subject rapidly increased and in 1796 Herholdt and Rafn published a monograph which has been translated into English by Poulsen (1960). The use of bellows for resuscitation was advocated by John Hunter, who invented a two-way bellows for the purpose (Hunter, 1776). The Royal Humane Society continued to recommend this method until 1837, when it was abandoned in favour of artificial ventilation by manual compression of the thoracic cage. This method persisted until Safar *et al.* (1958) showed that intermittent positive-pressure inflation of the lungs produced more efficient ventilation than manual compression.

The possibility that artificial inflation of the lungs by positive pressure might be applicable to respiratory failure during anaesthesia was missed by Hewitt (1901) who advocated the use of Sylvester's method and it was not until Gale and Waters (1932) suggested that pulmonary collapse during thoracic operations might be prevented by positive-pressure ventilation achieved by intermittent inflation of the reservoir bag, that the method was used in anaesthesia. Since the introduction of muscle relaxants it has become a standard technique. This method was first used to treat patients with long-term respiratory failure during the great epidemic of poliomyelitis in Copenhagen in 1952. Lassen (1953) working with Ibsen, used a Waters' canister and reservoir bag to give intermittent positive-pressure ventilation. This was continued for periods of up to three months by relays of·medical students who were paid 30 shillings (Krone) per 8-hour shift to squeeze the bag. He described the method as "bag ventilation" and it was applied via an endotracheal tube, or cuffed tracheostomy tube. During the subsequent years the method was extensively developed and medical students replaced by mechanical ventilators.

Artificial ventilation by intermittent positive pressure (IPPR) applied mechanically via a cuffed tracheostomy tube or endotracheal tube has now become the standard method of acute treatment for respiratory failure from many causes, some of which are outlined below. Manual manipulation of the thoracic cage was used mainly for emergency resuscitation by the methods of Holger Nielsen, Silvester and Schafer. These techniques are now obsolete. Pressure changes applied to the trunk but not the head, and displacement of subdiaphragmatic structures are still useful methods of assisting the ventilation of certain patients with permanent weakness of the muscles of respiration (see below); electrical stimulation of the respiratory muscles has rarely been found to be a useful practical procedure and has been abandoned.

FIRST AID METHODS

Resuscitation of partly drowned or asphyxiated subjects is often necessary when apparatus and equipment are not to hand. External cardiac massage by chest compression combined with simple methods of artificial ventilation has very greatly increased the chances of success in emergency resuscitation. Safar et al. (1958) and Poulsen et al. (1959) showed convincingly that expired air or mouth-to-mouth respiration is more effective in maintaining normal, or even increased, volumes of ventilation than manual compression of the chest. Subsequent work has confirmed these findings and the following methods are now widely accepted, taught and practised. The World Federation of Societies of Anaesthesiologists (Poulsen, 1968) produced an excellent manual on which teaching should be based.

Mouth-to-Mouth Resuscitation

The rescuer approaches the subject's head from the side and supports the upper airway by inserting his thumb between the teeth, grasping the mandible and pulling it forcefully upwards. The rescuer's mouth is placed on the subject's mouth and the subject's lungs are inflated by forcible expiration which the rescuer repeats 10–15 times per minute. An alternative technique in which the rescuer inflates via the subject's nose has been described. A possible advantage of this route is that there is less likelihood of inflating the stomach and therefore of regurgitation.

In addition to the observation that ventilation is more efficient by these methods, other advantages over manual compression methods are claimed:

1. If the airway becomes obstructed, the rescuer senses resistance.
2. If secretions or vomit accumulate, he feels and hears gurgling.
3. Expansion of the chest during inflation can be watched.
4. The return of spontaneous respiration can be felt.
5. Both the rescuer's hands are available for airway toilet and jaw support.
6. Positive pressure during inflation may make ventilation possible in patients with a high airway resistance caused by foreign material in the lungs.
7. It is suitable for neonates and children.

The disadvantages of mouth-to-mouth resuscitation are:

1. If the airway is not perfectly clear, or if the airway resistance is high, air may pass into the subject's stomach, thus increasing the likelihood of regurgitation or vomiting.
2. With the patient in the supine position, fluid or vomitus may enter the lungs before its presence is appreciated.
3. It is usually aesthetically unpleasant and in some circumstances may be sufficiently unacceptable to cause serious delay in starting resuscitation.
4. It cannot usually be maintained for more than 15 minutes without producing fairly severe dizziness in the rescuer.
5. It cannot be used on subjects who have inhaled noxious vapours.

It is now generally recognised that mouth-to-mouth or mouth-to-nose resuscitation is the most satisfactory method available for emergency use. Anaesthetists, therefore, have an important role to play in educating the lay public in these techniques, which should always be taught for preference.

ARTIFICIAL RESPIRATION USING SIMPLE APPARATUS

While it may be essential to perform artificial respiration at the scene of an accident with no apparatus at all, the use of simple apparatus can greatly increase the convenience and efficiency of the procedure and therefore the chances of a successful outcome. Apparatus of the type described below should be available in all hospital wards and departments, and as far as possible in ambulances, first aid posts, and general practitioners' bags.

The Brook Airway (Fig. 1a)

A wide variety of airways and connections have been developed in attempts to make mouth-to-mouth respiration less unpleasant to perform, and to make it easier for untrained operators to maintain a clear airway. Of these devices, the Brook airway has particular advantages and has maintained its place since it was first described by Brook et al., in 1962. It consists of an intra-oral section shaped like a pharyngeal airway. This is connected to a flange designed to maintain an airtight fit on the patient's lips. A tube projects from the airway section and flange. It contains a simple one-way valve, allowing expired air from the patient to pass out through a short side-arm rather than through the operator's mouthpiece. The apparatus is constructed of transparent plastic so that the presence of vomit can be easily seen. In use the operator stands above the patient's head and inserts the airway section into the patient's mouth until the flange fits closely over the lips (Fig. 1b). One hand is used to support the patient's jaw and the other to close the nostrils. The operator is then conveniently placed to watch the movements of the chest as he inflates the lungs by blowing down the tube section of the device rhythmically 10–15 times a minute.

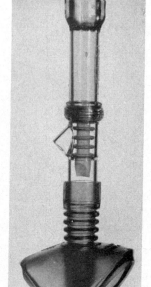

BLOW TUBE

NON-RETURN VALVE

FLEXIBLE NECK

MOUTH GUARD

ORAL AIRWAY

10/Fig. 1(a).—The Brook Airway.

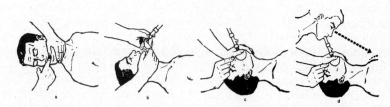

10/Fig. 1(b).—Mouth-to-mouth resuscitation using the Brook airway. (a) Place victim on back. Quickly clear mouth and throat of foreign matter with fingers. Tilt head fully back. (b) Insert airway over tongue until mouth-guard covers lips. (c) Raise the chin, and maintain this position with the same hand that holds the airway in place. Pinch nostrils closed to prevent air leakage. (d) Take a deep breath and blow into airway. Watch for chest rise. Between breaths listen for sound of air returning from the victim. Repeat every 3–4 seconds.

The Ambu Resuscitator (Fig. 2)

Ruben and Ruben (1957) have described a self-expanding bag attached to a Ruben non-rebreathing valve which enables intermittent positive-pressure respiration to be carried out with atmospheric air, which can be enriched with oxygen as required. The apparatus can be connected to an endotracheal or tracheostomy tube, or applied to the patient via an anaesthetic face-mask. When the bag is squeezed, a one-way valve at the distal end closes and air is forced into the patient via the Ruben non-rebreathing valve. During expiration, expired air passes out through the expiratory part of the non-rebreathing valve, and fresh atmospheric air is drawn into the self-expanding bag through the one-way valve at the distal end. Self-expansion of the bag is achieved by lining it with sponge rubber. The apparatus has two disadvantages:

1. It is sometimes difficult for untrained people to obtain an airtight fit of the mask on the patient's face, and the mask may conceal the presence of vomit.

2. If the resistance to inflation is high (50 cm H_2O; 4·9 kPa), air in the bag is compressed into the sponge rubber rather than forced into the lungs. This effect can be partly overcome by compressing the bag against the side of the patient's face.

Modifications of this apparatus are now available in which self-inflation of the bag is achieved without the need for sponge rubber.

The Ruben non-breathing valve. (Fig. 3). (Ruben, 1955).—This valve has a dead space of 9 ml and a resistance of 0·8 cm H_2O (0·08 kPa)

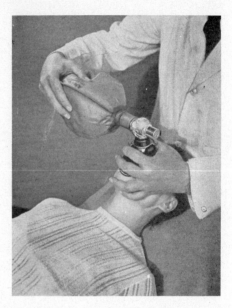

10/FIG. 2.—The Ambu resuscitator.

during inspiration and of 1 cm H_2O (0·1 kPa) during expiration at flow rates of 25 litres per minute. The expiratory resistance can be reduced to very low levels by removing the disc in the outlet channel when the valve is used for positive-pressure respiration. In this form the valve is not suitable for spontaneous respiration during anaesthesia because the patient will inspire air through the expiratory port.

The Ambu Hesse valve (Fig. 3).—This valve has advantages over the Ruben valve. It has a lower dead space and flow resistance. At 25 litres per minute the resistance during inspiration is 0·4 cm H_2O (0·04 kPa) and during expiration 0·6 cm H_2O (0·06 kPa). Excessive positive pressure will overcome the expiratory valve and allow excess gases to escape. In contrast to the Ruben valve it is quiet in operation and can be sterilised by autoclaving. A version of this valve which will permit spontaneous respiration is available.

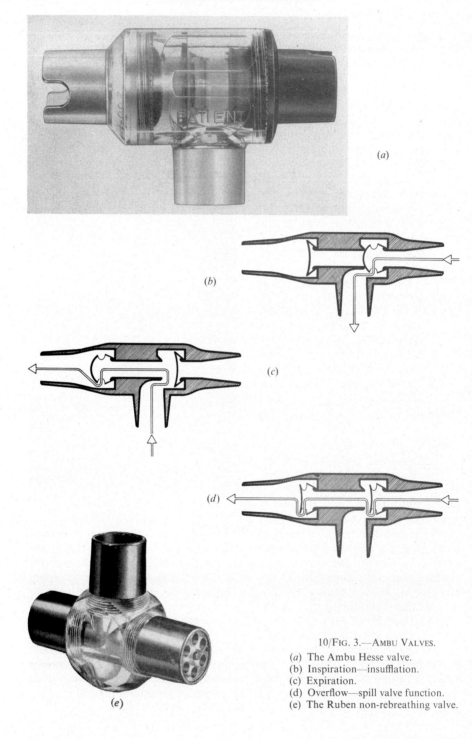

10/Fig. 3.—Ambu Valves.

(a) The Ambu Hesse valve.
(b) Inspiration—insufflation.
(c) Expiration.
(d) Overflow—spill valve function.
(e) The Ruben non-rebreathing valve.

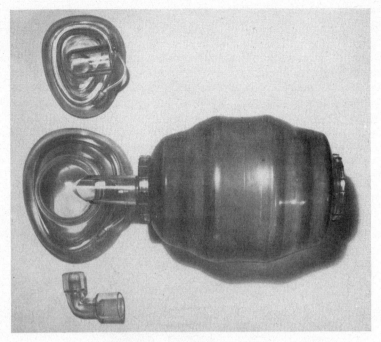

10/Fɪɢ. 4(*a*).—The Resusci Folding Bag.

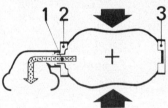

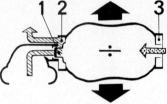

10/Fɪɢ. 4(*b*)—Inflation. The one-way lip valve (1) opens when the bag is compressed. The silicone flange (2) seals the perforations in the outer valve housing so that all the air from the bag is delivered to the patient. The intake valve (3) is closed by the positive pressure in the bag.

10/Fɪɢ. 4(*c*).—Expiration. The patient's exhaled air in closing the lip valve (1) presses the flange of the valve away from its perforated outer housing. This allows the exhaled air to escape into the atmosphere. The intake valve (3) is opened by the negative pressure in the bag.

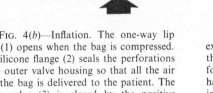

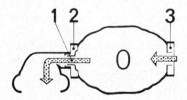

10/Fɪɢ. 4(*d*).—Spontaneous inspiration. Inhalation opens both the lip valve (1) and intake valve (3).

The Resusci Folding Bag (Mark I). (Figs. 4a–d)

This is a simplified version of the Ambu resuscitator which eliminates some of its disadvantages. The transparent, self-inflating, folding bag has a simple one-way valve at each end. These valves allow the recovering patient to make spontaneous inspiratory efforts as resuscitation proceeds. A supplementary oxygen point is incorporated into the distal valve, and the proximal valve has exhaust ports around its outer edge which prevent expired air from re-entering the bag (see Fig. 4a). The face-mask is transparent, allowing vomit to be seen at once, and mask and bag can be folded into a small box for storage and portability. A more sophisticated version of the Resusci Folding Bag, the Mark II, is also available. It is more suitable for hospital and anaesthetic use.

The Oxford Inflating Bellows (Fig. 5)

Macintosh (1953) designed a small hand-unit consisting of bellows with a pair of unidirectional valves for inflating the lungs. The concertina reservoir

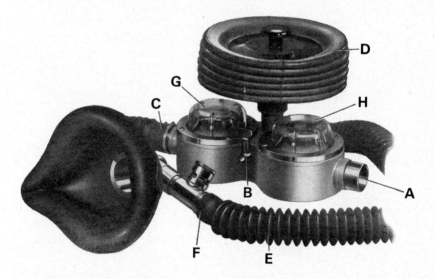

10/Fig. 5.—The Oxford inflating bellows.

A. Air inlet; B. Inlet tube and tap for oxygen; C. Air outlet to patient; D. Concertina reservoir bag; E. Corrugated tubing; F. Spring valve; G. and H. Gravity-operated unidirectional flow valves.

bag contains a spiral spring so that it automatically refills after each forced inspiration, while the valves prevent rebreathing. The unit can be used in anaesthesia in conjunction with an air draw-over inhaler such as the E.M.O. (see Chapter 6), with the patient breathing spontaneously. When used for positive-pressure ventilation for more than short periods it is necessary to include a non-rebreathing valve adjacent to the patient. These bellows formed the basis of the early version of the Radcliffe ventilator (Russell and Schuster, 1953). A weight was dropped on the bellows during inspiration, and lifted by an electric motor operating through a bicycle three-speed gear during expiration.

Mechanical Devices

In recent years a number of mechanical devices have been developed to assist ambulance and other paramedical personnel in maintaining artificial ventilation while patients are transported to hospital. They are usually pneumatically driven from an oxygen cylinder and are applied to the patient via a face-mask. This development is undesirable and should be condemned. Performing effective artificial respiration in an emergency requires the continuous attention of the rescuer. To apply and adjust a machine can only distract this attention and may delay the recognition of airway obstruction or the presence of vomit. If the airway is not perfectly clear these machines are liable to inflate the stomach and thus provoke vomiting.

ARTIFICIAL RESPIRATION WITH MECHANICAL VENTILATORS

There is no doubt that a mechanical apparatus properly used is the most efficient means of ventilating the lungs for long periods. Artificial respiration, by any known method, involves a disturbance to normal respiratory physiology. By altering intrathoracic pressure relations it also causes changes in circulatory physiology. Over short periods these changes may be insignificant, but their significance increases as their duration increases. Mechanical ventilators should be designed to cause the minimum possible upset to normal physiology, and the aim of medical and nursing care must be to correct or compensate for whatever disturbance is unavoidable.

Pressure to the Outside of the Body

Tank ventilators (Cabinet respirators, "Iron Lungs").—The first power-driven tank ventilator was invented by Professor P. Drinker, an engineer of Harvard University, and although modern tank ventilators have been modified in attempts to make them more convenient to use, and a positive phase added to the negative phase, the principles of operation remain the same. The patient is placed in a rigid tank from which only his head protrudes. Access to his body is

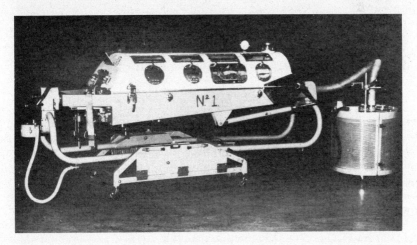

10/Fig. 6.—The Kelleher rotating tank ventilator (Kelleher, 1961).

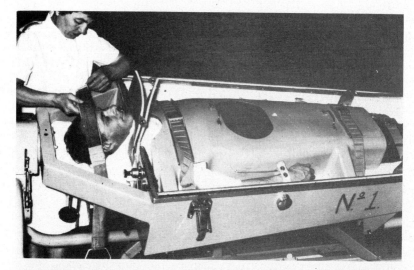

(a)

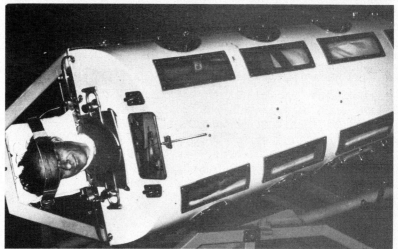

(b)

10/Fig. 7 (*see opposite*).

obtained either by placing him on a couch which can be slid out of the tank, or by using a tank whose upper half will hinge open like an alligator's jaws. An air-tight fit is obtained round the patient's neck using a flexible collar split into two sections. It must be carefully padded to prevent pressure sores developing and a tracheostomy is best avoided if a tank ventilator is to be used. Minor nursing attention can be carried out through ports in the side of the tank. The tank is connected to large mechanically operated bellows.

During inspiration the bellows expand, creating a subatmospheric pressure of 15–30 cm H_2O (1·5–2·9 kPa) within the tank. Air is drawn into the patient's lungs until the elastic resistance of the lungs and chest wall equals the pressure

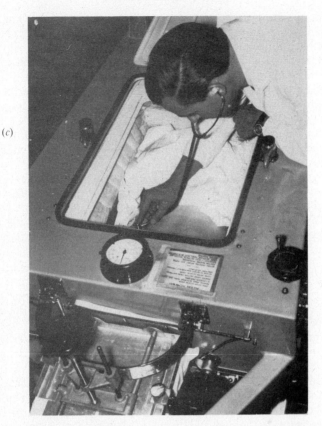

(c)

10/FIG. 7.—THE KELLEHER ROTATING TANK VENTILATOR IN USE.

(a) To rotate the patient into the prone position a shell, shaped to the body, is strapped into position inside the tank.

(b) The tank is rotated around its long axis with a forehead strap holding the patient's head.

(c) A section of mattress is removable allowing ausculation and physiotherapy to the posterior thorax.

difference between the inside and outside of the tank. Inspiration must be maintained for long enough to allow equilibration to occur. This usually takes 1–2 seconds, but if the airway resistance is high due to bronchial narrowing, accumulation of secretions, or partial obstruction of the upper airway as may occur during sleep, equilibration takes longer and may not be obtained. Ventilation may therefore be seriously reduced. During expiration the bellows contract, pressure in the tank rises to atmospheric, and air flows out of the lungs passively due to their elastic recoil. Expiration may be assisted by applying a positive pressure to the inside of the tank.

With the advent of intermittent positive pressure to the upper airway, the use of tank ventilators has declined. Their disadvantages are that they are cumbersome and difficult to use. Pulmonary atelectasis and accumulation of secretions can be difficult to prevent, although this problem can be largely overcome by using the Kelleher rotating ventilator (Kelleher, 1961) (Fig. 6). The tank section of this machine can be rotated through a complete circle on its long axis. A section of mattress can then be removed and the posterior aspect of the thorax is accessible for auscultation and physiotherapy (Figs. 7*a*–*c*).

The collar of a tank ventilator makes a tracheostomy difficult to manage. Thus, if the muscles of the pharynx and larnyx are paralysed, or if the patient is unconscious, vomiting and regurgitation become a desperate hazard. The supine patient is powerless to prevent pharyngeal contents being drawn into the lungs by the inspiratory stroke of the bellows. Even for the conscious patient with a normal pharynx, vomiting in a tank ventilator is hazardous. Should it occur, an access port should be opened immediately to equalise pressures and prevent aspiration.

Despite these disadvantages, there is no doubt that tank ventilators still retain a place in clinical practice (Kelleher, 1969; Spencer, 1969; Beaver, 1969). They are primarily used in the long-term management of patients with severe weakness of the respiratory muscles, but whose laryngeal and pharyngeal muscles are intact (see below under Poliomyelitis). Many such patients can breathe adequately while conscious, using techniques such as glossopharyngeal breathing (Ardran *et al.*, 1959), but require assistance during sleep. Tank ventilators may also be of value to these patients in tiding them over an acute respiratory infection. Their great advantage is that tracheostomy is avoided, normal use of the voice and the ability to perform glossopharyngeal breathing are retained, and subsequent machinery dependence is not increased.

Tank ventilators are also occasionally necessary for patients in whom tracheostomy and tracheal catheter suction are impossible, for example in haemophiliacs.

Cuirass ventilators.—The cuirass ventilator consists of a rigid shell held over the thorax and abdomen. It makes contact with the skin only at its edges with a padded rubber rim, which must fit sufficiently well to form an airtight seal. A bellows is connected to the shell and produces a subatmospheric pressure during inspiration. Unfortunately, the presence of the shell along the lateral side of the thoracic cage tends to splint the ribs laterally, preventing the "bucket-handle" movement. Inspiration is therefore limited to movements achieved by the "pump-handle" movement.

A modification of the cuirass which overcomes this difficulty to some extent is the Tunnicliffe breathing jacket. It incorporates a similar rigid shell, which is somewhat smaller in size than that of the cuirass. An airtight fit is achieved by enclosing the whole of the upper half of the body, except the head, in a soft jacket, with elastic tapes round the elbows, neck and waist. The Tunnicliffe jacket will produce greater ventilation for a given subatmospheric pressure than the cuirass (Spalding and Opie, 1958), but neither is as efficient as the tank and they can only be used as respiratory assistors in partly paralysed patients.

Belt ventilators.—The Bragg Paul Pneumobelt is the most widely used type and consists of an inflatable belt applied to the patient's abdomen. Inflation causes the diaphragm to rise, thus assisting expiration. Inspiration occurs by gravity, if the patient is sitting, or by what muscle power is available if the patient is lying. A belt ventilator is unobtrusive and portable, but somewhat limited in the amount of respiratory assistance which it can produce. Assisting expiration is physiologically unsound, in that it reduces functional residual capacity and increases ventilation perfusion inequalities in the lung. Despite this disadvantage, pneumobelts are still useful in a minority of patients (see Poliomyelitis, p. 416).

DISPLACEMENT OF SUBDIAPHRAGMATIC STRUCTURES

Schuster and Fischer-Williams (1953) described a motor-driven rocking bed which will produce an arc of swing of a little more than 40°; Bryce-Smith and Davis (1954) using a similar bed on a paralysed apnoeic patient in the supine position, were unable to obtain a tidal volume above 282 ml. Despite its inefficiency, some patients prefer this method of respiratory assistance to any other, because it leaves them unencumbered. Rocking beds are primarily suitable for patients with diaphragmatic paralysis. They are sometimes useful in weaning from IPPR a patient whose diaphragm has been paralysed.

PRESSURE APPLIED TO THE UPPER RESPIRATORY TRACT—INTERMITTENT POSITIVE-PRESSURE RESPIRATION (IPPR)

This is now much the most widely used form of artificial ventilation. Its short term use by manual squeezing of the reservoir bag has been practised in anaesthesia for at least forty years, and many ventilators have been designed for use during anaesthesia. Although this relieves the anaesthetist of his duties in bag squeezing, the value of mechanical ventilators during anaesthesia remains debatable. Intermittent positive-pressure respiration has become a vast subject in its own right, and as always in such instances has generated its own jargon, not all of which is either intelligible to the outsider or a credit to the English language. The peripatetic correspondent of *The Lancet* recently quoted from a published paper: "The patient was trached and respiratored machinewise".

The principle of IPPR is that the patient's upper airway is connected by tubing to a machine containing bellows. During inspiration the bellows contract —either mechanically or by gas pressure from without—and air is forced into the patient's lungs. Expiration is either passive, due to the elastic recoil of the patient's lungs and chest wall, or is assisted by applying a subatmospheric phase to the upper airway. Although the latter may be of benefit to the circulation of certain patients by reducing the intrathoracic pressure and aiding venous return, it carries a respiratory cost in that physiological dead space is increased and a larger inspiratory volume must be used.

The advantages of IPPR are that the patient is free of apparatus—apart from the connecting tubes—and can be easily nursed and cared for. Fully adequate ventilation can be produced for patients with all but the most severe forms of lung disease. Even here the limiting factor is usually circulatory embarrassment from high intrathoracic pressure, rather than an inability to achieve full ventilation (Bradley *et al.*, 1964). Although the presence of an endotracheal or tracheostomy tube is a disadvantage in some respects, it allows adequate removal of secretions by catheter suction to be carried out more efficiently than is possible with any other form of artificial respiration. There is no reason why, if treatment is properly carried out, the lungs should not remain clear and fully expanded throughout.

The disadvantages of IPPR all lie in the means by which the patient is connected to the ventilator. For long-term IPPR a tracheostomy is essential and a cuffed tracheostomy tube must be used. The patient is thus exposed to all the potential dangers and complications of tracheostomy, and in most cases is unable to use his voice. For shorter periods of IPPR, such as during and after anaesthesia, an endotracheal tube may suffice, but this cannot be left in place for longer than a few days, or damage to the larynx may result. An endotracheal tube is poorly tolerated by many conscious patients and secretions may only be removed through it with difficulty. In certain circumstances it may be possible to administer IPPR through a mouthpiece or anaesthetic face-mask, but this technique is only suitable for short-term or intermittent use. The presence of a face-mask is often as distressing for the patient as that of a tracheostomy or endotracheal tube, while gastric inflation may occur if a high inspiratory pressure is needed, and inhalation of pharyngeal contents is likely if the laryngeal and pharyngeal reflexes are absent. Where the reflexes are present, the efficiency of ventilation may be impaired by the patient's inability to co-operate.

Triggered Ventilators (Assistors)

Many ventilators now available incorporate a device which allows the patient's respiration to be assisted rather than fully controlled. The inspiratory effort of the patient produces a slight subatmospheric pressure in the connecting tubing which—provided that the tubing is of small volume and non-expansile—can be made to trigger off the inspiratory phase of the ventilator and thereby augment the patient's respiratory efforts. To be effective, the pressure and flow rate from the ventilator must rise rapidly following the start of inspiration. In the absence of this pressure pattern the ventilator may follow the patient too slowly and resist the patient rather than assist him. Furthermore, there is evidence showing that a rapid pressure and flow rise at the start of inspiration is not the most efficient pressure pattern, particularly for a patient with chronic lung disease, yet it is for acute exacerbations of chronic lung disease that assisted respiration is most advocated. Many studies have been made of its use in this condition, and those which include arterial gas tension estimations indicate that the ventilatory benefit may be marginal.

Despite this lack of ventilatory gain there is no doubt that patient-triggered respiratory assistors often appear to be of great benefit to many patients. The benefit is greatest in conditions such as status asthmaticus, where the work of breathing is greatly increased. The early use of a triggered ventilator may stave off exhaustion and further deterioration, thus avoiding more radical therapeutic methods. Further, patients with heart or lung disease usually have a strictly limited total oxygen uptake. A reduction in respiratory work by the use of an assistor may thus have a double benefit in allowing oxygen, which would otherwise be consumed in breathing, to be available to other tissues.

Patient-triggering of the ventilator is also used in anaesthesia, where it may provide a useful guide to the degree of curarisation. However, when a patient continues to make respiratory efforts during an anaesthetic which may well have included the use of respiratory depressant drugs, as well as muscle relaxants, it suggests that carbon dioxide retention is present. Assisted positive-pressure respiration is valuable during the phase of weaning a patient suffering from respiratory paralysis from artificial ventilation. It often enables the patient to regain the use of his respiratory muscles more quickly than is possible by the alternative method of intermittent short bouts of spontaneous respiration.

An important requirement of a triggered—or patient-cycled—ventilator is that, should the patient cease to make respiratory efforts, the machine will continue to ventilate him, though usually at a slower rate than his spontaneous one. Some of the early patient-cycled ventilators did not include this feature and stopped altogether if the patient ceased to make spontaneous efforts.

PHYSIOLOGY OF ARTIFICIAL RESPIRATION

Before the 1952 Copenhagen Poliomyelitis epidemic (Lassen, 1953), IPPR was used almost exclusively for maintenance of respiration during open chest surgery. It was thought that the high mean intrathoracic pressure which is inevitable when IPPR is applied with an intact chest wall would severely reduce venous return and therefore cardiac output. Lassen (1954) and Ibsen (1954) were obliged to try IPPR for the prolonged treatment of severe poliomyelitis because they had insufficient tank respirators to deal with the epidemic. Their results showed an immediate reduction from around 80 per cent to around 40 per cent in the mortality of patients suffering from acute bulbar poliomyelitis. This improvement was mainly due to improved secretion control resulting from tracheostomy but it also established conclusively that IPPR *per se* did not seriously depress cardiac output.

During subsequent years the physiological consequences of IPPR were intensively studied, notably by Price *et al.* (1954), and Watson (1961). Most of these studies, however, were made on subjects whose lungs were essentially normal and who were receiving IPPR for poliomyelitis or general anaesthesia with muscle relaxants. The success of IPPR as a therapeutic technique lead inevitably to its use for patients with respiratory failure, due to abnormal lungs (Bradley *et al.*, 1964). The pathophysiology of IPPR in obstructive airways disease is a special problem which will be considered later (p. 387).

In recent years it has come to be recognised that acute respiratory failure commonly occurs in patients who are critically ill from a wide variety of non-pulmonary causes. Various supposedly clinical entities have been postulated including "wet" lung, "post-perfusion" lung, "shock" lung, "oxygen toxicity" lung and "respiratory" lung. The subject has been well reviewed by Pontoppidan *et al.* (1972 *a*, *b* and *c*). Although this clinical picture may embrace several separate entities, for example, pulmonary oxygen damage, the pathophysiology in most cases is remarkably similar and probably represents a common end-result. The lungs show an abnormal pattern of gas distribution with closure of alveoli and airways and an increase in pulmonary extravascular water. These two conditions cause:

   (i) a reduction in functional residual capacity which may come to lie below the critical closing volume.

   (ii) A decrease in total pulmonary compliance.

   (iii) Maldistribution of ventilation and perfusion within the lung.

Pontoppidan calls this condition simple "Acute respiratory failure". This term, although perfectly correct, is misleading because it fails to distinguish it from other equally acute states of respiratory failure which have not progressed sufficiently to show these characteristic features. As it certainly represents a common end-point of many conditions, it will be referred to as terminal respiratory failure throughout this chapter. It must be recognised, however, that if skilfully applied, IPPR is now so efficient that this terminal condition is sometimes reversible provided the underlying cause or causes are themselves remediable. The value of IPPR is simply to buy time in which to treat these underlying causes. If they are irremediable the sooner IPPR is discontinued, the quicker can the patient be allowed to die with some semblance of dignity.

The techniques of IPPR which are necessary to treat this condition are often the reverse of those used to treat respiratory failure due to neuromuscular paralysis or obstructive airways disease. This must be borne in mind in reading the brief summary of the physiology of IPPR which follows.

Intrathoracic Pressure

During normal inspiration air is drawn into the lungs by expansion of the thoracic cage, which creates a subatmospheric pressure within the thorax. The subatmospheric pressure is made greater by the elastic properties of the lungs, and is transmitted to the right atrium, which is a lax-walled structure. This has the effect of assisting venous return. All forms of artificial respiration impede venous return to some extent by raising intrathoracic pressure relative to the atmosphere; the only exception being electrophrenic respiration.

It is sometimes stated that tank ventilators are more physiological than positive-pressure ventilators because the patient's lungs are expanded by producing a subatmospheric pressure within the tank. This argument is fallacious, because the subatmospheric pressure is applied everywhere, except the head. The intrathoracic pressure is higher than the pressure in the tank, due to the elastic recoil of the lungs and chest wall. The pressure gradient between the right atrium and peripheral veins therefore remains reversed, despite the subatmospheric pressure within the tank. It is clear that the same argument applies, though rather less forcibly, to the cuirass ventilator and Tunnicliffe breathing jacket, where subatmospheric pressure is applied to the chest and abdomen during inspiration.

During IPPR, the intrathoracic pressure is raised considerably, while the surface of the patient's body remains at atmospheric pressure. A marked pressure gradient therefore exists which tends to impede venous return. Attempts have been made to overcome this disadvantage by designing ventilators which apply a subatmospheric pressure to the lungs during expiration. This is known as negative phase. Opie et al. (1961) have shown that if a negative phase is applied throughout expiration it is possible to maintain mean intrathoracic pressure almost within normal limits. The use of a negative phase unfortunately reduces the efficiency of ventilation (see below, Physiological dead space). Opie also showed that the greatest rise in mean intrathoracic pressure occurs with ventilators which have a long inspiratory phase and slow rate of flow rise during inspiration.

Elastic Resistance during IPPR

In a paralysed unanaesthetised patient receiving IPPR the elastic resistance of the lungs is about three times normal (Smith and Spalding, 1959). In an anaesthetised patient Howell and Peckett (1957) found that the elastic resistance of the lungs was greater during paralysis than during spontaneous respiration, a finding which is in general agreement with those of Foster *et al.* (1957). Changes in elastic resistance occur within a few minutes of the start of IPPR (Watson, 1962*c*), suggesting that they are due to alterations in the distribution of air in the lungs, rather than to bronchial blockage by secretions. This is supported by the fact that during IPPR the fall in compliance is greatest when the duration of inspiration is less than one second (Watson, 1962*a*), the rapid introduction of air increasing its abnormal distribution within the lung.

During IPPR the chest wall, instead of producing inspiration, acts as an elastic resistance to it. In a totally paralysed subject this resistance is equal to about half that provided by the lungs themselves (Smith and Spalding, 1959). A patient with some respiratory power, however, often learns to assist the ventilator by expanding his chest wall during inspiration, and is more likely to do so when artificial respiration is less than adequate. Clinically such assistance is often impossible to detect.

Airway Resistance During IPPR

The greater part of the non-elastic resistance to inflation during IPPR is due to frictional resistance to the flow of air along the air passages which must include the resistance of the tracheostomy or endotracheal tube. The resistance to flow of air through a tube varies inversely with the fourth power of its diameter so that halving the diameter of a tracheostomy or endotracheal tube increases its resistance about sixteen times. This fact is of great importance during positive-pressure respiration in neonates and small babies. The fall in pressure between the ventilator and the alveoli is very large and accounts for the high pressures which must be applied if a significant ventilatory volume is to be achieved. Studies of oesophageal pressure during IPPR in babies show a considerably greater pressure gradient between the trachea and oesophagus than occurs in adults. A similar situation exists in patients with chronic obstructive airways disease. The walls of the small air passages are weakened by disease and can close completely during expiration, a phenomenon known as air trapping (Campbell, 1958). The airway resistance is further increased by the presence of copious secretions in the bronchial tree. Raised airway resistance may account for the clinical observation that high tracheal pressures used to ventilate bronchitics and babies do not often produce damage to the lung parenchyma. In paralysed patients with normal lungs it has been found by Opie *et al.* (1961) that during IPPR the non-elastic resistance of the lungs is about half that of normal subjects. This may be because the airways are dilated by the positive pressure from the ventilator (see section on PEEP).

Physiological Dead Space During IPPR

In normal subjects breathing spontaneously, physiological dead space (V_D) is less than a quarter of the tidal volume (V_T), i.e. the V_D/V_T ratio is less than 25 per cent. Watson (1962*b*) has shown that during IPPR the V_D/V_T ratio can be kept within normal limits if the inspiratory phase lasts more than 1·5 seconds. Using shorter durations of inspiration the V_D/V_T ratio rises. When inspiration lasts half a second it may be as high as 50 per cent. This observation is in line with Watson's findings for compliance during rapid inflation, and suggests that ventilation perfusion ratios are altered under these conditions (see also Chapter 3). A negative (subatmospheric) phase during IPPR also produces a rise of 10–15 per cent in the V_D/V_T ratio. It must be emphasised that the above observations apply only to patients with relatively normal lungs and do not necessarily hold for patients with chronic lung disease, or terminal respiratory failure.

Circulatory Effects of IPPR

Each inspiration during IPPR constitutes a mild Valsalva's manoeuvre. The effect of this upon the circulation depends upon the integrity of the patient's venous reflexes and whether there is a normal response to the raised intrathoracic pressure (see Chapter 13). Patients with normal venous reflexes (Sharpey-Schafer, 1961) are able to compensate for increases in intrathoracic pressure of the magnitude and duration used in IPPR by increasing their venous tone. Thus in most patients venous return is not seriously impeded by IPPR and a negative phase is unnecessary and a disadvantage since it serves only to increase the V_D/V_T ratio, necessitating a larger ventilatory volume to overcome this effect.

It is sometimes suggested that a negative phase is useful when IPPR has to be used on a patient in cardiac failure. The argument is that further obstruction to venous return is undesirable and may cause circulatory collapse. But this is an erroneous theory since a patient in cardiac failure shows a square wave response to Valsalva's manoeuvre (Sharpey-Schafer, 1955) and IPPR will therefore increase the stroke output of the heart and raise the blood pressure. Clinical experience confirms that IPPR is often beneficial to patients in heart failure. The benefit is obvious although Grenvik (1966) has shown that in these patients the start of IPPR is often accompanied by a small reduction in cardiac output. This effect appears to be secondary to reduced oxygen consumption resulting from the reduction in the work of breathing, in that the mixed venous oxygen saturation is unchanged and the oxygen available to the tissues is therefore greater.

Certain patients requiring artificial ventilation show a blocked response to Valsalva's manoeuvre since they are without reflex control of venous tone. As a result the capacitance vessels of the circulation behave mechanically, and a rise in intrathoracic pressure produces a proportional fall in venous return, stroke output and blood pressure. A negative phase during expiration may therefore maintain cardiac output and prevent severe hypotension. These patients include those with severe polyneuritis, cervical cord lesions, drug overdosage, oligaemia and other severe disorders (Barraclough and Sharpey-Schafer, 1963).

Unfortunately conflicting results have been obtained in studying the effect of a negative phase on cardiac output (Andersen and Kudriba, 1967; Prys-Roberts et al., 1967). Most of the information comes from animal studies or fit patients undergoing anaesthesia and although impressive improvements in cardiac output in man have been claimed using a negative phase, this has not been confirmed by the comprehensive study of Auchinloss and Gilbert (1967). Comparisons are difficult as many reports do not contain enough detail of the physical characteristics of the negative phase (Norlander, 1968).

Clinical experience suggests that the beneficial effects of a negative phase are marginal. This probably accounts for both the undoubted decline in its use and the difficulty in interpreting studies on negative phase.

The effects of IPPR on the pulmonary circulation are complex because it is a low pressure system and great variations exist in different parts of the lungs. During inspiration right ventricular stroke output falls and left ventricular stroke output rises (Morgan *et al.*, 1966). This effect is reversed during expiration and accounts for the cyclical variation in systemic arterial pressure, and the axis changes on the ECG seen during IPPR.

The circulatory effects of IPPR on patients with acute exacerbations of chronic lung disease and cor pulmonale are interesting and require further elucidation. During the first hours of treatment hypotension is usual (Bradley *et al.*, 1964). Unfortunately it is not possible to use Valsalva's manoeuvre in such patients as a means of obtaining information about circulatory reflexes. This is because air trapping prevents the sudden release of intrathoracic pressure which is necessary to demonstrate an overshoot. It seems unlikely, however, that hypotension in such patients is due to blocked reflexes. A more probable explanation may be the effect on the peripheral circulation of the rapid fall of carbon dioxide tension which accompanies the start of IPPR.

Inspired Gases during IPPR

Physiological dead space and venous admixture are always increased during IPPR and for this reason it is usually necessary to enrich the oxygen content of the inspired air if hypoxia is to be avoided (Nunn *et al.*, 1965). These changes, however, appear to lessen as IPPR is continued and patients with muscular paralysis and apparently normal lungs, who have been maintained on IPPR with air for months or years, often have an unusually high arterial oxygen tension. One patient who has received IPPR via a tracheostomy for seventeen years persistently maintains a Pao_2 of between 100 and 110 mm Hg (13·3 and 14·7 kPa). The mechanism of this long-term adjustment is unknown but it is clear that an increased alveolar-arterial oxygen gradient normally accompanies the start of IPPR (Pontoppidan *et al.*, 1965) and it is probably for this reason that artificial ventilation is rarely of value in pneumonia.

An excessive inspired oxygen concentration during IPPR is also harmful. Nash *et al.* (1967) studied the lungs of 70 patients who died after prolonged artificial ventilation. Lungs ventilated with high oxygen concentrations showed severe histological changes characterised by alveolar oedema, intra-alveolar haemorrhage and fibrin exudate. The mechanism of these changes is not known but they are now widely recognised and have led to the use of the term "respirator lung" (Fig. 8).

The oxygen concentrations necessary to produce these changes are uncertain but experience suggests that they are almost inevitable if concentrations above 80 per cent are used for more than a few hours. Clinically they are manifested by a progressively falling arterial oxygen tension and an increasing "white out" on radiological examination of the lung fields. Once established, this condition is almost universally fatal and it is therefore of the utmost importance never to use an inspired oxygen concentration higher than is necessary to produce an arterial tension between 100 and 150 mm Hg (13·3 and 20 kPa).

The use of nitrous oxide during prolonged IPPR is also undesirable. Despite its safety for short-term use during anaesthesia, if administration is prolonged for more than three to four days, serious bone marrow depression and leuco-penia results (Parbrook, 1967).

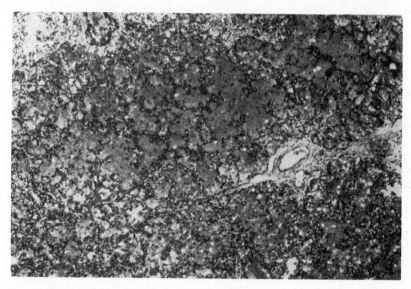

10/FIG. 8.—The "respirator lung" syndrome. Microscopic section of a lung following 5 days of IPPR with high oxygen concentration. Intra-alveolar haemorrhage is clearly seen.

POSITIVE END-EXPIRATORY PRESSURE (PEEP)

In 1948, Cournand *et al.* showed that cardiac output fell during IPPR as mean intrathoracic pressure rose. For a constant tissue oxygen consumption a reduction in cardiac output must cause a fall in mixed venous oxygen content and probably, therefore, a fall in arterial oxygen content. Thus for many years clinicians have been cautious about raising mean intrathoracic pressure during IPPR. Interest has centred rather on reducing it by introducing a sub-atmo-spheric expiratory phase. However, following the observations of McIntyre *et al.* (1969) and Russell *et al.* (1971), it has been recognised that in certain patients with very severe lung disturbances arterial oxygenation and carbon dioxide elimination can be usefully improved by maintaining a positive pressure of 5–15 cm H_2O (0·5–1·5 kPa) during the expiratory phase. The technique is described as positive end-expiratory pressure or PEEP. To be effective, the desired positive pressure has to be held constant throughout the expiratory pause. Delayed expiration, achieved by introducing a restriction into the expira-tory pathway does not achieve the same effect—though it may be of value in managing patients with emphysema when true PEEP is usually harmful and undesirable (Barrat and Asvero, 1975).

The use of PEEP may be particularly valuable in patients who would other-wise need unacceptably high inspired oxygen concentrations (over 80 per cent) if reasonable arterial oxygen tensions are to be achieved. These patients usually need a large minute volume and PEEP may also reduce the minute volume necessary to obtain a normal arterial carbon dioxide tension.

The decision when and how much PEEP should be used can only be reached by careful and sophisticated cardiopulmonary measurement in each individual patient. This is rarely possible in routine clinical practice and it has been suggested that the point of maximum compliance is the best single pointer to the end-expiratory pressure likely to result in optimal cardiopulmonary function.

In a comprehensive study and review, Suter *et al.* (1975) showed that the effects of PEEP may be both good and bad at different levels in the same patient. By raising functional residual capacity and increasing the lung volumes at which tidal exchange is performed, PEEP may prevent the lungs from deflating to below the critical closing volume and thus increase compliance and arterial oxygen tension. Conversely it may overdistend alveoli and decrease compliance, thereby increasing physiological dead space. If too much PEEP is used it may seriously obstruct venous return and so decrease cardiac output. In a study of 15 normo-volaemic patients, Suter *et al.* showed that what they termed "best PEEP" varied between 0 and 15 cm H_2O (0 and 1·5 kPa). In general, the lower the initial functional residual capacity in their patients, the higher the value of "best PEEP". An important observation was that arterial oxygen tension could continue to rise even after high levels of PEEP had started to cause falls in cardiac output and total oxygen transport. Arterial oxygen tension increase alone is therefore not an indication that PEEP is exerting a beneficial effect. The studies of Barrat and Asvero (1975) confirm the findings of Suter *et al.* that PEEP is likely to be harmful, or at least unnecessary, in patients with obstructive airways disease.

Finally, it is important to distinguish between PEEP and continuous positive airway pressure (CPAP). CPAP is used during spontaneous respiration by making a patient expire against a resistance. The benefits of CPAP are less well established and, as its use may be likened to the trick of pursed-lip breathing employed by victims of emphysema, the indications for CPAP are probably different from those for PEEP.

MANAGEMENT OF PATIENTS RECEIVING ARTIFICIAL RESPIRATION

Tracheostomy (see also Long-term Endotracheal Intubation in Children, p. 1422).

The indications for tracheostomy may be summarised as follows:

1. **Upper airway obstruction.**—This applies to acute and chronic obstruction above the level of the trachea. The obstruction is bypassed and the indication is usually clear-cut, although it may be difficult to distinguish between stridor and wheeze.

2. **Suction.**—Tracheostomy is indicated for patients who are unable, through muscular weakness or other debility, to cough up their bronchial secretions adequately. The situation can be temporarily relieved by bronchoscopy, but unless the cause of secretion retention is fairly rapidly self-limiting, or can be kept pace with by suction down an endotracheal tube, tracheostomy is necessary.

3. **Isolation of the lower respiratory tract.**—When, for any reason, the pharyngeal or laryngeal reflexes are lost, the lungs must be isolated from the pharynx and larynx by tracheostomy. This does not, of course, apply to short-term causes such as occur during anaesthesia, but to conditions in which reflexes

are absent for a significant period. Isolation can be maintained for several days using an endotracheal tube. As a result of improvements in the management of patients receiving IPPR via an endotracheal tube and improvements in the tubes themselves, it is now possible to leave them in position for up to one week (see below).

It is important to remember that this indication for tracheostomy may be present in neoplastic conditions of the pharynx, larynx and oesophagus, where mechanical interference with swallowing may be severe enough to necessitate isolation of the trachea and lungs.

4. **To maintain artificial ventilation.**—If artificial ventilation by intermittent positive pressure is necessary for more than a few days, tracheostomy is essential.

Tracheostomy is sometimes said to be of value in that it reduces respiratory dead space. This argument is fallacious, and has probably arisen from confusion between anatomical and physiological dead space. Tracheostomy has been shown in several studies to reduce anatomical dead space by 10–50 per cent. Immediately after it has been performed, the proportion of tidal volume which is effective in producing gaseous exchange, i.e. the alveolar ventilation, rises, the arterial P_{CO_2} falls, the central stimulus to ventilation is decreased, and the volume of ventilation falls until the arterial P_{CO_2} has become re-established at its previous level. The converse applies if anatomical dead space is increased by breathing through a face-mask. Ventilation rises and P_{CO_2} remains at almost its original level. These theoretical arguments have been confirmed by Froeb and Kim (1964) who showed that both in normal subjects and in patients with emphysema there is little alteration in arterial gas tensions and a reduction in respiratory minute volume following tracheostomy. The same authors found a small increase in arterial oxygen saturation following tracheostomy in subjects with a level below normal. This increase was not significant and was within the limits both of experimental error and normal variations in oxygen saturation due to alterations of the alveolar/arterial oxygen gradient within the lung. These results were confirmed in the studies of Grant et al. (1964).

It has also been suggested that, by reducing dead space, tracheostomy may postpone the need for artificial ventilation, but this is not so. In practice it is always found that due to hypoxia, clinical distress and possibly carbon dioxide retention, artificial ventilation is needed when vital capacity is still two or three times greater than mean tidal volume. If dead space reduction were to have any effect in avoiding artificial ventilation, vital capacity and tidal volume would have to be both equal and reduced. This situation represents a patient in extremis who should have been receiving respiratory assistance considerably earlier.

To summarise, tracheostomy produces a 10–50 per cent reduction in anatomical dead space, alveolar ventilation is unchanged, and dead space reduction per se is of little value to the patient.

Tracheostomy Tubes

A wide variety of tracheostomy tubes is available but none is completely satisfactory for all purposes.

Cuffed tracheostomy tubes.—A cuffed tube exposes the patient to a number of additional hazards (see below—Complications). It should not be used unless indications 3 or 4 (above) are present. The requirements of a cuffed tube are as follows:—It must have as wide a bore as possible to provide an airway with low resistance to airflow. The lumen must be smooth-walled to prevent crusting of secretions and to allow easy introduction of suction catheters. The curve of the tube must be gentle to facilitate suction. The cuff must be smooth-surfaced and inflate evenly to maintain an airtight fit in the trachea and minimise the risk of herniation. The inflatable section of the cuff should be not less than $1\frac{1}{4}$ inches (3 cm) long to ensure a wide area of gentle contact with the tracheal mucosa, and reduce the risk of tracheal damage. It must possess a suitable flange or neck to allow it to be securely tied in position. The connection to the ventilator tubing must be light in weight and not liable to become detached in use. At the same time it must be easily disconnected to facilitate suction.

Few, if any, tubes meet all these requirements completely. Two are illustrated which come near to it.

The Portsmouth tracheostomy tube (Hodges *et al.*, 1956) (Fig. 9) is built up from a Magill cuffed endotracheal tube. A silver lining piece is inserted to maintain a suitable curve and a plastic Cobb suction union (Portex Ltd.) used as a connection. It has been found (Bradley *et al.*, 1964) to be particularly suitable for use when high inflation pressures are needed. Although this tube may be regarded as somewhat old-fashioned today, it is useful in countries where disposable plastic apparatus is difficult to maintain in steady supply. Apart from the endotracheal tube, the remainder of its components can be home-made.

The Bassett tracheostomy tube (Whittard and Thomas, 1964) (Fig. 10) is disposable, plastic throughout and supplied sterile in a two-layered plastic container bag. It is convenient to use and non-irritant but the cuff is somewhat short and the connection tends to become insecure in use. Unfortunately, this tube is being withdrawn and replaced by one with a larger "floppy" cuff. In theory the benefits of a large volume floppy cuff are clear. Not only can it conform more easily to the shape of the tracheal wall and therefore maintain an airtight fit with less mucosal pressure, but the intracuff pressure can be further lowered until it is below the peak pressure applied in the trachea during inspiration. As the tracheal pressure rises during inspiration, back pressure is exerted on the wall of the cuff facing down the trachea. As the cuff is floppy, this wall can be compressed backwards up the trachea, thus reducing the cuff volume, increasing the pressure inside it and maintaining an airtight fit with the tracheal wall (Crawley and Cross, 1975). In practice, however, these benefits are offset by disadvantages. Floppy cuff tubes are more difficult to insert and painful and traumatic to change (Dinnick, 1975); this particularly applies to long-term tracheostomy with a tight stoma, when general anaesthesia may even be necessary to make the procedure tolerable. Floppy cuffs are also more likely to herniate over the end of the tracheostomy tube with potentially serious results. The cuff does not necessarily locate the tube in the centre of the tracheal lumen, so that the tube tip may remain in contact with the tracheal wall and the cuff may not be airtight under all conditions.

Non-cuffed tracheostomy tubes.—The requirements of a non-cuffed tracheostomy tube are not exacting and designs are well-established. The Negus silver tube with optional speaking flap is the most widely used, but recently silastic

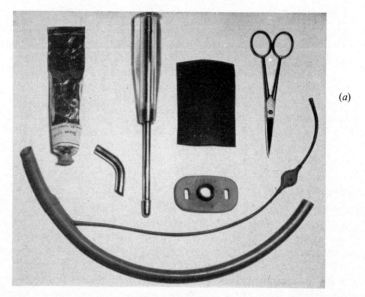

Component parts.

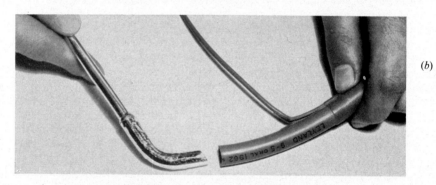

Introducing the silver lining tube.

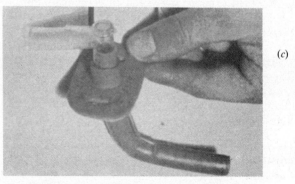

10/Fig. 9.—Portsmouth tracheostomy tube.

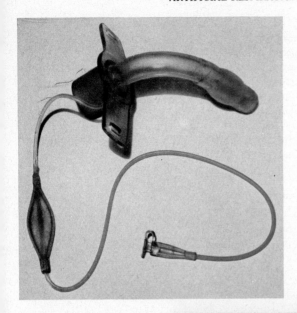

10/Fig. 10.—Bassett tracheostomy tube. A pre-sterilised, all
plastic, disposable tube.

10/Fig. 11.—Neonatal
tracheostomy tube (Frank-
lin). A silastic version of this
tube, called "The Aberdeen"
is also available at greater
cost.

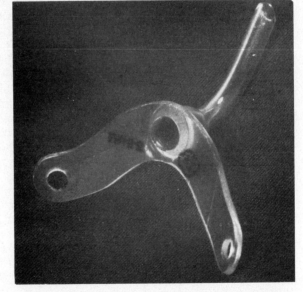

non-cuffed tracheostomy tubes have been introduced which, though relatively
thick-walled, may offer real advantages.

Neonatal tracheostomy tube (Glover, 1965). (Fig. 11).—This tube is specially
shaped for infants. To maintain as large a lumen as possible it is cuffless and
an airtight fit is obtained by selecting a size large enough to fit snugly into the
trachea. The funnel shaped enlargement below the flange serves both to maintain an airtight fit at the site of the tracheostome and to hold in position the

catheter mount connection. The flange is angled upwards to accommodate the anatomical differences of the neonate. The management of neonatal tracheostomy requires special precautions all of which are related to the small size of the bronchial tree. Serious blockage occurs more quickly than in adults and is more difficult to treat. Tracheal narrowing following decannulation is commoner and more likely to be clinically significant.

It is also clear from clinical experience and experimental studies (Okmian, 1966) that it is wrong to try to reproduce the same pattern of respiratory frequency during artificial ventilation that the infant maintains spontaneously. More efficient ventilation is achieved using frequencies of between 20 and 25 breaths per minute.

Anaesthesia for Tracheostomy

Tracheostomy is best performed under general anaesthesia with an endotracheal tube in place, and it should be an elective, planned procedure so far as is possible. Local analgesia is only justifiable when it is impossible to introduce an endotracheal tube beforehand, or when an experienced anaesthetist is not available.

Complications of Tracheostomy

Most of the complications of tracheostomy can be avoided provided great care is taken to see that management is always perfect. Nevertheless, complications are surprisingly common. McClelland (1965) found evidence of complications in over 50 per cent of tracheostomies performed in a general hospital.

Obstruction of the tube.—This is usually due to inadequate humidification of the inspired gases and the accumulation of inspissated secretions.

Displacement of the tube.—This can occur if the tubes from the ventilator are allowed to pull on the tracheostomy tube during nursing attentions. In the first few days following tracheostomy it may be a serious matter since replacement may be difficult until a track has become established. Certain patterns of tube, such as the Durham metal tube, are more liable to dislodge, owing to a short intratracheal section. If it is necessary to change a tracheostomy tube during the first 48 hours, a laryngoscope and endotracheal tube must always be immediately available. If it is difficult to insert the new tube an oral endotracheal tube should be passed and the new tube inserted under good vision, possibly in the operating theatre. If this procedure is not followed, a false passage may be created (Fig. 12).

Damage to surrounding structures.—Erosion into the oesophagus or innominate artery can occur. The former is most common when metal tracheostomy tubes are used, and the latter is usually associated with a cuffed tracheostomy tube and IPPR.

Infection.—Infection, either at the tracheostome or in the tracheobronchial tree, is difficult to prevent. A meticulous aseptic technique should be used at all times. The tracheostomy wound should be kept exposed and secretions removed from around it as soon as they appear.

Granulomata.—Granulomata of the trachea (Pearce and Walsh, 1961) can occur and they may cause respiratory difficulty when the tube is removed. Infection at the tracheostome is possibly a predisposing factor.

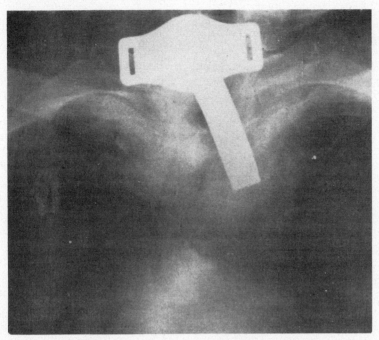

10/Fig. 12.—X-ray showing a tracheostomy tube in a false passage. This was caused by forceful tube replacement following a recent tracheostomy.

Dilatation of the trachea.—Some enlargement of the trachea at the site of the cuff is probably inevitable. If the cuff is too short, or over-inflated, the dilatation may be considerable (Lloyd and McClelland, 1964). Mucosal damage, due to cuff pressure is usual, but of no permanent significance. If cuff pressure is excessive or uneven, however, the cartilaginous rings of the trachea may be eroded, leading to tracheal collapse and stricture following decannulation (Figs. 13 and 14). Regular cuff deflation is widely advocated in an attempt to minimise tracheal damage. This technique usually does more harm than good. Unless the cuff is deflated with a suction catheter *in situ*, debris lodged in the trachea above the cuff can pass down into the lungs. More seriously, unless the tube is held carefully in the correct position during deflation it can easily be reinflated in the wrong place. Finally, unless the cuff is sucked flat and the pilot tube clamped, some air may remain in the cuff and when the same volume of air is replaced in the cuff the volume it contains may creep up at each deflation, thus actually causing tracheal dilation. The best protection against tracheal damage is meticulous management, with the tube lying in the neck without ventilator tubes pulling on it, and inflation with the minimum quantity of air only when the tube is inserted or changed. Given this care, it is doubtful whether floppy cuffs will reduce the overall incidence of tracheostomy complications, and Bradbeer *et al.* (1976) have described a stricture at cuff level following the use for a comparatively short period of a floppy cuffed endotracheal tube.

Tracheal stricture.—This is a late complication of tracheostomy. Strictures may occur:

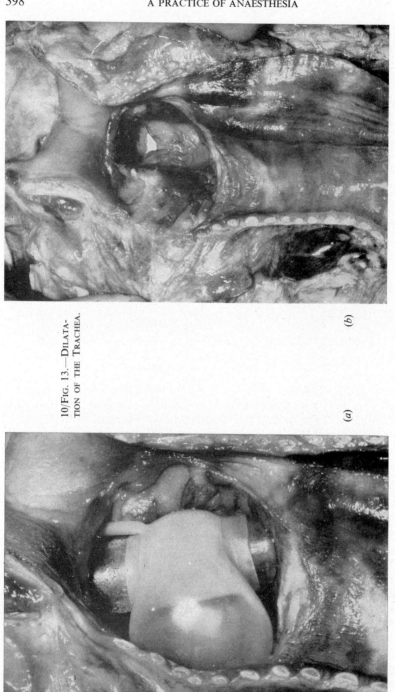

10/Fig. 13.—Dilata-
tion of the Trachea.

(a)

(b)

A trachea at autopsy, opened from behind. (a). Tracheostomy tube *in situ*. Excessive and uneven pressure from the cuff has caused a sacular dilatation of the trachea. The open end of the tracheostomy tube is completely obstructed by the wall of the sac. (b). Trachea with tracheostomy tube removed. The cartilaginous rings of the trachea can be seen in the walls of the dilatation. They are eroded and broken.

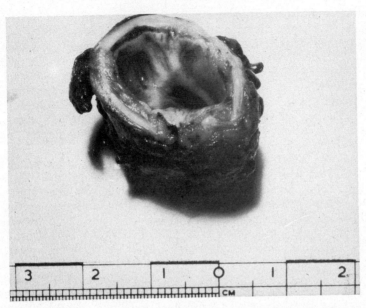

10/Fig. 14.—Tracheal Stricture. A section of the lower trachea removed at operation. The tracheal lumen is seen to be severely narrowed by a fibrous structure probably due to a tracheostomy tube cuff.

(i) At the cricoid ring if the tracheostomy has been performed too high.

(ii) At the site of the stoma; this is particularly common in babies or when a large stoma has developed due to infection or careless handling of ventilator tubing. Long-term tracheostomy with epithelialisation of the stomal track also predisposes to late stomal stricture if allowed to close spontaneously. Tracheostomies of more than three months duration are best treated by formal surgical closure.

(iii) At the cuff site; due to cartilaginous erosion (see above).

(iv) At the tube tip; due to cartilaginous damage by pressure from the tube tip.

Despite steady improvement in tracheostomy management, most follow-up studies continue to report an incidence of late stricture of up to 50 per cent (Aass, 1975). Friman *et al.* (1976), however, have shown that detectable strictures occur in virtually every patient subjected to tracheostomy but that the majority do not cause significant symptoms unless respiratory function from underlying disease remains substantially impaired.

Humidification (see also Chapter 1, p. 6).

In normal respiration inspired air is warmed and moistened during its passage through the nose and upper air passages. By the time it reaches the trachea the air is at 32–36° C, even when breathing cold air through the nose, and has a relative humidity of over 90 per cent (34–35 mg/litre at 32° C). Dry air passing straight into the trachea produces marked changes in the tracheal mucosa which becomes hyperaemic; and excessive mucus is formed which becomes dry and crusted. Cilial action is depressed or abolished (Burton, 1962). These effects can be avoided if the air or gas drawn in or blown through a tracheostomy is warmed to body temperature and adequately humidified. Most ventilators include a water bath humidifier in the inspiratory limb of the patient circuit. When a patient is breathing spontaneously through a tracheostomy tube, warm wet air can be supplied from a blower humidifier. Full humidification is needed for the first few weeks after tracheostomy, but after this time the trachea appears to become adapted to some extent and the mucosa undergoes squamous metaplasia. A metal-gauze condenser humidifier or "artificial nose" may then be adequate (Mapleson *et al.*, 1963).

An alternative method of humidification is to provide at the tracheostomy a fine mist of water droplets. Nebulisers for this purpose are included in some ventilators. Most operate on the venturi principle and produce water droplets of varying sizes up to 10μ in diameter. Many of these droplets are too large to reach the smaller bronchi and are deposited on the walls of the ventilator tubing and trachea. Although it may be difficult by this method to provide full humidification of the inspired air at all stages of the respiratory cycle, it has proved satisfactory in use and is often more comfortable for the patient.

Probably the best method of humidification is that which has been described by Herzog *et al.* (1964). An aerosol is generated by dripping water on to the metal plate of a transducer head which is made to vibrate at ultrasonic frequency by an electrical generator. Using this system, the particle size is a direct function of the vibration frequency. In the system described 70 per cent of the particles produced have diameters between 0.8 and 1.0μ. A gas-tight plexi glass container with a volume of 150 ml is included in the inspiratory limb of the ventilator. The vibrating transducer is incorporated in the base of the chamber and water or saline dripped on to it from an intravenous infusion set connected through the lid of the chamber. Aerosol is generated throughout the respiratory cycle as an almost invisible mist. At the start of inspiration, accumulated aerosol is carried into the patient, ensuring supersaturation (i.e. a relative humidity above 100 per cent) of the inspired air. The particle size is sufficiently small to prevent accumulation of water in the ventilator tubing. It has been found that using this system it is possible to add several hundred grams of water to the patient per 24 hours. This is in contrast to all other methods of humidification which involve a net water loss from the circulation and airways. The system is simple to use, and the only drawback at present is the cost of the apparatus. It has the additional advantage that it can be used for ventilator sterilisation. For a review of humidification requirements and techniques the reader is referred to Chamney (1969).

Prolonged Endotracheal Intubation (see also Chapter 45)

It is easier to manage a patient with a tracheostomy than a similar patient with an orotracheal or nasotracheal tube. Until recently this fact, reinforced by anxiety about laryngeal damage, was the paramount consideration in deciding whether to leave an endotracheal tube in place or to perform a tracheostomy. When nursing care is less than excellent it is still the paramount consideration. In recent years the segregation of patients receiving artificial ventilation into special care units has done much to improve the standard of nursing care they receive, and this fact, coupled with the introduction of plastic tubes which appear to lessen the risks of vocal cord damage have reawakened interest in prolonged endotracheal intubation. Given a high standard of nursing care the advantages and disadvantages of the two techniques can be compared as below. It cannot be too often repeated, however, that if nursing standards are not perfect, tracheostomy is safer.

The *advantages* of prolonged endotracheal intubation compared with tracheostomy are:

1. Endotracheal intubation is simple, repeatable and quick.
2. Immediate operative complications of tracheostomy are avoided. These risks include: haemorrhage, surgical emphysema, pneumothorax, air embolism and cricoid cartilage damage.
3. Stricture of the trachea at the stomal site is avoided.
4. Cross infection of a surgical wound adjacent to a tracheostomy, e.g. a median sternotomy, does not occur.
5. Even using a horizontal incision a tracheostomy scar does not heal well. This uncosmetic scar may be a serious disadvantage to some patients, e.g. young women who require short-term IPPR following suicidal drug overdosage. A tracheostomy scar is an unwelcome reminder of an unhappy incident in their lives. An endotracheal tube avoids this problem.
6. The incidence of complications is lower than those of tracheostomy (Lindholm, 1969).

The *disadvantages* of prolonged endotracheal intubation compared with tracheostomy are:

1. Laryngeal damage can occur although usually the effects of this are limited to transient hoarseness of the voice.
2. An endotracheal tube is less well tolerated by the patient than a tracheostomy. This may increase the need for sedation and make weaning more difficult.
3. Fixation of an oral endotracheal tube is difficult. A Nosworthy connection extending between the teeth is essential to prevent the patient biting the tube.
4. The tube may become kinked in the pharynx. This difficulty is better avoided by the use of smooth-walled plastic rather than nylon reinforced latex tubes, down which suction catheters can be difficult to pass.
5. Owing to the difficulties of fixation the tube may be easily displaced into the right main bronchus.
6. Though the incidence of complications is lower, when they do occur they are more severe, and approximately 1 per cent of patients need permanent tracheostomy (Tonkin and Harrison, 1966; Harrison and Tonkin, 1967, 1968; Fearon and Cotton, 1972).

Some of these disadvantages can be overcome by the use of a nasotracheal tube. This technique is particularly suitable for neonates and young children because the internal diameter of the nose is greater than that of the larynx. A suitable tube has been developed by Rees and Owen-Thomas (1966). Unfortunately nasotracheal intubation is less suitable for adults and can cause damage to the external nares. Effective aspiration of tracheal secretions is even more difficult owing to the greater length and narrower bore of the tube.

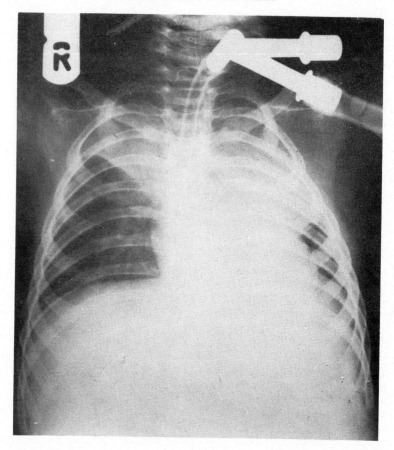

10/Fig. 15(a).—Chest X-ray of a child *before* physiotherapy.

In summary, prolonged endotracheal intubation has real advantages for selected patients, provided that the standard of nursing care is high. The naso-tracheal route is the most suitable for babies and the orotracheal route for adults. The subject has been comprehensively reviewed by Lindholm (1969).

Care of the Lungs

Adequate care of the lungs during artificial ventilation is the key to success. Bronchial secretions must be aspirated whenever they can be felt or heard and certainly never less than two-hourly. As far as possible an aseptic technique should be employed and a fresh sterile catheter must be used for each insertion. Ideally catheters should be individually packed and sterilised by autoclaving. Despite improvements in plastic suction catheters, soft rubber whistle-tipped catheters still remain the most satisfactory for use in prolonged IPPR. The whistle-tip pattern appears to be the least traumatic. In the words of one Doctor/ patient, after four years of artificial ventilation in several hospitals: "It's the only type which doesn't feel like a red hot wire thrust down my trachea!—single

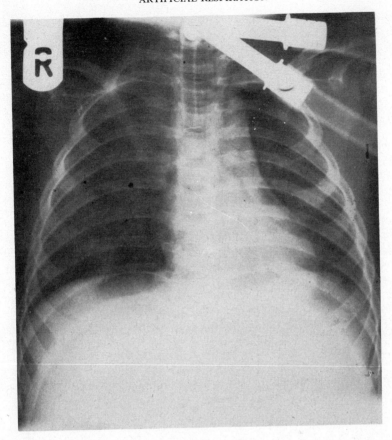

10/Fig. 15(*b*).—Chest X-ray of a child taken half an hour after physiotherapy by "artificial coughing".

hole catheters do a series of mucosal biopsies as they're hauled out!".

Plastic suction catheters frequently cause tracheal bleeding if they are used repeatedly. They are difficult to manipulate down plastic tracheostomy and endotracheal tubes because the two plastic surfaces tend to adhere. In a busy unit up to 500 suction catheters may be used per day. In the interests of cost, resterilisation is usually necessary and plastic catheters withstand this less well than rubber ones at present. Angulated suction catheters which can be made to enter the left main bronchus are not routinely necessary and their use has declined following improvements in physiotherapy techniques during IPPR.

Physiotherapy.—Transference of secretions from the periphery of the lungs to the trachea or main bronchi usually has to be assisted during the first months of artificial ventilation by postural drainage and physiotherapy. The most effective form of physiotherapy is the technique of artificial coughing described by Sykes *et al.* (1969). The lung is hyperinflated with oxygen by means of a reservoir bag and the squeeze on the bag is suddenly released. The moment of pressure release is made to coincide with an external squeeze and vibration produced by the physiotherapist. This procedure is repeated several times for each area of the chest until it is clear to auscultation.

If skilfully performed this technique is well tolerated even by severely ill patients and may need to be repeated several times a day. It is remarkably effective. Figure 15 *a* and *b* shows radiographs of the chest of a 3-year-old child taken half an hour apart, before and after physiotherapy. It has been suggested that physiotherapy by this technique may cause a subsequent reduction in arterial oxygen tension (Gormezano and Branthwaite, 1972). Fortunately these findings have not been confirmed by subsequent more detailed investigations (Brock-Vine *et al.*, 1975).

Periodic deep breaths.—During normal spontaneous breathing Bendixen *et al.* (1964) have shown that tidal volume varies greatly, and sighs (breaths larger than three times the average tidal volume) occur regularly about ten times per hour. These writers consider that periodic deep breaths are of physiological importance, because atelectatic air spaces are reinflated and pulmonary compliance, the work of breathing and venous admixture kept within the normal range. In relating these findings to artificial ventilation Bendixen *et al.* (1963) showed a mean fall of Pao_2 during controlled ventilation of 22 per cent and suggested that the cause might be small areas of pulmonary collapse not necessarily visible on X-rays. They postulated that these changes could be avoided during IPPR by the use of automatic periodic sighs built into the ventilator. A variety of devices have been developed to produce this effect (Feychting and Settergren, 1966). The changes described by Bendixen *et al.* have not been confirmed by subsequent work (Morgan *et al.*, 1970) and are ascribed by Norlander *et al.* (1968) to inefficient ventilators. Certainly artificial sighs have not been shown to be beneficial. Improved techniques of ventilation and physiotherapy are preferable.

Assessment of Respiration in Muscular Weakness

When are muscular paralysis and respiratory weakness severe enough to justify mechanical assistance? Generalisations on this question are no more accurate than most other clinical generalisations but individual clinical assessment of each patient remains the most valuable method for arriving at the correct answer. As respiratory paralysis progresses, a patient becomes anxious and restless, the accessory muscles of respiration are used, and frequent feeble attempts at coughing may be made. Carbon dioxide accumulation is a late sign of respiratory inadequacy due to muscular weakness. Hypoxaemia and cyanosis occur much earlier and minute volume may actually be increased from this cause, possibly due to increased venous admixture from maldistribution of ventilation and perfusion in the lung. The fact that respiratory assistance is often needed when vital capacity is still at least twice the average tidal volume may be due to the loss of this sigh mechanism. Measurements of peak expiratory flow rate may also be valuable in assessing the need for respiratory assistance, for when this flow is less than 100 litre/minute, coughing is inefficient and pulmonary complications are likely.

Volume of Ventilation

The only completely satisfactory way to ensure that a patient is receiving the correct volume of ventilation is to measure his arterial P_{CO_2} and preferably his arterial P_{O_2} as well. For patients who start off with normal lungs, respiration nomograms such as those of Engström and Herzog (1959) may be helpful. It is preferable to err on the side of overventilation rather than underventilation.

Patients receiving artificial ventilation for pulmonary disease present a special problem, since nomograms are of no value and measurement of arterial gas tensions is essential. In the early stages, however, it may be necessary to accept a less-than-ideal ventilatory volume. Ventilation may have to be set to the largest volume which does not lead to serious hypotension (Bradley *et al.* 1964).

SOME CONDITIONS IN WHICH ARTIFICAL RESPIRATION MAY BE REQUIRED

Artificial respiration has become an established form of therapy in an increasing range of conditions. It remains, nevertheless, a complicated and potentially dangerous treatment unless it is properly carried out in specially adapted units by staff experienced in the techniques involved. Like all forms of therapy, it cannot be considered in isolation without due consideration of the conditions for which it is being used and the indications for its use.

These conditions can be conveniently divided into four types, depending on which of the structures involved in normal respiration have failed.

Some of these conditions are now discussed, but only in respect of the need for artificial respiration in their treatment. Clinical details are not intended to be comprehensive since, in fact, many of the diseases are described more fully elsewhere in this book.

Failure of muscles or neuromuscular junction	*Failure of the lungs*	*Failure of the nervous system*		*Failure of bony structures*
		Central nervous system	*Peripheral nerves*	
General anaesthesia using muscle relaxants	Chronic bronchitis and emphysema	Drug over-dosage	Polio-myelitis	Crush injury to thorax
Tetanus	Neonatal respiratory distress syndrome	Status epilepticus	Poly-neuritis	Scoliosis
Myasthenia gravis				
Dystrophia myotonica	Status asthmaticus (Pneumonia)	Head injury		
		Cervical cord injury		
	Post-operative pulmonary complications	After neurosurgery		After thoracotomy
	Drowning "Terminal" respiratory failure			

It should be appreciated that in addition to the table on p. 405, artificial ventilation commonly has to be used for what are primarily cardiovascular reasons. These may also apply to some of the above conditions, for example in respiratory distress syndrome and status asthmaticus where the work of breathing is enormously increased and up to 30 per cent of the cardiac output may be used in this work. In addition, if the cardiac output is severely reduced as occurs after cardiac surgery or myocardial infarction, the oxygen demands of spontaneous respiration may be too great for the patient to perform satisfactorily and artificial ventilation is of great benefit (Norlander, 1968).

Artificial Respiration in General Anaesthesia

Two separate questions must be answered when the decision to use artificial respiration during general anaesthesia is being made. Firstly, will the patient's best interests be served by allowing him to breathe spontaneously, or by controlling his respiration? Secondly, if artificial respiration is used, is it best performed manually, or by a mechanical ventilator? The first question is much the more difficult one to answer satisfactorily. For thoracic surgery and operations requiring full muscular relaxation the answer is easy. For short operations, requiring little more than the abolition of painful stimuli, the answer is equally easy. Most operations lie between these two extremes, and it is in this large intermediate group that the answer is difficult. It is doubtful whether in most cases there would be any difference in the ultimate results after either method. Many schools of anaesthesia exist which hold strongly opposed opinions concerning the benefits of one technique over the other. It is obviously impossible for widely divergent views to be held if a highly significant advantage were offered by either method in a particular situation. Nevertheless, today, when satisfactory anaesthesia can be assured by so many methods, it is important to elucidate the marginal advantages offered by a particular technique. Due to the many variables involved, these advantages may be exceedingly difficult to establish. It seems reasonable to assume that the best anaesthesia is that which involves the least disturbance to normal physiology. It is therefore necessary to compare the physiological changes which accompany artificial respiration properly performed in paralysed patients, with those accompanying equivalent anaesthesia by narcotic and inhalational agents, but with spontaneous respiration. It may be that in the long run the most significant difference will be found to be in the post-operative effects on ventilation caused by a respiratory acidosis or alkalosis existing during anaesthesia (Semple, 1965) (see Chapter 3). When artificial respiration is used, it can be performed manually or mechanically. A ventilator frees the anaesthetist's hands, so that he is able when single-handed to attend to other duties, while at the same time ensuring efficient ventilation. However the feel of the anaesthetic reservoir bag is still a valuable adjunct in clinical practice. Its loss divorces the anaesthetist from his patient and makes it harder to observe and anticipate minor variations in the patient's condition. It is probably true that manual ventilation, no matter how conscientiously carried out, cannot hope to provide at all times throughout an operation the constant and physiological respiratory cycling of a good machine which has been correctly adjusted.

Tetanus (See also Chapter 28, p. 941)

Knott and Cole (1952) describe six types of tetanus.

Type I: Purely local, usually mild, which often occurs in people who have been immunised.

Type II: Generalised tonic rigidity which intensifies and then passes off without spasm.

Type III: Tonic rigidity, intensifying and leading to reflex spasms. These too increase and finally relax if the patient has not succumbed during the crescendo.

Type IV: Involvement of the muscles of deglutition and respiration with less emphasis on generalised spasms.

Type V: Cephalic tetanus, involving principally the cranial nerves.

Type VI: Infantile tetanus from infection of the umbilical cord.

In types I and II management by sedation and hypnotic drugs such as diazepam and chlorpromazine (Kelly and Laurence, 1956; Vassa et al., 1974) is usually sufficient. The use of these drugs has been accompanied by slight reduction in mortality during tetanus (Adams, 1958), whereas the value of curarisation and intermittent positive-pressure respiration—at least in types III to VI—is clearly established (Shackleton, 1954; Ablett, 1956; Wright et al., 1961; Pearce, 1961). In these groups death is most commonly due to respiratory failure, either from asphyxia during a spasm, or from chest complications following hypertonicity of the respiratory muscles or loss of the ability to swallow. Death may occur during the first major tetanic spasm, and such a spasm is a certain indication for tracheostomy, curarisation, and IPPR. When chest complications occur in tetanus it is usually necessary to perform a tracheostomy because hypertonicity prevents the patient from coughing. The irritation caused by the tube however may precipitate generalised spasms, and then curarisation and IPPR become essential.

Mortality in neonatal tetanus is very high. A substantial reduction has been achieved by using curarisation and IPPR (Wright et al., 1961; Ganendran, 1974). That the reduction in mortality was not greater was because the treatment is technically difficult and requires a higher standard of care than usually exists in areas where the disease is common. Tetanus is a self-limiting condition although curarisation may have to be maintained for 4–5 weeks. For this reason tubocurarine has usually been found to be the most satisfactory relaxant. It can be given intramuscularly in doses of 15 mg as often as is necessary to maintain flaccidity. Pancuronium has been advocated as an alternative to tubocurarine for the treatment of tetanus. Although it appears to have pharmacological advantages, in practice these advantages are theoretical rather than real.

In 1967 a symposium on tetanus in Great Britain was held in Leeds (Ellis, 1967) and the results of treatment in several centres were reviewed. The best series showed an overall mortality of 4 per cent in all cases. In most published series the mortality is well above this figure.

Sympathetic overactivity, characterised by tachycardia, dysrhythmias, raised blood pressure, sweating, severe vasoconstriction and raised catecholamines in the blood are occasional features of the disease that may be related to, or aggravated by, undersedation during IPPR and curarisation.

In an attempt to suppress these manifestations, the β-blocking drug, propranolol, has been used with some benefit (Kerr et al., 1968; Keilty et al., 1968; Benedict and Kerr, 1977).

Prys-Roberts *et al.* (1969) suggested that an adrenergic neurone blocking drug such as bethanidine might be beneficial. However, it will not block the effects of circulating catecholamines. Thus, to treat hypertension or peripheral vasoconstriction, an α-receptor blocker or a ganglion blocker (which will reduce catecholamine release from the adrenal medulla) would be a more logical choice. At present there is insufficient experience of these methods of treatment to make it possible to decide whether any reduction in mortality due to sympathetic overactivity will outweigh increased mortality from side-effects and secondary complications from the drugs themselves. To administer β-adrenergic blocking drugs to a paralysed patient receiving IPPR is a serious step. Should inadvertent disconnection from the ventilator occur, cardiac arrest follows more rapidly and is much more difficult to reverse.

It is encouraging that sympathetic overactivity is not universally noted in all reported series. Cole and others in an extensive clinical experience over many years have never seen sympathetic overactivity (Cole and Youngman, 1969). In a previous paper they point out that most patients find tetanus and its treatment a frightening and painful ordeal (Cole and Youngman, 1968). For this reason they have used paraldehyde freely as the drug of choice for central sedation throughout their experience.

These results raise the interesting possibility that sympathetic overactivity may be due to awareness and stress. Large doses of *d*-tubocurarine, used to maintain flaccidity in severe cases, may make it more difficult to detect wakefulness.

Myasthenia Gravis

This disease is described in Chapter 28. The past five years have seen a dramatic improvement in the morbidity and mortality of myasthenia gravis due to early thymectomy followed by prolonged administration of high dosage alternate day steroids. This has increased the number of severe cases, often with extensive malignant thymomata presenting for thymectomy as well as the numbers needing careful, often prolonged, post-operative management involving tracheostomy or prolonged intubation to prevent pulmonary contamination from bulbar weakness and to permit controlled or assisted respiration. Loach *et al.* (1975) showed that a low pre-operative vital capacity is likely to necessitate post-operative artificial ventilation but it is important to remember that post-operative improvement may be considerably delayed. Tracheostomy may have to be maintained for many months in a few cases before swallowing returns.

Dystrophia Myotonica (see also Chapter 28, p. 936)

Myotonia of the respiratory muscles commonly occurs in dystrophia myotonica. This may lead to a large reduction in the patient's vital capacity and maximum breathing capacity (Kaufman, 1960). It has been stated by Dundee (1952) that patients with dystrophia myotonica are particularly susceptible to thiopentone, possibly due to a specific peripheral action of the drug, but further studies have not substantiated this cause. While it is true that patients suffering from dystrophia myotonica are sensitive to thiopentone—100 mg may cause apnoea for twenty minutes—the effect is probably a central one and common to all respiratory depressant drugs. Weakness of the muscles of respiration may lead to respiratory inadequacy when depressant drugs are given, or when the work of breathing is increased.

Patients with dystrophia myotonica are sometimes presented for anaesthesia, particularly because premature cataract is one of the features of the disease. A period of artificial respiration may be necessary post-operatively, but myotonia of the respiratory muscles may make ventilation extremely difficult, if not impossible. The reaction to muscle relaxants is variable because the abnormality is in the muscle fibre itself. Quinine hydrochloride in doses of 300–600 mg may be useful, as it is said to prolong the refractory period of the muscle fibre after contraction (Harvey, 1939).

Chronic Bronchitis and Emphysema

Pulmonary changes in chronic bronchitis and emphysema are irreversible and progressive. The progression is not uniform, however. Successive bouts of superadded acute infection occur with increasing frequency. Patients usually die during these acute exacerbations from carbon dioxide retention leading to narcosis with further secretion retention. Severe ventilation-perfusion inequalities exist in the lung and give rise to marked hypoxaemia. Possibly due to the accumulation of bicarbonate in the cerebrospinal fluid, the respiratory centre, via its chemoreceptors, becomes less sensitive to increases in carbon dioxide tension and hypoxia forms the main drive to respiration. If hypoxia is relieved, respiration is further depressed, carbon dioxide accumulates and unconsciousness supervenes. In an attempt to prevent this sequence of events, Campbell (1960) described a method by which oxygen can be given to these patients in a controlled concentration which can be varied between 24 and 35 per cent. A special mask, working on the venturi principle, is used (p. 199). This has two advantages. The high flow rate produced prevents any rebreathing from the mask and minimises a further rise in arterial carbon dioxide tension. The oxygen lack is only partly corrected and the hypoxic drive to ventilation is thereby maintained. Owing to the shape of the oxygen dissociation curve for blood this relatively small increase in inspired oxygen tension produces a much larger rise in arterial oxygen content, and with careful supervision a course can be steered between dangerous hypoxia and narcosis from carbon dioxide. In severely ill patients this method is not always successful (Satinder Lal, 1965; Warrell et al., 1970). Furthermore, it seems reasonable to assume that it is best, if possible, to correct the hypoxia completely in patients so seriously ill. When this leads to severe carbon dioxide retention and narcosis, the alternatives are either to use a lower inspired oxygen concentration or to perform tracheostomy and artificial respiration. Their comparative merits cannot be finally decided until there are more data on the survival rate of patients treated by each of these two methods (Bradley et al., 1964). The aim of tracheostomy and fully controlled respiration under these conditions is to produce a normal arterial P_{CO_2} during treatment. Over physiological ranges the carbon dioxide dissociation curve for blood is virtually a straight line. It is therefore possible to compensate for under-ventilated or non-ventilated alveoli by hyperventilating the remainder, and normal arterial P_{CO_2} can usually be achieved by using large ventilatory volumes and high inflation pressures. This may necessitate the use of a volume-cycled machine. Unfortunately, it is not possible to relieve the hypoxia by hyperventilation, as a glance at the oxygen dissociation curve for blood will show. In fact, arterial oxygen tensions may even be reduced by artificial ventilation, due to increased maldistribution of ventilation and perfusion. It is, therefore, essential in these patients to measure the arterial oxygen tension frequently to ensure that adequate arterial tensions are maintained with the lowest possible concentration of oxygen in the inspired air.

There is an alternative way in which artificial ventilation can be used in acute exacerbations of chronic bronchitis (Sheldon, 1963). Assisted respiration using a patient-triggered ventilator is applied via an anaesthetic face-mask, mouthpiece or endotracheal tube. This technique can only be used for relatively short periods and rarely achieves a normal arterial Pco_2, but it may be sufficient to enable the patient to survive his acute exacerbation. Assisted respiration may prevent respiratory failure by reducing the work of breathing, which is much increased in obstructive lung disease.

A two to three week period of fully controlled artificial ventilation via a tracheostomy, may, if the volume of ventilation is sufficient to produce a normal arterial Pco_2, actually improve the patient's respiratory function after treatment is discontinued. Two mechanisms may be involved here. Rigidity of the thoracic cage, which is a common sequel to chronic bronchitis and emphysema, may be reduced by a period of forcible ventilation. After chronic carbon dioxide retention it may require several weeks of fully adequate ventilation for normal ionic concentrations in the cerebrospinal fluid to be restored (Semple, 1965). If this can be achieved, the patient may be able to maintain near-normal carbon dioxide tensions when artificial ventilation is stopped. This is possibly because the respiratory centre has been resensitised to carbon dioxide.

Weaning from artificial ventilation may be particularly difficult in these patients, so that it is well to decide in advance which patients are liable to become ventilator-dependent cripples. Munck et al. (1961) suggested that a useful guide might be obtained by assessing the patient's exercise tolerance and respiratory history prior to the acute exacerbation. Bradley et al. (1964) found a well-marked correlation between difficulty in weaning and the degree of emphysema detectable on the chest X-ray. This can be assessed by signs of attenuation of the peripheral pulmonary arteries and increased transradiancy of the lung fields (Fletcher et al., 1963).

Jessen et al. (1967) in a ten-year follow-up of 111 patients with chronic lung disease treated with IPPR divided their patients into three groups based on their physical states before treatment. These important results are summarised in the table below:

Patients		Survival rates on discharge	Survival rates three years after discharge
		%	%
Patients able to work to some extent	A	85	58
Patients unable to work but able to leave home for personal needs	B	70	31
Patients confined to their homes	C	50	0

They concluded that if artificial ventilation is undertaken for patients in group C they can be expected to require lifelong intermittent or constant artificial ventilation.

Status Asthmaticus

Reports have suggested that mortality from asthma may be increasing (Speizer *et al.*, 1968) and that this may be associated with increased use of corticosteroids and pressurised aerosols. Lung pathology in asthma has also been studied and it is now recognised that in severe asthma bronchial plugs are formed. These plugs are tenacious and persistent and completely obstruct many of the smaller bronchi. Mechanical ventilation combined with efficient humidification, possibly by bronchial lavage, have been used to overcome this problem. The results of Marchand and Van Hasselt (1966) and Ambiavagar and Sherwood Jones (1967) testify to the effectiveness of these methods in skilled hands.

The indications for mechanical interference are still under discussion. Once collapse, coma or respiratory arrest have occurred, interference is obligatory, but more difficult and less likely to be successful. It is therefore important to recognise clinical signs which may herald a life-threatening deterioration. Death in asthma can occur suddenly and unexpectedly (Earle, 1953). A rising Pa_{CO_2} is a late sign of deterioration but it is possible that taken in conjunction with the respiratory effort the patient is capable of generating, it may be helpful. A useful clinical measure of this effort is the magnitude of paradoxical arterial pressure swings with breathing. In severe asthma the systolic arterial pressure can vary by as much as 40 mm Hg (5·3 kPa) with respiration. The work involved in generating such pressure swings is great and few patients can sustain it for long. Decreasing arterial paradox and a rising Pa_{CO_2} would therefore seem, at present, to be the most useful criteria for judging when mechanical assistance is necessary.

Mechanical ventilation in asthma presents many problems and requires great care. The chest is already hyperinflated due to air trapping and efforts by the patient to increase bronchial calibre. Over-enthusiastic IPPR can easily worsen this state and cause severe embarrassment to the right ventricle. Ventilation must be set to the maximum which will not cause unacceptable hypotension and increasing chest distension. It is seldom possible to achieve anything approaching a normal Pa_{CO_2} during the early stages and for this reason heavy sedation or curarisation are needed to prevent the patient from fighting the machine.

Bronchial lavage by repeated instillation of 10 ml of sterile isotonic saline has been used successfully and certainly produces a good harvest of bronchial casts from the smaller bronchi with consequent easing of the difficulties of ventilation (Ambiavagar and Sherwood Jones, 1967). There are theoretical and practical objections to this technique. In normal lungs, saline lavage has been shown to cause a sustained decrease in lung compliance and a fall in Pa_{O_2} due to increased venous admixture (Colebatch and Halmagyi, 1961; Simenstad *et al.*, 1963). Further hypoxaemia in already hypoxic patients, even though temporary, may be dangerous and the technique must therefore be used with speed, skill and caution. Provided an efficient ventilator is available it may be that other methods of humidification, using ultrasonic vibrators to generate a finely divided aerosol, are better though slower (Herzog *et al.*, 1964; Stevens and Albregt, 1966).

Neonatal Respiratory Distress Syndrome (Hyaline Membrane Disease)

Advances in the understanding of the nature of this condition and improvement in apparatus and techniques of artificial ventilation in neonates have recently enabled an improvement in mortality to be achieved.

Artificial ventilation is still the mainstay of supportive treatment though the indications for its use vary in different reports. The most important indications are:

1. Recurrent apnoeic attacks in the small premature baby.
2. Continued deterioration despite adequate conservative therapy including complete correction of fluid and acid base disturbances (Reid *et al.*, 1967).

The techniques of artificial ventilation required are similar to those used in other neonatal conditions. Opinion varies as to whether it is best performed via an endotracheal tube or tracheostomy (Reid and Tunstall, 1966; Glover, 1965). (See also p. 400, Prolonged endotracheal intubation.)

Pneumonia

Artificial respiration has occasionally been advocated as a treatment for severe lobar pneumonia. It is rarely effective and the additional hazards to which the patient is subjected are not justified by the results obtained. The consolidated area of lung acts as an A-V shunt, producing severe arterial desaturation. The drive to ventilation is increased by this hypoxia and respiratory minute volumes of 10–20 litres are usual. Arterial Po_2 and Pco_2 are both low. Under these conditions the patient is usually able to do better for himself than a machine can do for him.

IPPR in the Post-operative Period

The effects of pre-existing pulmonary disease are usually increased by surgery and anaesthesia since coughing is impaired by pain, and a tracheostomy may be needed to remove secretions. The ability of severely ill and debilitated patients to prevent pharyngeal contents from entering their lungs is greatly impaired (Gardner, 1958) and a cuffed tracheostomy tube is of value in isolating the lungs from the pharynx. Nunn and Payne (1962) showed that hypoxaemia in the post-operative period is common, even in patients with normal lungs. This effect is probably due to an increase in ventilation-perfusion inequalities. It is likely to be greater in patients with pre-existing pulmonary disease and may precipitate respiratory failure.

After cardiac surgery artificial respiration may be particularly valuable. Signs of respiratory distress, an increasing tachycardia, circulatory failure or neurological damage are the most important indications for its use. The work of breathing is removed, oxygen demands reduced and despite the potentially adverse circulatory effects of IPPR most patients are improved by its use (Zeitlin, 1965). Some authorities use artificial respiration routinely after open cardiac surgery (Dammann *et al.*, 1963). The place of artificial respiration in the post-operative period has been reviewed by Norlander (1968) and for further reading reference should be made to *Respiratory Failure* by Sykes *et al.* (1976).

Drowning

Experimental study of human drowning and semi-drowning is virtually impossible, but various mechanisms have been postulated following animal experiments. Their relevance to human drowning is open to some doubt. The remarkable recovery of several children after lengthy immersion in icy fluids (Theilade, 1977) exemplifies this doubt. Apparently, in these patients, ventricular fibrillation did not occur, although experimental evidence from animals suggests that it should have been present for a considerable period before resuscitation was started.

From animal experiments, different consequences have been suggested following salt and fresh water drowning.

Salt water.—Being hypertonic, inhalation of sea water causes plasma water to be drawn into the alveoli, thus the lungs increase in weight and widespread peripheral haemorrhages occur. There may follow contraction of the endothelial cells, due to osmotic gradients between intracellular fluid and the sea water in the alveoli (Halmagyi, 1961). Pulmonary compliance decreases and arterial oxygen saturation falls, due to increased venous admixture (Halmagyi and Colebatch, 1961). Haemoconcentration has been said to occur, but the experimental evidence is doubtful. It is possible that blood volume may rise as water is drawn from the tissues. Serum sodium and potassium rise, and death is probably due to ventricular fibrillation following hypoxia and electrolyte disturbance.

Fresh water.—The sequence of events in fresh water drowning is somewhat clearer. Inhaled water is rapidly lost from the alveoli and a 50 per cent rise in blood volume may occur in 2–3 minutes, which accounts for the phenomenon known as "dry drowning". Lungs free of fluid have often been noticed at postmortem and this finding has previously been attributed to protection of the lungs by laryngeal spasm. Haemodilution causes rupture of red cells and liberation of potassium, so that death is due to ventricular fibrillation from hyperkalaemia and anoxia.

Modell (1968) cast doubt on the validity of these dogmatic distinctions between salt and fresh water drowning. In a review of data from several published series Rivers *et al.* (1970) concluded that there are no significant differences in the clinical pathology that can be attributed to the salinity of the drowning fluid.

The clinical picture presented by partly drowned subjects is due primarily to secondary effects such as hypoxaemia, aspiration pneumonitis and pulmonary oedema, rather than to the type of water aspirated.

In the clinical management of victims of near drowning, emphasis must be placed on correcting these disturbances and the electrolyte disorders which are usually present. Victims of drowning are frequently seriously hypothermic—a condition all too easy to miss in clinical practice, when body temperature is too low to register on a standard clinical thermometer. Rewarming of the near drowned is less hazardous than rewarming victims of air exposure, though ventricular fibrillation frequently occurs during rewarming. The mechanism of ventricular fibrillation during rewarming is probably that surface warming places unacceptable demands on the still cold myocardium, and it has been suggested that rewarming by preferential microwave heating of the heart might avoid this problem. In practice this technique is rarely available but an effective and safe alternative is to immerse one forearm and hand in a thermostatically heated stirred water bath at 41° C. This apparatus is widely available in most laboratories and allows the heart to warm first. Cardiac output rises and general rewarming is accelerated. It is important that the water in the bath be continuously stirred if rapid rewarming is to be achieved. This technique of rewarming is unfortunately not mentioned in an otherwise excellent review of the treatment of immersion by Golden and Rivers (1975).

Pulmonary damage following drowning may be considerable and artificial ventilation with the addition of PEEP may be needed for some days. The development of necrotising bronchopneumonia some days after apparent recovery is a serious risk as is well illustrated in a recent case report by Marshall Barr and Taylor (1976). The pathophysiology of the lungs in drowning is remarkably similar to that of terminal respiratory failure (see p. 386) and artificial respiration needs to be managed similarly.

Hyperventilation and drowning.—Hyperventilation and breath-holding prior to underwater swimming are dangerous. Hyperventilation causes only a small increase in arterial oxygen tension, but a considerable reduction in carbon dioxide tension. Cerebral blood flow is thereby reduced. Valsalva's manoeuvre may be maintained unintentionally during breath-holding, causing a fall in cardiac output, and a further fall in cerebral blood flow. During swimming a muscle oxygen debt is built up and glucose metabolism only proceeds to the lactic acid stage, so little carbon dioxide is formed. Cerebral hypoxia sufficiently severe to cause unconsciousness may then occur before sufficient carbon dioxide has accumulated to produce in the swimmer the desire to breathe (Dumitru and Hamilton, 1963).

Drug Overdosage

Massive overdosage with any sedative or hypnotic drug can cause respiratory or circulatory failure. Until recently barbiturates were the commonest group of drugs used for suicidal attempts. Following the decline in their use as sleeping pills, in favour of drugs such as benzodiazepines, most suicidal attempts today are made with other drugs such as tranquillisers and antidepressants. Salicylate overdosage has increased and its treatment is much more difficult than that of barbiturate overdosage. At least, however, it can be said that due to the variety of drugs now involved, decrease in the use of barbiturates has made the treatment of drug overdose more interesting. Experience has shown conclusively that the best treatment is to support respiration and circulation rather than to rely on antidotes, but it is also possible to hasten normal excretion of the drug (see also Chapter 22, p. 771). With many drugs gross oral overdosage causes gastric irritation which predisposes to vomiting and inhalation. Partial obstruction of the airway may have existed for some hours, and this makes regurgitation even more likely (O'Mullane, 1954). The first step is to pass an endotracheal tube and perform bronchial toilet. Only when this has been done is it safe to wash out the stomach. Gastric lavage is probably desirable when there is evidence that drug ingestion has been recent. It carries the risk however of diluting the drug in the stomach and upper intestine and increasing absorption. If the patient is sufficiently deeply unconscious to permit passage of an endotracheal tube without difficulty, it is best to assume that pharyngeal contents have already entered the lungs. This is often confirmed by bronchial toilet. If it is suspected, bronchoscopy should follow gastric lavage. Under these conditions bronchoscopy itself is not without hazard, since it may provoke further regurgitation during introduction or removal of the bronchoscope. The initial stages of the treatment of drug overdosage are most important and may greatly affect the chances of a successful outcome. It is easy to underestimate the severity of the condition, and unless vigorous treatment is started at the earliest possible moment, the patient may die from bronchopneumonia or other pulmonary complications a few days later.

Drug overdosage is one of the conditions in which a subatmospheric phase during IPPR may be of real value, since poisoning with many drugs appears to depress, probably centrally, the reflex mechanisms responsible for maintaining venous tone, with resultant hypotension.

Head Injury with or without Cervical Cord Injury

In the majority of moderately severe head injuries, the passage of a cuffed endotracheal tube may be all the respiratory treatment necessary. A clear airway is maintained and the trachea is isolated from pharyngeal contents. In some severe head injuries respiratory assistance may be needed. This usually indicates a grave prognosis, unless respiratory failure is precipitated by a rapid rise in intracranial pressure which it is possible to relieve surgically.

Head injury is sometimes accompanied by fracture dislocation of the cervical spine. Damage to the spinal cord resulting from this may cause respiratory failure and quadraplegia. In the presence of a head injury, this condition may be missed for some time, respiratory failure being attributed to the head injury. This is particularly likely if the cord is damaged below the origin of the phrenic nerve. The diaphragmatic component of respiration continues to function, but ventilation may become inadequate and require augmentation.

Tracheostomy in head injury.—Unless there is some evidence of inhalation of pharyngeal contents, the decision to perform tracheostomy is probably best left for at least 48 hours. An endotracheal tube can be used in the interim period, provided that the inspired air is efficiently humidified and it is possible to keep the lungs clear. At the end of this time many patients have recovered sufficiently to make further measures unnecessary. The presence of a tracheostomy tube irritates the trachea and increases coughing, intracranial pressure is raised and cortical damage may be increased.

Artificial respiration and cerebral oedema.—The place of artificial respiration and therapeutic hypothermia in the treatment of cerebral oedema following head injury is still the subject of debate. Hyperventilation reduces intracranial pressure and is widely used for this purpose during neurosurgery. Its value in cerebral oedema is more doubtful as blood flow to oedematous tissue may be seriously reduced thereby increasing hypoxic oedema. Hypoventilation, however, is harmful and artificial respiration may be necessary to prevent it. Hyperthermia is also harmful and active steps, involving artificial respiration, may be helpful in preventing it. Whether, by reducing cerebral oxygen needs, hypothermia is beneficial is debatable. The value of dexamethasone as an anti-oedema agent is well-established and the present trend is to combine its use with mild hyperventilation and slight hypothermia. It should be remembered that similar considerations apply to the treatment of cerebral oedema following anoxic cerebral insults due to all causes.

Status Epilepticus

Most patients with status epilepticus can be satisfactorily controlled by sedation and general measures, but artificial ventilation may occasionally be needed in severe cases. It must be considered if sedation fails to control the patient's fits. Under these conditions, the combination of heavy sedation, persistent unconsciousness between fits and respiratory arrest during each fit, may produce dangerous underventilation and pulmonary complications. Violent muscular activity increases the body's oxygen requirements and predisposes to respiratory insufficiency.

Poliomyelitis

Until a few years ago, poliomyelitis was the commonest single condition in which artificial respiration was needed for long periods. Many of the details of technique and management were worked out on patients with poliomyelitis. With the widespread use of effective vaccines, new cases of paralytic poliomyelitis are rare, at least in countries where the facilities for effective artificial ventilation are available.

Many patients, who contracted the disease some years ago, are still alive and remain extensively paralysed. In the acute phase of spinobulbar poliomyelitis the ability to swallow is usually lost and a tracheostomy must be performed. Swallowing commonly returns when the acute phase of the disease is over. If so, the cuff of the tracheostomy tube can be deflated, and the patient is able to talk during the inspiratory period.

The indications for artificial respiration are the same in all the paralysing diseases, and have been conveniently considered together under the section on general management of artificial ventilation. Today, the most commonly seen patients with poliomyelitis are those who have reached the chronic stage of the disease and who suffer a temporary set back due to such things as an upper respiratory infection. Respiratory assistance, physiotherapy and antibiotics are usually sufficient to help the patient over the acute episode. A tracheostomy is rarely indicated, and to perform one may seriously handicap the subsequent management of the condition. Many patients, who are afflicted with long term respiratory weakness, become expert in the management of their state, and the best advice on the therapeutic needs can often be obtained from the patient himself. Heroic efforts have been made in rehabilitating these severely handicapped patients and astonishing results achieved in the face of an almost overwhelming disability.

For rational clinical management it is convenient to divide patients with respiratory impairment after poliomyelitis into the following four categories:

Grade 1

Those patients who need respiratory assistance during minor ailments, particularly upper respiratory tract infections, but who breathe spontaneously without assistance at all other times.

Grade 2

Those patients who regularly need respiratory assistance during sleep, but are normally able to maintain adequate spontaneous respiration during the day.

Grade 3

Those patients who need full artificial respiration during sleep and who require some degree of mechanical respiratory assistance during waking hours.

Grade 4

Those patients who need totally artificial respiration at all times and who therefore rapidly succumb if this fails and immediate support is not available.

Patients in Grade 1 usually have vital capacities over 800 ml and are able to cough adequately when well by inflating their lungs using glossopharyngeal breathing. During upper respiratory tract infections, secretions are increased and they are best treated in a rotating tank ventilator (see Figs. 6 and 7).

Patients in Grade 2 usually use a cuirass ventilator or rocking bed for sleeping and adopt the same techniques as those in Grade 1 during waking hours. They have vital capacities in the 400–800 ml range.

Grade 3 patients commonly need a tank ventilator for sleeping and use pneumobelts during the day. These can be battery driven and incorporated into a wheel chair. Hamilton *et al.* (1970) showed that periodic deep inflations using a simple positive-pressure source such as a reversed portable domestic vacuum cleaner may be helpful in maintaining normal arterial gas tensions in these patients. Their vital capacities are in the 150–400 ml range.

Grade 4 patients have a spontaneous vital capacity below 150 ml. Permanent tracheostomy and IPPR is usually essential, though it is best avoided in the less severe grades as it is liable to increase their degree of machinery dependence.

A number of patients in this severe category have succeeded in rehabilitating themselves from hospital and leading independent lives at home. They have developed combined wheel-chair respirators (Fig. 16a and b) and talk intermittently during the inspiratory stroke of the ventilator.

Polyneuritis

This term includes what is probably a group of similar diseases. Names such as acute toxic polyneuritis, infective neuronitis and Guillain Barré syndrome have been used. When the disease is severe enough to involve the muscles of respiration, the management is similar to that of poliomyelitis, but a number of important distinctions exist. The onset of paralysis is sometimes slower and more insidious. Daily measurements of vital capacity are particularly important in assessing the need for artificial ventilation. Owing to the gradual onset and slow increase in paralysis, the patient is often less disturbed by his weakness and marked respiratory insufficiency can exist without the patient appearing distressed. In polyneuritis it is less usual for the muscles of respiration to be affected without involvement of the muscles of deglutition. A tracheostomy is therefore essential, and treatment in a tank ventilator rarely indicated. Polyneuritis sometimes affects the autonomic nervous system (Watson, 1962d). This may produce circulatory disturbances wholly or partly due to interruption of the autonomic reflex arcs which control the circulation, and a subatmospheric phase during the respiratory cycle is often necessary if an adequate circulation is to be maintained. Facial involvement in these patients may prevent them from closing their eyes, and protection may be needed to avoid corneal ulceration.

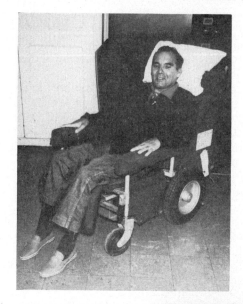

(a)

(b)

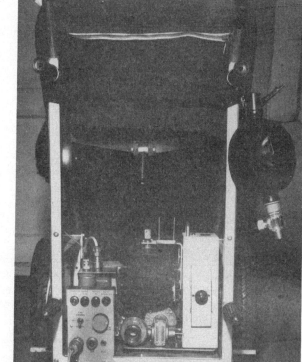

10/Fig. 16(a) and (b).—
The "Cavendish" wheel-
chair/ventilator.

The prognosis in polyneuritis is usually excellent. Virtually complete recovery is usual. These patients are some of the most rewarding to treat, and to lose one must be regarded as a tragedy. The presentation and management of polyneuritis has been well reviewed recently by McCleave *et al.* (1976) and evidence has been presented suggesting that patients severely affected by this condition show signs of sympathetic overactivity similar to that seen in severe tetanus (Dingle, 1969).

Chest Injuries

Chest injuries, involving sufficient disruption of the thoracic cage to cause serious interference with breathing, are difficult to treat. This is partly because the injury is rarely an isolated one, but is associated with a head or neck injury. Concurrent abdominal injuries, such as a ruptured spleen or liver, frequently present additional complications. Despite the theoretical disadvantage of IPPR, that of converting a pneumothorax or haemopneumothorax into a tension pneumothorax, it has proved of great value and is often life-saving. The indications for artificial respiration include pain and clinical distress on breathing, retention or inhalation of secretions and signs of paradoxical movement of the chest. Hypoxaemia may be present, due to increased venous admixture in areas of damaged, non-ventilated lung. This must be corrected at once. Endotracheal intubation, curarisation and positive-pressure ventilation using a high inspired oxygen concentration is the most effective method. Paradoxical movements of the chest are stopped, and the work of breathing which may be abnormally great if the airways are partly obstructed by foreign material, is eliminated.

Accumulation of carbon dioxide is usually a late sign of respiratory insufficiency in chest injuries. Its presence indicates that artificial ventilation is long overdue (Hunter, 1964).

It is probable that in assessing these complicated problems too much emphasis has been placed on the anatomical damage to the thoracic cage and not enough on damage to the underlying lung and the physiological disturbances resulting from this damage. Ambiavagar *et al.* (1966) showed that minor rib trauma in patients with pre-existing lung disease often constitutes a severe injury whereas, if pulmonary function is previously good and little new lung trauma results from the injury, respiratory function may be surprisingly little impaired, even after extensive rib injury.

Continuous thoracic epidural analgesia has been tried as a method of pain relief in these patients. Apart from localised chest injuries, in which pain and cough impairment may be slight, it is surprisingly ineffective. The source of pain extends over too many spinal cord segments for effective relief to be possible without producing unacceptable circulatory side-effects.

Scoliosis

Severe scoliosis is accompanied by deformity of the thoracic cage. Vital capacity is greatly reduced and coughing impaired by the structural deformity. Caro and Dubois (1961) have shown that chest wall compliance is progressively reduced as age advances. Lung compliance is also reduced. The patient is prone to recurrent pulmonary infections and eventually succumbs during an acute attack.

Artificial respiration by intermittent positive pressure is difficult to perform in scoliosis because vital capacity is so small. Tracheostomy is both difficult to perform and difficult to close. Its permanent presence is a severe handicap to a patient with respiratory insufficiency (see under poliomyelitis, p. 416). The pattern of respiratory failure in scoliosis is remarkably similar to that in poliomyelitis in that it is restrictive rather than obstructive and characterised by nocturnal hypoventilation. Until the disease has been present for many years the lungs remain essentially normal and the hypoxaemia commonly present appears to be due to reduced functional residual capacity rather than obstructive airway disease. It is therefore potentially reversible and the use of the techniques of respiratory assistance developed for the treatment of poliomyelitis are particularly appropriate though technically difficult due to the anatomical deformities. Carefully applied these methods can completely correct respiratory failure in scoliosis and the prognosis is considerably better than that in respiratory failure due to obstructive airways disease (Spencer, 1977).

APPENDIX TO CHAPTER 10

AUTOMATIC VENTILATORS

PRINCIPLES OF VENTILATORS

Ventilators can be conveniently classified by the patterns of flow, volume and pressure which they produce in the patient's lungs. Unfortunately, this classification does not define function fully and the method by which the machine is cycled has to be considered. Thus the respiratory cycle of a ventilator can be divided into four parts:

1. The inspiratory phase.
2. The change-over from the inspiratory to the expiratory phase.
3. The expiratory phase.
4. The change-over from the expiratory to the inspiratory phase.

(Mapleson, 1969).

1. The Inspiratory Phase

Flow generators.—These are ventilators which deliver a predetermined flow during the inspiratory phase. The flow may be generated by a compressor which pumps out a fixed volume at each stroke or revolution. The flow is not necessarily constant as many ventilators deliver a near sinusoidal flow. This can be generated by a bag or bellows which is compressed directly by a cam or crank, or indirectly by pneumatic compression of a bag in a bottle.

The volume delivered by a flow generator is independent of the resistance caused by the ventilator tubing, the patient's airway or the pulmonary compliance. An increase in any of these variables will produce a rise in inflation pressure rather than a fall in ventilatory volume. Flow generators are therefore particularly suitable for ventilating patients with pulmonary disease in whom they will maintain a constant minute volume despite variations in airway resistance or compliance. They are susceptible, however, to leaks in the circuit, because air so lost causes a corresponding loss to the inflation volume.

Compression volume.—Not all of the flow generated by the ventilator enters the patient's lungs and some is absorbed by air compression in the ventilator circuit. If the inflation pressure is high, or the volume of the humidifier or ventilator circuit large in relation to the tidal volume, losses from compression may be significant. Both these factors combine when small babies are being ventilated. Under these conditions the compression volume may be several times greater than the tidal volume.

Pressure generators.—These are ventilators which generate a constant pressure during the inspiratory phase. The pressure may be generated by the release of gas or air from a pressure source, or by a weight acting on a concertina bag.

The volume delivered by a pressure generator is dependent on the resistance of the ventilator circuit, the patient's airways and the pulmonary compliance. Regular measurements of minute volume will therefore provide an indication of changes in these variables, such as occur when secretions accumulate.

Pressure generators will to some extent compensate for leaks in the ventilator circuit. A leak acts as a loss of resistance, and a correspondingly greater volume will be delivered by the predetermined pressure. Equally, volume loss due to compression in the tubing will be constant and therefore less significant than when a flow generator is used.

Owing to the limits of pressure available it may be impossible, when airway resistance is high, to achieve the desired volume of ventilation. Maximum difficulty is encountered when ventilating small babies with pulmonary abnormalities.

2. The Change-over from the Inspiratory to the Expiratory Phase

Cycling at the end of inspiration may occur in three ways.

(*A*). *Time cycling.*—In time cycled ventilators the change-over from inspiration to expiration occurs after a fixed time and is uninfluenced by the state of the patient's lungs. The timing mechanism may be operated pneumatically, electrically or mechanically.

(*B*). *Pressure cycling.*—Here, the change-over occurs when a predetermined pressure is reached. The time taken to reach the critical pressure is influenced by the resistance offered by the patient's lungs, and will be reached more quickly when the resistance is high. An alteration in airway resistance is detectable by the alteration in respiratory rate which accompanies it.

(*C*). *Volume cycling.*—In volume-cycled ventilators, the change-over occurs when a fixed volume has been delivered from the machine. It occurs mechanically when the cam operating the bellows reaches the end of its stroke. It can also be made to occur by limiting the stroke of the bellows by a mechanical trip.

3. The Expiratory Phase

It is possible to apply the same terminology to the expiratory phase as has been used above to describe the inspiratory phase. This is cumbersome, however, as ventilators vary a lot in their expiratory phase characteristics and several different patterns may exist in the same ventilator at different stages of the expiratory phase. The simplest method of expiration is to connect the patient's lungs to the atmosphere. Most ventilators are now capable of exerting a subatmospheric pressure during the expiratory phase, which may last throughout it or only for part of it. The greatest negative pressure may occur at the start of expiration, and thereafter decline, or the pressure may become increasingly negative as the expiratory phase continues. At present no data is available to suggest which is the best pattern, and a functional analysis is therefore valueless. It can be argued that it is best to apply the greatest negative pressure at the start of expiration when bronchial calibre is larger and air trapping less likely to occur. It can be argued with equal force that a sudden change from maximum positive to maximum negative pressure may predispose to air trapping, and subatmospheric pressure is therefore best applied in a gradually increasing pattern. In certain patients (see p. 390) it is thought beneficial to maintain a slight positive pressure during the expiratory phase. This is called Positive End-Expiratory Pressure (PEEP). It can be achieved by introducing a restriction into the expiratory limb of the ventilator, in which case the flow will remain more nearly constant throughout expiration but positive pressure will steadily decline. It has been held to be preferable to aim for a constant pressure during expiration. This necessitates the use of a combination of a variable flow with a pressure sensor which is usually only possible in electronically controlled ventilators.

4. The Change-over from the Expiratory to the Inspiratory Phase

In practice only two methods are used for this change-over:

Time-cycling.—Here, the changeover from the expiratory phase to the inspiratory phase occurs at a pre-set time. In some ventilators, the timing of the expiratory cycle can be varied independently of the inspiratory cycle. In others, the two cycles cannot be varied independently, and the proportions of the respiratory cycle occupied by inspiration and expiration are fixed.

Patient cycling.—Ventilators which include this feature are commonly known as triggered ventilators, or assistors. A slight inspiratory effort by the patient produces a subatmospheric pressure in the ventilator tubing, which triggers off the change-over from the expiratory phase to the inspiratory phase, and the patient's spontaneous inspiration is augmented. A simple patient-cycling device of this type suffers from the disadvantage that, if the patient stops making inspiratory efforts, the machine stops cycling. In modern electronically-controlled ventilators it is therefore more usual to incorporate a patient-cycled over-ride system so that the machine will follow and augment an occasional, spontaneous, inspiratory effort, while at the same time maintaining a constant lower level of controlled ventilation. The lower this level is set, the more will the patient cycling over-ride operate. This has been called Intermittent Mandatory Ventilation (IMV).

In addition to assessing its function, a number of other factors have to be taken into account in choosing the most suitable ventilator for a particular purpose or hospital.

Motive Power

This may be provided by an electric motor or by a pressure input of gas or air, or by a combination of the two. No source of motive power is completely reliable and an ideal machine should, therefore, be capable of manual operation in the event of power failure. Ventilators driven mechanically by an electric motor usually provide this facility and should be capable of entraining their own room air in the event of gas input failure. Some also incorporate an alternative electrical supply or motor which will continue to operate the machine for a limited period following mains failure. Gas powered machines cannot operate if the gas pressure source fails. This may be an important consideration in hospitals with an incomplete or unreliable pipeline system.

Many modern ventilators are electronically cycled with flow sensors in the patient circuit. This system allows great flexibility in use but usually means that the machine is dependent upon both a reliable electrical and gas pressure source.

In the absence of these facilities, such machines are a liability.

BACTERIAL CONTAMINATION AND STERILISATION OF VENTILATORS

The bacterial contamination of automatic lung ventilators is a common occurrence during prolonged artificial respiration, and the possibility of transferring bacteria from one patient to another via the ventilator has been recognised for some time (Phillips and Spencer, 1965). Nevertheless the number of adequately documented instances are few (Phillips, 1967; Wright *et al.*, 1961; Bishop *et al.*, 1962). The organism concerned is usually *Pseudomonas aeruginosa*, which rapidly colonizes the upper respiratory tract of many patients following prophylactic antibiotic therapy and endotracheal intubation (Redman and Lockey, 1967). Although Helliwell *et al.* (1967) showed experimentally that bacteria introduced into the inspiratory limb of a ventilator did not spread in a retrograde direction, their results are in conflict with the experience of Phillips and Spencer (1965) and Reinarz *et al.* (1965). Multiplication of vegetative micro-organisms in the water bath humidifier of a ventilator can occur rapidly. This can be prevented either by filling the humidifier with a solution of 0·1 per cent chlorhexidine in distilled water, or by maintaining the water in the humidifier at a pasteurizing temperature of 60° C (Glover, 1966).

Filters

An absolute bacterial filter has been described by Bishop *et al.* (1963) for attachment to the air intake of ventilators. This is useful in cleaning incoming air, but it does not prevent contamination of the ventilator by the patient. Ideally, filters should be placed in the inspiratory and expiratory tubing to the patient, isolating him from the ventilator. The filter described above cannot be used in this position as it becomes blocked by water droplets condensed from the humidifier and the expired air. Blockage can be overcome by a suitable filter design (Pyle *et al.*, 1969), but unfortunately, when a volume cycled ventilator is used, filters in this position add substantially to the compression volume of the circuit.

Although filters are useful in delaying ventilator contamination by the patient, there is general agreement that they do not obviate the need to sterilise the ventilator between patients if it has been in action for more than a few days (Spencer *et al.*, 1968).

DISINFECTION OF VENTILATORS

A variety of methods of disinfecting ventilators between use has been described. These methods have been compared by Fisher and Kyi Kyi (1969). None is completely satisfactory and all have disadvantages. The only ideal solution is to design autoclavable ventilators (Norlander *et al.*, 1968).

Ethylene Oxide

This is a highly toxic and explosive gas which is heavier than air, freely soluble in water and rubber, and has only a faint smell. It can be used to sterilise apparatus which would be damaged by heat. Sterilisation is efficient provided the conditions are carefully controlled. It has been advocated as an agent for sterilising ventilators by Bishop *et al.* (1962), who enclosed the ventilator in a polyvinyl chloride bag containing a mixture of 10 per cent ethylene oxide in carbon dioxide—a mixture which is non-explosive. Ethylene oxide passes freely through polyvinyl chloride (Thomas, 1960) and a "Polythene" bag is preferable. It is doubtful whether the use of ethylene oxide in a plastic bag is either efficient or safe, and it is probably best restricted to specialised plant designed for the purpose.

Formaldehyde

Formaldehyde vapour can be used to sterilise ventilator circuits by intro-ducing 100 ml formaldehyde B.P. into the water bath humidifier and running the machine for a period. Although this method is effective, formalin can remain in the ventilator and contaminate the patient's lungs when next the machine is in use (Sykes, 1964). Residual formalin can be neutralised with ammonia vapour blown through the ventilator in a similar manner. A sophisticated sterilising chamber using this method is now available (Phillips *et al.*, 1974). Although relatively expensive to purchase and install, it is probably the most efficient method of disinfection at present available.

Alcohol Aerosol

This method was described by Peterson and Rosdahl (1966) and has proved satisfactory throughout considerable clinical experience (Spencer *et al.*, 1968; Gullers *et al.*, 1969). It has been suggested by Judd *et al.* (1968) that the alcohol method carries an explosion risk, but Herzog *et al.* (1970) have shown convincingly that this is not so.

The method depends on the generation of a finely divided mist of 70 per cent ethyl alcohol or 70 per cent isopropyl alcohol by an ultrasonic nebulizer (Herzog *et al.*, 1964). It can only be used for ventilators which are capable of conversion to a closed circuit system. It is desirable, though not essential, to fill the circuit with nitrogen before starting. The process is completed in two hours, and residual alcohol is not harmful to the next patient. It does, however, require very careful supervision by the user if reliable results are to be achieved.

Hydrogen Peroxide

This method was described by Judd *et al.* (1968). A finely divided mist of 20 vol. per cent H_2O_2 B.P. is generated by an immersed plate ultrasonic DeVilbis nebulizer or Monaghan ultrasonic nebulizer. It is effective and probably less limited in its application than the alcohol method, although only the expiratory limb of some ventilators is disinfected. It is potentially harmful to the skin of the operator and unless the ventilator is allowed to stand for long enough to allow residual hydrogen peroxide to break down, can desquamate the trachea of the subsequent patient.

Picloxydine

This method was described by Meadows *et al.* (1968) and simplified by Nancekievill and Gaya (1969). Clinical experience is limited at present and its use has so far been confined to the Radcliffe ventilator. It appears to be effective, cheap and fairly rapid, but the disinfectant may cause damage to mechanical parts of the ventilator. It is somewhat messy in use, but residual disinfectant is probably harmless to the patient.

REFERENCES

AASS, A. S. (1975). Complications to tracheostomy and long-term intubation: a follow-up study. *Acta anaesth. scand.*, **19**, 127.

ABLETT, J. J. L. (1956). Tetanus and the anaesthetist. A review of the symptomatology and the recent advances in treatment. *Brit. J. Anaesth.*, **28**, 258.

ADAMS, E. B. (1958). Clinical trials in tetanus. *Proc. roy. Soc. Med.*, **51**, 1002.

AMBIAVAGAR, M., ROBINSON, J. S., MORRISON, I. M., and JONES, E. S. (1966). Intermittent positive pressure ventilation in the treatment of severe injuries of the chest. *Thorax*, **21**, 359.

AMBIAVAGAR, M., and SHERWOOD JONES, E. (1967). Resuscitation of the moribund asthmatic. *Anaesthesia*, **22**, 375.

ANDERSEN, M. N., and KUDRIBA, K. (1967). Depression of cardiac output with mechanical ventilation. Comparative studies of intermittent positive, positive negative and assisted ventilation. *J. thorac. cardiovasc. Surg.*, **54**, 182.

ARDRAN, G. M., KELLEHER, W. H., and KEMP, F. H. (1959). Cineradiographic studies of glossopharyngeal breathing. *Brit. J. Radiol.*, **32**, 322.

AUCHINLOSS, J. H., and GILBERT, R. (1967). An evaluation of the negative phase of a volume limited respirator. *Amer. Rev. resp. Dis.*, **95**, 66.

BARRACLOUGH, M. A., and SHARPEY-SCHAFER, E. P. (1963). Hypotension from absent circulatory reflexes. *Lancet*, **1**, 1121.

BARRAT, G., and ASUERO, M. S. (1975). Positive end-expiratory pressure. *Anaesthesia*, **30**, 183.

BEAVER, R. A. (1969). Respirators in respiratory failure. *Brit. med. J.*, **4**, 494.

BENDIXEN, H. H., HEDLEY-WHYTE, J., and LAVER, M. B. (1963). Impaired oxygenation in surgical patients during general anaesthesia with controlled ventilation. *New Engl. J. Med.*, **269**, 991.

BENDIXEN, H. H., SMITH, G. M., and MEAD, J. (1964). Pattern of ventilation in young adults. *J. appl. Physiol.*, **19**, 195.

BENEDICT, C. R., and KERR, J. H. (1977). Assessment of sympathetic overactivity in tetanus. *Brit. med. J.*, **2**, 806.

BISHOP, C., POTTS, M. W., and MOLLOY, P. J. (1962). A method of sterilization for the Barnet respirator. *Brit. J. Anaesth.*, **34**, 121.

BISHOP, C., ROPER, W. A. G., and WILLIAMS, S. R. (1963). The use of an absolute filter to sterilize the inspiratory air during intermittent positive pressure respiration. *Brit. J. Anaesth.*, **35**, 32.

BRADBEER, T. L., JAMES, M. L., SEAR, J. W., SEARLE, J. F., and STACEY, R. (1976). Tracheal stenosis associated with a low pressure cuffed endotracheal tube. *Anaesthesia*, **31**, 504.

BRADLEY, R. D., SPENCER, G. T., and SEMPLE, S. J. G. (1964). Tracheostomy and artificial ventilation in the treatment of acute exacerbations of chronic lung disease. *Lancet*, **1**, 845.

BROCK-VINE, J. G., WINNING, E., BOTHA, E., and GOODWIN, N. M. (1975). Chest physiotherapy during mechanical ventilation. *Anaesthesia and Intensive Care*, **3**, 234.

BROOK, M. H., BROOK, J., and WYANT, G. M. (1962). Emergency resuscitation. *Brit. med. J.*, **2**, 1564.

BRYCE-SMITH, R., and DAVIS, H. S. (1954). Tidal exchange in respirators. *Curr. Res. Anesth.*, **33**, 73.

BURTON, J. D. K. (1962). Effects of dry anaesthetic gases on the respiratory mucous membrane. *Lancet*, **1**, 235.

CAMPBELL, E. J. M. (1958). Mechanisms of airway obstruction in emphysema and asthma. *Proc. roy. Soc. Med.*, **51**, 108.

CAMPBELL, E. J. M. (1960). A method of controlled oxygen administration which reduces the risk of carbon dioxide retention. *Lancet*, **2**, 12.

CARO, G. C., and DUBOIS, A. B. (1961). Pulmonary function in kyphoscoliosis. *Thorax*, **16**, 282.

CHAMNEY, A. R. (1969). Humidification requirements and techniques, including a review of the performance of equipment in current use. *Anaesthesia*, **24**, 602.

COLE, L., and YOUNGMAN, H. (1968). An attack of tetanus. *Lancet*, **2**, 567.

COLE, L., and YOUNGMAN, H. (1969). Treatment of tetanus. *Lancet*, **1**, 1017.

COLEBATCH, H. J. H., and HALMAGYI, D. F. J. (1961). Lung mechanics and resuscitation after fluid aspiration. *J. appl. Physiol.*, **16**, 684.

COURNAND, A., MOTLEY, H. L., WERKO, L., and RICHARDS, D. W., Jnr. (1948). Physiologic studies of the effects of intermittent positive pressure breathing on cardiac output in man. *Amer. J. Physiol.*, **152**, 162.

CRAWLEY, B. E., and CROSS, D. E. (1975). Tracheal cuffs. A review and dynamic pressure study. *Anaesthesia*, **30**, 4.

DAMMANN, J. F., THUNG, M., CHRISTLIEB, I. I., LITTLEFIELD, J. B., and MULLER, W. H. (1963). The management of the severely ill patient after open heart surgery. *J. thorac. cardiovasc. Surg.*, **45**, 80.

DINGLE, H. R. (1969). Sympathetic overactivity in tetanus (in discussion). *Proc. roy. Soc. Med.*, **62**, 664.

DINNICK, O. P. (1975). Tracheal cuffs (letter). *Anaesthesia*, **30**, 553.

DUMITRU, A. P., and HAMILTON, F. G. (1963). A mechanism of drowning. *Anesth. Analg. Curr. Res.*, **42**, 170.

DUNDEE, J. W. (1952). Thiopentone in dystrophia myotonica. *Curr. Res. Anesth.*, **31**, 257.

EARLE, B. V. (1953). Fatal bronchial asthma. A series of fifteen cases with a review of the literature. *Thorax*, **8**, 195.

ELLIS, M. (1967). Editor: *Proceedings of a Symposium on Tetanus in Great Britain*, Leeds.

ENGSTRÖM, C.-G., and HERZOG, P. (1959). Ventilation nomogram for practical use with the Engström respirator. *Acta chir. scand.*, Suppl. **245**, 37.

FEARON, B., and COTTON, R. (1972). Surgical correction of subglottic stenosis of the larynx. *Ann. Otol. (St. Louis)*, **81**, 508.

FEYCHTING, H., and SETTERGREN, G. (1966). Automatic sighing device. *Lancet*, **1**, 26.

FISHER, M. F., and KYI KYI, K. (1969). Contamination and disinfection of lung ventilators. *Brit. Hosp. soc. Serv. J.*, 1404.

FLETCHER, C. M., HUGH-JONES, P., MCNICOL, M. W., and PRIDE, N. B. (1963). The diagnosis of pulmonary emphysema in the presence of chronic bronchitis. *Quart. J. Med.*, **32**, 33.

FOSTER, C. A., HEAF, P. J. D., and SEMPLE, S. J. G. (1957). Compliance of the lung in anaesthetised and paralysed subjects. *J. appl. Physiol.*, **11**, 383.

FRIMAN, L., HEDENSTIERNA, G., and SCHILDT, B. (1976). Stenosis following tracheostomy. A quantitative study of long term results. *Anaesthesia*, **31**, 479.

FROEB, H. F., and KIM, B. M. (1964). Tracheostomy and respiratory dead space in emphysema. *J. appl. Physiol.*, **19**, 92.

GALE, J. W., and WATERS, R. M. (1932). Closed endobronchial anaesthesia in thoracic surgery: A preliminary report. *J. thoracic Surg.*, **1**, 432.

GANENDRAN, A. (1974). Intensive therapy in neonatal tetanus. *Anaesthesia*, **29**, 356.

GARDNER, A. M. N. (1958). Aspiration of food and vomit. *Quart. J. Med.*, **27**, 227.

GLOVER, W. J. (1965). Mechanical ventilation in respiratory insufficiency in infants. *Proc. roy. Soc. Med.*, **58**, 902.

GLOVER, W. J. (1966). *Pseudomonas aeruginosa* cross infection (letter). *Lancet*, **1**, 203.

GOLDEN, F. St. C., and RIVERS, J. F. (1975). The immersion incident. *Anaesthesia*, **30**, 364.

GORMEZANO, J., and BRANTHWAITE, M. A. (1972). Effects of physiotherapy during intermittent positive pressure ventilation. *Anaesthesia*, **27**, 258.

GRANT, J. L., COOK, J., and MOULTON, P. P. (1964). Effects of tracheostomy in chronic pulmonary disease. *Amer. Rev. resp. Dis.*, **90**, 424.

GRENVIK, A. (1966). Respiratory, circulatory and metabolic effects of respirator treatment. *Acta anaesth. scand.*, Suppl. **19**.

GULLERS, K., MALMBORG, A.-S., NYSTRÖM, B., NORLANDER, O. P., and PETERSON, N. (1969). Clinical experience of disinfection of the Engström respirator by ultrasonic nebulized ethyl alcohol. *Acta anaesth. scand.*, **13**, 247.

HALMAGYI, D. F. J. (1961). Lung changes and incidence of respiratory arrest in rats after aspiration of sea and fresh water. *J. appl. Physiol.*, **16**, 41.

HALMAGYI, D. F. J., and COLEBATCH, J. H. (1961). Ventilation and circulation after fluid aspiration. *J. appl. Physiol.*, **16**, 35.

HAMILTON, E. A., NICHOLS, P. J. R., and TAIT, G. B. W. (1970). Late onset of respiratory insufficiency after poliomyelitis. *Ann. phys. Med.*, **10**, 223.

HARRISON, G. A., and TONKIN, J. P. (1967). Some serious laryngeal complications of prolonged endotracheal intubation. *Med. J. Aust.*, **1**, 605.

HARRISON, G. A., and TONKIN, J. P. (1968). Prolonged (therapeutic) endotracheal intubation. *Brit. J. Anaesth.*, **40**, 241.

HARVEY, A. M. (1939). Mechanism of action of quinine in myotonica and myasthenia. *J. Amer. med. Ass.*, **112**, 1562.

HELLIWELL, J., JEANES, A. L., WATKIN, R. R., and GIBBS, F. J. (1967). The Williams bacterial filter. *Anaesthesia*, **22**, 497.

HERHOLDT, J. D., and RAFN, C. G. (1796). *Life Saving Measures for Drowned Persons*. Copenhagen: Acta Anaesth. Scandinav. English translation by Henning Poulsen (1960).

HERZOG, P., NORLANDER, O. P., and ENGSTRÖM, C.-G. (1964). Ultrasonic generation of aerosol for the humidification of inspired gas during volume controlled ventilation. *Acta anaesth. scand.*, **8**, 79.

HERZOG, P., NORLANDER, O. P., and NYSTRÖM, B. (1970). Physical principles of ultrasonic aerosol generation for disinfection. *Proc. roy. Soc. Med.*, **63**, 911.

HEWITT, F. W. (1901) *Anaesthetics and their Administration*, p. 468, 2nd edit. London: Macmillan & Co.

HODGES, R. J. H., MORLEY, R., O'DRISCOLL, W. B., and McDONALD, I. (1956). A tracheostomy tube for use in acute poliomyelitis. *Lancet*, **1**, 26.

HOWELL, J. B. L., and PECKETT, B. W. (1957). Studies of the elastic properties of the thorax of supine anaesthetised paralysed human subjects. *J. Physiol. (Lond.)*, **136**, 1.

HUNTER, A. R. (1964). Artificial ventilation of the lungs in combined head and chest injuries. *Lancet*, **2**, 279.

HUNTER, J. (1776). Proposals for the recovery of people apparently drowned. *Phil. Trans. roy. Soc. Lond.*, **66**, 412.

IBSEN, B. (1954). The anaesthetist's viewpoint on the treatment of respiratory complications in poliomyelitis during the epidemic in Copenhagen. *Lancet*, **1**, 37.

JESSEN, O., SUND KRISTENSEN, H., and RASMUSSEN, K. (1967). Tracheostomy and artificial ventilation in chronic lung disease. *Lancet*, **2**, 9.

JUDD, P. A., TOMLIN, P. J., WHITBLY, J. L., INGLIS, T. C. M., and ROBINSON, J. S. (1968). Disinfection of ventilators by ultrasonic nebulisation. *Lancet*, **2**, 1019.

KAUFMAN, L. (1960). Anaesthesia in dystrophia myotonica. *Proc. roy. Soc. Med.*, **53**, 183.

KEILTY, S. R., GREY, R. C., DUNDEE, J. E., and McCULLOUGH, H. (1968). Catecholamine levels in severe tetanus. *Lancet*, **2**, 195.

KELLEHER, W. H. (1961). A new pattern of iron lung for the prevention and treatment of airway complications in paralytic disease. *Lancet*, **2**, 1113.

KELLEHER, W. H. (1969). Respirators in respiratory failure. *Brit. med. J.*, **3**, 528.

KELLY, R. F., and LAURENCE, D. R. (1956). Effect of chlorpromazine on convulsions of experimental and clinical tetanus. *Lancet*, **1**, 118.

KERR, J. H., CORBETT, J. L., PRYS-ROBERTS, C., CRAMPTON-SMITH, A., and SPALDING, J. M. K. (1968). Involvement of the sympathetic nervous system in tetanus. *Lancet*, **2**, 236.

KNOTT, F. A., and COLE, L. (1952). "Tetanus". In: *British Encyclopaedia of Medical Practice*, Vol. 12, p. 40. London: Butterworth & Co.

LASSEN, H. C. A. (1953). A preliminary report on the 1952 epidemic of poliomyelitis in Copenhagen with special reference to the treatment of acute respiratory insufficiency. *Lancet*, **1**, 37.

LINDHOLM, C. E. (1969). Prolonged endotracheal intubation. *Acta anaesth. scand.*, Suppl., **33**.

LLOYD, J. W., and McCLELLAND, R. M. A. (1964). Tracheal dilatation. *Lancet*, **2**, 83.

LOACH, A. B., YOUNG, A. C., SPALDING, J. M. K., and CRAMPTON-SMITH, A. C. (1975). Post-operative management after thymectomy. *Brit. med. J.*, **1**, 309.

McCLEAVE, D. J., FLETCHER, J., and CRUDEN, L. C. (1976). The Guillain-Barré syndrome in intensive care. *Anaesthesia and Intensive Care*, **4**, 46.

McCLELLAND, R. M. A. (1965). Complications of tracheostomy. *Brit. med. J.*, **2**, 567.

MACINTOSH, R. R. (1953). Oxford inflating bellows. *Brit. med. J.*, **2**, 202.

McINTYRE, R. W., LAWS, A. K., and RAMACHANDRAN, P. R. (1969). Positive expiratory pressure plateau: improved gas exchange during mechanical ventilation. *Canad. Anaesth. Soc. J.*, **16**, 477.

MAPLESON, W. W. (1969). In: *Automatic Ventilation of the Lungs*. Edit. Mushin, W. W. *et al.* Oxford: Blackwell Scientific Publications.

MAPLESON, W. W., MORGAN, J. G., and HILLARD, E. K. (1963). Assessment of condenser-humidifiers with special reference to a multiple-gauze model. *Brit. med. J.*, **1**, 300.

MARCHAND, P., and VAN HASSELT, H. (1966). Last-resort treatment of status asthmaticus. *Lancet*, **1**, 227.

MARSHALL BARR, A., and TAYLOR, M. (1976). A case of drowning. *Anaesthesia*, **31**, 651.

MEADOWS, G. A., RICHARDSON, J. C., FISH, E., and WILLIAMS, A. (1968). A method of sterilization for the East-Radcliffe ventilator. *Brit. J. Anaesth.*, **40**, 71.

MODELL, J. H. (1968). The pathophysiology and treatment of drowning. *Acta anaesth. scand.*, Suppl., **29**, 263.

MORGAN, B. C., MARTIN, W. E., HORNBEIN, T. F., CRAWFORD, E. W., and GUNTHEROTH, W. G. (1966). Haemodynamic effects of intermittent positive pressure respiration. *Anesthesiology*, **27**, 584.

MORGAN, M., LUMLEY, J., and SYKES, M. K. (1970). Arterial oxygenation and physiological deadspace during anaesthesia: effects of ventilation with a pressure preset ventilator. *Brit. J. Anaesth.*, **42**, 379.

MUNCK, O., KRISTENSEN, H. S., and LASSEN, H. C. A. (1961). Mechanical ventilation for acute respiratory failure in diffuse chronic lung disease. *Lancet*, **1**, 66.

NANCEKIEVILL, D. G., and GAYA, H. (1969). Disinfection of the East-Radcliffe ventilator. *Anaesthesia*, **24**, 42.

NASH, G., BLENNERHASSETT, J. B., and PONTOPPIDAN, H. (1967). Pulmonary lesions associated with oxygen therapy and artificial ventilation. *New Engl. J. Med.*, **276**, 368.

NORLANDER, O. P. (1968). The use of respirators in anaesthesia and surgery. *Acta anaesth. scand.*, Suppl. **30**.

NORLANDER, O. P., HERZOG, P., NORDEN, I., HOSSLI, G., SCHAER, H., and GATTIKER, R. (1968). Compliance and airway resistance during anaesthesia with controlled ventilation. *Acta anaesth. scand.*, **12**, 135.

NORLANDER, O. P., NORDEN, I., OLOFSSON, S., and HERZOG, P. (1968). The new Engström Respirator 300. *Acta anaesth. scand.*, **12**, 213.

NUNN, J. F., BERGMAN, N. A., and COLEMAN, A. J. (1965). Factors influencing the arterial oxygen tension during anaesthesia with artificial ventilation. *Brit. J. Anaesth.*, **37**, 898.

NUNN, J. F., and PAYNE, J. P. (1962). Hypoxaemia after general anaesthesia. *Lancet*, **2**, 631.

OKMIAN, L. G. (1966). Artificial ventilation by respirator for newborn and small infants during anaesthesia. *Acta anaesth. scand.*, Suppl. **20**.

O'MULLANE, E. J. (1954). Vomiting and regurgitation during anaesthesia. *Lancet*, **1**, 1209.

OPIE, L. H., SPALDING, J. M. K., and SMITH, A. C. (1961). Intrathoracic pressure during intermittent positive-pressure respiration. *Lancet*, **1**, 911.

PARBROOK, G. D. (1967). Leucopenic effects of prolonged nitrous oxide treatment. *Brit. J. Anaesth.*, **39**, 119.

PEARCE, D. J. (1961). Experiences in a small respiratory unit of a general hospital with special reference to the treatment of tetanus. *Anaesthesia*, **16**, 308.

PEARCE, D. J., and WALSH, R. S. (1961). Respiratory obstruction due to tracheal granuloma after tracheostomy. *Lancet*, **2**, 135.

PETERSON, N. O. A., and ROSDAHL, K. G. (1966). Ultrasonic nebulized ethanol for the disinfection of respiratory equipment. *Opusc. med.* (*Stockh.*), **11**, 278.

PHILLIPS, I. (1967). *Pseudomonas aeruginosa* cross infection in patients receiving mechanical ventilation. *J. Hyg.* (*Lond.*), **65**, 228.

PHILLIPS, I., JENKINS, S., KING, A., and SPENCER, G. (1974). Control of respirator-associated infection due to *Pseudomonas aeruginosa*. *Lancet*, **2**, 871.

PHILLIPS, I., and SPENCER, G. (1965). *Pseudomonas aeruginosa* cross infection due to contaminated respiratory apparatus. *Lancet*, **2**, 1325.

PONTOPPIDAN, H., GEFFIN, B., and LOWENSTEIN, E. (1972). Acute respiratory failure in the adult. *New Engl. J. Med.*, (I) **287**, 690; (II) **287**, 743; (III) **287**, 799.

PONTOPPIDAN, H., HEDLEY-WHITE, J., BENDIXEN, H. H., LAVER, M. B., and RADFORD, E. P. (1965). Ventilation and oxygen requirements during prolonged artificial ventilation in patients with respiratory failure. *New Engl. J. Med.*, **273**, 401.

POULSEN, H., (1968). *Cardiopulmonary Resuscitation*. World Fed. Soc. Anaesth., Aarhus, Denmark.

POULSEN, H., SKALL-JENSEN, J., STAFFELDT, I., and LANGE, M. (1959). Pulmonary ventilation and respiratory gas exchange during manual artificial respiration and expired air resuscitation on apnoeic normal adults. *Acta anaesth. scand.*, **3**, 129.

PRICE, H. L., CONNOR, E. H., and DRIPPS, R. D. (1954). Some respiratory and circulatory effects of mechanical respirators. *J. appl. Physiol.*, **6**, 517.

PRYS-ROBERTS, C., CORBETT, J. L., KERR, J. H., CRAMPTON-SMITH, A., and SPALDING, J. M. K. (1969). Treatment of sympathetic overactivity in tetanus. *Lancet*, **1**, 542.

PRYS-ROBERTS, C., KELMAN, G. R., GREENBAUM, R., and ROBINSON, R. H. (1967). Circulatory influences during artificial ventilation during nitrous oxide anaesthesia in man. *Brit. J. Anaesth.*, **39**, 534.

PYLE, P., DARLOW, M., and FIRMAN, J. E. (1969). A heated ultra-high efficiency filter for mechanical ventilators. *Lancet*, **1**, 136.

REDMAN, L. R., and LOCKEY, E. (1967). Colonisation of the upper respiratory tract with gram-negative bacilli after operation, endotracheal intubation and prophylactic antibiotic therapy. *Anaesthesia*, **22**, 220.

REES, G. J., and OWEN-THOMAS, J. B. (1966). A technique of pulmonary ventilation with a nasotracheal tube. *Brit. J. Anaesth.*, **38**, 901.

REID, D. H. S., and TUNSTALL, M. E. (1966). The respiratory distress syndrome of the newborn. *Anaesthesia*, **21**, 72.

REID, D. H. S., TUNSTALL, M. E., and MITCHELL, R. G. (1967). A controlled trial of artificial respiration in the respiratory distress syndrome of the newborn. *Lancet*, **1**, 532.

REINARZ, J. A., PIERCE, A. K., MAYS, B. B., and SANFORD, J. P. (1965). The potential role of inhalation therapy equipment in nosocomial pulmonary infection. *J. clin. Invest.*, **44**, 831.

RIVERS, J. F., ORR, G., and LEE, H. A. (1970). Drowning. Its clinical sequelae and management. *Brit. med. J.*, **2**, 157.

RUBEN, H. (1955). A new non-rebreathing valve. *Anesthesiology*, **16**, 643.

RUBEN, H., and RUBEN, A. (1957). Apparatus for resuscitation and suction. *Lancet*, **2**, 373.

RUSSELL, W. J., MORGAN, M., and LUMLEY, J. (1971). Application of an end-expiratory pressure in the management of three cases of pulmonary oedema. *Brit. J. Anaesth.*, **43**, 705.

RUSSELL, W. R., and SCHUSTER, E. (1953). Respiration pump for poliomyelitis. *Lancet*, **2**, 707.

SAFAR, P., ESCARRAGA, L. A., and ELAM, J. O. (1958). A comparison of the mouth to mouth and mouth to airway methods of artificial respiration with the chest-pressure arm-lift methods. *New Engl. J. Med.*, **258**, 671.

SATINDER LAL (1965). Blood gases in respiratory failure. *Lancet*, **1**, 339.

SCHUSTER, E., and FISCHER-WILLIAMS, M. (1953). A rocking bed for poliomyelitis. *Lancet*, **2**, 1074.

SEMPLE, S. J. G. (1965). Respiration and the cerebro-spinal fluid. *Brit. J. Anaesth.*, **37**, 262.

SHACKLETON, R. P. W. (1954). The treatment of tetanus. Role of the anaesthetist. *Lancet*, **2**, 155.

SHACKLETON, R. P. W. (1962). In my end is my beginning. *Ann. roy. Coll. Surg. Engl.*, **30**, 229.

SHARPEY-SCHAFER, E. P. (1955). Effects of Valsalva's manoeuvre on the normal and failing circulation. *Brit. med. J.*, **1**, 693.

SHARPEY-SCHAFER, E. P. (1961). Venous tone. *Brit. med. J.*, **2**, 1589.

SHELDON, G. P. (1963). Pressure breathing in chronic obstructive lung disease. *Medicine (Baltimore)*, **42**, 197.

SIMENSTAD, J. O., GALWAY, C. T., and MACLEAN, L. D. (1963). The treatment of aspiration and atelectasis by tracheobronchial lavage. *Anesth. Analg. Curr. Res.*, **42**, 616.

SMITH, A. C., and SPALDING, J. M. K. (1959). Intermittent positive pressure respiration. Some physiological observations. *Proc. roy. Soc. Med.*, **52**, 661.

SPALDING, J. M. K., and OPIE, L. (1958). Artificial respiration with the Tunnicliffe breathing jacket. *Lancet*, **1**, 613.

SPEIZER, F. E., DOLL, R., and HEAF, P. (1968). Observations on recent increase in mortality from asthma. *Brit. med. J.*, **1**, 335.

SPENCER, G. (1977). Respiratory insufficiency in scoliosis: clinical management and home care. In: *Scoliosis*, p. 315. Ed P. A. Zorab. London: Academic Press.

SPENCER, G., RIDLEY, M., EYKYN, S., and ACHONG, J. (1968). Disinfection of lung ventilators by alcohol aerosol. *Lancet*, **2**, 667.

SPENCER, G. T. (1969). (Indications for tank ventilators.) Respirators in respiratory failure. *Brit. med. J.*, **3**, 780.

STEVENS, H. R., and ALBREGT, H. B. (1966). Assessment of ultrasonic nebulization. *Anesthesiology*, **27**, 648.

SUTER, P. M., FAIRLEY, H. B., and ISENBERG, M. D. (1975). Optimum end-expiratory airway pressure in patients with acute pulmonary failure. *New Engl. J. Med.*, **292**, 284.

SYKES, M. K. (1964). Sterilizing mechanical ventilators (letter). *Brit. med. J.*, **1**, 561.

SYKES, M. K., MCNICOL, M. W., and CAMPBELL, E. J. M. (1976). In *Respiratory Failure*, 2nd edit., p. 153. Oxford: Blackwell Scientific Publications.

THEILADE, D. (1977). The danger of fatal misjudgement in hypothermia after immersion. *Anaesthesia*, **32**, 889.

THOMAS, C. G. A. (1960). Sterilization by ethylene oxide. *Guy's Hosp. Rep.*, **109**, 57.

TONKIN, J. P., and HARRISON, G. A. (1966). The effect on the larynx of prolonged endotracheal intubation. *Med. J. Aust.*, **2**, 581.

VASSA, N. T., DOSHI, H. V., YAJNIK, U. H., SHAH, S. S., JOSHI, K. R., and PATEL, S. H. (1974). Comparative clinical trial of diazepam with other conventional drugs in tetanus. *Postgrad. med. J.*, **50**, 755.

WARRELL, D. A., EDWARDS, R. H. T., GODFREY, S., and JONES, N. L. (1970). Effect of controlled oxygen therapy on arterial blood gases in acute respiratory failure. *Brit. med. J.*, **2**, 452.

WATSON, W. E. (1961). Physiology of artificial respiration. (D. Phil. Thesis submitted to Oxford University.)

WATSON, W. E. (1962a). Some observations on dynamic lung compliance during intermittent positive pressure respiration. *Brit. J. Anaesth.*, **34**, 153.

WATSON, W. E. (1962b). Observations on physiological dead space during intermittent positive pressure respiration. *Brit. J. Anaesth.*, **34**, 502.

WATSON, W. E. (1962c). Observations on the dynamic lung compliance of patients with respiratory weakness receiving intermittent positive pressure respiration. *Brit. J. Anaesth.*, **34**, 690.

WATSON, W. E. (1962d). Some circulatory responses to Valsalva's manoeuvre in patients with polyneuritis and spinal cord disease. *J. Neurol. Neurosurg. Psychiat.*, **24**, 19.

WHITTARD, B. R., and THOMAS, K. E. (1964). A new polyvinyl chloride cuffed tracheostomy tube. *Lancet*, **1**, 797.

WHITTENBERGER, J. L. (1955). Artificial respiration. *Physiol. Rev.*, **35**, 611.

WRIGHT, R., SYKES, M. K., JACKSON, B. G., MANN, N. M., and ADAMS, E. B. (1961). Intermittent positive pressure respiration in tetanus neonatorum. *Lancet*, **2**, 678.

ZEITLIN, G. L. (1965). Artificial respiration after cardiac surgery. *Anaesthesia*, **20**, 145.

FURTHER READING

MUSHIN, W. W., RENDELL-BAKER, L., THOMPSON, P. W., and MAPLESON, W. W. (1977). *Automatic Ventilation of the Lungs*, Oxford: Blackwell Scientific Publications.

POULSEN, H. (1968). *Cardiopulmonary Resuscitation*. Aarhus, Denmark: World Fed. Soc. Anaesth.

SYKES, M. K., MCNICOL, M. W., and CAMPBELL, E. J. M. (1976). *Respiratory Failure*, 2nd edit. Oxford: Blackwell Scientific Piblications.

Chapter 11

SPECIAL CARE UNITS

THE general hospital ward has proved a durable and flexible unit in which to care for patients and on which to base the medical and nursing staff. From an early stage in hospital development general wards have tended to become less general and more specialised in the type of patient they cater for. This has largely resulted from specialisation within the medical profession. Traditionally, therefore, wards have become restricted by the specialised work of the doctor in charge and patients have been sited in hospital by virtue of their disease rather than by the amount of attention and treatment they need. The development of complex methods of treatment which are necessary and effective in only a minority of patients has resulted in a small number of very ill patients requiring more attention, facilities and space than can conveniently be provided in a normal ward if they are to have the best chance of recovery. On the other hand, many patients require less attention and facilities than a normal ward provides.

Recognition of these developments has led to the concept of Progressive Patient Care. Under this system patients are grouped in hospital according to the severity of their illness rather than its nature. The stimulus to this development has its origin in staff shortage. By adopting progressive patient care it is hoped to make more efficient use of staff, concentrating expertise where it is really needed and thus avoiding wasteful staff deployment. In practice, progressive patient care has been found to have many disadvantages and the claimed advantages have rarely been fully realised. The provision of special areas in hospital where severely ill patients can be treated intensively has been more successful. This is the one aspect of progressive patient care which is becoming widely adopted. Such units are called, for want of a better term, Intensive Therapy Units (Planning Unit Report No. 1, 1967).

Parallel with these developments has come the recognition that many patients cannot safely be returned to a general ward immediately upon completion of any but the most trivial operation or anaesthetic. Special recovery units have been developed in an attempt to overcome this problem. They can be staffed by experienced nurses and thus effectively bridge the gap between the continuous individual medical attention inevitable during surgery and anaesthesia, and the more sporadic nursing care in a general ward (Jolly and Lee, 1957). Such areas are termed "recovery rooms" or "post-operative observation rooms".

Patient monitoring is an important function of all types of special care units and will be discussed briefly before the different types of unit are described.

Patient Monitoring

Although monitoring schemes have now reached a high level of sophistication (Hill and Dolan, 1976) one should remain aware of their limitations. Perhaps the most obvious limitation is that the assessment of a patient involves more than an analysis of physiological variables; the importance of human observation of the whole being is in no way reduced by the advent of electronics. It is generally agreed that these monitoring systems do not reduce the number of trained staff required, but they ease the burden of routine measurement and, at the same time, reduce observer error. The monitor can be set so that an alarm is given if a variable exceeds the pre-set range and may in this way draw attention to an abnormality sooner than it would otherwise be detected, so enabling a greater stability of that particular variable to be achieved. One advantage of digital computer systems is the greater versatility of their alarms. For each of the monitored variables the computer can calculate a "tracking signal" and sound an alarm when a change occurs which is statistically significant at the 5 per cent level. It is also possible to reduce the number of false alarms by linking the signals from, for example, an ECG and pulse monitor in such a way that "alarm incidents" are required in both channels before the alarm will sound.

In general, there is much to be said for using the least complicated equipment necessary for a particular task. It is vital that the use of the equipment is properly understood and that it is accurately calibrated and well maintained. Pitfalls, such as an amplifier gain set to the wrong range, await the unwary and it should be remembered that the more electrical equipment in contact with the patient the greater the risk of electrocution.

Which variables are monitored will depend upon the condition of the patient and the facilities available. It is not proposed to describe all the techniques of monitoring now in use, but a few recent developments are mentioned.

The management of some neurosurgical patients has been aided by monitoring intracranial pressure (McDowall, 1976; Turner and McDowall, 1976) and this technique is also of use in cases of severe head injury when it can give early warning of brain compression. Obviously, it will not indicate whether the cause is haemorrhage or oedema, but this distinction can often be made by computer-assisted tomography. In the management of cerebral oedema, intracranial pressure monitoring enables the optimum combination of techniques such as hyperventilation, steroids, and posture to be adopted, as well as giving warning of dangerous peaks of pressure which may occur when the patient is disturbed.

EEG monitoring has received relatively little attention because of the complexity of the wave-forms recorded. Computer analysis of the frequency content of a 30 second record has produced promising results (Lack, 1974) and the EEG has been monitored during anaesthesia using on-line telephonic computer analysis (Myers *et al.*, 1973). One of the main problems in EEG monitoring is that of reducing the huge amount of information contained in the trace to manageable proportions. Maynard *et al.* (1969*a* and *b*) produced a "cerebral function monitor", which records at a slow paper speed, the trace appearing as a solid band. Cerebral hypoxia causes a reduction in amplitude (voltage) of the EEG and the band is depressed and narrowed. To date, clinical experience with this device is encouraging (Schwarz *et al.*, 1973).

An interesting development in the field of blood gas analysis is that of non-invasive, transcutaneous methods of Po_2 and Pco_2 measurement. The oxygen electrode is fixed to the skin and contains three platinum cathodes and $Ag/AgCl_2$ anodes. Vasodilatation is produced by a heating coil incorporated into the electrode (Huch *et al.*, 1975). This method is still at the development stage, but if it becomes a reliable alternative to arterial blood sampling it will be a welcome means of avoiding the complications of long-term arterial cannulation or repeated arterial puncture.

RECOVERY UNITS

Recovery Units can be divided into two types with different advantages and disadvantages.

Recovery Rooms

These are usually small rooms which form an integral part of an operating suite. They are conveniently sited alongside the anaesthetic room so that the patient enters the operating room via the anaesthetic room and leaves it via the recovery room. Their particular advantage is that being close to the theatre, they allow easy supervision of the patient by the surgeon and anaesthetist who have performed the operation, and thus achieve the best possible continuity of medical responsibility. They are only suitable for short-stay patients because the facilities which can be provided in a single room are space-limited. If a patient is not ready to leave the recovery room by the time the subsequent operation is completed, serious congestion and disruption of the work of the theatre can result. Nurse staffing is difficult because the work load is irregular and dispersed. It is sometimes necessary to release a theatre nurse with limited experience to supervise the patient. This may seriously deplete staffing of the operating theatre.

Recovery rooms are most suitable for small hospitals with single theatre units, or for departments such as X-ray or out-patients where occasional anaesthetic services only are required.

Recovery Areas (Post-anaesthetic recovery units: Post-operative Departments)

In an attempt to overcome these disadvantages, larger recovery areas have been developed which are common to a number of operating theatres. They can be more extensively equipped than a recovery room and patients can remain in them for longer periods. A separate nursing and medical staff is needed, and if the area serves four or more theatres the work load may be sufficiently sustained to justify a night staff and twenty-four hour service. While this is always desirable, it is inefficient unless regularly used.

The disadvantage of a recovery area often lies in its siting. Unless it has been included from the outset in the centre of a multiple theatre suite it may have to be sited at a considerable distance from some of the operating theatres feeding it. Transport of patients from theatre to recovery area may then be hazardous or disruptive to the work of the theatre if an anaesthetist has to accompany them.

A centrally sited recovery area in a multiple theatre suite is ideal for patient admission and supervision during the working day, but suffers from the disadvantage of being in the clean area of modern theatre design. Access to the recovery area is inconvenient once medical staff have left the theatre suite and continuity of medical and nursing care may therefore suffer. Probably the best compromise is to site the area in the junction zone near the entrance to a multiple theatre suite. Even in this situation the area may, in large theatre complexes, be at an inconvenient distance from some of the theatre suites it serves.

SPECIAL FUNCTION UNITS

These units are designed to meet the needs of patients suffering from a particular disease, or type of disease (Bell et al., 1974).

Respiratory Units

Respiratory Units were the prototype for all special care units and many have been adapted to cater for a wider variety of conditions. Lassen (1953) was among the first to recognise the need to set aside special areas for the treatment of respiratory poliomyelitis, and the requirements of such units have now become clearly established. Their design can be specialised and their needs are well exemplified by the unit which has been described by Hercus et al. (1962, 1964).

Coronary Care Units

In recent years there has been considerable interest in reducing the mortality following myocardial infarction by prevention and treatment of dysrhythmias and ventricular fibrillation, which are liable to occur in the first few days. Brown et al. (1963) and Julian et al. (1964) showed that deaths following myocardial infarction are mainly due to electrical disturbances of cardiac rhythm which are potentially reversible if appropriate resuscitative measures can be promptly undertaken. If treatment is to be successful, it is clear that patients who have suffered an infarct must be admitted to a unit staffed and equipped to provide continuous electrocardiographic monitoring as soon as possible after the acute episode (Pantridge and Geddes, 1976). The design and organisation of typical units have been described by Shillingford and Thomas (1964) and Lawrie et al. (1967).

In theory, therefore, the problem is simple and the benefits obvious. In practice, coronary care has raised as many problems as it has solved and the benefits are less than had been hoped. In one study (Mather et al., 1971) the mortality of patients treated at home after myocardial infarction was no greater than that of those treated in intensive care units. Although doubts have been expressed about the design of this study, any reduction in mortality due to coronary care units is modest. Most deaths due to heart attack occur outside hospital and many of the deaths in hospitals are caused by "pump failure" due to massive infarction.

Medical resources.—Myocardial infarction in Western countries is a distressingly common condition, and full intensive care for all cases is economically unrealistic. Statistical surveys have suggested that up to 30 per cent of the occupants of acute medical beds in general hospitals are there either directly or indirectly as a result of ischaemic heart disease. It is costly to equip so many beds with ECG monitors, and virtually impossible to provide enough staff to interpret the information displayed.

It can be argued that the research benefit from intensive coronary care is considerable. This is true but it is not an argument for its universal adoption as a routine therapeutic measure. Moreover it is important not to concentrate too much research effort on end-stage disease (Miller, 1969) thereby deflecting it from studying the underlying causes of atherosclerosis.

Case selection.—Approximately 90 per cent of patients with myocardial infarction who reach hospital alive exhibit rhythm disorders during the first 72 hours, and the incidence declines steadily with the passage of time (Lown *et al.*, 1967). Thus it is common practice to limit the period of continuous monitoring to about 72 hours unless there is evidence that serious dysrhythmias are still present or a pacemaker is *in situ*. Although it is reasonable to place a time limit on continuous monitoring in this way, it has the disadvantage that a small proportion of patients with minor infarcts do not develop serious dysrhythmias for a week or more after infarction. Since attempts to select cases at particular risk have rarely been successful, it has been suggested that graded coronary care with telemetric monitoring continued for a longer period may help to overcome this problem. At present there is little information concerning long-term electrocardiography in normal subjects and in a recent study of apparently normal subjects monitored for 24 hours, 12 per cent had disturbances of rhythm which are widely believed to be of serious prognostic significance, including R-on-T ventricular ectopics and ventricular tachycardia (Clarke *et al.*, 1976).

Staffing.—Although the staff requirements of a coronary care unit are less than those of an intensive therapy unit, they still present a major problem. Coronary care units tend to be particularly unpopular with nurses because the work is unvarying and the mortality is high. Continuous observation of one or more oscilloscopes is impossible to perform efficiently for long periods and machinery capable of pattern recognition is complex and not yet generally available. In practice, the establishment of coronary care units is limited by the availability of suitable staff.

Psychological effects of coronary care.—A doctor who believes that monitoring will help a patient can usually quite readily persuade the patient to accept the minor discomforts involved (Crook, 1970). Most patients are reassured by monitoring equipment once their initial fears have been overcome. Nevertheless, there is evidence suggesting that a proportion of the rhythm disturbances observed during coronary care are caused by the patient's fear of the circumstances in which he finds himself. It has even been suggested that the indications for hospital admission in myocardial infarction are social rather than medical; provided he can be cared for at home, he is just as well off in his own familiar environment. Telemetric ECG monitoring is of value because it is less obtrusive to the patient, and reassurance at all times is of vital importance. One death in a coronary care unit can have a devastating effect on the other patients who know they are suffering from the same disease. The psychological problems of intensive care have been reviewed by Baxter (1974).

Pre-hospital coronary care.—The majority of deaths from myocardial infarction occur soon after the onset of symptoms, 40 to 60 per cent being in the first hour. McNeilly and Pemberton (1968) showed that the mean time interval between onset of symptoms and hospital admission was more than eight hours. In an attempt to reduce this massive death rate, Pantridge and Adgey (1969) have established a mobile coronary care unit based on an extensively equipped ambulance. The benefits of pre-coronary care were discussed at a symposium in 1969, and the proceedings published (Goldstein and Moss, 1969). Although encouraging results were described, it is too early to assess the overall benefits to be expected from pre-hospital coronary care.

Conclusions.—Intensive coronary care is undoubtedly a therapeutic advance.

Properly applied it can usefully save lives, though the economic outlay and staff requirements are heavy. The danger of needlessly and officiously prolonging the act of dying is ever present and it is vitally important to preserve a sense of proportion. It is no substitute for efficient care and adequate resuscitation services for the hospital as a whole (see Chapter 17).

INTENSIVE THERAPY UNITS

The essential difference between an intensive therapy unit (ITU) and the various special function units from which the concept emerged is that it is a multi-discipline, and preferably central, service area.

An intensive therapy unit has been defined as a special unit providing the following:

(1) A *Facility* available to all medical staff giving more space, staff and equipment for the care of a patient than can be provided in the ordinary wards.

(2) A *Service* which provides continuous observation of the vital functions and can support these functions more promptly and efficiently than could be done elsewhere in the hospital.

Both the facility and the service can be developed within a specialist division or ward, but the essence of the ITU is that, like most operating theatres, it is communal (Planning Unit Report No. 1, 1967).

Size of Unit

The optimum size for an intensive therapy unit is 6–8 beds. Units of less than four beds are rarely viable because the work load is so variable that at many times the unit is empty, the staff become dispersed to other duties and are unavailable when a need suddenly arises (Jørgensen, 1966). Units of over ten beds are unwieldy and incoherent; it is impossible for one person to be aware of what is happening to all the patients at all times.

One per cent of acute beds in a general hospital has usually been found adequate to meet the need for intensive therapy (Lees, 1965). Thus it is more difficult to justify a unit in a hospital of less than 400 beds. Where a district service is shared between several smaller hospitals it is preferable to transfer patients to a single central unit. A hospital of over a thousand beds will tend to need more than one unit. In such hospitals there is usually at least one speciality or division which has sufficient need for intensive therapy to justify having its own special function unit of four or more beds (Spencer, 1970).

Cross Infection

Cross infection in an intensive therapy unit is a serious problem. The more diverse the work of the unit, the more critical it becomes. There are three main reasons for this: firstly, the patients are critically ill and any infection may tip the balance between survival and death. Secondly, patients are often unduly susceptible to bacterial infection, either as a result of their disease or the treatment they are receiving. Thirdly, the unit is bound to admit some patients whose basic problem is bacterial infection, often wildly out of control. These patients are a potent source of bacterial infection (Ridley, 1970).

Airborne cross infection can be largely eliminated by adequate air conditioning, allowing parts of the unit to be isolated. Sterilisation of equipment between use is essential. Within limits dictated by staff numbers and the needs of observation, movement of staff between patients should be discouraged, if necessary by physical barriers. Cross infection is most likely to occur when the unit is overworked or understaffed, or both. The problem of control of infection in intensive care units has been discussed recently by Gaya (1976).

Layout of Unit

Many layouts have been described for intensive therapy units (Rosen and Secher, 1963; Hamilton, 1964; Spencer, 1970; Verner, 1974). None has been shown to have particular advantages provided certain basic requirements are met.

Adequate space is essential (Fig. 1). 25–30 sq metres per bed is necessary in single-bed areas, and 20 sq metres in multiple-bed areas. The service area should be at least equal to the bed area. 30–50 per cent of the beds should be in single areas. Units accepting a wide variety of patients may need to be separated into clean and dirty areas. An open plan unit is easy to staff but bacteriologically unsatisfactory, except for short-stay patients. A unit of single cubicles is bacteriologically ideal but extravagant to staff and sometimes undesirable for conscious patients, who may feel unduly isolated.

Staffing

This really is the heart of the matter. An intensive therapy unit succeeds if its staff have the confidence and goodwill of the hospital—whatever formal arrangements are made. Without these intangibles, the advantage of a communal site in providing a common ground for staff of all disciplines is replaced by the disadvantage of incomplete consultation, with failure to define or accept responsibility leading to illwill and indecision which endangers the life of the patient (Planning Unit Report No. 1, 1967).

Senior medical staff commitment to the unit is essential, though it should probably take the form of an administrative rather than a clinical responsibility. The development of intensive therapy as a medical speciality is not desirable (Hunter, 1967). No single doctor can be competent in all aspects of treatment of the severely ill. If the medical staff running the unit become too involved with clinical responsibility the unit tends to develop into an elite organisation separate from the rest of the hospital, and thereby loses goodwill and service function. It is also helpful if administrative responsibility rests in the hands of a doctor who does not have a vested interest in bed allocation.

Junior medical staff commitment to the unit is equally important. One doctor must be available at all times to act as the final common path for medical orders. This is essential in order to prevent conflicting instructions being issued to nursing staff. The chain of medical command must be clearly understood by all concerned if misunderstandings are to be avoided.

Nurse staffing is the greatest problem, and the work of most units is limited by the availability of adequate experienced staff. Overall nurse shortage, however, is only part of the problem. The work load of a unit can vary several hundred per cent over the space of a few hours; if the unit is kept fully staffed at all times there will inevitably be periods of inefficient under-employment, and if it is not fully staffed it may be unable to meet a sudden demand. Holmdahl

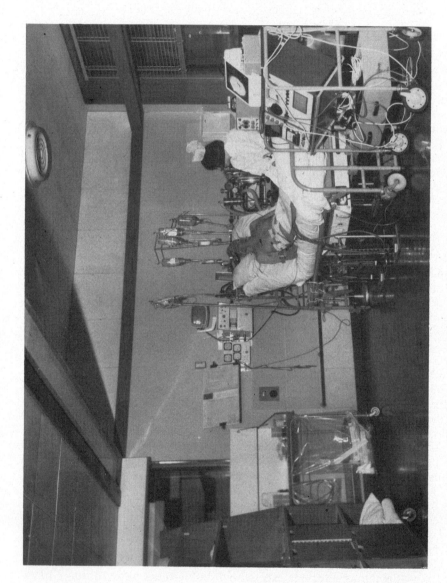

11/Fig. 1.—The Intensive Therapy Unit: space is the essential requirement.

(1962) has described a method of "on call" duties for specially trained nursing auxiliaries which goes some way towards resolving this dilemma.

Conclusions.—Intensive therapy units undoubtedly save lives and make possible techniques of therapy which would otherwise be impossible. Due mainly to its staffing needs, the cost of running a unit is high, and medical priorities have to be considered. Over-energetic treatment may be encouraged; the fact that it is possible to maintain and prolong life does not inevitably mean that to do so is justifiable or even desirable. Patients should only be admitted to an intensive therapy unit after individual consideration, and not simply because they belong to a particular diagnostic category.

REFERENCES

BAXTER, S. (1974). Psychological problems of intensive care. *Brit. J. hosp. Med.,* **2,** 875.

BELL, J. A., BRADLEY, R. D., JENKINS, B. S., and SPENCER, G. T. (1974). Six years of multi-disciplinary intensive care. *Brit. med. J.,* **2,** 483.

BROWN, K. W. G., MACMILLAN, R. L., FORBATH, N., MEL'GRANO, E., and SCOTT, J. W. (1963). Coronary Unit. An Intensive Care Centre for acute myocardial infarction. *Lancet,* **2,** 349.

CLARKE, J. M., HAMER, J., SHELTON, J., TAYLOR, S., and VENNING, G. R. (1976). The rhythm of the normal human heart. *Lancet,* **2,** 508.

CROOK, J. (1970). User needs of patients and nurses in clinical monitoring. *Postgrad. med. J.,* **46,** 374.

GAYA, H. (1976). Infection control in intensive care. *Brit. J. Anaesth.,* **48,** 9.

GOLDSTEIN, S., and MOSS, A. J. (1969). Eds. Symposium on the pre-hospital phase of acute myocardial infarction. *Amer. J. Cardiol.,* **24,** 609.

HAMILTON, M. K. (1964). Workshop on Intensive Care Units. *Anesthesiology,* **25,** 192.

HERCUS, V. (1962). Planning a Respiratory Unit. *Brit. med. J.,* **2,** 1604.

HERCUS, V., JOHNSTON, J. B., ROLLISON, R. A. A., and HACKETT, R. E. (1964). The place of a respiratory unit in a general hospital. *Lancet,* **1,** 1265.

HILL, D. W., and DOLAN, A. M. (1976). *Intensive Care Instrumentation.* London: Academic Press.

HOLMDAHL, M. H. (1962). The Respiratory Care Unit. *Anesthesiology,* **23,** 559.

HUCH, R., LUBBERS, D. W., and HUTCH, A. (1975). The transcutaneous measurement of oxygen and carbon dioxide tensions for the determination of arterial blood-gas values with control of local perfusion and peripheral perfusion pressure. Theoretical analysis and practical application. In: *Oxygen Measurements in Biology and Medicine,* pp. 121–137. Eds. J. P. Payne and D. W. Hill. London: Butterworth & Co.

HUNTER, A. R. (1967). Intensive care as a specialty. *Lancet,* **1,** 1151.

JOLLY, C., and LEE, J. A. (1957). Post-operative observation ward. *Anaesthesia,* **12,** 49.

JØRGENSEN, C. C. (1966). Establishment of, and experience gained in, an intensive care unit in a Danish Regional Hospital. *Acta anaesth. scand.,* Suppl. **23,** 108.

JULIAN, D. G., VALENTINE, P. A., and MILLER, C. G. (1964). Disturbances of rate, rhythm and conduction in acute myocardial infarction. A prospective study of 100 consecutive unselected patients with the aid of electrocardiographic monitoring. *Amer. J. Med.,* **27,** 915.

LACK, J. A. (1974). Computerized measurements in anaesthesia. In: *Measurement in Anaesthesia,* pp. 201–213. Eds. S. A. Feldman, J. M. Leigh and J. Spierdijk. Leiden University Press.

LASSEN, H. C. A. (1953). A preliminary report on the 1952 epidemic of poliomyelitis in Copenhagen, with special reference to the treatment of acute respiratory insufficiency. *Lancet,* **1,** 37.

LAWRIE, D. M., GREENWOOD, T. W., GODDARD, M., HARVEY, A. C., DONALD, K. W., JULIAN, D. G., and OLIVER, M. F. (1967). A Coronary Care Unit in the routine management of myocardial infarction. *Lancet*, **2**, 109.

LEES, W. (1965). In: *Hospital Management, Planning & Equipment*, p. 690. London: H.M.S.O.

LOWN, B., VASSAUX, C., HOOD, W. B., FAKHRO, A. M., KAPLINSKY, E., and ROBERGE, G. (1967). Unresolved problems in coronary care. *Amer. J. Cardiol.*, **20**, 494.

McDOWALL, D. G. (1976). Monitoring the brain. *Anesthesiology*, **45**, 117.

McNEILLY, R. H., and PEMBERTON, J. (1968). Duration of last attack in 998 fatal cases of coronary artery disease and its relation to possible cardiac resuscitation. *Brit. med. J.*, **3**, 139.

MATHER, H. G., PEARSON, N. G., READ, K. L. Q., SHAW, D. B., STEED, G. R., THORNE, M. G., JONES, S., GUERRIER, C. J., ERAUT, C. D., McHUGH, P. M., CHOWDHURY, N. R., JAFARY, M. H., and WALLACE, T. J. (1971). Acute myocardial infarction: Home and hospital treatment. *Brit. med. J.*, **3**, 334.

MAYNARD, D., PRIOR, P. F., and SCOTT, D. F. (1969*a*). A continuous monitoring device for cerebral activity. *Electroenceph. clin. Neurophysiol.*, **27**, 672.

MAYNARD, D., PRIOR, P. F., and SCOTT, D. F. (1969*b*). Device for continuous monitoring of cerebral activity in resuscitated patients. *Brit. med. J.*, **4**, 545.

MILLER, H. (1969). Real goals for medicine. *Sci. J.*, **5a**, 90.

MYERS, R. R., STOCKARD, J. J., FLEMING, N. I., FRANCE, C. J., and BICKFORD, R. G. (1973). The use of on-line telephonic computer analysis of the E.E.G. in anaesthesia. *Brit. J. Anaesth.*, **45**, 664.

PANTRIDGE, J. F., and ADGEY, A. A. J. (1969). Pre-hospital coronary care; The Mobile Coronary Care Unit. *Amer. J. Cardiol.*, **24**, 666.

PANTRIDGE, J. F., and GEDDES, J. S. (1976). Diseases of the cardiovascular system: Management of acute myocardial infarction. *Brit. med. J.*, **2**, 168.

Planning Unit Report No. 1 (1967). *Intensive Care*. London: British Medical Association.

RIDLEY, M. (1970). Cross-Infection in Intensive Therapy Units. In: *Progress in Anaesthesiology* (Proc. 4th World Congr. of Anaesthesiologists). Amsterdam: Excerpta Medica Foundation.

ROSEN, J., and SECHER, O. (1963). Intensive Care Unit at University Hospital, Copenhagen. *Anesthesiology*, **24**, 855.

SCHWARTZ, M. S., COLVIN, M. P., PRIOR, P. F., STRUNIN, L., SIMPSON, B. R., WEAVER, E. J. M., and SCOTT, D. F. (1973). The cerebral function monitor. *Anaesthesia*, **28**, 611.

SHILLINGFORD, J. P., and THOMAS, M. (1964). Organisation of unit for intensive care and investigation of patients with myocardial infarction. *Lancet*, **2**, 1113.

SPENCER, G. T. (1970). Planning and construction of Intensive Therapy Units. In: *Progress in Anaesthesiology* (Proc. 4th World Congr. of Anaesthesiologists). Amsterdam: Excerpta Medica Foundation.

TURNER, J. M., and McDOWALL, D. G. (1976). The measurement of intracranial pressure. *Brit. J. Anaesth.*, **48**, 735.

VERNER, I. R. (1974). The organisation, design and staffing of intensive therapy units. *Brit. J. hosp. Med.*, **2**, 828.

FURTHER READING

Planning Unit Report No. 1 (1967). *Intensive Care*. London: British Medical Association.

Intensive Therapy Units. A Symposium (1970). *Progress in Anaesthesiology* (Proc. 4th World Congr. of Anaesthesiologists), p. 477 *et seq*. Amsterdam: Excerpta Medica Foundation.

SPALDING, J. M. K., and SMITH, A. C. (1963). *Clinical Practice and Physiology of Artificial Respiration*. Oxford: Blackwell Scientific Publications.

Chapter 12

THORACIC ANAESTHESIA

INCLUDING

POST-OPERATIVE PULMONARY COMPLICATIONS

A GENERAL clinical examination of the patient is a valuable aid to the diagnosis of most ailments of the respiratory tract, and an essential preliminary for assessment of any patient's fitness to undergo operation and anaesthesia. Particularly in diseases affecting the lungs and bronchi, specific investigations may be necessary to establish a precise diagnosis before operation is undertaken, and some of these may need anaesthesia for their successful accomplishment. The three commonest special investigations in thoracic disease are examination of the sputum, radiography of the chest, and direct examination of the respiratory tract by laryngoscopy and bronchoscopy. From the anaesthetist's point of view, the importance of sputum examination lies not only in any possible contamination of the anaesthetic apparatus but in the theoretical and practical possibilities that follow upon the presence of considerable quantities in the respiratory tract during anaesthesia. A great deal of practical information—which may be of value in choosing a particular anaesthetic or technique—can be gleaned from macroscopical examination of the sputum, and from a knowledge of the quantity expectorated during the course of 24 hours.

In the following section a description is given of both anaesthesia and chest disease which will not be commonly seen in the United Kingdom today. It is, however, representative of the kind of chest medicine which was common a few years ago and the detailed descriptions given are necessary both to help the anaesthetist when he meets the occasional case in this country and because the diseases described are still common in many other parts of the world.

The three main alterations in current chest anaesthesia practice are:

1. A decrease in the number of operations for carcinoma of the bronchus. There are fewer exploratory thoracotomies because the degree of operability is more correctly assessed by modern diagnostic techniques. Further, there is a tendency for carcinoma of the bronchus to present in an older age group in whom operation may be precluded by the deterioration in lung function which goes with age.

2. In Britain there is virtually no surgery performed for pulmonary tuberculosis. It is, however, still common in the underdeveloped countries.

3. A decrease in the incidence of surgery for infection in the chest. The incidence of bronchiectasis has diminished with the decline in whooping cough and primary tuberculosis while the prompter recognition and correct treatment of pneumonia have decreased the complications of lung abscess and empyema. At the same time, there remains a high incidence of chronic bronchitis and emphysema in the population although this will remain a problem in respect of incidental surgery rather than during a direct attack on the chest.

RADIOGRAPHIC INVESTIGATIONS

The interpretation of X-rays of the chest in the standard posterior-anterior, oblique and lateral views, particularly in relationship to the normal anatomy of the lungs, is important and in most instances is sufficient for accurate diagnosis. The lungs and their normal subdivisions are illustrated in Figs. 1 to 6 inclusive. Bronchography (see below) is a method of determining the state of the bronchial tree and is nowadays infrequently used in the United Kingdom, being largely replaced by the use of fibre-optic bronchoscopy. Good standard X-rays of the lungs provide almost as much, and usually sufficient, information for accurate diagnosis, while there are fewer and fewer patients with diseases such as bronchiectasis for whom bronchographic investigation may be essential. Bronchography has, too, its own morbidity which may result from plugging of the bronchi and bronchioles or from reactions to the substances used for the investigation.

Bronchography

The bronchial tree can be outlined either by instillation of a radio-opaque liquid or by insufflation of a radio-opaque powder.

Radio-opaque liquids.—An aqueous, rather than an oily, suspension of contrast medium is preferred because it is less irritating to the bronchial tree, does not require much reflex suppression during instillation and mixes with bronchial secretions.

Propyliodone (Dionosil) is a suspension of the n-propyl ester of 3:5 diodo-4-pyridone-n-acetic acid. The iodine is in firm organic combination so that there is no breakdown to iodides or free iodine. It is available either as a 50 per cent aqueous suspension or as a 60 per cent suspension in arachis oil. Propyliodone is less irritant to the bronchial mucosa than most other media but it is absorbed and hydrolysed and finally excreted by the kidneys within a short period. Iodism may therefore follow its use. Unlike some other contrast media no interaction with volatile anaesthetic agents such as halothane have been reported.

Iodism.—Reactions to iodine during or following bronchography' are extremely uncommon. An acute reaction is most likely to be anaphylactic in type and will require immediate emergency therapy. Treatment includes the rapid infusion of large amounts of fluids (particularly those likely to remain in the circulation for some time) in an attempt to combat the severe hypotension due to generalised vasodilatation: dexamethasone or hydrocortisone to achieve bronchial dilatation, and isoprenaline or a vasoconstrictor (with an inotropic action) to support the myocardium and circulation. However, in the early stages of a reaction it is almost impossible to forecast its probable extent. Thus, treatment must be undertaken in all suggestive cases, and should consist of attempts to remove any residual contrast medium by posturing with encouragement to cough, and by aspiration from the stomach. Next the patient may usefully be given sodium chloride to enable the free iodine to attach itself to a sodium ion, thereby assisting renal excretion.

Radio-opaque powders.—The bronchial tract can be outlined by the insufflation of particles of a heavy metal in the form of a powder. Tantalum oxide has been used for this purpose (Nedel *et al.*, 1968). It has a particle size of 3—4μm. The technique requires manipulation of a catheter into a major bronchus with the aid of fluoroscopy. A few squeezes of an insufflator distribute the powder,

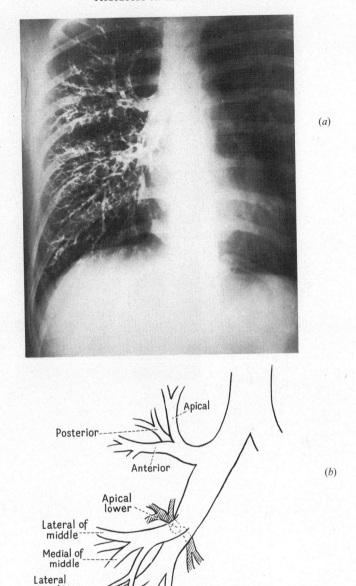

12/Fig. 1.—Normal right bronchogram—anterior-posterior.

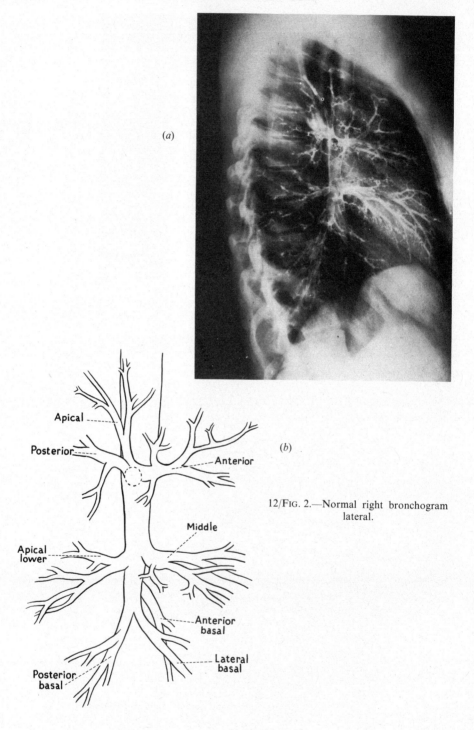

(a)

Apical

Posterior

Anterior

(b)

Apical
lower

Middle

Anterior
basal

Lateral
basal

Posterior
basal

12/Fig. 2.—Normal right bronchogram
lateral.

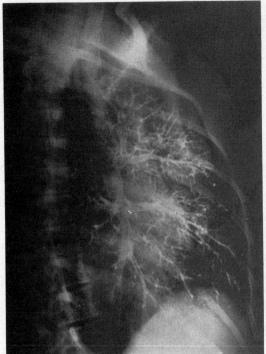

(a)

(b)

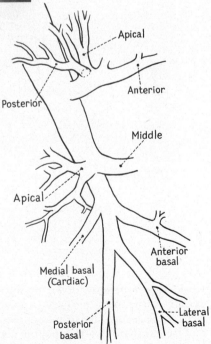

12/FIG. 3.—Normal right bronchogram—
oblique.

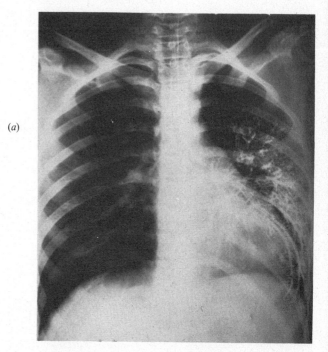

(a)

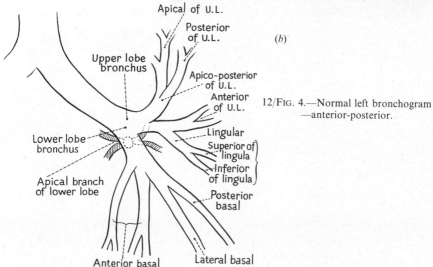

(b)

Apical of U.L.

Posterior of U.L.

Upper lobe bronchus

Apico-posterior of U.L.

Anterior of U.L.

Lower lobe bronchus

Lingular

Superior of lingula

Inferior of lingula

Apical branch of lower lobe

Posterior basal

Anterior basal

Lateral basal

12/Fig. 4.—Normal left bronchogram —anterior-posterior.

which is non-irritant, down to secondary bronchi and because of the high density of the metal particles, low concentrations of tantalum oxide contrast well on the X-rays. This method does not block the smaller bronchi, but it does require fluoroscopy and probably general anaesthesia.

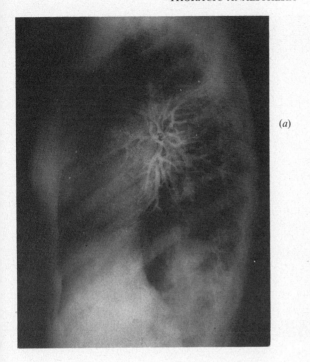

(a)

12/FIG. 5.—Normal left bronchogram—lateral.

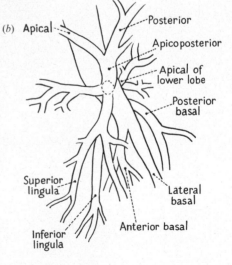

(b) Apical — Posterior
Apicoposterior
Apical of lower lobe
Posterior basal
Superior lingula — Lateral basal
Inferior lingula — Anterior basal

Technique for bronchography with a radio-opaque liquid.—Adequate postural drainage should be carried out for some time before bronchography in wet cases, in order to reduce the sputum as much as possible; this not only makes for safety, but also gives the contrast medium a chance to reach the smaller bronchi.

(a)

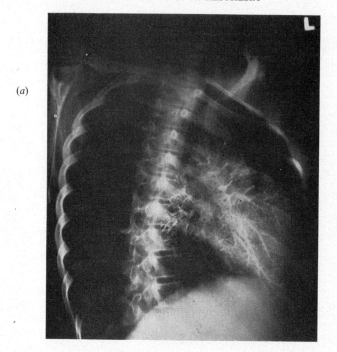

(b)

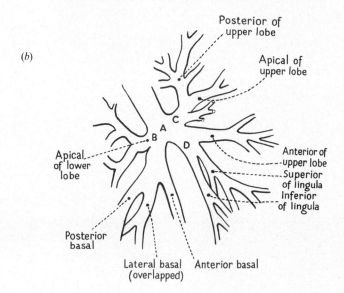

12/FIG. 6.—NORMAL LEFT BRONCHOGRAM—OBLIQUE

A = Upper lobe bronchus.   C = Apico-posterior bronchus (of upper lobe).
B = Lower lobe bronchus.   D = Lingular bronchus.

The contrast medium is introduced into the bronchial tree either through a rubber catheter passed via the nose or over the back of the tongue, or by direct injection through the cricothyroid membrane. A third method, now used as a rule only under general anaesthesia, is to pass an endotracheal tube, down which a small rubber catheter is introduced. In adults and co-operative children local analgesia is perfectly satisfactory for bronchography, which is at the most an uncomfortable procedure. In the young, up to about the age of 6 years, and in older children who are unco-operative, general anaesthesia may be necessary, and this permits good pictures being taken with safety. Indeed, from the practical point of view, general anaesthesia for all children may save a lot of time and lead to better overall results, since a slight movement or a bout of coughing can easily spoil the final result.

Adults.—Premedication is unnecessary unless the patient is particularly nervous, when a barbiturate such as pentobarbitone (100 to 200 mg) is helpful. Surprisingly little surface analgesia is needed, since it is not essential to anaesthetise the tracheal or bronchial mucosa, the contrast medium usually running smoothly without producing any marked irritation.

When the catheter is to be passed over the back of the tongue some surface analgesia of this area and perhaps of the glottis itself may be helpful—although if the operator is skilled the whole procedure can be done without it. Effective analgesia can be quickly produced by spraying the area with 4 per cent lignocaine a minute or two beforehand. The patient then sits up in a chair with his neck extended, and grasping his tongue with a piece of gauze between finger and thumb holds it firmly forward. He is told to breathe deeply and the appropriate amount of contrast medium to outline the particular lobe is then injected over the back of the tongue. A similar technique is used for the nasal route.

When a needle of the requisite bore is to be inserted through the cricothyroid membrane, local anaesthesia of the skin and tissues down to the membrane is necessary. The patient lies on his back with his head extended on a pillow, and when the membrane has been located by palpation a skin weal is raised over it and the deeper tissues also infiltrated with 2 per cent lignocaine. After the patient has been warned that it will make him cough, 1 ml of 2 per cent lignocaine is squirted through the membrane during inspiration, and the needle immediately withdrawn to avoid breakage. When the coughing has subsided a special flanged needle of 12 or 14 gauge is pushed through the same track into the trachea, and attached by its bayonet fitting to the syringe already charged with contrast medium. The careful aspiration of a little air to show that the trachea has been entered is essential before making the injection. Dangers are the production of a haematoma, intravascular injection, and breakage of the needle. The subcutaneous injection of propyliodine is not dangerous. The suspension is non-irritant to the tissues, but it will remain *in situ* for up to eight weeks. The cricothyroid route is potentially a hazardous and complicated method but it gives great control of the instillation and enables a more deliberate positioning of the patient between the intermittent injections, and therefore more accurate localisation of the contrast medium. An alternative to direct injection is to thread a fine catheter through the needle and then with the aid of fluoroscopy to manipulate the tip of it into the desired bronchus.

Positioning for bronchography.—Three distinct positions are necessary to

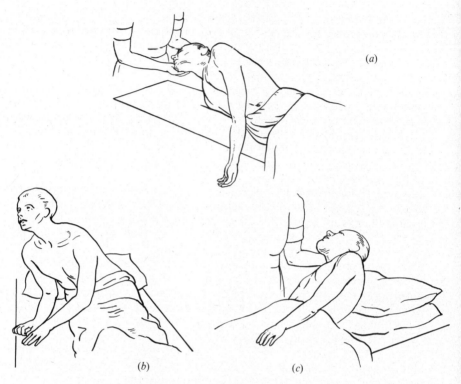

12/Fig. 7.—The Three Positions for Bronchography
(a) Upper lobe; (b) Middle lobe; (c) Lower lobe.

fill the lower lobe, middle (or lingular) lobe and upper lobe respectively (Fig. 7). It is preferable to fill each in turn and to instil into the trachea a small quantity of contrast medium—3 to 5 ml—on each occasion. For the lower lobe the patient is partially sitting, inclined about 20° posteriorly and to the side to be filled, and a minute is allowed for the contrast medium to reach the branches of the lower lobe bronchus. The patient then lies on the side to be filled in the horizontal plane, and if an X-ray shows no reflux of contrast medium from the lower lobe bronchus to the upper lobe, a further 5 ml are added with the head raised during the injection.

The upper lobe bronchus may be filled by alternative methods. First, after the instillation of 5 ml of contrast medium in the lateral, horizontal position, the patient is turned almost into the prone position and the table tilted head-down. Secondly, provided a catheter lies in the trachea, the patient is placed in the Trendelenburg position on the side to be filled and 5 ml of contrast medium is injected. In this method, if the lower and middle lobes have just been filled, it is worth waiting a minute and then taking an X-ray, before adding more contrast medium, to see whether the upper lobe will fill by reflux from the lower.

Pictures of each lobe should be taken in postero-anterior, lateral and oblique views. It is generally better to restrict a bronchogram to one side at a time in order to avoid overlap of structures in lateral views. If localisation of disease is unimportant, and the bronchogram is being performed for purely diagnostic reasons (Fig. 8), both sides can be done at the same time since a good oblique will often show all branches of the bronchi in both lungs. Bronchography should be restricted to one lung at a session when the patient has a very reduced pulmonary function.

Children.—If the child is co-operative, any of the techniques described for adults can be used, though the nasal route is the least satisfactory owing to the smallness of the passage and the likely presence of adenoid tissue. Careful training is a wise precaution, not only to gain the confidence of the child but to accustom him to the X-ray department, the various procedures, and the positions needed. This may take a week or longer, and should be carried out along with postural drainage and breathing exercises. The quantity of local analgesic and contrast medium must be proportionate to the size of the child. The dose of lignocaine should not exceed 2·6 mg/kg. Bronchography under topical analgesia in children is not always successful, particularly when they are unco-operative, and it can be dangerous. The hazard of too much local analgesic drug has been referred to, but there is also a danger of respiratory obstruction (Atwood, 1965). It is best to limit bronchography under topical analgesia in children to one lung at a session.

General anaesthesia.—Preparation designed to drain as much of the secretions away prior to the bronchogram is just as important before general anaesthesia as local analgesia. Premedication depends upon the size and age of the child, but in general, basal anaesthesia to ensure that the child arrives in the X-ray department asleep is our preference. This can be achieved in several ways (see Chapter 45, p. 1432) and should be followed by atropine sulphate 0·6 mg subcutaneously.

If the child has a considerable quantity of sputum such preliminary sedation may introduce the dangers of respiratory obstruction, both in the pre-investigation period and during post-investigation recovery. For such cases kindness must give way to safety, and either atropine only be ordered, or a combination of opiate and atropine suited to the child's size.

The child is brought to the radiological department in his cot and anaesthesia induced. When a barbiturate or phenothiazine has been given for premedication, nitrous oxide and oxygen followed by halothane is the best, but after atropine alone, or atropine with an opiate, a small dose of thiopentone may be used. Relaxation is procured by intermittent injections of suxamethonium or by a single injection of a non-depolarising relaxant, the object being complete control of respiration during the whole procedure. After intubation with an endotracheal tube attached to a Cobb's suction connection piece, as much sputum as possible is sucked out of the lungs. It is undesirable to inflate the lungs by intermittent positive-pressure before suction when a fair quantity of sputum is present; when this is the case, after induction and before the muscle relaxant is given, the child must be allowed to breathe a high concentration of oxygen for a minute or so in order to prevent hypoxia occurring during suction. Anaesthesia is maintained for this period by the combined effects of any sedative premedication and the residue of halothane or thiopentone left over from the induction.

After the sputum has been removed, the child is inflated with oxygen and the

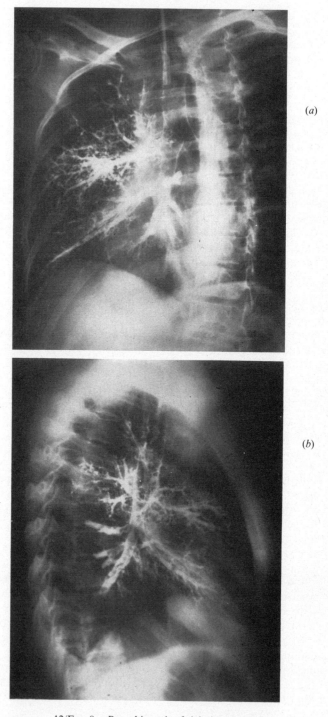

(a)

(b)

12/Fig. 8.—Bronchiectasis of right lung.

contrast medium is injected through a separate rubber catheter passed down the endotracheal tube. The child is then placed in the required positions for filling the various lobes on one side, but only kept in each position for a few seconds since the contrast medium flows more quickly under general anaesthesia. The pictures are taken while the child is still apnoeic, and if oxygenation has been properly performed before the injection of the contrast medium, cyanosis will not occur. After the completion of one side, as much contrast medium as possible is quickly aspirated and then the child is ventilated.

Positioning of an anaesthetised child is basically the same as that for the adult, but the whole of the contrast medium for one side should be injected into the trachea at once, with the child held in the sitting position but inclined 40° to that side. Immediately after the injection the child, while inclined laterally, is moved backwards and forwards so that the middle (or lingular) and lower lobe bronchi are entered by the contrast medium, and after a few seconds it is held on its side head-down over the end of the table so that the upper lobe bronchus can be filled. X-ray pictures are then taken as soon as the child has been returned to the horizontal.

If both lungs are to be outlined at the same session the views should be restricted, and taken in the following order:

1. *Right lung.*   Right lateral followed by an antero-posterior view.
2. *Left lung.*   Right antero-oblique followed by antero-posterior view.

Atwood (1965) strongly recommends that bilateral bronchography at the same session should be avoided in a child under 18 months of age. For such an infant, airway obstruction is a particular hazard, bearing in mind the relative sizes of the bronchial tree, the endotracheal tube and the catheter for the contrast medium. Removal of the contrast medium by suction is difficult, and an infant has a relatively poor power of coughing (Freifeld and Zalvendo, 1964; Atwood, 1965).

Respiration should be spontaneous at the end of the whole procedure, but after using a non-depolarising relaxant, neostigmine and atropine may be needed. The child should be nursed on one or other side and with his head and thorax tilted downwards until fully conscious to facilitate some lung drainage.

The essential requirements of any general anaesthetic technique for bronchography are control of the airway with adequate oxygenation at all times and a brief suppression of the cough reflex. The return of reflex activity must be rapid at the end of the procedure. There must be no explosion hazard. Although individual drugs, depending upon personal preference, are used to procure the necessary conditions, a clear distinction can be made between methods entailing the use of an endotracheal tube, and those in which the glottic reflexes are depressed by general anaesthesia and opaque oil poured into the trachea over the back of the tongue. Complete safety and control of secretions can only be achieved by intubation of the trachea and the use of suction, but these procedures and the associated depression of reflexes by relaxants or deep anaesthesia complicate the anaesthetist's work. A further advantage of endotracheal intubation is that the whole examination can be carried out deliberately and smoothly without undue haste, while the use of explosive and inflammable agents is easily excluded. Good team work between radiologist, anaesthetist and nurse is an essential prerequisite for safety and perfect pictures.

LARYNGOSCOPY AND BRONCHOSCOPY

Indirect Laryngoscopy

Indirect inspection of the glottis, even though performed by someone other than the anaesthetist, may provide information valuable to the anaesthetist concerning the type and extent of any laryngeal lesions, the degree of obstruction present, if any, and how the vocal cords move. These facts are of considerable importance when choosing an anaesthetic sequence for any form of operation, but more particularly when an operation in the neighbourhood of the glottis is contemplated, or intubation of the trachea intended.

Method.—A small circular laryngeal mirror set at an angle on the end of a metal stem is used. The mirror must be warmed by dipping in hot water just before use to prevent steaming up when the larynx is visualised. The patient sits opposite the operator with his mouth wide open and pulls his tongue well forward between a piece of gauze with his right hand. The back of the mirror is gently pushed up against the soft palate while a light is shone on the glass so that an inverted vision of the glottis is shown. In sensitive patients who tend to gag during the procedure, it is helpful to spray the soft palate and back of the tongue with a little 4 per cent lignocaine a few minutes before starting.

Direct Laryngoscopy and Micro-Laryngoscopy

All anaesthetists are familiar with the two principal types of laryngoscope— the straight and the curved (Macintosh) blade. The straight blade exposes the vocal cords by lifting the epiglottis itself; whereas the curved blade, which was designed to avoid stimulation of this sensitive structure, indirectly raises the epiglottis and brings the larynx into view by pressing upon the base of the tongue. Several variations of these two styles are described. Some of those that are commonly used by anaesthetists are illustrated in Fig. 9. For diagnostic purposes, particularly when biopsy is necessary, the straight bladed type is essential, not only to fix a particular cord, but also to evert it so that its inferior surface can be inspected. In the new technique of micro-laryngoscopy a straight blade including a small side-vent for insufflation is essential. Once the laryngoscope is fixed in a suitable position the surgeon can then focus a microscope on the vocal cords and observe any lesion. The anaesthetic technique is similar to that described for bronchoscopy (below).

Bronchoscopy

Bronchoscopy may be performed for diagnostic reasons, for purposes of treatment when it is necessary to remove excessive or troublesome secretions, or as an essential part of an anaesthetic technique when it is desirable to use a bronchial blocker.

Satisfactory conditions for performing a bronchoscopy can be achieved with either local or general anaesthesia.

Local anaesthesia.—The nerve supply to the larynx is principally derived from the glossopharyngeal and vagus nerves (9th and 10th cranial nerves). The glossopharyngeal, through its pharyngeal, tonsillar and lingual branches, sup-

LARYNGOSCOPE BLADES

MAGILL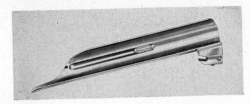

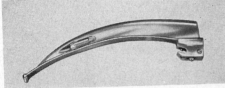 MACINTOSH

GUEDEL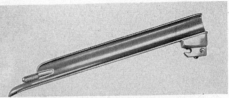

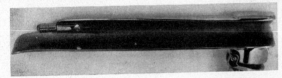 FOREGGER

SOPER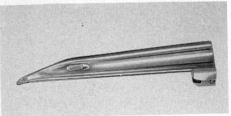

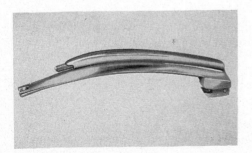 B-J (Bowen-Jackson)

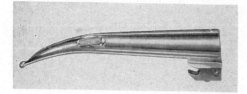

SEWARD

OXFORD INFANT

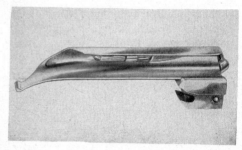

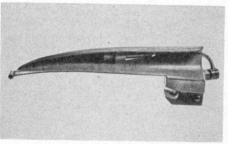

ROBERTSHAW

12/FIG. 9.—SOME STYLES OF LARYNGOSCOPE BLADES.

The Magill, Macintosh, Guedel, Foregger and Soper blades were designed primarily for adults, though each is available in a size suitable for children. The Soper blade combines the "Z" part of the Macintosh design with a straight blade. The B-J (Bowen-Jackson) is a compromise, and can be used for children and adults. The blade has a cleft at the end which enables it to straddle the glosso-epiglottic fold and enter the depths of the vallecula. It also has a marked curve at the distal end, while its depth is shallow so that it can be easily inserted between large teeth. The Seward, Oxford Infant and Robertshaw blades were all produced for infants and children. The Oxford Infant has an overhang on the open side to prevent the lips obscuring vision, and a broad, flat lower surface which is helpful for a child with a marked degree of cleft palate.

plies the sensory innervation of the pharynx, tonsils and posterior third of the tongue; while the vagus through the internal branch of the superior laryngeal nerve innervates both surfaces of the epiglottis, the aryepiglottic folds and the mucous membrane of the larynx down to the false cords. The recurrent laryngeal nerves (branches of the vagus) supply the rest of the mucous membrane and the upper part of the trachea.

In a suitably premedicated patient the back of the throat is first sprayed with 2 ml of 4 per cent lignocaine. It is then necessary to pass a small pledget of cotton-wool soaked in 4 per cent lignocaine into each pyriform fossa. This is done slowly with the aid of suitably curved forceps (Krause). Once satisfactory anaesthesia of the mucous membrane has been achieved a similar swab is passed centrally, with the tongue pulled forward, until after passing over the posterior surface of the tongue and epiglottis it comes to lie between the false cords. If required, an injection of 2 ml of 4 per cent lignocaine can be given through the cricothyroid membrane to reach the trachea and under-surface of the true vocal cords; alternatively a curved spray can be passed into the trachea.

General anaesthesia.—General anaesthesia for bronchoscopy requires good oxygenation, effective carbon dioxide elimination, complete paralysis and an unconscious patient. There are a number of techniques available. Unconsciousness is usually attained with thiopentone and complete paralysis with intermittent doses of suxamethonium. The various methods of producing oxygenation and eliminating carbon dioxide are discussed below:

(a) *Apnoeic oxygenation.* A fine catheter is passed into the trachea and oxygen is insufflated throughout the bronchoscopy. Experience has shown that despite adequate oxygenation the flow of gas is not sufficient to remove the carbon dioxide satisfactorily. Although sometimes adequate for short periods, an increased incidence of dysrhythmia is experienced as time progresses.

(b) *Occasional ventilation through the bronchoscope* using an endotracheal tube together with a high flow of oxygen has proved satisfactory. However, this method requires repeated interruption of the surgeon—which is not always appreciated!

(c) *Ventilating bronchoscope.* Anaesthetic gases are administered through a side-arm and the proximal lumen of the bronchoscope is occluded by a glass window in order to contain the gases. Apart from problems of misting, the window often needs to be removed for suctioning and the taking of a biopsy.

(d) *The fibre-optic bronchoscope.* This instrument can be passed through the rubber seal of a Cobb's suction connector and through the endotracheal tube into the distal bronchi. This has the advantage that anaesthesia can be continued with positive-pressure ventilation through the endotracheal tube at the same time.

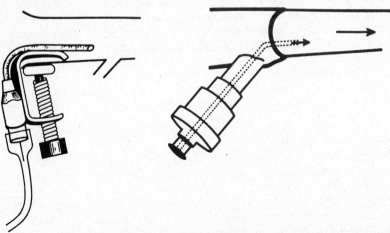

12/Fig. 10.—Diagram of two types of injector using venturi principle that can be attached to either a laryngoscope or a bronchoscope.

(e) *Venturi jet principle.* Sanders in 1967 proposed the use of the venturi principle for intermittent pressure breathing by attaching a jet injector to the bronchoscope (Fig. 10). In an adult the diameter of the jet needle is usually 0·9 mm and it is attached to a source of oxygen with a pressure of 60 p.s.i. (414 kPa). With this attachment the lungs can be regularly inflated without interfering with the activities of the surgeon. In normal adults, it is possible not only to improve on the Pao_2 but also to keep the $Paco_2$ within normal limits (Baraka and Muallem, 1972).

THORACOTOMY

GENERAL CONSIDERATIONS

Patients about to undergo a pulmonary operation need a careful explanation of what they are expected to do in the immediate post-operative period. Particular attention must be paid to the fitting and practical use of an oxygen mask or tent, and instruction must be given in breathing exercises and postural drainage, although the latter may not be necessary pre-operatively. When employed for these purposes a physiotherapist must have a clear understanding of the different operations which are likely to be performed and their individual requirements.

Breathing Exercises and Postural Drainage (see also p. 402)

Ventilatory movement, even of sound areas, is often diminished in pulmonary disease, partly because these patients are often confined to bed for relatively long periods and partly because they find that shallow breathing reduces the tendency to cough. A further specific factor is the effect of retraction of the lung on the side of the operation; and following a thoracoplasty respiration may be further embarrassed by strapping to prevent paradoxical movement.

Breathing exercises are designed to increase the capacity of all areas of the lungs, including those affected by disease. Excessive or sudden movements may be harmful to an area of healing tuberculosis, but movement and increased capacity of the normal parts is important. With the exception of tuberculous patients, the aim should be good and equal movements on *both* sides of the thorax. The emphasis should be on the affected side to bring it up to the standard of the good. Even after pneumonectomy, bilateral chest movements help to prevent deformity and keep the mediastinum central.

In wet cases postural drainage must be continued until the sputum can be reduced no further in quantity. Amounts of 30 ml or less, in a twenty-four hour period should be aimed at, and although such a result might be expected after a week of treatment, it may be necessary to persevere for a month in some patients.

Blood Gas Tensions

Impaired arterial gas tensions may be expected in patients with severe disease of the lungs. When a patient with pre-existing impairment of gas exchange in the lungs undergoes a pulmonary operation there will be a further deterioration and some degree of consequential hypoxia unless positive steps are taken to avoid this. It has been suggested that in such circumstances the oxygen-fraction of the inspired gas mixture should not fall below 50 per cent (Nilsson *et al.*, 1965; Lunding and Fernandes, 1967).

Antibiotics

Although anaesthetists are most likely to be concerned with the administration of these drugs for respiratory tract infections, certain general principles determining the use of antibiotics are worthy of discussion. It must first be emphasised that when problems do exist they are best solved by close co-operation between the clinician and the bacteriologist. The need for this co-operation stems largely from the increasing number of bacterial strains hitherto sensitive, but now resistant, to certain antibiotics, and from the many new antibiotics that have been produced to cope with the resistant bacterial strains.

All specimens should whenever possible be obtained from the patient before treatment is started with any antibiotic. The choice of a particular antibiotic, or combination of antibiotics, may then be made on the basis of a clinical judgement, but it is preferable whenever possible to wait until *in vitro* sensitivity tests have been carried out in the laboratory. These, however, though normally reliable when translated to the patient are not always so. When there is an apparent discrepancy of this nature, other possible causes of failure—such as inadequate dosage, lack of absorption, organisms isolated in an abscess, and inactivation of the antibiotic—should be sought. Furthermore, it is important to be sure that sufficient time has elapsed for the antibiotic given to be effective, since the patient's response may be delayed. Changing from one antibiotic to another too rapidly is unhelpful.

Generally speaking, the penicillins, streptomycin and the cephalosporins are bactericidal, while the tetracyclines are notably bacteriostatic. The former group should always be used when it is important to kill organisms, rather than merely stop their multiplication and allow the patient's natural resistance to do the rest. An overwhelming infection—particularly in the very young or the very old—is the sort of absolute indication for a bactericidal drug. Although there are exceptions, it is best not to combine a bactericidal with a bacteriostatic antibiotic.

There is good evidence that the prophylactic use of antibiotics may cause a higher rather than a lower incidence of infection, although, of course, this risk may have to be taken in certain instances. It is important to remember that in hospital practice resistant bacteria stem from the previous use of antibiotics. To put a patient on an antibiotic (particularly one of the broad-spectrum variety) will increase the risk of superinfection of that patient with resistant bacteria.

Non-tuberculous pulmonary infections.—As already outlined, antibiotics are best prescribed on the basis of bacterial sensitivity and there is good evidence that they are most valuable when started early in an infection (Malone *et al.*, 1968). When the occasion demands speedy action, such as an acute post-operative infection or a pre-operative acute bronchitis in a patient needing an operation urgently, then either ampicillin or tetracycline can be used. The adult dose of the former is from 250 mg to 1 g 6-hrly and of the latter 200 mg 6-hrly. Both are broad-spectrum antibiotics, but tetracycline is less so than when it was originally introduced, due to the appearance of strains of bacteria resistant to it. A recent broad-spectrum drug of value is trimethoprim sulphamethoxazole (Bactrim).

Empyema, lung abscess and other infected cases will need a systemic cover of a specific antibiotic depending on the sensitivity of the particular organism. Such a drug may also be usefully given intrapleurally to a patient with an empyema, but this is not a substitute for drainage by rib resection once the pus is too thick for aspiration, or when the lung stops expanding before closing the infected space.

Tuberculous pulmonary infections.—Pulmonary tuberculosis is still a major infectious disease in many parts of the world. Treatment will take from one to two years depending on the severity of the condition. The principal drugs used are streptomycin (1·0 g/day I.M.), isoniazid (100 mg 8-hrly) and the latest and most effective bactericidal agent rifampicin (450–600 mg by mouth, once a day). Once the diagnosis is established all three drugs are used whilst antibiotic sensitivity is established. After this is known, treatment is adjusted accordingly. Streptomycin cannot be given over a long period as it is liable to cause damage to the VIII cranial nerve. Rifampicin is relatively free from side-effects but cases of jaundice with liver damage and thrombocytopenia have been reported.

ANAESTHESIA

Controlled respiration is the most practicable method of ensuring adequate oxygenation and elimination of carbon dioxide in the presence of an open thorax. It also offers considerable advantages to the surgeon in terms of pulmonary and diaphragmatic movements suited to the practical procedure. Occasionally there are contra-indications to intermittent positive-pressure respiration for the whole or part of an anaesthetic, while some diseases, or the physical condition of the patient, may make a particular procedure or choice of drugs more valuable than the general routine. These points, as they arise, are mentioned in the pages that follow during the discussion of the specific conditions. The common routine—provided the sputum is not excessive—is suitable premedication, then an intravenous induction and intubation with the aid of suxamethonium or a longer acting muscle relaxant after ventilation with oxygen. Anaesthesia is maintained with nitrous oxide and oxygen and doses of a longer acting muscle relaxant, such as d-tubocurarine, are added when required. Pethidine and phenoperidine may be helpful to make up for the lessening effect of the premedication. They help the maintenance of controlled respiration by central depression so that the total dose of muscle relaxant need not be so great, and they also ensure that after a lengthy operation, some analgesia extends into the immediate post-operative period—an important point when the patient is fully conscious so soon after nitrous oxide. The principal disadvantage of pethidine and phenoperidine is the risk of overdosage, with inactive respiratory tract reflexes and respiratory depression during the early post-operative period. Any such depression can be overcome by the judicious use of a specific analgesic antagonist (naloxone) or a central nervous system stimulant (doxapram).

Replacement of blood loss can be a very important factor in some pulmonary operations, particularly if there has been any chronic sepsis with the formation of adhesions in the pleural space. Even with minimal loss it is probable that an average thoracotomy requires at least some blood to cover the operation and immediate post-operative period.

Normally, spontaneous breathing is allowed to return as soon as the skin suturing is started. On occasions when the chest is closed without drainage, however, controlled respiration must be continued because the thorax cannot be considered airtight until after the skin has been sutured; were spontaneous breathing to start before this, there is the possibility that the lung might collapse and be difficult to re-expand.

Basal pleural drainage with an under-water seal is, overall, an asset to the anaesthetist and the patient—many surgeons use one routinely whenever the pleural cavity is opened. It has three advantages:

(i) The anaesthetist can force air out of the pleural cavity after the skin of the operation wound is closed. Post-operatively, the patient does this when he coughs. Both these factors militate against pulmonary collapse.

(ii) Blood will not accumulate in the pleural cavity, so that bleeding can be quickly and simply assessed by looking at the contents of the drainage bottle.

(iii) After lobectomy or segmental lung operations, suction—at about minus 5 cm H_2O (0·5 kPa)—can be applied from a pump to the drain to encourage expansion of the remaining lung tissue. For such cases, basal and apical drains are normally used. Suction removes air from any leaks in the lung tissue, but may tend to keep such holes open. It should not be used after pneumonectomy, since it increases the risk of bronchial fistula and it may pull the mediastinum and its contents unduly into the thoracotomy cavity. In the latter instance the cardiac action can be hampered.

The disadvantage of pleural drainage is the increased risk of introducing sepsis into the operation site. Basal drains are normally removed after one or two days, depending on the amount of blood that is draining. Following a lobectomy or segmental removal, one or other of the drains should be left in place for at least four days.

Tracheobronchial suction down the endotracheal tube is a wise precaution at the end of operation. Bronchoscopy is rarely necessary and may do far more harm than good because the anaesthetic conditions for its performance at this stage are not ideal, and to produce them specially is rarely to the patient's advantage.

CONTROL OF SECRETIONS

With proper preparation few, if any, patients should come to operation with large quantities of infected sputum, although this may occasionally be loculated in the form of a lung abscess. The production of anaesthetic conditions adequate for thoracic surgery depresses all protective reflexes in the tracheobronchial tract so that secretions, squeezed by the manipulation of the surgeon, may easily spread to normal parts of the pulmonary tree during operation and are even likely to do so as soon as the patient is placed on the operating table in the lateral position. In this position (Fig. 11), the most commonly used for pulmonary operations because of the excellent approach which it affords to the hilar vessels, the diseased lung is uppermost, and draining both towards the normal lung below and its own upper lobe which is also frequently normal. No amount of head-down tilt can prevent this risk of spread (see Fig. 12), though it is valuable as an aid towards some drainage down the trachea.

Obstruction to respiration with consequent hypoxia, lung collapse, and spread of infection is a likely complication, so that special precautions must be taken to deal with secretions from the moment that anaesthesia is induced.

Simple Suction

This is the mainstay in the control of secretions in the respiratory tract, whether excessive or normal in amount. It must be to hand at all times and used not only intermittently throughout the operation when there are suggestive signs of mucus being present, but also at more specific moments during both the

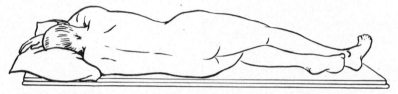

12/Fig. 11.—The lateral position for thoracic operations.

production of anaesthesia and certain surgical manipulations when large quantities are most likely to be released from the diseased areas. The presence of secretions in the trachea or major bronchi is usually apparent from an increased resistance to positive-pressure respiration, or from audible râles transmitted to and amplified in the rebreathing bag. The use of a stethoscope attachment incorporated in the anaesthetic system just above the endotracheal tube helps in their early recognition. Nevertheless a considerable amount of material can collect without very obvious clinical evidence, so that suction must be carried out at regular intervals throughout the operation in wet cases.

Thin, watery sputum or blood may easily pass, or indeed be forced with positive-pressure respiration, into the small bronchioles and eventually into the alveoli of normal lung. Apart from the risk of pulmonary collapse and infection, fluid of either type may coat the alveoli and effectively prevent the normal gaseous interchange.

The specific occasions when suction must be carried out are immediately after intubation of the trachea and—when secretions are excessive—before any positive-pressure respiration is used, as soon as the patient is turned from the

12/Fig. 12.—Diagram to illustrate how, in the right lateral position, the uppermost and diseased left lung may drain into its own upper lobe, despite a steep head-down tilt, and empty into the dependent right lung.

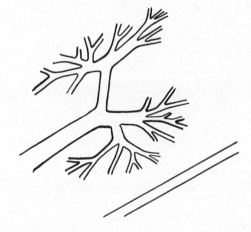

supine to the lateral position on the operating table, when the pleural cavity is opened, and whenever the surgeon manipulates the lung. Since suction may stimulate some reflex activity such as coughing, the surgeon must be warned before it is performed while surgery is in progress, but in the presence of large quantities of secretions there must be no delay.

Suction Combined with a Bronchus Clamp

A useful addition to suction is occlusion by the surgeon of the main bronchus of the affected side with a non-crushing clamp. This can only be carried out after the chest has been opened, but it is a valuable technique for producing not only control of secretions but also one lung anaesthesia (see also p. 472).

Bronchial Block

Secretions may be isolated in the affected area by blocking the bronchus concerned, or if it is impracticable to block the actual bronchus to a particular lobe, less specific control may be produced by blocking that which serves the whole lung. Block may be produced by placing in the bronchus a blocker of the Thompson, Magill or Macintosh-Leatherdale inflatable cuff type or by plugging this area with a strip of gauze (Fig. 13).

Complete block is unsatisfactory because it shuts the lobe or lung off completely from the rest of the pulmonary tree and delays its collapse. In these circumstances not only does the lung tend

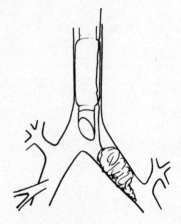

12/Fig. 13.—Crafoord's tampon.

to obscure the surgeon's field of vision, but a proportion of the pulmonary circulation passes through the non-functioning area without either elimination of carbon dioxide or uptake of oxygen. For this reason blockers consist of a drainage or central suction tube surrounded by an inflatable cuff. A further objection to tamponage of the bronchus (now out-dated) is the difficulty in carrying it out accurately even under direct vision, particularly when the smaller bronchi are concerned. There was always a risk of movement of the gauze during the operation even though it was held down by a wire stilette.

The actual *blocking* of a main bronchus or one leading to a particular lobe is not commonly practised nowadays. Isolation of one or other bronchus is generally achieved by selection of either an endobronchial or a double-lumen tube.

Blockers (Figs. 14 and 15).—The Thompson blocker consists of a gauze-covered cuff which can be inflated through a narrow tube. This tube is fused with a larger tube running through the cuff to provide drainage from the blocked lung (Fig. 14a). The gauze cover tends to keep the cuff securely fixed by friction against the bronchial mucous membrane and prevents over-inflation with the risk of rupture. The covered cuff, even when deflated, will only pass with ease down a large bronchoscope. The Magill blocker is designed on a

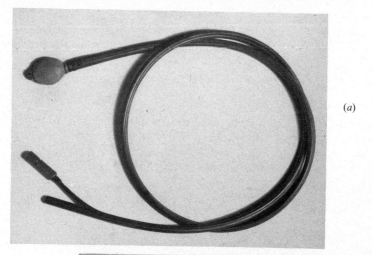

(a)

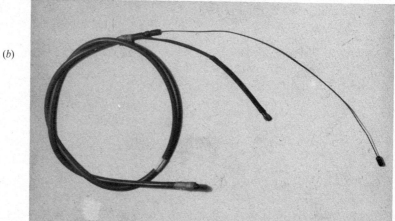

(b)

12/FIG. 14.—ENDOBRONCHIAL BLOCKERS
(a) Thompson's endobronchial blocker. (b) Magill's endobronchial blocker.

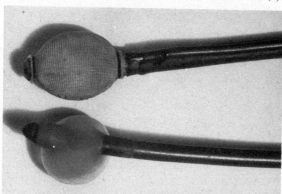

12/FIG 15.—Comparison of
inflated cuffs on the Thompson
(above) and Magill blockers.

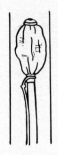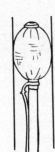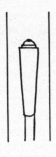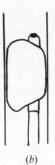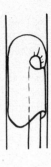

(a)   (b)

12/Fig. 16.—Diagrammatic Illustration to Show how a Blocker may Lie in the Bronchus

   (a) Thompson. Uninflated and inflated.
   (b) Magill. Note how over-inflation blocks the lumen of the tube.

similar principle but without a gauze cover, so that the deflated cuff is small and adaptable for passing down a small bronchoscope—minimum size 8 mm—and placing in the small bronchi. However, the cuff ruptures easily and there is a danger of over-inflation with ballooning over the end of the drainage tube (Fig. 16). For routine use the Thompson blocker is most favoured, but for upper lobes and children large enough for consideration of the technique the Magill,

or modified Magill (see p. 469), being smaller, is more valuable. The Macintosh-Leatherdale bronchus blocker (Fig. 17) has two cuffs, one to lie in the trachea and the other in the left main bronchus. This tube is passed without the aid of a bronchoscope and combines the advantages of an endotracheal tube and a bronchus blocker.

Technique for passing blockers.—Prior to use the cuff must be tested for leaks and the blocker must be pushed down the bronchoscope until the deflated cuff is just beyond the distal end (with the Thompson blocker and large bronchoscope this will be felt as a definite give). An ink mark is then made on the tubing at the level of the proximal end of the bronchoscope so that when the actual operation is performed there will be no doubt that the

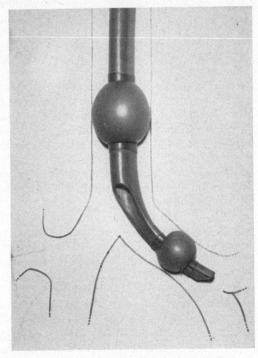

12/Fig. 17.—Macintosh-Leatherdale bronchus blocker.

cuff has reached the bronchus. This is very important, since, although the place in the bronchus is first visualised down the bronchoscope, the actual positioning of a blocker cannot be done under direct vision. The blocker is fitted with a wire stilette which runs down the drainage tube and this must be greased with a little water-soluble lubricant immediately before use so that it can be easily withdrawn once the blocker is in position. A little pasta lubricans should also be put on the cuff.

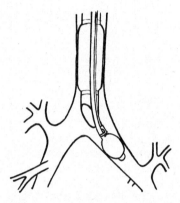

12/Fig. 18.—Diagram to show relationship of blocker to endotracheal tube.

The patient is bronchoscoped, the carina and both main bronchi visualised, and any obvious secretions removed by suction. The tip of the bronchoscope is then placed in the appropriate bronchus just above the level required and the blocker passed to the measured distance so that the cuff lies in the bronchus. The cuff is then inflated, and first the stilette and then the bronchoscope removed. It is usual to inflate the cuff of a Thompson blocker with water and the quantity needed is approximately 3 ml. Water offers a more even pressure than air, and its volume is not dependent upon temperature. Magill blockers are inflated with air, since they hold more and the risk of rupture and leakage of water into the lung is greater. At this stage the patient is intubated with a large endotracheal tube which can be most easily passed with the tubing of the blocker lying posteriorly in the glottis.

A glance at Fig. 18 will show that this method of bronchial blocking is particularly useful for block of the left main bronchus just past the carina and of the left lower lobe or right middle and lower lobes. Upper lobe bronchus block is a more specialised technique which is described below. The distance of 5 cm between the carina and the orifice of the left upper lobe bronchus leaves plenty of room for the cuff when it is desired to collapse the left lung, and block of the lower lobe bronchus on this side is no more difficult, since plenty of room is available below the opening of the upper lobe bronchus. However, on this side the lingula is frequently removed at the same time as the lower lobe, but since its bronchus arises from the upper lobe bronchus it cannot be blocked separately or in conjunction with the lower lobe. On the right side the problem is more difficult. There is only 2·5 cm between the carina and the upper lobe bronchus, so that the cuff must be placed very accurately (Fig. 19). The principal difficulty is to avoid direct block of the upper lobe bronchus by the side of the cuff. This may be useful sometimes (Fig. 20), but not only prevents drainage of secretions from the upper lobe but also the escape of air, and leaves a partially inflated lobe in the surgeon's way. Furthermore, a ball valve may be produced leading to marked distension of the lobe as the anaesthetic progresses.

A much commoner mistake is to place the blocker too far down the right bronchus, leaving the upper lobe bronchus partially or completely open so that this lobe is not affected. Block of the middle and lower lobes is not difficult to

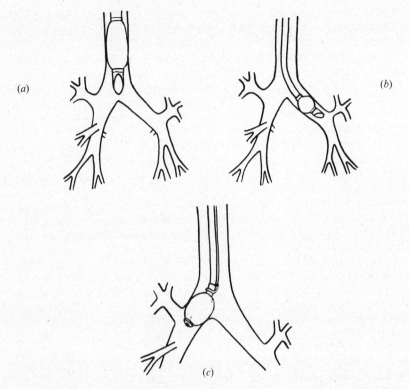

(a)

(b)

(c)

12/Fig. 19.—(a) Endotracheal cuffed tube. (b) Left endobronchial tube. (c) Right endobronchial blocker.

accomplish, but attempted block of the lower lobe by pushing the blocker well down to avoid the middle lobe bronchus usually leaves the apical lower lobe bronchus open. These several practical disadvantages of the right bronchial tree will be discussed further in the comparison of contralateral bronchial block and endobronchial anaesthesia.

Upper lobe blocking (Stephen, 1952).—A special Magill blocker with a small cuff of approximately half the normal length is necessary for this procedure, since the upper lobe bronchus frequently subdivides soon after leaving the main bronchus. This leaves very little room for insertion of a blocker, and the difficulty may be further accentuated by disease. Upper lobectomies are most often performed for tuberculosis, which more than other lesions is likely to lead to fibrosis with narrowing of the lumen and distortion of the angle formed between this bronchus and the

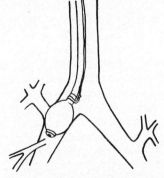

12/Fig. 20.—Diagram to show blocker placed to occlude right upper lobe bronchus completely.

parent stem. An acute angle makes the procedure difficult, if not impossible. With the stilette in position the cuff end of the blocker is slightly angulated so as to increase the ease of insertion, without preventing its free passage down the bronchoscope. When the bronchoscope is passed an attempt must be made to get it and the orifice of the particular upper lobe bronchus in a straight line by bending the patient's head as far as possible to the opposite side. Such a position is only practicable under general anaesthesia. The chances of success are greater on the right side where the upper lobe bronchus lies nearer the carina. This avoids the necessity of introducing more than the tip of the bronchoscope into the main bronchus, and makes for greater flexibility. When the bronchoscope is correctly positioned the rest of the bronchial tree is automatically shut off so that passage of the blocker should lead easily to intubation of the upper lobe bronchus.

Checking the position.—Once the blocker is placed its position should be checked. In the case of block of one or other main bronchus, particularly after suction down the blocker, there are usually obvious signs of pulmonary collapse present, such as the absence of thoracic movement on that side and of breath sounds on auscultation during inflation. When the bronchus to a lobe is blocked these signs may be equivocal, due to aeration of the remaining lobes, but unless there are other reasons for doubting a good position this should not be taken as an indication for repeating the procedure. The true test of success can only be made when the thorax is open and movement of the lung can be watched during positive-pressure respiration.

It might be expected that the sudden dependence on one lung would lead to obvious evidence of hypoxia—particularly during the first few minutes after block when pulmonary collapse is incomplete and a considerable quantity of blood is still circulating without aeration. In practice, visible cyanosis or evidence of circulatory upset are rare provided the remaining lung is sound and the patient is properly anaesthetised. Under anaesthesia, and particularly with controlled respiration, the oxygen saturation of the blood should be normal.

There is a risk of the blocker slipping if the patient coughs, after sudden movement—such as might occur when positioning on the operating table—or when the surgeon handles the lung near it. In these circumstances the whole cuff may come back into the trachea and perhaps cause obstruction to respiration. If there is any difficulty in inflating a patient after inserting a blocker, particularly in the absence of other more obvious factors, the blocker must be deflated and removed at once. But a blocker may slip back into the trachea without causing complete obstruction and its dislodgement will only be appreciated when suction is applied to it. This will lead to rapid removal of gas from the lungs and anaesthetic system.

Removal.—The blocker must be removed just before the surgeon clamps the bronchus. The cuff is deflated by sucking out the water or air and the whole tube pulled out of the tracheobronchial tree. This can be done without removing the endotracheal tube, but its cuff must be momentarily deflated. During removal of the blocker, constant suction should be applied to its lumen in an attempt to aspirate any residual secretions in the trachea or bronchus.

Endobronchial Intubation

A diseased lung may be isolated by intubating the bronchus of the normal lung. The affected area remains in communication with the atmosphere but not with the anaesthetic system, and as it is not ventilated pulmonary collapse follows. Secretions will drain from it with posture into the trachea and oropharynx. The endobronchial tube is normally placed in the main bronchus.

Endobronchial tubes are made in several sizes, the essential points being a narrow cuff and beyond this a very brief length of tube and short bevel. They are placed in position under direct vision with an intubating bronchoscope of the Magill (Fig. 21) or modified Magill type. The latter is adapted to take the standard light fitting of a Negus bronchoscope (Mansfield, 1957).

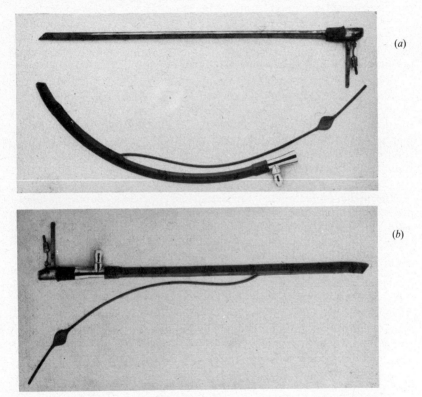

(a)

(b)

12/FIG. 21.—(a) Magill's intubating bronchoscope with Machray's endobronchial tube.
(b) Bronchoscope and endobronchial tube ready for bronchial intubation.

Technique for endobronchial intubation.—The bronchoscope is greased with a little sterile lubricant paste and then placed within the endobronchial tube. This must be stretched to its full length, so that the bevel of the bronchoscope and of the tube correspond in position. There is no advantage in attempting to cut the tube to the exact distance between the major bronchi and the front teeth, and it is better to have the tube a little too long than too short. Bronchoscopy is performed and any secretions in the tracheobronchial tree are removed. For left endobronchial intubation the beak of the bronchoscope is placed well within the main bronchus, the cuff is inflated, and the bronchoscope slid from within the tube while this is firmly held in position at the mouth. On the right side the opening of the upper lobe bronchus must first be visualised and then the cuff of the endobronchial tube placed between this and the carina with the bevel facing towards it. This ensures that ballooning of the cuff is unlikely to block off the upper lobe. In practice right endobronchial anaesthesia with the Machray tube is unsatisfactory, since it is difficult to avoid impinging on the upper lobe bronchus in some degree (Fig. 22).

Special endobronchial tubes have been designed for either right lung surgery (Macintosh-Leatherdale, Fig. 23a and Brompton triple cuff, Fig. 23b), or left lung surgery (Green and Gordon, Fig. 23c).

There is a risk of the Machray endobronchial tube slipping from its position, particularly on the right side, though this is less than with a blocker because of the relative sizes of tube and cuff. The cuff on the endobronchial tube only expands a little and gives a firmer fit.

Removal.—Endobronchial anaesthesia is usually performed for pneumonectomy so that the question of removal does not arise until the operation is over. However, the surgeon may decide to do only a lobectomy and this will require the tube being withdrawn to the trachea so that the remaining lobe can be reinflated. The small bore of the tube constitutes a marked disadvantage in this situation—particularly if the remainder of the operation is going to take long. It may be better to remove it altogether and intubate with a full-sized tube, but the position of the patient does not make laryngoscopy easy.

Discussion on the relative merits of blockers and endobronchial tubes.—The distance between the orifice of the upper lobe bronchus and the carina on the right side leaves so little room for an inflated cuff that whenever possible it is wiser to use the left main bronchus, either for a blocker to isolate the left lung or for an endobronchial tube to isolate the right lung.

The correct placing of an endobronchial tube or blocker, but particularly of the latter, is a skilled manoeuvre which only practice can make effective on every occasion. It must be remembered that the physical factors present in the bronchus all militate against the success of the procedure. Inflation of the cuff tends to push it out of the bronchus, which is itself a fluted tube becoming progressively smaller in diameter. Failure of the cuff to stick is often accentuated by a mucous membrane made slippery by purulent secretions, and by movement from ventilation and surgical manipulation in that region. It is a good maxim to be satisfied with an apparently reasonable or partially effective result, rather than to go on making more attempts while the patient's condition deteriorates; it is best to remove the tube completely if it is impossible to aerate the patient adequately after its insertion. Even when correctly placed, endobronchial tubes and blockers slip at the crucial moment during operations in a proportion of cases, so that complete reliance can never be placed on them and suction must be available on all occasions. Ideally in all wet cases this method of controlling secretions should be looked upon as a temporary expedient until the surgeon can clamp the bronchus himself. It is usually feasible to clamp the main bronchus very soon after entering the pleural cavity, and there does not appear to be any

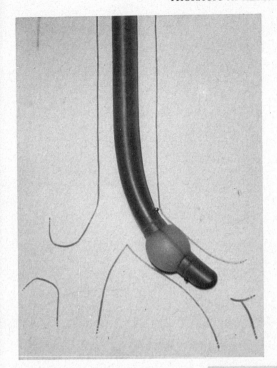

12/Fig. 22.—Machray endobronchial tube.

12/Fig. 23(a).—Macintosh-Leatherdale left endobronchial tube.

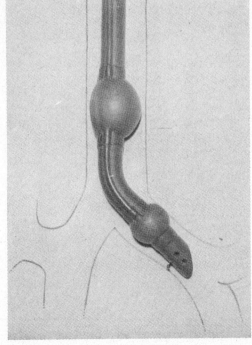

12/FIG. 23(*b*).—Brompton triple-cuffed endobronchial tube. This tube was designed for wedge resection of part of the right lung. The cuff in the left main bronchus is duplicated so that accidental puncture during operation of the outer cuff is not a disaster.

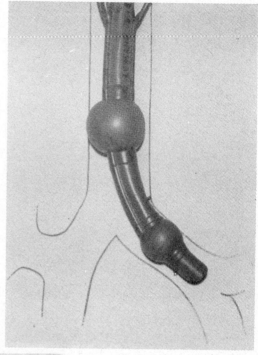

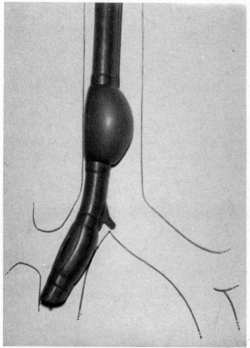

12/FIG. 23(*c*).—Green and Gordon's right endobronchial tube. The lower cuff lies in the right main bronchus. A small opening at the level of the right upper lobe bronchus prevents this lobe of the lung being obstructed. This tube is suitable for left lung surgery.

practical objection to this procedure even though the projected operation is for lobectomy alone. In theory, to clamp the main bronchus and leave normal lung tissue collapsed for the greater part of an operation will lead to an increased incidence of spread of infection to these areas and a greater tendency to their post-operative collapse. In practice, this has not been proved to be the case, provided toilet of the remaining bronchi is performed by the surgeon before reinflation, since collapse of the whole lung with loss of air movement greatly diminishes the chance of spread from one lobe to another. The benefits in terms of a trouble-free anaesthesia performed through the sound lung are very great and the relatively short time the cuff remains in the bronchus in these circumstances decreases the chance of mucosal sloughs from pressure anaemia.

The overall advantages of endobronchial anaesthesia or bronchial blocking are not in doubt provided they are used with care and not looked upon as being fool-proof. They can be used with great advantage not only in the handling of excessive secretions, but to control or limit bleeding in the lower respiratory tract; to localise slight but infected sputum as in tuberculosis; to facilitate surgical access by collapsing the lung prior to removal for a neoplasm or other disease; and to control a broncho-pleural fistula. They may also be useful during the removal of an air cyst from the lung (see p. 483).

Anaesthesia for Endobronchial Intubation or Bronchial Blocking

When selective lung collapse is to be performed to control either excessive secretions, bleeding, or small amounts of sputum infected with tubercle bacilli, the mode of anaesthesia must allow for adequate removal of visible secretions by suction and the placing of the blocker or endobronchial tube before positive-pressure respiration in any form is carried out. Moreover, until this is accomplished it is axiomatic that the posture of the patient must be such as to retain the secretions in the affected areas once the protective cough reflexes of the patient are removed. Under local analgesia there is no need to bother about positive-pressure respiration and the patient oxygenates himself throughout the procedure. But placing either a blocker or endobronchial tube is uncomfortable for a conscious patient, puts some strain on his already diminished circulatory and respiratory reserves when the lung collapses, and is not easy to perform correctly unless the patient breathes very quietly. It does, however, encourage gentleness and avoids the need to hurry. The conditions produced by general anaesthesia with a relaxant make the procedure easier and considerably quicker, but in inexperienced hands and for those patients in whom there is little margin for error, local analgesia is less likely to lead to a dangerous situation if the procedure fails at the first attempt.

The essentials for general anaesthesia are inhalation of oxygen for about 3–4 minutes followed by induction of anaesthesia with a small dose of thiopentone and then the production of total paralysis with suxamethonium or pancuronium. Pre-operative oxygen inhalation can be dispensed with in dry cases, but inflation with oxygen must then be carried out after the onset of paralysis and before bronchoscopy so that the period of apnoea does not lead to anoxia. The tracheo-bronchial tree should also be well sprayed with topical analgesic to prevent coughing with possible dislodgement of the tube on recovery from the paralysis. An alternative method of general anaesthesia is to use oxygen and halothane and to maintain spontaneous respiration until the blocker or tube is in position. Patients with broncho-pleural fistula or air cysts present special problems and must usually be treated the same way as wet cases (see p. 482 *et seq.*).

"Sleeve" Resection

The treatment of a neoplastic growth in the upper lobe of a lung cannot be effected by simple lobectomy when there is invasion of the main bronchus. A "sleeve" resection involves removing a length of the main bronchus together with the affected lobe. Following this, on the right side the end of the right bronchus is anastomosed to the trachea, while on the left side the bronchus is restored in continuity. The anaesthetist may encounter difficulty as the cut bronchus must remain open for a considerable period, but this can be overcome by the use of a blocker or double-lumen tube. However, it is important to remember that a blocker or tube may be displaced due to manipulation of the bronchus and that the cuff of either may be accidentally deflated by the surgeon's knife. A reserve cuff is therefore an advantage (Pallister, 1959).

Double-Lumen Tubes

There are three principal tubes which are now widely used in thoracic anaesthesia and permit selective control of either lung to be carried out during anaesthesia. These are the Carlens, Bryce-Smith and Robertshaw double-lumen tubes, and they are illustrated in Figs. 24 *a–d.* The Carlens tube was not designed for use during operations and in many centres has been superseded by the Bryce-Smith and Robertshaw tubes which are both made in right and left forms. They are easier to manipulate than the Carlens and have a proportionately larger lumen which makes suction easier.

The double-lumen tube will probably be the method of choice in most cases as it has the advantage of allowing both lungs to be inflated except when one-lung anaesthesia is desired. This is obviously more physiological than the use of single-lumen endobronchial tubes or bronchial blockers. Two other advantages are that the wide lumen permits easy passage of a suction catheter and that the tube is fairly easy for the inexperienced to pass into the correct place.

The Robertshaw is the most commonly used. The Carlens tube is less robust, has a smaller diameter lumen and the hook is a disadvantage when a pneumonectomy is to be performed.

For operations in the chest, when one-lung anaesthesia is required to facilitate surgical access (for example, oesophagectomy), the left tube is preferred and the right tube is only needed when the left lung is being operated upon.

Robertshaw tubes come in three sizes, small, medium and large, and the diameter increases simultaneously with the length. Occasionally this gives rise to difficulty if the patient is unusual in the proportion of laryngeal diameter to tracheal length.

Technique for insertion.—The PA penetrated chest X-ray should be carefully inspected prior to anaesthesia to confirm that the anatomy of the trachea, carina and main bronchi are normal, as distortion of these structures may make the correct placement of the tube impossible. Both cuffs should also be tested.

The tube is passed after the patient has been paralysed with suxamethonium. The larynx is exposed with a Macintosh curved-blade laryngoscope and the tip of the tube engaged in the cords. Sometimes the tube will then slide straight in, otherwise it should be rotated through 180° or 360°, moving forward as it is rotated. It is pushed until it obviously settles in the correct position.

The catheter mount to the tracheal lumen is clamped and the bronchial lumen is inflated while the bronchial cuff is blown up until the air leak ceases. Now, only the single lung should inflate. Next, the tracheal lumen is inflated while the bronchial catheter mount is clamped and the tracheal cuff inflated until the leak ceases, as for a normal endotracheal tube. Only the contralateral lung inflates. Finally, the clamp is removed and both lungs are inflated, and the tube is tied securely. Once the patient has been positioned for the operation, the chest should again be auscultated to ensure that either lung can be inflated at will and that the tube has not become dislodged.

If the tube is incorrectly placed, inflation of the bronchial cuff is not followed by unilateral lung inflation and, commonly, when the tracheal cuff is inflated, ventilation of the lungs becomes impossible. Both cuffs should be deflated, the tube partially withdrawn and then reinserted. If correct positioning is still not achieved, it may be worth turning the head to one side or the other, or perhaps trying a different size tube. It is most certainly unsatisfactory, and perhaps dangerous, to allow surgery to start if the tube is not correctly positioned. In fact, it is far better to substitute an ordinary endotracheal tube and ask the surgeon to make some alternative arrangement to isolate the lung.

One-Lung Anaesthesia and Hypoxaemia

The advantages of a collapsed lung in the operative field during thoracic surgery are obvious to all. With controlled respiration (IPPR), before the pleural

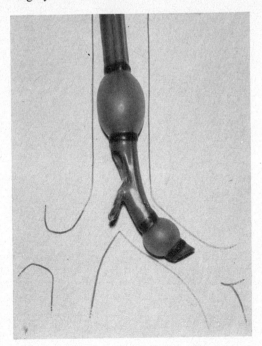

12/Fig. 24(a).—Carlens double-lumen endobronchial tube.

12/Fig. 24(b).—Bryce-Smith right endobronchial double-lumen tube. The lower cuff has an opening opposite the origin of the right upper lobe bronchus.

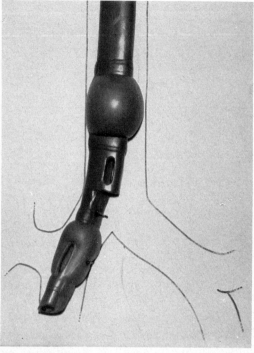

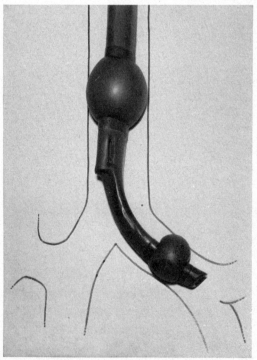

12/Fig. 24(c).—Bryce-Smith left endobronchial double-lumen tube.

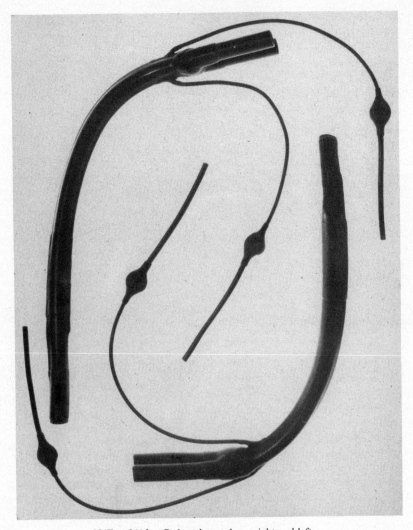

12/Fig. 24(*d*).—Robertshaw tubes—right and left.

cavity is entered and with the patient in the lateral position, the underlying lung will receive a preferential flow of pulmonary blood due to gravity whilst the uppermost lung receives the lion's share of the ventilation. This is in contrast with the situation when the patient breathes spontaneously as then the lower lung gets a preferential blood supply *and* greater ventilation. Again during IPPR, on entering the pleural cavity the lung is allowed to collapse but there is little or no reduction of the blood flow through the atelectatic lung. In fact, Torda and his co-workers (1974) observed shunts varying from 21 to 65 per cent of the cardiac output during one-lung anaesthesia with a double-lumen tube. These authors concluded that patients undergoing a thoracotomy with one-lung anaesthesia may have only marginal arterial oxygen tensions.

Khanam and Branthwaite (1973 *a* and *b*) undertook an extensive study in an attempt to determine the most beneficial respiratory pattern for patients undergoing a thoracotomy. In their control series the "ideal" ventilatory pattern which enabled the Pa_{CO_2} to be kept within the range of 30 to 40 mm Hg (4·0–5·3 kPa) with one-lung anaesthesia using a mixture of 40 per cent oxygen and 60 per cent nitrous oxide was achieved with:—

         Tidal volume   7 ml/kg body weight
         Respiratory rate   20 per minute

Attempts to vary this "ideal" ventilation either by increasing or decreasing the rate or tidal volume did not improve the arterial oxygen tension. The introduction of a positive end-expiratory pressure (PEEP) also did not improve oxygenation. However, they observed that when using an endobronchial tube, if the cuff to the affected lung was *not* inflated until the pleura was opened then both lungs could continue to be inflated with the aid of the tracheal cuff. The use of an endobronchial or double-lumen tube, therefore, led to significantly higher values for arterial oxygen tension. They concluded that once ventilation to the defective lung ceased, it was advisable to occlude the pulmonary vessels to that lung at the earliest possible opportunity. Prior to the opening of the pleura both lungs should continue to be ventilated.

The insufflation of oxygen through a small catheter into the affected lung during the period of collapse and before the arrest of the pulmonary circulation would seem a wise precaution to diminish the hypoxaemia.

The Prone Position with Drainage of Secretions

This position was designed to allow free drainage from the diseased areas to the trachea and into the mouth without soiling the sound lung (Parry Brown, 1948). It has the further advantage of avoiding mediastinal displacement when the pleural cavity is opened. The basic position is obtained by putting two padded supports beneath the prone patient, one at the level of the pelvis and one under the lower chest extending up to the manubrium sterni. The side for operation is placed at the edge of the table with that arm hanging down (Fig. 25), and keeping the scapula away from the operation field. The upper dorsal and cervical vertebrae are flexed over the chest support and should be tilted downwards, while the lower dorsal and lumbar vertebrae are made horizontal. The head is extended at the atlanto-occipital joint and with the neck rotated to face the side of the lesion so that the trachea and bronchus of the affected lung are in a straight line. There is a danger that the bronchus on the sound side may become kinked during hilar traction at operation when the head is slanted in the opposite direction.

The principal objection to this position is the more limited surgical exposure which it allows. There is adequate freedom for diaphragmatic movement and the hanging arm does not suffer. The position has marked advantages in allowing free drainage of secretions. This is particularly important in children where other methods of control, such as blocking or suction, may be impracticable or inadequate, though posture alone cannot be relied upon when the secretions are copious and intermittent suction must be carried out. There is, however, a slight risk of spread either to the dependent middle or lingula lobe bronchus. Induced hypotension is dangerous in the prone position as an abnormally low systemic pressure may follow its use.

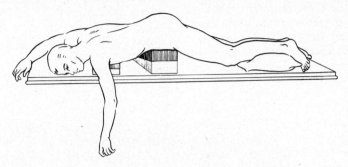

12/FIG. 25.—Prone position (Parry Brown) for drainage of secretions.

Prone Position with Retention of Secretions

In this position the patient is supported at the head, shoulders and hips so that there is no restriction of respiratory movement. The diseased side, although the patient is tilted head-downwards, is dependent to keep secretions from spreading (Overholt *et al.*, 1946).

With this method, if the secretions are copious, manipulation of the lung may cause periodic overflow. It is better, therefore, to have them flowing freely during the whole operation, as is the case in Parry Brown's position, and to aid their removal by intermittent suction.

Upright Retention Position

The flow of large quantities of secretions in young children may seriously affect the airway despite repeated suction, and even in the prone position there is a possibility of spread to the dependent middle or lingula lobe. In patients with bilateral disease this risk is greatly increased and may constitute an indication for the use of an upright retention method. Anaesthesia must be induced with the child upright, and suction used to clear as much sputum as possible from the respiratory tract.

The advantage of the method is that the secretions remain in the affected areas, thus limiting the need for suction: there is also less risk of respiratory obstruction.

EMPYEMA

Empyemata offer many dangers to the unwary anaesthetist and for reasons of safety should be drained under local anaesthesia with the patient sitting in an upright position. The line of the proposed incision should be infiltrated, and the intercostal nerves of the ribs to be resected, and those immediately above and below, should be blocked with 1 per cent lignocaine.

The presence of an active cough reflex, and avoidance of the lateral, supine and prone positions, diminishes the danger of pus flooding from the infected pleural cavity into the bronchial tree. The absence—proved or presumed—of a broncho-pleural fistula makes no difference and is no excuse for neglecting elementary precautions, since the surgeon's manipulations may well make a fistula. Should factors—such as the mental state of the patient or the surgeon's desire to do more than simple drainage—make local anaesthesia insufficient, a method of general anaesthesia must be selected and administered as described in the next section. The most recent thinking on the treatment of empyema comprises excision of the whole empyema cavity under general anaesthesia with removal of the pleura. The remaining lung tissue then adheres directly to the interior of the thoracic cage.

BRONCHO-PLEURAL FISTULA

A broncho-pleural fistula may follow a pulmonary resection, rupture of a lung abscess or may result from the spread of an untreated empyema. Whatever the origin an operation may be necessary and the presence of the fistula complicates anaesthesia and increases its dangers.

Diagnosis.—Post-operatively fistulae usually develop within the first two weeks, though they may occur after several months of convalescence when they are perhaps symptomatic of an unsuspected empyema. In their mode of onset the majority are undramatic; the usual suggestive signs are a cough which—especially after changes of position—is productive, the sputum being often blood-stained. If there is much fluid in the pleural cavity the sputum may be copious. Occasionally the onset is dramatic, as when after a bout of coughing the patient suddenly brings up large quantities of fluid. Sometimes when the fistula is small it has a valvular action—each cough forcing air into the pleural space. In this event the rising pleural pressure leads to collapse of the lung and mediastinal shift, with consequent dyspnoea, tachycardia, cyanosis and engorged neck veins—all signs of a tension pneumothorax.

In all cases the danger of a broncho-pleural fistula is overflow of infected pleural fluid into normal lung, and this risk is greatly increased by anaesthesia unless special precautions are taken. Surgical treatment usually takes one of three forms—a simple rib resection and drainage of the pleural space, thoracoplasty for chronic or grossly infected cases, or thoracotomy with closure of the fistula in early post-operative cases. A fistula occurring soon after lung resection is not necessarily associated with an infected pleural space, but this complication will soon follow unless the fistula is quickly closed.

Anaesthesia.—It is important when considering anaesthesia for simple drainage of an empyema, to have in mind the possibility that a fistula may be already present or be caused during the operation. This operation should, therefore, be performed with the patient sitting up. In the presence of a fistula the risk of spread under local analgesia is minimal, and in view of the comparatively minor nature of the operation, this technique is preferable to general anaesthesia which necessitates, in this instance, a complicated procedure.

When general anaesthesia is essential—as for instance when sepsis of the chest wall contra-indicates local injections—three points must be considered. First, that placing the patient supine, or worse still in the lateral position with the diseased side uppermost, will lead to flooding of the normal lung. These positions must never be used for the induction of general anaesthesia for this type of case. Secondly, that even with positive-pressure respiration it may be

impossible to oxygenate the patient adequately in the presence of a large fistula
—particularly when the surgeon enters the thorax; and thirdly, that if the hole
is very small, continued positive pressure may lead to a tension pneumothorax.
The choice of technique therefore depends to some extent on a clinical evaluation
of the type and size of the fistula; but unless the surgeon is prepared to guard
against contralateral spread by operating in the prone position, one lung
anaesthesia or the use of a double-lumen tube is to be preferred. Indeed, one or
other of these may be essential to ensure efficient ventilation even in the prone
position when the fistula is large. A particular advantage of a double-lumen tube
is that when an attempt is being made to close a broncho-pleural fistula, the
efficacy of the repair can be tested easily, whereas in similar circumstances an
endobronchial tube would need to be withdrawn into the trachea.

Since both tubes and blockers may slip, their use should be combined with
as much anti-Trendelenburg position on the operating table as possible in a
further attempt to localise all fluid to the lower part of the diseased pleura. The
surgeon must be prepared to clamp the bronchus as soon as he enters the thorax,
or to occlude the fistula temporarily if it is a large one.

The choice between local and general anaesthesia for placing the blocker or
tube must be made for reasons similar to those already described under wet lung
cases. The margin of safety is so narrow with a broncho-pleural fistula and an
infected pleural space that if there is any doubt about the practical problem,
bronchoscopy and placing of the blocker or tube should be done under local
analgesia and general anaesthesia induced afterwards. When general anaesthesia
with a muscle relaxant is proposed, it must be preceded by the inhalation of
oxygen as described for wet lung cases, so that positive-pressure respiration can
be avoided until the affected lung has been isolated. An alternative method is to
use oxygen and halothane, maintaining spontaneous respiration until the tube
or blocker is in position (Francis and Smith, 1962). The induction of anaesthesia,
bronchoscopy and the passage of the tube or blocker must be performed with
the patient sitting up.

Lung Cysts

Gray and Edwards (1948) note that cysts of the lung occasionally have a
one-way valvular mechanism (Fig. 26). Such cysts are usually congenital, but
some may be acquired in emphysematous patients. As previously mentioned
above, a similar valvular mechanism sometimes occurs at the site of a small
broncho-pleural fistula, or when an endobronchial blocker is incorrectly placed;
if intermittent positive-pressure respiration is used in such circumstances the
tension of the gases in the cyst (the pleural space or the isolated lobe as the
case may be) will rise, and may eventually cause enough distension to collapse
the surrounding lung tissue and displace the mediastinum and its contents with
serious impairment of the patient's gaseous exchange and circulation.

When such a condition is suspected pre-operatively, spontaneous respiration
must be maintained until the valve can be isolated either by a blocker or endobronchial tube, or by the surgical operation. If it is only discovered after
respiration has been controlled as a result of deterioration in the patient's
condition, increased pressure needed for inflation, and loss of gases in the
anaesthetic breathing bag, then speedy treatment may be necessary. Either the

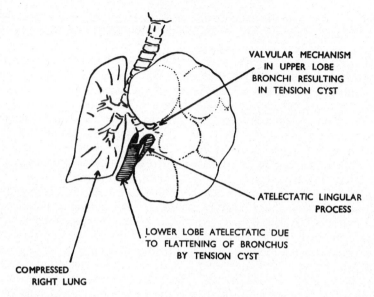

VALVULAR MECHANISM
IN UPPER LOBE
BRONCHI RESULTING
IN TENSION CYST

ATELECTATIC LINGULAR
PROCESS

LOWER LOBE ATELECTATIC DUE
TO FLATTENING OF BRONCHUS
BY TENSION CYST

COMPRESSED
RIGHT LUNG

12/FIG. 26.—Tension cyst of lung.

surgeon must quickly open the pleural cavity or, if he is not prepared, a large-bore needle must be passed into it to let off the pressure.

POST-OPERATIVE PULMONARY COMPLICATIONS

General Considerations

Despite the great improvement in anaesthetic techniques and an increased understanding of the mechanism of post-operative pulmonary complications, most studies have shown that there has been little decrease in their incidence over the past thirty years. Wightman (1968) in an extensive survey of 785 patients suggests that the reason why the advances in chemotherapy, antibiotics and surgical anaesthetic techniques appear to have had so little effect on the overall incidence of pulmonary complications is that patients are now operated on who would formerly have been rejected on grounds of age, chronic respiratory or other disease. It would seem almost certain that this explanation is correct. So much is now known about the varying and numerous aetiological factors that not only is avoidance of many of them simple, but active preventive therapy can be almost routinely carried out. In fact the key to the problem is drainage, and although infection can and does occur as a primary and acute event, it is more commonly secondary to inadequate drainage.

Normally secretions are removed from the lower to the upper bronchial tree by ciliary activity, while at the higher level an active cough reflex leads to effective expulsive efforts. Free drainage is also dependent upon aeration of all parts of the lung and hence upon an adequate minute volume of respiration. Disease, personal habits, climatic changes, surgery and anaesthesia, and indeed many other factors, can totally upset or alter these normal relationships in the lungs. It is unfortunate that in spite of all that is known about the causes of post-operative chest complications, so little is done to minimise the likelihood of their occurrence. Few patients are admitted long enough before an operation to allow pre-existing respiratory disease to be detected and treated. Improvement will probably only come from the more widespread adoption of already well-known therapeutic measures.

Factors Concerned in the Aetiology of Pulmonary Complications

The patient.—Post-operative pulmonary complications occur more frequently in men than in women, but no satisfactory explanation of this discrepancy has yet been found. They are particularly likely to occur in the winter months. This fact has a connection with the seasonal incidence of respiratory tract infection, since there is no doubt that pre-existing pulmonary disease increases the incidence. Smoking is a contributing factor, probably on account of the sputum that it causes, and it has been suggested that the occurrence of chest complications is six times more frequent in smokers than in non-smokers (Morton, 1944). Although it is widely assumed that pulmonary complications are commoner in the older age groups, recent studies (Wightman, 1968) have failed to confirm this and suggest that it is little more than a reflection of the higher incidence of pre-existing respiratory disease in the elderly. The same probably applies to obesity.

The operation.—Site of operation is the most important factor affecting the incidence of pulmonary complications. Most series show an overall incidence of 5 per cent. This rises to 21 per cent for operations on the gastro-intestinal and biliary tract, but only to 6 per cent for other abdominal operations. Non-abdominal operations are followed by a much lower incidence of pulmonary complications, usually below 1 per cent. The pain that high abdominal incisions cause in the post-operative period is a principal factor in reducing vital capacity and effective coughing, but the proximity of the operative site to the diaphragm and the way in which the operation is performed are factors of great importance. Thus retraction and handling of the bowel will lead to some post-operative swelling, while a slight leak at an anastomosis will markedly aggravate the situation. In either event there is some diaphragmatic splinting, and Mimpriss and Etheridge (1944) showed a connection between the complications of gastric surgery and post-operative pulmonary complications. Anscombe (1957) reports that pulmonary mechanical function may be decreased by 50–70 per cent after upper abdominal operations and by 25–35 per cent after lower abdominal ones. Collins and his co-workers (1968) reported a reduction of 50 per cent or more in vital capacity, peak expiratory flow rate, and forced expiratory volume in 1 second, on the first post-operative day in 132 male patients who had undergone upper abdominal surgery.

Prolonged surgery, and the effects of posture, particularly the steep Trendelenburg and lithotomy positions, which limit total lung capacity because of the pulmonary venous engorgement they cause, are potentiating factors (Hamilton and Morgan, 1932).

The anaesthetic.—Pre- and post-operative medication must be considered here. Morphine, atropine, and their analogues can be effective instruments in the prevention of pulmonary complications if used in judicious dosage, but overdosage or underdosage can equally mitigate against the patient. All drugs of these types depress ciliary activity and therefore the normal clearing mechanism of the lower bronchial tract, but the beneficial effects of atropine in preventing excessive secretions, and morphine in relieving pain, are paramount. Excessive medication may produce viscous mucus which is difficult to expectorate and a too-sleepy patient with depressed respiration and a depressed cough reflex. Movement of mucus in the trachea is slowed if dry gases are inhaled (Forbes, 1974) probably due to the drying of secretions and slowing down of ciliary activity. Furthermore, some volatile anaesthetic agents may depress ciliary activity (Nunn et al., 1974).

Individual anaesthetic agents and sequences, including local analgesia, are of little importance, provided there is no pre-existing chest disease. Lucas (1944) has shown in a comparable series of cases that the incidence of post-operative pulmonary complications is the same, whatever the anaesthetic. On the other hand, the way in which the anaesthetic is administered can, like the performance of the surgical operation, be decisive. Depth of anaesthesia, inadequate ventilation and a prolonged post-operative recovery during which reflex activity is markedly depressed or absent, must be avoided. Infected foreign material, such as blood, vomit or pus, should not be allowed to reach the lower respiratory tract either fortuitously or because of bad technique, while excessive secretions, which are often present in the lungs or the pharynx at the end of operation, and particularly after the use of neostigmine, must be removed.

A subsidiary factor is the rate of absorption of gases from the alveoli. The elimination of nitrogen during a long anaesthetic and the substitution of rapidly absorbed anaesthetic gases will increase the risk of pulmonary collapse distal to complete—or, in certain circumstances, incomplete—bronchial obstruction. If ventilation is depressed or inadequate—as in partial curarisation without assisted respiration—gases may be absorbed from peripheral lung segments more quickly than they can be replaced from above a partially blocked bronchus. Many inhalational anaesthetics, in depressing ciliary activity, may contribute to bronchial obstruction.

Post-operative pain relief.—Abdominal pain is a potent cause of a diminished tidal volume and vital capacity. The patient is reluctant to make a maximum inspiratory effort and the experience of pain suppresses the cough reflex. Bromage (1967) and Spence and Smith (1971) have shown that epidural anaesthesia provides better post-operative pain relief than systemic analgesic drugs. However, whilst the latter can depress the respiratory centre with excessive dosage, continuous epidural anaesthesia is not without the hazard of hypotension and motor paresis (Hewlett and Branthwaite, 1975).

Post-operative hypoxaemia.—It is now generally accepted that a fall in arterial oxygen tension may follow even a minor general anaesthetic involving peripheral tissues. There are a number of aetiological factors some of which are discussed below:

1. *Age*. Nunn (1965) demonstrated a close correlation between increasing age and the degree of hypoxaemia after anaesthesia. In conscious patients it is known that the greater the age of the subject, the lower the arterial Po_2 falls (Raine and Bishop, 1963; Marshall and Miller, 1965). It seems likely, therefore, that anaesthesia merely represents an extension of this process.

2. *Diffusion hypoxia*. This is the term used to describe the situation im-

mediately after a general anaesthetic when a highly soluble agent like nitrous oxide is excreted into the alveoli, thereby diluting the other alveolar gases—particularly oxygen (Fink *et al.*, 1954). This situation is only important in the very early part of the post-operative period lasting with diminishing influence only over the first 30 minutes (Marshall and Miller, 1965).

3. *Depletion of total body carbon dioxide stores*. After a prolonged period of passive hyperventilation the total stores of carbon dioxide may be reduced leading to a period of underventilation whilst these are replenished.

4. *Increased mismatch or true shunting in the lungs.* All general anaesthetics increase the proportion of the cardiac output that fails to be exposed to oxygen during its passage through the lungs. In the conscious state only about 4 per cent of the total cardiac output is not oxygenated, whilst under general anaesthesia this figure may rise as high as 20 to 30 per cent. Possible reason for this are:

(*a*) *Reduction in ventilation to parts of the lung.*—Beecher (1933) was the first person to point out that a laparotomy was followed by a fall in the functional residual capacity (FRC) of the lung during the post-operative period. Bromage (1967) has shown that abdominal pain results in an increase in transpulmonary pressure. This can lead not only to a decrease in FRC but also will encourage airway closure in the dependent parts of the lung. Spence and Alexander (1972) postulated that spasm of the expiratory muscles was the principal cause of the reduction in functional residual capacity. The raised transpulmonary pressure resulting from this spasm is believed to lead to closure of the small airways. The lung volume at which airway closure occurs is described as the Closing Volume (CV). In young conscious subjects this closure only takes place when the lung has nearly emptied (i.e. near to the residual volume); but, in old age, pulmonary disease and like states, the closing volume may come to lie within the range of the tidal volume itself so that now there is a great increase in the mismatch of ventilation and perfusion.

The original suggestion that a progressive atelectasis occurs during anaesthesia due to the suppression of the intermittent deep breath or "sigh" (Bendixen *et al.*, 1963) has not been confirmed by other authors (Sykes *et al.*, 1965; Panday and Nunn, 1968; Alexander *et al.*, 1973). Recently, however, Hewlett and his colleagues (1974 *a, b, c*) have shown that following the induction of anaesthesia there is a stepwise reduction in the FRC of the lungs and consequently an increase in the alveolar-arterial oxygen tension difference. This process takes place whether ventilation is spontaneous or controlled and cannot be explained solely on the basis of a high inspired oxygen concentration. The precise reason for this reduction in FRC is not clear but its significance in terms of hypoxaemia is obvious. Similarly, additional factors which alone are capable of reducing FRC (e.g. obesity, secretions, abdominal distension, restrictive bandaging) will further aggravate the situation.

(*b*) *Changes in pulmonary blood pressure.*—In certain circumstances a reduction in pulmonary blood flow may be even more important than the reduction in ventilation. The lung normally comprises three areas. One where blood flow exceeds ventilation, one where ventilation exceeds blood flow and one where they are perfectly matched. In the low-pressure pulmonary vasculature the blood flow distribution is strongly affected by gravity and only small reductions in pulmonary artery pressure result in a large increase in the amount of unperfused but overventilated lung.

At the same time, any reduction in cardiac output and, therefore, pulmonary blood flow will have a much more significant effect on arterial oxygenation in the presence of any degree of veno-arterial shunt within the lung. In the normal patient with a 4 per cent physiological shunt, the A–a (alveolar–arterial) oxygen tension difference is small but it may become significant either if the cardiac output is reduced or alternatively if the shunt is increased, but the greatest production of hypoxaemia will be by the combination of low cardiac output and lung shunt together. Similarly, intravascular debris such as aggregates of white cells, platelets and fibrin as are found in stored blood (Mossely and Doty, 1970) can clog the pulmonary capillaries, particularly after massive transfusion (Reul et al., 1973). Amniotic and fat emboli can do likewise.

To summarise, post-operative hypoxaemia has many aetiological factors. The precise cause of the reduction in functional residual capacity during anaesthesia still remains to be elucidated. However, in the post-operative period pain represents one of the principal factors and probably leads to a spasm of the muscles of expiration. This causes a rise in transpulmonary pressure and closure of some of the smaller airways. The increase in mismatch or true shunt leads to hypoxaemia.

BRONCHITIS

A brief note is needed of the several post-operative pulmonary complications which are not infrequently lumped together under the general term of "bronchitis". In fact the pathology may vary from the minimal but normal accumulation of secretions that follows most operations and anaesthetics, albeit for a brief period of time, to the presence of an acute infective process with the production of purulent and excessive quantities of sputum. Moreover it may be difficult, if not impossible, to differentiate on purely physical examination between bilateral bronchial infection with associated bronchial spasm and congestion, and the presence of multiple and scattered areas of peripheral lobular lung collapse (see below). Indeed the bronchitis may be a potent cause of the latter. More often than not bronchitis is a trivial complication of anaesthesia, being little more than a slight exacerbation of a pre-existing condition. Phillips (1966) has shown that the use of contaminated endotracheal tubes and unsterile analgesic lubricant may precipitate bronchial infections.

COLLAPSE OF LUNG

In this disease there is an area of collapse which may vary in size from a small lobule to that of a segment, lobe, or whole lung.

Lobular collapse is of particular interest, not only because it may occur more often than clinical diagnosis can confirm, but because untreated it could be a precursor of more extensive lung collapse by diminishing the compliance, increasing airway resistance and therefore the work of breathing. Since there is an inter-alveolar gaseous interchange via the pores of Kohn, many people have argued that lobular collapse cannot occur; but although this may be so in normal people, under abnormal conditions, particularly when respiration is depressed, such a gaseous exchange is absent (Van Allen *et al.*, 1931).

Sooner or later in the collapsed area infection supervenes, and indeed it is probable that in the smaller lesion until this occurs there is neither constitutional upset nor even pyrexia to suggest a complication. Infection also accounts for the fact that many cases of post-operative pulmonary collapse are mistakenly diagnosed as pneumonia.

It is difficult to say when the process of collapse begins, for although most cases present clinically between 24 and 48 hours after operation there is some evidence that the disease starts much earlier—perhaps even on the operating table during the anaesthetic. Stringer (1947) found that five out of thirteen patients who developed radiological evidence of collapse had abnormal pictures as early as four hours after operation.

The processes of infection in a collapsed area of lung may lead to a sequence of events which ultimately terminate in a bronchiectatic area. But even without treatment there is a tendency for the disease to cure itself, since with infection there is liquefaction of the mucus which blocks the bronchus and a better opportunity, therefore, for the patient to clear the obstruction and aerate the distal alveoli. In less fortunate cases the process may be severe enough to lead to a mistaken diagnosis of primary pneumonia, while gross destruction of lung tissue is a rare cause of lung abscess.

Bronchiectasis is the long-term result of incomplete and delayed re-expansion of lung tissue. The walls of the bronchi or bronchioles are weakened by infection since healing is by fibrosis, while during the period of collapse the negative pressure in the pleural space is greatly increased and thus exerts traction on the lung and air passages. Peribronchial fibrosis also exerts a pull which can lead to bronchial dilatation.

Diagnosis.—The diagnosis of a sizeable area of collapse is usually readily made from an examination of the patient. The onset is often acute and associated with pain in one or other side of the chest, a dry cough and dyspnoea. It usually occurs within the first forty-eight hours after operation.

On examination temperature, pulse and respiration rate are all increased, and indeed a clinical chart which shows the sudden onset of this classical triad of signs in the immediate post-operative period is itself almost pathognomonic of the condition. Although the increase in pulse and respiratory rate can easily be accounted for by the sudden change in respiratory mechanics, no satisfactory explanation has yet been given for the high rise in temperature at this early stage. Cyanosis may be present if the area of collapse is large.

Classical physical signs of collapse will be found on physical examination of the patient, while substantiation of the diagnosis may be aided by radiography (see Figs. 27 *A* and *B*).

PREVENTION AND TREATMENT OF BRONCHITIS AND PULMONARY COLLAPSE

Prevention

The most essential component of the treatment of post-operative pulmonary

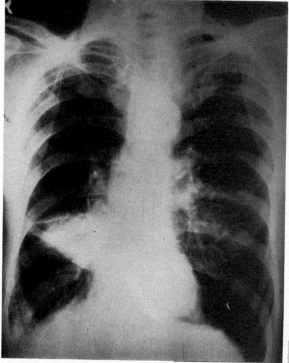

(a)

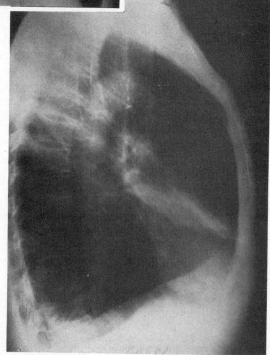

(b)

12/FIG. 27(A).—Right middle lobe
collapse.
(a) Antero-posterior view.
(b) Lateral view.

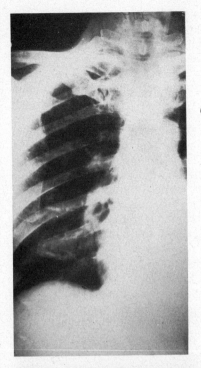
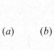
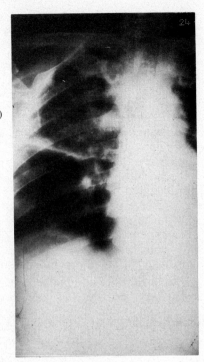

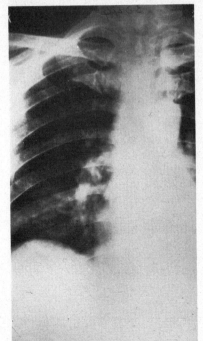

12/FIG. 27(*B*).—ACUTE POST-OPERATIVE PULMONARY
COLLAPSE

(*a*) Lung expanded before operation.

(*b*) Right upper and middle lobe collapse (X-ray
taken ½ hour after end of operation because patient
had tracheal tug and was breathing inadequately).

(*c*) Lung expanded again after bronchoscopy
and removal of small amount of mucus.

complications is undoubtedly the wise use of preventive measures. In the first place a thorough understanding of the aetiological factors and the systematic avoidance of all possible ones should be a routine part of anaesthetic practice.

No patient should be submitted to non-emergency surgery unless an effort has been made to clear pre-existing respiratory tract disease. If cure is impossible then the patient should be presented for anaesthesia in the best possible conditions. It is sometimes preferable to wait until spring or summer rather than operate on a "chesty" patient in the winter. Ellis (1955) suggests that many operations can be carried out with little increase in the risk by the presence of a common cold, although he excludes abdominal operations and those on the chest and respiratory tract itself. Upper respiratory tract infection, irrespective of operation and anaesthesia, is a not uncommon cause of aspiration pneumonia —a condition of collapse and pneumonia of a broncho-pulmonary segment from aspiration of infected secretions—which in turn can lead to bronchiectasis in as high a proportion as 5 per cent of all such cases (Morle and Robertson, 1953). There can be little excuse for increasing such a risk by the administration of an anaesthetic if the operation can safely be delayed. This dictum applies equally to the use of general anaesthesia or local analgesia.

Loder (1955) has advocated that a chest X-ray should be taken routinely before non-emergency surgery. In a series of 1000 pre-operative chest radiographs, 29 patients were found to have chest disease sufficient to necessitate postponement of their operation. Advanced pulmonary tuberculosis was discovered for the first time in six of these patients. However, random preoperative chest X-rays in the apparently healthy individual have now been largely abandoned. This investigation is reserved for the elderly and in those known to have chest disease.

In the prevention of pulmonary complications the pre- and post-operative use of breathing exercises and postural drainage is of considerable importance, particularly for thoracic and upper abdominal operations. In the two subsequent sections these forms of therapy are described in some detail, although it will be apparent to the reader that in their entirety neither is necessary for every case submitted to operation and anaesthetic.

Breathing exercises.—Most post-operative patients, particularly those accustomed to a sedentary occupation, rely upon upper thoracic movement for aeration of their lungs and the diaphragmatic element is small. In the post-operative period ventilation is reduced as a result of pain and analgesic drugs, while other factors which have already been discussed, such as an alteration in the secretion of mucus and a reduction in ciliary action, are at work.

The object of breathing exercises is to increase the vital capacity and aid drainage of the respiratory tract. This implies an increase in the capacity of all areas of the lung, including those affected by disease. Vital capacity does not in itself give an indication of respiratory efficiency, but an increase in it, with improved chest measurements, indicates that greater ventilation can take place.

More specifically, breathing exercises should be carried out with three purposes in mind:

(a) To encourage diaphragmatic movement so that the lung bases are well ventilated.

(*b*) To teach the patient how to produce good and controlled movement in all parts of the chest.

(*c*) To teach the patient how to cough effectively, particularly in the presence of a surgical wound.

Method.—The patient should be lying in a comfortable position in bed with the head and chest supported by pillows. Each breath should be taken quietly and slowly and no emphasis should be placed on expiration which should be purely passive. Excessively deep inspiration is not necessary. Throughout the exercises care must be taken to avoid movement of the shoulder girdle and also postural changes such as rotation or arching of the thoracic spine, all of which mitigate against effective respiration, especially when localised breathing is being practised. The maintenance of a good posture should be taught coincidentally with breathing exercises, so that any tendency to deformity which may arise as a result of disease or operation is prevented.

Progression to exercises for localised expansion should not overshadow the importance of bilateral movements. Localised breathing should be practised so that all parts of the thorax can be used individually or collectively. This is important after thoracic operations.

Localised breathing.—Adequate diaphragmatic breathing needs relaxation of the abdominal muscles during inspiration. Descent of the diaphragm can be roughly marked if the attendant's hand is placed over the substernal angle on the lower ribs. Lateral costal breathing should be practised in the direction of a hand placed in the mid-axillary line, either over the lower or upper ribs, while for apical breathing the hand must be just beneath the clavicle. Lateral costal breathing should be carried out unilaterally, and, when abdominal surgery is contemplated, postero-lateral expansion again in the direction of a hand behind the mid-axillary line may be included. This latter movement is less painful than lateral costal breathing in the presence of an upper abdominal incision, though its efficiency is open to some doubt.

Postural drainage.—The object of postural drainage is not only to drain a diseased area, but also all segments of the lungs, since clinical and radiographic investigations are not invariably correct in limiting the site of the disease, and to allow sputum to accumulate in the main bronchi, where the cough reflex is active and will lead to expulsion. The segments are illustrated diagrammatically

12/TABLE 1

Lobe	Segment	Position of patient	
Upper	Anterior	Horizontal	Supine
	Apical	Vertical	Sitting
	Posterior	Inclined forward	Sitting
Middle of Lingula		35° head-down tilt	Inclined to normal side
Lower	Apical	Horizontal	Pillow at hips. Supine
	Posterior	45° head-down tilt	Inclined to normal side
	Lateral	45° head-down tilt	Lying on normal side
	Anterior	45° head-down tilt	Supine

in Fig. 28. The positions needed to drain each individual segment have been described by Gaskell and Webber (1973).

Each position should be maintained for a few minutes while the secretions are encouraged to flow—by percussion over the affected area—with localised breathing exercises and periodic coughing. Physiotherapy should be continued until an optimum reduction in sputum is obtained or the collapsed area completely re-expanded.

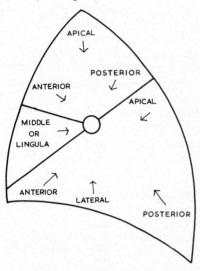

12/Fig. 28.—Composite picture to show the eight areas of the lung requiring separate postural drainage.

Combined physiotherapy and "bag-squeezing".—Some patients may require continuous pulmonary ventilation. Routine physiotherapy combined with the appropriate distension of the lung via an endotracheal tube has proved effective both in prevention and treatment of areas of pulmonary collapse. The technique involves placing the intubated patient in a suitable position of postural drainage, then applying external vibratory movements to the chest wall in an attempt to shift any mucous secretions within the bronchi. (Clement and Hubsch, 1968). The effect of such physiotherapy on blood gas tension was studied by Gormezano and Branthwaite (1972), who cautioned about its use in patients with circulatory failure or in the presence of severe airways obstruction. However, a more recent haemodynamic analysis on cardiac patients showed the treatment to have negligible effect on the circulation when properly carried out.

The treatment of pain.—The influence of post-operative pain in reducing vital capacity and preventing coughing is well-known. The use of respiratory depressants such as morphine may, paradoxically, improve the situation when used in moderate dosage by allaying pain, and, with the possible exception of morphine and morphine-antidote combinations, no other agents have yet proved so satisfactory when all factors are taken into consideration.

Nevertheless, mention must be made of local infiltration of the operation wound with a local analgesic, and of epidural analgesia.

The former method has fallen into disrepute because a safe long-acting local analgesic has not yet been discovered, while irrigation of the wound through a plastic catheter with a short-acting drug is cumbersome and unsatisfactory. Several people have claimed success for the use of an intravenous procaine drip after upper abdominal operations for the control of pain without further decreasing pulmonary ventilation. But contrary to expectations this method does not lead to an increase in vital capacity over the normal post-operative figures (Pooler, 1949).

The benefits of epidural anaesthesia are most marked in patients who have undergone upper abdominal surgery. Improvements in arterial oxygen tension

(Spence and Smith, 1971; Holmdahl and Modig, 1975; Miller *et al.*, 1976) and reduction in arterial carbon dioxide (Miller *et al.*, 1976) have been demonstrated as compared with narcotic analgesia. The evidence as to an effect on static or dynamic lung volumes is less clear, though it seems that an increase in tidal volume and reduction in respiratory rate follows satisfactory epidural blockade. Miller *et al.* (1976) showed that the vital capacity in patients given pethidine post-operatively fell to 36·5 per cent of pre-operative values, whilst in patients with epidural blockade, the vital capacity was only reduced by 50 per cent. Spence and Logan (1975) report a reduction in FRC of 16 per cent following an epidural as compared with 21·7 per cent for patients given morphine. However, further studies have failed to demonstrate any significant improvement in those other components of respiratory function investigated.

Epidural anaesthesia for operations at sites away from the upper abdomen has not been clearly demonstrated to have any beneficial effects on respiratory function (e.g. Drummond and Littlewood, 1977) though Modig (1976) showed some improvement in arterial oxygen tension after major hip surgery.

A reduction in the post-operative changes in arterial blood gases which follows upper abdominal surgery may also be achieved by intercostal nerve block (Moore, 1975).

Other drugs.—Palmer and Sellick (1953), in a survey of 180 patients undergoing abdominal operations, were able to show a remarkable decrease in the incidence of pulmonary complications by the adoption of isoprenaline inhalation combined with postural drainage and with vibratory and clapping percussion to the chest wall before and after operation. In 90 patients treated in this way the incidence of lung collapse was 9 per cent compared with 43 per cent in 90 similar patients treated with breathing exercises alone before and after operation. All these patients had procaine penicillin before and after operation.

Salbutamol is now used in preference to isoprenaline. It acts principally on the β-2 receptors in the bronchi and is virtually devoid of effect on the β-1 receptors in the heart when used in the correct dosage. 2·5 mg salbutamol is usually diluted with normal saline and is then nebulised for inhalation.

Although obviously bronchodilators will be most useful in patients in whom reversible airway obstruction has been clearly demonstrated, they are probably of value prior to physiotherapy in all patients who have infected sputum as these patients will have oedematous bronchial mucosa and will usually have some element of small airway obstruction.

The use of specific antibiotics should be reserved for cases with pre-existing respiratory tract diseases when they help to avoid the risk of exacerbation, or for part of the treatment of post-operative purulent bronchitis or infected areas of collapsed lung. Although Collins *et al.* (1968) showed a reduction of over 50 per cent in the incidence of pulmonary complications following the use of prophylactic antibiotics, this method is not generally accepted in view of the well-recognised disadvantages which accompany the administration of antibiotics on a prophylactic basis. Such drugs can never be a substitute for active treatment of the type described to deal with the mechanical factors concerned in these post-operative pulmonary complications. Expectorants are more likely to increase secretions than to aid in their efficient elimination at this stage, and the inhalation of carbon dioxide and oxygen mixtures is of little value.

Tracheostomy and Artificial Ventilation (see Chapter 10, p. 391)

PNEUMONIA

Although both lobar and broncho-pneumonic forms may occur, pneumonia is a very rare primary complication of anaesthesia. So-called pneumonia occurring in the immediate post-operative period is usually infection in an area of collapse, although the acuteness of the onset and the gravity of the patient's state—particularly in aspiration cases—causes the essential basic pathology to be overlooked. Hypostatic broncho-pneumonia occurs as a terminal phenomenon in seriously ill and bedridden patients.

LUNG ABSCESS

Post-operative lung abscess is an uncommon complication which is usually due to the aspiration of septic material or to an acute infection in a collapsed area of lung. More rarely this complication may arise as a secondary blood-borne infection in a case of pyaemia, or as a result of lung destruction in a suppurative primary pneumonia, such as is sometimes caused by Friedländer's bacillus. The onset of symptoms and signs may be delayed for as long as three weeks from the time of operation and anaesthetic.

Sources of infection for aspiration abscesses are commonly found in septic teeth and gums, and the upper respiratory tract—particularly the sinuses. Indeed Brock (1946), reporting on 316 non-malignant lung abscesses, states that 25, or 7 per cent, followed dental extractions. He considered that the offending material was the tartar masses on the septic teeth. Abscesses may also follow the inhalation of larger and more obvious foreign bodies during anaesthesia, such as pieces of food.

Prevention should be aimed at by attending to oral hygiene and nasal sepsis before anaesthesia—particularly prior to major surgery. Endotracheal anaesthesia and the use of packs and cuffs will prevent aspiration during operation, but particular care must be taken during induction and in the immediate post-operative period. The indications for intubation might well be enlarged to include cases with sepsis in the pharynx or sinuses, particularly if the operation is likely to be prolonged. Dental operations merit special attention, since under normal out-patient conditions, even though the period of anaesthesia may be less than two or three minutes, the opportunities for aspiration are considerable. Here the use of the sitting position, the inadequate control of the airway, the frequency of multiple extractions and the common use of nitrous oxide are factors of importance.

Fry and Earl (1950) made an investigation into the incidence of inhalation of blood and other debris during dental operations under these conditions. They injected a radio-opaque liquid into the buccal sulcus on the side of the majority of the extractions and were able to demonstrate that conditions were favourable for aspiration despite the use of a dental pack. Indeed, the liquid could be seen in the lungs on radiography in one patient who had a prolonged and difficult anaesthetic with hypoxia and struggling, which led to deep breaths at the end of anaesthesia. Although aspiration under these conditions is possible and is probably more frequent than generally supposed, the incidence of resulting lung complications is very small indeed. Nevertheless, preventive measures must be taken. The patient's head should be kept upright, so that blood is likely to pool in the front of the mouth and not run back into the pharynx. Only a brief simple anaesthesia should be allowed; struggling and hypoxia, both of which—though for different reasons—are likely to lead to excessively deep breaths, must be avoided. More prolonged procedures must be accepted as an indication for intubation and the use of an efficient pack or cuff on the tube.

ASPIRATION PNEUMONIA AND EXUDATIVE OEDEMA

Aspiration of stomach contents into the bronchial passages can occur at any time during the operative period. It is particularly common in elderly patients awaiting surgery for intestinal obstruction, in those recovering from anaesthesia, and in the later post-operative period following gastro-intestinal surgery. Gardner (1958) in a comprehensive review has shown that the administration of oral fluid to debilitated patients by the traditional ward feeding cup, with a partly covered top, is particularly liable to cause aspiration. The presence of a nasogastric tube does not necessarily prevent it; indeed it may predispose to regurgitation and aspiration by rendering the cardia and cricopharyngeal sphincters incompetent and impede swallowing. The discomfort caused to a patient by an indwelling nasogastric tube is often underestimated.

The most fulminating type of aspiration pneumonia is that which follows inhalation of vomit during the induction of anaesthesia in patients with a full stomach undergoing obstetric procedures. Mendelson (1946) described the principal features of this condition, which has come to be known as "Mendelson's syndrome". He conducted animal experiments from which he suggested that the irritant effect of gastric hydrochloric acid is the causal factor. Subsequent experimental work has not entirely confirmed this explanation (Halmagyi, 1961; Halmagyi and Colebatch, 1961; Alexander, 1968) and the aetiology of this irregularly occurring but serious condition remains in doubt.

Clinically the disease presents with the onset of dyspnoea, cyanosis and tachycardia, while examination of the patient shows no localised signs of lung collapse, but generalised adventitious sounds, often with evidence of bronchial spasm. Very high pulse and respiratory rates are common, while gross pulmonary oedema may supervene with death from cardiac failure. Radiography may show irregular mottling scattered through the lung fields, but no evidence of lung collapse. Should death occur, examination of the lungs will reveal gross swelling of tissue and a pink frothy oedema fluid throughout the trachea, bronchi, bronchioles and alveoli. On microscopy peribronchiolar haemorrhages and exudate, areas of necrosis of bronchiolar epithelium, and a marked leucocytic reaction, can be seen. Free hydrochloric acid can often be demonstrated by staining.

In such cases only small quantities of fluid may be concerned; in fact there may be no obvious history of vomiting or regurgitation and still less evidence of actual aspiration, while in several reported instances the patients have recovered full consciousness after the causative episode and before the onset of symptoms. Thus the connection between vomiting and this pulmonary complication may conceivably be disregarded or lost. As a syndrome it seems most commonly to occur in obstetrics, although cases have been met in other branches of surgery. This is surprising because equal opportunities for aspiration occur in general surgical emergencies, and it may be that the susceptibility of the obstetric patient to the effects of gastric inhalation is greater than others. Indeed Hausmann and Lunt (1955) have suggested that acute adrenal failure accounts for the difference. They consider that after delivery the loss of the placenta, an organ which is partly responsible for the increase in ACTH and glucocorticoids normally found in pregnancy, the patient is in no state to stand a sudden and severe stress, such as that produced by the effects of gastric inhalation.

Treatment.—Treatment should first be aimed at prevention (see Chapter 37).

TUBERCULOSIS

Cross-infection from anaesthetic apparatus contaminated through previous use on a case of pulmonary tuberculosis has not been shown to occur in practice, although, as might be expected, clinical records which could be correlated back to such an incident would be difficult, if not impossible, to obtain. Careful bacteriological examination of apparatus used on infected cases has demonstrated, however, how remarkably difficult it is to show any evidence of tubercle bacilli at all. Nevertheless, precautions must be taken to prevent any chance of cross-infection and all apparatus must be properly sterilised after use.

Pulmonary tuberculosis occurring in the post-operative period is almost always due to a latent lesion becoming active. The points concerned are not so much the use of local or general anaesthesia, nor of actual individual agents, as the impact of a large number of individual factors, such as are at work in the picture of post-operative pulmonary collapse, on a patient with latent tuberculosis. Care must be exercised in the use of intermittent positive-pressure respiration for cases with recently healed foci, since it is presumably possible to break down adhesions by excessive movement and pressure. The natural resistance of the patient is diminished in the immediate post-operative period, while any area of collapsed lung is a potential source of spread from infected sputum. Cases with known active pulmonary tuberculosis are potential candidates for spread of the disease, but it must not be supposed that the risk is greater should general anaesthesia be used in preference to local analgesia. The latter may be a more expedient method in certain circumstances, but the incidence of tuberculosis-spread, like that of all pulmonary complications, does not differ after either form of anaesthesia, provided each is competently administered.

REFERENCES

ALEXANDER, I. G. S. (1968). The ultrastructure of the pulmonary alveolar vessels in Mendelson's (acid pulmonary aspiration) syndrome. *Brit. J. Anaesth.*, **40**, 408.

ALEXANDER, J. I., HORTON, P. W., MILLER, W. T., PARIKH, R. K., and SPENCE, A. A. (1973). The effect of upper abdominal surgery on the relationship of airway closing point to end-tidal position. *Clin. Sci.*, **43**, 137.

ANSCOMBE, A. R. (1957). *Pulmonary Complications of Abdominal Surgery*, p. 56. London: Lloyd-Luke (Medical Books).

ATWOOD, J. M. (1965). Respiratory obstruction during bronchography. *Anesthesiology*, **26**, 234.

BARAKA, A., and MUALLEM, M. (1972). Use of oxygen bypass button of the Boyle machine to trigger venturi ventilation during bronchoscopy. *Brit. J. Anaesth.*, **44**, 413.

BEECHER, H. K. (1933). Effect of laparotomy on lung volume. Demonstration of a new type of pulmonary collapse. *J. clin. Invest.*, **12**, 651.

BENDIXEN, H. H., HEDLEY-WHYTE, J., and LAVER, M. B. (1963). Impaired oxygenation in surgical patients during general anaesthesia with controlled ventilation. *New Engl. J. Med.*, **269**, 991.

BROCK, R. C. (1946). Studies in lung abscess. *Guy's Hosp. Rep.*, **95**, 40.

BROMAGE, P. R. (1967). Extradural analgesia for pain relief. *Brit. J. Anaesth.*, **39**, 721.

CLEMENT, A. J., and HUBSCH, S. (1968). Chest physiotherapy by the "bag-squeezing" method. *Physiotherapy*, **54**, 355.

COLLINS, C. D., DARKE, C. S., and KNOWELDEN, J. (1968). Chest complications after upper abdominal surgery: their anticipation and prevention. *Brit. med. J.*, **1**, 401.

DRUMMOND, G. B., and LITTLEWOOD, D. G. (1977). Respiratory effects of extradural analgesia after lower abdominal surgery. *Brit. J. Anaesth.*, **49**, 999.

ELLIS, G. (1955). Anaesthesia and the common cold. *Anaesthesia*, **10**, 78.

FINK, B. R., CARPENTER, S. L., and HOLADAY, D. A. (1954). Diffusion anoxia during recovery from nitrous oxide/oxygen anaesthesia. *Fed. Proc.*, **13**, 354.

FORBES, A. R. (1974). Temperature, humidity and mucus flow in the intubated trachea. *Brit. J. Anaesth.*, **46**, 29.

FRANCIS, J. G., and SMITH, K. G. (1962). An anaesthetic technique for the repair of broncho-pleural fistula. *Brit. J. Anaesth.*, **34**, 817.

FREIFELD, S., and ZALVENDO, P. (1964). A technique for anesthesia in pediatric bronchography. *Anesth. Analg. Curr. Res..*, **43**, 45.

FRY, I. K., and EARL, C. J. (1950). Report on preliminary investigation into incidence of inhalation of blood and other debris during dental extraction under general anaesthesia in upright position. *Guy's Hosp. Rep.*, **99**, 41.

GARDNER, A. M. N. (1958). Aspiration of food and vomit. *Quart. J. Med.*, **27**, 227.

GASKELL, D. V., and WEBBER, B. A. (1973). *The Brompton Hospital Guide to Chest Physiotherapy.* Oxford: Blackwell Scientific Publications.

GORMEZANO, J., and BRANTHWAITE, M. A. (1972). Effects of physiotherapy during intermittent positive pressure ventilation. *Anaesthesia*, **27**, 258.

GRAY, T. C., and EDWARDS, F. R. (1948). The anaesthetic problems associated with giant tension cysts of the lung. *Thorax*, **3**, 237.

HALMAGYI, D. F. J. (1961). Lung changes and incidence of respiratory arrest in rats after aspiration of sea and fresh water. *J. appl. Physiol.*, **16**, 41.

HALMAGYI, D. F. J., and COLEBATCH, J. H. (1961). Ventilation and circulation after fluid aspiration. *J. appl. Physiol.*, **16**, 35.

HAMILTON, W. F., and MORGAN, A. B. (1932). Mechanism of postural reduction in vital capacity in relation to orthopnea and storage of blood in lungs. *Amer. J. Physiol.*, **99**, 526.

HAUSMANN, W., and LUNT, R. L. (1955). The problem of the treatment of peptic aspiration pneumonia following obstetric anaesthesia (Mendelson's syndrome). *J. Obstet. Gynaec. Brit. Emp.*, **62**, 509.

HEWLETT, A. M., and BRANTHWAITE, M. A. (1975). Post-operative pulmonary function. *Brit. J. Anaesth.*, **47**, 102.

HEWLETT, A. M., HULANDS, G. H., NUNN, J. F., and HEATH, J. R. (1974a). Functional residual capacity during anaesthesia. II: Spontaneous respiration. *Brit. J. Anaesth.*, **46**, 486.

HEWLETT, A. M., HULANDS, G. H., NUNN, J. F., and MILLEDGE, J. S. (1974b). Functional residual capacity during anaesthesia. III: Artificial ventilation. *Brit. J. Anaesth.*, **46**, 495.

HEWLETT, A. M., HULANDS, G. H., NUNN, J. F., and MINTY, K. B. (1974c). Functional residual capacity during anaesthesia. I: Methodology. *Brit. J. Anaesth.*, **46**, 479.

HOLMDAHL, M. H., and MODIG, J. (1975). The role of regional block versus parenteral analgesics in patient management with special emphasis on the treatment of post-operative pain. *Brit. J. Anaesth.*, **47**, 264.

KHANAM, T., and BRANTHWAITE, M. A. (1973*a*). Arterial oxygenation during one-lung anaesthesia (1). A study in man. *Anaesthesia*, **28**, 132.

KHANAM, T., and BRANTHWAITE, M. A. (1973*b*). Arterial oxygenation during one-lung anaesthesia (2). *Anaesthesia*, **28**, 280.

LODER, R. E. (1955). Routine pre-operative chest radiography: analysis of 1,000 cases. *Lancet*, **1**, 1150.

LUCAS, B. G. B. (1944). Pulmonary complications following simple herniorrhaphy. *Proc. roy. Soc. Med.*, **37**, 145.

LUNDING, M., and FERNANDES, A. (1967). Arterial oxygen tension and acid-base status during thoracic anaesthesia. *Acta anaesth. scand.*, **11**, 43.

MALONE, D. N., GOLD, J. C., and GRANT, I. W. B. (1968). A comparative study of ampicillin, tetracycline hydrochloride and methacycline hydrochloride in acute exacerbations of chronic bronchitis. *Lancet*, **2**, 594.

MANSFIELD, R. (1957). Modified bronchoscope for endobronchial intubation. *Anaesthesia*. **12**, 477.

MARSHALL, B. E., and MILLER, R. A. (1965). Some factors influencing post-operative hypoxaemia. *Anaesthesia*, **20**, 408.

MENDELSON, C. L. (1946). Aspiration of stomach contents into lungs during obstetric anesthesia. *Amer. J. Obstet. Gynec.*, **52**, 181.

MILLER, L., GERTEL, M., FOX, G. S., and MACLEAN, L. D. (1976). Comparison of effect of narcotic and epidural analgesia on postoperative respiratory function. *Amer. J. Surg.*, **131**, 291.

MIMPRISS, T. W., and ETHERIDGE, F. G. (1944). Post-operative chest complications in gastric surgery. *Brit. med. J.*, **1**, 466.

MODIG, J. (1976). Respiration and circulation after total hip surgery. A comparison between parenteral analgesics and continuous lumbar epidural block. *Acta anaesth. scand.*, **20**, 225.

MOORE, D. C. (1975). Intercostal nerve block for postoperative somatic pain following surgery of thorax and upper abdomen. *Brit. J. Anaesth.*, **47**, 284.

MORLE, K. D. F., and ROBERTSON, P. W. (1953). Segmental aspiration pneumonia and bronchiectasis. *Brit. med. J.*, **1**, 130.

MORTON, H. J. V. (1944). Tobacco smoking and pulmonary complications after operation. *Lancet*, **1**, 368.

MOSELY, R. V., and DOTY, R. B. (1970). Changes in the filtration characteristics of stored blood. *Ann. Surg.*, **171**, 329.

NEDEL, J. R., WOLFE, W. G., and GRAF, P. D. (1968). Tantalum oxide. *Invest. Radiol.*, **3**, 229.

NILSSON, E., SLATER, E. M., and GREENBERG, J. (1965). The cost of the quiet lung: fluctuations in Pa_{O_2} when the Carlens tube is used in pulmonary surgery. *Acta anaesth. scand.*, **9**, 49.

NUNN, J. F. (1965). Influence of age and other factors on hypoxaemia in the post-operative period. *Lancet*, **2**, 466.

NUNN, J. F., STURROCK, J. E., and WILLS, E. J. (1974). The effect of inhalational anaesthetics on the swimming velocity of *Tetrahymena Pyriformis*. *J. cell. Sci.*, **15**, 537.

OVERHOLT, R. H., LANGER, L., SZYPULSKI, J. T., and WILSON, N. J. (1946). Pulmonary resection in the treatment of tuberculosis. *J. thorac. Surg.*, **15**, 384.

PALLISTER, W. K. (1959). A new endobronchial tube for left lung anaesthesia. *Thorax*, **14**, 55.

PALMER, K. N. V., and SELLICK, B. A. (1953). The prevention of post-operative pulmonary atelectasis. *Lancet*, **1**, 164.

PANDAY, J., and NUNN, J. F. (1968). Failure to demonstrate progressive falls of arterial Po_2 during anaesthesia. *Anaesthesia*, **23**, 38.

PARRY BROWN, A. I. (1948). Posture in thoracic surgery. *Thorax*, **3**, 161.

PHILLIPS, I. (1966). Postoperative respiratory-tract infections with *Pseudomonas aeruginosa* due to contaminated lignocaine jelly, *Lancet*, **1**, 903.

POOLER, H. E. (1949). The relief of post-operative pain and its influence on the vital capacity. *Brit. med. J.*, **2**, 1200.

RAINE, J. M., and BISHOP, J. M. (1963). "A—a difference" in O_2 tension and physiological dead space in normal man. *J. appl. Physiol.*, **18**, 284.

REUL, G. J., GREENBERG, S. D., LEFRAK, E. A., McCOLLUM, W. B., BEALL, A. C., Jr., and JORDAN, G. L., Jr. (1973). Prevention of post-traumatic pulmonary insufficiency. *Arch. Surg.*, **106**, 386.

SANDERS, R. D. (1967). Two ventilating attachments for bronchoscopes. *Delaware med. J.*, **39**, 170.

SPENCE, A. A., and ALEXANDER, J. I. (1972). Mechanism of post-operative hypoxaemia. *Proc. roy. Soc. Med.*, **65**, 6.

SPENCE, A. A., and LOGAN, D. A. (1975). Respiratory effects of extradural nerve block in the postoperative period. *Brit. J. Anaesth.*, **47**, 281.

SPENCE, A. A., and SMITH, G. (1971). Postoperative analgesia and lung function: a comparison of morphine with extradural block. *Brit. J. Anaesth.*, **43**, 144.

SPOEREL, W. E., and GRANT, P. A. (1971). Ventilation during bronchoscopy. *Canad. Anaesth. Soc. J.*, **18**, 178.

STEPHEN, E. D. S. (1952). Problem of "blocking" in upper lobectomies. *Curr. Res. Anesth.*, **31**, 175.

STRINGER, P. (1947). Atelectasis after partial gastrectomy. *Lancet*, **1**, 289.

SYKES, M. K., YOUNG, W. E., and ROBINSON, B. E. (1965). Oxygenation during anaesthesia with controlled ventilation. *Brit. J. Anaesth.*, **37**, 314.

TORDA, T. A., McCULLOCH, C. H., O'BRIEN, H. D., WRIGHT, J. S., and HORTON, D. A. (1974). Pulmonary venous admixture during one-lung anaesthesia. *Anaesthesia*, **29**, 272.

VAN ALLEN, C. M., LINDSKOG, G. E., and RICHTER, H. G. (1931). Collateral respiration, transfer of air collaterally between pulmonary lobules. *J. clin. Invest.*, **10**, 559.

WIGHTMAN, J. A. K. (1968). A prospective study of the incidence of postoperative pulmonary complications. *Brit. J. Surg.*, **55**, 85.

FURTHER READING

ANSCOMBE, A. R. (1957). *Pulmonary Complications of Abdominal Surgery*. London: Lloyd-Luke (Medical Books).

NUNN, J. F. (1977). *Applied Respiratory Physiology*, 2nd edit. London: Butterworth & Co.

SYKES, M. K., McNICOL, M. W., and CAMPBELL, E. J. M. (1976). *Respiratory Failure*, 2nd edit. Oxford: Blackwell Scientific Publications.

Section Two

THE CARDIOVASCULAR SYSTEM

Chapter 13

THE CARDIOVASCULAR SYSTEM

THE ANATOMY OF THE CORONARY VASCULATURE

THE heart is supplied with blood by two coronary arteries which arise from the root of the aorta immediately above the aortic valve (Fig. 1). Their detailed anatomy is variable, but the left coronary artery always gives rise to the left anterior descending branch which supplies the anterior wall of the left ventricle and a major portion of the interventricular septum. The continuation of the left coronary, now called the circumflex, is more variable but usually supplies the lateral part of the left ventricle. In ten per cent of the population the left coronary is dominant and the circumflex supplies the inferior and posterior parts of the left ventricle, but in 90 per cent of the population this territory, including the atrioventricular node, is supplied by the right coronary, another smaller branch of the right supplying the right ventricle.

The main venous return from the heart is via the coronary sinus which drains to the right atrium. Some myocardial drainage does occur directly into the ventricles and that direct to the left ventricle accounts for part of the right-to-left shunt which exists normally.

THE CORONARY BLOOD FLOW AND MYOCARDIAL OXYGEN CONSUMPTION

Under most circumstances coronary arterial autoregulation adjusts the coronary blood flow (CBF) according to the myocardial oxygen demand. Autoregulation, however, only occurs at arterial pressures between 70 and 160 mm Hg (9·3 and 21·3 kPa). At pressures less than this the flow may be inadequate

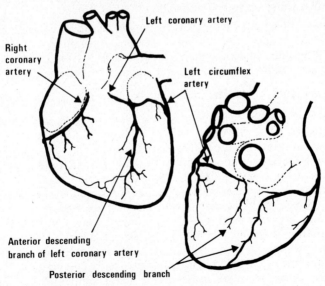

13/FIG. 1.—The coronary arteries.

while at higher pressures the oxygen consumption rises disproportionately. The flow may be insufficient even within the normal pressure range in the presence of coronary artery disease or if the left ventricular wall tension is high. The major portion of coronary flow takes place during diastole when the ventricular tension is low and at high heart rates the diastolic interval may become a limiting factor, particularly if there is associated coronary artery disease or a high myocardial oxygen consumption. As high cardiac rates themselves increase oxygen consumption they should be avoided in the presence of coronary artery disease and the rationale for the use of β-adrenergic blockade (i.e. cardiac slowing) is obvious.

Both α and β-receptor sites exist in the coronary arterial tree but the systemic administration of vasoactive drugs affects coronary blood flow mainly by their indirect effects on myocardial oxygen consumption, subsequent to changes in arterial pressure and ventricular work. The most effective drug in the treatment of angina, glyceryl trinitrate, is ineffective when given directly into the coronary artery unless the dose is large enough to reduce the systemic vascular resistance.

Coronary Blood Flow

Accurate measurement of the CBF is difficult and requires coronary sinus cannulation. The classic method is that of Katz using nitrous oxide uptake but more recently thermodilution has been used. These methods give a coronary blood flow of approximately 250 ml/minute and an oxygen consumption of 25 ml oxygen/minute. Thus the myocardial blood flow is approximately 5 per cent of the cardiac output whereas the myocardial oxygen consumption is about 10 per cent of the minute oxygen uptake. This implies a high oxygen extraction by the heart and coronary sinus blood is more desaturated than other venous blood.

The Myocardial Oxygen Consumption

There are three main factors which affect myocardial oxygen consumption:

1. *Left ventricular wall tension.*—Oxygen consumption is related to the wall tension; under Laplace's law the wall tension (T) is a function of the ventricular pressure (P) and the size of the chamber (radius = r) such that $T = \dfrac{Pr}{2}$. The important implications of this are that tension and therefore oxygen consumption increase (i) as ventricular pressure increases, (ii) as the ventricle dilates (bigger radius), even if the pressure stays constant as in the failing heart and (iii) if the ventricle hypertrophies since "r" is compounded both of the cavity radius and the wall thickness.

2. *Myocardial contractility.*—Increase in the rate of rise of ventricular pressure and hence in the acceleration of blood flow may have little effect on the size of the cardiac output but produce striking increase in myocardial oxygen consumption. β-adrenergic blocking drugs reduce myocardial contractility and, without necessarily affecting the cardiac output, decrease myocardial oxygen consumption except in the presence of cardiac failure with left ventricular dilatation (see above).

3. *Heart rate.*—Increases in heart rate are accompanied by shortening of diastolic period, particularly in the diseased heart, and thus at high heart

rates the proportion of time that the wall tension is high is greater. This may be quantified as a tension-time index which is shown to be directly related to myocardial oxygen consumption. As coronary blood flow occurs principally in diastole and depends on the diastolic perfusion pressure the ratio of the tension-time index to the product of the filling-time and pressure is a useful method of assessing the adequacy of the myocardial oxygen supply.

The Measurement of Cardiac Output

In the experimental animal and during human cardiac surgery it is possible to measure cardiac output by electromagnetic flow probes placed around the aorta. Under most other circumstances cardiac output is determined either by the direct Fick method or by indicator dilution. Non-invasive methods are now becoming more accurate and therefore more popular.

(a) **The direct Fick method** is the most accurate method and remains the standard by which other methods are judged. The information required is the oxygen uptake from the lungs in unit time and the oxygen content of arterial and mixed venous blood. The technique implies right heart catheterisation to obtain mixed venous blood from the pulmonary artery and requires considerable skill with the van Slyke apparatus for the measurement of oxygen content in blood. The relationship of flow to oxygen consumption is then given by the equation:

$$Q = \frac{O_2 \text{ consumption}}{(A\text{-}V)O_2 \text{ content difference}}$$

The technical difficulties of the Fick method have resulted in a general acceptance of less accurate but easier methods of which the commonest are the indicator dye and thermal dilution methods. Both involve a bolus injection of indicator proximal to the heart and the measurement of a concentration-time curve distal to the heart which is assumed to be a uniform mixing chamber.

(b) **Indocyanine green** has superceded other dyes. It has the advantage that the concentration is measured by spectrophotometry in the infrared region at 805 Å (80.5 nm) at which wave length both oxygenated and reduced haemoglobin have identical optical densities. The value is therefore unaffected by changes in the haemoglobin saturation. The arterial sample may be drawn from any artery and passed through a cuvette densitometer. More recently an end-catheter densitometer has been evolved which measures the concentration within the artery.

(c) **The thermodilution** technique uses room temperature saline or dextrose and its negative heat (relative to body temperature) as the indicator. The advantages of thermodilution as a method are that the problems of recirculation on the concentration-line curve are insignificant and that the harmless indicator is speedily excreted making frequent estimations possible. The accuracy of the method is greatest when the injection is made just proximal to the right atrium and the change of temperature monitored by a thermistor in the pulmonary artery. The transit time is thus kept to a minimum and extravascular heat loss diminished.

Of the non-invasive methods *thoracic impedance plethysmography* is the

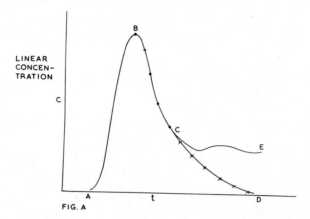

13/FIG. 2(a).—Curve A B C E is that produced by the output of a cuvette densitometer.

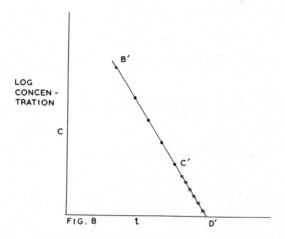

13/FIG. 2(b).—This is the downslope portion of the curve in Fig. 2(a) redrawn on semi-logarithmic paper.

The concentration of dye (C) in Fig. 2(a) does not fall to zero after one passage through the body due to the effect of recirculation of the dye. The effect of recirculation is ignored by re-plotting the downslope portion of the curve (BC) on a semi-logarithmic scale (B′C′). Since the downslope is an exponential decay, B′C′ will be linear and may be extrapolated to D′. Points along the line CD on the original curve may thus be obtained by reference to the semi-logarithmic plot. Thus the area beneath the curve A B C D may be obtained, free of the effects of recirculated dye.

most acceptable although variable correlation has been shown with the standard methods. Two electrodes are placed at neck level and two round the lower thorax. A constant sinusoidal current is passed between the outer electrodes and voltage fluctuations which reflect cardiac output are observed on the inner electrodes. A different approach is to measure aortic flow utilising the Doppler ultrasound system with the transducer placed over the suprasternal notch so that the beam is almost co-axial with the ascending aorta.

THE ASSESSMENT AND MANIPULATION OF THE CIRCULATION

This section briefly reviews the circulatory physiology which must be understood by the anaesthetist so that he can (1) correctly interpret the circulatory signs that he observes and (2) manipulate the circulation either to correct some alteration that has occurred or to produce some new situation. A comprehension of the normal circulation is an essential basis for dealing with the abnormal circulation described in the next chapter.

CIRCULATORY ASSESSMENT

Although much cardiovascular physiology is concerned with the heart, the primary function of the system is to satisfy the metabolic needs of the body, and the circulation might be more correctly assessed by looking at either whole body or individual organ function. A normal whole body oxygen consumption suggests that oxygen supply, and therefore blood flow, is normal. Inadequate perfusion of the brain usually results in loss or clouding of consciousness and while this is a sign not normally available to the anaesthetist, there are other easily made observations such as the EEG, ECG, and urine production which may give some indication of organ function. Skin colour and temperature are often assessed both for their satisfactory state and for the absence of signs of vasoconstriction or sweating. While these signs are all essential and important observations which contribute to the assessment of the circulatory state, most measurement and recording is centred around the circulatory variables, being based on the inference that the body requirements will be satisfied by an adequate flow of well-oxygenated blood at a suitable pressure—the adequate flow of oxygenated blood being necessary to supply essential substrates, particularly oxygen and to remove waste products including heat, and the suitable pressure being necessary to provide a background against which local changes in resistance can alter flow distribution. Cardiac output not being a commonly measured variable (see p. 507) the other more easily measured variables are taken with a knowledge of the circulatory determinants to make an estimate of circulatory well-being—an estimate which may not have much absolute value but which is useful in assessing change.

In considering circulatory variables and the various determinants of function, it has to be remembered that:

(a) When more than one variable affects a particular function the separate variables may have very different quantitative effects (e.g. pulse rate and filling pressure on cardiac output).

(b) The relationship between a variable and the function it affects may not be linear or may be linear only over a limited range (e.g. pulse rate and cardiac output).

(c) In the intact circulation, the effect of alteration of a variable on a given function is frequently confused by the compensating effects of the rest of the circulation which usually alters in a way designed to counteract or minimise the effect of the primary change (e.g. baroreceptor response to hypertension producing bradycardia). This effect is frequently modified by the action of anaesthetic agents.

The Determinants of Cardiac Output

The cardiac output is a function of heart rate and stroke volume (the output per beat). The stroke volume is itself the consequence of three variables, the preload, the myocardial contractility and the afterload.

Heart Rate and Rhythm

When in sinus rhythm the cardiac rate is determined by the rhythmicity of the sino-atrial node. Other sites in the heart also exhibit this rhythmicity but under normal circumstances the sino-atrial node has the fastest rate and the quickest transmission route enabling it to over-ride the other slower sites. In the sinus node there is a steady continuous decay of resting-membrane potential resulting from an increase of cell membrane conductivity for potassium and an influx of sodium. This phase IV depolarisation (Fig. 3) continues until the

13/Fig. 3.—The action current of a pacemaker fibre recorded by an intracellular electrode.

potential has declined from -90 mV to a threshold at around -40 mV, when a rapid spontaneous depolarisation spike occurs. This intrinsic rhythmicity is enhanced by factors such as increased stretch, pyrexia and hyperthyroidism but is depressed by cold, hypothyroidism and by ischaemia. The sinus node is strongly influenced by nervous impulses. The rate of the denervated sinus is about 120/min and most variation in pulse rate below this level, that is most normal rate control, is the result of variations in the dominant parasympathetic influence. Under normal circumstances the sympathetic system plays little part in the control of rate, although catecholamines are known to increase the rate of phase IV depolarisation. In heart failure, the adrenergic control is more important.

The input to the centre which supplies the innervation to the sinus node is from higher centres, from the vascular reflexes originating in the stretch receptors in the aorta and great vessels, which give rise to the inverse relationship between blood pressure and cardiac rate, and from the chemoreceptors. The significance of cardiac rate as an influence in cardiac output is demonstrated by those patients who have fixed heart rates. Despite a normal myocardium with a capacity for increase in stroke volume, they are incapable of raising their cardiac output appropriately (Braunwald, 1972).

Although cardiac rhythm is commonly considered with rate since abnormal rhythms frequently result in abnormal rates, it is equally important in the consideration of ventricular preload. Firstly, because of the contribution which atrial contraction makes to ventricular filling and secondly, because in abnormal rhythms the atrial pressure may no longer accurately reflect the ventricular end-diastolic pressure (see below).

Preload

Ventricular stroke work or stroke output is related to the initial or end-diastolic fibre length—the greater the initial fibre length, the greater the shortening and therefore the output. Initial fibre length is not a practical clinical measurement but initial or end-diastolic pressure is. The alinear relationship between these two is an expression of ventricular compliance. Under most circumstances end-diastolic pressure changes accurately reflect changes in initial fibre length but compliance can change after extracorporeal circulation or myocardial infarction when changes in end-diastolic pressure may not represent an alteration in initial fibre length. Provided the atrioventricular valve is open, and unobstructed, the diastolic pressures in the atrium and ventricle are the same and under most clinical circumstances the mean atrial pressure is a sufficiently accurate reflection of ventricular preload. This relationship is true for both sides of the heart and the cardiac output can normally be increased by raising the preload usually by transfusion. The limits to which preload can be increased are placed on the right side of the heart by dilatation of the right ventricle with development of tricuspid incompetence and, on the left side of the heart by increases in pulmonary blood volume leading to a progressive decrease in lung compliance and the eventual development of pulmonary oedema.

The determinants of ventricular preload.—If it is accepted that mean atrial pressure is a good reflection of ventricular preload, the factors which determine its value are:

1. Blood volume
2. Venous tone
3. Ventricular compliance
4. Myocardial contractility
5. Ventricular afterload.

If the other factors are kept constant the atrial pressure will reflect the ability of the ventricle to contract, thus when the heart develops left ventricular failure, the left atrial pressure rises and when the right ventricle fails the right atrial pressure rises. Interpretation of a venous pressure value must, therefore, include some consideration of the state of the myocardium.

The preload is also affected by acute changes in afterload. The right atrial pressure is commonly raised in pulmonary embolism and the left atrial pressure raised in the hypertension caused by the administration of a pure vasopressor, such as phenylephrine, both of which represent increased afterload on the respective ventricle. When the acute load is relieved, the atrial pressure necessary for the ventricle to produce a normal cardiac output falls.

Under clinical conditions, both myocardial contractility and ventricular compliance may alter. Myocardial contractility is depressed by most anaesthetic agents and ventricular afterload may be altered by vasopressor agents or by the action of hypoxia on the pulmonary vascular resistance. The effect of endogenous catecholamine secretion is complex as not only may it raise the afterload but it will also affect cardiac rate, myocardial contractility and venous tone.

However, the commonest causes of variation in ventricular preload during anaesthesia and surgery are alterations either in blood volume or venous tone.

Blood volume may be depleted either by haemorrhage or by fluid loss due to fluid restriction, diuresis, sweating, gastro-intestinal losses or losses from raw surfaces. The commonest cause of increased blood volume is undoubtedly over-enthusiastic fluid replacement particularly when not accurately monitored and when given to a vasodilated patient. If the anaesthetic-induced vasodilatation wears off, the blood volume may then be much too great and the atrial pressure rises excessively.

The Venous System

The large capacity venous reservoir contains approximately 70 per cent of the total blood volume and the greater proportion of this is accommodated in the splanchnic bed. The compliance of this system is determined by venomotor tone which, like arterial tone, is controlled by autonomic impulses from the vasomotor centre in the floor of the fourth ventricle. This centre receives inputs from higher and other centres and from the carotid sinus and aortic arch baroreceptors, cardiopulmonary baroreceptors, the carotid and aortic body chemoreceptors and from skeletal muscle receptors. The effect of sympathetic stimulation on the venous capacitance is to increase the venous tone and, therefore, to increase the ventricular preload by producing a transient disequilibrium between the venous return and the cardiac output. Under normal circumstances, variations in venous tone will cope with the effect of altered posture and increases in venous tone will maintain ventricular filling pressure when blood volume falls due to haemorrhage. This compensatory ability may be affected by disease or by drugs. In certain conditions which affect the nervous system (diabetes, peripheral neuritis) the vasomotor outflow is inactive and the patient suffers from postural hypotension due to venous pooling in the unconstricted veins in the upright condition. Autonomic neuropathy often results in a failure to increase the venous tone during positive-pressure respiration so that the effective filling pressure and thus the cardiac output falls. Both these effects may be mimicked by anaesthetic agents, particularly ganglion-blocking agents, which produce vasomotor paralysis and impair the ability of the patient to compensate either for alterations in posture or reversal of intrathoracic pressures. The integrity of the circulatory reflex may be tested by the Valsalva manoeuvre (see Figs. 4–6). In patients with blocked cardiovascular reflexes the Valsalva produces a progressive fall in blood pressure with a slow recovery and no overshoot when the expiratory pressure is withdrawn. During cardiac failure, the sympathetic activity is increased and the venous tone high, hence paralysis of the vasomotor response by anaesthesia in patients with cardiac failure produces dramatic falls in blood pressure and cardiac output.

The ability of changes in venous tone to compensate for changes in blood volume, and body posture, may be inadequate if the alterations in the latter are excessive. The effective ventricular preload will also be affected by factors affecting venous flow, such as venous compression by skeletal muscle, intrapleural and intrapericardial pressure and the atrial contribution to ventricular filling.

The Relationship Between Left- and Right-Sided Filling Pressures

The filling pressure of each ventricle depends on the venous pressure (blood volume/venous tone), the ventricular compliance, the myocardial contractility and the afterload. The left ventricle is less compliant with a greater afterload than the right ventricle and the left-sided filling pressure is normally higher than the right. If the right-sided filling pressure is raised by transfusion the increase in pressure is greater on the left than on the right. Under all normal circumstances the right side of the heart and the lungs are merely passive conduits for the blood and it is possible to discern a relationship between right-sided filling pressure (central venous pressure) and left-sided cardiac output. This is the common clinical situation in which the circulation is manipulated by transfusion according to measurements of central venous pressure and if the left atrial pressure was measured it would alter passively, reflecting left ventricular compliance, contractility and afterload.

In Fig. 7 at a right-sided filling pressure of 3 mm Hg (0·4 kPa) the right ventricle has a stroke output of 55 ml/beat while the left ventricle has the same stroke output from an initial filling pressure of 6 mm Hg (0·8 kPa). If the patient is transfused to raise the right ventricular filling pressure to 5 mm Hg (0·7 kPa) the stroke output rises to 76 ml/beat. There is a transient disequilibrium with

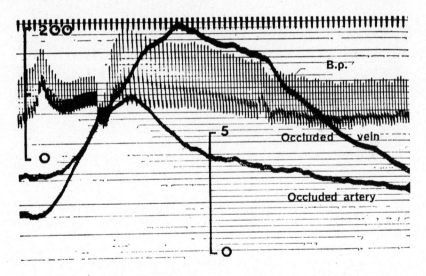

13/Fig. 4.—Effect of Valsalva Manoeuvre on Arterial and Venous Pressure.

Upper margin: time-scale (sec.).

Upper record (B.p.) is that of the arterial pressure in the left brachial artery and shows the usual changes with the Valsalva manoeuvre in a subject with a normal circulation.

The two curves are the right brachial artery pressure (occluded artery) and the right antecubital venous pressure (occluded vein). The limb has been cut off from the rest of the circulation by a high-pressure cuff on the upper arm, so that only nervous impulses can influence the vessels. The blood is stationary in the limb. After seven seconds of the Valsalva manoeuvre, reflex arterial and venous constriction is shown by the rise of pressure in both sets of vessels. Reflex dilatation occurs after the overshoot.

Calibrations in mm Hg.

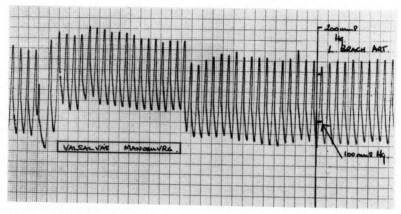

13/FIG. 5.—Square wave response to the Valsalva manoeuvre in a patient with left ventricular failure.

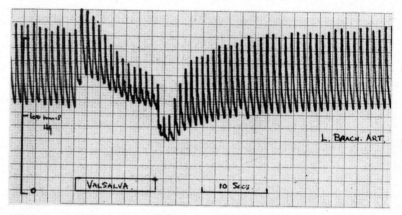

13/FIG. 6.—Effect of Valsalva manoeuvre in a patient with blocked circulatory reflexes.

the right ventricular output higher than the left, resulting in an increase in central blood volume. The left ventricular output rises until a new equilibrium is reached with left and right ventricular outputs the same, but now the left ventricular end-diastolic pressure is 12 mm Hg (1·6 kPa) and the pulmonary blood volume is higher than it was. As the left atrial pressure rises, there is a progressive increase in lung stiffness, a progressive diminution in arterial oxygen tensions due to the development of interstitial oedema (Szidon et al., 1972) and ultimately pulmonary oedema. The disadvantage of manipulating the circulation according to measurements of the central venous pressure is that it presupposes knowledge of the relationship between left and right ventricular compliance, contractility and afterload. In health it may be possible to make reasonable assumptions about these relationships and it is probably true that any patient whose central venous pressure is less than 5 cm H$_2$O (0·5 kPa) relative to the sternal angle is not overfilled. However, in disease, no such assumptions can be made and under the conditions of anaesthesia and surgery, when the heart may be modified by anaesthetic and other drugs and by the effects of blood/gas, electrolyte and autonomic nervous system disturbances, conclusions about the left heart based on measurements of the central venous pressure may well be invalid. In this case it is much safer to manipulate the circulation according to the left-sided filling pressure measured either directly by a catheter inserted at cardiac surgery or through the atrial septum or by indirect measurement using the pulmonary capillary wedge pressure which may be determined through a Swan-Ganz flow-directed catheter.

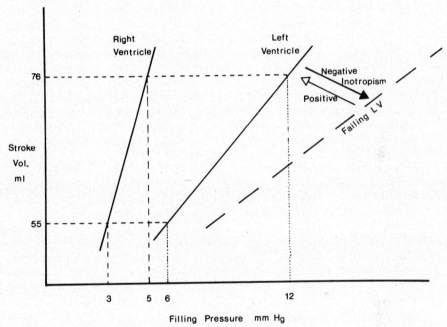

13/FIG. 7.—Diagrammatic representation of relationship between left- and right-sided filling pressures of the heart.

Myocardial Contractility

This controversial subject refers to the intrinsic muscle fibre shortening property of the myocardium. The simplest approach is to consider that an increase in cardiac output with an unchanged filling pressure represents increased contractility, but this takes no account of the effect of afterload which must also remain constant. Because afterload is itself a function of the ventricle (see below) this is a difficult concept to apply in practice and among the many efforts made to quantitate contractility an important approach is to consider the ventricle only during its isovolaemic phase before the aortic valve opens and the fibres start to shorten. In the non-experimental situation of clinical anaesthesia the simpler concept of the slope of the curve defining the relationship between stroke work and ventricular filling pressure usually suffices as an index of cardiac performance, as it represents the integrated response of the heart in its role of the central component of the intact circulation (Jenkins *et al.*, 1973). A steep slope implies good myocardial performance, a flatter curve a worse ventricle, but there is no doubt that this seriously understates the complexity of the relationship between contractility and cardiac output. Anaesthetic agents in general depress myocardial contractility, an action which can be reversed by β stimulation or drugs such as digoxin or calcium.

Afterload

After the isovolaemic phase is over and the aortic valve opens, the left ventricle is interacting with the peripheral circulation which now becomes an important determinant of the rate of rise of aortic pressure, the size, duration and velocity of ejection and the shape and volume of the ventricles during systole. The afterload is a function both of the impedance to blood flow (see below) and the anatomy of the ventricle. Intraventricular tension is dependent not only on the intracavity pressure but on mean ventricular radius, itself dependent on the size and thickness of the ventricle. This of course means that afterload changes as the heart contracts and the ventricle changes size. During heart failure, when the heart dilates, myocardial wall tensions (and afterload and oxygen consumption) increase above normal. Hypertrophy of the ventricle reduces the stress on each unit of the myocardium and tends to maintain the afterload of each myocardial cell close to normal.

It is a common observation that, during the production of induced hypotension after a ganglion blocker has been given but before the filling pressure has been reduced by posturing the patient, the cardiac output often rises as the afterload decreases. This ability to increase cardiac output secondary to a reduction in afterload does not depend on a normal heart but can also be observed in the failing heart and in patients with aortic or mitral incompetence.

Afterload, by being both a determinant and a consequence of stroke volume, plays an important role in circulatory equilibrium. The normal heart continually adjusts its contractile state to compensate for changes in afterload (Anrep effect).

The Arterial System and Blood Pressure

The arterial system, which contains 15 per cent of the blood volume, is the distributive and resistive element of the circulation. The interaction between this resistive element and the cardiac output results in the development of the blood pressure whose function is to ensure a forward flow of blood to all parts of the body and to provide a general pressure background against which local alterations in resistance can affect the distribution of flow.

During exercise, blood pressure may change very little although cardiac output increases enormously implying a large drop in total vascular resistance and hence in afterload. Most of this occurs in the vessels supplying the exercising muscle and if the rise in cardiac output is inadequate to supply the demand for flow in the muscle then resistance rises in those areas, such as the mesenteric bed, which are uninvolved in the exercise.

Control Mechanism of the Arterial Bed

The control of individual arteriolar resistance is both by intrinsic and extrinsic mechanisms. The intrinsic mechanism is the inherent myotonic activity of the smooth muscle in the precapillary resistance vessels which accounts for most of the basal vascular tone. This activity is modified by the dilator influences of hypoxia and metabolites and by the constrictor effect of the distending blood pressure within the lumen. If extrinsic factors are abolished the intrinsic factors tend to maintain appropriate tissue flow despite wide perfusion pressure changes. The extrinsic factors are neural and humoral, of which the latter is less important. The innervation is predominantly sympathetic but, depending on the tissue, may be vasoconstrictor or vasodilator. The contribution which the constrictor fibres make to basal vascular tone is minimal provided the heart is normal. The main function of the neural extrinsic mechanism is to provide speedy or even anticipatory response to an instantaneous demand for increased blood flow as part of the general neural control of the circulation.

Determinants of Blood Pressure

When blood is ejected into the aorta the derived pressure depends partly on the stroke volume and partly on the impedance. Impedance is defined as the ratio of the instantaneous rate of change of aortic pressure to the instantaneous aortic pressure. It depends on the compliance of the aorta and large arteries and the rate of run off from the arterial bed during systole. This explains the systolic hypertension of slow heart rates (large stroke volume) of senile athero-sclerosis (decreased aortic and large vessel compliance) and of essential hyper-tension (decreased run off). While resistance is mainly a function of arteriolar radius which may be altered structurally or by variations in muscle tone, it is also influenced by blood viscosity which is frequently changed during anaesthesia and surgery by infusions of different solutions. The factors affecting diastolic pressure are related but not identical so that the two pressures normally vary independently of each other.

THE MANIPULATION OF THE CIRCULATION

The common situation in which the anaesthetist finds himself is needing to improve the circulation because he believes the blood pressure or the cardiac output or both are too low to provide the adequate circulation of well-oxygen-ated blood at a suitable perfusion pressure.

If the cardiac output is satisfactory, but the perfusion pressure so low that certain organs, particularly brain, kidneys and heart, may be in jeopardy then the pressure might logically be treated with a pure vasopressor. The resulting increase in afterload may reduce the cardiac output particularly if the ventricle is depressed and a good general principle is to use a vasopressor with some β-stimulating properties (metaraminol).

The more common and worrying situation is when the cardiac output is thought to be low and the blood pressure either inadequate or temporarily sustained by vasoconstriction. The methods for increasing the cardiac output are (1) control of rate and rhythm; (2) alterations in ventricular preload; (3) alterations in myocardial contractility and obviously consideration of all three proceeds simultaneously.

(a) *Rate and rhythm.*—As cardiac output is largely dependent on rate, the restoration of a normal rate from bradycardia or even the production of a mild tachycardia will improve output. Heart rate may be altered with drugs such as atropine, isoprenaline or adrenaline or by electrical pacing.

The atrial transport mechanism plays an important part in producing effective ventricular filling and sinus rhythm may be necessary for a good cardiac output. Any other rhythm may be associated with a reduction in cardiac output (see p. 564).

(b) *Alterations in ventricular preload.*—A low cardiac output may be associated with a low filling pressure, usually the consequence either of haemorrhage or peripheral vasodilatation, or with a high filling pressure the commonest cause of which is cardiac failure. Having resolved this diagnostic problem the low filling pressure group can be treated either by infusions of suitable fluid, by posture or (if it is due to pure vasodilatation and is unresponsive to fluid therapy) by vasoconstriction. The latter has the disadvantage of also raising the afterload and should be avoided if possible. It is important to distinguish early those patients whose ventricular function is inadequate and who will not respond to increased preload because in this group quite modest increases in central venous pressure may result in large increases in left atrial pressure leading to pulmonary oedema.

(c) *Improvement in myocardial contractility.*—Myocardial contractility is most easily improved by a slow intravenous infusion (1–4 µg/min) of iso-prenaline. This has the added advantage of increasing cardiac rate, of tending to preserve or restore sinus rhythm and by its peripheral dilator action, of reducing ventricular afterload. It does have the disadvantage of increasing myocardial oxygen consumption which may be deleterious if the low cardiac output and hypotension is due to a myocardial infarct when it may increase the eventual size of the infarct. In some circumstances the tachycardia of isoprenaline may be excessive and can result in a reduction in coronary flow (see below) whereas intravenous salbutamol will give the inotropic effect without the chronotropic response. Finally, in some circumstances isoprenaline may not result in any increase in cardiac output and the peripheral vasodilator action produces a fall in blood pressure below that necessary to perfuse the essential organs. In this extreme circumstance it may be necessary to preserve pressure at the expense of flow and use adrenaline rather than isoprenaline. Changing from isoprenaline to adrenaline may result in a fairly large increase in the left and right atrial pressures. Isoprenaline dilates blood vessels and in an effort to raise the ventricular pressure the patient will have been well-transfused. Adrenaline, however, constricts the capacitance vessels so that the combined effect of the transfused fluid and the increase in venous tone is to raise the cardiac filling pressure, sometimes to excessive levels. The converse will of course occur if the adrenaline is diminished or discontinued.

The Electrocardiogram

The electrocardiogram (ECG) is a graphic display of the electrical activity of the heart as detected on the surface of the body, in which the major deflections represent the depolarisation of atrial and ventricular muscle. The activity of the specialised conducting tissue is deduced from the timing and spatial orientation of the electrical activity but no such similar deduction can be made from the ECG about the ability of the heart to contract and to generate pressure.

The 12-lead standard ECG (Fig. 8) consists of 3 bipolar limb leads, 3 uni-polar limb leads and 6 chest leads positioned as in Fig. 9. The six chest leads lie

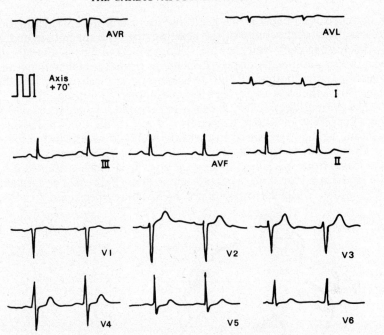

13/Fig. 8.—Normal standard 12-lead ECG.

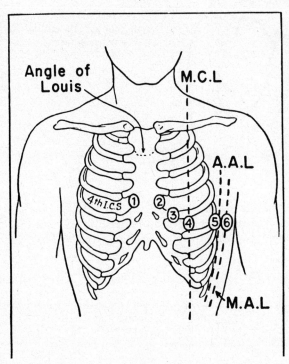

13/Fig. 9.—The Location of
the Six Precordial Leads
M.C.L., midclavicular line;
A.A.L., anterior axillary line;
M.A.L., midaxillary line.

in the horizontal plane of the heart and are useful for considering horizontal vectors—electrical activity of the heart having both magnitude and direction is a vector quantity—but they are seldom practical during anaesthesia. However the six limb leads display principally frontal vector activity and as the normal vector of both the P and QRS complex lies close to lead II in the frontal plane this is the most useful lead for continuous monitoring.

The normal electrocardiograph is recorded at a paper speed of 2·5 cm/sec and a sensitivity of 10 mm deflection = 1 mV. If the ECG is displayed on an oscilloscope the sweep speed and sensitivity should be adjusted to these values.

The normal electrocardiogram.—The impulse that initiates a normal heart beat arises from specialised tissue—the sino-atrial node—situated at the junction of the superior vena cava and right atrium (Fig. 10). The specialised conducting tissue of the heart comprises the SA node, specialised atrial pathways,

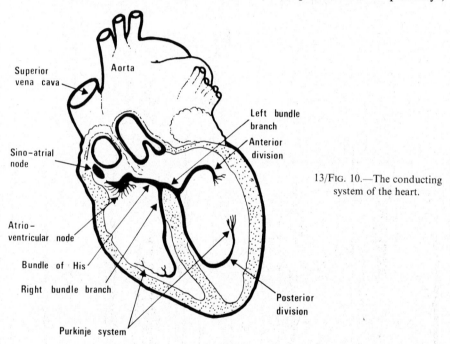

13/Fig. 10.—The conducting system of the heart.

the atrioventricular node, the bundle of His, the right and left bundle branches and the distal Purkinje fibres. The time taken for an impulse to traverse this pathway is seen in the P-R interval which in adults varies between 0·12 to 0·20

13/Table 1
SHOWING POSITION OF BIPOLAR AND UNIPOLAR LIMB LEADS

Lead	I	Right arm—left arm	aVR	.	Right arm lead
	II	Right arm—left leg	aVL	.	Left arm lead
	III	Left arm — left leg	aVF	.	Left leg lead
		Right leg lead—earth lead			

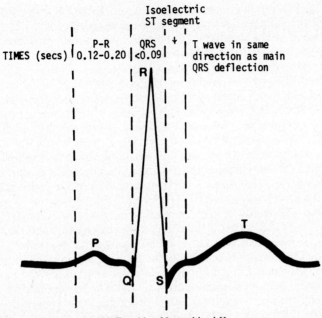

13/Fig. 11.—Normal lead II.

The normal ECG is defined by:
(1) P waves of normal size, direction and shape at an appropriate rate and each followed by a QRS complex.
(2) The PR interval less than 0·20 seconds (0·18 seconds in children).
(3) A QRS of less than 0·09 seconds and with a frontal axis between −30° and +100°.
(4) An isoelectric S-T segment.
(5) The T waves in the limb leads in the same direction as the corresponding QRS complex.
(For discussion of the abnormal ECG see p. 566 *et seq.*).

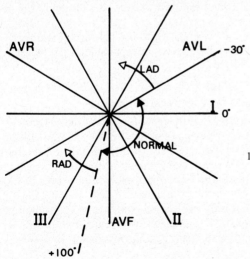

13/Fig. 12.—Frontal QRS vector diagram.

seconds (Fig. 11), but in children the time is shorter (0·10–0·18 seconds). To a small extent the value varies inversely with the heart rate.

The P wave is the resultant of the electrical current produced by atrial muscle depolarisation. Atrial hypertrophy increases the size of this wave and delays in its passage across the atrium will prolong it.

Sinus rhythm may be inferred from the finding of normal P waves (indicating the expected pattern of atrial muscle depolarisation) and their constant relationship with the QRS complexes. During sinus rhythm the cardiac rate will show minor variations in response to a variety of normal physiological stimuli and in particular may show a periodic variation with respiration. This sinus arrhythmia results from the increase in vagal tone which accompanies inspiration producing cardiac slowing, the heart speeding up again during expiration.

The QRS complex represents the depolarisation of the ventricular muscle. In a normal heart the mean frontal QRS vector lies between $-30°$ and $+100°$ (Fig. 12) and the width of the complex is narrow (less than 0·09 second). Widening of the QRS occurs if the conduction velocity through the specialised pathways is slower than normal or if the pathway is abnormally long. The height of the QRS complex represents the net resultant of the electrical forces generated by the muscle in a number of different directions. When in a normal heart the muscle depolarises simultaneously in all areas, a considerable cancellation of electrical forces occurs and the QRS is relatively small. An increase in the size of the QRS occurs not only in the presence of ventricular hypertrophy but also when conduction is altered. Thus in right or left bundle-branch block, or in a ventricular ectopic beat, not only is the QRS prolonged but it is larger than usual.

The ST segment of the ECG is usually iso-electric. It corresponds to the plateau phase of the intracardiac action potential (Fig. 13). A shift in the ST segment reveals the presence of an abnormal current in the heart.

The T wave portrays the repolarisation (phase 3) of the ventricular muscle and is normally orientated in the same direction in the frontal plane as the preceding QRS complex. Abnormalities of repolarisation either flatten or invert this T wave.

The duration of depolarisation and repolarisation (Q-T interval) is directly related to cardiac rate becoming shorter at faster rates provided the heart is normal.

(For discussion of the abnormal ECG see Chapter 14, p. 566 *et seq.*).

Effect of Electrolyte Changes upon the Electrocardiogram

(*a*) *Calcium.*—Changes in the serum calcium level often accompany those of serum potassium. The normal range for serum calcium is 2·25–2·55 mmol/l. The Q-T interval varies inversely with the calcium level of the blood. Thus, when the calcium level is high the Q-T interval is shortened; when it is low, the interval is lengthened (Fig. 14). These changes are not accompanied by alterations in the height or shape of the T wave as seen in hypokalaemia. A low serum calcium level occurs in hypoparathyroidism or after prolonged vomiting. A high calcium level may be encountered after the intravenous injection of calcium chloride or gluconate following massive blood transfusion therapy—or in hyperparathyroidism.

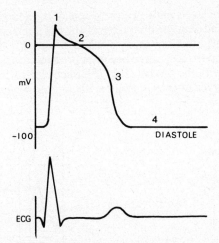

13/Fig. 13.—The action current of a ventricular muscle fibre recorded by an intracellular electrode and simultaneous external ECG.

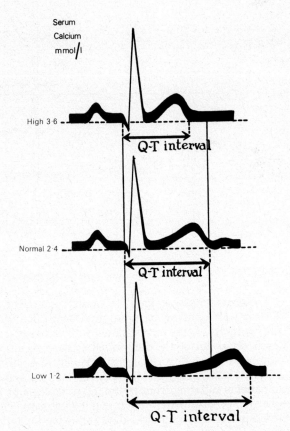

13/Fig. 14.—Effect of alteration in serum calcium level on ECG.

(b) *Potassium* levels influence the whole of the action potential and direction of the T wave and also the character of the S-T segment. Under normal conditions the serum potassium level is 3·5 to 5 mmol/l. When the level drops to 3·0 mmol/l or lower the T wave becomes broader and flatter, and a U wave may be seen to fuse with the T wave (Fig. 15). Such electrocardiographic patterns are sometimes observed in patients with acute or chronic intestinal obstruction with hypovolaemia.

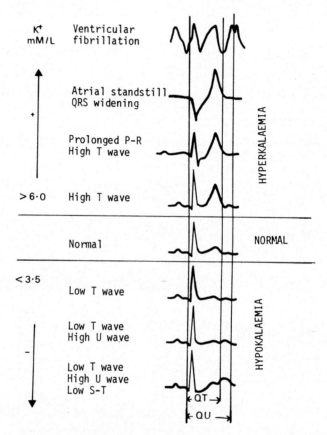

13/Fig. 15.—Effect of serum potassium levels on ECG.

A serum potassium level of 7 mmol/l and over leads initially to a tall, peaked T wave with a narrow base. An increasing QRS width is a danger sign and any further increase may be associated with ventricular fibrillation. High potassium levels occur during the diminished urinary excretion of renal failure, dehydration, and adrenal cortical insufficiency (e.g. Addison's disease or bilateral adrenalectomy). Sudden increases in serum potassium levels have been reported in patients suffering from traumatic paraplegia or burns immediately after the injection of suxamethonium (see p. 869 *et seq.*). The highest levels are believed to occur between 15 and 75 days following the injury.

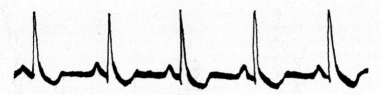

13/Fig. 16.—Effect of digitalis. Note that S-T segment is depressed and "sagging" is present. There is a low-voltage T wave.

Effect of Drugs upon the Electrocardiogram

Digitalis principally produces alterations in the S-T segment and the T wave. With early digitalisation there is a depression of the S-T segment in all leads in the opposite direction to the main deflection of the QRS complex. As digitalis therapy proceeds, first the T wave becomes reduced in amplitude and then the S-T segment moves above or below the base line in the opposite direction to the QRS complex. The result is an ECG with a typical "sagging" effect (Fig. 16).

These changes can be observed within a few minutes of an intravenous dose of digoxin during anaesthesia. Over-digitalisation affects not only the rate and the rhythm of the heart by means of vagal stimulation and a direct depressant action on the conductive system, but it is capable of reproducing every known type of dysrhythmia and heart block. The effects of digitalis therapy may be observed in some cases 2–3 weeks after cessation of therapy and they are exaggerated in the presence of a low serum potassium.

Quinidine tends to depress the electrical activity of the heart. The P wave and the QRS are increased in duration. The S wave widens and the T wave is lowered and widened (Fig. 17). In excessive dosage all types of cardiac irregularities may be observed.

Adrenergic drugs, adrenaline, ephedrine, etc. lower the amplitude of T waves and may reverse their direction. Cholinergic drugs may have the same effect.

Amyl nitrite produces marked tachycardia and reversal of the direction of the T wave.

THE EFFECTS OF ANAESTHESIA ON THE CARDIOVASCULAR SYSTEM

The effects of anaesthetic agents may be considered in relation to the heart, to the peripheral circulation or to the integrated response of the whole cardio-vascular system in the intact patient. When anaesthetising patients it is obviously the latter which is of concern but this is the area where responses are most individual depending so much on the balances, not least between sympathetic and parasympathetic influence, which exist between the different parts of the circulation.

Most early and some quite recent investigatory work of the effect of anaes-thetics on the heart reflects different concepts about the circulation to those ob-taining today and shows the limitation of investigatory methods then available. The fundamental contractile property of the myocardium must be quantitated in a manner which is independent of those variables such as preload, afterload and heart rate which cannot be kept constant and which may themselves be influenced by anaesthesia. Other variables such as carbon dioxide tension and the effects of pre-anaesthetic medication need to be rigidly controlled. A further problem lies in how far results obtained in isolated heart or heart lung preparation, together with the problems of species difference, are applicable to the human. Accepting these limitations (Merin, 1975) it appears that inhalational anaesthetic agents and most intravenous agents produce true depression of myocardial contractility but that with ether, cyclopropane and fluroxene the effect is offset by increased sympathetic drive.

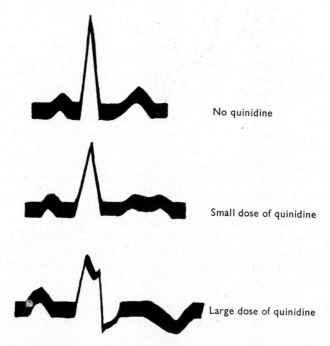

13/Fig. 17.—Effect of quinidine. Changes produced in the ECG with varying doses.

While anaesthetic agents depress contractile force they do so to a degree not critical under normal circumstances (Price and Pauca, 1969). The three other and more important ways in which anaesthetic agents affect the circulation are by affecting the heart rate, the afterload and the preload. The cardiac output during anaesthesia is very rate-dependent up to a limit beyond which the output falls again. Dilatation of the resistance vessels either by reduction of sympathetic tone or by direct effect on the smooth muscle may lead to a rise in cardiac output despite a fall in blood pressure provided the filling pressure is maintained. It is, however, perhaps in their effects on the capacitance vessels, and thus on the ventricular filling pressure, that anaesthetic agents may exert their most significant, and unfortunately least investigated, effect.

CIRCULATORY INNERVATION

Central control of the circulation is exerted both via the autonomic nervous

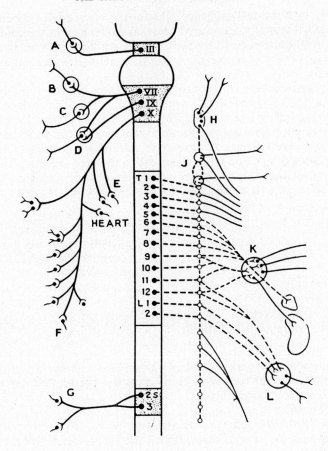

13/FIG. 18.—THE AUTONOMIC NERVOUS SYSTEM

On left: Cranial and sacral autonomic (parasympathetic) system. Thick lines from III, VII, IX, X, and S2, 3 are pre-ganglionic (connector fibres).

A—ciliary ganglion.

B—sphenopalatine ganglion.

C—submaxillary and sublingual ganglia.

D—otic ganglion.

E—vagus excitor cells in nodes of heart.

F—vagus excitor cells in wall of bowel.

G—sacral autonomic ganglion cells in pelvis. Thin lines beyond—post-ganglionic (excitor) fibres to organs.

On right: Sympathetic nervous system. Dotted lines from T 1–12, L 1, 2 are pre-ganglionic fibres.

H—superior cervical ganglion.

J—inferior cervical and 1st thoracic ganglia (stellate ganglion).

K—coeliac and other abdominal ganglia (note pre-ganglionic fibres directly supplying the adrenal medulla).

L—lower abdominal and pelvic sympathetic ganglia. Continuous lines beyond—post-ganglionic fibres.

system and by hormonal influence. The former obviously provides a quicker response but the totally denervated heart, as in the human transplanted heart recipient, will function perfectly satisfactorily within a wide range of activity. In this situation the heart is responding to variations in circulating catechol-amine levels.

The parasympathetic outflow to the heart is the dominant influence in the normal rate control of the heart, increase in activity slowing the heart, decrease in activity producing tachycardia. The alterations in ventricular contractility caused by variations in vagal tone are almost entirely the consequence of changes in cardiac rate. The sympathetic adrenergic outflow to the cardiovascular system may be stimulatory or inhibiting according to the area supplied. The receptor components of the effector system are divided pharmacologically into two groups, alpha and beta, on the basis of their response to adrenergic stimuli.

Tissue	Receptor	Effect
The heart	Beta	Sympathetic adrenergic stimulation increases cardiac rate, atrioventricular conduction and force of ventricular contraction.
Coronary vessels	Alpha	Coronary vasoconstriction
Blood vessels:		
of the skeletal muscle	Beta	Dilatation
of the skin and mucosa	Alpha	Constriction

The autonomic nerves are the final pathway for a number of reflexes which are fundamental to the control of blood pressure. The centre from which they arise is subject to influences from:

(a) *Higher centres*

(b) *The sino-aortic reflexes.*—In the dog the baroreceptor in the carotid sinus and aortic arch have different thresholds and different ranges, the sinus receptors working at a lower threshold (80 mm Hg; 10·7 kPa) and a lower range (80–180 mm Hg; 10·7–24·0 kPa). The aortic reflex is ineffective in combating hypotension and it appears to be involved mainly in the control of high blood pressure (Shepherd, 1974).

(c) *Chemoreflexes.*—The chemoreceptors in the carotid and aortic body produce stimulation leading to vasoconstriction when the oxygen tension falls or when the carbon dioxide tension rises.

(d) *Cardiopulmonary baroreceptors.*—Sensory bodies exist in the heart, great vessels and lungs whose response appears to be evoked by mechanical deformation and which exert a continuous restraint on the cardiovascular centre.

(e) *Skeletal muscle.*—Contraction of even small muscle groups produces an almost instantaneous rise in cardiac output and blood pressure.

The particular significance of these reflexes for the anaesthetised patient is that those anaesthetic techniques which depress or inhibit circulatory adapta-tion such as vasoconstriction of the arteries and capacitance vessels, increase in heart rate, increase in force of contraction of the heart—which are the response to haemorrhage—place the anaesthetist with his judgement of blood volume and ventricular filling pressure as the only defence the patient has against life-threatening falls in blood pressure and cardiac output, whether this be produced by haemorrhage, posture or the mechanical effects of positive-pressure respiration.

REFERENCES

BRAUNWALD, E. (1972). Myocardial function. *Anesth. Analg. Curr. Res.*, **51,** 489.

JENKINS, B. S., BRANTHWAITE, M. A., and BRADLEY, R. D. (1973). Cardiac function after open heart surgery: Relation between the performance of the two sides of the heart. *Cardiovasc. Res.*, **7,** 297.

MERIN, R. G. (1975). The effects of anaesthetics on the heart. *Surg. Clin. N. Amer.*, **55,** 759.

PRICE, H. L., and PAUCA, A. L. (1969). The effects of anaesthesia on the peripheral circulation. In: *Clinical Anaesthesia* Series 3/1969, "A Decade of Clinical Progress", Ed. L. Fabian. Oxford: Blackwell Scientific Publications.

SHEPHERD, J. T. (1974). The cardiac catheter and the American Heart Association. *Circulation.* **50,** 418.

SZIDON, J. P., PIETRA, C. G., and FISHMAN, A. P. (1972). The alveolar capillary membrane and pulmonary oedema. *New Engl. J. Med.*, **286,** 1200.

FURTHER READING

BRAUNWALD, E. (1974). Regulation of the circulation (in two parts). *New Engl. J. Med.*, **290,** 1124 and 1420.

COHN, J. N. (1973). Blood pressure and cardiac performance. *Amer. J. Med.*, **55,** 351.

GUYTON, A. C. (1973). Central venous pressure: Physiological significance and clinical implications. *Amer. Heart J.*, **86,** 431.

Chapter 14

ANAESTHESIA AND CARDIAC DISEASE

CARDIAC disease covers a wide spectrum of both anatomical and physiological disturbance. How cardiac disease affects and is affected by anaesthesia and surgery is discussed in the following pages. However, the basic principles for successful management of cardiac patients derive, in the first place, from a proper understanding of the haemodynamic effects and complications of the patient's lesion. The anaesthetist needs, therefore, to be able to diagnose the lesion and to assess correctly the effect that it has had on the patient's haemodynamic state.

THE ASSESSMENT OF THE PATIENT WITH CARDIAC DISEASE

Objects.—The main objects in the assessment of patients with cardiac disease are:

(a) to determine the capability of the heart and circulation to withstand the stresses which accompany anaesthesia and surgery, not only during the operative period but equally in the post-operative period;

(b) to make a logical choice of anaesthetic techniques and supportive therapy, based on an understanding of the patient's haemodynamic state.

Diagnosis.—Assessment involves firstly the diagnosis of the nature and severity of the specific lesion present. From this the haemodynamic consequences and likely complications can be predicted and therefore sought. The complications of a lesion are often more important than the actual disease itself.

An assessment, therefore, includes consideration of:

(a) the state of the myocardium—which may be shown by low cardiac output, congestive cardiac failure, or by the occurrence of dysrhythmias;

(b) the state of the systemic vessels—particularly in respect of coronary artery disease or systemic hypertension;

(c) the condition of the lungs—both the ventilatory function which may be impaired by pulmonary oedema, chronic bronchitis and emphysema, and the pulmonary vascular tree in which pulmonary arterial obstructive disease can occur;

(d) the function of other organs—particularly of the liver and kidneys— which may be affected by tricuspid valve disease, venous engorgement or a low cardiac output.

Clinical assessment.—A thorough history and clinical examination of the patient will provide most of the information needed in the assessment of the fitness of patients to withstand the operation and post-operative period.

Observation of the Patient

A simple estimation of what the patient can do is valuable. The ability to carry out housework normally in the case of a woman, to climb a flight of stairs without stopping, to walk up a hill or even to dress, in some measure gives an indication of whether or not the heart can increase its output in response to demand.

Symptoms.—The symptoms of cardiac disease result from physiological disturbances. The likely symptoms can be predicted if the diagnosis is known and the patient specifically questioned for them. The haemodynamic alterations are:

i. *Raised left atrial pressure* gives rise to dyspnoea, cough and recurrent bronchitis and may be due to left heart failure, mitral or aortic valve disease.

ii. *Raised systemic venous pressure* giving rise to peripheral oedema. This is due to right heart (congestive) failure, itself the consequence of lesions of the pulmonary valve, or pulmonary hypertension, or secondary to left ventricular failure. Hepatic pain occurs particularly if there is associated tricuspid incompetence. A raised systemic venous pressure, without right ventricular failure, may also be the result of pericardial disease or tricuspid stenosis.

iii. *Low cardiac output* which produces the symptoms of fatigue. This results from cardiac failure, valvular stenosis, raised pulmonary vascular resistance, tamponade or constrictive pericarditis.

iv. *Myocardial ischaemia*, of which the principal symptom is angina, and which is usually due to coronary artery disease.

v. *Dysrhythmias* felt by the patients as palpitations. These result principally from ischaemia or electrolyte disturbances and may be provoked by drug therapy.

Angina.—Angina is due to inadequate oxygen supply to the myocardium. This may follow narrowing of the coronary arteries, severe anaemia, thyrotoxicosis, or increased myocardial demands for oxygen which exceed the supply, as may occur in the hypertrophic ventricle of aortic stenosis or in the rapid heart rates of paroxysmal tachycardia. There are four major features of anginal pain:

i. it is situated maximally behind the sternum or across the front of the chest;

ii. the pain is described as "crushing" or as a "tight constricting sensation";

iii. it radiates characteristically to the angle of the jaw and down the inside of the left arm, but may also spread into the shoulders and neck and down the other arm to the hand;

iv. the pain comes on during exertion, anger or excitement, and when the stimulus is discontinued the pain wears off in two to three minutes.

Dyspnoea.—Dyspnoea is probably the most common symptom of cardiac disease and is usually the result of a raised pulmonary venous pressure. Rises of pressure in the left atrium and pulmonary veins are transmitted back to the pulmonary capillaries increasing the transudation of fluid from the capillaries into the interstitial tissues of the lungs. These spaces drain via the lymphatics which can be seen to be engorged both at operation and in the chest X-ray. This reduces the ventilation and increases the effort needed to inflate and deflate the lungs.

Orthopnoea and paroxysmal nocturnal dyspnoea are specific types of dyspnoea. Orthopnoea means dyspnoea which occurs when lying flat and which is relieved by sitting up. Paroxysmal nocturnal dyspnoea is orthopnoea which wakens the patient from sleep forcing him to sit upright or stand out of bed for relief. In either case the effect is due to the increased output from the right heart secondary to the increased right atrial pressure in the horizontal position. The left ventricle is unable to cope with the increased supply of blood, so the left ventricular end-diastolic, left atrial and pulmonary capillary pressures rise.

Should the pressure in the pulmonary veins rise above the osmotic pressure of the plasma proteins pulmonary oedema will occur; dyspnoea is then acute and is accompanied by a cough and copious pink or white frothy sputum. The upright position lowers the right atrial pressure which in turn diminishes the right ventricular output and leads to a decrease in pulmonary congestion and consequently ventilation becomes easier with less dyspnoea. Chronic congestion leads to fibrosis in the interstitial tissue of the lung between the alveoli and the capillaries, and tends to prevent transudation into the alveoli so that frank pulmonary oedema is less evident at this stage. Pulmonary oedema thus occurs essentially early in the progress of cardiac disease and is often precipitated by the stress of effort or emotion or by uncontrolled atrial fibrillation or tachycardia.

Useful information about the severity of heart disease is obtained by grading the severity of the dyspnoea:

Grade 1. Dyspnoea while undertaking unusual exertion (running, walking up hill, scrubbing).

Grade 2. Moderate walking on the level causes dyspnoea.

Grade 3. Unable to continue walking, even slowly, on the level. All but the lightest housework has to be given up.

Grade 4. The slightest effort produces breathlessness: the patient is practically confined to bed by dyspnoea.

A history of nocturnal dyspnoea or acute pulmonary oedema places the patient in grade 4 irrespective of effort tolerance. Dyspnoea may also occur in conditions which give rise to a low cardiac output when tissue anoxia may be responsible for mild dyspnoea. Breathlessness on exertion is present in all right-to-left intracardiac shunts as the reduced oxygen content of the arterial blood stimulates the chemoreceptors at the carotid body. Dyspnoea occurring in patients with cardiac disease may also be due to some incidental lung disease.

Cough may be precipitated by a rise in pulmonary venous pressure during exertion, causing engorgement of the bronchial mucosa. This gives rise to a troublesome dry cough. Recurrent bronchitis is a common symptom of raised left atrial pressure or increased pulmonary blood flow.

Haemoptysis.—Haemoptysis is an important symptom in cardiac disease. It commonly occurs from the rupture of a small engorged vein in conditions which give rise to a raised left atrial pressure. The source of bleeding may be a pulmonary infarct and haemoptysis is common in chronic bronchitis. The patient may also describe "coughing up blood" when suffering from acute pulmonary oedema.

"Palpitations".—This is a commonly used term for any increased awareness of the heart beat. The sudden onset of fast palpitations may represent the onset of an attack of paroxysmal tachycardia or of atrial fibrillation.

Syncope.—This symptom arises from more than one mechanism. Syncope on effort occurs as a symptom of a low fixed cardiac output due to severe aortic or pulmonary stenosis or to mitral stenosis with severe pulmonary hypertension.

Syncope also occurs as Stokes-Adams attacks during rhythm changes, particularly at the onset of complete heart block. Sudden loss of consciousness is not uncommon in children with Fallot's tetralogy. These attacks are often precipitated by emotional stress when they are thought to be due to spasm of the infundibulum of the right ventricle. If the attack is prolonged, death may occur.

Peripheral oedema.—Congestive cardiac failure is one of the causes of peripheral oedema and is due to an abnormal retention of salt and water. The fluid tends to settle under the influence of gravity into the most dependent parts of the body.

Hepatic pain follows the enlargement and distension of the hepatic capsule which is secondary to a high systemic venous pressure in right heart failure. It causes a dull ache in the epigastrium and right hypochondrium and is often aggravated by exertion which further increases the systemic venous pressure.

Examination of the Patient

Examination of the cardiovascular system is carried out in a standard order so that no detail is missed. The patient is placed reclining against the pillows of the bed so that the thorax is at an angle of 45° to the horizontal and the head is supported so that the sternomastoid muscles are relaxed.

General appearance.—The general appearance of the patient is noted, especially emaciation which might accompany chronic heart failure, stunted growth which may be the result of congenital cyanotic heart disease, or obesity which may aggravate cardiac disease. Patients with a chronically low cardiac output have a dusty mauve flush with telangiectases on their cheeks known as a malar flush, most commonly seen in mitral valve disease complicated by pulmonary hypertension.

Cyanosis indicates an excess of reduced haemoglobin in the blood and the critical distinction must be made between peripheral and central cyanosis. Peripheral cyanosis due to increased oxygen extraction by the tissues as a compensation for low cardiac output is best seen in the lobes of the ear, the nose, and in the fingers. Central cyanosis, which is caused by reduction in oxygen content of the systemic arterial blood due to intracardiac or pulmonary right-to-left shunts, is characteristically seen in warm mucous membrane, such as the tongue, lips and conjunctivae. Although clubbing of the fingers occurs with a variety of diseases, it may be seen in cyanotic heart disease, bacterial endocarditis or left atrial myxoma.

The signs of anaemia and thyrotoxicosis are sought for as these two conditions both aggravate cardiac disease or may even precipitate cardiac failure.

Arterial pulse.—The arterial pulse is analysed for the four characteristics of rate, rhythm, amplitude and wave form. The brachial is a larger and more convenient artery for study than the radial, but wave form is best appreciated in the carotid. At the same time the quality of the vessel wall is noted. The main peripheral pulses are palpated to confirm their presence and to exclude the diagnosis of a coarctation of the aorta. A very rapid rate is likely to lead to cardiac failure, whereas a slow rate of 60 per minute or less in the absence of heart block is the most frequent precursor of ventricular extrasystoles, and this may slow even further after anaesthetic premedication. If a dysrhythmia is present it will require ECG confirmation of its type. Pulsus alternans should be

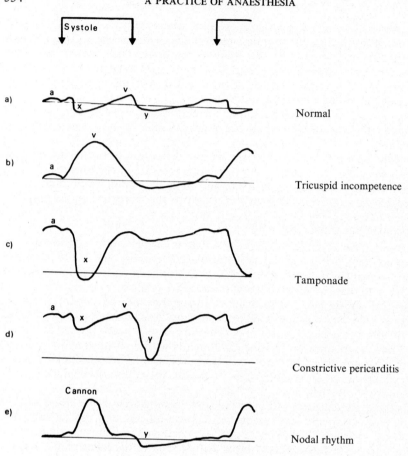

14/Fig. 1.—Characteristic jugular venous wave forms.

sought as this is good evidence of left ventricular failure. Pulsus paradoxus, in the absence of an increased inspiratory effort due to asthma or laryngeal stridor, is an indication of tamponade or constrictive pericarditis.

Blood pressure.—The blood pressure, systolic and diastolic, is measured with particular attention being paid to the width of the sphygmomanometer cuff which has to be appropriate to the circumference of the arm.

Jugular venous pressure.—The jugular venous pressure is assessed with the patient lying at 45° to the horizontal and the pulsations in the internal jugular vein are sought. The venous pulse is analysed for its height above the sternal angle and for its wave form (Fig. 1). The normal mean pressure is −5 to +3 cm of water above the sternal angle and the wave form reveals both "a" and "v" waves of approximately equal heights. A raised JVP will be apparent in right ventricular failure. The "a" and "v" waves may be replaced by fast flutter waves in atrial flutter. Large "v" waves will occur if there is tricuspid incompetence and these may be confused with "cannon waves" which will be regular if due to nodal rhythm or irregular if due to atrioventricular dissociation. A high venous pressure occurs with cardiac tamponade (note the systolic descent) and constrictive pericarditis (note the post-systolic descent). Non-pulsatile veins may simulate a raised central venous pressure and result from superior vena caval obstruction, perhaps due to bronchial or thyroid carcinomas.

Palpation.—The most reliable evidence of cardiac enlargement comes from the chest radiograph, but a good estimate of the heart size can be made by palpating the apex beat which should lie in the fifth intercostal space within the mid-clavicular line. Apex beats outside these boundaries indicate cardiac enlargement provided the heart is not displaced by pulmonary disease or thoracic deformity. The characteristic of the apical impulse is assessed to estimate left ventricular hypertrophy while the left sternal edge is palpated to assess right ventricular hypertrophy. Loud murmurs may be felt as palpable vibrations (thrills) which are maximal where the murmur is loudest. Loud heart sounds can also be felt—in mitral stenosis the loud first sound (the tapping impulse) and the second sound in the pulmonary area if the pulmonary arterial pressure is raised.

Auscultation.—In each area the appropriate heart sound is listened to individually and separately and additional heart sounds—ejection click, opening snap, third and fourth heart sounds—are sought. When the timing and characteristics of the heart sounds have been clearly established, murmurs are sought. A full description of any murmur includes its timing—systolic or diastolic (Fig. 2), the site of its maximal intensity and conduction, its loudness and quality, and the influence on it of respiration. Mitral murmurs are heard loudest in the region of the apex beat with the patient turned on the left side with the breath held in expiration. Tricuspid murmurs are localised to the fourth left interspace at the sternal edge and are accentuated by inspiration which increases flow across the valve. Aortic murmurs are heard loudest in the aortic area, at the apex and over the carotid arteries in the neck. The diastolic murmur of aortic regurgitation is heard at the left sternal edge during full expiration with the patient leaning forward. Sounds from the pulmonary valve are usually localised and heard best over the pulmonary area and are accentuated during inspiration with the increased blood flow into the lungs.

Lungs.—The lungs are examined for the presence of a pleural effusion, which is not uncommon in heart failure, and for the presence of crepitations or râles at the lung bases. Left ventricular failure does not always give rise to crepitations and the absence of these sounds does not exclude the diagnosis. Sounds will also frequently be suppressed by positive-pressure respiration. Increased bronchial secretions caused by a high left atrial pressure may cause widespread rhonchi. Widespread crepitations caused by fluid in the bronchi and alveoli are heard in pulmonary oedema.

Liver.—The liver is palpated to determine whether it is enlarged below the costal margin and whether it is tender as well as enlarged. The oedema fluid of cardiac failure settles under the influence of gravity and is most commonly found as pitting oedema of the ankles and feet in ambulant patients, or as a pad of oedema overlying the sacrum in patients who have been confined to bed.

Signs of Cardiac Failure

(a) *Left ventricular failure.*—The physical signs of early left ventricular failure are sinus tachycardia, a slightly raised jugular venous pressure and a third sound at the apex. The congestion of the pulmonary capillaries leads to dyspnoea and orthopnoea and, on auscultation, moist sounds can be heard at the bases of the lungs. More severe left ventricular failure may be associated with pulsus alternans and Cheyne-Stokes respiration.

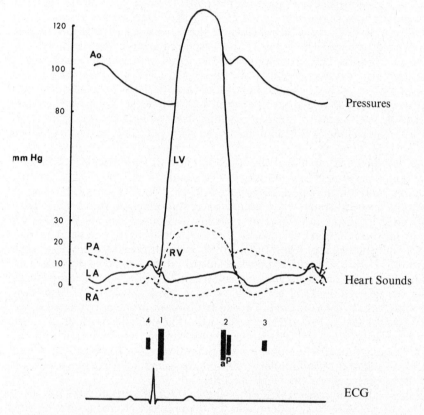

14/Fig. 2.—Typical normal pressure tracings for the various chambers of the heart superimposed on a common scale. From the relative pressures, the time of aortic and pulmonary valve movement and the opening and closing of the atrioventricular valves can be predicted. The diagram also enables the timing of murmurs in the heart to be understood.

(b) *Right ventricular failure.*—The signs of right ventricular failure may exist by themselves or be superimposed on those of left ventricular failure. The main sign of right-sided failure is a raised jugular venous pressure with a large "v" wave. A right ventricular third sound may be audible. The liver is enlarged, and may be tender. Oedema collects at the ankles and sacrum, and pleural effusions and ascites may be present.

Chest Radiography

Clinical examination of the patient continues with an interpretation of the straight X-ray of the heart in the standard posterior-anterior view. Penetrated

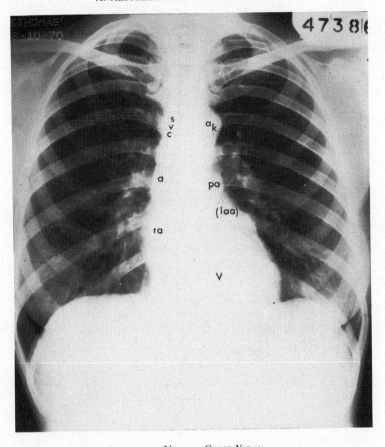

NORMAL CHEST X-RAY

V—Ventricular mass
r.a.—Right atrium
a—Ascending aorta
S.V.C.—Superior vena cava

a.k.—Aortic knuckle
p.a.—Pulmonary artery
(laa)—Position of left atrial
appendage

14/FIG. 3.

posterior-anterior and penetrated left lateral chest X-rays may also be valuable for the detection of valvular or pericardial calcification, or left atrial enlargement.

Having checked that the patient is not rotated and that the film is straight, the heart is scrutinised in an orderly fashion. First, the right border working from above downwards. The superior vena cava is seen as a vertical line at the upper border of the heart medial to the sterno-clavicular angle. Below this lies the ascending aorta which if dilated projects to the right and distorts the normal smooth line of the SVC. This suggests post-stenotic dilatation, due to aortic valve disease, or an aneurysm of the ascending aorta. Below the ascending aorta the right atrium forms the right border of the heart, terminating at the diaphragm. A prominent or bulging right wall of the heart may be due to right atrial enlargement, to enlargement of the left atrium or to a pericardial effusion.

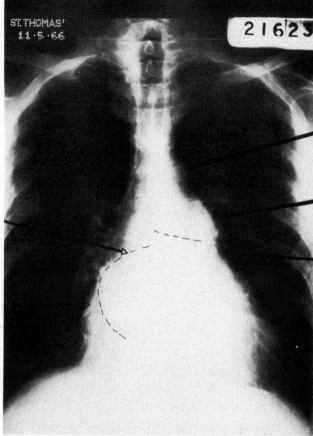

ST. THOMAS'
11·5·66

2 1 6 2 3

Aortic knuckle
normal

Large left atrium
seen through the
right atrium in the
penetrated view,
which is displacing
the left main
bronchus
horizontally

Large pulmonary
artery

Concavity produced
by amputation of
left atrial appendage
at previous
operation

Moderately enlarged
right atrium

MITRAL STENOSIS
14/FIG. 4.

Normal ventricular
mass

Second, the left border of the heart. At the top, this is composed of the arch of the aorta, seen as a rounded knuckle at the upper left margin of the cardiac silhouette. This may be prominent in aortic incompetence or lesions causing dilatation of the aorta, or it may be inconspicuous in low cardiac output states such as severe mitral stenosis. The pulmonary trunk lies immediately below the aortic knuckle and is dilated in pulmonary valve stenosis or in conditions leading to an increased flow or pressure in the pulmonary artery. Below the pulmonary artery is the atrial appendage and this is not normally visible on chest radiography unless enlarged. Enlargement of the left atrium usually accompanies enlargement of the appendage and this chamber can usually be seen as a circular shadow lying centrally behind the heart or to the right of the right atrium and of a slightly higher density. This is seen best on a penetrated posterior-anterior picture.

Differentiation of left and right ventricular hypertrophy is not easy on a chest

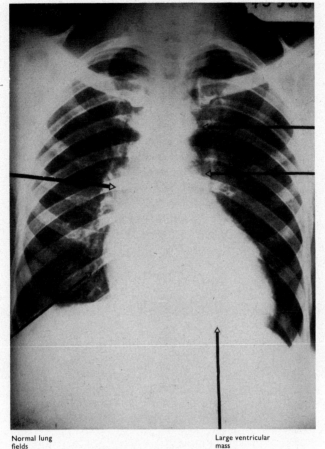

Post-stenotic
dilatation of the
ascending aorta

Small aortic knuckle

Normal pulmonary
artery

Normal right atrium

Normal lung
fields

Large ventricular
mass

AORTIC STENOSIS
(with slight incompetence)
14/FIG. 5.

X-ray, being better appreciated by palpation of the precordium and on the ECG.

Examination of the chest radiograph is completed by consideration of the lung fields. The larger branches of the pulmonary arteries and main pulmonary veins responsible for the normal lung markings dilate and the smaller vessels become visible when the blood flow through the lungs is increased. This is a characteristic of a left-to-right cardiac shunt.

If the pulmonary vascular resistance is raised (pulmonary hypertension) the proximal pulmonary arteries are large but the peripheral vessels become almost invisible leaving the lung fields abnormally clear and translucent. With decreased pulmonary blood flow (pulmonary atresia, pulmonary stenosis, Fallot's tetralogy) the vascular markings are small and sparse and the lung fields abnormally clear. In pulmonary venous congestion, secondary to a raised left atrial pressure, the veins are dilated and the upper lobe pulmonary veins more easily

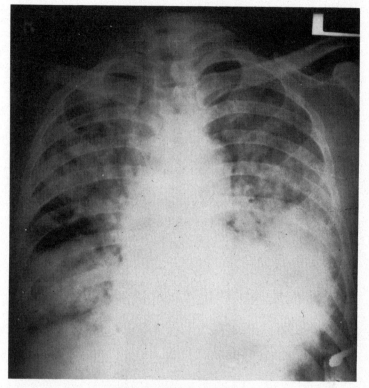

Severe bilateral pulmonary oedema, particularly marked in the lower lobes, following a myocardial infarction. Note that the heart is quite small. Physical signs at this time:

Patient dyspnoeic, sweating, confused, cyanosed, hypotensive.
Moist sounds all over chest.
Copious pink frothy sputum.
pH 7·31, Pa_{CO_2} 30 mm Hg (4·0 kPa), Pa_{O_2} 46 mm Hg (6·1 kPa)

14/Fig. 6.

seen. The increased interstitial fluid and engorgement of the lymphatics produces an overall ground-glass appearance, a peri-hilar flare and fine horizontal lines in the costophrenic angle (Kerley B lines). Pulmonary oedema represents extreme pulmonary venous congestion and patchy shadowing is seen around the hilum extending out into the surrounding lung.

In certain circumstances, the clinical examination is supplemented by special investigations such as electrocardiography or cardiac catheterisation and angiocardiography.

Electrocardiography

After the clinical examination and examination of the chest radiograph, the assessment is completed by consideration of the electrocardiograph. This is inspected principally for evidence of myocardial disease, ventricular hypertrophy, conduction defects or dysrhythmias, remembering that a normal ECG does not exclude cardiovascular disease. (The normal ECG is described on page 518 *et seq.*, the diagnosis and treatment of dysrhythmias on page 564 *et seq.*, the ECG appearances of acute myocardial infarction on page 552).

Right ventricular hypertrophy: during early childhood the right is the dominant ventricle. However, after this period, the following are the signs of pathological right ventricular hypertrophy (Fig. 7*a*):

Tall peaked P waves in lead II (right atrial hypertrophy).

Right axis deviation—that is, a mean frontal QRS greater than 100°.

Dominant R waves in leads V_{1-3}.

Left ventricular hypertrophy: this cannot be diagnosed on the ECG in the presence of left bundle-branch block. The signs suggestive of left ventricular hypertrophy are (Fig. 7*b*):

Bifid P waves in lead II (left atrial hypertrophy).

Large voltage R waves in leads I, aVL,V_{2-7}.

More severe disease results in the appearance of abnormal repolarisation and the development of a strain pattern evidenced by depression of the ST segments and T wave inversion (Fig. 7*c*). Ischaemia is suggested by flat ST depression greater than 1 mm in any lead (Fig. 8), while an old infarct may be recognisable by Q waves greater than 0·3 mm.

CARDIAC CATHETERISATION AND ANGIOCARDIOGRAPHY

A thorough history and clinical examination supplemented by examination of the ECG and chest radiograph will enable the precise diagnosis to be made in most cases of cardiovascular disease. In some instances, however, the diagnosis may remain in doubt and in other cases the diagnosis may be known but its quantitative effects not be clearly apparent. Cardiac catheterisation and angiocardiography are undertaken to confirm the diagnosis accurately and to provide the information on which future treatment can be based. There is a small but definite morbidity and mortality with cardiac catheterisation, higher when the left side of the heart is entered than the right and it is therefore a procedure which should not be undertaken unless there is likely to be obvious benefit to the patient.

In right heart catheterisation a catheter is passed through a vein, usually in the groin or elbow via the vena cava to the right atrium. It can then be passed through the tricuspid valve to the right ventricle and out through the pulmonary valve into the pulmonary arteries. If the catheter is pushed as far as possible into the lung fields the tip will wedge and it is then possible to make an indirect measurement of left atrial pressure. The coronary sinus can also be entered from the right atrium.

Left heart catheterisation can be performed in three ways. The left heart may be entered in the presence of a septal defect during right-sided cardiac catheterisation. If there is no communication it is possible to perforate the inter-atrial septum with a special needle during right-sided catheterisation and a catheter can then be threaded over the needle into the left atrium and thence to the left ventricle. Alternatively, aortic catheterisation can be performed by the retrograde passage of a catheter up the aorta and thence across the aortic valve and into the left ventricle.

The coronary arteries can be entered from the aorta. During cardiac

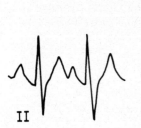
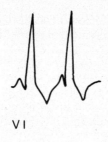

II   V I   (a) Right ventricular hypertrophy

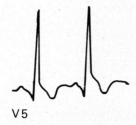

V 5   (b) Left ventricular hypertrophy

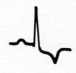

                                             (c) Strain

14/Fig. 7.

14/Fig. 8.—(a) Patient at rest; (b) Same patient after exercise. Note the development of flat ST depression denoting cardiac ischaemia.

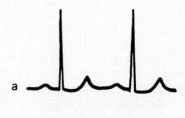

a

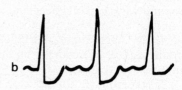

b

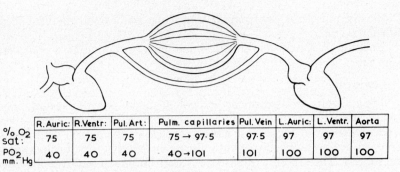

% O₂ sat:	R.Auric:	R.Ventr:	Pul.Art:	Pulm. capillaries	Pul.Vein	L.Auric:	L.Ventr.	Aorta
%O₂ sat:	75	75	75	75 → 97·5	97·5	97	97	97
PO₂ mm. Hg	40	40	40	40→101	101	100	100	100

14/FIG. 9(*a*).—Oxygen saturation and tension figures in a normal person breathing air. The fall in saturation and tension between pulmonary vein and left auricle is due to pulmonary shunting. (Adapted from Comroe *et al*., 1962).

catheterisation and angiocardiography the information derived is either anatomical or physiological. Anatomical information includes the outlining of abnormal communications or anatomy in the heart, the configuration of the chambers, the size and flexibility of the valves and the size and regularity of the coronary arteries.

Physiological information includes measurement of cardiac output, pressure measurements within chambers and measurement of oxygen content or tension (Fig. 9). From these numbers it is possible to calculate the size of the various valves. Oxygen values enable shunts to be detected and cardiac output confirmed.

Recently techniques have been developed which are designed to assess the function of the ventricle so that a distinction can be made between the effects of valvular incompetence or stenosis and the effects of the consequent myocardial deterioration.

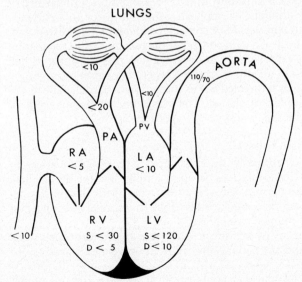

14/FIG. 9(*b*).—Normal mean intracardiac and major vessel pressures in mm Hg.

Finally, muscle biopsy from the ventricular wall can be obtained at cardiac catheterisation.

Anaesthesia for cardiac catheters and angiocardiography is considered on page 586.

Comment

The difficulty in assessment lies not in diagnosing the specific lesion or complication, nor perhaps in estimating its anatomic severity. The problems lie in deciding how far the disease has encroached on the patient's cardiovascular reserves and how much the patient's disease increases his risk during anaesthesia and surgery. The presence or absence of heart failure, pulmonary hypertension or angina and the patient's response to exercise may help resolve the first problem and enable some comparison to be made with the stresses of anaesthesia, surgery and the post-operative period.

At the extremes of cardiac disability, severe heart failure, fixed low cardiac output, or recent myocardial infarction, the risks are obvious, but there is evidence that any form of cardiovascular disease, even asymptomatic changes in the ECG, increase the risk over the normal population (Mauney *et al.*, 1970; Arkins *et al.*, 1964). The quantitation of this risk in the individual patient remains imprecise and Kitte *et al.* (1969), in a survey designed to determine the significant factors in risk, ended with the conclusion that the physician's estimate of risk provides the best predictive value for mortality.

The other benefit in careful pre-operative assessment is in ensuring that the patient presents for surgery in his optimum condition having received the correct therapy for his disease, suitably modified for surgery.

Pre-operative Treatment

Pre-operative treatment depends both on the nature of the cardiac disease and the nature of the operation to be performed. Treatment prior to cardiac or major vascular surgery is different in emphasis from that prior to some incidental operations. All treatment should be considered under two headings: first, the treatment which is necessary to gain control of the patient and to render him in the best possible condition for surgery, and second, how this treatment should be modified in the immediate operative and post-operative period.

In general, such treatment is directed to the correction of cardiac failure, the prevention or treatment of dysrhythmias, the symptomatic management of coronary artery disease, and the treatment of hypertension.

The Treatment of Cardiac Failure

Cardiac failure should normally be considered a contra-indication to anaesthesia and the operation postponed to allow ample time for the medical treatment of the patient. Sometimes the operation is so urgent that postponement is not possible but even then much can be done to improve the condition of the patient in the short interval available.

(*a*) **Bed rest** is the mainstay of treatment. As long as failure continues there should be strict bed rest and the patient only allowed up very cautiously once control has been gained.

(*b*) **Low salt diet.**—A normal diet contains 50 to 60 mEq (mmol) of salt per day. Patients being treated for cardiac failure are advised not to add salt to their food and to avoid salty dishes. This reduces the intake to around 40 mEq (mmol) per day. Only as a last resort, when digitalis and diuretics are unable to control the failure, is a low salt diet (less than 10 mEq (mmol) per day) prescribed.

(c) **Digoxin.**—*Action.*—The main action of digoxin is to increase the force of ventricular contraction both in failing and normal hearts. The cardiac output of the failing heart is improved and pulmonary congestion and oedema are diminished.

Conduction through the A–V node is slowed and vagal activity enhanced. Digoxin also shortens the refractory period of atrial muscle and has a variable effect on the Purkinje fibres.

Indications.—The established indications for digoxin are overt heart failure and atrial fibrillation or flutter.

In the treatment of cardiac failure the principle is to digitalise the patient fully, raising the dose until the desired effect is achieved or the patient develops signs of digoxin toxicity, at which point the drug is stopped until the symptoms cease and started again at a lower dose. Normally the initial digitalising dose is 0·03 mg/kg given as tabs. digoxin in divided doses over 24 hours. The intravenous route is more dangerous, and is reserved for use in emergencies when the drug should be given slowly because its initial vasopressor action precedes the inotropic effect and may aggravate the cardiac failure. In the control of atrial fibrillation, the dose is maintained at that level which controls the ventricular rate.

Pre-operative digitalisation (Deutsch and Dalen, 1969) may be considered in order to prevent intra- or post-operative cardiac failure or supraventricular dysrhythmias. Prophylactic digitalisation has been suggested in patients with a previous history of cardiac failure, and for patients who show signs of cardiac disease (enlarged heart on X-ray, cardiac hypertrophy in the ECG) to prevent heart failure secondary to the stress of anaesthesia and to facilitate the mandatory increase in cardiac output in the post-operative period. Patients liable to develop supraventricular dysrhythmias are those with a past history of such dysrhythmias, patients undergoing cardiac or pulmonary surgery (particularly if over 50 years old) and patients with mitral stenosis. The prophylactic administration of digoxin will also reduce the negative inotropic effect of anaesthetic agents.

The danger of digoxin is that the margin between the therapeutic and toxic dose is small and great care is needed in the elderly, those with renal impairment or myxoedema, or if the serum potassium is not normal.

In hospital patients receiving digoxin, toxicity is not uncommon and the mortality from that toxicity is considerable (*Lancet*, 1971). Furthermore, the diagnosis of digitalis toxicity is difficult as many of the symptoms could be due to some other cause or to the disease itself. Cardiac toxicity appears either as a worsening of the heart failure or the development of a dysrhythmia or a conduction defect. This difficulty is now somewhat resolved by the development of quick accurate methods of measuring blood digoxin levels. Digoxin toxicity during anaesthesia may be precipitated by changes in catecholamine level, potassium or calcium levels, alteration in pH consequent on changes in ventilation and by drugs such as suxamethonium, which alter potassium flux.

For these reasons we agree with Harrison and colleagues (1970) who advise that digoxin should only be used pre-operatively to treat established cardiac failure or dysrhythmias. In the quickly changing conditions of the operative period, sudden cardiac failure is more precisely treated with a short-acting inotropic agent such as isoprenaline or adrenaline, while life-threatening dysrhythmias usually respond to DC cardioversion (see p. 572).

Patients for major cardiac surgery who present already digitalised will usually have their digoxin stopped 2 days pre-operatively, their cardiac failure being controlled by bed rest, and the opportunity is also taken to stop diuretics and increase potassium supplements. It may, however, be more difficult to stop digoxin when this is given to control ventricular rate in atrial fibrillation.

Patients having minor or incidental surgery will often only omit the dose due on the morning of operation but note should be taken of the dose the patient has been receiving, the resting pulse rate and any symptoms which might suggest digoxin toxicity so that the treatment may be amended. As a general rule, when in doubt about the advisability of continuing digoxin, the best course is to withhold it.

(*d*) **Diuretics.**—The other mainstay in the treatment of cardiac failure is the use of diuretics. The best index of fluid retention is the weight of the patient, and daily weighing is the most accurate chart of progress in the treatment of cardiac failure. The jugular venous pressure and ankle or sacral oedema are less reliable because pure left ventricular failure can exist in the presence of an almost normal right atrial pressure, although sinus tachycardia and apical gallop (3rd sound) may point to the diagnosis. Diuretics are prescribed initially to reduce the weight and thereafter to maintain it constant, while keeping the haematocrit, serum sodium and blood urea at normal levels.

Thiazides.—These are potent non-mercurial diuretics which are well tolerated and which can be given by mouth. Their mode of action is to inhibit proximal tubular reabsorption of sodium and chloride, in contrast to mercurials which act primarily by inhibiting chloride reabsorption. There are now a number of these drugs whose effectiveness is comparable and which differ only in dose and price. *Bendrofluazide* is cheap and effective. The dose is initially 5–10 mg with a maintenance of 2·5–5·0 mg daily. Diuresis starts two hours after ingestion and lasts for twelve hours.

Frusemide is a monosulphanyl diuretic which acts similarly to the thiazides but is much more potent. It is both quicker-acting and of shorter duration and possesses the advantage that it can be given intravenously. The initial oral dose is 40 mg but up to 160 mg can be given daily. The intravenous dose is 20 mg.

Bumetamide is an alternative diuretic for patients who are unresponsive to frusemide. Given orally the dose is up to 10 mg daily.

Ethacrynic acid is a desulphanyl compound which is even more potent and can be given intravenously in a dose of 50 mg.

Both frusemide and ethacrynic acid have been advocated for use in the treatment of acute pulmonary oedema. Given intravenously, both produce a response within 10 minutes which may be very effective. Their potency gives rise to two dangers—the diuresis is accompanied by potassium loss and the very size of the diuresis after intravenous ethacrynic acid may produce hypovolaemic hypotension. Hypovolaemia is a danger with all diuretic therapy and care must be taken that, in encouraging the excretion of excess fluid, the filling pressure of the heart is not reduced below that level necessary to produce a good cardiac output.

(e) **Potassium and diuretics.**—All the above diuretics, besides causing inhibition of salt and water retention, lead to excessive loss of body potassium. This may be a chronic state following long-continued diuretic therapy, an acute response to a sudden diuresis, or, most dangerously, an acute loss superimposed on a chronic deficiency. Many patients who have been on continued diuretic therapy will have a total body potassium content which may be reduced by 30–50 per cent despite replacement therapy and a normal serum potassium level. A low serum potassium or an otherwise unexplained metabolic alkalosis suggests a very severe deficiency. Potassium depletion potentiates dysrhythmias due to digoxin and may lead to ventricular tachycardia or fibrillation.

Patients who are receiving diuretic therapy should receive potassium supplements in some form which contains chloride, such as "Slow K" (8 mmol/tablet) or "Kloref" (6·7 mmol/tablet). The dose depends slightly on diet, but because not all is absorbed and the minimum loss in urine is about 30 mmol/day, patients may require 50–100 mmol daily. If the potassium level falls below 3·5 mmol/l as a result of an acute diuresis and the patient develops ventricular dysrhythmias, intravenous potassium is given in 5 mmol increments until the dysrhythmia disappears, when a slow infusion of potassium 50–100 mmol/day can be used to restore the potassium balance. Because of the loss of potassium which accompanies the use of the diuretics already described, three other diuretics—spironolactone, triamterene and amiloride—which promote potassium reabsorption are sometimes prescribed in conjunction with the thiazides.

Spironolactone is an aldosterone antagonist. Aldosterone, secreted by the adrenal cortex, promotes the retention of sodium and excretion of potassium. Spironolactone reverses this effect and when used in conjunction with the thiazides, frusemide or ethacrynic acid, increases the diuresis as well as reducing the potassium loss. The minimum effective dose is 100–150 mg daily, but due to its blocking action further increments do not enhance its effect.

Triamterene which is an aminopteridine, increases excretion of sodium and chloride but it also acts on the distal tubule to decrease potassium loss, but not by antagonism of aldersterone (dose 50 mg b.d.).

Amiloride acts on the distal tubule producing potassium retention. A more powerful diuretic than spironolactone it is sometimes given in combination with frusemide, dose 5–10 mg daily.

Effusions.—In the medical treatment of cardiac failure, pleural effusions or ascites are rarely tapped. However, large pleural effusions may embarrass cardiac and pulmonary function, particularly if the patient is to be placed in the lateral position on the operating table. These are best removed the day before operation so that the patient has 24 hours to readjust, as on rare occasions acute pulmonary oedema may develop when the fluid is removed too quickly.

BETA-ADRENERGIC BLOCKADE

There are now considerable numbers of β-adrenergic blocking drugs available some of which are cardioselective, blocking predominantly the β-1 receptors in the heart and which may or may not show intrinsic sympathomimetic activity.

The most frequent cardiac indications for the use of these drugs are the treatment of hypertension and of angina pectoris. They are also used in left and right ventricular outflow tract obstruction (Fallot's tetralogy, hypertrophic obstructive cardiomyopathy), phaeochromocytoma and in the control of dysrhythmias.

The effect of β-blockade in the normal healthy patient is small: there is only a mild drop in blood pressure and cardiac rate. However, the magnitude of the effect depends as much on the degree of sympathetic tone prevalent at the time of the administration as it does on the dose administered (Shand, 1975). This has a particular relevance both to anaesthesia and to heart failure. During anaesthesia the response to beta-adrenergic blockade is much more unpredictable, reflecting the variations in sympathetic activity which are accentuated by alterations in carbon dioxide level (Foex and Prys-Roberts, 1974) and by the effects of the anaesthetic agents (particularly ether and cyclopropane) and techniques (Merin, 1972).

In cardiac failure, the cardiac output is maintained by reflex sympathetic stimulation which increases both rate and force of myocardial contraction as well as raising venous tone in the capacitance vessels. Because such patients require this sympathetic stimulation to maintain their precarious haemostatic balance, even a small degree of β-blockade may be sufficient to precipitate dramatic heart failure and life-threatening hypotension.

During cardiac surgery, the prior existence of β-blockade may be hazardous. Vilgöen and his colleagues (1972) who were using methoxyflurane as their anaesthetic agent recommended that propranolol be withheld two weeks prior to coronary artery surgery. The half-life of oral propranolol after a single dose is 3–6 hours, although the duration of action does depend on the size of dose administered, and Coltart and colleagues (1975) suggest that stopping the drug for 24–48 hours is probably sufficient.

With certain specific exceptions, the discontinuation of β-blockade before cardiac surgery or cardioversion would appear advisable. Before minor and non-cardiac surgery the argument may be less strong, and as with digoxin or anti-hypertensive agents the indications for continued therapy may be dominant. The exacerbation of angina to the point of myocardial infarction has been reported in patients whose propranolol has been suddenly stopped (Alderman et al., 1974). The choice of anaesthetic agents for a patient who is receiving β-blocking drugs now appears more complicated than was originally thought. Obviously, ether and cyclopropane which owe their benign effect on the heart to concomitant sympathetic stimulation, in the presence of β-blockade will produce myocardial depression. However, the benign effect of β-blockade in nitrous oxide halothane anaesthesia, both under routine anaesthesia and during response to the stress of haemorrhage is not duplicated under trichloroethylene anaesthesia (Roberts et al., 1976), nor particularly during methoxyflurane anaesthesia (Saner et al., 1975), when there is a large rise in systemic vascular resistance and drop in cardiac output. Similar effects occur with enflurane (Horan et al., 1976). β-receptor blockade induced with propranolol does not appear to cause any serious interaction with isoflurane (Horan et al., 1977).

A further point about β-blockade is that both hypoxia and hypercarbia are directly depressant on the heart, although initially this depressant effect is countered by sympathetic stimulation. Hence hypercarbia and hypoxia are even more undesirable when the patient is under β-blockade, and this may represent a particular risk in the post-operative period.

The dangers of β-blockade may have been exaggerated because the effect may be countered by drugs producing inotropic and chronotropic stimulation via alternative pathways. Atropine will speed the heart, while calcium, glucagon, aminophylline and digoxin will all still improve cardiac contractility. β-adrenergic blockade is produced by competitive inhibition at the receptor site and it is of course possible to produce an effect by a higher dose than usual of the agonist.

HYPERTENSION

The hypertensive patient represents an increased risk for anaesthesia and surgery (Hickler and Vandam, 1970). This is the result of two factors, the much greater lability of the blood pressure which is due to the systemic vascular resistance changing markedly for small alterations in vessel tone and the fact that patients with hypertension show earlier and more widespread arteriosclerosis than do comparable normotensive patients (Deming, 1968). The two particular dangers to which the hypertensive subject is liable under anaesthesia are hypotension and an exacerbation of hypertension. Hypotension produces serious reduction in flow in the arteriosclerotic renal, cerebral and myocardial vessels with the danger of renal failure, cerebrovascular accidents and myocardial infarction. Hypertension may precipitate cardiac failure, cause myocardial ischaemia, or lead to a cerebrovascular accident.

Assessment and Treatment

Patients with hypertension need careful assessment before anaesthesia and surgery. This should include a full medical history and examination together with chest X-ray and an ECG. An attempt must also be made to assess the extent of arteriosclerosis in the important vessels; myocardial ischaemia may be apparent from the history or the ECG; laboratory tests may demonstrate renal impairment; the fundal vessels should be inspected by ophthalmoscopy for direct evidence of arteriosclerosis. Any cardiac failure should be treated prior to surgery.

Prys-Roberts and his colleagues (1971) in their study showed a high incidence of myocardial ischaemia in patients with high initial arterial pressure exposed to anaesthesia, and suggested that even symptom-free hypertensive patients should receive therapy to lower their pressure before anaesthesia and surgery. Mauney and his colleagues (1970) and Breslin and Swinton (1970) also concluded that pre-operative stabilisation of high arterial pressures should be achieved before elective surgery.

The usual aim of medical treatment is to produce a standing diastolic pressure of 100 mm Hg (13·3 kPa) or lower although this aim is not always possible.

According to the severity of the hypertension, different drug combinations are employed.

Diuretics.—The thiazide diuretics promote salt and water excretion and, by reducing plasma volume, may be sufficient therapy for some mild hypertensives. It is possible that they have some direct vasodilator action because the blood pressure remains low when the plasma volume returns to normal. In mild hypertension, diuretics alone may be used but in more severe cases they may also be employed to potentiate the anti-adrenergic drugs.

Considerable reductions in whole body potassium occur without production of definite symptoms or signs (Edmonds and Jasani, 1972) although hypochloraemic alkalosis and ECG changes may be seen (Breslin and Swinton, 1970). More commonly, trouble arises if the patient develops cardiac failure or requires digitalisation for some other reason when digoxin toxicity is easily provoked.

Beta-adrenergic blockade.—Both propranolol and oxprenolol are widely used in the treatment of hypertension, frequently in combination with a diuretic. Beta-adrenergic blockade sometimes reveals a high degree of spontaneous α-adrenergic vasoconstrictor activity which may be treated with a vasodilator such as hydrallazine. By their negative chronotropic and inotropic effects, and by the lowering of plasma renin activity, the β-blockers lower blood pressure both in the standing and lying positions.

Methyldopa.—More severe hypertension is treated with methyldopa which inhibits vasoconstrictor impulses both by a central action and by interrupting the normal synthesis of noradrenaline and depleting the adrenergic neurones of noradrenaline. After oral administration an effect is achieved in three to five hours and lasts up to twenty-four hours. Renal blood flow and glomerular filtration are well maintained but fluid retention, tiredness and depression are complications and drug tolerance often develops. A diuretic is usually added to combat fluid retention.

Anti-adrenergic drugs.—Bethanidine, guanethidine and debrisoquine all block post-ganglionic adrenergic neurones and deplete catecholamine stores. They have different rates of onset and duration of action but all produce a postural hypotension which may be troublesome in the morning and on exercise. Hot weather and factors which deplete blood volume will potentiate their effects. Side-effects are bradycardia, dry mouth, impotence, diarrhoea and fluid retention.

Other drugs.—*Rauwolfia* is rarely used now due to its undesirable side-effects, particularly psychiatric depression.

Clonidine is a centrally-acting hypotensive drug which may have two disadvantages. Firstly, sudden withdrawal of clonidine may lead to an exacerbation of the hypertension. Secondly, when given with digitalis it provokes digitalis toxicity.

Diazoxide is a thiazide derivative which causes hypotension and hyperglycaemia. It is only used intravenously in the acute treatment of uncontrolled hypertension where it has tended to replace pentolinium and trimetaphan. Intravenous anti-adrenergic drugs should not be used for this purpose as they produce an initial transitory rise in blood pressure.

Antihypertensive drugs and anaesthesia.—Once antihypertensive drugs have been started, even temporary discontinuation may be dangerous. Discontinuation may precipitate renal failure, cardiac failure or a cerebrovascular accident and the patient with a high blood pressure is much more liable to large alterations in blood pressure with the particular danger of producing myocardial ischaemia or infarction. Ominsky and Wollman (1969) consider that most intra-operative hypotension is related to the patient's disease or the anaesthetic and not to the antihypertensive therapy which most authorities (Dingle, 1966; Hickler and Vandam, 1970; Prys-Roberts et al., 1972) consider should be continued throughout the operative period.

Fortunately, with the wide variety of anaesthetic techniques available, continued therapy is quite compatible with anaesthesia. At the same time, care must be taken to avoid those drugs which will potentiate the hypotensive action, particularly by direct depression of the myocardium, and the circulation must be properly monitored and supported. An ECG is an obvious requirement. Blood loss is measured and replaced to maintain an adequate ventricular filling pressure.

Should a vasopressor be required, it must be one which is effective in the face of the antihypertensive therapy (Smith and Corbascio, 1970), and the dose must be restricted to that necessary to restore the blood pressure to its previous level since, in excess, it may impose an overwhelming afterload on a potentially depressed myocardium (Prys-Roberts et al., 1972) particularly if the anaesthetic includes such direct myocardial depressants as halothane. In this case a pressor drug may precipitate cardiac failure.

Extreme variations in pressure are a particular hazard to the arteriosclerotic hypertensive due to the dangers of ischaemia or thrombosis, and Prys-Roberts and his colleagues (1972) have shown that whereas the well-controlled hypertensive patient tends to behave like his normotensive counterpart, the untreated or badly treated hypertensive patient is at considerable risk during anaesthesia. This risk occurs not only during steady state anaesthesia but is accentuated during induction, when severe hypotension may be precipitated by intravenous agents including tubocurarine, and during laryngoscopy and intubation which usually cause hypertension. A hypertensive episode may also follow the use of pancuronium which must be used with caution in these patients. The immediate awakening period may also provoke a hypertensive reaction. Although an increase in blood pressure might be expected to improve coronary flow, the resulting increase in intracavity pressure in the ventricle raises myocardial oxygen consumption and diminishes circulation in the subendocardial collaterals which may cause subendocardial ischaemia or necrosis. S–T segment deviation may often be seen on the ECG under these circumstances.

The Treatment of Coronary Artery Disease

Drug therapy aimed at producing coronary vasodilatation is unsatisfactory. Hypoxia itself is the most potent vasodilator but the diseased vessels are incapable of response. Symptomatic relief of angina can be produced by reducing the work of the heart either by lowering the peripheral resistance with glyceryl trinitrate or by diminishing the ventricular contractility with β-adrenergic blockade.

Glyceryl trinitrate tablets are normally sucked and absorption occurs through the oral mucosa. Because of the time taken for absorption their main value is in prophylactic use before exercise. Direct vasodilatation of the diseased coronary artery is unlikely and the effect is probably due to reduction in cardiac output and blood pressure which reduces myocardial work.

β-blockade reduces the heart rate and the velocity of contraction of the myocardial fibres. This reduces cardiac work and myocardial oxygen requirements so that the limited coronary blood flow is used to the best advantage. It also prevents the rise in work associated with exercise or emotion. There is, however, a risk of producing cardiac failure in patients with serious disease of the left ventricle.

Current surgical treatment of coronary artery disease consists mainly of inserting a length of saphenous vein between the aorta and the coronary artery below the block. This is sometimes coupled with coronary endarterectomy or resection of ventricular aneurysm (for anaesthetic management, see p. 582).

MYOCARDIAL INFARCTION AND ANAESTHESIA

Several studies have been published which relate the incidence of post-operative complications to the pre-operative cardiac state and in particular to pre-operative myocardial infarction (Topkins and Artusio, 1964; Mauney *et al.*, 1970; Tarhan *et al.*, 1972; Knapp *et al.*, 1962). Comparison between these papers is not easy as they are usually unmatched in respect of factors such as age and sex, which are known to affect the incidence of myocardial infarction. There is also a wide variety in the type and duration of anaesthesia, the type of operation performed and national differences in disease patterns and medical attitudes.

Those patients who do not die immediately from an infarct present with either severe chest pain which lasts more than half-an-hour in the absence of exertion or emotion, with sudden left ventricular failure, with severe dysrhythmias or in cardiogenic shock. The diagnosis of myocardial infarction is made primarily on the history supported by serial electrocardiograms and enzyme studies, although the changes in the ECG may take several hours to develop. (McGuiness *et al.*, 1976).

It is generally believed that patients who have had a previous infarct are more likely to have a second one at the time of surgery. The time incidence of a second infarct may well be higher than the figures suggest as infarction in the post-operative period is difficult to diagnose. It is frequently silent and may present only as sudden heart failure or hypotension.

The electrocardiographic changes of myocardial infarction are variable in their time of appearance. The earliest change is elevation of the T wave over the site of the infarct. This is followed by ST segment elevation, T wave inversion and, if the infarct is transmural, the development of a Q wave (Fig. 10). If the infarct is not full thickness the Q wave does not appear but the amplitude of the R wave is diminished.

The site of the infarct is revealed by the leads in which the changes are best seen:

Left Coronary Artery Disease   — anteroseptal: V_{1-3} anterior: V_{1-5}
                                                    anterolateral: V_{5-7} High lateral: I, aVL

Right Coronary Artery Disease — inferior: II III aVF
                                                 — posterior: V_{1-2} (tall R waves).

It is probably untrue that patients having myocardial infarcts in the operative period are more likely to die than "medical" infarcts, as the figures are artificially loaded against the surgical cases because a large proportion of patients who die from "medical" infarction do so before they reach hospital. However, the mortality from post-surgical infarcts will only be lowered to the same level as those reported from coronary care units if the patients are monitored and nursed under the same conditions. A general surgical ward is not the correct place to care for a peri-operative infarct.

14/Fig. 10.—Developed transmural myocardial infarct. Note Q wave, ST segment elevation and T wave inversion.

How soon after a myocardial infarct is it safe for a patient to undergo anaesthesia and surgery? In the absence of diagnostic criteria for the infarct no precise answer is available. Tarhan and his colleagues (1972) found that the re-infarction rate stabilises after six months, while Knapp and colleagues (1962) found an increased risk for up to two years. All authorities are agreed that only very urgent operations should be undertaken on patients who have had a myocardial infarction in the previous three months (*Lancet*, 1972).

Much depends not only on the type and extent of the prior infarction but also on the patient's condition since that time and Papper (1965) comments that if a patient has a healed myocardial infarction of more than three months' duration, if his ECG is stable and resembles his pre-infarct pattern and there is no angina or signs of cardiac failure, he is an essentially normal risk for anaesthesia and surgery.

FIXED LOW CARDIAC OUTPUT

A common end-point to cardiac failure, myocardial ischaemia, valvular lesions, constrictive pericarditis and pulmonary vascular disease is that the patient enters a condition of fixed low cardiac output. Prior to this the patient will have had depressed ventricular function curves but will have managed to maintain a fairly normal cardiac output although at higher than normal ventricular filling pressures and with a restricted capacity for increase. Ultimately the cardiac output declines below that necessary to supply the metabolic demands of the body despite strong sympathetic stimulation and intense vasoconstriction. In this state he is particularly vulnerable to certain effects of anaesthesia:

(1) *Bradycardia or dysrhythmias*—the stroke output is small and the cardiac rate must be maintained.

(2) *Myocardial depression*—myocardial contractility must not be further reduced by depressant anaesthetics.

(3) *Vasodilatation*—particularly that affecting the capacitance vessels causing a drop in ventricular filling pressure.

(4) *Hypotension*—which may further reduce myocardial oxygen supply.

At the same time, skilful anaesthesia which avoids these hazards may improve the patient by reducing ventricular afterload and by reducing total body oxygen consumption by abolishing the work of breathing.

Raised pulmonary vascular resistance (Pulmonary hypertension).—The pulmonary artery pressure may be raised, with no change in the pulmonary vessels, as a result of a raised left atrial pressure. A raised pulmonary vascular resistance is due to medial hypertrophy and intimal thickening in the walls of the pulmonary arterioles. This change, which may be irreversible, occurs in 30 per cent of those conditions which are characterised by a chronically raised left atrial pressure or a large left-to-right shunt. A similar effect may be produced by recurrent pulmonary emboli. Pulmonary hypertension is aggravated by anoxia or respiratory acidosis. These patients are existing at the limits of their right ventricular function and need a high right ventricular end-diastolic pressure to maintain their output. They are, therefore, if anything, even more sensitive to vasodilatation than patients whose fixed cardiac output is due to left ventricular limitation.

CHANGES IN VENTILATORY FUNCTION ASSOCIATED WITH HEART DISEASE

Patients with cardiac disease frequently suffer from associated respiratory problems. The cardiac disease itself may be secondary to chronic lung disease. The lungs may have interstitial oedema from acute rise in left atrial pressure or long-standing congestion may have led to thickening and fibrosis in the lung. The effect is that the work of breathing is increased but at the same time, owing to abnormal ventilation-perfusion relationships within the lung, arterial oxygenation may be incomplete. Reductions in cardiac output will increase the arterial hypoxaemia (Kelman *et al.*, 1967).

Norlander and colleagues (1969) have shown that their patients undergoing cardiac surgery had an increased V_D/V_T ratio, a low cardiac output and a substantial amount of venous admixture. This, combined with the increased oxygen consumption in the post-operative period, indicates a need for a high inspired oxygen consumption, and the frequent continuation of ventilation in the post-operative period.

Positive-pressure ventilation is usually beneficial to these patients. The work of breathing ceases and the inspired oxygen tension can be raised (up to 50 per cent O_2) to compensate for the ventilation-perfusion abnormalities. The cardiac output may become depressed if the carbon dioxide level is lowered excessively (Prys-Roberts *et al.*, 1967) or if, because of a non-compliant chest, excessive inflation pressures are necessary. The restricted pulmonary blood flow in pulmonary stenosis and pulmonary hypertension is very vulnerable to right ventricular depression secondary to drug action and to the mechanical effects of increased airway pressure. Rarely, in patients with tabes, diabetes or drug overdosage, the circulatory reflexes may be blocked and positive-pressure ventilation will reduce the cardiac output. Rises in carbon dioxide tension increase the work of the heart and add to the incidence of dysrhythmias. The principal danger of these effects is that although they may be only transitory in themselves, the reduction in cardiac output which they cause leads to arterial hypoxaemia and decrease in ventricular performance. The patient then enters a vicious circle of increasing hypoxia and metabolic acidosis which is now independent of its original cause.

If there is confusion as to whether the patient's dyspnoea is of pulmonary or cardiac origin it may be necessary to perform pre-operative lung function tests both to define the respiratory limitation and to show to what extent it can be reversed by bronchodilator drugs or alterations in inspired oxygen tension.

ANAESTHESIA FOR PATIENTS WITH CARDIAC DISEASE

To a certain extent the management of patients with cardiac disease undergoing anaesthesia and surgery depends on the particular operation being performed. Open cardiac surgery with extracorporeal circulation is the extreme example and this consideration is discussed later in this chapter.

To a much greater extent the choice of anaesthesia, of monitoring, of circulatory management depends on the cardiac state of the patient. The pre-operative assessment defines the nature and severity of the haemodynamic alteration in the patient's cardiovascular system. The consequences of anaesthesia and surgery on the normal circulation are known. The difficulty lies in predicting how the intact but abnormal circulation, which is limited in its physiological reserves, will respond to the stresses imposed upon it.

There is some evidence concerning the effects of anaesthetic agents on the abnormal heart. Measurements of the effect of halothane on the contractility of isolated heart muscle with experimentally produced ventricular hypertrophy and failure showed that the additive effects of the anaesthetic combined with the cardiac muscle pathology produced very severe depression of myocardial contractility (Shimosato et al., 1973). The state of the heart may of course vary during the operation; at rest or during uncomplicated anaesthesia no depression of myocardial contractility may be evident. However, increases in preload or afterload, during the operative period, may reveal the true functional state of the heart (Shimosata and Etsten, 1969).

Some conclusions can be drawn from knowledge of the patient's lesion. Specific lesions are considered in detail later in this chapter but a few examples may be cited in brief here. In mitral stenosis a long diastolic period is needed for adequate ventricular filling and anaesthetic-induced tachycardia will depress cardiac output, while at the same time, due to the relatively small left ventricle in mitral stenosis, bradycardia will also reduce cardiac output.

In aortic stenosis the thick-walled left ventricular cavity needs the extra distension of atrial contraction to produce a good cardiac output. Rhythm disturbances and slow rates will severely depress the cardiac output while the cardiac output will be enhanced by increased filling pressure, tachycardia and by inotropic stimulation. In the apparently similar subaortic stenosis of hypertrophic obstructive cardiomyopathy, inotropic stimulation will however aggravate the obstruction and in this condition which is commonly treated with β-adrenergic blockade, a reasonable case can be made for the use of a myocardial depressant anaesthetic to prevent endogenous catecholamine secretion exacerbating the ventricular obstruction. In subaortic stenosis a well-maintained filling pressure is important to reduce the obstruction and the effect of a maintained blood pressure and afterload is to prevent the ventricle contracting down at the end of systole and aggravating the obstruction. A similar effect may be seen in severe right ventricular infundibular stenosis. When this is associated with a ventricular septal defect in Fallot's tetralogy, the magnitude of the right-to-left shunt will depend on the relative resistances to the outflow down the pulmonary artery and aorta. A reduction in systemic vascular resistance will alter the magnitude of the shunt and in a delicately balanced situation may even reverse it.

Thus the haemodynamic effects of the patient's lesion may suggest that some particular state, perhaps tachycardia or low filling pressure or catecholamine secretion, is undesirable and the anaesthetic technique chosen to avoid this factor, whether it be produced by the anaesthetic agent itself, by ventilatory or reflex effects or by any other way. And similarly the correct supportive measures, the ideal cardiac rate, the state of the preload and afterload are defined by an understanding of the patient's cardiovascular state.

The other factor of importance in dealing with the abnormal circulation and particularly with the failing heart, is the extent to which the maintenance of such a circulation depends on elevated sympathetic drive. Any interference by anaesthesia with this increased activity, either by depressing it or by depressing the ability of the end-organ to react to it, will have much more profound effects than in the normal circulation.

This small amount of information when set against the infinite variety of patient response dictates the two principles of successful cardiac anaesthesia:

(a) Meticulous continuous accurate monitoring of the patient's circulation (Siegel, 1969).
(b) A choice of anaesthetic agents and techniques which produces the least alteration in cardiovascular performance (Shimosata and Etsten, 1969).

MONITORING DURING ANAESTHESIA FOR CARDIAC PATIENTS

The minimum acceptable monitoring for any patient with cardiac disease is frequent recording of the pulse and blood pressure and a continuous electro-cardiographic display. Perhaps, considering the ease with which it can be measured, the central venous pressure could be added to this list.

For cardiac surgery or major general surgery in cardiac patients, full monitoring would include:

ECG: pulse rate: arterial blood pressure: central venous pressure and perhaps left atrial pressure: arterial oxygen and carbon dioxide tension: acid-base state: urine output: temperature: serum potassium: blood loss and replacement.

In monitoring one only measures "what one measures" (Kirklin). This truism implies that even with accurate measuring apparatus the greatest care must be taken in the interpretation of values obtained. For example, the numerical value of the central venous pressure is just that, of itself, it conveys no information whatsoever about the left atrial pressure, the function of the left ventricle, the need for blood replacement or the size of the circulating volume. Some of this information may be deduced by comparison with earlier values for CVP and considered in relation to the other information about the patient, but of itself, a numerical value is only evidence about that value. Further when taken by itself with no other knowledge of the patient's condition, the value may suggest therapy which is wrong or even dangerous.

The second point of importance about monitoring is that the evidence must fit together logically and no piece of information must be discarded on the grounds that it must be wrong unless the most careful scrutiny shows this to be so. Otherwise the first sign of some disorder will frequently be overlooked.

Most measurements have to be interpreted both against the patient's general condition and all the factors known to affect that measurement. Thus the arterial oxygen and carbon dioxide tensions are relevant only when considered against the cardiac output, the patient's metabolic state, the composition of the inspired gas, the mechanical factors of ventilation (tidal volume, airway pressure, expiratory pressure, ventilatory pattern) and the anatomical state of the patient's heart and lungs.

The difficulty in monitoring and assessing the cardiovascular system is that there is no one measurement of cardiovascular well-being. Because of the ease with which it is measured, the blood pressure has always been accorded a degree of importance (Cullen, 1974). Certainly, extremes of blood pressure are potentially lethal in hypertension, coronary artery and other vascular disease or aortic valve disease but, equally, the blood pressure can be substantially normal a few seconds before terminal cardiovascular collapse. It is often assumed that the cardiac output is a more important value and inferences are made about the output from the appearance of the patient's skin and temperature, the urine output, the arterial pressure and the blood gas values. Again, the cardiac output can be normal at a time when the blood pressure or the ECG suggest a far from normal state. Only very limited inferences can be made about ventricular function from the blood pressure and the left atrial pressure and these are invalidated by the presence of valvular disease and probably nothing can be said about the left ventricle from knowledge of arterial and central venous pressure. Absolute circulatory assessment is therefore difficult but if all the measurements and observations are taken together in the context of the patient's lesion, it is fairly easy to monitor change. Fortunately, this is more important than the absolute state and most circulatory support during anaesthesia and surgery is directed toward maintaining the *status quo*.

Technical Considerations

All monitoring techniques must be carefully examined to ensure that they do not add to the risks to the patient, particularly in relation to electrical hazards and to sepsis. Because much monitoring relies on electricity (ECG, EEG, pressure monitoring, temperature) it brings the dangers of electric shock producing ventricular fibrillation and a potential for burns, particularly in conjunction with faulty diathermy apparatus. With the increasing tendency to leave monitoring catheters in for several days, sterility at the time of insertion and whenever fluids are added, particularly through 3-way taps, must be maintained. A potential hazard exists if foreign material, air, sterilising fluids or caustic substances (KCl, $CaCl_2$) are injected, particularly with arterial cannulae.

ECG.—Ideally the ECG amplifier should have an electrically isolated power supply. Although this will render unnecessary subsequent precautions it is good practice to use them due to the frequency of mixed electrical apparatus in use. The precautions include large ECG plates rather than needle electrodes, a common earth (right leg lead) attached to the diathermy plate, and the use of high-resistance leads.

Lead II is the most useful for long-term observation of cardiac rhythm.

Central venous pressure.—Accurate values for central venous pressure can only be obtained if the tip of the catheter is within the thorax. It must be possible to aspirate blood, the level must fall freely and, once settled, must fluctuate with respiration before the readings are taken as valid. Access to an intrathoracic site can be via an antecubital, jugular, subclavian or femoral vein. Using the antecubital vein, 36 per cent of catheter tips were found not to be intrathoracic (Johnston and Clark, 1972) and one can only be certain of its site after a confirmatory X-ray (Lumley and Russell, 1975).

The femoral vein below the inguinal ligament is easily punctured and on the right side the catheter usually runs up freely. If the catheter catches in the bifurcation or a renal vein, it kinks and goes up with a loop which can be detected by difficulty in aspirating blood. Partial withdrawal usually straightens the loop and the catheter can be readvanced. Perhaps sterility is more difficult in the inguinal region and there is an increased risk of venous thrombosis in the leg.

In the head and neck, percutaneous puncture is described of the subclavian, external and internal jugular veins. The external jugular is easily seen but once punctured the catheter often fails to pass into the thorax and the most satisfactory vessel to use is the right internal jugular (English *et al.*, 1969) (Fig. 11).

The interpretation and significance of CVP is discussed in the previous chapter.

Arterial Pressure

If the arterial pressure is measured with a cuff and stethoscope or palpation, the size of cuff must be appropriate for the arm; the thicker the arm, the wider the cuff, or spurious readings will be obtained. The oscillotonometer, although very accurate in conditions associated with peripheral vasodilatation (induced hypotension) is more difficult to read if the circulation is inadequate and, for most ill patients requiring major surgery, the preference is for intra-arterial cannulation and continuous display on an oscilloscope after amplification in an electrically isolated amplifier.

Although the ulnar, dorsales pedes, femoral, brachial or other arteries are sometimes recommended, the commonly chosen artery is the left radial. Allen's test is normally undertaken to demonstrate the presence of collateral circulation to the hand. With practice, arterial cannulation is no more difficult than venepuncture and there is no need to puncture the back wall of the artery as this could result in an unnecessary haematoma. Teflon catheters are reputed to be less irritant. If tapered catheters are used, they should not be advanced so that the lumen is totally obstructed. There is now a considerable quantity of literature on the complications of radial artery cannulation (Oh and Davis, 1975) and while the advantages of continuous display and availability of arterial blood samples may be necessary in the severely ill, complications must be kept minimal by meticulous technique.

Drips and Drug Administration

Blood loss during cardiac surgery is often less than in many other forms of major surgery, however when it occurs it can be quick and massive. For this

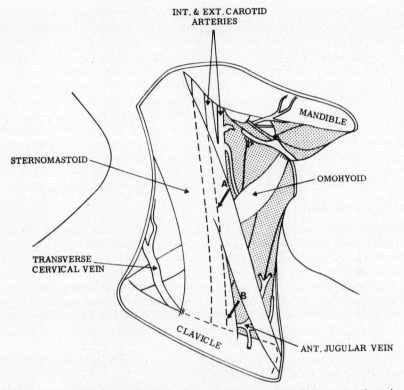

14/Fig. 11.—Relations of the right internal jugular vein in the neck. Skin puncture is made at A, the midpoint of a line joining the mastoid process and the medial edge of the clavicular head of the sternomastoid, and the needle directed laterally and backward.

reason, an absolute requirement is a large intravenous cannula connected to the drip bottle through a blood-warming coil.

At critical moments during surgery, it may be necessary to transfuse quickly, measure the central venous pressure and administer drugs simultaneously. There are disadvantages to injecting irritant drugs (KCl, CaCl$_2$) into peripheral veins and to injecting potent drugs into lines whose rate of flow is dependent on some other factor. For these reasons there is much in favour of an extra central venous line reserved for the administration of drugs.

CHOICE OF ANAESTHETIC AGENTS AND TECHNIQUES

(a) Anaesthetic Agents

Anaesthetic agents may possess one or more of several actions which are undesirable. The most important actions are depression of myocardial contractility and reduction in peripheral venous tone, and when these two are combined together in a drug such as thiopentone, its quick administration can be lethal to severely incapacitated patients. Reduction in venous tone is perhaps less dangerous than myocardial depression as it can be compensated for by fluid infusion, provided the venous pressure is monitored. Myocardial depression caused by anaesthetic agents could be treated with inotropic drugs but this would postulate an unnecessarily complicated anaesthetic technique, very dependent on accurate monitoring and prompt correction of anaesthetic side-effects with other potent drugs. The better rule in the choice of drugs for cardiac patients is to select those agents which produce minimal myocardial depression and which do not significantly alter peripheral venous tone. Within these restrictions the actual choice of drugs probably does not matter and it is the skill of the administrator in the careful maintenance of the circulation which is important. The many papers which attest to the value of one technique over another and the difficulty in substantiating the claims, confirm this view. The most popular techniques are nitrous oxide-oxygen-relaxant techniques, neuroleptanalgesia, nitrous oxide-oxygen-minimal halothane (or methoxyflurane) and, in the United States rather than the United Kingdom, "morphine anaesthesia".

(b) Premedication

Mental sedation is necessary for patients with cardiac disease. Fear or emotional upset may induce an attack of angina or precipitate acute pulmonary oedema. Although careful pre-operative psychological support and explanation should always be given, this does not obviate the need for premedicant drugs.

Morphine is particularly suitable and the dose given can usually be generous as large doses can be safely used in patients with minimal cardiac reserves (Lowenstein et al., 1969). It will produce some dilatation of capacitance vessels and caution may be needed if the patient is very vasoconstricted or dependent on a high ventricular filling pressure. Morphine or papaveretum will usually be given in combination with hyoscine as an antisialogogue which has the advantage of some sedative amnesic property.

Atropine has the disadvantage of producing no sedative action and producing a tachycardia. This is particularly undesirable in coronary artery disease or mitral valve disease. The use of atropine as a sole premedicant in cardiac patients may be positively harmful.

If the effect of the premedication is very unsatisfactory, either markedly depressant or absolutely ineffective, on rare occasions the operation may have to be postponed.

(c) Induction

Except in the most ill patients, induction is usually performed in the anaesthetic room and it is usually easier to bring the operating table into the anaesthetic room and place the patient on it before induction. Some patients, particularly children, may be better induced in bed and patients in incipient or actual failure may need to be induced sitting up. These patients should be moved from their ward in a sitting up position and not forced to lie down on a trolley. In children who have been inadequately premedicated, making them lie down often causes them to cry.

The ECG should be attached before induction. For very ill patients, arterial and venous pressure monitoring will need to be established under local anaesthesia before induction. However, most patients will be presented in their optimum condition, not in cardiac failure, and then provided manual measurement of pulse and blood pressure is normal, arterial, venous and central venous cannulation can be more speedily and conveniently performed after induction.

In the extremes of low fixed cardiac output, the use of the intravenous barbiturates is potentially lethal and induction must be performed either with morphine anaesthesia, neuroleptanalgesia or gaseous induction with cyclopropane, perhaps accompanied by intravenous diazepam.

Cyclopropane has enjoyed a popularity for the induction of high-risk cardiac patients as its potency ensures a quick induction in a high oxygen atmosphere. It has the advantage of not producing vasodilatation and its myocardial depressant activity is counteracted by the sympathetic stimulation it produces. Kemmotsu and colleagues (1974) have shown that when the combined negative inotropic effects of cardiac failure and equipotent doses of anaesthetic agents are compared, cyclopropane has the least depressant effect; halothane, enflurane, isoflurane and fluroxene all produce an approximately 20 per cent reduction in myocardial performance. The main cardiac disadvantage of cyclopropane is that it raises the pulmonary vascular resistance (Price *et al.*, 1970) and is therefore contra-indicated in pulmonary hypertension accompanied by a fixed low cardiac output.

For the great majority of cardiac patients with well-compensated disease, a small sleep dose of thiopentone will not be dangerous, particularly if it is combined with pancuronium when this combination is more likely to raise than to drop the blood pressure. Pancuronium appears to increase the blood pressure mainly by raising the cardiac rate rather than by affecting the peripheral resistance (Kelman and Kennedy, 1971). The combination of tachycardia and hypertension may be disadvantageous in coronary artery disease when perhaps curare is a better drug.

Harrison and Sellick (1972) found induction of cardiac patients with Althesin caused tachycardia and hypotension.

Preoxygenation is advisable in most cardiac cases. Intubation is not performed until the patient is well oxygenated and fully relaxed, due to a high incidence of dysrhythmias or hypertension with difficult premature intubation.

(d) Ventilation during Anaesthesia

Respiratory dysfunction is commonly found in association with cardiac disease, particularly that which causes high left atrial pressure or increased pulmonary blood flow. These patients may exhibit mechanical difficulties with respiration (decreased compliance, airway obstruction) or have clinical or subclinical hypoxia when breathing room air. The carbon dioxide tension may be altered in either direction. For these reasons, intermittent positive-pressure ventilation, using an increased inspired oxygen content is advisable. Normally, IPPV will have little effect on the cardiovascular system (Conway, 1975) provided the inspiratory-expiratory time ratio is short, the airway pressures low and the carbon dioxide tension not excessively reduced. In the presence of high pulmonary capillary pressures, a small amount of end-expiratory positive pressure may improve oxygenation without impairing the cardiac output. Positive-pressure ventilation can be hazardous in those states in which pulmonary blood flow is severely reduced such as pulmonary embolism, severe pulmonary stenosis, and right-to-left shunts, such as Fallot's tetralogy, although rises in pulmonary vascular resistance secondary to hypercapnia may produce equally severe difficulties for the pulmonary blood flow.

COMPLICATIONS

1. **Hypotension.**—Mild hypotension by itself, if the cardiac output is maintained, may not be serious. In cardiac failure, dilatation of the resistance vessels by reducing the afterload may improve cardiac output while diminishing the oxygen consumption of the ventricle (Cohn, 1973). However, a falling output with systemic hypotension must not be tolerated without a diagnosis of its cause. A slight, but frequently progressive, deterioration can be expected during the manipulative part of a cardiac operation in patients with severe disease. More noticeably marked and successive falls in pressure may occur after the establishment of controlled respiration—particularly if the pulmonary vascular resistance is already high—during the thoracotomy with its attendant haemorrhage and trauma, and when the heart is handled at the time of examination and cardiotomy. The results of surgical manipulation of the heart are often especially disturbing, particularly when rotation or retraction of the organ and its great vessels from their normal position is essential. Dysrhythmias are very likely to occur at this stage and, should they be persistent, increase the hypotension.

The distinction must be made between hypotension secondary to cardiac failure, in which case the filling pressure (central venous pressure) will be high, and that secondary to a low filling pressure. The latter may be due to peripheral vasodilatation with a normal blood volume or to inadequately replaced blood loss. In either case the correct treatment is to restore the filling pressure to normal with the appropriate fluid.

The treatment of low cardiac output secondary to cardiac failure is directed firstly to removing the cause of the failure if possible. It may be secondary to trauma and manipulation of the heart by the surgeon, in which case a rest period is indicated. Progressive slow deterioration is to be feared more than sudden transitory deterioration which accompanies some manipulation. Abnormal cardiac rates and dysrhythmias may reduce the output (see below). Metabolic acidosis, itself a consequence of low output, will depress cardiac response to sympathetic stimulation.

Initial treatment is to restore the filling pressure to normal if it is low. It can then be raised further to see if the heart is capable of increasing its output. This must be performed cautiously as, if the left ventricle has failed, infusion of fluid can provoke pulmonary oedema with little or no rise in right atrial (central venous) pressure (see p. 513).

The cardiac output may have been depressed by an alteration in rate, usually bradycardia, but sometimes excessive tachycardia or an alteration in rhythm. The most common cause of a sudden change in pressure and output is a change from sinus into nodal rhythm or atrial fibrillation.

Finally, the cardiovascular depression may be due to a decrease in myocardial contractility. This may be the response of a potentially failing heart to depressant anaesthetic agents and will be aggravated by hypoxia, acidosis or hyperkalaemia. If elimination of the precipitating causes and correction of hypoxia and acidosis is ineffective, then an inotropic drug is indicated. Isoprenaline (1 mg in 500 ml dextrose, infused via a microdrip set) is the most frequently chosen drug. It has a strong β-stimulating action on the heart, it increases the cardiac rate and produces peripheral vasodilatation, reducing the afterload on the left ventricle. It will frequently convert nodal rhythm back into sinus control. Isoprenaline (and other sympathomimetic drugs) are inactive in the presence of a severe metabolic acidosis. The disadvantages of isoprenaline are that the tachycardia may be excessive or there may be an increased incidence of dysrhythmia; it produces a marked rise in myocardial oxygen consumption; in cases where it does not improve the output (severe mitral stenosis; complete heart block with fixed rate) the reduction in systemic vascular resistance results in a further drop in blood pressure and coronary and cerebral perfusion may become inadequate. In these cases, salbutamol, dopamine or adrenaline may be preferred. Adrenaline produces β-cardiac stimulation but also raises systemic vascular resistance and blood pressure. By constricting the capacitance vessels it will raise the filling pressure of the heart whereas isoprenaline produces vasodilatation and isoprenaline infusion will usually need to be accompanied by additional fluid replacement to maintain filling pressure.

The use of vasopressors is not recommended for hypotension secondary to a reduced cardiac output except in an emergency situation when, either as a result of a very low pressure or abnormal systemic arteries, coronary artery perfusion is reduced to a life-threatening level. In these circumstances a vasopressor may be necessary to support the circulation until the other measures have had time to work; choice should be made of a drug such a metaraminol which has a β-stimulating activity as well as vasoconstrictor action.

2. **Pulmonary oedema.**—The pressure in the pulmonary artery during diastole is only 8 mm Hg (1·1 kPa) rising to 20 mm Hg (2·7 kPa) during systole, but by the time the capillaries are reached these pressures have dropped even further (2–8 mm Hg or 0·3–1·1 kPa).

Pulmonary oedema is a late effect of a serious rise in pulmonary capillary pressure and is preceded by a progressive increase in lung blood volume and in the volume of interstitial fluid in the lung (Szidon *et al.*, 1972). This is accompanied by a decrease in pulmonary compliance and a falling arterial oxygen tension (see Fig. 6, p. 540).

The mechanism of pulmonary oedema following cerebral injury may be similar. Cerebral injury may be accompanied by a sympathetic discharge causing constriction of the capacitance vessels leading to a mass movement of fluid from the systemic to the pulmonary vascular bed.

Pulmonary oedema will occur at lower levels of pulmonary capillary pressure if the osmotic effect of the plasma protein is lowered. This may occur either as a result of a true reduction in plasma proteins or a relative reduction due to their dilution by the infusion of excessive amounts of clear fluid. Once pulmonary oedema has occurred, local anoxia damages the pulmonary endothelium and causes the breakdown of the semipermeable membrane so that plasma proteins and electrolytes pass into the alveolar spaces.

The Treatment of Acute Pulmonary Oedema During Anaesthesia

1. Reduction in the output of the right ventricle:
   (a) Anti-Trendelenburg position to encourage venous pooling in the dependent parts.

    (b) Vasodilator drugs to enlarge the capacitance vessels—morphine.

    (c) Positive-pressure ventilation with an end-expiratory pressure to reduce effective right ventricular filling by raising the intrathoracic pressure.

    (d) Venesection—the removal of fluid which may have been infused in excess.

2. Enhancement of the excretion of the excess fluid:
Diuretics—frusemide or ethacrynic acid intravenously (see p. 546).

3. Improvement in the function of the left ventricle:
Isoprenaline or digoxin (see p. 545).

Removal of the oedema fluid by suction is quite useless. Fluid merely accumulates as fast as it is removed and the action of sucking impairs ventilation. Continuous positive-pressure ventilation must not be discontinued until the measures to lower left atrial pressure have had time to work.

In general, good anaesthesia decreases the risk of acute pulmonary oedema, but in those patients whose circulatory equilibrium is finely balanced, even a change of posture—from the upright to the lateral horizontal—may induce failure. Patients who are on the borderline of pulmonary oedema may need to be induced in the upright position when the blood pressure will require continuous monitoring. Pregnant women with cardiac disease are especially liable to this complication after delivery of the placenta at the moment when the contracting uterus displaces a large volume of blood into the general circulation. The intravenous use of ergometrine enhances the risk.

Cardiac arrest.—This is discussed in Chapter 17.

The Diagnosis and Treatment of Cardiac Dysrhythmias Occurring During Anaesthesia

Cardiac dysrhythmias are common during anaesthesia and operation. They occur most frequently during induction and intubation, and less frequently during stable anaesthesia. Somewhat surprisingly they are equally common during regional anaesthesia but the overall incidence of serious dysrhythmias is low; Vanik and Davis (1968) found that only 0·9 per cent of 5012 patients had a serious rhythm disturbance.

The significance of dysrhythmias is twofold. Firstly the presence of dys-rhythmias may be the only indication of underlying cardiovascular disease, when they may be either the cause or the effect of progressive deterioration in myocardial performance. Secondly, whereas the normal myocardium will tolerate dysrhythmias well and maintain a reasonable output in the face of a continued abnormal rate, even minor dysrhythmias may be haemodynamically significant in the presence of myocardial or valvular disease (Samet, 1973).

Haemodynamic Implications

Dysrhythmias produce alterations in the haemodynamic state whose impor-tance varies with the underlying disease.

1. *Lack of atrial transport mechanism.* Atrial contraction is important for ventricular filling under three circumstances:

    (a) Where obstruction exists between atrium and ventricle. Commonly mitral stenosis, rarely tricuspid stenosis.

    (b) Where the ventricle is hypertrophied or non-compliant and requires extra filling pressure to distend it adequately, e.g. aortic or pulmonary stenosis, systemic or pulmonary hypertension, cardiac ischaemia, post-myocardial infarction.

(c) Where the unhypertrophied ventricle is suddenly stressed, e.g. pulmonary embolism.

2. *Effects of bradycardia.* Patients with low fixed stroke volumes depend on an adequate rate for their cardiac output. Bradycardia causes a serious drop in cardiac output in constrictive pericarditis and cardiac tamponade, pulmonary hypertension and cardiac failure. It is also deleterious in both aortic incompetence and stenosis.

3. *Effects of tachycardia.*

(a) Lack of time for diastolic filling of ventricle. This is most obvious in patients with mitral stenosis but even normal hearts are embarrassed if the rate is fast enough.

(b) An increase in the tension-time index demonstrating an increase in myocardial oxygen consumption, usually unaccompanied by any increase in coronary blood flow. Tachycardia is thus bad both in coronary artery disease and in ventricular hypertrophy.

4. *Effects of abnormal pattern of ventricular contraction.* The abnormally propagated excitatory impulse in ventricular dysrhythmias produces a less efficient contraction. This is particularly disadvantageous in aortic and pulmonary stenosis, systemic and pulmonary hypertension.

Predisposing Factors

Dysrhythmias may result from a simple cause such as direct stimulation of the heart by surgical instruments or cardiac catheter, but more commonly, rhythm disturbances are produced by the summation of a number of factors which, taken singly, would not cause the same effect. During anaesthesia dysrhythmias are common in patients with heart disease and in patients with pre-existing dysrhythmias. Predisposing factors include:

Increased catecholamine levels may be due to exogenous catecholamines from local infiltration or intravenous inotropic agents, or to excessive endogenous catecholamine liberated in response to painful stimuli under too light anaesthesia, ether or cyclopropane anaesthesia, hypercarbia or hypoxia.

Hypoxia, besides stimulating catecholamine secretion, has a direct action on the heart muscle cells. While general hypoxia may result from ventilatory or circulatory defects, local areas of hypoxia in the heart arise from discrepancies between oxygen delivery and oxygen consumption.

Reflex stimulation can arise from pharynx, larynx, abdominal and thoracic organs and the eye muscles. It may both provoke catecholamine secretions and stimulate the vagus so that the development of escape beats is more likely. At the same time, excessive parasympathetic blockade with atropine leaves the way for unopposed sympathetic action and a higher incidence of dysrhythmias.

Electrolyte changes—disturbances, particularly of extracellular potassium, predispose to the development of dysrhythmias (Fisch, 1973). Alterations in potassium may follow direct administration or result from alterations in pH, usually the consequence of change in ventilation or metabolic state, or occur following the administration of intravenous succinylcholine.

Drugs—certain anaesthetic agents are associated with the development of dysrhythmias particularly cyclopropane and the halogenated hydrocarbons. Other drugs include digoxin and the tricyclic antidepressants.

Physical factors—ventricular dysrhythmias are more common if the arterial pressure rises while atrial tachycardias are more common when the atrial pressures are high.

Mechanism of Dysrhythmias

There are two mechanisms of dysrhythmia production:

(a) *Enhancement of phase 4 depolarisation* (see 13/Fig. 3, p. 510). This may occur in any part of the heart which has rhythmic activity. It is characteristic of the rhythm disturbances caused by hypoxia or over-distension.

(b) *Electrical re-entry* in tissues where there are disparities in refractory period. This occurs in cardiac disease, digoxin toxicity and at slow heart rates.

Classification and Diagnosis of Dysrhythmias

Dysrhythmias are most conveniently considered under the headings of those which arise above the atrioventricular node, at the node and below the node. The particular diagnosis is made on the ECG appearance although this will not identify the cause. Diagnosis may be assisted by a knowledge of the pulse rate and its rhythm and by the appearance or disappearance of normal or abnormal wave forms in the venous pulse. If the heart is exposed during cardiac surgery, direct observation may help elucidate the time relationship between atrial and ventricular contraction.

SUPRAVENTRICULAR DYSRHYTHMIAS

1. **Atrial ectopic beats.**—These are due to premature atrial depolarisation in some site other than the sinus node. Isolated atrial ectopics are not particularly common but multiple ectopics may herald the onset of atrial fibrillation. The P wave configuration is abnormal and different to the existing P wave shape. It is followed by a normal QRS complex (Fig. 12a).

2. **Atrial tachycardias.**—(a) *Atrial fibrillation* is due to totally disorganised atrial depolarisation which results in the atrioventricular node being bombarded with impulses which are irregular both in time and strength. The ventricular response is, therefore, irregular and ECG diagnosis depends on irregular QRS complexes and the absence of P waves. The recognition of atrial electrical activity is not necessary for diagnosis (Fig. 12e).

(b) *Atrial flutter* is due to regular atrial depolarisation at some site other than the sinus node. The atrial rate is usually near 300/min and is commonly associated with 2:1 block giving a ventricular rate of 150, although other fixed block may occur and variable block is common in the presence of digoxin. The diagnosis may be difficult but is suggested by the absence of P waves, a regular fixed ventricular rate of approximately 150/min having normal QRS complexes. Flutter waves, so-called saw tooth appearance, may or may not be obvious (Fig. 12b and c).

(c) *Paroxysmal atrial tachycardia* is due to fast depolarisation at a site other than the sinus node which has a rate between 140–200/min (faster in children) and which is not accompanied by block so that the ventricles have the same rate. ECG shows normal QRS at approximately 140–200 beats/min preceded by an abnormal P wave.

A varying degree of block with paroxysmal atrial tachycardia is suggestive of digoxin toxicity (Fig. 12d).

a   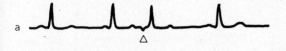   Isolated atrial ectopic beat

b   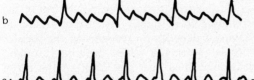   Atrial flutter with 3:1 block.

c   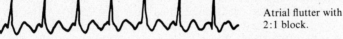   Atrial flutter with 2:1 block.

d   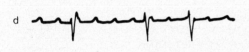   Paroxysmal atrial tachycardia with varying block.

e   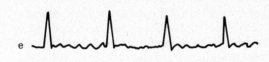   Atrial fibrillation.

14/Fig. 12.—Supraventricular dysrhythmias.

3. **Atrial bradycardias.**—(a) *Sinus bradycardia* may occur as a continuing pathological state or may result from strong vagal stimulation. The extreme example is sinus arrest with no electrical activity until it is terminated by a junctional or lower escape beat.

(b) *Sino-atrial block*: the activity of the SA node is not transmitted to the atrium and no P wave occurs. Some lower rhythm establishes itself.

JUNCTIONAL DYSRHYTHMIAS

1. **Nodal ectopics** are isolated beats arising in the atrioventricular node and which are premature, in contrast to escape beats which occur after a long pause. P waves may not be recognisable, being buried in the QRS complex which is normal.

Inverted P waves due to retrograde atrial activation may be seen immediately before or after the ventricular complex (see Fig. 13).

2. **Tachycardia.**—(*a*) *Nodal tachycardia*: regular depolarisation at approximately 120–150/min arising in the AV node and faster than the natural sinus rate. P waves are either buried in the normal QRS or appear inverted before or after the ventricular complex. It is a common rhythm after cardiac surgery and in digoxin intoxication. The diagnosis may be assisted by the observation of regular cannon waves in the venous pulse.

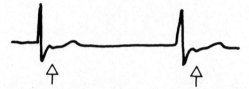

14/FIG. 13.—Nodal rhythm; note inverted P waves following the ventricular complex side.

(*b*) *Atrioventricular dissociation* between the atria under the control of the sinus node and the ventricles responding to a slightly faster rate arising in the atrioventricular node. ECG diagnosis depends on recognising the regular but differing atrial and ventricular rates. (Normal P waves "walking through" normal QRS complexes). An occasional sinus beat may capture the atrioventricular node and thus the ventricles (interference) causing an occasional irregularity in the ventricular rate. The venous pulse will show irregular cannon waves.

3. **Nodal bradycardia** has the same ECG characteristics of a nodal rhythm but occurs at between 40–60/min. Spontaneous sinus node activity must be absent or slower than the nodal rate. Cannon waves are apparent in the venous trace.

VENTRICULAR DYSRHYTHMIAS

1. **Ventricular ectopics**: premature beats arising somewhere within the ventricle. The ECG is characterised by a wide QRS complex whose voltage is usually greater than the normal complexes and which is not preceded by an associated P wave. The ectopic may or may not be followed by a compensatory pause. The shape of the QRS complex may suggest the site of origin (left bundle-branch block configuration suggests origin in right ventricle) and different shaped complexes suggest more than one site of origin (Fig. 14*a*).

Ventricular ectopic beats are very common and often benign. Those arising in the left ventricle may, perhaps, be more serious than those from the right ventricle. Features of ventricular ectopic beats which give rise to concern are:

   i. Multifocal origin shown by varying QRS shapes which suggest more widespread disease.

   ii. Runs of two or more which may herald ventricular tachycardia or ventricular fibrillation.

   iii. Ectopics which are close to the preceding beat. Should the ectopic fall on the peak of the preceding T wave, ventricular fibrillation may occur.

   iv. Frequency: less significant than the first three factors, but ventricular ectopics predispose to further dysrhythmias, therefore the more frequent the ectopics the greater the possibility of some other rhythm disturbance. This is the particular significance of bigeminy in digitalis therapy.

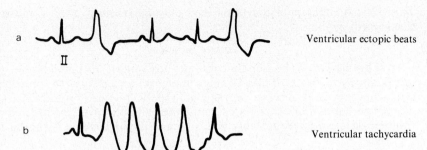

a   Ventricular ectopic beats

II

b   Ventricular tachycardia

c   Ventricular fibrillation.

14/Fig. 14.—Ventricular dysrhythmias.

2. **Ventricular tachycardia.**—This is always a dangerous rhythm. It drops the cardiac output and frequently precedes ventricular fibrillation. The ECG diagnosis is given by wide bizarre complexes occurring at 150–200/min, which may be slightly irregular. The P waves are usually not seen being buried in the ventricular complex from which they are dissociated, although regular retrograde activation of the atria may occur (Fig. 14b). This condition is often confused with supraventricular tachycardia with abnormal QRS complexes (see below).

3. **Ventricular fibrillation** is due to multiple areas of re-entry in the ventricular muscle. Diagnosed on the ECG by the totally random appearance (Fig. 14c). The bigger the amplitude of the complexes the better the prognosis for restarting the heart.

Supraventricular or nodal tachycardia may be associated with wide QRS complexes leading to confusion with ventricular tachycardia. The widening of the QRS complex may be due to right or left bundle-branch block or to aberrant conduction secondary to drugs or hyperkalaemia, or to the fast rate, overloading the normal conduction system causing it to be refractory to the next impulse.

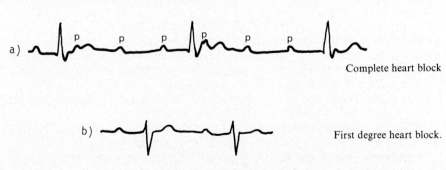

a)   p   p   p   p   p   p   Complete heart block

b)   First degree heart block.

14/Fig. 15.—Conduction defect.

This difficult differential diagnosis may only be resolved after intracardiac electrocardiography.

HEART BLOCK

1. **First degree.**—The bundle continues to conduct all impulses but at a slower rate than normal. It may be a sign of digoxin toxicity or of the presence of atrioventricular node disease. On the ECG the PR interval is greater than 0·22 seconds in adults only changing slightly with alterations in cardiac rate. In children there is more variability with rate and the upper limit is shorter (see Fig. 15b).

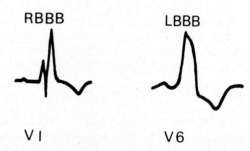

14/FIG. 16.—Right and left bundle-branch block.

2. **Second degree.**—(a) *Wenckebach phenomenon.* There is a progressive increase in the PR interval until an impulse is not transmitted. This pause allows the AV node time to recover and the cycle is repeated starting with the shortest PR interval. It may occur in digoxin therapy or as a result of atrioventricular node ischaemia.

(b) *Regular 2 to 1 or 3 to 1 heart block.* ECG shows normal P waves and QRS complexes but only alternate (or third etc.) P waves are followed by the ventricular complex.

3. **Complete heart block.**—The electrocardiographic appearance is one of complete dissociation of atrial and ventricular complexes, with the ventricular rate slower than the atrial rate. If the block is high the QRS complex will appear normal and confusion may exist with 2:1 heart block as the sinus rate is often 80/min and the idioventricular rate 40. If the block is lower, the QRS complex will appear widened (see Fig. 15a).

BUNDLE-BRANCH BLOCK

If one or two of the three main fasciculi (see p. 520, 13/Fig. 10) are interrupted, although the electrical impulse down the unaffected bundles will activate its related area of ventricle normally, the part of the ventricle no longer supplied by its bundle will be activated by some other slower route. The QRS will therefore be widened and the bundle that is interrupted can be recognised by the complex shape in different leads (see Fig. 16).

Right bundle-branch block.—QRS greater than 0·12 seconds. Delay in right ventricular activation produces a late R wave in leads V_1, V_2.

Left bundle-branch block.—QRS greater than 0·12 seconds. Delay in right ventricular activation produces late R wave in leads 1, AVL, V_{5-7}.

Left anterior hemiblock.—QRS up to 0·10 seconds with the appearance of left axis deviation.

Left posterior hemiblock.—QRS up to 0·10 seconds with appearance of right axis deviation.

Hence the association of either left or right axis deviation with right bundle-branch block suggests that two of the three fasciculi are interrupted and that there is a danger of complete heart block.

Prevention and Treatment

The prevention of dysrhythmias lies in the avoidance of those factors known to predispose towards their production and the first stage in the treatment of any dysrhythmia is the elimination of predisposing factors before proceeding to further therapy.

If a dysrhythmia occurs during anaesthesia it must be decided if the disturbance is immediately life-threatening because of inadequate cardiac output either because the heart is arrested (asystole, ventricular fibrillation) or because the cardiac output has been severely lowered by one or more of the haemodynamic consequences of the dysrhythmias listed above. The second possibility is that the dysrhythmia is the precursor of a rhythm which is life-threatening. The tachycardias are particularly dangerous in the presence of coronary artery disease. In either case, immediate treatment is needed to restore the rhythm to normal and, if necessary to support the circulation until that happens.

The great majority of dysrhythmias will not fall into these categories (Katz and Bigger, 1970), in which case specific treatment may not be needed and care must be taken that therapy does not introduce a greater hazard.

Once the predisposing factors have been eliminated, the number of serious dysrhythmias remaining is small and in the short term, as during anaesthesia, the selection of drugs for their treatment is relatively limited.

Ventricular fibrillation and ventricular tachycardia associated with an inadequate cardiac output are both emergency situations requiring immediate DC cardioversion. Ventricular ectopics are treated in two ways. In patients already on digoxin, a high proportion are due to hypokalaemia and will disappear if a small amount (up to 5 mmol) KCl is given intravenously over one minute. This may need to be repeated. If, however, the patient is not hypokalaemic, then the treatment is to suppress ventricular excitability. The drug of first choice is lignocaine (1 mg/kg intravenously) which can, if necessary, be given as a continuous intravenous infusion (Aps *et al.*, 1976). A small proportion of intractable ventricular dysrhythmias will be suppressed only by β-adrenergic blockade but under normal circumstances this should certainly not be used before all predisposing factors have been corrected. Under certain conditions of halothane anaesthesia, associated with sympathetic hyperactivity, the administration of β-adrenergic blocking drugs may cause a large fall in cardiac output (Stephen *et al.*, 1971). In anaesthetic practice droperidol may be a useful drug having been shown to have an antidysrhythmic effect at a dose which does not depress myocardial contractility. In larger doses it has an α-blocking effect in addition (Bertolo *et al.*, 1972). In the treatment of ventricular ectopic beats one must be certain that the ectopics are not, in fact, ventricular escape beats secondary to supraventricular bradycardia for which the treatment is stimulation of the sinus or atrium, usually with isoprenaline rather than the use of myocardial depressants. The sudden onset of any supraventricular tachycardia may be treated either by DC cardioversion or with digoxin. If the rate has a very deleterious effect on the cardiac output and if the factors provoking it are temporary, then cardioversion is the treatment of choice. This may be accompanied by digitalisation to control the rate of ventricular response should it recur. If, however, the cardiac output is adequate and it is thought that cardioversion is unlikely to be successful, then digitalisation alone is indicated.

Sinus arrest, sinus or nodal bradycardia, will usually revert to sinus rhythm after intravenous atropine or an infusion of isoprenaline. Isoprenaline may be useful in nodal tachycardia, the rate seldom increases, but P waves appear, capture the node, and when the infusion is slowed, the patient continues in sinus rhythm. Rarely, cardioversion of nodal tachycardia may be necessary.

Heart block may respond to isoprenaline infusion. Extreme fixed bradycardia may respond only to transvenous pacing. Paroxysmal atrial tachycardia may respond to vagal-stimulating action. Finally, perhaps the commonest rhythm disturbance is sinus tachycardia which is often a sign that there is some defect in anaesthetic or circulatory management.

Cardioversion.—Cardioversion is used to terminate both supraventricular and ventricular tachycardias. Conversion of ventricular tachycardia and ventricular fibrillation are considered elsewhere, only supraventricular dysrhythmias being considered here.

Cardioversion may be performed as an emergency procedure when some rhythm is life-threatening and other treatment will take too long to be effective. Thus the sudden onset of fast atrial fibrillation in a patient with heart disease may reduce cardiac output severely and cardioversion is performed while digitalisation takes effect.

More commonly, cardioversion is performed where a dysrhythmia has persisted after the precipitating cause has been removed and it is thought likely that sinus rhythm, if restored, will be stable. Thus it is sometimes performed postoperatively after cardiac surgery, or after pneumonia or thyrotoxicosis which have been treated. Quinidine is no longer used to attempt conversion of atrial fibrillation to sinus rhythm. Digoxin is normally stopped 24 to 48 hours prior to cardioversion.

The contra-indications to attempted cardioversion are when the tachycardia is sinus in origin and when the patient is suffering from digoxin toxicity. Fast atrial fibrillation itself, paroxysmal atrial tachycardia with block, and nodal tachycardia may all be manifestations of digoxin toxicity and further administration of digoxin or cardioversion may be dangerous as they may precipitate ventricular fibrillation which on further attempted cardioversion changes to a refractory asystole. If a shock is deemed life-saving it is preceded by intravenous lignocaine (1 mg/kg) and is of smaller amplitude than usual. Sometimes reversion to sinus rhythm may bring out latent digoxin toxicity and rapid administration of intravenous potassium and lignocaine is then necessary. β-adrenergic blockade is normally considered a contra-indication to attempted cardioversion as a refractory asystole may follow the shock.

Cardioversion is not usually performed if the patient has had a recent history of systemic embolism unless he has been anticoagulated for a month. A large heart, long-standing fibrillation and ischaemic heart disease are relative contra-indications and decrease the chance of successful reversion.

A DC shock of 75–300 joules is administered with two electrodes so positioned that the shock passes through the atria. The principal danger is the production of ventricular fibrillation should the shock fall on the T-wave upstroke although this should be avoided by proper synchronisation with the R wave. Other complications are the appearance of digoxin toxicity, sudden development of cardiac failure with acute pulmonary oedema and electrical failures which can lead to the patient's attendants being shocked should they be touching him.

(Anaesthesia for cardioversion is considered on p. 585).

The Post-operative Care of Cardiac Patients

The immediate post-operative period is perhaps the commonest time for patients to suffer serious complications. These can only be anticipated and prevented if the standard of care post-operatively is as high as during the operation.

After major surgery, and particularly after cardiac surgery, the journey between theatre and intensive care or recovery area is frequently hazardous—monitoring is temporarily discontinued, the supervision of blood balance and potent inotropic drugs may be less than adequate and the movement of the patient encourages venous pooling. For these reasons the journey should be speedy and planned in advance. The ECG can be displayed on a battery-operated portable instrument and the blood pressure measured on an aneroid gauge connected to the arterial line or assessed by the movement of an air bubble in the arterial line. Other monitoring is discontinued last and reconnected first on arrival in the ITU. There is seldom any need to extubate the patient before he has been allowed to restabilise and ventilation during the journey from theatre to recovery is facilitated by the use of Entonox (50 per cent N_2O/50 per cent O_2).

Once the patient has an adequate and stable cardiovascular system, circulatory support may be slowly withdrawn by a process of incremental reduction allowing adequate time between each reduction for reassessment and taking care not to change more than one factor at a time. Only after the circulation has demonstrated its capability for adequate function over some time without circulatory support should monitoring be discontinued.

Post-operative ventilation.—After surgery there is a mandatory increase in cardiac output to satisfy the rise in oxygen consumption caused by increased metabolism. This rise in oxygen consumption may be aggravated by catecholamine secretion secondary to hypoxia, hypercapnia, pain or fear.

At the same time the efficiency of ventilation and gas exchange may be impaired. Lung compliance is decreased by high left atrial pressures causing pulmonary engorgement, by retention of secretions causing bronchial obstruction and segmental lung collapse and by the mechanical effects of surgery on the thoracic cage. Oxygen uptake is reduced by the development of areas of arteriovenous shunt within the lungs which in severe cases may account for up to 30 per cent of the cardiac output.

In such patients the rise in oxygen consumption when spontaneous ventilation is restored is not the normal 3·5 per cent but may be as high as 30 per cent (Thung *et al.*, 1963). Even if the gas transfer is adequate the compromised circulation may be unable to raise the cardiac output proportionately to satisfy this demand and the patient becomes hypoxic.

While it is possible to improve the cardiac output with inotropic drugs, to reduce the pulmonary engorgement with diuretics and to treat lung collapse with physiotherapy, the immediate improvement of the hypoxic low cardiac output patient is best achieved by removing the excessive but unproductive work of breathing and employing positive-pressure ventilation until the other measures have had time to work.

Treatment of Post-operative Ventilatory Inadequacy

(*a*) *Prophylactic.*—Post-operative ventilatory problems are reduced if the patient presents in his optimum respiratory and cardiovascular state. Smoking should be stopped and adequate time allowed for pre-operative physiotherapy to clear the lungs of excess secretions. Cardiac failure, particularly left venticular failure, must be correctly treated.

(*b*) *Pulmonary venous engorgement.*—Lung compliance and oxygen transfer is facilitated if pulmonary venous congestion is minimised by keeping the left atrial pressure low. This implies that if the cardiac output is low, it is increased by the early introduction of an inotropic agent rather than by transfusion and elevation of the left-sided filling pressure.

(*c*) *Pain relief.*—Inadequate pain relief increases oxygen consumption and cardiac output, while at the same time inhibiting respiration and discouraging deep breathing so that retained secretions and lung collapse become more likely. The catecholamine secretion which accompanies pain raises venous tone and, transferring blood from the systemic to the pulmonary vascular tree, tends to raise the left atrial pressure.

Pain relief tends to be inadequate for a number of reasons:
  (i) the "time rule"—analgesia is better given in frequent small doses rather than by adhering to a 3- or 4-hour rule;
 (ii) carbon dioxide tension—an undue obsession with maintaining a normal arterial carbon dioxide tension may cause analgesia to be withheld. Provided the patient is not hypoxic and has a good cardiovascular function, free from dysrhythmias, then it is probably unimportant if the Pco_2 rises to 50 or even 55 mmHg (6·7–7·3 kPa). Sometimes the administration of morphine may result in a reduction in CO_2 tension following the relaxation of the inhibition of breathing caused by pain.
(iii) Hypotension. A fall in blood pressure may follow the administration of morphine and is usually due to a relaxation of tone in the venous capacitance vessels resulting in a fall in cardiac filling pressure. It responds to transfusion. There are two implications of this effect. The capacitance vessels must have been constricted previously, perhaps due to lack of analgesia or to hypovolaemia and secondly if the analgesia is allowed to wear off and pain recurs the vessels will again constrict and the left atrial pressure rise, perhaps this time even higher due to the infused fluid. This "yo-yo" effect of analgesia on the cardiovascular system dictates that stability is best achieved by frequent small or

continuous doses of analgesia with careful maintenance of the blood volume.

Ventilator Support

Now that ventilator support can be performed via an endotracheal tube for several days rather than depending on the performance of a tracheostomy, the decision to continue ventilation is much easier. If ventilator support is needed it is better to control ventilation rather than merely to assist it although the provision of a trigger mechanism even when ventilation is controlled is valuable, so that endotracheal suction or movement of the tube does not provoke the patient to fight the ventilator. In patients with interstitial pulmonary oedema, a small amount of positive end-expiratory pressure usually increases arterial oxygen tension without adversely affecting cardiovascular function, but there is no apparent benefit derived from PEEP in patients with good pulmonary and cardiovascular function after open-heart surgery (Drugge *et al.*, 1973). Control and sedation are achieved by mild hyperventilation and the use of narcotics supplemented if necessary with a tranquilliser such as diazepam. The only indications for the use of muscle relaxants during post-operative ventilation are:

(*a*) If the patient is severely hypoxic and his respiratory drive comes not from his CO_2 tension but from his hypoxia, when control may be very difficult to achieve without paralysis. This hypoxia may be the result of a ventilatory derangement or the consequence of a severely reduced cardiac output.

(*b*) If due to neurological damage the patient has either excessive CNS drive to respiration or uncontrollable fits which make mechanical ventilation impossible.

Inspired oxygen content seldom needs to be above 50 per cent. If this still results in hypoxaemia it is probable that either the cardiac output is too low or that gross lung collapse has occurred. The commonest cause of a patient "fighting" the ventilator or being "impossible" to sedate is underventilation, and measurement of the carbon dioxide tension will suggest that a greater minute volume is required.

If the patient has been properly prepared violent chest physiotherapy should not be needed but lung collapse can be treated or prevented with moderate "bag-squeezing" (see Chapter 12, page 494). In contrast to normovolaemic chronic chest patients, the post-operative cardiac patient who normally has a high venous pressure shows very little cardiovascular change to "bag-squeezing" provided the periods of high inspiratory pressure are short.

Criteria to be Reached Before Extubation

Although each case needs to be considered individually, or for some reason may be considered to differ from the usual (e.g., pulmonary hypertension), the normal criteria for discontinuing ventilatory support are:

1. *An intact neurological system.* If it is thought that the patient has suffered neurological damage at the time of operation, ventilatory support tends to be continued because of the risk to recovery of the neurological system by any degree of hypoxia or hypercarbia.

2. *A stable cardiovascular system.* This implies a reasonable cardiac output

adequately perfusing all organs, free from dysrhythmias and working at a suitably low left atrial pressure. If the circulation is still receiving inotropic support, the continuous reduction in this support should be temporarily stopped during the immediate post-extubation period until the response of the circulation to extubation has been established.

3. *Adequate mechanical and gas exchange function in the lung.*
   (*a*) Alveolar-arterial oxygen tension gradient should be small. The patient must be capable of an arterial oxygen tension greater than 100 mm Hg (13·3 kPa) when receiving 40 per cent oxygen in the inspired air—this being the concentration he will get from the mask after extubation.
   (*b*) The minute volume of ventilation to produce a normal carbon dioxide tension should be approximately that expected for the size of the patient.
   (*c*) The tidal volume should be achieved at a low inflation pressure implying a compliant chest so that the work of breathing will be small.

4. *The chest X-ray should be clear and the patient pain-free.*
   Because a patient is on a ventilator there may be a tendency to reduce the analgesic dose and once he is extubated the pain of breathing with a chest wound, particularly a lateral thoracotomy, will be such that considerable amounts of narcotics may be needed. The gas tensions should be carefully monitored in the post-extubation period and deterioration in their values or in the cardiovascular state (as evidenced by dysrhythmias, tachycardia, rising venous pressure, falling blood pressure and diminution in urine output) or the appearance of respiratory distress (tiredness, the use of the accessory muscles of respiration) are indications to reintubate the patient.

The problem of long-term nutrition after cardiac surgery is reviewed by Manners (1974).

SOME ASPECTS OF DIFFERENT CARDIAC DISEASES IN RELATION TO ANAESTHESIA AND OPERATION

It is not intended to describe all the individual diseases comprehensively but rather to pick out some and to discuss their special aspects which are of prime concern to the anaesthetist. The principles of anaesthesia previously described apply irrespective of the particular disease in the heart, but certain lesions may suggest a variation of technique or the use of an ancillary such as induced hypotension, hypothermia, or the extracorporeal circulation. Moreover, increasing experience of the behaviour of patients with certain lesions during anaesthesia and operation gives a clue to expected morbidity and mortality. Such facts as these and brief descriptions of those rarer diseases and operations, which are only likely to be seen in specialised clinics, are included to give the anaesthetist a broad background to the subject.

The particular problems of infants and children are not discussed here.

The reader is referred to the paediatric section of this book (Chapter 45) and to Seelye (1973).

Coarctation

Coarctation is a common form of congenital heart disease occurring once in every 1500 births. When it occurs proximal to the ductus arteriosus (pre-ductal) it is almost always associated with an open duct and the lower limbs are perfused with desaturated blood from the pulmonary artery. The children usually have other congenital cardiac abnormalities and present in cardiac failure.

Adult (post-ductal) coarctation has a very varied anatomy and 25 per cent of all cases have associated lesions. The patients have a labile hypertension above the constriction with a lower pressure below. The left ventricle is hypertrophied and the dilated aorta above the coarctation is thick-walled.

The lower part of the body is supplied by a collateral circulation, principally via the internal mammary, subscapular and intercostal arteries. These anastomotic vessels are thin-walled, tortuous and easily damaged at operation, particularly the intercostals which are often aneurysmal at their origins from the aorta.

If the disease is untreated, premature death occurs due to heart failure, aortic rupture, intracranial haemorrhage from the commonly associated berry aneurysm, or bacterial infection. Most patients fall in the age group 10–30 years, but prophylactic resection is now advocated at any age over 5 years unless uncontrollable cardiac failure makes earlier operation necessary.

The choice of operation lies between resection of the stricture with end-to-end anastomosis, insertion of a dacron gusset or tube grafting if the gap between the ends, after resection, is too great. Unless heart failure has already ensued, the patient will be physically fit and the mortality rate low.

The special factors to be noted are:

1. Excessive bleeding may be encountered from the chest wall during the thoracotomy.
2. The intercostal arteries are easily torn during the mobilisation of the aorta.
3. The left subclavian may be anatomically abnormal or may be clamped during the operation and cannot be used for blood pressure measurements. On rare occasions, the right subclavian may come off the aorta below the coarctation.
4. During the period of resection and anastomosis the aorta is clamped above and below the coarctation. The proximal blood pressure may rise depending on the adequacy of the collateral circulation. If the subclavian, which through its branches normally carries a large proportion of the anastomotic flow, is also clamped, the proximal hypertension is aggravated.
5. When the clamps are removed the sudden decrease in resistance causes a considerable drop in blood pressure.
6. Haemorrhage is likely to occur to some degree from the anastomosis in the period immediately after the clamps are removed.

The foregoing factors strongly favour the use of induced hypotension to reduce haemorrhage, to facilitate the surgery by reducing the tense pulsation in the vessels as they are mobilised and anastomosed, and to prevent excessive proximal hypertension when the clamps are applied. In view of the danger of hypotension when the clamps are removed the induced hypotension is produced with a short-acting agent which can be discontinued just before the anastomosis is opened. The drop in blood pressure can also be minimised by more than adequate fluid replacement prior to this moment.

If the coarctation is mild and hypertension only develops on exercise, or if the patient is being re-operated upon for restenosis or inadequate primary resection, the anastomatic vessels may be inadequate and clamping of the aorta, besides producing dangerous hypertension in the upper part of the body, will endanger the spinal cord and kidneys (Brewer *et al.*, 1972). In these patients, left atrio-femoral bypass or a temporary jump graft will be needed to protect the spinal cord.

In the post-operative period the patients commonly develop temporary hypertension (Bennett and Dalal, 1974). The blood pressure ought not to be allowed to rise above the pre-operative value and if adequate sedation and a head-up posture do not produce sufficient control, a long-acting agent, such as pentolinium, may be needed.

Left-to-Right Shunt

The three common congenital conditions which lead to an increased flow through the lungs are patent ductus arteriosus, atrial septal defect and ventricular septal defect. The enhanced pulmonary blood flow results in rapid uptake of oxygen and inhalational anaesthetic agents. As any left-to-right shunt may have a small right-to-left component at certain moments in the cardiac cycle, intravenous injections must be scrupulously sterile and free from air bubbles. Patent ductus leads to an overload of the left ventricle, atrial septal defect to an overload of the right ventricle, while a ventricular septal defect loads both ventricles. Anaesthesia for all three types of case presents no problem unless the patient is suffering from a complication and they can be treated as relatively healthy patients with good cardiorespiratory reserve.

The complications which may occur are:

(i) *Cardiac failure.* This may often be precipitated by the patient changing from sinus rhythm to atrial fibrillation or flutter. Failure must be treated with the appropriate measures before surgery. Sometimes in neonates the size of shunt is so large that only repair of the defect will enable the failure to be controlled. Frequently severe cardiac failure in neonates with left-to-right shunts is complicated by the presence of multiple circulatory abnormalities.

(ii) *The development of pulmonary hypertension.* When the pulmonary vascular resistance exceeds that of the systemic circuit the shunt will be reversed (Eisenmenger syndrome) and corrective surgery is no longer possible. With lesser degrees of pulmonary hypertension anaesthesia must be conducted with care (see above).

(iii) *Chest infections.* The vascularity of the pulmonary circulation leaves these patients very prone to recurrent chest infections and bronchitis.

Although most left-to-right shunts are congenital in origin, there are acquired lesions. A ventricular septal defect may appear after myocardial infarction involving the septum. Aorto-atrial shunts may follow rupture of an aneurysm of sinus of Valsalva.

Atrial and ventricular septal defects accompanied by a significant left-to-right shunt are repaired during extracorporeal circulation at an early age to prevent the development of complications.

Patent ductus arteriosus.—A narrow or long ductus is easily ligated but a broad short one requires careful dissection to avoid a tear, and its tense pulsations can be reduced at the time of ligation with a short-acting hypotensive agent. After ligation the patient develops a rise in diastolic pressure and a brady-cardia (Bramham phenomenon). The left recurrent laryngeal nerve may be damaged at the time of operation and give rise to post-operative respiratory problems.

Right-to-left Shunts

This group includes Fallot's tetralogy, pulmonary stenosis with atrial septal defect and transposition of the great vessels. The common features are central cyanosis, which is unrelieved by increasing the inspired oxygen concentration, and an increased haemoglobin concentration. They frequently have a metabolic acidosis.

Due to their reduced lung blood flow, the rate of rise of the arterial concentration of poorly soluble anaesthetics is much reduced, although the more soluble agents are less affected (Stoelting and Longnecker, 1972). The speed of induction will, of course, still depend to a large extent on the potency of the inhalational agent used and, despite its poor solubility, cyclopropane will produce a speedy induction. High concentrations of inhalational induction agents are well tolerated because of the slow rise of blood level. Arm-brain circulation time is very short and intravenous agents act quickly. Meticulous care is required both in sterile technique and in preventing air from being accidentally injected.

Fallot's tetralogy.—In this combination of pulmonary stenosis, patent ventricular septal defect, overriding aorta and enlarged right ventricle, the defect between the ventricles is usually large and the pressures in the right and left ventricles are identical. The degree of shunt, which is normally right to left, depends on the balance between the resistance due to the obstruction in the pulmonary outflow and the systemic vascular resistance. The pulmonary obstruction will be fixed if due to valve stenosis but pulmonary infundibular stenosis may be aggravated by hypoxic or catecholamine secretion. The shunt will be increased if the systemic vascular resistance drops on induction of anaesthesia and the resulting hypoxia will further reduce pulmonary flow, therefore hypotension must be promptly treated with a peripheral vasoconstrictor such as metaraminol. Positive-pressure ventilation will further reduce pulmonary blood flow and aggravate the shunt.

Normally the packed cell volume (haematocrit) is high, leading to a marked rise in viscosity of the blood. There is a danger of spontaneous thrombosis occurring if the patient becomes dehydrated. As a consequence of the small plasma volume there is a low renal plasma flow and renal problems occur. To compensate for the danger of spontaneous thrombus formation these patients develop a very active fibrinolytic mechanism and blood loss is higher and coagulation difficulties more common at surgery.

In the management of cyanotic patients with a high haematocrit fluid balance must be well maintained to avoid dehydration. Initially, lost blood can be replaced with plasma or plasma-substitute with frequent checks made of the packed cell volume, although the oxygen carrying capacity of the blood must not be seriously reduced until the haemodynamic defect is corrected. Coagulation difficulties are best dealt with by meticulous surgical haemostasis, as use of antifibrinolytic drugs may be accompanied by serious thrombus formation in the vascular tree.

VALVE DISEASE

Pulmonary Stenosis

Pulmonary stenosis produces little effect until it becomes severe, the cardiac output being maintained by a higher than normal right ventricular pressure. Once cardiac failure occurs or the rhythm changes from sinus to nodal or atrial fibrillation then the cardiac output falls. Normally the non-compliant hypertrophied right ventricle requires a high filling pressure and the additional filling of atrial contraction to distend it adequately in diastole. The right ventricular output can be increased with inotropic drugs (isoprenaline, adrenaline, and digoxin) if the stenosis is valvular but these drugs must be given cautiously if the obstruction is infundibular, as the increase in right ventricular tone aggravates the obstruction. Under this circumstance, a high filling pressure is particularly important. The output is better sustained at faster heart rates.

Once the stenosis is severe or cardiac failure occurs, anaesthetic management falls under the heading of fixed low output (q.v.) and operative intervention at this stage is associated with a high mortality. Patients with severe pulmonary stenosis are very vulnerable to right ventricular depression secondary to anaesthetic or drug action and to the mechanical effects of positive-pressure respiration.

Mitral Valve Disease

Mitral stenosis is undoubtedly a more difficult problem for the anaesthetist than mitral incompetence. Dyspnoea is the main symptom caused by elevation of the left atrial pressure with pulmonary venous engorgement. With time the pulmonary artery and right ventricular pressures rise, ultimately the right ventricle fails and the patient develops a fixed low cardiac output state.

The left ventricular output is very dependent on the cardiac rate, fast rates reduce the time available for ventricular filling across the stenosed valve but as commonly the left ventricle is small, bradycardia also produces a low output.

In the early stages of haemodynamically significant mitral stenosis the problem is to maintain the cardiac output without provoking pulmonary oedema either by overtransfusion or by increasing the right ventricular output. During anaesthesia, hypotension at this stage of the disease is perhaps best treated with a vasoconstrictor such as metaraminol rather than isoprenaline which may provoke a tachycardia and reduce systemic vascular resistance, thus lowering the blood pressure if the cardiac output does not improve. Once severe right ventricular failure has occurred, particularly if associated with pulmonary hypertension, then hypotension and low output may respond to cautious inotropic stimulation of the right ventricle together with increasing the right-sided filling pressure, the likelihood of pulmonary oedema now being much less. Thiopentone as an induction agent is particularly dangerous in this late fixed cardiac output stage of the disease.

Mitral valvotomy is performed to relieve the stenosis once it has become haemodynamically significant as shown by a raised left atrial pressure. The stenosed valve is split with a dilator passed through the apex of the left ventricle. At the time of cardiac manipulation clot may be thrown off and the anaesthetist is called on to compress the carotid arteries temporarily. Cardiac manipulation produces acute falls in blood pressure, particularly when the surgeon's fingers or the dilator are blocking the stenosed orifice and the pulse must be kept under continual observation and the blood pressure frequently recorded. Immediately the valvotomy has been performed the circulation usually improves but, if not, the surgeon is requested not to manipulate the heart further until the cardiac output, which is now more responsive to inotropic drugs, has improved. Digoxin can be safely given if the ventricular rate is too fast provided the serum potassium is normal. Before awakening the patient the peripheral pulses should be palpated to exclude embolism at the time of surgery.

Mitral incompetence is a disease of the left ventricle and although the patients develop cardiac failure they seldom present for surgery in the low output state seen with the stenotic valve. The mean left atrial pressure is lower in mitral incompetence than in a comparable degree of mitral stenosis and the heart is less embarrassed by increases in right ventricular output or by tachycardia. Mitral incompetence will, however, produce severe pulmonary congestion when it is of sudden onset, as following ruptured chordae tendinae or infarction of the papillary muscle. Under these conditions, left atrial pressure is high and pulmonary oedema common. Myocardial depressant anaesthetic agents will depress cardiac output but vasodilatation is less hazardous than increases in systemic vascular resistance, which aggravates the mitral regurgitation. Goodman and his colleagues (1974) have demonstrated an improvement in left ventricular dynamics and forward flow, when patients with mitral incompetence have their afterload reduced with sodium nitroprusside.

Again, the development of pulmonary hypertension or the presence of other lesions, particularly aortic valve disease, increase the danger.

Aortic Valve Disease

Aortic stenosis.—Aortic stenosis occurs as a congenital abnormality, as the result of rheumatic fever, or as the result of calcification in a congenital bicuspid valve. Outflow obstruction to the left ventricle also occurs in hypertrophic obstructive cardiomyopathy.

Patients develop a thickened hypertrophied ventricle which is called on to perform more work. Despite this, cardiac output and coronary filling are depressed resulting in myocardial ischaemia with angina, syncopal attacks and left ventricular failure leading to pulmonary oedema.

The small cavity of the thickened ventricle is only filled with difficulty to produce an adequate cardiac output and it is essential to maintain a good filling pressure and sinus rhythm. The development of dysrhythmias, particularly nodal rhythm, may result in an acute drop in cardiac output and is a common cause of sudden death in these patients. If cardiac arrest occurs, resuscitation is difficult due to the ineffectiveness of external cardiac compression in producing a good coronary flow.

Myocardial depressant drugs and vasodilators will reduce coronary perfusion. If the blood pressure falls during anaesthesia, despite a good filling pressure and a fairly fast heart rate in sinus rhythm, the output may be improved with isoprenaline although this will increase the myocardial oxygen consumption. Alternatively, adrenaline may be necessary to restore the arterial pressure and hence coronary blood flow.

Reflex hypertension due to hypoxia, catecholamine secretion or injudicious administration of vasopressor agents during anaesthesia in patients with aortic stenosis, is dangerous and by increasing the work load of the heart can precipitate acute myocardial ischaemia.

Hypertrophic obstructive cardiomyopathy produces a subvalvar stenosis and hypovolaemia, β-adrenergic stimulation or reduction in systemic vascular resistance will aggravate its effects. Hence filling pressure and systemic vascular resistance must be well maintained and inotropic drugs are contra-indicated. Patients are commonly treated with propranolol which should be continued during anaesthesia and surgery.

Aortic incompetence.—Aortic incompetence normally leads to a dilated left ventricle with a rise in left ventricular end-diastolic pressure which causes breathlessness. The decreased cardiac output and arterial diastolic blood pressure result in diminished coronary filling but as the ventricle is only slightly hypertrophied and the afterload is not increased, angina only occurs in 5 per cent of cases of pure aortic incompetence and then only when the leak is severe. These patients are vulnerable to changes in rate and rhythm and to the effects of myocardial depressants. Reduction in systemic vascular resistance is less important than in aortic stenosis and, as in mitral incompetence, tends to promote forward flow although the already low diastolic pressure, if reduced further, will impair coronary filling.

Cardiac Valve Prosthesis

Many patients with cardiac valve disease will present subsequently for surgery after the insertion of a valve prosthesis. Maillé *et al.* (1973) review their anaesthetic problems and comment that they will still have many of the problems associated with their original disease. Further, they will have acquired new restrictions and problems (e.g. anticoagulation) and will still require careful management. Before surgery, prophylactic antibiotics should be started at the time of the premedication.

CORONARY ARTERY DISEASE

Patients with coronary artery disease may present for incidental surgery or for operation designed to improve the blood supply to the myocardium. Sympathectomy, the creation of adhesions in the pericardium and the implantation of the internal mammary artery (Vineberg's operation) have entirely given way to saphenous vein bypass grafting in which a length of saphenous vein is anastomosed between the aorta and the coronary artery distal to the block. The advantage of this operation compared with those which preceded it is that, provided the distal coronary vasculature is good, the operation produces immediate benefit and the post-operative care is uncomplicated. The operation is performed during cardiopulmonary bypass as a motionless heart is necessary for the delicate distal anastomosis.

The management of patients with coronary artery disease undergoing surgery have been well described by Viljöen and Gindi (1971) and by Wynands and his colleagues (1970) who comment that these are frequently fitter patients than those with acquired valvular disease and may require more anaesthesia to maintain unconsciousness during extracorporeal circulation. The morbidity and mortality are significantly raised when patients with this disease are exposed to the stress of operation. The oxygen requirements of the myocardium are raised if the blood pressure rises or if the heart rate increases. Intravenous atropine in patients with multiple vessel coronary disease may provoke ischaemia as myocardial blood flow does not rise proportionally with rate, as it does in normal subjects (Massumi et al., 1972) and its use to treat sinus bradycardia in ischaemic patients may precipitate ventricular fibrillation (Knoebel et al., 1974). There is a danger of producing myocardial anoxia in patients with coronary artery stenosis if an attempt is made to stimulate the heart with isoprenaline or glucagon. If the arterial pressure falls due to peripheral dilatation the coronary flow declines. In contrast noradrenaline raises myocardial oxygen tension (Furuse et al., 1973).

Potent coronary vasodilators may produce overperfusion of normal areas at the expense of the diseased areas. Recently, nitroglycerin has been reported to reduce resistance to coronary collateral flow in patients undergoing operation for severe coronary artery disease (Goldstein et al., 1974). Complications are best prevented by maintaining a normal systolic and diastolic blood pressure and cardiac rate. Hypertension and tachycardia in response to anoxia, carbon dioxide retention, too light anaesthesia and pain make excessive demands on the myocardium, but hypotension is dangerous. It may be that in some circumstances the use of a myocardial depressant drug such as halothane to block these responses under anaesthesia may be needed.

PULMONARY EMBOLISM

Patients with massive pulmonary embolism may present for anaesthesia for pulmonary embolectomy.

With major degrees of block to the pulmonary circuit these patients represent the extreme examples of a fixed low output state and are highly vulnerable to all forms of myocardial depressant, vasodilatation and to the mechanical effects of positive-pressure ventilation.

For pulmonary embolectomy it is unwise to start the anaesthesia unless the theatre is ready and the surgeon is scrubbed ready to continue should the patient arrest on induction. Everything that can be done, positioning of drips, pressure monitoring lines, both venous and arterial, should be performed under local anaesthesia before induction which may have to be preceded by the injection of a vasopressor agent such as phenylephrine. The filling pressure of the right ventricle must be maintained by adequate transfusion. Isoprenalin may reduce the blood pressure if it produces vasodilatation without improving the output and in experimental pulmonary embolism has been shown to increase mortality. Adrenaline or noradrenaline are the inotropic agents of choice (Rosenberg *et al.*, 1971). In the extreme case supportive bypass after cannulation of the femoral vein and artery under local anaesthesia may be necessary.

Pulmonary angiography is frequently associated with acute deterioration due to the toxic effect of the contrast medium and is best performed without anaesthesia. Preferably it is carried out in the operating theatre so that the patient does not have to be moved before surgery is commenced.

CONSTRICTIVE PERICARDITIS

The essential effect of this disease is to limit the diastolic expansion of all the chambers of the heart. The stroke output of both ventricles is reduced. Eventually the pressure rises in the atria and systemic venous congestion occurs. Pulmonary congestion is, however, rare. Because of the limitation on stroke volume, the cardiac output is very dependent on cardiac rate.

The risk during anaesthesia is essentially similar to that of other diseases in which the cardiac output is reduced to a stage when compensation for sudden falls in peripheral resistance cannot take place. These patients must be treated in a manner similar to those with mitral stenosis and great caution exercised in the use of thiopentone.

Central venous pressure monitoring is essential during pericardectomy, both for the maintenance of right ventricular filling pressure and to enable the surgeon to see that relief of the constriction has been adequate. Haemorrhage during the operation may be considerable. The rotation of the heart necessary during the approach to the pericardium around the base of the heart and right atrium results in frequent dysrhythmias and hypotension. Besides an ECG, a continuous display of arterial pressure is valuable. The left ventricle is normally decompressed before the right, otherwise there is a danger of pulmonary oedema.

In the pre-operative preparation, despite their high venous pressure and frequent oedema, patients with constrictive pericarditis must not be given an excessive diuresis as they are very dependent on an adequate right-sided filling pressure to maintain the cardiac output.

TAMPONADE

Cardiac tamponade is an acute and often life-threatening event. The cardiac output is severely limited and is only maintained by a tachycardia and a high right ventricular filling pressure.

The diagnosis is made on the discovery of a low cardiac output with pulsus paradoxus in association with a high right atrial pressure showing a marked systolic descent. The immediate treatment of tamponade is the percutaneous aspiration of the accumulation in the pericardial sac. Then anaesthesia and surgery can be more safely performed. If, however, anaesthesia is required before pericardial decompression as for instance in stab wounds of the heart, the cardiac rate and sinus rhythm must be maintained and vasodilatation actively prevented if necessary with a vasopressor. Anaesthesia for patients with cardiac tamponade ranks with severe pulmonary hypertension and pulmonary embolism as a dangerous procedure.

EXTRACORPOREAL CIRCULATION

The general principles for anaesthesia and management of patients with cardiac disease, paying particular attention to the problems of specific lesions, apply to operations performed with the aid of extracorporeal circulation. The peculiar problem posed is that of keeping the patient unconscious during the period of bypass.

The technique chosen will usually be the same as that used to anaesthetise the patient before and after the bypass as this makes for ease in understanding and supporting the circulation at the beginning and end of bypass. While hypothermia will depress consciousness, it may not be sufficient to produce anaesthesia. If an inhalational technique has been used, small quantities of the agent can be vaporised in the gas flow to the oxygenator.

Narcotics, principally morphine, are the most commonly used agents. They may form part of a narcotic/muscle relaxant/nitrous oxide technique which has the advantage of flexibility in that doses can be altered or other drugs introduced as the state of the circulation indicates, without the danger that essential circulatory reflexes have been blocked by a long-acting drug. Morphine anaesthesia has been widely advocated (White and Tarhan, 1974), principally in America where Dalton (1972) in a survey of 54 open-heart units found it to be the second commonest technique after halothane. The benign effect of large doses of morphine on the circulation is markedly altered when the α-receptor stimulating action of nitrous oxide is introduced, particularly when the patient is suffering from myocardial or valvular disease (Stoelting and Gibbs, 1973; Wong et al., 1973). Conahan et al. (1973) in a prospective randomised comparison of halothane and morphine anaesthesia (in which both groups also received curare and 50 per cent nitrous oxide:oxygen) found the incidence of hypotension to be similar but hypertension was more frequent and more severe with morphine. These authors concluded that their data did not justify a claim for the superiority of either technique.

Narcotics may be also used as part of the neuroleptanalgesia technique. The adrenergic blocking effect of droperidol suppresses the peripheral vasoconstriction which accompanies long bypass and encourages good tissue perfusion. Morgan and colleagues (1974) report on its use in bypass surgery and Jacobsen (1970) in a comparative study of 400 cases between halothane and neuroleptanalgesia says that the latter is the method of choice.

The diversity of claims and the lack of strong evidence for the superiority of one technique over another suggests that the total understanding and management of the patient's circulation, the speed and quality of the surgery, the preservation of the myocardium and the selection of patients are more important factors than the choice of anaesthetic agent.

CARDIOVERSION

Electrical countershock for the conversion of tachyarrhythmias may be performed as an elective procedure or as an emergency if the cardiac output is severely depressed. Unless the patient is already unconscious, it is too painful to be performed without anaesthesia. The cardioversion of chronic atrial fibrillation to sinus rhythm is a relatively safe procedure provided there is no danger of digoxin toxicity and the serum potassium is normal.

Wagner and McIntosh (1969) have reviewed the likelihood of successful cardioversion in relation to the sympathetic and parasympathetic influences of different forms of anaesthesia. Neither premedication nor succinylcholine are necessary. Although inhalational amnesia/analgesia with methoxyfluorane has been described, intravenous anaesthesia with thiopentone, methohexitone, Althesin or diazepam is commoner. Because more than one shock may be required, it is worth continuing with nitrous oxide and oxygen so as to reduce the total dose of intravenous agent.

In the doses used, diazepam produces virtually no effect on the cardiovascular system, although in larger doses, it produces a transient decrease in left ventricular function (Bianco *et al.*, 1971). Due to its respiratory depressive effect, it should not be given unless facilities for artificial ventilation are at hand. The dose range for diazepam is very variable (Somers *et al.*, 1971; Vinge *et al.*, 1971), but low dosage may result in inadequate amnesia. Drowsiness usually lasts half-an-hour, but occasional patients remain somnolent for several hours. Due to the pain of injection and the danger of venous thrombosis, diazepam must be given into a large vein.

Post-conversion dysrhythmias may occur and atropine, potassium chloride, lignocaine and β-blockers should be to hand. Pulmonary oedema is a rare post-conversion complication.

Cardiac Catheterisation and Angiocardiography

Cardiac catheterisation is not a painful procedure except for the introduction of the catheter through the skin and this can be adequately covered by local anaesthesia. The passage of the catheter through the veins should provide no sensation but the mental strain and the discomfort of lying continuously in the dark X-ray room on a hard table for any length of time may make it unacceptable to the patient. Angiocardiography may be less pleasant, the injection of the dye is followed by a warm sensation spreading over the body.

The choice for cardiac catheterisation is either local analgesic, local analgesic combined with basal sedation, or general anaesthesia (Manners, 1971). The argument in favour of avoidance of general anaesthesia is mainly on the grounds that changes in cardiorespiratory function during anaesthesia are unpredictable and that unpremedicated, unanaesthetised patients breathing air are likely to be in a more physiological condition. The technique of cardiac catheterisation without sedation is well described (Mendel, 1974) and produces satisfactory results, if the staff work hard at reassuring the patient beforehand and avoid upsetting him during the procedure.

Sedation or anaesthesia tends to be indicated for the following groups of patients:

1. Those patients in whom catheterisation without sedation is impossible due to the presence of a language barrier or the patient having such a low mentality that one is unable to communicate with him properly.

2. If the patient has had a previous catheterisation of which he has unpleasant memories, he may express unwillingness to have a second performance without the benefits of general anaesthesia.

3. Children (see Adams and Parkhouse, 1960).

Moffit and colleagues (1970) reviewing eleven years' experience of anaesthesia in children, found it satisfactory both for child and physician. The exposure to the process of diagnosis made the anaesthetist better able to manage the same child at the subsequent operation.

Special considerations

(a) A steady state is required because the various measurements at different sites are often made consecutively, not simultaneously.

(b) The cardiovascular state (pulse, resistance, cardiac output, etc.) should be altered as little as possible. Although output is often measured at some time during the catheterisation, this is not always so. Deductions can only be made from the measurements on the assumption that the cardiovascular state is substantially unchanged by the anaesthetic technique.

(c) Ventilation. Alterations in oxygen or carbon dioxide tension have circulatory effects as do the mechanical factors of positive-pressure respiration. Again, the requirement is to maintain the patient as near normal as possible.

(d) In small children, the temperature is monitored to guard against hypothermia.

(e) Fluid balance. Blood samples and unnoticed haemorrhage may add up to large fluid deficits while enthusiastic flushing of catheters can result in considerable fluid administration.

(f) Contrast medium. The dye used for angiography has a transient depressive action on the heart and is also a powerful vasodilator. Although the volume is usually strictly limited, the fluid is hypertonic and leads to an expansion in the circulatory blood volume which may overload the heart.

(g) Acidosis. A metabolic acidosis may develop if the cardiac output is low, particularly if the reduction is aggravated by dysrhythmias provoked during the catheterisation. The acidosis will itself impair cardiac contractility.

Techniques

Sedation.—The principal advantage of sedation is that patients breathe air spontaneously. The obvious danger is respiratory depression to the point of hypoxia with changes in the circulation secondary to hypoxia and hypercapnia. Manners and Codman (1969) showed that properly applied positive-pressure respiration did not significantly alter the haemodynamic findings.

Up to the age of about 12 years, good results with heavy sedation can be obtained for catheterisation and angiocardiography using the schedule recommended by Nicholson and Graham (1969). Sodium phenobarbitone 2 mg/kg given the previous evening and again three hours before the procedure. Half an hour before the procedure an intramuscular injection of 1 ml/10 kg body weight of a compound injection of pethidine, of which 1 ml contains chlorpromazine 6·25 mg, promethazine 6·25 mg and pethidine 25 mg.

The dose is halved in very small or ill children. If the child becomes restless towards the end of a long procedure the sedation is supplemented with small doses of intravenous diazepam.

Neuroleptanalgesia.—Innovar (droperidol-fentanyl) has been shown to have minimal effects on the cardiac output and work, although the blood pressure and vascular resistance declined. However, in their study (Tarhan *et al.*, 1971) all patients had decreases in arterial oxygen tension, sometimes to hypoxic levels and the effects of hypercapnia and hypoxia may have masked cardiovascular depression. Graham and colleagues (1974) recommend Innovar 0·025 ml/kg body weight to a maximum of 1 ml. This gave good results but the does must not be exceeded.

Ketamine.—Bovill and colleagues (1971) regard cardiac catheterisation as being a specific indication for the use of ketamine, although Tweed *et al.* (1972) describe it as unsuitable in the presence of coronary artery disease, severe myocardial disease or aortic stenosis. There is respiratory depression and rise in blood pressure which usually returns to normal after 15 minutes. It does not appear to affect the pulmonary vascular resistance (Gassner *et al.*, 1974). Atropine premedication is necessary and Brandus and colleagues (1971) recommend ketamine intramuscularly 5 mg/kg in children, 3–4 mg/kg in infants, 1–2 mg/kg in neonates and thereafter adjusting the dose to the response of the patient. The use of ketamine does not dispense with the need to have an anaesthetist present.

General anaesthesia.—Our preference is to ventilate patients with nitrous oxide and 25 per cent oxygen after paralysis with pancuronium, or to control ventilation with nitrous oxide, oxygen and minimal halothane (less than ½ per cent) after intubation under suxamethonium. Inspired oxygen content is maintained at 25 per cent and ventilation adjusted to produce only a slight reduction in carbon dioxide tension. The minor deviations of cardiorespiratory performance induced by positive-pressure ventilation are more than offset by the avoidance of other agents which affect myocardial contractility, peripheral resistance and the likelihood of dysrhythmias.

HEART BLOCK

Complete heart block is defined as a condition in which there is atrioventricular dissociation and the ventricular rate is slower than the atrial rate.

Complete atrioventricular block most commonly results from degeneration of the conducting tissue of the heart. It may also be the result of surgery or drug therapy, occur as a congenital abnormality, or be due to ischaemic disease. Block may be complete or affect only one or two of the three main fasciculi. Complete block occurring high in the bundle produces a fairly fast ventricular rate and Stokes-Adams attacks are unusual. Low block is associated with slow and unreliable spontaneous ventricular activity.

Stokes-Adams attacks occur:

(*a*) When partial block becomes complete.

(*b*) During established block with unreliable ventricular activity (low block).

(*c*) As attacks of ventricular tachycardia or fibrillation.

Partial or unstable block is a more dangerous condition than stable complete block and a history of Stokes-Adams attacks, giddiness, collapse or fainting suggests an unstable block.

Patients present for anaesthesia in two states:

1. They may present in partial or complete block for pacemaker insertion or for incidental surgery.

2. Patients may appear for anaesthesia and surgery with an indwelling pacemaker already in use.

Patients with stable complete block have a very fixed cardiac output which can only be altered marginally by increases in stroke volume. They are, therefore, very vulnerable both to myocardial depressant drugs and to vaso-dilatation, although it may be possible to increase their rate with atropine or isoprenaline. If isoprenaline does not speed up the heart the blood pressure is liable to fall due to its vasodilator action. Provided the patient's cardiac output is sufficient to sustain him normally, he can probably be safely anaesthetised using techniques which avoid myocardial depression or peripheral dilatation.

Patients with block of recent onset or with unstable block and a history of Stokes-Adams attacks need a temporary transvenous pacemaker inserted prior to anaesthesia and surgery. This will probably apply to patients presenting for their first permanent pacemaker insertion.

When any patient with a conduction defect is being anaesthetised, a continuous ECG display is mandatory. A pacing box and sterile transvenous leads must also be available in the theatre. If a transvenous pacemaker is in use any sudden or violent movement may dislodge the pacing contact. Failure to pace may also arise from increases in pacemaker threshold due to alterations in serum electrolytes or myocardial depression due to anaesthetic agents. The efficacy of pacing must be judged not by the ECG but by an adequate peripheral pulse. Sudden cessation of pacing is an emergency and if the spontaneous cardiac output is inadequate and shows no response to isoprenaline, external cardiac compression may be necessary until the defect is repaired.

Diathermy and the Pacemaker

The dangers of diathermy used on a patient with a pacemaker are twofold. The diathermy may affect the rate of pacemaker discharge—most commonly this is apparent as total inhibition of demand pacing but it may also result in high discharge rate (200–600 impulses/min) which will cause an inadequate cardiac output (Orland and Jones, 1975). Alternatively diathermy may induce currents in the circuit at an inappropriate moment and provoke ventricular fibrillation. The safest course if a patient has an indwelling pacemaker, is to forbid the use of the diathermy. If the patient is being paced with an external box, the pacer can be disconnected briefly each time the diathermy is used—it may not be sufficient merely to turn it off. As the ECG will also be inhibited by the diathermy at this moment, the pulse must be monitored continuously while the diathermy is used.

REFERENCES

ADAMS, A. K., and PARKHOUSE, J. (1960). Anaesthesia for cardiac catheterisation in children. *Brit. J. Anaesth.*, **32**, 69.
ALDERMAN, E. L., COLTART, D. J., WETTACH, G. E. and HARRISON, D. C. (1974). Coronary artery syndromes after sudden propranolol withdrawal. *Ann. intern. Med.*, **81**, 625.
APS, C., BELL, J. A., JENKINS, B. S., POOLE-WILSON, P. A., and REYNOLDS, F. (1976). Logical approach to lignocaine therapy. *Brit. med. J.*, **1**, 13.
ARKINS, R., SMESSAERT, A. A., and HICKS, R. G. (1964). Mortality and morbidity in surgical patients with coronary artery disease. *J. Amer. med. Ass.*, **190**, 485.

BENNETT, E. J., and DALAL, F. Y. (1974). Hypotensive anaesthesia for coarctation. *Anaesthesia*, **29**, 269.

BERTOLO, L., NOVAKOVIC, L., and PENNA, M. (1972). Antiarrhythmic effects of droperidol. *Anesthesiology*, **37**, 529.

BIANCO, J. A., SHANAHAN, E. A., OSTHEIMER, G. W., GUYTON, R. A., POWELL, W. J., and DAGGETT, W. M. (1971). Cardiovascular effect of diazepam. *J. thorac. cardiovasc. Surg.*, **62**, 125.

BOVILL, J. G., COPPELL, D. L., DUNDEE, J. W., and MOORE, J. (1971). Current status of ketamine anaesthesia. *Lancet*, **2**, 1285.

BRANDUS, V., BENOIT, C., and KOCH, L. (1971). Ketamine anaesthesia. *Lancet*, **2**, 543.

BRESLIN, D. J., and SWINTON, N. W. (1970). Elective surgery in hypertensive patients—pre-operative considerations. *Surg. Clin. N. Amer.*, **50**, 585.

BREWER, L. A., FOSBURG, R. G., MULDER, G. A., and VERSKA, J. J. (1972). Spinal cord complications following surgery for coarctation of the aorta. *J. thorac. cardiovasc. Surg.*, **64**, 368.

COHN, J. N. (1973). Vasodilator therapy for heart failure. The influence of impedance on left ventricular performance. *Circulation*, **48**, 5.

COLTART, D. J., CAYEN, M. N., STINSON, E. B., GOLDMAN, R. H., DAVIES, R. O., and HARRISON, D. C. (1975). Investigation of the safe withdrawal period for propranolol in patients scheduled for open heart surgery. *Brit. Heart. J.*, **37**, 1228.

COMROE, J. H., JR., FORSTER, R. E. (II), DUBOIS, A. B., BRISCOE, W. A., and CARLSON, E. (1962). *The Lung*, 2nd edit. Chicago: Year Book Medical Publishers, Inc.

CONAHAN, T. J., OMINSKY, A. J., WOLLMAN, H., and STROTH, R. A. (1973). A prospective random comparison of halothane and morphine for open heart surgery. *Anesthesiology*, **38**, 528.

CONWAY, C. M. (1975). Haemodynamic effects of pulmonary ventilation. *Brit. J. Anaesth.*, **47**, 761.

CULLEN, D. J. (1974). Interpretation of blood pressure measurements in anaesthesia. *Anesthesiology*, **40**, 6.

DALTON, B. (1972). Anaesthesia for cardiac surgery. *Anesthesiology*, **36**, 521.

DEMING, Q. B. (1968). Blood pressure: its relation to atherosclerotic disease of the coronaries. *Bull. N.Y. Acad. Med.*, **44**, 968.

DEUTSCH, S., and DALEN, J. E. (1969). Indications for prophylactic digitalization. *Anesthesiology*, **30**, 648 (and correspondence **31**, 583).

DINGLE, H. R. (1966). Antihypertensive drugs and anaesthesia. *Anaesthesia*, **21**, 151.

DRUGGE, U., NORLANDER, O., ULSSON, P., and KADEGRAM, K. (1973). Positive and expiratory pressure ventilation after open heart surgery. *Acta anaesth. scand.* (Suppl.), **53**, 81.

EDMONDS, C. J., and JASANI, B. (1972). Total body potassium in hypertensive patients during prolonged diuretic therapy. *Lancet*, **2**, 8.

ENGLISH, I. C. W., FREW, R. M., PIGOTT, J. F., and ZAKI, M. (1969). Percutaneous catheterisation of the internal jugular vein. *Anaesthesia*, **24**, 521.

FISCH, C. (1973). Relation of electrolyte disturbances to cardiac arrhythmia. *Circulation*, **47**, 399.

FOËX, P., and PRYS-ROBERTS, C. (1974). Interactions of beta-receptor blockade and Pco_2 levels in the anaesthetized dog. *Brit. J. Anaesth.*, **46**, 397.

FURUSE, A., BRAWLEY, R. K., and GOTT, V. L. (1973). Effects of isoproterenol, l-norepinephrine and glucagon of myocardial gas tensions in animals with coronary artery stenosis. *J. thorac. cardiovasc. Surg.*, **65**, 815.

GASSNER, S., COHEN, M. AYGEN, M., LEVY, E., VENTURA, E., and SHASHDI, J. (1974). The effect of ketamine on pulmonary artery pressure. *Anaesthesia*, **29**, 141.

GOLDSTEIN, R. E., STINSON, E. B., SCHRERER, J. L., SENINGEN, R. P., GREHL, T. M., and EPSTEIN, S. E. (1974). Intraoperative coronary collateral function in patients with coronary occlusive disease. *Circulation*, **49**, 298.

GOODMAN, D. J., ROSSEN, R. M., HOLLOWAY, E. L., ALDERMAN, E. L., and HARRISON, D. C. (1974). The effect of nitroprusside on left ventricular dynamics in mitral regurgitation. *Circulation*, **50**, 1025.

GRAHAM, T. P., ATWOOD, G. F., and WERNER, B. (1974). Use of droperidol-fentanyl sedation for cardiac catheterisation in children. *Amer. Heart, J.*, **87**, 287.

HARRISON, D. C., KERBER, R. E., and ALDERMAN, E. L. (1970). Pharmacodynamics and clinical use of cardiovascular drugs after cardiac surgery. *Amer. J. Cardiol.*, **26**, 385.

HARRISON, S. G. C., and SELLICK, B. A. (1972). Cardiovascular effects of Althesin in patients with cardiac pathology. *Brit. J. Anaesth.*, **44**, 1205.

HICKLER, R. B., and VANDAM, L. D. (1970). Hypertension. *Anesthesiology*, **33**, 214.

HORAN, B. F., PRYS-ROBERTS, C., FOEX, P., and ROBERTS, J. G. (1977). Interaction of isoflurane anaesthesia, β-receptor blockade and blood loss in the dog. *Brit. J. Anaesth.*, **49**, 187.

HORAN, B. F., PRYS-ROBERTS, C., HAMILTON, W. K., and ROBERTS, J. G. (1976). Interaction of enflurane anaesthesia, β-receptor blockade and blood loss in the dog. *Brit. J. Anaesth.*, **48**, 817.

JACOBSEN, F. H. (1970). A comparison between halothane and neuroleptanalgesia in open heart surgery. *Anaesthesist*, **19**, 16.

JOHNSTON, A. O. B., and CLARKE, R. G. (1972). Malpositioning of central venous catheters. *Lancet*, **2**, 1395.

KATZ, R. L., and BIGGER, J. T. (1970). Cardiac arrhythmias during anesthesia and operation. *Anesthesiology*, **33**, 193.

KELMAN, G. R., and KENNEDY, B. R. (1971). Cardiovascular effects of pancuronium in man. *Brit. J. Anaesth.*, **43**, 335.

KELMAN, G. R., NUNN, J. F., PRYS-ROBERTS, C., and GREENBAUM, R. (1967). The influence of cardiac output on arterial oxygenation. *Brit. J. Anaesth.*, **39**, 450.

KEMMOTSU, O., YASHIMOTO, Y., and SHIMOSATA, S. (1974). The effects of fluroxene and enflurane on the contractile performance of isolated papillary muscles from failing hearts. *Anesthesiology*, **40**, 252.

KITTLE, C. F., DYE, W. S., GERBODE, F., GLENN, W. W. L., JULIAN, C., MORROW, A. G., SABISTON, D. C., and WEINBERG, M. (1969). Factors influencing risk in cardiac surgical patients: Cooperative study. *Circulation*, **39** and **40**, Suppl. I, 169.

KNAPP, R. B., TOPKINS, M. J., and ARTUSIO, J. F. (1962). The cerebrovascular accident and coronary occlusion in anaesthesia. *J. Amer. med. Assn.*, **182**, 332.

KNOEBEL, S. B., McHENRY, P. L., PHILLIPS, J. F., and WIDLANSKY, S. (1974). Atropine induced cardio-acceleration and myocardial blood flow in subjects with and without coronary artery disease. *Amer. J. Cardiol.*, **33**, 327.

Lancet (1971). Editorial. Digitalis intoxication. **2**, 362.

Lancet (1972). Editorial. Postoperative myocardial infarction. **2**, 472.

LOWENSTEIN, E., HALLOWELL, P., LEVINE, F. H., DAGGETT, W. M., AUSTEN, W. G., and LAVER, M. (1969). Cardiovascular response to large doses of intravenous morphine in man. *New Engl. J. Med.,* **281**, 1389.

LUMLEY, J., and RUSSELL, W. J. (1975). Insertion of central venous catheters through arm veins. *Anaesth. Intens. Care*, **3**, 101.

McGUINESS, J. B., BEGG, T. B., and SEMPLE, T. (1976). First electrocardiogram in recent myocardial infarction. *Brit. med. J.*, **2**, 449.

MAILLÉ, J., DRYDA, I., PAIEMENT, B., and BOULANGER, M. (1973). Patients with cardiac valve prosthesis: subsequent anaesthetic management for non-cardiac surgical procedures. *Canad. Anaesth. Soc. J.*, **20**, 207.

MANNERS, J. M. (1971). Anaesthesia for diagnostic procedures in cardiac disease. *Brit. J. Anaesth.*, **43**, 276.

MANNERS, J. M. (1974). Nutrition after cardiac surgery. *Anaesthesia*, **29**, 675.

MANNERS, J., and CODMAN, V. A. (1969). General anaesthesia for cardiac catheterisation in children. *Anaesthesia*, **24**, 541.

MASSUMI, R. A., MASON, D. T., AMSTERDAM, E. A., DEMARIA, A., MILLER, R. R., SCHEINMAN, M. M., and ZELLIS, R. (1972). Ventricular fibrillation and tachycardia after intravenous atropine for treatment of bradycardias. *New Engl. J. Med.*, **287**, 336.

MAUNEY, F. M., EBERT, P. A., and SABISTON, D. C. (1970). Post-operative myocardial infarction: a study of predisposing factors, diagnosis and mortality in high risk group of surgical patients. *Ann. Surg.*, **172**, 497.

MENDEL, D. (1974). In: *A Practice of Catheterisation*. 2nd edit. Oxford: Blackwell Scientific Publications.

MERIN, R. G. (1972). Anaesthetic management problems posed by therapeutic advances. III. Beta-adrenergic blocking drugs. *Anesth. Analg. Curr. Res.*, **51**, 617.

MOFFIT, E. A., MCGOON, D. C., and RITTER, D. G. (1970). The diagnosis and correction of congenital cardiac defects. *Anesthesiology*, **33**, 144.

MORGAN, M., LUMLEY, J., and GILLIES, I. D. S. (1974). Neuroleptanaesthesia for major surgery. *Brit. J. Anaesth.*, **46**, 288.

NICHOLSON, J. R., and GRAHAM, G. R. (1969). Management of infants under six months of age undergoing cardiac investigation. *Brit. J. Anaesth.*, **41**, 417.

NORLANDER, O., BERNHOFF, A., and NORDEN, I. (1969). Dead space, compliance and venous admixture during heart surgery. *Acta anaesth. scand.*, **13**, 143.

OH, T. E., and DAVIS, N. J. (1975). Radial artery cannulation. *Anaesth. Intens. Care*, **3**, 12.

OMINSKY, A. J., and WOLLMAN, H. (1969). Hazards of general anaesthesia in the reserpinised patient. *Anesthesiology*, **30**, 443.

ORLAND, H. J., and JONES, D. (1975). Cardiac pacemaker induced ventricular fibrillation during surgical diathermy. *Anaesth. Intens. Care*, **3**, 321.

PAPPER, E. M. (1965). Selection and management of anaesthesia in those suffering from diseases and disorders of the heart. *Canad. Anaesth. Soc. J.*, **12**, 245.

PRICE, H. L., COOPERMAN, L. H., WARDEN, J. C., MORRIS, J. J., and SMITH, T. C. (1970). Pulmonary hemodynamics during general anaesthesia in man. *Anesthesiology*, **30**, 629.

PRYS-ROBERTS, C., FOËX, P., GREENE, L. T., and WATERHOUSE, T. D. (1972). Studies of anaesthesia in relation to hypertension: IV. The effect of artificial ventilation on the circulation and pulmonary gas exchanges. *Brit. J. Anaesth.*, **44**, 335.

PRYS-ROBERTS, C., KELMAN, G. R., GREENBAUM, R., and ROBINSON, R. H. (1967). Circulatory influences of artificial ventilation during nitrous oxide anaesthesia in man. II. Results. *Brit. J. Anaesth.*, **39**, 533.

PRYS-ROBERTS, C., MELOCHE, R., and FOËX, P. (1971). Studies of anaesthesia in relation to hypertension: I. Cardiovascular responses of treated and untreated patients. *Brit. J. Anaesth.*, **43**, 122.

ROBERTS, J. G., FOËX, P., CLARKE, T. N. S., BENNETT, M. J., and SANER, C. A. (1976). Haemodynamic interactions of high dose propranolol pretreatments and anaesthesia in the dog. III. The effects of haemorrhage during halothane and trichloroethylene anaesthesia. *Brit. J. Anaesth.*, **48**, 411.

ROSENBERG, J. C., MUSSAIN, R., and LENAGHAN, R. (1971). Iso-proterenol and norepinephrine therapy for pulmonary embolus shock. *J. thorac. cardiovasc. Surg.*, **62**, 144.

SAMET, P. (1973). Hemodynamic sequelae of cardiac arrhythmias. *Circulation*, **47**, 399.

SANER, C. A., FOËX, P., ROBERTS, J. G., and BENNETT, M. J. (1975). Methoxyflurane and practolol: a dangerous combination. *Brit. J. Anaesth.*, **47**, 1025.

SEELYE, E. (1973). Anaesthesia for children with congenital heart disease. *Anaesth. Intens. Care*, **1**, 512.

SHAND, D. G. (1975). Propranolol, *New Engl. J. Med.*, **293**, 280.

SHIMOSATO, S., YASUDA, I., KEMMOTSU, O., SHANKS, C., and GAMBLE, C. (1973). Effect of halothane on altered contractility of isolated heart muscle obtained from cats with experimentally produced ventricular hypertrophy and failure. *Brit. J. Anaesth.*, **45**, 2.

SHIMOSATO, S., and ETSTEN, B. E. (1969). Effects of anaesthetic drugs on the heart. A critical review of myocardial contractility and its relationship to haemodynamics. In: *A Decade of Clinical Progress* (Clinical Anaesthesia Series, 3/1969, 60) Ed. Fabian, L. W. Oxford: Blackwell Scientific Publications.

SIEGEL, J. H. (1969). The myocardial contractile state and its role in the response to anaesthesia and surgery. *Anesthesiology*, **30**, 519.

SMITH, N. T., and CORBASCIO, A. N. (1970). The use and misuse of pressor-agents. *Anesthesiology*, **33**, 58.

SOMERS, K., GUNSTAVE, R. F., PATEL, A. K., and D'ARBELA, P. G. (1971). Intravenous diazepam for cardioversion. *Brit. med. J.*, **4**, 13.

STEPHEN, G. W., DAVIE, I. T., and SCOTT, D. B. (1971). Haemodynamic effects of beta-receptor blocking drugs during nitrous oxide/halothane anaesthesia. *Brit. J. Anaesth.*, **43**, 320.

STOELTING, R. K., and GIBBS, P. S. (1973). Hemodynamic effects of morphine and morphine-nitrous oxide in valvular heart disease and coronary artery disease. *Anesthesiology*, **38**, 45.

STOELTING, R. K., and LONGNECKER, D. E. (1972). The effect of right to left shunt on the rate of increase of arterial anaesthetic concentrations. *Anesthesiology*, **36**, 352.

SZIDON, J. P., PIETRA, G. G., and FISHMAN, A. P. (1972). The alveolar capillary membrane and pulmonary oedema. *New Engl. J. Med.*, **286**, 1200.

TARHAN, S., MOFFITT, E. A., LUNDBORG, R. O., and FRYE, R. L. (1971). Hemodynamic and blood-gas effects of "Innovar" in patients with acquired heart disease. *Anesthesiology*, **34**, 250.

TARHAN, S., MOFFITT, E. A., TAYLOR, W. F., and GIULIANI, E. R. (1972). Myocardial infarction after general anaesthesia. *J. Amer. med. Assn.*, **220**, 1451.

THUNG, N., HERZOG, P., CHRISTLIES, I., THOMPSON, W. M., and DAMMANN, J. (1963). The cost of respiratory effort in postoperative cardiac patients. *Circulation*, **28**, 552.

TOPKINS, M. J., and ARTUSIO, J. F. (1964). Myocardial infarction and surgery. *Anesth. Analg. Curr. Res.*, **43**, 716.

TWEED, W. A., MINUCK, M. and MYMIN, D. (1972). Circulatory responses to ketamine anaesthesia. *Anesthesiology*, **37**, 613.

VANIK, P. E., and DAVIS, H. S. (1968). Cardiac arrhythmias during halothane anaesthesia. *Anesth. Analg. Curr. Res.*, **47**, 299.

VILJÖEN, J. F., ESTAFANOUS, F. G., and KELLNER, G. A. (1972). Propranolol and cardiac surgery. *J. thorac. cardiovasc. Surg.*, **64**, 826.

VILJÖEN, J. F., and GINDI, M. Y. (1971). Anaesthesia for coronary artery surgery. *Surg. Clin. N. Amer.*, **51**, 1081.

VINGE, L. N., WYANT, G. M., and LOPEZ, J. F. (1971). Diazepam in cardioversion. *Canad. Anaesth. Soc. J.*, **18**, 166.

WAGNER, G. S., and MCINTOSH, H. D. (1969). The use of drugs in achieving successful D.C. cardioversion. *Progr. cardiovasc. Dis.*, **11**, 431.

WHITE, R. D., and TARHAN, S. (1974). Anaesthetic aspects of cardiac surgery. A review of clinical management. *Anesth. Analg. Curr. Res.*, **53**, 98.

WONG, K. C., MARTIN, W. E., HORNBEIN, T. F., FREUND, F. G., and EVERETT, J. (1973). The cardiovascular effects of morphine sulfate with oxygen and with nitrous oxide in man. *Anesthesiology*, **38**, 542.

WYNANDS, J. E., SHERIDAN, C. A., BATRA, M. S., PALMER, W. H., and SHANKS, J. (1970). Coronary artery disease. *Anesthesiology*, **33**, 260.

Chapter 15

HYPOTENSION IN ANAESTHESIA

THE problem of a patient with a low blood pressure may confront the anaesthetist at any time. Hypotension may be present pre-operatively, it may occur during anaesthesia and surgery, sometimes being deliberately induced by the anaesthetist and finally, the commonest yet least recorded occasion is during the early post-operative period.

PRE-OPERATIVE HYPOTENSION

The absolute value of a patient's immediate pre-operative blood pressure must be considered against the patient's general condition and knowledge, if any, of his previous blood pressure. Thus a "normal" blood pressure may represent hypotension, as may occur following a myocardial infarct in a hypertensive patient, or alternatively, a "normal" blood pressure may be being sustained only by extreme vasoconstriction when the abolition of this compensatory mechanism by anaesthesia will result in a profound fall in pressure.

The induction of anaesthesia in a patient with a naturally low systemic pressure presents no special problems beyond the normal precaution against the too rapid intravenous injection of drugs which are likely to lower it still more.

When the pre-operative hypotension is due to a low filling pressure, either the result of hypovolaemia or of peripheral vasodilatation, steps can be taken to correct this before embarking on anaesthesia. Replacement of the appropriate fluid while monitoring the central venous pressure usually restores the situation to normal. If hypotension is the result of extreme vasodilatation, which may be the sequel to infection or to drug therapy, provided the cardiac output is good and the peripheral tissues well perfused, it may be better to accept a low pressure than to administer vasopressor drugs, remembering that any further fluid losses will have to be promptly replaced.

Where the hypotension is the result of a fixed low-output cardiac disease, which is usually associated with vasoconstriction in the peripheral vessels, the induction of anaesthesia and the consequent peripheral vasodilatation may be fatal, particularly when it is sudden.

HYPOTENSION DURING ANAESTHESIA AND OPERATION

During normal sleep, blood pressure falls. In a small series of patients who had normal blood pressure when awake (Richardson *et al.*, 1964) it was demonstrated that systolic pressures of 90 or 80 mm Hg (12·0 or 10·7 kPa) were normal while asleep. Littler and his colleagues (1975) investigated 18 subjects and found an almost equal fall of about 20 per cent in both systolic and diastolic pressure in normotensive, hypertensive and treated hypertensive groups although they did not elucidate the mechanism of this fall. A blood pressure lower than the pre-operative value might perhaps be considered physiological during anaesthesia. A satisfactory blood pressure is not the cardinal sign of circulatory well-being and it needs to be correlated with other physical signs in an attempt to judge the state of the circulation. The systolic blood pressure is, however, a good index upon which the anaesthetist can calibrate his impression of circulatory change (Prys-Roberts, 1974).

Moderate falls in blood pressure with the body performing its own regulation of distribution of flow are preferable to a blood pressure sustained at an arbitrary level by drugs which alter the distribution of blood flow, often in a deleterious manner.

Surgical stimulation in the early stages of an operation in the lightly anaesthetised patient frequently induces a rise in the systemic pressure, but during abdominal and thoracic surgery a fall in blood pressure may follow various manipulations and this has always been believed to be due to a visceral reflex. A more common cause is obstruction to the flow of blood in the inferior vena cava due to a retractor, a gall-bladder bridge or indirect pressure in the prone position. A reduction in blood volume is, however, probably by far the commonest cause of hypotension. This may be acute and obvious enough to warrant immediate notice but more commonly the loss is either insiduous or concealed. Proper estimation of blood loss, by weighing of the swabs or the colorometric estimation of haemoglobin, added to the sucker loss plus the blood observed on the towels and surgeons' gowns should help prevent this complication. Measurement of the right atrial pressure with a saline manometer connected to a catheter fed from the neck or arm to the superior vena cava is technically easy and will add useful information. Prompt treatment of blood loss is advisable as up to one fifth of the total blood volume may be lost before significant changes in the systemic pressure of an anaesthetised patient are produced. Thus hypotension represents a late stage in the body's reaction to haemorrhage.

The action of drugs and the institution of intermittent positive-pressure ventilation, even if the carbon dioxide level remains normal, can both result in hypotension—this is considered below in greater detail.

Hypotension from a sensitivity reaction due to the injection of a foreign protein is believed to be rare during anaesthesia. There is insufficient information available to permit a dogmatic statement on the subject, but reports of reactions under such conditions are few. An incompatible blood transfusion may even pass unnoticed until the patient recovers consciousness.

Bleeding during Surgery

One of the functions of anaesthesia and the anaesthetist is to provide optimum operating conditions for the surgeon. Blood loss, by obscuring the surgical field, or even by the sheer magnitude of the loss, may make surgery difficult or even impossible and it is a part of good anaesthesia to provide as bloodless a field as possible. In the past this has too often been considered under the heading of "induced hypotension". Eckenhoff (1966) has described the term "deliberate hypotension" as being both misleading and poorly descriptive, because in the production of a bloodless field a specific degree of hypotension is not required, nor is ganglionic blockade always necessary. It also obscures the concept that much blood loss is venous in origin and he therefore suggests the use of the term "circulatory control" to cover all those points of technique which are used to ensure a good operating field.

The factors which give rise to increased wound bleeding usually result in either venous engorgement or an increased cardiac output.

(a) **Hypercapnia.**—In this instance, the raised carbon dioxide tension increases both the blood pressure and cardiac output by stimulation of the sympathetic nervous system whilst the capillaries are dilated by a local effect of the carbon dioxide on the vessel wall itself.

(b) **Hypoxia.**—A low arterial oxygen tension produces vasodilatation and chemoreceptor stimulation increases the cardiac output.

Anaesthesia tends to produce deleterious alterations in the lung ventilation-perfusion ratios, changes which are accentuated by reduction in blood pressure or cardiac output. The anaesthetist must compensate for these alterations, if necessary with controlled ventilation with an increased oxygen content of the inspired mixture.

(c) **Respiratory obstruction.**—Besides the effect on blood oxygen and carbon dioxide levels the alterations in intrathoracic pressure can result in a raised central venous pressure. With spontaneous respiration any resistance to expiration can increase venous pressure and the amount of bleeding.

(d) **Improper posture** is the most important factor in promoting venous bleeding (see below).

(e) **Inadequate analgesia** results in a raised cardiac output as a consequence of peripheral somatic stimulation causing an increase in catecholamines.

(f) **Ether and cyclopropane** both cause secretion of catecholamines and a raised cardiac output.

(g) **Very deep anaesthesia,** now seldom used, to the point of myocardial depression produces hypoxia and venous engorgement.

(h) **Certain drugs** employed in anaesthesia may produce tachycardia (gallamine; atropine) or cause hypertension (pancuronium, pentazocine, ketamine) both of which may increase surgical blood loss.

Reduction in Bleeding during Surgery

In seeking to reduce the amount of bleeding during surgery the first principle is to avoid those factors, discussed above, which give rise to an increase in haemorrhage.

The good anaesthetist thus provides adequate unobstructed ventilatory exchange, a light but fully analgesic anaesthetic avoiding those agents which provoke catecholamine secretion in a patient who is properly postured. Larson (1964), in an excellent review, comments that induced hypotension must never be considered a panacea for indifferent anaesthesia but rather that anaesthesia must first be perfect in all respects and hypotension induced as a complementary measure only.

Further reduction of blood supply to the operative field can then be produced in a number of different ways.

(a) *Tourniquet.*—Obviously restricted in its application but producing complete ischaemia for a limited period.

(b) *Use of local vasoconstrictor solutions.*—Used mainly for skin infiltration before operation (thyroidectomy) or topically, during eye or ear, nose and throat operations.

(c) *The use of induced hypotension.*

INDUCED HYPOTENSION AND CIRCULATORY CONTROL

The reduction of blood pressure and cardiac output must be considered together because of their interdependence. The blood pressure can be reduced by lowering the systemic vascular resistance but if the patient remains flat the cardiac output is usually unchanged or may even rise due to the removal of the afterload on the heart. Of itself, this hypotension will not necessarily produce a good operating field, but if the part being operated upon is elevated, blood flow and loss is reduced.

Enderby (1954b) stressed the importance of taking into account the effect on the brain of any tilt away from the horizontal. For example, the blood pressure is usually measured in the arm, with the limb on a level with the heart; if the patient is tilted into the head-up position the pressure in the arm may remain the same, but the effect of the weight of the column of blood must be taken into account on both the head and the feet. Thus, in this position, the pressure in the feet may be 180 mm Hg (24·0 kPa) or more yet in the head it may be only 80 mm Hg (10·7 kPa).

As a general rule the difference in pressure in a particular area may be calculated on the basis of allowing + or − 2 mm Hg (0·25 kPa) for every one inch (2·5 cm) vertically below or above the level of the heart. This is one reason why posture has come to play such an important part in reducing bleeding during surgery. If the operation site is raised above the level of the heart the effect of gravity reduces the pressure in the arterial system and also empties the venous channels.

This may reduce bleeding insufficiently and the optimum operating conditions are only produced if the hypotension is accompanied by a reduction in cardiac output.

A reduction in cardiac output is achieved by:
(1) decreasing cardiac preload by a combination of reduction in venous tone and posture;
(2) decreasing cardiac contractility;
(3) blocking sympathetic stimulation;
(4) utilising mechanical and chemical changes of controlled ventilation (Blackburn et al., 1973).

Reduction in Venous Tone

This can be produced by specific ganglionic blockade, by spinal or epidural analgesia or by the effects of some anaesthetic drugs. Paralysis occurs in the arteriolar resistance vessels leading to a drop in systemic vascular resistance, but more importantly paralysis occurs in the capacitance vessels on the venous side and blood can be made to pool in different parts of the body. The decreased filling pressure of the heart then leads to a reduction in the cardiac output.

The basic mechanism of this technique results in a vascular tree which is unresponsive to the effects of low cardiac output or haemorrhage. With dilated inelastic capacitance vessels quite small blood losses can produce large alterations in the filling pressure of the heart, and thus the cardiac output. More prompt action is required than in the normal patient to raise the filling pressure by alteration in posture or by blood transfusion in the event of haemorrhage.

1. Subarachnoid and epidural block.—For many years some anaesthetists and surgeons have favoured "high" spinal analgesia not only for the excellent muscular relaxation but also for the relatively bloodless field which ensues. A "high" spinal extending from the first thoracic segment downward leads to total sympathetic paralysis.

The technique and choice of drug is discussed elsewhere (Chapter 36).

The mechanisms whereby spinal and epidural block produce a fall in blood pressure are similar because both block pre-ganglionic sympathetic fibres.

Although continuous epidural analgesia is technically more difficult, it greatly extends the usefulness of the technique.

Normally the patient is anaesthetised before the block is induced because the position and the fall in blood pressure produce considerable discomfort. Also, as inadequate respiration and hypoxia are so dangerous during hypotension, respiration is usually controlled.

Immediately after the injection the patient is turned on his back in a fairly steep Trendelenburg position until the systolic pressure has fallen to 80–90 mm Hg (10·7–12·0 kPa) and then the patient is suitably postured.

Two facts sometimes adduced in favour of the technique are that with suitable analgesic concentration only the sympathetic fibres can be blocked and secondly, that compensatory vasoconstriction and reduction in bleeding occurs in those vessels whose sympathetic supply is not blocked. In practice it seems logical, when other methods of vascular relaxation are available, to use the techniques of spinal and epidural analgesia only when surgery is being performed on those areas which are rendered analgesic by the block.

A clinical impression exists that epidural analgesia produces a reduction in bleeding due to the qualities of the block itself and this belief often accounts for surgical requests for epidural analgesia in those patients in whom induced hypotension is contra-indicated. Donald (1969) showed that in pelvic floor surgery induced hypotension produced a highly significant reduction in blood loss, irrespective of whether respiration was spontaneous or controlled, and that this reduction was similar whether the hypotension was produced with trimetaphan or by epidural block. As epidural analgesia always produced some fall in blood pressure as compared to the standard technique, it was impossible to isolate the effect of the epidural alone. In two further papers, a series by Bond (1969) has no correlation between mean operative systolic blood pressure and blood loss, while Moir (1968) did not quote blood pressures. This emphasises the many factors which influence surgical haemorrhage and the difficulty in controlling these variables in an experimental study.

2. **Drug induced.**—Reduction in venous tone may be produced by sympathetic ganglion-blocking drugs, whose action may be short or long, or by drugs which cause peripheral vasodilatation by direct action.

Opinions differ about the technique for induced hypotension by ganglion blockade. There are those who recommend posturing the patient for the surgical operation—even though this necessitates the use of the head-up position—before giving any hypotensive drug, and there are others who induce vasodilatation in the horizontal position and only make use of posture should it be needed to reduce the cardiac output. The latter technique is safer and to be preferred, and should normally be combined with an initial small dose of the hypotensive drug to assess the reaction of the patient.

Young, normotensive people are more resistant to induced hypotension than the aged or those with hypertension. An initial fall in blood pressure may be quickly followed by a rise to the normal level in the former; further doses of ganglion-blocking agent may then have little effect even with the aid of posture. For such people halothane or controlled respiration can assist in controlling the level of blood pressure. It is essential to have some reliable method of measuring the blood pressure and most anaesthetists, in the absence of direct intra-arterial manometry, prefer the use of the oscillotonometer. A reliable intravenous infusion is also essential.

Hexamethonium is usually given initially in a small intravenous test dose (10 mg) in the horizontal position before proceeding with the main injection, as occasionally a patient will be found to be hypersensitive, in which case the hypotension will be profound. Provided this is not so an intravenous dose of 25–50 mg should be given. Thereafter these doses can be repeated after five minutes if the extent of the fall in systolic pressure is not sufficient. Enderby and Pelmore (1951) have described how in fit, young, healthy adults, it may be difficult to induce or maintain hypotension with hexamethonium on account of a tachycardia which often follows the use of this drug.

Pentolinium, or pentamethylene-1:5 bis-(1-methylpyrrolidinium hydrogen tartrate), has about five times the activity of hexamethonium bromide (Wien and Mason, 1953) and a longer duration of action. The initial intravenous dose varies from 3 to 20 mg depending upon the age and physical state of the patient. Enderby (1954a) notes that pentolinium causes a slow fall in blood pressure, that the hypotension it produces is more easily potentiated by posture and controlled respiration than that of hexamethonium, and that a single dose is effective for up to 45 minutes and rarely leads to tachycardia. But in fact the blood pressure may take several hours to return to normal.

Trimetaphan, one of the short-acting thiophanium group of drugs, has a marked ganglion-blocking effect (Randall *et al.*, 1949) but it also has a direct vasodilator action in dogs (McCubbin and Page, 1952), while its intravenous injection leads to the release of histamine both in man (Payne, 1956) and in dogs (Randall *et al.*, 1949). Histamine release could account for some of the hypotension that trimetaphan produces. The extremely short length of action of this drug is believed to be partly due to its destruction by the enzyme cholinesterase. It can be given either as a continuous steady infusion (1 mg/ml) or by the intermittent injection of 2·5 to 5 mg. The latter technique has the small advantage that it obviates the use of a drip and also allows each successive dose to wear off before the next one is repeated. One of the principal disadvantages of the continuous drip technique is that a "base-line" may be reached in which the systolic pressure will fall no further unless the posture or blood volume of the patient are altered. If the drug is then continuously infused, the final recovery of blood pressure will be very much prolonged. It is important, therefore, periodically to stop the infusion and check that the blood pressure does soon start to rise again. Rarely it may appear from the rate of administration that the total dose of trimetaphan is likely to exceed 1 g due to the patient's resistance. Prolonged neuromuscular blockade has been described as following this dose of trimetaphan and if it appears that the patient is probably resistant (usually due to tachycardia) a β-blocker should be added or a change made to another drug.

Sodium nitroprusside.—Although sodium nitroprusside has been known for over 100 years and its basic pharmacology since 1930, it has only recently been used clinically. Its primary action is to produce smooth muscle relaxation. The onset is rapid—within 90 seconds—and its action evanescent. These features have made it popular both for induced hypotension in anaesthesia and for reduction in afterload in diseased or post-operative hearts (Palmer and Lasseter, 1975). Its very profound effect means, however, that it is a drug not to be used by the inexperienced. Verner (1974) has detailed the theory and practice of its use.

Sodium nitroprusside is normally given as an intravenous infusion of 0·01 per cent solution. In an adult between 20–50 mg are usually required in the first hour. Cyanide accumulation leading to death has been reported in patients who have received large doses and for this reason McDowall *et al.* (1974) have suggested limiting the dose to 1·6 mg/kg/hour, while Merrifield and Blundell (1974) suggest a total dose not exceeding 3 mg/kg and Davies and colleagues (1975) a total dose not exceeding 3·5 mg/kg.

Larger doses have usually been given in an attempt to lower the pressure in a fit adult who has responded by producing a tachycardia. This is better treated with 0·5 mg increments of propranolol and once the tachycardia is controlled, the requirements for nitroprusside will be within the safe limits.

Sodium nitroprusside is contra-indicated in liver failure, Leber's optic atrophy and patients with low plasma vitamin B_{12} concentrations (Vesey *et al.*, 1974).

Halothane.—Halothane is now a commonly used adjuvant in various hypotensive techniques, where it is used to achieve a degree of fine control or to potentiate the action of other agents. While initially a number of mechanisms were described as being responsible for its hypotensive action, it is now believed that myocardial depression is its predominant effect with little overall change in systemic vascular resistance (Hughes, 1973), although distribution is altered. The different effects reported earlier of halothane on the cardiovascular system may have been the consequence of variations in the carbon dioxide tension (Weaver, 1971).

Sympathetic Stimulation and Tachycardia

Tachycardia can be a troublesome complication of drug-induced hypotension particularly in younger fit patients in whom the tachycardia may be sufficient to prevent much fall in the blood pressure. The exact mechanism of this response is not clear. It may represent an attenuation of vagal control by the ganglion blocker or more probably be the result of carotid and aortic baroreceptor stimulation. Other causative factors are atropine premedication, gallamine used as a muscle relaxant, surgical stimulus under too light anaesthesia, and carbon dioxide retention or hypoxia. In a healthy patient the tachycardia may be troublesome only in that it prevents much fall in the blood pressure. In the presence of coronary artery disease or certain cardiac diseases—when induced hypotension is probably contra-indicated anyway—tachycardia in the face of a lowered blood pressure may be dangerous and must be promptly controlled.

Halothane may control tachycardia and facilitate the reduction of the blood pressure in the middle-aged and elderly but in the young and particularly in children the cardiac rate can only be controlled by the use of β-blockade.

β-Adrenergic Blockade During Hypotensive Anaesthesia

Propranolol (Hellewell and Potts, 1966; Hewitt *et al.*, 1967) was the first drug used in this way but practolol which has a longer duration of action and is more cardioselective is now often preferred (Enderby, 1974). In old patients (55 years or more) these drugs are seldom necessary and when used the dose should be small (propranolol 0·25–0·50 mg; practolol 0·5–1·0 mg). There is an increasing requirement for these drugs in younger patients and the dose is increased to 1·0–2·5 mg, repeated as necessary. In children and young adults below the age of 25, Enderby (1974) has recommended that both drugs (propranolol 0·035 mg/kg and practolol 0·14 mg/kg) be given slowly intravenously before the production of ganglionic blockade. Labetalol, which possesses both alpha- and beta-adrenergic blocking properties, has also been used (Scott *et al.*, 1978).

Controlled Ventilation and Hypotensive Anaesthesia

During hypotensive anaesthesia in a 30° head-up posture, Eckenhoff and his colleagues (1963) demonstrated a markedly increased respiratory physiological dead space with values up to 80 per cent of the tidal volume. Similar results were shown in dogs by Leigh and Tyrrell (1969). Also, if the cardiac output is reduced, the effect of any degree of pulmonary venous admixture to produce a decrease in arterial oxygen tension is increased.

For these reasons, meticulous attention to arterial oxygenation is necessary, utilising increased inspired oxygen concentrations and some authors consider hypotensive anaesthesia an indication for controlled ventilation. This has the advantage that the mean airway pressure can be varied to provide a fine control over the cardiac output and the systemic arterial pressure (Conway, 1975). The level of carbon dioxide also affects myocardial function and hypocapnia is associated with a reduction in cardiac output (Prys-Roberts *et al.*, 1967).

Sellery and colleagues (1973) reporting on hypotensive anaesthesia specifically for neurosurgery consider spontaneous respiration preferable because hypocarbia, with its deleterious effect on cerebral and coronary blood flows, is prevented and the respiratory pattern can be monitored. Abnormalities in respiratory pattern, gasping or Cheyne-Stokes respiration may indicate cerebral ischaemia. These authors do, however, continuously monitor blood gas levels.

Dangers of Induced Hypotension

The most serious complications are those involving the brain, heart and kidneys. While the circulation to these organs is usually capable of adaptation to alterations in blood pressure and cardiac output, these compensatory mechanisms may fall down in the face of abnormally low perfusion pressures or in the presence of diseased unreactive blood vessels. Autoregulation of the cerebral blood vessels becomes inadequate when the mean arterial pressure falls below 60–70 mm Hg (8·0–9·3 kPa) and cerebral blood flow declines rapidly below these levels (Locke *et al.*, 1971). The level at which cerebral ischaemia becomes manifest depends on the patient's previous blood pressure. In conscious man, signs of ischaemia (confusion, etc.) appeared at mean arterial pressure of 29 mm Hg (3·9 kPa) in normotensive subjects, but at mean arterial pressure of

90 mm Hg (12·0 kPa) in patients with severe hypertension (Finnerty *et al.*, 1954). Cerebral thrombosis is sometimes encountered, and this may either prolong unconsciousness, appear as a hemiplegia, or even develop after consciousness has been regained. Thrombosis of the central artery of the retina, leading to unilateral blindness, may also occur. These cerebrovascular complications are almost all confined to patients with signs of arteriosclerosis, and the few in normal patients only occur when excessive degrees of hypotension (i.e. 60 mm Hg (8·0 kPa) and below) have been produced.

Again, Bedford (1955) has drawn attention to the possible psychological changes that may occur in the elderly after the use of this technique. Unfortunately, such changes are known to occur even in the absence of hypotension, when old people undergo major surgical operations, and therefore it is difficult to assess the precise part played by the low blood pressure.

Coronary thrombosis has been reported but the fact that the generalised vasodilatation reduces the work of the heart will in some measure compensate for any reduction in blood flow. This may however be offset by the development of a tachycardia. In the presence of any doubt about the state of the myocardium, the ECG should be monitored continuously.

Oliguria suggests a renal lesion, but one of the fundamental points that must be borne in mind when assessing the complications of hypotension is that these lesions may arise from other causes such as the surgical trauma, haemorrhage, or the anaesthetic itself. The complete absence of figures on a well-controlled series of cases with and without induced hypotension makes it difficult to arrive at any definite conclusions. If the patient has been observed to have an excessive drop in blood pressure during hypotensive anaesthesia and then shows signs of a delayed return to consciousness it is advisable to assume that he is suffering from cerebral oedema and institute appropriate treatment.

Reactionary haemorrhage may arise if particular care is not taken to ligate any vessel seen to be bleeding; the use of induced hypotension does not excuse the surgeon the task of tying all bleeding-points, but by removing the persistent ooze it makes this work much easier.

McLaughlin (1961), using meticulous haemostasis at the time of operation, reports an incidence of only one reactionary haemorrhage in 1,000 cases of controlled hypotensive anaesthesia.

Much depends on the rate of rise of the blood pressure in the post-operative period. In some cases only a transient fall in systemic pressure is required at particular stages of an operation as during resection of coarctation of the aorta or ligation of a big patent ductus arteriosus. Much more commonly, the beneficial effects are required for some time afterwards and a sustained fall in blood pressure with a gentle protracted return to normal values reduces the incidence of reactionary haemorrhage and haematoma formation.

Indications for Induced Hypotension

In one sentence the indication for induced hypotension has been described as where the advantages are of certain benefit and likely to outweigh the accepted risks (Gillies, 1959). That is to say that there are no absolute indications. McLaughlin (1966) has emphasised that the technique needs to be considered in relation to each patient and that both surgeon and anaesthetist must understand the implications of the technique and that if either feels incapable of mastering these, hypotension should not be induced.

The claimed benefits of induced hypotension are a reduced blood loss, thus avoiding the dangers of massive blood transfusion, a more accurate surgical technique, and in cases where large raw areas are produced, as in reconstructive surgery, better wound healing. Cancer surgery is an indication as any improvement in operating conditions may directly benefit the patient. At one time or another every operation has been advocated as suitable for induced hypotension but the decision must be made consciously each time.

Contra-indications to Induced Hypotension

Most contra-indications are not particularly well substantiated and depend on logical thought rather than positive evidence.

Any patient with a history of coronary ischaemia, hypertension or cerebrovascular disease is unsuitable for this technique. Sudden or profound changes in blood pressure are unwise in patients with obvious disease of any vital organ. Diabetes, asthma and pre-existing neurological disease have been cited as contra-indications.

Conditions which interfere with the transport of oxygen, such as anaemia, respiratory insufficiency, hypovolaemia and cardiac failure, are all contra-indications. Obstructive airway disease is probably also a contra-indication as the high inflation pressures required may severely reduce the cardiac output. Due to the need for special post-operative care (see below) absence of good immediate post-operative supervision may well be a contra-indication.

Post-operative Care after Induced Hypotension

To avoid the danger of reactionary haemorrhage, blood pressure is usually allowed to rise gently, although the return to consciousness normally causes some elevation. If the cardiac output and blood pressure are low, pain and restlessness may increase the body oxygen demand above the level of supply, a situation which is aggravated by respiratory obstruction or lung dysfunction in a patient breathing air.

With a vascular system still unresponsive to haemorrhage quite small blood losses will result in acute drops in blood pressure. Blood loss and replacement need to be as carefully monitored and controlled, using central venous pressure measurement if necessary, as they were during the operation.

Combining the results of 16 papers representing 13,264 cases of induced hypotension, 110 deaths (97·3 per cent of the total deaths) were reported to have occurred in the post-operative period (Larson, 1964).

Discussion

The arguments for and against induced hypotension (Enderby, 1958; Armstrong Davison, 1958) have continued unabated since its introduction. Many feel that this technique only adds an unjustifiable risk to the patient's life and intellectual capacity. Others argue that in skilled hands it carries no great risk. Wyman (1953) reported on its use in 1,000 patients with 5 deaths. Two were believed to be due to the patient's disease and three to faulty technique. If the technique is understood he claims it should not offer any additional risks at an operation. Larson (1964) in a comprehensive review of controlled hypotension points out that though the complication risk is higher than normal, in skilled hands a very high degree of proficiency with a low morbidity can be obtained. Among the factors which he lists as militating against success are inexperience with the technique and lack of teamwork between surgeon and anaesthetist. The best results are obtained by careful selection of patients, control of ventilation, sustained gentle changes in blood pressure, the careful maintenance of blood volume and adequate post-operative care.

One of the great difficulties in assessing results is that like is not always compared with like. Ideally, we should consider operations with and without hypotension performed by the same surgeon and anaesthetist, using the same technique for blood loss measurement and replacement, but, as was discussed at the start of this chapter, the aim of the technique is to produce good operating conditions by reducing haemorrhage and with so many other factors influencing wound bleeding there is no constant relationship between blood pressure and the amount of haemorrhage. As Eckenhoff (1966) has pointed out, there is very little data on the surgical benefits of hypotension so it is hard to know how much one can offset an increased morbidity.

Figures for mortality and morbidity need to be accepted with caution. If some of the early large series are examined in the light of current thought about technique, about monitoring of blood loss and blood replacement, about the relationship of flow and pressure, about proper selection of cases and post-operative care, then one may arrive at quite different conclusions from the original authors.

Eckenhoff and his colleagues (1969) have compared 18 patients undergoing hypotension with 18 patients operated on at normal pressures and have been unable to show any change in brain function as demonstrated by psychometric testing. This study was on young patients but Rollason et al. (1968) reached a similar conclusion in a group of elderly men undergoing prostatectomy. In another comparison involving 301 patients Eckenhoff and Rich (1966) demonstrated an appreciable saving in blood loss with no death directly attributable to deliberate hypotension.

Later, Rollason et al. (1971) compared mental function assessed by psychometric tests in elderly patients who were given spinal anaesthesia with or without a vasopressor to prevent hypotension and could find no difference.

In a recent review Lindop (1975) pooled data using an incidence of non-fatal complications of 1 in 39, and of fatal complications of 1 in 167 cases, although adding a rider that no conclusion could be drawn as to whether these complications were directly caused by the hypotensive technique. However, unreported personal series by anaesthetists with much experience of the technique suggest a low complication rate is attainable.

The final assessment and decision on the use of induced hypotension must rest with a balance of the relative risks and merits to a particular patient. The size of that risk depends on the state of that patient's vascular tree, the degree of hypotension attained, and the skill of the administrator. It would be unwise however, to dismiss completely a most useful adjunct to the anaesthetist's armamentarium, but it is imperative to proceed with circumspection.

POST-OPERATIVE HYPOTENSION

One of the most illogical situations in present day anaesthesia is the immense amount of expert skill and care that is lavished upon the patient in the operating theatre, often only to be abruptly abandoned the moment the anaesthetic is stopped. During a period when a rapid physiological transition is taking place, the patient may be submitted to major alteration in posture and environment and transported to some far corner of the hospital where, although observed for the gross complication, he is rarely tested for the earliest premonitory signs of them (*Lancet*, 1958).

Hypotension in the post-operative period is common. Its occurrence should lead to a careful appraisal of the patient's circulation (see pp. 509 and 659) and the appropriate therapy instituted.

Probably the two commonest causes of hypotension are hypovolaemia and the residual action of anaesthetic agents—the two frequently combining. The amount of blood lost is frequently underestimated and in the event of post-operative hypotension the blood loss and replacement figures should be re-examined, consideration also being given to concealed losses, and the central venous pressure measured. Most patients respond to correct replacement therapy although the residual action of drugs such as halothane or chlorproma-zine may result in a low pressure despite a normal blood volume. In this case, when oligaemia has been treated or excluded, moderate hypotension can be safely treated expectantly by keeping the patient flat or by raising the foot of the bed. Hypotension may be precipitated if the patient is rolled over onto his side or sat up prematurely before the return of his vascular control.

Myocardial insufficiency due to cardiac disease will produce hypotension secondary to a low cardiac output, while quite severe hypotension may follow an operation and anaesthetic when a patient fails to compensate by the normal output of adrenocortical hormones (see Chapter 40). This is particularly liable to happen after previous treatment with cortisone or related steroids, or it may occur in patients who have been suffering from prolonged or severe disease.

Unrelieved pain will cause hypotension, but before administering potenti-ally hypotensive drugs other causes of hypotension should be eliminated. The essentials of post-operative care therefore are the proper relief of pain, the correct replacement of fluid and the ensuring that respiration, both oxygenation and CO_2 elimination, is adequate.

A condition termed "cyclopropane shock" used to be seen following spon-taneous respiration under cyclopropane anaesthesia when hypercarbia was severe. When the carbon dioxide was eliminated in the post-operative period the artificially sustained blood pressure fell. It is possible that a similar condi-tion may be seen after closed-circuit halothane anaesthesia with spontaneous ventilation.

REFERENCES

BEDFORD, P. D. (1955). Adverse cerebral effects of anaesthesia on old people. *Lancet*, **2**, 259.

BLACKBURN, J. P., CONWAY, C. M., DAVIES, R. M., ENDERBY, G. E. H., EDRIDGE, A. W., LEIGH, J. M., LINDOP, M. J., PHILLIPS, C. D., and STRICKLAND, D. A. P. (1973). Valsalva responses and systolic time intervals during anaesthesia and induced hypotension. *Brit. J. Anaesth.*, **45**, 704.

BOND, A. G. (1969). Conduction anaesthesia, blood pressure and haemorrhage. *Brit. J. Anaesth.*, **41**, 942.

BROMAGE, P. R. (1967). Physiology and pharmacology of epidural analgesia. *Anesthesiology*, **28**, 592.

CONWAY, C. M. (1975). Haemodynamic effects of pulmonary ventilation. *Brit. J. Anaesth.*, **47**, 761.

DAVIES, D. W., GREISS, L., KADAR, D., and STEWARD, D. J. (1975). Sodium nitroprusside in children. Observations on metabolism during normal and abnormal responses. *Canad. Anaesth. Soc, J.*, **22**, 553.

DAVISON, M. H. A. (1958). The disadvantages of controlled hypotension in surgery. *Brit. med. Bull.*, **11**, 52.

DONALD, J. R. (1969). The effect of anaesthesia, hypotension and epidural analgesia on blood loss in surgery for pelvic floor repair. *Brit. J. Anaesth.*, **41**, 155.

ECKENHOFF, J. E. (1966). Circulatory control in the surgical patient. *Ann. roy. Coll. Surg.*, **39**, 67.

ECKENHOFF, J. E., CROMPTON, J. R., LARSON, A., and DAVIES, R. M. (1969). Assessment of the cerebral effects of deliberate hypotension by psychological measurements. *Lancet*, **2**, 711.

ECKENHOFF, J. E., ENDERBY, G. E. H., LARSON, A., EDRIDGE, A., and JUDEVINE, D. E. (1963). Pulmonary gas exchange during deliberate hypotension. *Brit. J. Anaesth.*, **35**, 750.

ECKENHOFF, J. E., and RICH, J. C. (1966). Clinical experiences with deliberate hypotension. *Anesth. Analg. Curr. Res.*, **45**, 21.

ENDERBY, G. E. H. (1954a). Pentolinium tartrate in controlled hypotension. *Lancet*, **2**, 1097.

ENDERBY, G. E. H. (1954b). Postural ischaemia and blood pressure. *Lancet*, **1**, 185.

ENDERBY, G. E. H. (1958). The advantages of controlled hypotension in surgery. *Brit. med. Bull.*, **14**, 49.

ENDERBY, G. E. H. (1974). Pharmacological blockade. *Postgrad. med. J.*, **50**, 572.

ENDERBY, G. E. H., and PELMORE, J. F. (1951). Controlled hypotension and postural ischaemia to reduce bleeding in surgery. Review of 250 cases. *Lancet*, **1**, 663.

FINNERTY, F. A., WITKINS, L., and FAZEKAS, J. F. (1954). Cerebral hemodynamics during cerebral ischaemia induced by acute hypotension. *J. clin. Invest.*, **33**, 1227.

GILLIES, J. (1959). In: *General Anaesthesia*, p. 55. Ed. by Evans, F. T. and Gray, T. C. London: Butterworth.

HELLEWELL, J., and POTTS, M. W. (1966). Propranolol during controlled hypotension. *Brit. J. Anaesth.*, **38**, 794.

HEWITT, P. B., LORD, P. W., and THORNTON, H. L. (1967). Propranolol in hypotensive anaesthesia. *Anaesthesia*, **22**, 82.

HUGHES, R. (1973). Haemodynamic effects of halothane in dogs. *Brit. J. Anaesth.*, **45**, 416.

Lancet (1958). Post-operative hypotension (Annotation). **1**, 575.

LARSON, A. G. (1964). Deliberate hypotension. *Anesthesiology*, **25**, 682.

LEIGH, J. M., and TYRRELL, M. F. (1969). Some haemodynamic effects of induced hypotension in dogs. In: *Progress in Anaesthesiology* (Proc. IVth World Congr. of Anaesthesiologists). Ed. by T. B. Bolton, R. Bryce Smith, M. K. Sykes, G. B. Gillet, and A. L. Revell. Amsterdam: Excerpta Medica.

LINDOP, M. J. (1975). Complications and morbidity of controlled hypotension. *Brit. J. Anaesth.*, **47**, 799.

LITTLER, W. A., HONOUR, A. J., CARTER, R. D., and SLEIGHT, P. (1975). Sleep and blood pressure. *Brit. med. J.*, **3**, 346.

LOCKE, G. E., YASHON, D., and HUNT, W. E. (1971). Cerebral tissue lactate in trimetaphan induced hypotension. *Amer. J. Surg.*, **122**, 818.

MCCUBBIN, J. W., and PAGE, I. H. (1952). Nature of hypotensive action of thiophanium derivative (Ro 2-222) in dogs. *J. Pharmacol. exp. Ther.*, **105**, 437.

MCDOWALL, D. G., KEANEY, N. P., TURNER, J. M., LANE, J. R., and OKUDA, Y. (1974). The toxicity of sodium nitroprusside. *Brit. J. Anaesth.*, **46**, 327.

MCLAUGHLIN, C. R. (1961). Hypotensive anaesthesia in plastic surgery: a surgeon's view. *Brit. J. plast. Surg.*, **14**, 39.

MCLAUGHLIN, C. R. (1966). Hypotensive anesthesia. A surgeon's view. *Anesthesiology*, **27**, 239.

MERRIFIELD, A. J. and BLUNDELL, M. D. (1974). Toxicity of sodium nitroprusside. *Brit. J. Anaesth.*, **46**, 324.

MOIR, D. D. (1968). Blood loss during major vaginal surgery. *Brit. J. Anaesth.*, **40**, 233.

PALMER, R. F., and LASSETER, K. C. (1975). Drug therapy: sodium nitroprusside. *New Engl. J. Med.*, **292**(6), 294.

PAYNE, J. P. (1956). Histamine release during controlled hypotension with Arfonad. *Proc. World Congress of Anesthesiologists, 1955*, p. 180. Minneapolis: Burgess Pub. Co.

PRYS-ROBERTS, C. (1974). Editorial. *Anesthesiology*, **40**, 1.

PRYS-ROBERTS, C., KELMAN, G. R., GREENBAUM, R., and ROBINSON, R. H. (1967). Circulatory influences of artificial ventilation during nitrous oxide anaesthesia in man. II. Results. *Brit. J. Anaesth.*, **39**, 533.

RANDALL, L. O., PETERSEN, W. G., and LEHMANN, G. (1949). The ganglionic blocking action of thiophanium derivatives. *J. Pharmacol. exp. Ther.*, **97**, 48.

RICHARDSON, D. W., HONOUR, H. J., FENTON, G. W., STOTT, F. N., and PICKERING, G. W. (1964). Variation in arterial pressure throughout day and night. *Clin. Sci.*, **26**, 445.

ROLLASON, W. N., ROBERTSON, G. S., and CORDINER, C. M. (1968). Effect of hypotensive anaesthesia on mental function in the elderly. *Brit. J. Anaesth.*, **40**, 477.

ROLLASON, W. N., ROBERTSON, G. S., CORDINER, C. M., and HALL, D. J. (1971). A comparison of mental function in relation to hypotensive and normotensive anaesthesia in the elderly. *Brit. J. Anaesth.*, **43**, 561.

SCOTT, D. B., BUCKLEY, F. P., LITTLEWOOD, D. G., MACRAE, W. R., ARTHUR, G. R., and DRUMMOND, G. B. (1978). Circulatory effects of labetalol during halothane anaesthesia. *Anaesthesia*, **33**, 145.

SELLERY, G. R., AITKEN, R. K., and DRAKE, C. C. (1973). Anaesthesia for intracranial aneurysms with hypotension and spontaneous respiration. *Canad. Anaesth. Soc. J.*, **20**, 468.

VERNER, I. R. (1974). Sodium nitroprusside: theory and practice. *Postgrad. med. J.*, **50**, 576.

VESEY, C. J., COLE, P. V., LINNELL, J. C., and WILSON, J. (1974). Some metabolic effects of sodium nitroprusside in man. *Brit. med. J.*, **2**, 140.

WEAVER, P. C. (1971). A study of the cardiovascular effects of halothane. *Ann. roy. Coll. Surg.*, **49**, 114.

WIEN, R., and MASON, D. F. J. (1953). The pharmacological actions of a series of phenyl alkane p-ω-bis-(trialkylammonium) compounds. *Brit. J. Pharmacol.*, **8**, 306.

WYMAN, J. B. (1953). Discussion on hypotension during anaesthesia. *Proc. roy. Soc. Med.*, **46**, 605.

Chapter 16

EXTRACORPOREAL CIRCULATION AND HYPOTHERMIA

The Place of Hypothermia and Extracorporeal Circulation in Cardiac and Vascular Surgery

SOME operations can be performed on the heart or arterial system without the need for any special ancillary technique. Ligation of patent ductus arteriosus or femoral disobliteration is carried out under normal anaesthesia and mitral valvotomy is performed on the beating heart which continues to supply the circulation throughout the operation.

Other operations may interrupt the circulation either in its entirety as in a heart operation, or locally as in thoracic aneurysm, for periods which, in the absence of some support technique, would lead to the death of an organ or of the whole patient. The techniques used are:

1. **Simple hypothermia.** Body temperature is reduced to approximately 30° C resulting in a 25 per cent decrease in metabolic rate which enables whole body or organ circulatory interruption to be prolonged proportionately.

2. **Deep or profound hypothermia.** Body temperature reduced to approximately 15–20° C in a technique which usually necessitates some form of extracorporeal circulation and which allows much longer circulatory arrest.

3. **Bypass techniques.**
   (*a*) Simple bypass—the temporary insertion of a conduit, e.g. into the carotid artery, while a segment supplying a vital organ is disobliterated.
   (*b*) Extracorporeal circulation—
   i. without a gas-exchange apparatus (e.g. left atriofemoral bypass in surgery of the descending thoracic aorta).
   ii. with a pump oxygenator with or without some degree of hypothermia (e.g. most open heart surgery).

HYPOTHERMIA

Introduction and Historical Note

During hypothermia the body temperature is reduced below its normal value so that therapeutic use can be made of the concomitant reduction in metabolic rate. Hypothermia is described as mild (35–28° C), moderate (27–21° C) and deep or profound (below 20° C) and is further divisible into surface cooling and core cooling—the latter implying the use of some extracorporeal circuit.

Cold therapy for a variety of conditions attracted the intermittent attention of physicians from the 15th century onwards until in 1940 Smith and Fay reported on the use of general hypothermia in the treatment of malignant disease. This followed their histological findings that cold led to a regression and degeneration of neoplastic tissue. The importance of this contribution did not lie in its effectiveness as a cancer cure but rather it revealed the essential secret of hypothermia, namely that sedation or anaesthesia (including muscle relaxants) must be used to control shivering.

In 1950, Bigelow and his colleagues demonstrated survival in experimental dogs after 15 minutes circulatory arrest at 20–25° C and this observation was applied clinically by Lewis and Tauffic (1953) during the correction of an atrial septal defect. Surface hypothermia became widely applied in cardiac surgery but its usefulness was limited by the incidence of ventricular fibrillation at temperatures below 28° C. The safe temperature limit of 30° C allows only ten minutes of circulatory interruption which restricts the surgery to easily repaired defects. Despite experiments with various drugs to depress myocardial irritability, no reliable method of surface cooling to deeper levels was found and the impetus to further research was diminished by the successful development of the pump-oxygenator for extracorporeal circulation. Later, mild and moderate hypothermia were introduced into bypass practice but dissatisfaction with the pump oxygenator system and its results led Drew and colleagues (1959) to develop the technique of profound hypothermia to 13–15° C. The unsuccessful results of conventional bypass in neonates caused a group of Japanese surgeons (Horiuchi et al., 1963) to re-examine the possibilities of surface-induced deep hypothermia and a technique developed which enabled 50–60 minutes circulatory interruption (Mohri et al., 1966). In many hands this has now been modified to include some degree of extracorporeal circulation particularly in the rewarming phase.

The late 1950s were probably the heyday of surface-induced hypothermia when it was widely applied in cardiac and great vessel surgery, in neurosurgery, as an ancillary technique to induced hypotension, and as a treatment for anoxic cerebral damage. The last is no longer considered an indication and McDowall (1971) found that 12 of 31 British neurosurgery centres had abandoned surface hypothermia altogether and in another 13 it was used only rarely. Currently the commonest indication is to protect the brain during induced hypotension for surgery of vascular lesions.

Physiology of Hypothermia

Temperature Regulation and Shivering

Heat production in the body comes from two main sources; the metabolism in ordinary cells, particularly the very active ones (e.g. liver) and from the effect of muscle contraction, most of which is voluntary, but some of which (e.g. heart) is continuous and involuntary. This heat is dissipated through the skin and exhaled air and there is a temperature gradient between the body core and the surface. The amount of heat dissipation through the skin is controlled by variations in skin blood flow and this is normally sufficient to maintain the body temperature within its physiological range. Major decreases in environmental temperature may be too great for the adaptive power of the skin and blood temperature falls. When the temperature of the blood reaching the brain is reduced by about 0·5° C the thermal nucleus in the hypothalamus is stimulated. This nucleus is concerned with co-ordinating the peripheral response to changes in skin and blood temperature. The effect of this stimulation is to provoke the shivering reflex producing a massive increase in metabolism and cardiac output.

It is not possible to induce hypothermia in man unless the shivering reflex is obtunded either by central depression of the thermal nucleus or by preventing the muscle activity by the use of muscle relaxants.

Metabolic Rate: Oxygen Consumption and Utilisation

Experimental work on metabolic rate during hypothermia has been confused by:

1. Difficulties in temperature measurement—the temperature measured (e.g. oesophageal) may not accurately reflect the temperature of the whole body.
2. Temperature gradients within the body—calculations have been based on the assumption that the body has been uniformly cooled whereas a steady state has not been achieved and some highly metabolic organs are still not hypothermic.
3. Drug and metabolic effects: early work was often made with the patient breathing spontaneously. The effects of hypercarbia and of anaesthetic agents in stimulating the autonomic nervous system were not eliminated.

When these defects are corrected it appears that the oxygen consumption and metabolic rate are depressed to 75 per cent of basal at 30° C to 45 per cent at 25° C and to 17 per cent at 20° C (Watanabe *et al.*, 1959).

The possibility exists that this reduction in oxygen consumption represents a failure in supply and utilisation rather than a true depression of metabolism. This could result from inhibition of enzymatic processes by hypothermia, changes in the oxygen dissociation curve or alterations in the circulation. The latter two effects may be offset by increased dissolved oxygen in plasma at low temperatures, which might be enough to supply the metabolic needs of the cells. The effect of hypothermia is to displace the oxygen dissociation curve to the left (p. 151 *et seq.*) producing a reduction in oxygen release by haemoglobin at the periphery, although this effect can be offset by the creation of a respiratory acidosis. Depression of the circulation consequent on hypothermia may depress oxygen availability to the cells. However, if the circulation is interrupted at a low temperature so that an oxygen debt occurs, when the circulation is restored there is a rise in oxygen consumption until the oxygen debt is paid off. This effect occurs even if the patient is maintained hypothermic suggesting that the capacity for utilisation of oxygen at these temperatures is not the limiting factor.

Acid-base Balance

Interpretation of acid base during hypothermia is complicated by the problem of measurement. Most acid-base machines are maintained at normal blood temperatures and if blood from a hypothermic patient is put into the electrode, the increased dissolved carbon dioxide becomes less soluble as the temperature rises and so the carbon dioxide tension increases. A similar change occurs in the pH electrode. The results must either by interpreted allowing for this effect or temperature correction factors applied. The quantitation of fixed acids will be affected only to an insignificant degree.

Respiratory effects.—During spontaneous respiration the minute volume progressively decreases and ventilation will cease at about 23° C. Gas transfer is not impaired but an increase in anatomical and physiological dead space occurs due to cold-induced bronchial dilatation. The overall effect is the development of a respiratory acidosis. Respiration is normally controlled during hypothermia and with the decreased carbon dioxide production and increased carbon dioxide solubility, a respiratory alkalosis is easily produced. This has deleterious effects on the cardiac output, the oxygen dissociation curve and the cerebral blood flow, and is usually associated with the development of a metabolic acidosis. The minute volume of artificial ventilation during hypothermia must therefore be reduced according to the blood gas tension values.

Metabolic effects.—The development of a metabolic acidosis is common, although less so during surface hypothermia than during core cooling. It results from the availability of oxygen being reduced by depression of the cardiovascular system, by the breakdown of autoregulatory systems and by the increase in blood viscosity with intracapillary sludging so that the reduction in blood flow is greater than the reduction in cellular metabolism. Lactic acidosis is inevitable during periods of circulatory occlusion, but may not become apparent until rewarming when tissue blood flow is re-established. If the circulation is intact and liver function returned to normal, this acidosis is often self-correcting and the administration of sodium bicarbonate leads subsequently to a severe alkalosis.

Carbohydrate Metabolism

Hypothermia causes an increase in plasma glucose. This is thought to be due to reduced insulin activity, depressed liver function and inhibition of enzymes concerned with glucose metabolism. If glucose is given intravenously the blood sugar rises steeply and exerts an osmotic effect on the cells, increasing blood volume and depressing serum electrolyte levels. Small infants undergoing surface hypothermia who receive no intravenous glucose during the procedure show satisfactory and stable blood glucose levels throughout (Mohri and Merendino, 1969).

Fluid Balance and Electrolytes

Studies of water balance and electrolyte levels during hypothermia often show completely divergent findings due either to methodological differences or to alterations in respiratory or circulatory function predominating over the minor changes consequent on the effects of hypothermia itself.

Circulatory System

Heart.—Myocardial oxygen uptake is reduced as temperature falls and this facilitates longer periods of interruption to the coronary circulation with better preservation of myocardial function. During surface cooling there is a small fall in blood pressure and a more marked slowing of the pulse until about 25–26° C. Below 26° C the blood pressure falls more quickly as the cardiac output declines and then at 20° C, as the peripheral vascular resistance, which has initially increased, gives way to vasodilatation with venous pooling the blood pressure drops more quickly.

Once the temperature falls below 32° C–30° C dysrhythmias are common of which the most frequent are ventricular extrasystoles and there is a progressive increase in the development of atrioventricular dissociation. In the ECG, prolongation of P–R, QRS and QT intervals are seen and below 25° C ST segment and T wave changes occur. It is common for patients to develop ventricular fibrillation below 28° C. The cause of this increased myocardial irritability is unknown. It occurs later in children who can often be cooled below 25° C particularly if the serum potassium level is carefully controlled (Brown *et al.*, 1973). Possible factors are temperature or pH gradients in the myocardium and disproportion in alteration of conduction velocities. A large number of apparently contradictory methods have been advocated for its prevention.

Blood Elements and the Microcirculation

Blood viscosity increases and platelets and white cells diminish during hypothermia but these changes are small above 28° C. However, at temperatures below this the alteration in the blood and in haemodynamics result in poor tissue perfusion. These effects can be reversed by mechanical augmentation of the circulation, by the use of vasodilator drugs, and most importantly by the reduction in blood viscosity in the hemodilution technique which significantly increases tissue blood flow and oxygen availability.

Liver

Hypothermia reduces splanchnic blood flow and liver metabolism in direct proportion to the fall in body temperature. The detoxication of drugs such as barbiturates, morphine and adrenaline is reduced and the coagulation time of the blood is prolonged. However, the liver will then tolerate increased periods of circulatory occlusion provided these are not accompanied by a high venous pressure with consequent engorgement of the liver parenchyma.

Kidneys

Blood flow, oxygen consumption and glomerular filtration decrease during hypothermia and urine production usually ceases around 20° C. Hypothermia appears to protect the kidneys well against circulatory interruption both in the intact patient during cardiac and great vessel surgery where post-operative renal failure is uncommon, and in the isolated kidney where hypothermia is used to protect the organ during the interval between removal from a donor and implantation in a recipient.

The Central Nervous System and Tolerance to Cold and Circulatory Interruption

It was suggested initially that cold itself might induce damage in brain and nerve. In many of the early experiments it is possible to incriminate either low-flow perfusion or the existence within the brain of temperature gradients usually the result of too rapid cooling. The large body of recent clinical evidence suggests that reducing brain temperature to 10° C *per se* is not a cause of brain injury. Nervous tissue metabolism appears to fall with temperature in the normal way and, despite the absence of any stored metabolic substrate, the brain appears to be able to tolerate circulatory arrest for periods which are proportionate to the reduction in temperature. The practitioners of deep hypothermia, by paying meticulous attention to cerebral blood flow and to slow cooling with an absence of temperature gradients, allow 60 minutes total arrest at 15° C with apparent complete recovery. Fisk and his colleagues (1974) when examining the brains of piglets which had clinically shown no lesions after experimental deep hypothermia with circulatory arrest, found histological evidence to suggest that damage had occurred and with other authors have cautioned that circulatory interruption times during hypothermia should be the minimum possible, not the longest practicable.

CLINICAL TECHNIQUE OF MILD SURFACE HYPOTHERMIA

(i) **Anaesthesia.**—The anaesthetic requirement is that the shivering reflex is prevented so that the patient allows his temperature to fall. Due to the inadequacy of spontaneous ventilation during hypothermia, patients will normally be intubated and ventilated, thus muscle relaxants will assist in the prevention of shivering. The volume of ventilation is adjusted to maintain the carbon dioxide tension approximately at normal values after the appropriate temperature correction has been made. The natural response to a cold environment is vasoconstriction and the drop of body temperature is facilitated by the production of vasodilatation.

Ether was originally a popular drug, both for its vasodilatory action and for its benign effect on the circulation, but is contra-indicated with the widespread use of the diathermy and vasodilatation is usually achieved with drugs such as chlorpromazine, which can be given intravenously at the time or may be included in the premedication. The latter should also include a vagal blocking drug to prevent the cold-induced bradycardia.

(ii) **Monitoring.**—Temperature is best monitored with an electric thermometer which can display mid-oesophageal temperature as representative of heart temperature and nasopharyngeal temperature as representative of brain temperature. The heart temperature is obviously important in respect of the development of dysrhythmias while the brain temperature dictates the safe duration of circulatory arrest. Rectal temperature is useful as an index of temperature gradient within the body and, particularly during rewarming, to indicate when this can be safely discontinued without danger of recooling. An electrocardiogram is mandatory and most anaesthetists would prefer direct arterial and venous pressure monitoring in addition to a reliable infusion site. Arterial cannulation also provides easy access for samples for blood gas and electrolyte estimation.

(iii) **Cooling Techniques.**

    (a) *Immersion.*—Once anaesthetised, the patient is lowered on a canvas stretcher into a bath of water at 4° C. The toes and fingers are normally held out of the bath to guard against frostbite. Sudden movement, particularly elevation of a cold limb, may lead to the arrival of a quantity of supercooled blood at the heart causing ventricular fibrillation. The limbs must either be left stationary or massaged continuously. This will speed the cooling process and reduce the amount of "afterdrop" and the average adult will cool from 37° to 30° C in an hour.

    (b) *Evaporation.*—Although less efficient than immersion, it is easier to perform. The patient is positioned on the operating table. Ice bags are placed over the groin, neck and axilla, but not over the precordium. The skin is thoroughly wetted and heat loss by evaporation is encouraged by creating a wind tunnel with fans around the patient. Although the rate of cooling is slightly slower, this method has the advantage that the patient is positioned for surgery before cooling commences and unlike the immersion method, there is not the danger of having to move the patient once the temperature is low.

(c) *Cooling blanket.*—This is the least satisfactory. The area of contact between patient and blanket is often small but the solution in the pipes must not be below 0° C for danger of localised ice-burns. Cooling is therefore slow.

Level of Hypothermia and Rate of Cooling

In simple hypothermia, cooling is usually to a temperature of not less than 30° C which will protect the brain from up to ten minutes circulatory interruption. The rate of cooling is such that the temperature usually falls to this level in about an hour. Active cooling stops some way above 30° C because the peripheral tissues are cooled below this level and their continued perfusion causes the central temperature to continue to drop. This "afterdrop" or "overshoot" depends partly on the speed of cooling, being greater when the temperature has dropped rapidly, and partly on the size and shape of the patient. It is unwise to allow the surgeon to start operating until one is quite certain that the temperature drop has plateaued. In the cool environment of the theatre, the patient will usually stay cold unless active rewarming is undertaken. The most satisfactory solution is to have a water blanket under the patient and this can be circulated to provide fine control of the temperature, to check the afterdrop or to prevent rewarming. However, it is important to be thinking and planning well ahead as the application of warmth under such conditions is rarely followed by a rise in body temperature for at least half-an-hour. At the same time, the warm water must not exceed the skin temperature by too much because of the danger of skin burns.

Safety in a hypothermia technique depends on continued careful monitoring. If the electrocardiogram shows signs of dysrhythmias which are not due to hypoxia, acid-base or electrolyte disturbance, then the technique must be stopped at a temperature short of that which gives rise to the disturbance.

Infusion.—Care is needed both in the type of solution and its temperature. During hypothermia glucose metabolism is inhibited and glucose administration leads to high blood sugar levels. Quite satisfactory levels are maintained if Ringer lactate is used and its temperature should be adjusted to that of the patient. In particular, very cold blood should not be given quickly to already hypothermic patients. Metabolic destruction of citrate is retarded and ACD blood must be carefully covered with the correct quantities of calcium salts.

Rewarming.—There is usually no hurry about rewarming which can be allowed to occur slowly with a hot water blanket over the top of several normal blankets. This will prevent localised areas of heating which might lead to burns. If speedy rewarming is very necessary re-immersion in a warm bath is quickest. The anaesthesia must not be discontinued until the temperature has returned to normal otherwise shivering will occur placing a tremendous load on the still hypothermic cardiovascular system.

Indications

Simple surface hypothermia was at one time widely practised, but today the commonest indication is probably vascular surgery to protect a distal organ from damage during operation on its arterial supply. Hypothermia is sometimes used during coarctation of the aorta or aneurysm surgery to protect the kidneys or spinal cord, or during carotid disobliteration to protect the brain. McDowall (1971), in his questionnaire to neurosurgery centres, listed the indications as aneurysm surgery, and surgery of arteriovenous malformations and vascular tumours. His correspondents added reduction in brain volume, protection against retractor anaemia and as an ancillary to induced hypotension as other indications. All but one anaesthetist felt their usage of surface hypothermia was declining.

When used in cardiac surgery the technique was to expose the heart after cooling to 30° C then to clamp off both vena cava and aorta thus isolating the heart from the rest of the circulation. Within an eight-minute period, the heart was opened, the defect repaired, the heart closed and all air evacuated from it. Few intracardiac lesions can be repaired in this time and the better operating conditions provided by extracorporeal circulation, together with the comparable operative risk has resulted in inflow occlusion with mild hypothermia being generally abandoned in favour of extracorporeal circulation.

THE EXTRACORPOREAL CIRCULATION

Extracorporeal circulation has now progressed to the point where it is undertaken routinely in many centres with a very low morbidity and mortality attributable to the technique itself. Unfortunately, this good clinical result has been the consequence of greater technical dexterity by the surgeon, anaesthetists and perfusionists and stricter manufacturing tolerances in the apparatus rather than the consequence of a more profound understanding of the physiological effects of bypass. It is to be hoped that now most clinical problems can be solved on the empirical basis of experience, time can be taken to study scientifically the unexplained problems. Perhaps in the field of post-operative care this generalisation is untrue and thanks to a greater understanding of circulatory physiology and its interaction with respiratory physiology, many patients can be carried through the difficult immediate post-operative period.

HISTORICAL NOTE

In 1812 Legallois wrote "If one could substitute for the heart a kind of injection of artificial blood, either naturally or artificially made, one would succeed in maintaining alive indefinitely any part of the body whatsoever." This armchair experimentation became a near-reality nearly fifty years later, when the physiologist Brown-Séquard (1858) attempted, with moderate success, to perfuse the decapitated head of a dog. He was one of the first workers to emphasise the importance of cerebral blood flow and, in fact, showed that a period of five minutes' ischaemia of the brain was sufficient to cause death in dogs.

The development of the various methods of oxygenating blood has been a slow process and those in use today are similar to many that were tried over eighty years ago. The difference between the present-day success and the failures of yesterday seems to lie in the realisation of the enormous surface of blood that must be exposed if adequate oxygenation is to occur. Amongst the first reports of a mechanical oxygenator is that of Ludwig (1865), who tried shaking blood in a balloon filled with air. Later, other workers tried bubbling air through blood but although they achieved adequate oxygenation they were hampered by foaming (Schroder, 1882; Jacoby, 1890; Brodie, 1903).

Frey and Gruber (1885) were amongst the first to exploit the idea of a thin film of blood exposed to oxygen. Their apparatus consisted of a cylinder and the blood was allowed to flow along the inner walls and thus take up oxygen on its way. This principle of a thin film of blood was brilliantly adapted by Gibbon (1937) and became the basis of one of the most successful heart-lung machines.

Discovery and Development of Heparin and Protamine

An inability to prevent clotting of the blood was one of the principal causes of failure in the early experiments on the extracorporeal circulation. The discovery of *heparin* represents one of the rare "accidental finds" in modern medicine. Before 1916 there was no known substance which could prevent coagulation of the blood. Howell, who is well-known for his contribution to the theories on the clotting mechanism, assigned the task of purifying certain phosphatides to a second-year medical student—one Jay McLean—at Johns Hopkins University, Baltimore. At that time, Howell was looking for a substance that would speed up rather than slow down the clotting process. McLean found that one phosphatide (cuorin) extracted from the heart muscle of dogs actually prevented coagulation. Howell recognised immediately the importance of this substance and in the following year, at an Harveian Oration in London, he described this substance as an anti-prothrombin. Later, it was found that this substance could be extracted in abundance from dog's liver, and thus it came to be called *heparin*.

More recent work has shown that heparin originates in the granules of mast cells of both animals and man; these cells are found not only in the liver and lungs, but also in the connective tissue surrounding capillaries and in the walls of blood vessels throughout the body.

The role of protamine in restoring the coagulating mechanism after the use of heparin was soon identified. As long ago as 1880 Schmidt-Mulheim described the effect of "peptone shock" in dogs; this condition is characterised by circulatory collapse followed by a temporary loss of clotting power in the blood. This later effect is believed to be due to the release of heparin from the mast cells. Waters and his colleagues (1938) conclusively demonstrated the value of protamine when they showed that it prevented the failure of clotting which is the characteristic of this condition.

BYPASS PUMPING CIRCUITS AND CANNULATIONS

The pumping circuits to be considered are:
  (i) Normal extracorporeal circulation with a pump oxygenator.
 (ii) Supportive bypass.
(iii) Left atriofemoral bypass.
(iv) Profound hypothermia techniques
      —with normal extracorporeal circulation
      —with homologous lung gas exchange.

Normal Extracorporeal Circulation with a Pump Oxygenator

This is currently the commonest method of choice for supporting the circulation during the performance of open intracardiac and great vessel surgery (Fig. 1).

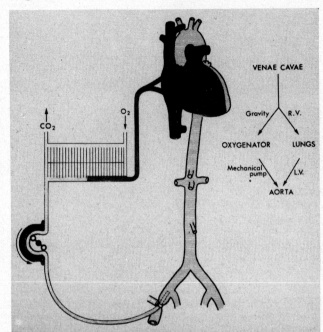

16/Fig. 1.—Partial bypass.

The heart is most commonly approached through a midline sternal split incision although rarely a left or right thoracotomy may be specially indicated.

Venous cannulation.—The superior vena cava and inferior vena cava are normally cannulated with catheters passed through the right atrium although when operating on the left heart a simple tube in the right atrium can be used.

The size of the venous catheters is chosen by prior calibration to be adequate for the drainage of blood through them during bypass but, at the same time, to be not so large as to obstruct the venous return before the onset of perfusion (Fig. 2). Once bypass has commenced, venous drainage is achieved with a gravity siphon, the rate of flow being controlled by an adjustable clamp on the main venous line. If the venae cavae of the patient are 20–30 cm higher than the oxygenator or venous reservoir, siphonage produced by this difference in height is sufficient to maintain a good flow. In some cases, the siphonage may become excessive when it only defeats its own end by collapsing the vessel walls against the orifice of the tubes. If the right side of the heart, or the left side in the presence of a septal communication, is opened air will enter the tubes and stop the siphon flow. This is prevented by two snares around the two cavae once bypass is established (Fig. 3), a condition termed "total" bypass. It has the advantage that venous pressure can be maintained at normal in the rest of the patient without the heart being flooded with blood.

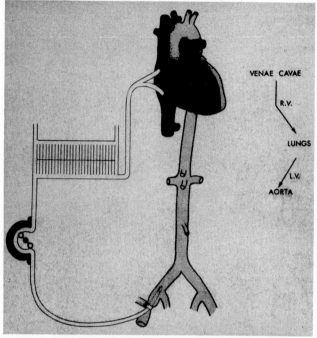

16/FIG. 2.—Before cardiopulmonary bypass.

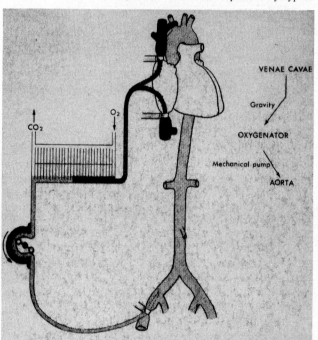

16/FIG. 3.—Total bypass.

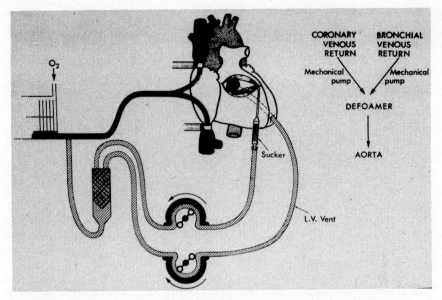

16/Fig. 4.—Return of blood from bypassed heart.

Blood also enters the heart from three other possible sources (Fig. 4).

1. Coronary venous return mostly re-enters the heart through the coronary sinus which drains into the right atrium. If the venous pressure is low, this blood then flows backwards into the venae cavae and down the main tubes. Alternatively, if the venous pressure is high or the venae cavae are snared up, this blood is aspirated with coronary suckers.

2. The bronchial arteries, which in Fallot's tetralogy can take up to 20 per cent of cardiac output, anastomose with the pulmonary circulation and drain to the left side of the heart where the blood is aspirated with suckers or with the left ventricular vent (see below).

3. In the presence of aortic incompetence, blood can also pass retrogradely across the aortic valve and will have to be aspirated from the left ventricle by the vent.

During the period that the patient is heparinised the blood aspirated by the suckers is passed with the venous return to the oxygenator.

Arterial cannulation.—Direct return of blood to the aorta is standard except where special consideration indicates use of the femoral or iliac vessels. Size is less critical than for the venous cannula because the arterial cannula is unlikely to obstruct the aorta. It must, however, be large enough that the pressure drop across it at the expected flow is small. Thus damage to the red cells caused by high velocity flow is decreased and the possibility of cavitation with bubble formation in the flow after entry to the aorta is avoided.

Left heart venting.—The left heart vent (which is usually in the ventricle) has two functions. Firstly it acts as a simple sucker in keeping the field clear of blood (e.g. aortic valve surgery). Secondly, in some circumstances (myocardial failure, ventricular fibrillation) blood enters the left heart but is not ejected from it. This leads to overdistension of the ventricle with damage to the myocardium. Back-pressure effects are transmitted via the left atrium to the pulmonary capillaries where they cause pulmonary engorgement and, ultimately, pulmonary oedema. The left ventricular vent by decompressing the ventricle prevents these effects. The blood is returned to the pump oxygenator. The vent must be clamped or removed before attempting to discontinue bypass.

Supportive Bypass

Some intracardiac operations, particularly mitral valvotomy in the presence of pulmonary hypertension, can be performed with the heart supporting the circulation but owing to the delicate condition of these patients the manipulations which accompany surgery may cause profound hypotension. The low output and its consequent metabolic acidosis worsens the pulmonary hypertension which further reduces the output of the right ventricle. This vicious circle can only be broken with the use of extracorporeal circulation to transfer a proportion of the cardiac output from the right atrium to a systemic artery. This technique is termed supportive bypass (Fig. 5).

Two other situations in which this technique may be useful are
  (i) in difficult repeat operations when there is a danger of damaging the heart while opening the chest; the femoral vein and artery can be cannulated before starting the main incision and bypass instituted if the circulation is jeopardized by manipulation or haemorrhage;
 (ii) in life-threatening pulmonary embolism, supportive bypass can be established after cannulating the femoral vessels under local anaesthesia. If necessary this can be performed before pulmonary angiography which frequently causes a severe deterioration to the point of cardiac arrest.

Left Atriofemoral Bypass

During operations for aneurysms of the descending thoracic aorta (or coarctation of the aorta) the arterial supply to the kidneys and spinal cord may be temporarily interrupted, leading to renal failure or paraplegia. These organs can be supported by taking oxygenated blood from the left atrium and returning it, at arterial pressure levels, to the aorta below the clamp. The blood pressure is measured continuously in the major vessels of the upper part of the body which are supplied normally by the beating heart (Fig. 6).

The pump is run at such a speed that the arterial pressure remains constant. If there is proximal hypertension the pump is speeded up to lower left atrial pressure and thus reduce the output of the left ventricle to the upper part of the body and vice versa. With adequate flow the pressure in the lower half of the body seems unimportant. Gas exchange occurs normally in the patient's lungs.

Profound Hypothermia Techniques

In 1963, Horiuchi and his colleagues described a technique for inducing profound hypothermia in neonates by surface cooling. Profound hypothermia, in which the aim is to reduce the body temperature to 10–15° C permitting circulatory arrest for up to an hour, is more commonly achieved with extracorporeal circulation in one of two ways.

(*a*) In a normal extracorporeal circuit removing blood from the right side

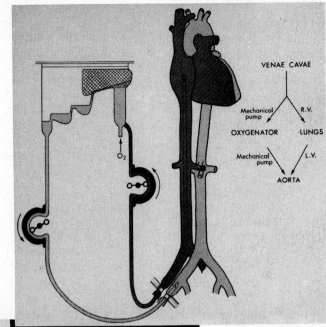

16/Fig. 5.—Supportive bypass without thoracotomy.

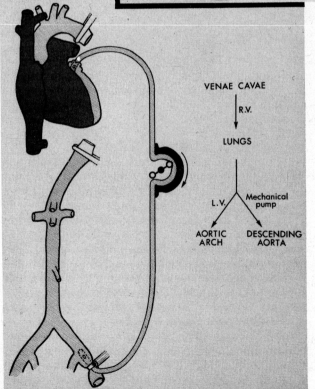

16/Fig. 6.—Left atrio-femoral bypass.

of the heart, passing it through an oxygenator and a heat exchanger, and returning it to a systemic artery. This method has the advantage of considerable flexibility. It is sometimes indicated for operations on the great vessels where continuous perfusion would involve multiple cannulations of the aorta, carotid and subclavian arteries, and it is particularly suitable for complex congenital heart surgery.

(*b*) The Drew technique (Drew *et al*., 1959; Feldman 1971) (Fig. 7) involves

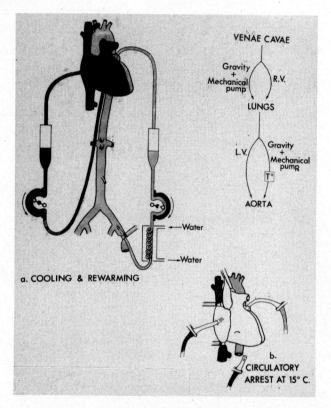

16/Fig. 7.— Profound hypothermia (Drew technique).

cannulation of the right atrium and pulmonary artery to bypass the right ventricle and of the left atrium and a systemic artery to bypass the left ventricle. The patient's own lungs are used for oxygenation and carbon dioxide elimination. This method has achieved considerable success, particularly in the treatment of congenital heart disease. It has the disadvantages of requiring multiple vessel cannulations, of being time-consuming, as both cooling and rewarming are slow to avoid the development of temperature gradients within the body and yet, at the same time, placing a restriction on intracardiac operating time. It is also technically difficult in the presence of severe aortic incompetence. The merit of this method lay in the very good oxygenation of the patient's blood when compared with the performance of early oxygenators but with the development of machines capable of fully oxygenating high flows of blood the need for this type of profound hypothermia has decreased and its popularity has waned. The Drew technique is not simple and requires good control and equipment. It should be regarded as an alternative to, not a replacement for, conventional extracorporeal circulation (Melrose, 1969).

APPARATUS

Anaesthetised adult patients consume approximately 110–130 ml O_2 per square metre of body surface area per minute, with a higher rate in infancy. To provide a full flow of completely oxygenated blood, an oxygenator needs to be capable of adding this quantity of oxygen to the venous blood for an indefinite period. Sufficient reserve capacity is also needed to cope with patients who initially are hypoxic or who develop an oxygen debt before bypass or during rewarming.

16/TABLE 1

DIFFERENCE BETWEEN NORMAL LUNG AND ARTIFICIAL OXYGENATORS

	Normal Lung	Artificial Oxygenator
Thickness of Blood Film	Monocorpuscular	20–60 r.b.c. thick (0·1–0·3 mm)
Surface Area	50–200 m^2	2–10 m^2
Plasma Diffusion Distance	Very short	Long (N.B. Turbulence)
Capillary Membrane Diffusion	Yes	No
Oxygen Gradient	$100 - 40 = 60$ mm Hg	$673 - 40 = 633$ mm Hg
	$(13·3 - 5·3 = 8·0$ kPa$)$	$(89·7 - 5·3 = 84·4$ kPa$)$
Time of Exposure	0·1–0·8 seconds	15–30 seconds
Blood/gas Interface	No	Yes
		(except membrane oxygenators)

In the human lung, blood is efficiently oxygenated because of the huge surface area and the very intimate contact between the red cells and the alveolus (Table 1). Thus oxygenation is achieved despite a low oxygen tension difference between alveolus and capillary ($100 - 40 = 60$ mm Hg or $13·3 - 5·3 = 8·0$ kPa), a short exposure time (0·1 sec to 0·3 sec) and a low lung blood volume. The principal problem in the design of oxygenators has been the production of a sufficiently thin film of blood. Most filming oxygenators have a film of 0·1 to 0·3 mm (30–60 r.b.c.) thick. As a consequence, if the surface area is large, considerable amounts of blood are held up in the oxygenator. Also, the distance oxygen has to diffuse through plasma to reach the red cells is great. These disadvantages are offset by increasing the oxygen gradient tenfold, by prolonging the time of exposure to 15–30 seconds and by producing turbulence in the blood so that the red cells are constantly carried up to the surface.

Oxygenators

Despite the large number of types of oxygenators which have been described and used at different times, today there are only three basic types in common use: those in which blood is dispersed in oxygen, those in which oxygen is dispersed in blood and those which seek to re-create normal lung relationships.

(a) Dispersal of Blood in Oxygen

This principle is exemplified by the first generation stationary screen and rotating disc oxygenators. Their popularity has declined due to their initial high cost, the difficulty in resterilisation and their high priming volume and thus they have been widely abandoned in favour of disposable bubble oxygenators.

(b) Dispersal of Oxygen in Blood

Blood and gas flow together at the bottom of a column which is thus filled with ascending froth and which has a very large area of blood gas interface. The size of the bubble is important. Small bubbles produce a large surface area and thus good oxygenation, but are difficult to eliminate before the blood is returned to the patient. A proportion of larger bubbles is necessary for the adequate elimination of carbon dioxide. At the top of the column the froth comes into contact with a large surface area coated with silicone-type anti-foam, which causes the bubbles to burst. Any residual bubbles are trapped at the surface of settling reservoirs or helices before the blood is returned to the patient. Modern bubble oxygenators are highly efficient and can cope with large flows of blood. They are slightly more traumatic to blood than the screen oxygenators. Bubble oxygenators are generally made of plastic, and are supplied pre-sterilised and designed to be used only once. Because of their small priming volume, the use of blood is frequently unnecessary. This oxygenator was originally described by De Wall and colleagues (1957) and is widely available in a variety of slightly different forms.

(c) Recreating Normal Lung Relationships—the Membrane Oxygenator

Both types of oxygenator described above depend for their efficiency on the existence of a large blood-gas interface to which the blood is repeatedly exposed, which is in direct contrast to the normal lung where blood and air are separated by pulmonary endothelium. Lee and his colleagues (1961) showed that the physical forces at the interface caused destruction of the plasma proteins with separation of the bound fat and that this caused an increase in the biological and chemical reactivity of the proteins and an alteration in their physical properties. Although other forms of damage—haemolysis, chemical trauma—occur during extracorporeal circulation, it is the effects of plasma protein destruction which limit the duration of successful bypass.

Attempts to design a successful membrane (Drinker, 1972) oxygenator were hampered in two ways.

(i) *Membrane availability.*—Early membranes were either too fragile and ruptured easily or were robust but had poor gas transfer characteristics. Current silicone elastomer membrane is thin but robust, can be unsupported over suitable surface areas and has good oxygen transfer properties.

(ii) *Haemodynamic design.*—As with film oxygenators the initial problem was that of obtaining a thin film, but later it became apparent that the limiting factor to diffusion is the existence of a stable boundary layer of plasma through which oxygen passes slowly.

Commercially available membrane oxygenators will transfer about 30–40 ml O_2 $min^{-1}m^{-2}$ membrane area with a blood flow of 1 l/minute although experimentally gas transfer rates of 200 ml O_2 $min^{-1}m^{-2}$ have been achieved in oxygenators which can effectively break up the plasma boundary layers.

There is no doubt that membrane oxygenation is a more benign process than interface oxygenation and the duration of successful bypass is measured in days or even weeks, not hours. Overall surgical mortality in short clinical perfusions is related to problems of surgical selection, myocardial preservation and quality of surgery rather than to the effects of the oxygenator and until the costs of membrane oxygenation are comparable, the cheaper bubble oxygenators will remain standard equipment.

PUMPS

Pumps are used in the extracorporeal circuit to return the oxygenated blood to the systemic arterial tree at high pressure levels and to provide suction to remove blood from the operative field. Pumps need to be simple, robust, easily calibrated and adjusted, and atraumatic to blood. Those parts actually in contact with the blood are usually disposable.

Of the many types of pump described, only the roller pump has survived for widespread use. These may have single, double (Fig. 8), or, less commonly, triple arms. Correctly adjusted for minimal occlusion with good quality tubing, they are relatively atraumatic to blood. The rate of haemolysis is directly related to the number of passages the roller makes over the tube and large-bore tubing in a slow running pump is to be preferred.

Blood flow, pulsatile or continuous.—Most pumps in use today, which are robust and simple, produce a predominantly continuous flow. Pulsatile flow can be produced by a pump which is more complicated and, in some cases, more traumatic to the blood. However, the principal difficulty in producing the pulsatile flow to the patient lies in the size of the arterial cannula. This is normally the smallest point in the arterial line and commonly imposes a large resistance if high flow rates are used. To produce a pulsatile flow distal to this restriction would entail very high pressure swings proximal to it and intermittent high velocity jets through it, both of which would result in substantial damage to the blood and plasma proteins. With pulsatile flow, whole body oxygen consumption is higher, acid metabolite production lower, systemic vascular resistance lower and renal function better preserved. However, in short term clinical perfusions the attendant problems more than outweigh the benefits.

Filters

A filter, often combining the function of a bubble trap, is usually incorporated into the circuit. A pore size of 40μm is necessary to catch the microaggregates of leucocytes and platelets which pass freely through the standard 200μm filters. As these emboli arise mainly in the oxygenator the filter needs to lie between the oxygenator and the patient.

Choice of Materials, Cleaning and Sterilisation

Though at first sight the matter of cleanliness of the machine would seem a relatively simple one, in practice it has been proved to be of the utmost importance in the development of the extracorporeal circulation. It can be shown that on almost every surface that has been in contact with blood a thin layer of

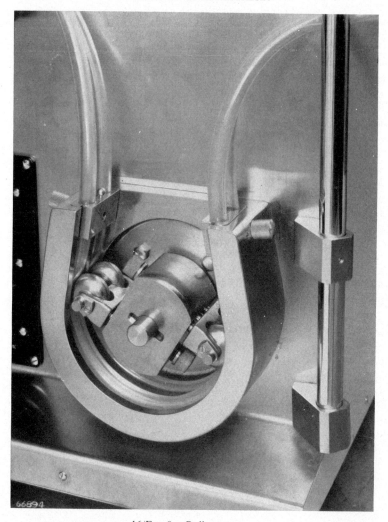

16/Fig. 8.—Roller pump.

protein substance remains. Minute scratches on the interior surface of the apparatus lead to the deposition of fibrin and platelets in this area which could be transferred from patient to patient.

One approach to the problem is to make as much of the apparatus disposable as possible. All tubing, both connecting and that used within the pumps, is normally used only once. The bubble oxygenators are usually supplied pre-sterilised by gamma radiation for single use only and other pieces of apparatus, heat exchangers, filters, even disc oxygenators, are following this pattern. This is a very expensive process because despite their short life they need to be manufactured with a high degree of precision to provide smooth atraumatic surfaces from high purity materials free from the danger of chemical toxicity (Duke and Vane, 1968).

Those parts of the circuit which are not disposable are commonly manufactured from stainless steel which can be given a highly polished and lasting surface that is chemically inert. This can be cleaned with haemolytic compounds, acids and alkalies, or ultrasonic vibrations.

Sterilisation varies with the facilities available. Disposable parts are commonly irradiated or exposed to ethylene dioxide gas. An autoclave technique is used for glass and stainless steel parts. The total circuit of separately sterilised parts is then assembled using a full sterile technique.

ANAESTHESIA AND MONITORING

Anaesthesia and monitoring for patients undergoing extracorporeal circulation is considered in greater detail in Chapter 14, Anaesthesia and Cardiac Disease.

Monitoring during Extracorporeal Circulation

It has been said that the more experienced the surgical team, the less the need for monitoring. Alternatively, if monitoring can be achieved with no increased morbidity the extra information is always available when needed for making decisions and for teaching or research. Melrose (1969) has expressed this viewpoint, saying "the maximum security of a perfusion system follows the meticulous monitoring of many parameters".

Percutaneous catheterisation by the anaesthetist of the radial artery, the internal jugular vein, and the femoral vein for cannulation of the inferior vena cava, are all technically easy. Indwelling catheters enable continuous display of arterial and venous pressures and samples are easily obtainable for blood gas, electrolyte and coagulation estimations. A display ECG is mandatory and an EEG is often included. Temperature is normally measured electrically at several sites, commonly the oesophagus, nasopharynx and rectum. Finally, the urine output is recorded hourly. The routine use of a wide but specific range of monitoring enables the anaesthetist continually to reassess the patient's condition on some basis other than mere clinical instinct.

PHYSIOLOGY OF THE EXTRACORPOREAL CIRCULATION

At first sight, the withdrawal of blood from a patient with subsequent oxygenation and then retransfusion would appear to be a simple matter, but in practice it is fraught with difficulties. Each machine has its own characteristics but the most important single factor for success is the organisation of the team, which is fully conversant with all the aspects of extracorporeal circulation. Some of these problems are considered individually below.

Clotting of Blood

When blood is removed from a patient, it starts to clot within a few minutes unless some steps are taken to prevent this process. Contact of blood with any part of the machine, even if it is thoroughly siliconised, is sufficient to start the coagulation process and may ultimately lead either to the infusion of a fatal embolus or to the complete defibrination of the blood, followed by intractable bleeding. Complete reversible inhibition of the coagulation process is required and this is produced with heparin. Before cannulation of the vessels, the patient is heparinised and a similar concentration put in the priming volume of the machine.

The response in terms of prolongation of clotting time to a standard dose of heparin is extremely variable in different patients and, furthermore, the duration of this effect is itself variable and bears no relation to the initial response. The only effective way of controlling heparin dose is to monitor an activated clotting time test which can be done quickly and easily in the theatre. By this method, incremental doses are less frequent, the total heparin dose smaller and its accurate reversal with protamine easier.

As soon as the cannulae are removed from the thoracic vessels, protamine sulphate is given. The quantity may be determined, prior to administration, by a protamine-heparin titration of the blood, or a predetermined amount (e.g. 6 mg per kg body weight) may be given, and the clotting time compared with the pre-bypass specimen. Protamine is always given slowly as a rapid injection can cause profound hypotension, particularly if the patient is slightly hypovolaemic. Unfortunately, the heparin-protamine complex is sometimes broken down by sulphases in the blood before it is excreted and an hour or so after protamine administration coagulation may again become prolonged and further administration of protamine is necessary. This reappearance of free heparin should always be proved before more protamine is given as a similar effect is produced clinically by the breakdown of fibrinogen. The continued exact correction of the coagulation mechanism is required for minimal blood loss. Only very rarely is major fibrinolysis a problem and then usually in patients with severe polycythaemic heart disease (Fallot's tetralogy). The anti-fibrinolytic agents (Trasylol and Aminocaproic acid) are best reserved for administration when major fibrinolysis is demonstrated by coagulation tests. Other substances involved in coagulation (e.g. fibrinogen, vitamin K) are sometimes administered, but usually on an empirical rather than scientific basis. Patients who have been on long-term anticoagulation prior to operation normally have their prothrombin time reduced to normal over the operative period.

Priming Solutions

(a) **Volume.**—It is possible to construct an oxygenator system with a minimal priming blood volume. In such a system, however, any interference with the venous return results either in the reduction of flow or in the almost instantaneous emptying of the oxygenator into the patient with consequent risk of air embolism. For safety, therefore, most open systems have a reserve volume of about 25 per cent of the minute volume flow over and above the volume in the connecting tubes, and thus priming volumes of between two and four litres for adults are usual.

(b) **Composition.**—The factors which have to be taken into consideration include oxygen carrying capacity, viscosity, tonicity, electrolyte balance and clotting ability.

Oxygen carrying capacity.—Provided the flow rate is adequate, it is quite possible to maintain a near-normal mixed venous oxygen tension in the face of a reduced oxygen carrying capacity. The lower limit for packed cell volume once mixing between patient and prime has occurred, is usually put at 28–30 per cent, although much lower levels are tolerated in those units which feel strongly about the need to avoid the use of stored blood. In an adult patient with, say, a blood volume of 4600 ml and 2000 ml r.b.c. it is possible to prime a machine with 2000 ml of clear fluid and still have enough oxygen carrying capacity.

Blood.—Whereas blood was originally thought to be the most physiological fluid to prime a heart lung machine, today the opposite view is more common. Blood is only used to raise the oxygen carrying capacity of the priming solution to an acceptable minimum. It has fallen out of favour, partly because of the immense difficulties of finding the quantities of blood required each day for the many operations performed. The homologous blood syndrome (Gadboys *et al.*, 1962), although seen only in dogs in its most florid form, also occurs to some extent in humans. Post-operatively there is a much greater incidence of poor lung function after a blood prime than if the prime is with non-sanguinous fluid. Coagulation difficulties are also provoked by the use of large quantities of blood. These dangers are added to all the normal problems (incompatibility, serum hepatitis, etc.) of blood transfusion in general.

When blood is required, and this occurs most commonly in infants in whom the ratio of priming volume to patient's blood volume is large, this is provided as normal ACD or CPD blood, usually one to two days old, which is heparinised and recalcified before use.

Haemodilution technique.—The reduction in viscosity achieved by using isotonic solutions leads, under the artificial conditions of extracorporeal circulation, to a better tissue perfusion: there is also very little difficulty in obtaining the venous return sufficient to attain the ideal flow rate. Where hypothermia is used, this decrease in viscosity also offsets the rise in viscosity which normally occurs when the temperature drops.

The very multiplicity of fluids advocated and actually used indicates that no one priming solution is ideal. The large molecular dextrans are not used because of the interference with the clotting mechanisms and this is true also of low molecular dextrans in amounts in excess of 20 ml/kg body weight. A lactated Ringer's solution or 5 per cent dextrose plus certain electrolytes (usually calcium and potassium) are the most common. If the solution is to be fully re-infused, the water load is usually restricted to 30–40 ml/kg body weight; this fluid is usually rapidly excreted and the haematocrit returns to normal in the early post-operative phase.

Control of Perfusion and Flow Rates

In the early days of heart surgery, due to the inadequacy of oxygenators, only a low flow of blood was used. With the advent of oxygenators capable of adding 250 to 300 ml of oxygen per minute to the blood flow, low flow has become unacceptable. As flow rate is increased the oxygen consumption rises until it reaches a near plateau at approximately $2.4 \ 1/\text{min}^{-1}\text{m}^{-2}$ body surface area. Further increase in flow rate does not increase oxygen consumption but causes more blood destruction in the oxygenator.

This rate of oxygen consumption is maintained or enhanced by haemo-dilution and may be increased by pulsatile flow. Perfusion at this rate should not result in an oxygen debt or the development of a metabolic acidosis but does depend on normal distribution of flow through the body. This tends to fail during hypothermia when a metabolic acidosis develops despite a high flow.

Tissue perfusion is impaired by excessive reduction in carbon dioxide tension and systemic vascular resistance rises with duration of bypass and with high oxygen tensions. Unfortunately, venous oxygen tension is not a good index of the quality of tissue oxygenation as a high venous oxygen tension may be associated with arteriovenous shunts and a low oxygen consumption.

Gas Flow

The gas flow through the oxygenator is only roughly predictable. In theory a relatively low oxygen flow should be adequate to oxygenate the blood and by careful monitoring to remove the carbon dioxide. In practice, the control of carbon dioxide tension is much easier if the oxygenator is flushed out with a flow of gas two to three times that of the flow of blood, and which contains approximately $2\frac{1}{2}$ to 3 per cent carbon dioxide. Fine adjustment of carbon dioxide tension to physiological values is made after blood gas measurements once bypass has achieved a steady state. The disadvantages of a low carbon dioxide tension in shifting the oxygen dissociation curve and in reducing tissue and cerebral blood flow are so great that a slightly raised carbon dioxide level is to be preferred during bypass.

Now that oxygenators are capable of producing oxygen tensions of the order of 300 mm Hg (40 kPa) the effect of high oxygen tension in raising peripheral vascular resistance and impairing tissue perfusion becomes relevant, and the oxygen tension should perhaps be limited to that which produces full oxygen saturation of the blood.

Arterial Pressure

During cardiopulmonary bypass, the arterial pressure is generally said to be less important than the flow rate. Low perfusion pressures, either accidental or deliberate, are not uncommon, the result partly of anaesthetic drugs and partly from the low viscosity of the blood in the haemodilution technique. It is desirable to maintain the mean arterial pressure between 50 and 100 mm Hg (6·7–13·3 kPa) depending slightly on the patient's previous blood pressure and tending towards the upper figure in coronary artery disease.

Blood Volume

In patients undergoing cardiac surgery, blood volume is much less important than the filling pressure in each ventricle. During full-flow bypass, the filling pressure is largely irrelevant and the venous pressure, and hence blood volume, can be altered to provide the optimum operating conditions for the surgery. These changes should be produced gradually so as not to invoke vasomotor reflexes which can produce a "faint" situation.

Induced Cardiac Arrest

In the early days of cardiac surgery, it was common practice to stop the action of the heart by injecting potassium into the root of the aorta after it had been cross-clamped. This provided a motionless field but had the disadvantage of being an anoxic technique. The current techniques of induced arrest are:

1. **Aortic cross-clamping**—an anoxic technique but one which appears not to do too much long-term damage to the myocardium provided the periods of

clamping are short compared with the periods of perfusion. Damage is also lessened if the heart is hypothermic.

2. **Electrically induced fibrillation**—the fibrillating heart has a high muscle tone and oxygen consumption. Coronary perfusion of the subendocardial region is impaired and if the mean arterial pressure is allowed to fall subendocardial infarction occurs. The fibrillating heart also loses potassium from its cells and develops interstitial oedema.

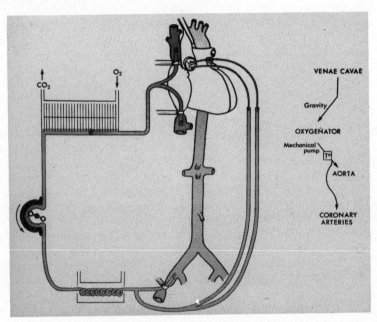

16/Fig. 9.—Circuit for aortic valve surgery.

3. **Cardioplegic solutions**—a re-examination of the technique of potassium arrest has shown that injection into the aortic root of a hypothermic solution containing potassium, magnesium and ATP will reduce myocardial metabolism to a very low level and the heart will not deteriorate despite prolonged coronary occlusion, particularly when this technique is combined with local topical hypothermia. An implied disadvantage of all cardiac arrest techniques is that during surgery in the region of the atrioventricular bundle the integrity of the conduction bundle cannot be monitored on the ECG.

Myocardial Preservation and Coronary Perfusion

During simple extracorporeal circulation the myocardium is perfused normally from the coronary arteries by the blood which is returned to the aorta by the heart-lung machine. This perfusion may be interrupted for two reasons:

(*a*) **Aortic valve surgery.**—To obtain access to the aortic valve, the aorta is cross-clamped and then opened between the clamp and the heart. This means that no perfusion of the coronary arteries can occur unless they are cannulated separately (Fig. 9). It would appear most physiological to perfuse the coronary arteries continuously with a normal flow of blood at normal temperatures. In practice this is not always easy and sometimes, to facilitate surgery, the coronary perfusion is interrupted and may occur only intermittently for, say, three in every thirteen minutes. To help preserve the myocardium during these anoxic periods, hypothermia is sometimes employed to reduce the myocardial metabolic demands. Alternatively, it may be felt that the unphysiological effects of hypothermia are worse than the transitory anoxia which obtains if the aorta is clamped continuously for a short period of, say, half an hour. Although the ideal solution to this problem ought to be apparent from theoretical arguments and the experience of research, this is not necessarily so. Much of the success of intracardiac operations depends on the precision with which the repair can be effected and sometimes this precision can only be obtained at the expense of transitory myocardial hypoxia. Therefore, a somewhat unphysiological technique may, in the long term follow-up, give rather better results than an apparently more physiological technique of coronary perfusion.

(b) **Aortic cross-clamping.**—Precision of surgery is important in all branches of cardiac surgery and, to facilitate this precision, the aorta is sometimes cross-clamped. The effects of this are:

   i. The cessation of coronary arterial perfusion stops blood pouring out of the coronary sinus to flood the operative field.

   ii. If there is any aortic incompetence present, it prevents blood regurgitating through the aortic valve to obscure the operative field.

   iii. As the heart becomes hypoxic, the muscle relaxes and the heart is more easily displaced and retracted to provide better access for surgery.

   iv. If there is any danger from air embolism from a beating heart, cerebral air complications can be prevented by the presence of an aortic clamp.

HYPOTHERMIA DURING EXTRACORPOREAL CIRCULATION

The aims of selective hypothermia of the heart and of mild hypothermia, i.e. down to about 30° C as a part of an extracorporeal technique, are the same, namely to reduce metabolic demands so that inadequate or interrupted perfusion can be better tolerated by the heart.

Although in theory greater reductions of temperature might be desirable as providing better protection, hypothermia itself produces complications. Vascular spasm occurs and leads to underperfusion of tissue, viscosity of the blood increases, and below 30° C there is a marked increase in the incidence of bleeding in the post-operative period.

Temperature control during extracorporeal circulation is normally effected by the passage of blood through heat exchangers, which are large surface areas of a high conductivity material over which the blood is filmed. The temperature in the water jacket can then be altered to affect the temperature of the blood. In some instances the heat exchanger is incorporated into some other piece of apparatus such as the oxygenator. Cooling can usually be effected more rapidly than rewarming because of the larger temperature gradient possible between blood (37° C) and the circulating fluid (0° C), whereas during rewarming the highest possible water temperature is approximately 40° C. Slow rewarming is desirable to avoid islets of cold tissue remaining in the body which cause the patient to cool again, perhaps dangerously, after bypass has been discontinued.

Renal Preservation

Disturbances of renal function during and after extracorporeal circulation are now uncommon. Under conditions of high flow, particularly when associated with haemodilution, urine output is normally sustained at a high level during cardiac surgery. This is particularly so if dextrose is used in the priming solution due to its osmotic effect. If the urine output falls below 30 ml of urine per hour, mannitol (25 g) is commonly added to the perfusate. A high urine output also helps to excrete the products of haemolysis. The urine production commonly ceases if the patient becomes acidotic and then returns to normal on correction of the metabolic acidosis. Post-operative renal problems appear to stem not so much from the bypass procedure but from a low cardiac output produced by the patient after surgery.

COMPLICATIONS

Haemolysis

Trauma to the formed elements of the blood can be a major complication of extracorporeal circulation. The most easily measurable result is the appearance of free plasma haemoglobin, but presumably other deleterious effects occur at the same time, particularly the denaturation of the plasma proteins which results from the presence of blood-gas interface in the oxygenator. Haemolysis can be reduced to a minimum by the use of high-quality tubing, by the siliconing of parts which come into contact with the blood, by the use of roller pumps which are carefully adjusted and which have large-bore tubing over which the roller only passes very slowly. Haemolysis is commoner in bubble oxygenators than in stationary screen and rotating disc oxygenators, but the principal source of haemolysis in fact lies in the suckers which are used to aspirate spilt blood from the heart. These should be of a wide bell-mouthed type and the surgical assistant should, wherever possible, suck pools of liquid blood, rather than a mixture of blood and air. Haemolysis normally increases almost linearly with the passage of time. However, with current-day well-maintained apparatus, it is rare for plasma haemoglobins to exceed approximately 100 mg per 100 ml blood even at the end of long perfusions. This is a level which is not normally associated with renal damage.

Air Embolism

Air embolism is one of the major hazards of open heart surgery. The air normally gains access to the heart during an intracardiac manoeuvre and is then ejected out into the systemic circulation when the heart is reconnected to the general circulation. Every effort, therefore, is made to ensure that the heart is free of air before the heart is reconnected to the circulation.

The following manoeuvres are employed:

   i. Whilst the aortic clamp is still applied, the venous pressure can be raised so that blood passes through the pulmonary capillaries, fills the left atrium and then the left ventricle, whilst the air passes outwards through a needle placed through the base of the aorta.

ii. Alternatively, air can be aspirated from the chambers of the heart, using a syringe and needle, from the left ventricle after up-ending the apex of the ventricle, or from the left atrium after the patient is positioned on his left side so that the left atrium lies above the ventricle and the mitral valve rendered incompetent.

Despite all these manoeuvres, air is commonly ejected into the aorta and the brain can be to some extent protected by positioning the patient with head downwards and also by making multiple holes or leaving needles through the arch of the aorta at its highest point. The bubbles then pass up the needles whilst the blood continues in the vessels.

During intracardiac manoeuvres, air commonly gains access to the pulmonary veins and this is often not dislodged until the pulmonary veins are perfused by raising the venous pressure and positive pressure ventilation begins. Before the aortic clamp is removed, the lungs should be inflated several times while aspirating the ventricle.

Flooding the operative site with carbon dioxide has been advocated on the grounds that if this gains access to the circulation, being highly absorbent, it will not cause significant embolism. In practice, with the motions of the heart, the patient's lungs and the surgeon's hands, it is virtually impossible to obtain local high concentrations of carbon dioxide.

Post-perfusion Lung

Post-perfusion lung is the name given to a collection of syndromes which result from different causes. The common feature is that lung function is disturbed and there is a large alveolar-arterial difference in oxygen tension. Whereas in normal lungs the venous admixture effect in the lung is approximately 3 per cent of the cardiac output, after extracorporeal circulation this figure may rise as high as 30 per cent (Fordham, 1965). In the face of a low cardiac output the alveolar-arterial (A–a) O_2 tension difference may be large enough to make the patient hypoxic despite ventilation with pure oxygen.

The causes of lung disturbance are:
  i. Simple lung collapse, usually of the left or right lower lobe and much commoner than usually thought. This will always respond to physiotherapy but is better prevented than treated.
 ii. Overdistension of pulmonary capillaries at operation. Before the routine use of a left heart vent to decompress the left heart at operation, damage used to occur to the lung capillaries and at post-mortem the lungs appeared liver-like with the alveoli filled with haemorrhagic exudate.
iii. High left atrial pressure. Gross damage to the pulmonary capillaries is now rare but pulmonary engorgement due to an excessively high left atrial pressure is common. This results from efforts to increase the cardiac output by raising the filling pressure of the ventricles while measuring only the right atrial pressure. Quite huge and unpredictable differences can exist between the functions of the two ventricles and quite small increases in right atrial pressure can produce increases in the left sided pressure which will result in pulmonary oedema (Sarin et al., 1970).
 iv. Blood prime. Sykes et al. (1966) have shown that lung function is much less affected after pure haemodilution prime than after a bypass with

a blood-containing prime. This is perhaps due to an immune response of white cells to the foreign protein in the donated blood.

If all these causes are eliminated, lung function is still altered in the post-operative period but to a much smaller extent. This small degree of change might properly be termed "post-perfusion lung" and is perhaps due to some alteration in the patient's own blood plasma proteins or lung surfactant.

REFERENCES

BIGELOW, W. G., CALLAGHAN, J. C., and TUPPS, J. A. (1950). General hypothermia for experimental intracardiac surgery. *Ann. Surg., 132,* 531.

BRIERLEY, J. B. (1967). Brain damage complicating open-heart surgery. *Proc. roy. Soc. Med., 60,* 858.

BRODIE, T. G. (1903). The perfusion of surviving organs. *J. Physiol. (Lond.), 29,* 266.

BROWN, T. C. K., DUNLOP, M. E., STEVENS, B. J., CLARKE, C. P., and SHANANAN, E. A. (1973). Biochemical changes during surface cooling for deep hypothermia in open heart surgery. *J. thorac. cardiovasc. Surg., 65,* 402.

BROWN-SÉQUARD, E. (1858). Du sang rouge et du sang noir, et de leurs principaux éléments gazeuses, l'oxygène et l'acide carbonique. *J. Anat. (Paris), 1,* 95.

DE WALL, R. A., WARDEN, H. E., VARCO, R. L., and LILLEHEI, C. W. (1957). Helix reservoir pump oxygenator. *Surg. Gynec Obstet., 104,* 699.

DREW, C. E., KEEN, G., and BENAZON, D. B. (1959). Profound hypothermia. *Lancet, 1,* 745.

DRINKER, P. A. (1972). Progress in membrane oxygenator design. *Anesthesiology, 37,* 242.

DUKE, H. N., and VANE, J. R. (1968). An adverse effect of polyvinylchloride tubing used in extracorporeal circulation. *Lancet, 2,* 21.

FELDMAN, S. A. (1971). Profound hypothermia. *Brit. J. Anaesth., 43,* 244.

FISK, G. C., WRIGHT, J. S., TURNER, B. B., BAKER, W. de C. HICKS, R. G., *et al.* (1974). Cerebral effects of circulatory arrest at 20° C in the infant pig. *Anaesth. Intens. Care, 2,* 33.

FORDHAM, R. (1965). Hypoxaemia after aortic valve surgery under cardiopulmonary bypass. *Thorax, 20,* 505.

FREY, M., and GRUBER, M. (1885). Ein Respirationsapparatus für isolirte Organe. *Arch. Anat. Physiol., 9,* 519.

GADBOYS, H. L., SLONIM, R., and LITWAR, R. (1962). Homologous blood syndrome. *Ann. Surg., 156,* 793.

GIBBON, J. H. (1937). Artificial maintenance of circulation during experimental occlusion of the pulmonary artery. *Arch. Surg., 34,* 1105.

HORIUCHI, T., KOYAMADA, K., MATAMO, I., *et al.* (1963). Radical operation for ventricular septal defect in infancy. *J. thorac. cardiovasc. Surg., 46,* 180.

JACOBY, C. (1890). Apparat zur Durchblutung isolirter überlebender Organe. *Naunyn-Schmiedeberg's Arch. exp. Path. Pharmak., 26,* 388.

JAVID, H., TUFO, H. M., NAJAFI, H., DYE, W. S., HUNTER, J. A., and JULIAN, O. C. (1969). Neurological abnormalities following open heart surgery. *J. thorac. cardiovasc. Surg., 58,* 502.

LEE, W. H., KRUMHAAR, D., FONKALSRUD, E. W., SCHJEIDE, O. A., and MANNEY, J. V. (1961). Destruction of plasma proteins as a cause of morbidity and death after intracardiac operations. *Surgery, 50,* 29.

LEGALLOIS, J. J. C. (1812). *Expériences sur le principe de la vie, notamment sur celui des mouvements du coeur, et sur le siège de ce principe.* Paris.

LEWIS, F. J. and TAUFFIC, M. (1953). Closure of atrial septal defects with the aid of hypothermia. *Surgery, 33,* 52.

LUDWIG, C. F. W. (1865). *Die physiologischen Leistungen des Blutdrucks.* Leipzig: S. Hirzel.

McDOWALL, D. G. (1971). The current usage of hypothermia in British neurosurgery. *Brit. J. Anaesth.*, **43**, 1084.

MELROSE, D. G. (1969). In: *Medical and Surgical Cardiology.* Ed. by Cleland, Goodwin, McDonald and Ross. Oxford: Blackwell Scientific Publications.

MOHRI, H., and MERENDINO, K. A. (1969). In: *Hypothermia With or Without a Pump Oxygenator in Surgery of the Chest.* Ed. by Gibbon, Sabiston and Spencer. Philadelphia: W. B. Saunders.

MOHRI, H., NESSEL, E. A., NELSON, R. J., MATANO, I., ANDERSON, N. H., DILLARD, D. H. and MERENDINO, K. A. (1966). Use of rheomacrodex and hyperventilation in prolonged circulatory arrest under deep hypothermia induced by surface cooling. *Amer. J. Surg.*, **112**, 241.

SARIN, C. L., YALAV, E., CLEMENT, A. J., and BRAIMBRIDGE, M. V. (1970). The necessity for measurement of left atrial pressure after cardiac valve surgery. *Thorax*, **25**, 185.

SCHMIDT-MULHEIM, A. (1880). Beitrage zur Kenntniss des Peptons und seiner physiologischen Bedeutung. *Arch. Anat. Physiol., Lpz.* (Physiol. Abt.). p. 33.

SCHRODER, W. (1882). Über die Bildungstatte des Harnstoffs. *Naunyn-Schmiedeberg's Arch. exp. Path. Pharmak.*, **15**, 364.

SMITH, L. W., and FAY, T. (1940). Observations on human beings with cancer maintained at reduced temperatures of 75–90° Fahrenheit. *Amer. J. clin. Path.*, **10**, 1.

SYKES, M. K., ROBINSON, B., MELROSE, D. G., and NAHAS, R. (1966). Pulmonary changes after extracorporeal circulation in dogs. *Brit. J. Anaesth.*, **38**, 432.

WATANABE, A., OKAMURA, N., TAKAHASHI, T., *et al.* (1959). Étude expérimentale de la réanimation cardiogne après interruption circulatorie prolongée practiqée à très basse température. *Path. et Biol.*, **7**, 1017.

WATERS, E. T., MARKOWITZ, J., and JAQUES, L. B. (1938). Anaphylaxis in the liverless dog, and observations on anticoagulant effect of anaphylactic shock. *Science*, **87**, 582.

Chapter 17

CARDIAC AND CIRCULATORY COMPLICATIONS

CIRCULATORY ARREST

HYPOXIA and haemorrhage are the most common causes of cardiac arrest during surgery. Occasionally cardiac disease or interference with the heart or great vessels may be responsible. In a small proportion of patients, circulatory arrest occurs when death is expected in the immediate future from some terminal illness. Then, even though temporary resuscitation may be possible, it is neither reasonable nor desirable. Most cases of circulatory arrest can be successfully treated provided action is efficient and prompt.

In general, cardiac arrest falls into two categories. It may be the end result of a progressive derangement of physiology which has gone unnoticed or unheeded for some time and which usually includes respiratory or metabolic acidosis and electrolyte disturbances. Alternatively, it may result from some sudden catastrophic event superimposed on an otherwise normal background. Camarata and colleagues (1971) confirmed the impression of intensive care physicians that in the latter group one may expect initial and long-term success but that in the former group success will be rare and that cardiac arrest is better prevented than treated.

Diagnosis

The most important point in the diagnosis is that no pulse can be felt in a large artery (femoral or carotid). In a surgical case this disappearance of an effective circulation may be noted by the sudden cessation of bleeding. An absent pulse indicates that the circulation is inadequate and that immediate treatment is needed.

Unconsciousness and cessation of respiration occur, and, usually within one minute, the pupils dilate. The absence of heart sounds is an unreliable sign and unless an ECG is already connected no time should be wasted in so doing before starting treatment.

The time interval between cardiac arrest and the death of tissue in the central nervous system is approximately three and a half minutes and there is ample clinical justification for accepting this period, though patients have survived intact for longer intervals. It can, however, only be completely acceptable on the basis that the patient is adequately oxygenated up to the moment of cardiac arrest. If hypoxia is present before this occurs, then severe neurological damage may result from even shorter periods of ischaemia than three and a half minutes.

Treatment

Once circulatory arrest has been diagnosed, whether the heart be in standstill, dysrhythmia or ventricular fibrillation, and whatever the initial cause, the immediate treatment must be aimed at providing an artificial circulation of oxygenated blood, followed by a rapid return to a normal circulation. Treatment, therefore, falls simultaneously under a number of headings:

(*a*) Artificial circulation of oxygenated blood.
   i. Artificial ventilation.
   ii. Closed chest cardiac massage.
(*b*) Restoration of cardiac function.
   i. Diagnosis—electrical activity, underlying causes.
   ii. Drug and fluid therapy.
   iii. Defibrillation.

Artificial ventilation.—Of the many methods of artificial ventilation advocated over the years, only those methods involving intermittent positive pressure ventilation produce sufficient volume exchange. In the hospital environment there will usually be to hand either a facemask or an endotracheal tube with oxygen supply, or an Ambu bag or Brook airway. Every anaesthetist should, however, be familiar with the technique of mouth-to-mouth or mouth-to-nose ventilation.

In all cases the first step is to clear the airway and then to maintain it clear, by endotracheal tube where possible, while ventilation is carried out. Intubation must be speedy so as not to interrupt ventilation and cardiac compression except briefly. If it is difficult the anaesthetist would do better to ventilate with a facemask until skilled assistance is at hand. Due to the low cardiac output produced by cardiac compression and the deranged ventilation-perfusion relationships in the lung, ventilation with 100 per cent oxygen will often not produce fully saturated arterial blood and despite apparent hyperventilation the carbon dioxide level rises. It is not possible to inflate the lungs at the same time as cardiac compression is carried out and ventilation normally alternates with cardiac compression in the ratio 1:5.

Closed chest cardiac massage.—The efficacy of closed chest cardiac massage in compressing the heart between the sternum and vertebral column was first reported by Kouwenhoven and his associates (1960). The technique is effective whether the heart is in asystole or ventricular fibrillation and produces a satisfactory central aortic pressure, although this is not a good index of the amount of flow. Ventricular fibrillation may cease spontaneously and a normal beat follow as a result of closed chest massage. Lateral displacement of the heart does not occur and while there may be some ventilation of the lungs it is not enough to obviate the need for simultaneous artificial respiration.

Technique.—Immediately the diagnosis is made and the airway has been cleared the patient is laid flat and external cardiac compression started. Although ideally the patient should lie on a firm surface, in practice it is more important to start the massage first and then, at a convenient moment, slip a wooden board, fracture board or even a tray under the patient during a pause while the patient is ventilated.

Compression is applied through the heel of one hand which is placed over the lower half of the sternum while the operator's other hand rests on the top of the hand directly on the chest. No force is transmitted through the fingers so that compression of the lateral part of the thorax, which produces rib fractures, is avoided. In an adult the sternum is depressed for 4–5 cm ($1\frac{1}{2}$–2 in) towards the spine—this requires a force of 50–70 lb (23–32 kg) and it is necessary for the operator to be well above the patient, kneeling on the bed if necessary, so as to use his body weight rather than the arm muscles alone, which is both fatiguing and ineffective. The cardiac output produced is only 20–40 per cent of normal and is rate-dependant. Cardiac compression is applied at a rate of 100 beats/min although after pauses for ventilation, only about 80 beats will be produced per minute. Slower rates than this produce an inadequate output.

In children compression is with one hand only, producing proportionately less sternal displacement, and is at a faster rate. In babies the whole chest may be grasped with one hand and the sternum displaced with the thumb while the fingers support the spine.

To be effective, external cardiac compression must produce a palpable pulse in the carotid or femoral artery. In cases where a direct arterial pressure recording is possible systolic pressures of 100 mm Hg (13·3 kPa) are commonly seen during massage, although of course this near normal pressure does not signify a near normal cardiac output. The pupils will diminish in size and sometimes consciousness and spontaneous respiration will return when the patient may have to be restrained so that resuscitation can continue.

External cardiac compression has to be interrupted to allow ventilation to occur, as it is impossible to inflate the chest while cardiac compression is occurring. Usually every sixth compression is missed to allow a positive-pressure ventilation to be performed. When working single-handed a ratio of two inflations to fifteen compressions is easier.

The exact technique of cardiac compression which produces the optimum output is unfortunately only learnt with experience. Too quick a compression while producing a good systolic pressure results in little forward flow, too slow a compression results in a low systolic pressure and too slow a rate, thus producing a low output. Practice on a "Ressussi-anne" or similar manikin with an experienced teacher is invaluable.

Internal cardiac massage.—External cardiac compression has replaced internal cardiac compression because of its greater feasibility and efficiency. In most cases when external compression is ineffective it is unlikely that direct cardiac compression will be any more so. There are, however, certain indications for the internal rather than the external technique if the latter fails.

(a) If the chest is already open during thoracic or cardiac surgery.

(b) In the presence of intrathoracic pathology, e.g., cardiac tamponade, pulmonary embolism, air embolism.

(c) Gross chest deformity or an excessively stiff rib cage which prevents effective external compression.

The incision is made in the fourth left interspace lateral to the internal mammary artery and the space pulled open with the hands. In the absence of a rib spreader an anaesthetic mouth gag can be used. After the pericardium has been incised, the heart is compressed, between two hands or, failing this, with the flat of one hand behind the heart and the thumb and thenar eminence in front, taking care not to perforate any of the chambers with the fingers.

If cardiac arrest occurs during abdominal surgery, closed chest massage is preferable to massage through the diaphragm.

Restoration of Cardiac Function

In cases of transient circulatory arrest such as Stokes-Adams attacks, or dysrhythmias associated with myocardial infarction, the prompt institution of external cardiac compression and artificial ventilation may result in the return of an effective spontaneous heart beat. In a coronary care unit with the patient already connected to an ECG, it may be possible to have one attempt at defibrillation as a first manoeuvre if this is within seconds of the arrest.

If the circulation is not restored immediately, definitive therapy is required as an emergency because the chances of success diminish as time passes.

First, the patient should be intubated and ventilated with pure oxygen with proper elimination of carbon dioxide.

A drip is set up which will provide a route for fluid and drug therapy. If possible the catheter should be advanced from the femoral or internal jugular vein to the vena cava so that it can be used to measure central venous pressure.

A diagnosis of cardiac rhythm is made by electrocardiography.

Arterial blood is withdrawn for estimation of acid/base state and for serum electrolytes, especially serum potassium.

Drug Therapy

1. **Correction of metabolic acidosis.**—The circulatory stagnation of cardiac arrest always leads to some degree of metabolic acidosis and this may be so severe that it depresses the circulatory effects of catecholamines or even prevents restoration of a normal beat. In an intensive care unit where cardiac arrest may be treated within thirty seconds and a normal circulation is quickly restored no alkalinising agent may be required, but generally an initial dose of 1–2 mEq/kg (mmol/kg) body weight of sodium bicarbonate is necessary. Thereafter the correction of metabolic acidosis is best controlled by serial estimations of the acid-base state of the arterial blood bearing in mind that the fluid compartment accessible for correction under the conditions of cardiac massage may be quite small. Excessive administration of sodium bicarbonate besides leading to an alkalosis which may itself depress the heart, leads to large shifts in potassium so that the patient may become severely hypokalaemic. The fluid and sodium load may also contribute to the development of pulmonary oedema. Once a normal beat is restored and the tissues become perfused a much larger acidosis is revealed which may often require correction.

2. **Inotropic drugs.**—Inotropic drugs are given both for cardiac asystole, in an attempt to provoke a return to a spontaneous heart beat, and for ventricular fibrillation, to improve the tone of the myocardium before attempting electrical defibrillation. The specific treatment of a dysrhythmia should precede the general use of inotropic drugs.

The drug of choice is adrenaline in a dose of 1 mg (10 ml of 1:10,000 solution) given intravenously, preferably into a central vein. Attempted intracardiac injection may produce a pneumothorax or an injury to a coronary artery and should be avoided whenever possible unless the heart is directly exposed at surgery. The adrenaline can be repeated every two to five minutes. Calcium is also frequently used and is best given as an intravenous injection of $CaCl_2$ in doses of up to 1 g (9 mmol), unless the arrest is thought to be hypokalaemic in origin. Adrenaline in this dosage is a vasopressor and the raised systemic vascular resistance will encourage coronary and cerebral blood flow, and augment venous return. Other vasopressors (methoxamine, metaraminol, ephedrine) are less effective while isoprenaline, due to its vasodilator action, may be positively harmful.

Cardiac standstill.—Asystole will usually respond to effective cardiac massage and ventilation together with correction of the acidosis and the administration of inotropic drugs. In cases of complete heart block or refractory bradycardia which do not respond to an infusion of isoprenaline it may be necessary to resort to electrical pacing. In the emergency this can be started using two electrodes applied over the precordium, although this is sufficiently painful that the patient must be anaesthetised if it is continued and, as soon as possible, internal pacing is substituted using a pacemaker placed in the right ventricle via an intravenous catheter.

Ventricular fibrillation.—Fibrillation may be present as the initial form of circulatory arrest or it may arise during the emergency treatment. Once the myocardial tone has been improved with adequate oxygenation by good massage, drug therapy and the correction of acid-base and electrolyte abnormalities, defibrillation is attempted preferably with a direct current machine. The two paddles are positioned so that the heart lies between them. One is placed over the apex, and it is convenient if the other can be placed under the right scapula as it can be left there during cardiac compression.

Direct current defibrillation through the closed chest requires an energy release of between 200–400 joules (50–200 joules in children). For direct defibrillation of the exposed heart 20–100 joules may be required according to the size of the heart.

In the event of defibrillation not occurring or the heart repeatedly refibrillating due to extreme irritability of the myocardium, this can be suppressed (without depressing myocardial contractility) by lignocaine given intravenously (dose 1 mg/kg). If defibrillation is subsequently successful but recurrent dysrhythmia is a problem, the lignocaine is continued as an infusion at a rate of 1 to 2 mg per minute. This drug has largely replaced the use of quinidine and procaine amide. In intractable ventricular fibrillation, β-blockade may be necessary before successful conversion. Intravenous practolol (1–2 mg increments to a maximum of 20 mg) is preferable to propranolol. While propranolol is used to suppress ventricular dysrhythmias after myocardial infarction, its use in the treatment of ventricular fibrillation is hazardous and if the patient is restored to normal rhythm the heart may not be capable of producing a sufficient output.

In cardiac patients or patients with electrolyte imbalance, disturbances of serum potassium may cause cardiac arrest, and defibrillation may not be possible until this has returned to normal. Hypokalaemia is easily treated with intravenous potassium. The effects of hyperkalaemia can be partially antagonised by administration of $CaCl_2$, or the level of serum potassium may be reduced by increasing the cellular uptake of $K+$ either by giving glucose and insulin intravenously (100 ml 50 per cent dextrose with 12·5 units soluble insulin) or by bicarbonate administration and hyperventilation, while cardiac massage is continued.

After Treatment

Once a normal beat has been restored the patient is carefully monitored to ensure that the circulation is adequate. This may necessitate further periods of external cardiac compression if the pulse becomes feeble. The cardiac output is then best supported by an infusion of isoprenaline (1 mg in 200 ml dextrose with a microdrop giving set), rather less importance being placed on vasopressor drugs and the actual value of the blood pressure. Lignocaine (1–2 mg/min) may be needed to control dysrhythmias, the rhythm being observed on an electro-cardioscope. The filling pressure of the heart is measured via a central venous line as a guide to fluid replacement, the acid-base state estimated on arterial samples, the urine output charted and the pulse and blood pressure recorded.

Frequently the respiration is inadequate after cardiac resuscitation, either because of damage sustained by the rib cage or because of poor lung function. Large shunts occur in the lung which, in the face of a low cardiac output, lead to arterial hypoxaemia despite a high inspired oxygen concentration. After an arrest, the patient must receive a high inspired oxygen content and artificial ventilation be maintained until blood gas measurement shows that the patient is capable of supporting his own ventilatory needs.

Comment

All too often, cardiac arrest is the end-result of a derangement of physiology which has been either unnoticed or untreated for some time. It is much better to prevent a cardiac arrest than to treat it, however effectively.

Also, the treatment defined above covers only the essential practical details of resuscitation. Resuscitation will often be ineffective if the precipitating cause is not recognised and treated. It requires a calm logical mind with a good under-standing of medicine to sort out and treat the underlying condition while at the same time performing emergency resuscitation.

However, accepting that cardiac emergencies may arise suddenly, the successful treatment must depend to some extent on the provision of proper facilities and the adequate training of personnel.

Basic resuscitation kits should be kept available in all wards and departments of the hospital. There should be a well-rehearsed plan of action so that no time is wasted on inessential manoeuvres. The ultimate result for a patient will depend on the brevity of the interval between cardiac arrest and the restoration of an effective circulation, and every anaesthetist should know what can and what should be done in that period.

POST-OPERATIVE VENOUS THROMBOSIS
AND PULMONARY EMBOLISM

Deep Vein Thrombosis

There has been a continuous absolute increase in deaths from pulmonary embolus since 1943 and it has been estimated that currently 21,000 patients die annually in the United Kingdom from this cause (Kakkar, 1975). Of these patients 60 per cent might have been expected to return to normal life had it not been for their embolus (Evans, 1971). Swollen legs and trophic changes are distressing complications of non-fatal deep vein thrombosis.

Aetiology.—The actual "trigger" mechanism of deep vein thrombosis is unknown. The thrombosis starts as a small area of platelet deposition and then propagates. Although the calf is the commonest site of thrombosis, it can begin in any part of the peripheral venous system and may develop in more than one site simultaneously (Browse and Lea Thomas, 1974).

Deep vein thrombosis is associated with bedrest, major surgical procedures, cerebrovascular accidents and malignancy. The middle-aged and elderly are more at risk than the young although the use of the contraceptive pill is tending to change this distribution. Chest, abdomen and hip operations have a greater incidence than head, neck and breast surgery.

Anaesthesia and operation are conducive to venous stasis. Certain positions on the operating table and some anaesthetic techniques favour venous pooling. The removal of all skeletal muscle tone and the direct effects of surgical trauma —as in pelvic operations—are normal accompaniments of many operations. These may be accentuated by oligaemia and by changes in coagulability which occur in the pre-operative period.

Deep venous thrombosis may start at the time of operation or in the first 24–48 hours after surgery but if the predisposing factors existed pre-operatively, the thrombotic process may already have been established by the time the patient comes to surgery. Pulmonary embolism may then be precipitated when the femur is manipulated or an Esmarch tourniquet applied.

Diagnosis.—The diagnosis is not obvious, 70 per cent of deep vein thromboses having neither signs nor symptoms. The most reliable sign when it occurs is ankle oedema; less reliable but much commoner are tenderness of the calf accompanied perhaps by an increase in calf diameter or a slight rise in temperature. Early diagnosis depends on a suspicious mind in the doctor.

The Doppler ultrasound technique, which has the merits of simplicity and cheapness, is accurate in diagnosing thrombosis from the level of the knee to the IVC. It cannot detect thrombosis in the calf veins which are best diagnosed using ^{125}I-labelled fibrinogen uptake (Kakkar *et al.*, 1970). Fortunately, calf vein thrombosis although commonest, seldom gives rise to pulmonary embolism. Ultimate definition of the clot is obtained by phlebography.

Prophylaxis.—The best treatment for deep vein thrombosis is obviously prophylactic, and there are two main approaches—prevention of stasis and alteration of blood coagulability.

Prevention of stasis.—This can be passive—elastic stockings and elevation of the leg—or active. There is only marginal evidence that passive measures are effective (Flanc *et al.*, 1969). The active measures include regular electrical stimulation of the calf muscle, mechanical movement of the feet and intermittent pneumatic compression of the calf muscles. These measures produce benefit except in high-risk patients and there are logistic difficulties about applying them in the post-operative period.

Alteration in blood coagulability.—The most popular and effective methods are small dose heparin and intravenous dextran-70. Infusion of dextran 70 reduces the incidence of deep venous thrombosis compared with control patients undergoing general surgery but not to the same extent as heparin (Vasilescu and Ruckley, 1974); troublesome side-effects have not been reported.

Low dose heparin is undoubtedly effective in reducing the incidence of calf vein thrombosis detectable by ^{125}I-labelled fibrinogen uptake. Several dose schedules are recommended, the commonest being 5,000 units twice daily for 5–6 days, starting two hours before operation. Because of the variability of effect of heparin in individual patients this schedule may be ineffective in some patients, particularly those undergoing hip operations, but may give rise to bleeding problems in others. Sharnoff recommends the modified Dale and Laidlaw coagulometer in monitoring the effect of subcutaneous heparin.

Pulmonary Embolism

The common sites of origin for a pulmonary embolism are the veins of the pelvis and lower extremities—small emboli arising from the calves while large emboli come from the ilio-femoral venous segment. In cardiac disease thrombi may originate on the right side of the heart. The total incidence of pulmonary embolism is very high—in unselected post-mortem examinations as many as 70 per cent of cases can be shown to have some degree of pulmonary emboli—but the incidence of clinically detectable pulmonary embolism in post-operative patients is probably less than 1 per cent. This incidence is of course much higher in groups of patients particularly at risk, notably those with a previous history of thrombo-embolism and those undergoing orthopaedic operations or splenectomy.

The common time of occurrence is some days—3 to 21—after an operation, but this depends on the patient being fit and well previously. If the predisposing factors have existed for some time pre-operatively the time scale is shifted—the embolism may even occur at the time of operation. Fractured neck of femur followed by late reduction in an elderly patient—a situation full of predisposing factors—may well result in a pulmonary embolus at the time of reduction.

Diagnosis.—Sudden pain in the chest and dyspnoea are the classical symptoms, and if the blood clot is large enough to obstruct the pulmonary arterial circulation materially, death may rapidly follow from acute cor pulmonale. Smaller degrees of obstruction produce a less catastrophic picture but evidence of right ventricular failure—dyspnoea, tachycardia, venous engorgement, hypotension—may be present to some degree. The ECG may show right ventricular strain and the chest X-ray shows "pruning" of the affected pulmonary vessels.

Small emboli usually cause little more than pain and dyspnoea in the first place, but these symptoms may be followed after twenty-four hours by haemoptysis, fever, and signs of pulmonary infarction. The ultimate circulatory result of a simple pulmonary embolus in a given patient is influenced partly by the size of the embolus and partly by the preceding state of the patient's heart and pulmonary vasculature—thus some patients may survive a single large pulmonary embolism, while others die from the effects of repeated small ones.

Prophylaxis.—While subcutaneous heparin has been shown to reduce the frequency of calf vein thrombosis, no study has so far provided evidence that it reduces the prevalence of pulmonary embolism (LeQuesne, 1974) and such evidence will only be obtainable from a very large prospective study (Kakkar, 1975).

Treatment of Simple Deep Vein Thrombosis

Once diagnosed, the treatment is with anticoagulants. Intravenous heparin is given either as 6,000 units 4-hourly or as a continuous infusion giving 40,000 units over 24 hours. At the same time oral warfarin or phenindione is started. The heparin is usually discontinued after 2–3 days but continued for 5–6 days if there is a pulmonary embolus. Oral anticoagulants are continued for at least 3 months with the blood prothrombin time increased two or threefold.

Surgical removal of vein clot in the upper femoral or iliac vein is only successful if there is recent non-adherent clot. Plication of the inferior vena cava or iliac vein, or ligation of the femoral vein below the profunda, may be indicated if anticoagulation fails to prevent recurrent pulmonary embolism.

Treatment of Deep Vein Thrombosis with Pulmonary Embolism

As with simple deep vein thrombosis the initial treatment is with heparin. A phlebogram is performed to define the thrombi. If the thrombus appears old and well fixed long-term anticoagulation is the only treatment necessary; if however the clot appears fresh and loose and is thought likely to cause further emboli then more radical treatment is required. Thrombectomy is possible for thrombi lying in the major vessels, but where the smaller vessels, such as the calf veins, are affected, then either peripheral vein ligation or streptokinase therapy are indicated, although recent surgery may prohibit the latter. Thrombectomy or peripheral vein ligation may be performed under general anaesthesia when the anaesthetist may be called upon to perform a Valsalva manoeuvre to reverse the flow in the inferior vena cava at the moment the vein is opened. The anaesthetist should also remember that positioning on the table, perhaps even the muscle fasciculations of succinylcholine, may precipitate a further larger pulmonary embolus during anaesthesia and careful monitoring of the patient is necessary despite the apparent simplicity of the surgical procedure.

Treatment of Pulmonary Embolism

The treatment of pulmonary artery embolism depends on the degree of pulmonary artery obstruction and the pre-existing state of the patient. The immediate treatment consists of the administration of heparin, the use of oxygen to prevent hypoxia, and the administration of digitalis and vasopressor drugs when indicated to support the circulation and in particular the right ventricle.

The extremes of pulmonary embolism provide no problem in treatment. The patient who is severely disabled, dyspnoeic, and in imminent danger of death, needs surgical removal of the embolus. This is preceded wherever possible by pulmonary angiography to define the affected vessels. It may be necessary to use supportive bypass, in addition to the other supportive measures, at the time of investigation, which is best carried out on an X-ray table in the theatre. It is then possible to continue the operation, with cardiopulmonary bypass if necessary, without delay. These patients are best investigated by pulmonary angiography without anaesthesia, but when anaesthesia is necessary it represents an extreme hazard for the patient and a most taxing demand on the anaesthetist.

Patients with small pulmonary emboli are treated with anticoagulants and the deep vein thrombosis considered separately for special treatment as defined above. The difficulty in choice of treatment lies in those patients who have had major pulmonary emboli but who are not so ill as to require immediate pulmonary embolectomy. These are probably best investigated with a pulmonary angiogram and then treated with streptokinase. Routine phlebography should always follow a pulmonary embolism to identify, and treat, the patient who remains at risk of a further, possibly fatal, embolism.

EMBOLISM

Embolus translated literally means a plug. Various substances may be carried along in the blood stream until they ultimately obstruct one or more blood vessels but those of particular interest are fat, air, tumour, blood clot, and amniotic fluid.

Fat Embolism

This usually follows fracture of a bone—typically a long bone or rib—or rupture of the liver or kidney. It may result from an operative procedure on a bone and rarely may follow sudden decompression in a deep-sea diver or high-altitude flier.

Sevitt (1960; 1962) has shown that pulmonary fat embolism is very common after injury and he believes it to be almost universal after fracture of a marrow bone. Clinically fat embolism can be divided into three groups; first the fulminating case, secondly the classical syndrome with cerebral, neurological and respiratory symptoms, and thirdly the incomplete or partial case. *A fulminating embolus* may occur within a few hours or days of a severe traumatic injury and is generally only diagnosed when the brain is sectioned after a post-mortem. Fat embolism may be suspected when the patient fails to respond to adequate resuscitation therapy, and when a period of normal consciousness subsequent to the injury is followed by coma. *The classical syndrome* can be expected to occur suddenly some twenty-four hours after an injury, and is typified by a mixture of mental confusion, often with localising neurological symptoms and signs, respiratory distress with pyrexia, and a petechial rash mainly over the upper chest, shoulders and lower neck. *An incomplete or partial case* is mild in course showing only some of the symptoms of the classical case.

In fracture patients with signs of fat embolism, hypoxaemia is often clinically important. Gurd and Wilson (1974) found the arterial oxygen tension below 50 mm Hg (6·7 kPa) in 24 of 50 cases and between 51 and 80 mm Hg (6·8 and 10·7 kPa) in another 17. Studies of other fracture patients with no other evidence of fat embolism frequently reveal subclinical hypoxaemia (Pao_2 circa 70 mm Hg–9·3 kPa), and although other causes such as post-traumatic pulmonary microthrombo-emboli may be responsible, fat embolism as the cause would accord with the high rate of histologically proven lung embolism after fractures.

The diagnosis is usually made on clinical grounds (Wright, 1971) but fat globules may be seen in the retinal vessels or in the urine or sputum. Histological examination of petechiae may demonstrate fat. The discovery of fat globules larger than 10μm in diameter in the serum is said to be pathognomonic of fat embolism (Harman and Ragaz, 1952).

The origin of the fat is generally considered to be the fat at the site of trauma. Hallgren and his colleagues (1966) showed that emboli recovered from the lungs of dogs with fractured legs have a similar triglyceride composition to bone marrow and depot fat but dissimilar to chylomicron fat.

The hypoxaemia following pulmonary fat embolism is due partly to an increase in alveolar dead space and to an increase in pulmonary veno-arterial admixture of between 20 and 50 per cent of the cardiac output (Prys-Roberts *et al.*, 1970). Sevitt (1973) has postulated two routes for the fat emboli to gain access to the systemic circulation and thus the brain. Minor systemic embolism may occur by small fat globules passing through the pulmonary capillaries but when there is serious blockage of the pulmonary vascular bed, blood might be diverted via pulmonary-bronchial anastomoses to the left side of the heart without passing through a fine capillary bed.

Treatment.—The efficacy of many of the advocated treatments is not proven. The respiratory system should be treated symptomatically which will usually mean a raised inspired oxygen concentration and sometimes positive-pressure ventilation. Circulatory support is not often needed provided the hypoxia is eliminated.

Air Embolism

The first recorded case of air embolism in the medical literature is that occurring in a French locksmith in 1818 (Magendie, 1821). Sporadic reports followed this and Hunter (1962) has remarked that air embolism as a complication during anaesthesia was not common until the advent of controlled respiration (for neurosurgery in the sitting position). Others (Michenfelder *et al.*, 1969) have felt that this increase was secondary to the introduction of muscle relaxants and the low venous pressure which followed their use in the upright patient. More recently the true and much larger incidence of air embolism has been revealed in prospective studies (Tateishi, 1972) and by the use of the Doppler ultrasound device (Michenfelder *et al.*, 1972).

Although air embolism has been most commonly described in relation to posterior fossa neurosurgery performed in the sitting position (O'Higgins, 1970) there are a large number of other situations in which it can occur (Table 1). Indeed when one considers how often a low central venous pressure and an open vein must exist, e.g. cervical laminectomy, the surprise is how seldom it actually gives rise to trouble (Leivers *et al.*, 1971) and that there must be other aetiological factors. There is a suggestion that children may be more at risk than adults in some circumstances. Gardner (1971) reports 13 cases of gas embolism during diagnostic radiology of which nine occurred in children. Perhaps this is due to the large volume of air used relative to the child's size.

Effects of Air Embolism

In some cases air enters the arterial system direct—usually during open heart surgery or extracorporeal circulation—and passes to the periphery causing effects according to the vessel entered and the position of the patient at the time. The air causes obstruction in flow in the arterioles and also acts as an endothelial irritant producing segmental arteriolar spasm. In the cerebral vessels air can be found 48 hours after experimental air embolism.

More commonly air enters the venous system. The effect depends partly on the total volume and perhaps more importantly on the rate of entry, although precise quantitation of these factors is lacking. The air bubbles may collect in the right atrium, from where they can often be aspirated, but, depending on the right atrial pressure, the flow rate of blood through it and the position of the patient, may be passed into the right ventricle and be churned up into froth before being ejected into the pulmonary artery. Pulmonary hypertension (with right ventricular strain) develops partly due to mechanical blockage of the pulmonary vessels and partly through a neurogenic effect. The churning action of the foam may lead to fibrin deposits in the pulmonary artery and damage may occur to blood elements at the blood gas interface. The cardiac output and blood pressure fall and dysrhythmias, including ventricular fibrillation, may be precipitated. Respiration is stimulated (becoming laboured) and respiratory efforts may break through controlled ventilation. The large inspiratory pressure swings thus generated may enhance the entrainment of air.

17/Table 1
The Principal Sources of Air Embolus

1. Surgical —danger increased by low central venous pressure.	Operations involving veins of head, neck, thorax, abdomen, pelvis Heart—particularly open heart operations.
2. Obstetric and Gynaecological	Delivery in presence of placenta praevia Insufflation of fallopian tubes. Criminal abortion.
3. Diagnostic	Air encephalogram. Angiocardiography. Air myelography.
4. Therapeutic	I.V. therapy. Antral washouts. Pneumothorax. Pneumoperitoneum. IPPV. Transfusion. Monitoring apparatus. Haemodialysis. Extracorporeal circulation.
5. Accidental	Rapid decompression.

Air will pass from the right side of the heart to the systemic circulation either through the pulmonary vascular bed or across intracardiac defects. Knowledge of an intracardiac defect in a patient demands even more scrupulous care about intravenous therapy than normal. The particular dangers of systemic air are that very small quantities of air entering the coronary arteries can provoke ventricular fibrillation and that air entering the cerebral vessels can produce permanent neurological damage.

The effect of air embolism is aggravated if the patient is receiving high concentrations of nitrous oxide at the time. Nunn (1959) was the first to suggest than N_2O which is thirty times more soluble than N_2, would diffuse quickly into the bubbles and appreciably increase their size, a complication which may be particularly important when air has reached the systemic circulation. Munson and Merrick (1966) have shown experimentally that venous air embolism is more likely to be fatal if a large percentage of nitrous oxide is being administered at the time, and Munson (1971) has shown that as the bubbles pass through the pulmonary capillaries very rapid direct gas exchange occurs between the alveolus and the bubble which emphasises the need to *discontinue* the N_2O if air embolism is suspected.

Monitoring Techniques

In an anaesthetic situation in which air embolism is an expected complication—such as posterior fossa neurosurgery, careful prospective monitoring using the techniques described below must be undertaken. In less likely situations if a patient suddenly develops hypotension, dysrhythmias, and irregular respirations, the possibility of air embolism should be considered and auscultation of the heart will confirm the diagnosis. Sometimes, of course, the noise of air entering the vein may have been heard.

1. Doppler ultrasound technique

Doppler cardiac auscultation (Edmonds-Seal and Maroon, 1969; Michenfelder et al., 1972) is the most sensitive qualitative method for detecting intravascular air embolism. The receiver is placed over the tricuspid valve and its function confirmed with a small injection of CO_2. "It is the only diagnostic technique which is not dependent on a pathophysiological alteration in vital functions and thus allows preventative and therapeutic measures to be instituted before cardiorespiratory collapse develops" (Maroon, 1973).

The Doppler is not a quantitative instrument, it being impossible to determine the volume of air from the character and loudness of the air artefact, but it will detect very small amounts of air. Thus vanguard bubbles which may herald a larger air embolism may be detected. Electrical interference occurs between the diathermy and the ultrasound device, which is worse with spark gap (rather than valve operated) diathermy, but this is a transient effect and could, if necessary, be excluded.

2. Auscultation

The first effect of air entering the heart is to produce faintly audible transitory high-pitched tinkling sounds; as the volume of air increases the heart sounds become resonant and drumlike. 30 ml of air produces the characteristic harsh mill-wheel murmur which denotes a worse prognosis. These changes are better and earlier appreciated through an oesophageal stethoscope than via a precordial instrument. Michenfelder et al., writing in 1969 before the use of the Doppler, reported that in 90 per cent of cases the first observed sign was a cardiac murmur.

The oesophageal stethoscope being simple and inexpensive, should be standard practice where air embolism is expected and will assist prompt recognition of changes in respiratory pattern (McComish and Thompson, 1968).

3. Electrocardiogram

Lewis and Rees (1964) have described the ECG changes which follow air embolism. These are best seen in lead V_1 and comprise signs of right heart strain (right bundle-branch block, inverted T waves and tall peaked P waves in the right chest leads) and the development of ventricular dysrhythmias and sometimes ventricular fibrillation. Small amounts of air may, on occasion, produce ECG abnormalities before alterations in heart sounds are noted.

4. Cardiovascular monitoring

(a) *Arterial pressure.* A fall in arterial pressure, secondary to a low cardiac output usually accompanied by tachycardia, and best seen on a continuous display of directly measured pressure, is a relatively late sign of a quite large air embolism.

(b) *Right atrial line.* A catheter whose tip is in the right atrium (Michenfelder et al., 1969)—confirmed by radiography or by intracardiac electrocardiography—can be used for therapy (see below) and diagnosis. The two diagnostic signs are that the central venous pressure rises when the right ventricle comes under strain, and it may be possible to aspirate air from the right atrium. The catheter needs to be long enough that it can be advanced into the right ventricle if necessary.

5. *End-expiratory carbon dioxide content*

Pulmonary air embolism results in a sudden fall in alveolar carbon dioxide content due to an increase in alveolar dead space secondary to the development of veno-arterial shunts in the lung and this can be picked up as a sudden diminution in the end-expiratory CO_2 content measured with an infra-red rapid CO_2 analyser (Brechner and Bethune, 1971).

Edmonds-Seal and his colleagues (1971) compared different methods of detecting air embolism and found the ultrasonic method to be the most sensitive, followed by the measurement of end-tidal CO_2. The latter technique tends to be rejected on grounds of cost and complexity. Changes in BP, ECG, CVP, and respiratory pattern occurred only after quite large emboli, and the changes in these variables due to small amounts of air may be indistinguishable from those due to alterations in surgical stimulation or level of anaesthesia.

Prevention.—There are a number of factors which either encourage or worsen air embolism. Obviously the first is a portal of entry for the air, and in those operations where air embolism is a known hazard, special care must be taken by the surgeon.

The next most important factor is a low central venous pressure, and while this applies particularly in respect of head and neck veins while in the upright posture it also applies during such conditions as lacerated liver. The low venous pressure may be caused by posture, haemorrhage, the effects of vasodilator drugs, and perhaps the effects of muscle relaxants. It will be aggravated by violent or obstructed respiratory movements. It has been suggested that the CVP should be maintained at a level which is just less than that which causes troublesome oozing. This may be achieved by infusion of plasma expanders, by the use of an antigravity suit, by the adjustment of the intrathoracic pressure with IPPV or expiratory resistance, and local venous congestion can be caused by intermittent compression with an inflatable collar or an intravenous balloon catheter.

The use of air as a contrast medium in radiology should be replaced by a more soluble gas such as carbon dioxide, or perhaps nitrous oxide.

In view of the diffusion of N_2O into air bubbles, with consequent increase in size, this gas should be avoided as part of the anaesthetic technique when the complication is considered likely. At the same time it has to be remembered that the mortality of air embolism is low and that the methods used for its detection and prevention must not introduce a greater hazard of their own.

Treatment.—The most important factor in treatment is speedy recognition of the complication. Treatment can be considered under three headings—prevention of entry of more air, removal of the embolised air, and support of the circulation.

(*a*) *Prevention of further entry of air*

The first act is to compress or ligate the open vessel: if it cannot be identified then flooding the wound with saline or packing it with saline-soaked swabs may suffice. Identification of the vessel may be helped, and further air entry prevented, if the central venous or local venous pressure can be raised by altering the posture of the patient, by inflation of a balloon catheter or antigravity suit, by local venous compression, or by raising the intrathoracic pressure using positive pressure applied to the airway.

(*b*) *Support of the circulation*

If the circulation is obviously inadequate, external cardiac massage is started and the patient placed with a left-hand tilt. Not infrequently these two measures are sufficient to restore a circulation. If not, massage must be continued, vasopressors administered, and acid/base imbalance corrected. Ventricular fibrillation will require electrical defibrillation. Ventilation is started with pure oxygen.

(*c*) *Removal of air*

The classical description is that turning the patient on the left side head down places the right atrium and tricuspid valve above the right ventricle and tends to delay the passage of air into the pulmonary artery. The foam stays uppermost with liquid blood flowing underneath it and the air can be aspirated through the right atrial monitoring catheter which can be advanced into the right ventricle if required. However, in Michenfelder's large series successful aspiration was usually performed with the patient still in the upright position and the table was lowered in only 13 per cent of cases. It is rare for direct aspiration of the heart to be necessary.

The natural absorption of the air is hastened by ventilation of the patient with pure oxygen which reduces the amount of nitrous oxide (and nitrogen) in the blood.

Whole body compression at greater than atmospheric pressures may be valuable to force the gas into solution, particularly in cases of systemic air embolism involving the brain, or when gas bubbles form in the blood following rapid decompression. Calverley and his colleagues (1971) discuss this in some detail and describe a technique which employs rapid compression to six ATA. If the patient responds favourably after 10–20 minutes the pressure is reduced to three ATA. At this level 100 per cent oxygen can then be used for progressive decompression over the next few hours.

Tumour Embolism

Tumour embolism may occur spontaneously or at operation, and, should the pieces of growth be big enough, can obstruct the pulmonary (arterial) or the systemic circulation, depending upon the site of the growth. Sudden death may occur from pulmonary obstruction or obstruction of the outflow tract of the left heart. Probert (1956) describes a patient who died suddenly during exploration of a carcinoma of the bronchus due to tumour embolism in the pulmonary veins.

Amniotic Fluid Embolism

This is considered on page 1386.

REFERENCES

BRECHNER, V. L., and BETHUNE, R. W. M. (1971). Recent advances in monitoring pulmonary air embolism. *Anesth. Analg. Curr. Res.*, **50**, 255.

BROWSE, N. L., and THOMAS, M. L. (1974). Source of non-lethal pulmonary emboli. *Lancet*, **1**, 258.

CALVERLEY, R. K., DODDS, W. A., TRAPP, W. G., and JENKINS, L. C. (1971). Hyperbaric treatment of cerebral air embolism. *Canad. Anaesth. Soc. J.*, **18**, 665.

CAMARATA, S. J., WEIL, M. H., HANASHIRO, P. K., and SHUBIM, H. (1971). Cardiac arrest in the critically ill. A study of predisposing causes in 132 patients. *Circulation*, **44**, 688.

EDMONDS, SEAL, J., and MAROON, J. C. (1969). Air embolism diagnosed with ultrasound. A new monitoring technique. *Anaesthesia*, **24**, 438.

EDMONDS-SEAL, J., and MAROON, J. C. (1969). Air embolism diagnosed with ultrasound. of various methods of detection. *Anaesthesia*, **26**, 202.

EVANS, D. S. (1971). The early diagnosis of thromboembolism by ultrasound. *Ann. roy. Coll. Surg. Engl.*, **49**, 225.

FLANC, C., KAKKAR, V. V., and CLARKE, M. B. (1969). Postoperative deep vein thrombosis. *Lancet*, **1**, 477.

GARDNER, L. G. (1971). Air embolism during arterial air myelography. *Brit. J. Anaesth.*, **43**, 807.

GURD, A. R., and WILSON, R. I. (1974). The fat embolism syndrome. *J. Bone Jt. Surg.*, **56B**, 408.

HALLGREN, B., KERSTELL, J., RUDENSTAN, C. M., and SVANBONG, A. (1966). Chemical analysis of fat emboli in experimental bone fractures. *Acta chir. scand.*, **132**, 613.

HARMAN, J. W., and RAGAZ, F. J. (1952). The pathogenesis of experimental fat embolism. *Amer. J. Path.*, **26**, 551.

HUNTER, A. R. (1962). Air embolism in the sitting position. *Anaesthesia*, **17**, 467.

KAKKAR, V. V. (1975). Deep vein thrombosis. Detection and prevention. *Circulation*, **51**, 8.

KAKKAR, V. V., NICOLAIDES, A. N., RENNEY, J. T. G., FRIEND, J. R., and CLARKE, M. B. (1970). ^{125}I-labelled fibrinogen test adapted for routine screening for deep vein thrombosis. *Lancet*, **1**, 540.

KOUWENHOVEN, W. B., JUDE, J. R., and KNICKERBOCKER, G. G. (1960). Closed chest cardiac massage. *J. Amer. med. Ass.*, **173**, 1064.

LEIVERS, D., SPILSBURY, R. A., and YOUNG, J. V. I. (1971). Air embolism during neurosurgery in the sitting position. *Brit. J. Anaesth.* **43**, 84 (with 25 references).

LEQUESNE, L. P. (1974). Relation between deep vein thrombosis and pulmonary embolism in surgical patients. *New Engl. J. Med.*, **291**, 1292.

LEWIS, J. M., and REES, G. A. D. (1964). Electrocardiography during posterior fossa operations. *Brit. J. Anaesth.*, **36**, 63.

MCCOMISH, P. B., and THOMPSON, D. E. A. (1968). Respiratory disturbances in air embolism. *Anaesthesia*, **23**, 259.

MAGENDIE, F. (1821). Sur l'entree accidentelle de l'air dans les veins. *J. de Physiologie Experimentale (Paris)*, **1**, 190.

MAROON, J. C. (1973). Venous air embolism. *Lancet*, **1**, 605.

MICHENFELDER, J. D., MARTIN, J. T., ALTENBURG, B. M., and REHOER, K. (1969). An evaluation of right atrial catheter for diagnosis and treatment of air embolism during neurosurgery. *J. Amer. med. Ass.*, **208**, 1353.

MICHENFELDER, J. D., MILLER, R. H., and GRONERT, G. A. (1972). Evaluation of an ultrasonic device (Doppler) for the diagnosis of venous air embolism. *Anesthesiology*, **36**, 164.

MUNSON, E. S. (1971). Effect of nitrous oxide on the pulmonary circulation during venous air embolism. *Anesth. Analg. Curr. Res.*, **50**, 785.

MUNSON, E. S., and MERRICK, H. C. (1966). Effect of N_2O on venous air embolism. *Anesthesiology*, **27**, 783.

NUNN, J. F. (1959). Controlled respiration in neurosurgical anaesthesia. *Anaesthesia*, **14**, 413.

O'HIGGINS, J. W. (1970). Air embolism during neurosurgery. *Brit. J. Anaesth.*, **42**, 459.

PROBERT, W. R. (1956). Sudden operative death due to massive tumour embolism. *Brit. med. J.*, **1**, 435.

PRYS-ROBERTS, C., GREENBAUM, R., NUNN, J. F., KELMAN, G. R. (1970). Disturbances of pulmonary function in patients with fat embolism. *J. clin. Path.*, 23, Suppl., **4,** 143.

SEVITT, S. (1960). The significance and classification of fat embolism. *Lancet,* **2,** 825.

SEVITT, S. (1962). *Fat Embolism.* London: Butterworth and Co.

SEVITT, S. (1973). The significance of fat embolism. *Brit. J. hosp. Med.,* **9,** 784.

TATEISHI, H. (1972). Prospective study of air embolism. *Brit. J. Anaesth.,* **44,** 1306.

VASILESCU, C., and RUCKLEY, C. N. (1974). A multi-unit trial of dextran and heparin in prophylaxis of deep vein thrombosis. *Brit. J. Surg.,* **61,** 320.

WRIGHT, B. D. (1971). Diagnostic features of fat embolism—results in six cases. *Anesthesiology,* **34,** 290.

Chapter 18

SHOCK

THE term "shock" is commonly used but ill-defined. Conditions to which it is applied vary in aetiology, pathology and presentation, so that the value of the term even as a clinical description is frequently challenged (Bloch *et al.*, 1966; Thal and Kinney, 1967). However, the most widely accepted definition is a state of generalised impairment of the function of vital organs due to acute circulatory inadequacy (MacLean, 1966; Dietzman and Lillehei, 1968). It is important to recognise that "circulatory inadequacy" includes abnormalities of pressure, flow or distribution of blood supply, and that there are circumstances in which excessive metabolic demand may render inadequate an otherwise normal circulation (Roe and Kinney, 1965).

The factors which initiate and perpetuate this imbalance between supply and demand have been the source of speculation and study for many years and both experimental work and clinical observation have contributed to the available knowledge. Before the First World War, emphasis was laid on the behaviour of the peripheral circulation and its response to nervous stimuli. Crile's theory (1899) of vasomotor paralysis was widely accepted. The high mortality of traumatic shock in the First World War led to further investigation, and intense vasoconstriction rather than vasodilatation was demonstrated in both animals and man (Erlanger *et al.*, 1919a; Ducastaing, 1919). The possible dangers of excessive amounts of circulating adrenaline were emphasised by Bainbridge and Trevan (1917) and Erlanger *et al.*, (1919b).

It was also shown that the circulating blood volume is decreased in traumatic shock even in the absence of external blood loss (Keith, 1919). This finding, together with the observation that restoration of circulation to a crushed limb was followed by the rapid development of shock led Cannon and Bayliss (1919) to postulate that wound shock could be defined as a discrepancy between blood volume and vascular capacity, and that toxic substances liberated from damaged tissues caused a generalised increase in capillary permeability with loss of fluid from the circulation and stagnation of blood in venous reservoirs. Subsequent work by Blalock (1930) emphasised the extent of fluid loss around the site of injury and challenged the concept of generalised vascular damage.

CURRENT CONCEPTS

The Peripheral Vasculature

Renewed interest in the behaviour of the peripheral vessels followed experimental work on the effects of haemorrhage and endotoxin administration in the dog. In this animal, haemorrhagic hypotension of four to five hours duration does not respond to the return of the shed blood but the blood pressure continues to fall until death occurs. Post-mortem examination reveals haemorrhagic necrosis of the bowel mucosa (Lillehei, 1957) and comparable changes are seen after the administration of bacterial endotoxin (Longerbeam *et al.*, 1962) or following prolonged infusions of adrenaline (Freeman *et al.*, 1951). Microscopy of the damaged gut shows capillary engorgement with arteriolar dilatation and venular contraction (Zweifach, 1958, 1961), possibly due to the differing ability of the pre- and post-capillary sphincters to maintain their tone during prolonged adrenergic stimulation (Lewis and Mellander, 1962). At first, both pre- and post-capillary sphincters are tightly constricted allowing little blood to enter the capillary bed. The pre-capillary sphincters then lose tone due to local anoxia and the accumulation of acid metabolites, while the post-capillary sphincters remain constricted. This leads to capillary engorgement and stagnation, with extravasation of fluid causing further depletion of the blood volume. Ultimately there is capillary destruction and loss of frank blood. According to Lillehei *et al.* (1964) the onset of this state during prolonged haemorrhagic hypotension or shock from any cause marks the change of the condition from "reversible" to "irreversible", in other words the point at which restoration of blood volume alone is insufficient to prevent progressive deterioration and death. The same authors point out that the organs showing most damage vary from one species to another but that this haemodynamic disturbance in the peripheral vascular bed is a common feature and is the result of prolonged and harmful vasoconstriction. Stimulation of the sympathetic nervous system and the liberation of adrenaline can accommodate quite considerable physiological demands on the circulation by increasing venous tone, increasing the rate and force of myocardial contraction and maintaining blood pressure by arteriolar constriction, but prolonged and intense sympathomimetic activity, either endogenous or exogenous, may be harmful (Nickerson, 1963; Lillehei *et al.*, 1962).

Haematological Disturbances

There is also evidence that flow patterns within the microcirculation are altered. Knisely (1965) and Gelin (1956) demonstrated aggregation and sludging of red cells in human conjunctival vessels following injury and Brill and Shoemaker (1960) showed experimentally that a similar process occurs in the liver of dogs given large doses of adrenaline.

The development of platelet thrombi with consequent plugging of small vessels was demonstrated by Robb in 1963 and the importance of widespread intravascular coagulation with subsequent coagulation defects in the circulating blood was emphasised by Hardaway *et al.* (1967) as part of the later stages of acute circulatory failure. The slow-flowing and therefore abnormally acid capillary blood is hypercoagulable, and disseminated intravascular coagulation is readily initiated by thrombogenic agents such as the products of haemolysis, bacterial toxins or the proximity of damaged tissue. Lysis of these clots *in situ* will ultimately follow but by this time there may be irretrievable cell death in the tissue beyond the obstructed vessels. The occurrence of widespread intravascular thrombosis depletes the circulating blood of a number of coagulation factors and haemorrhagic manifestations are sometimes seen. Unequivocal evidence of disseminated intravascular coagulation only occurs in a small percentage of patients with circulatory failure, particularly those suffering from sepsis. However, lesser degrees of the same abnormality are probably common although difficult to quantitate, and the formation of platelet micro-emboli by this process may be of particular importance in the genesis of pulmonary dysfunction (Blaisdell *et al.*, 1970).

Endotoxaemia

The administration of bacterial endotoxin is a potent cause of circulatory collapse and is widely used as an experimental model, although the cardiovascular sequelae in animals differ from those seen in clinical "septic shock" (Bhagat, 1974). Fine (1972) suggests that endotoxaemia can also be a feature of refractory *non-septic* shock, and postulates that prolonged visceral ischaemia permits the entry of intestinal bacteria and bacterial toxins. While this mechanism may be of importance in some species, particularly the dog, its relevance in man and other primates is questionable. Endotoxaemia is difficult to demonstrate and the only test available at present is the Limulus method in which protein-rich fluid derived from the blood cells of the horseshoe crab (Limulus) gels in the presence of endotoxin (Levin *et al.*, 1970). Using this test, endotoxaemia can be demonstrated in a high proportion of patients suffering from fulminant hepatic failure, in whom the normal clearance mechanisms of the liver are defective (Wilkinson *et al.*, 1974), and also in some patients suffering from septicaemia caused by Gram-negative organisms (*Brit. med. J.*, 1974). However, endotoxin cannot be detected in all cases of Gram-negative septicaemia and it is not a feature of infection with Gram-positive organisms, even though the clinical condition appears identical.

The damaging effects of endotoxin are generally attributed to two features: a direct action on capillaries causing an increase in permeability, and an indirect effect in which vaso-active substances are liberated either directly from the adrenal medulla and post-ganglionic sympathetic nerve endings (Bhagat, 1974), or by the interaction of endotoxin with various plasma factors and white cells (Reichgott and Melmon, 1972). Precise evaluation of changes in vaso-active peptides is notoriously difficult and their role in endotoxaemia and shock states in general remains uncertain. Sympathomimetic activity due to endotoxins can be demonstrated experimentally in kidney, lung and bowel (Hinshaw *et al.*, 1961; Kuida *et al.*, 1958; Motsay *et al.*, 1974) but evidence that this vasoconstriction is an important contributory factor in the development of septic shock is better for dogs than for man.

The Role of Lysosomal Enzymes and the Myocardial Depressant Factor

An alternative mechanism which may contribute to generalised cellular damage is the release of lysosomal enzymes (Janoff, 1964). Cellular biochemical activity in the absence of adequate supplies of oxygen results in an intracellular acidosis and depletion of ATP. Intracellular acidosis has been implicated in the lysis of lysosomal membranes, while ATP deficiency may produce alterations in biosynthesis around ribosomes, possibly leading to the formation of vaso-active peptides (Schumer, 1972). Many lysosomal enzymes are proteolytic and their activity therefore propagates tissue destruction. In particular, lysosomal hydrolysis may be responsible for the liberation of myocardial depressant factor, a peptide with a molecular weight of 800–1,000 which was first described by Brand and Lefer in 1966, and which is thought to originate from ischaemic pancreatic tissue. The deleterious effects of this peptide are listed as a negative inotropic effect on the myocardium, splanchnic vasoconstriction which may augment visceral ischaemia, and reticulo-endothelial blockade which can impair clearance of both lysosomal enzymes and the myocardial depressant factor itself (Lefer and Glenn, 1974).

Myocardial Function

Myocardial dysfunction during prolonged experimental haemorrhagic hypotension was described by Sarnoff *et al.* in 1954, and more recently by Gomez and Hamilton (1964). The contribution of some degree of cardiac failure to circulatory inadequacy in a variety of clinical disorders, often in young and previously healthy subjects, was documented by MacLean (1966), and the myocardial lesions which can be recognised in shock have recently been reviewed by Hackel *et al.* (1974). The possibility that these defects represent the action of a specific myocardial depressant factor has been discussed already but even without invoking the operation of such a mechanism, impaired cardiac function might be anticipated because the myocardial microvasculature is itself subject to damage by the systemic haemodynamic abnormality. The recognition and treatment of this aspect of circulatory failure is frequently life-saving.

The evidence presented so far has all emphasised deficiencies of blood flow: low cardiac output due to myocardial impairment, deficient blood volume, or poor tissue perfusion due to excessive vasoconstriction and abnormalities within the microcirculation. This is reflected in the conventional clinical description of the "shocked patient"—hypotensive with small pulse pressure, cold, pale or cyanosed sweating extremities, oliguria or anuria, rapid respiration, anxiety, restlessness or clouding of consciousness.

However, there are situations (some cases of septicaemia, some following myocardial infarction) where overall blood flow is normal or high and systemic vascular resistance low (MacLean *et al.*, 1967; Thomas *et al.*, 1966). Tissue perfusion may still be inadequate if blood flow is diverted through arteriovenous shunts, if blood pressure is lower than the critical closing pressure of small vessels (Burton, 1951) or if hypermetabolic states such as severe trauma, burns or sepsis impose an increased demand for oxygen supply.

These features underline the difficulty of applying the single term "shock" to such a variety of conditions. It is perhaps fair to accept shock or acute circulatory inadequacy as generic terms similar to respiratory or renal failure, realising that they cover a variety of conditions. Impairment of function of vital organs is a feature common to all; the circulatory defect which is responsible may differ according to the aetiology of the condition.

CLASSIFICATION

Attempts to classify shock (Tables 1 and 2) are generally based either on the initial precipitating event (Thal and Kinney, 1967; Dietzman and Lillehei, 1968) or on the haemodynamic diagnosis (MacLean, 1966).

The latter system is not fully comprehensive—for example, the septic patient with high cardiac output, low systemic vascular resistance and normal or low arteriovenous oxygen difference is not apparently suffering from a cardiac defect, hypovolaemia or peripheral pooling. The limitation of discussing conditions in terms of the precipitating event is that several factors may coexist or there may be a transition from one variety of shock to another—for example, the coexistence

18/TABLE 1

CLASSIFICATION OF SHOCK BASED ON AETIOLOGY. (From Thal and Kinney, 1967)

1. Hypovolaemic shock
   (a) pure
   (b) combined with sepsis or cardiac failure
2. Cardiogenic shock
   (a) failure of left ventricular ejection
   (b) failure of left ventricular filling
3. Septic shock
   (a) pure
   (b) combined with cardiac failure or hypovolaemia
4. Neurogenic shock (loss of vasomotor control).

18/TABLE 2

CLASSIFICATION OF SHOCK BASED ON HAEMODYNAMIC DIAGNOSIS. (From Maclean, 1966)

1. Cardiac deficit.
2. Hypovolaemia.
3. Peripheral pooling.

of sepsis and fluid loss with the subsequent development of impaired cardiac function. However, this aetiological system is the one most widely used. On this basis, it is necessary to consider hypovolaemia and the effective hypovolaemia of vasodilatation, together with the conditions of cardiac and septic shock.

Hypovolaemia is still one of the commonest causes of circulatory inadequacy, especially in surgical practice. Fluid loss may be overt or concealed, and consist of blood, plasma or extracellular fluid. Sympathomimetic activity is prominent, initially maintaining the cardiac output, venous and arterial pressures within the normal range but these indices fall with progressive fluid loss. Oliguria is present, due initially to hormonally mediated retention of sodium and water and subsequently to the damaging effects of hypotension and a lowered blood flow on renal function.

It is clinical custom to include in the consideration of shock conditions in which vasodilatation is accompanied by low venous and arterial pressures, although the cardiac output is relatively normal until vasodilatation is extreme. This can be described as "effective hypovolaemia"—a blood volume within the normal range but still inadequate to achieve normal filling of a dilated vascular bed. Such disorders include barbiturate overdosage, certain neurological injuries, anaphylaxis, acute adrenal steroid depletion and some cases of septicaemia. However, not all patients with these conditions can justifiably be classified as "shocked" defining the term as "impaired function of vital organs due to acute circulatory inadequacy."

Cardiogenic shock as a primary event is due most commonly to myocardial infarction. Other causes are dysrhythmias or extremes of cardiac rate, sudden obstruction to the pulmonary circulation (pulmonary embolism), regurgitation caused by a ruptured cusp, papillary muscle dysfunction, or acute septal perforation, cardiac compression (pericardial tamponade) or direct myocardial trauma.

The haemodynamic findings are variable. Hypotension, tachycardia and elevation of the venous pressure are common and in most cases there is a lowered cardiac output and a high systemic vascular resistance. In a few patients with myocardial infarction, there is hypotension with a normal cardiac output and low systemic vascular resistance, possibly due to vasodilating reflexes arising from afferents in the coronary bed (Dawes and Comroe, 1954) or left ventricle (Braunwald, 1968; Thomas *et al.*, 1965, 1966).

Septic shock is the group in which clinical and haemodynamic findings are most variable. Both Gram-positive and negative infections can be responsible (*Lancet*, 1963; Austen and Buckley, 1967) and the effects may be attributable to circulating endo- or exotoxins rather than true bacteraemia.

The haemodynamic changes are sometimes those of vasoconstriction with a low cardiac output and high systemic vascular resistance but the exact opposite, namely the combination of a high cardiac output and low systemic vascular resistance is also common. In these cases, metabolic demands are often supplied inadequately in spite of the high flow; hyperkalaemia is common and there is generally a gross metabolic acidosis. The arteriovenous oxygen content difference is normal or low and the acidosis does not respond to treatment with hyperbaric oxygen, suggesting either that blood is flowing through arteriovenous shunts, or that cellular utilisation of oxygen is impaired (Siegel *et al.*, 1967; Sardesai and Thal, 1966; Thal and Wilson, 1965). The increased cardiac output may be secondary to this defect at cellular level (Duff *et al.*, 1972), or alternatively, the hyperkinetic state may be an early response to bacterial toxins (Spink, 1962). The cardiac output is low when there is myocardial impairment or hypovolaemia, the latter caused by pre-existing fluid loss (such as often occurs when sepsis complicates intra-abdominal pathology), or by fluid loss associated with diarrhoea, sweating and excessive capillary permeability (Austen and Buckley, 1967; MacLean *et al.*, 1967).

Disseminated intravascular coagulation and secondary haemorrhagic phenomena are prominent features of septic shock in man and may be the result of a generalised Schwartzmann reaction (Rapaport *et al.*, 1964). This inevitably causes further impairment of tissue perfusion. Intravascular haemolysis may also develop and so diminish oxygen-carrying capacity.

Although the group of vasodilated, hyperkinetic patients sometimes remain alert initially and have a good urinary output in spite of hypotension, evidence of widespread organ failure (heart, kidney, liver, brain and gut) ultimately appears. There is a high mortality in this group and acute respiratory insufficiency is a common feature (see p. 665).

DIAGNOSIS AND ASSESSMENT

Although it is customary to subdivide "shock" into these three categories, it cannot be emphasised too strongly that these divisions are not absolute and that patients suffering from a single disease may manifest, together or sequentially, all three disorders; even more important is that both hypovolaemia and myocardial impairment are common features of the septic shock syndrome.

A further difficulty is the accurate recognition of "shock" bearing in mind the problems of definition. Most commonly the term is used clinically to describe hypotension, although the arterial blood pressure is a notoriously poor guide to the adequacy of circulatory function. Alternatively, patients are described as shocked when their skin is vasoconstricted, cold and sweating even though the arterial pressure is still within the normal range.

The two essential requirements for the management of such patients are to attempt some assessment of blood flow rather than pressure and to determine, by observing the height of the venous pressure, whether hypovolaemia is contributing to circulatory inadequacy. Some idea of blood flow may be gained by noting the level of consciousness, the rate of urine secretion, and the colour, temperature and degree of superficial venous filling of the peripheral tissues.

When flow is well maintained the limbs are warm and often dry, peripheral pulses are palpable, urine flow is not interrupted and consciousness is fully maintained in spite of arterial hypotension.

Poor flow is suggested if the skin is cold, sweating and cyanosed, urine secretion reduced or absent and consciousness impaired. Peripheral pulses are weak because the pulse pressure is low and the blood pressure is difficult to record using a sphygmomanometer. If recovery occurs, urine flow improves (provided the kidneys have not been too severely damaged) and warmth gradually spreads down the limbs until the skin is uniformly pink, warm and dry and the superficial veins are well-filled.

In addition to the clinical assessment of tissue perfusion, there must be a careful examination of the heart, lungs and abdomen, together with a brief neurological survey (for evidence of raised intracranial pressure, meningism or localising signs). Few patients are so desperately in need of therapeutic intervention that this initial examination cannot be made thoroughly, and an accurate diagnosis of the primary event is most likely to be reached only if this examination is carried out before therapy has modified the clinical features. It is important to realise however that some physical signs may be masked by the presence of shock. In particular, severe peritonitis can be present with few if any signs in the abdomen until the circulation has been restored towards normal.

In many patients, the history and initial clinical examination are sufficient to establish the diagnosis, but if this is not so the following assessment should be made.

Measurement of Venous Pressure

Unless the central venous pressure can be accurately determined by observation of the neck veins, it must be measured in a vessel in free communication with the intrathoracic veins. This is the most important single observation which can be readily made in general clinical practice because it reflects the adequacy of both cardiac filling and cardiac performance.

The right atrial or central venous pressure is a poor index of left atrial filling when there is a discrepancy between the performance of the two sides of the heart (Guyton et al., 1973) and fluid replacement therapy can be controlled with greater accuracy if the left atrial pressure is monitored as well. The advent of the Swan-Ganz catheter (Swan et al., 1970) has facilitated the measurement of pulmonary arterial wedge pressure which, in most patients, is a good index of pressure in the left atrium; the end-diastolic pressure in the pulmonary artery also correlates well with mean left atrial pressure, provided the pulmonary vascular resistance is normal (Jenkins et al., 1970). These techniques permit greater accuracy in the definition of cardiovascular function in patients with complex disorders and they are often combined with measurements of cardiac output, generally undertaken in acutely sick patients by the thermal dilution technique (Branthwaite and Bradley, 1968). However, monitoring pulmonary arterial or pulmonary wedge pressure requires a pressure transducer, amplifier and display system, and this apparatus is only available in a few centres whereas the central venous pressure can be monitored very simply using a saline column manometer.

Interpretation of the Venous Pressure

In the shocked patient, a value of less than zero (using the sternal angle as the reference point) indicates inadequate filling of the circulation. This may be due to fluid loss or to excessive vasodilatation of the capacitance vessels, and means that in these acute situations there is no absolute value for "normal blood volume" (MacLean *et al.*, 1965; Friedman *et al.*, 1966; Daintree-Johnson, 1966; Sampson and Hutchinson, 1967). Optimal blood volume is that which provides adequate cardiac filling at any particular level of venous tone. When venous tone is high (prolonged sympathetic stimulation, heart failure) a "normal" blood volume may result in a venous pressure so high that pulmonary oedema is produced (Fig. 1). Conversely, when venous tone is low (sympathetic paralysis, barbiturate overdosage) a "normal" blood volume may still result in such a low venous pressure that cardiac filling is inadequate and cardiac output low (Starling's law). This means that the measurement of venous pressure must be interpreted in conjunction with either a measurement of blood volume or an assessment of vascular tone. There are many sources of potential error which can invalidate measurements of blood volume in the shocked patient (Heath and Vickers, 1968), quite apart from the temptation to use the value obtained as the sole criterion of adequate circulatory filling. It is both safe and simple to interpret venous pressure in conjunction with the physical signs of vaso-constriction or vasodilatation.

An occasional difficulty is introduced when the central venous pressure is referred to atmospheric pressure (zero) in patients requiring intermittent positive-pressure ventilation, particularly those in whom positive end-expiratory pressure (PEEP) is being used. This technique of ventilation raises the mean intrathoracic pressure and the central venous pressure rises too, although not necessarily by a value numerically equal to the PEEP pressure. Ideally, the transmural cardiac filling pressure is determined by subtracting intrathoracic pressure (determined with an oesophageal balloon) from the apparent central venous pressure, both referred to atmospheric pressure. This is generally impractical and a normal transmural cardiac filling pressure can usually be assumed during controlled ventilation with positive end-expiratory pressure when the mean central venous pressure, referred to zero at the sternal angle, is at or a little above the upper limit of normal (e.g. 3–6 mm Hg or 0·4–0·8 kPa).

It is also important to note that there may be a considerable discrepancy between the pulmonary wedge pressure and the left atrial pressure when the intrapulmonary pressure has been elevated by the application of PEEP. Good correlation was reported by Lozman *et al.* (1974) when the end-expiratory pressure was 5 cm H_2O (0·5 kPa) or less, but the left atrial pressure may be con-

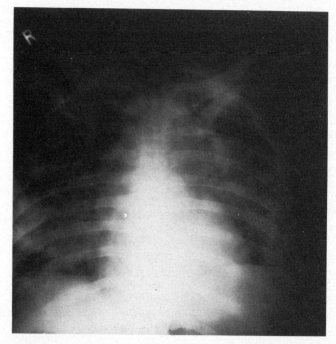

18/Fig. 1.—Chest X-ray of a 52-year-old patient with ischaemic heart disease in whom pulmonary oedema developed when the measured blood volume (3·1 litres) was increased to the predicted normal for age, height and weight (4·2 litres).

siderably lower than the pulmonary arterial wedge pressure when the end-expiratory pressure exceeds 10 cm H_2O (1·0 kPa).

Low venous pressure.—Vasoconstriction and a low venous pressure can only be produced by fluid loss. This loss may be whole blood (overt or concealed haemorrhage), plasma or protein-rich exudate (burns or inflammatory exudates) or protein-free fluid (intestinal obstruction, diabetic coma). Measurements of haematocrit, electrolytes and urea, plasma proteins and blood sugar as appropriate will help to differentiate these causes.

Vasodilatation with a low venous pressure is due to an increased vascular capacity such as may be seen in certain forms of neurological damage, barbiturate and other drug overdosage, fever and some patients with sepsis. These conditions are commonly associated with an abnormally low tone in resistance vessels so that arterial as well as venous pressure is low, but unless vasodilatation is extreme or the myocardium damaged, overall blood flow is normal or even elevated (Fig. 2).

High venous pressure.—Elevation of the venous pressure is most commonly due to cardiac disorders but it can also be produced by over-transfusion. An initial difficulty is to define what constitutes dangerous elevation of the venous pressure. The normal range is given by Paul Wood (1968) as minus 5 to plus 3 cm ($-0·5$ to $+0·3$ kPa) relative to the sternal angle. However, the fact that the venous pressure lies outside this range does not necessarily mean that

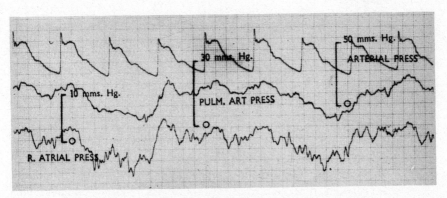

18/Fig. 2.—Haemodynamic and biochemical findings in a boy of 16 with Gram-negative septicaemia.

Cardiac output = 11·4 1/min	Pao$_2$ 62 mm Hg; 8·3 kPa (breathing oxygen)
Pulse rate = 130/min	Paco$_2$ 41·5 mm Hg; 5·5 kPa
Stroke output = 88 ml/beat	pH 7·29

(N.B. 10 mm Hg = 1·3 kPa; 30 mm Hg = 4·0 kPa; 50 mm Hg = 6·7 kPa)

circulatory function is impaired. If a normal heart is over-filled so that the venous pressure is above plus 3 cm (0·3 kPa) the cardiac output will rise (Starling's law; Fig. 3). This situation shows none of the features of shock or circulatory failure. Ultimately a point is reached where the venous pressures (both pul-

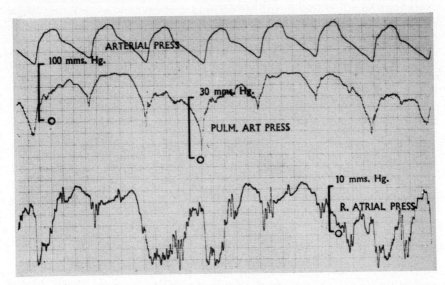

18/Fig. 3.—Haemodynamic findings in a young adult (19 years) with acute glomerulonephritis.

Cardiac outout = 12·0 1/min
Pulse rate = 120/min
Stroke output = 100 ml/beat

(N.B. 100 mm Hg = 13·3 kPa; 30 mm Hg = 4·0 kPa; 10 mm Hg = 1·3 kPa)

monary and systemic) are so high that oedema develops, and the combination of systemic and pulmonary oedema with elevation of the venous pressure is clinically labelled "heart failure". However, it is difficult to accept this in a physiological sense as the heart is still behaving normally in response to increased filling. Finally however, true cardiac failure is produced when the hypoxia of pulmonary oedema together with functional tricuspid and mitral regurgitation due to cardiac over-distension combine to lower the cardiac output so that the blood pressure falls and reflex vasoconstriction develops.

More commonly shock associated with a high venous pressure reflects impaired cardiac performance due to myocardial damage, valvular defects, obstruction or compression. The high venous pressure is produced by a combination of factors including fluid retention in situations where heart failure has been present for some time, an increase in venous tone (Sharpey-Schafer, 1961), and redistribution of blood volume.

When faced with the shocked patient in whom the venous pressure is elevated, overtransfusion must be excluded first. This can generally be done from the history and fluid-balance chart, although measurements of pulmonary arterial or left atrial pressure if available are more sensitive guides to the degree of fluid over-load (Hardaway, 1968; Sampson and Hutchinson, 1967).

A history of preceding heart disease, ECG or X-ray evidence of ventricular hypertrophy or recent cardiac damage and a careful clinical examination may reveal other causes of cardiac embarrassment such as pulmonary embolism, coronary thrombosis or tamponade, although again, in some instances, cardiac catheterisation is necessary to establish a complete diagnosis.

In the absence of specific cardiac pathology or over-transfusion, the combination of a high venous pressure with the signs of vasoconstriction and a low flow is indicative of impaired myocardial performance. This may be due to unsuspected underlying cardiac disease, or to the detrimental effects of prolonged hypotension and circulatory inadequacy on a previously normal heart (see page 657).

ASSESSMENT OF FUNCTION OF OTHER SYSTEMS

Respiratory Function

Abnormalities of respiratory function are common in shock from any cause. Clinically this is manifest by an increased respiratory rate and frequently dyspnoea. Biochemically there is most commonly hypoxia and hyperventilation, the latter occurring independently of the presence or absence of metabolic acidosis. The hypoxia is attributable to an increase in the mismatch of ventilation and perfusion within the lungs, together with a more marked effect on arterial Po_2 from the shunting of mixed venous blood of lower than normal oxygen content (Kelman et al., 1967). Hyperventilation is probably due to a number of factors which may include arterial hypoxaemia, metabolic acidosis, reflex response to stimulation of arterial or venous baroceptors, or possibly the direct effect of endotoxins on the medulla (MacLean et al., 1967).

Abnormalities of gas exchange have been documented following cardiac infarction (MacKenzie et al., 1964) and haemorrhagic hypotension (Gerst et al., 1959; Freeman and Nunn, 1963; Naimark et al., 1968). Cahill et al. (1965) also demonstrated decreased compliance with normal or increased airway resistance following endotoxin administration.

Great interest has developed during the last few years in the syndrome of "shock lung" or acute respiratory distress syndrome of adults (Moore *et al.*, 1969; Pontoppidan *et al.*, 1972). Characteristically, an episode of trauma is followed a few days later by dyspnoea, tachypnoea and cyanosis. Life-threatening hypoxia occurs and is difficult to relieve, even with controlled ventilation. A similar disorder can accompany septicaemia or experimental endotoxaemia, and comparable pulmonary dysfunction is caused in clinical practice by embolism of fat or amniotic fluid, blast injuries, pulmonary contusion, burns and the inhalation of noxious vapours or chemicals (including gastric acid). "Pump lung" or pulmonary dysfunction following cardiopulmonary bypass may represent a less florid form of the same condition (Wilson, 1972*a*), while oxygen toxicity and secondary infection developing during treatment may aggravate the pre-existing pathology.

It is important to appreciate that quite considerable abnormalities of respiratory function can exist without physical signs in the lungs or the production of appreciable quantities of sputum. In early cases, there may be no demonstrable pathology on the chest X-ray, but soon diffuse mottling occurs and later there is confluent shadowing with air-filled bronchi clearly visible ("negative bronchogram"). The pathogenesis of the syndrome is obscure. There appear to be considerable species differences in the response of the pulmonary vascular bed but experimentally there is evidence of pulmonary vasoconstriction affecting either the pulmonary arterioles or the pulmonary veins (Hyman *et al.*, 1974; Kusajima *et al.*, 1974). Vasoconstriction may be initiated by vasoactive substances which are liberated within the circulation or are derived from damaged lung tissue, and vascular obstruction is aggravated by the mechanical effects of platelet and white cell micro-emboli. These aggregates develop intravascularly or are derived from transfused blood and they are thought to disintegrate within the lungs, so liberating serotonin and lysosomal enzymes (Blaisdell, 1974) which perpetuate local damage. Milligan *et al.* (1974) suggested an association between haematological evidence of disseminated intravascular coagulation and defects in gas exchange.

Histologically, there is evidence of widespread damage to both pulmonary capillary endothelium and alveolar epithelium. A protein-rich exudate accumulates, caused by vascular damage rather than by an increase in pulmonary capillary pressure (Riordan and Walters, 1968), and alveolar collapse is facilitated by surfactant loss secondary to damage to type II alveolar pneumocytes.

Pulmonary oedema and atelectasis result in gross mismatch of ventilation and perfusion and arterial hypoxaemia is inevitable. The minute volume rises and this workload cannot be sustained easily because the pulmonary compliance is low. Controlled ventilation eliminates the work of breathing and improves gas exchange. Moreover there is some evidence which suggests that the prognosis is improved if this therapy is instituted early in the course of the disorder (Milligan *et al.*, 1974).

Renal function

Renal function is frequently deranged in shock and minor degrees of impairment, detectable by refined methods of investigation are more common than is appreciated if only urine volume and blood urea are observed (Hayes, 1957). Sustained decrease in blood flow is the initiating event in the renal damage, but the effects of hypotension, hypoxia, haemoconcentration and tubular obstruction are also important. A primarily glomerular defect can occur in endotoxaemia (Wilkinson *et al.*, 1974). Microscopy and simple analysis of the urine may provide early warning of renal damage, and if measurements of osmolality are not available, a useful empirical test of renal function in patients with oliguria and an increased blood urea is the urine to plasma ratio of urea concentration (U/P ratio) (Perlmuter *et al.*, 1959). A value of less than 14 suggests renal impairment (failure to concentrate) whereas a value of more than 14 suggests dehydration. The absolute amount of urinary urea excreted per day gives some idea of the degree of cell catabolism taking place.

Liver and Gastro-intestinal Tract Function

Paralytic ileus is common in shock, even though the appearance of haemorrhagic necrosis seen in shocked dogs does not occur in man. In Gram-negative septicaemia however, the illness may commence with profuse diarrhoea (Borden and Hall, 1951). Jaundice and impaired liver function tests are frequently seen in patients with sepsis or prolonged low tissue perfusion, although in some cases the jaundice may be partly haemolytic in origin (Eley *et al.*, 1965).

Blood

Changes in the blood reflect a variety of separate processes. Serial measurements of haemoglobin or haematocrit will document the net effect of red cell loss or destruction, haemoconcentration and haemodilution. Changes in the white cells may occur but are unpredictable and often of little diagnostic value. Abnormalities of clotting factors are common particularly in septic shock, and include defects in both the number and quality of platelets, depletion of other clotting factors and the presence of fibrinolysins or the end-products of clot lysis. Special tests may be necessary to elucidate the complete haematological situation (Ingram, 1966).

THERAPY

Therapy must include resuscitation and support of the shocked patient together with appropriate treatment for the precipitating condition. Speed in the provision of this specific therapy may be important, for example the prompt use of antibiotics in septicaemia, early pericardial drainage in cases of tamponade, and venesection when pulmonary oedema is due to over-transfusion.

The essential requirement for resuscitation is the restoration of an adequate oxygen supply at cellular level and an analysis of how this may be impaired is given in Tables 3 and 4.

Hypovolaemia, effective or absolute, must be corrected using the central venous or pulmonary wedge pressures in conjunction with signs of vasoconstriction or vasodilatation to assess the volume required. If hypovolaemia is the sole mechanism of circulatory inadequacy, the infusion of fluid will restore adequate tissue flow—vasodilatation will occur and the venous pressure will rise

18/Table 3 Factors Contributing to Tissue Oxygen Supplies

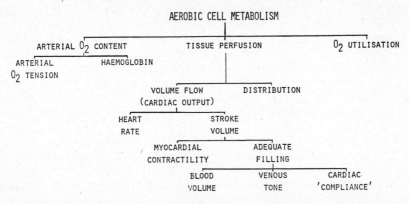

to normal. If in a patient suspected of hypovolaemia, central venous pressure is already normal but there is evidence of persistent vasoconstriction, it is safe to infuse small volumes of fluid (100–200 ml) in a short period of time (5–15 minutes) and observe the circulatory changes this produces. If hypovolaemia is still present, a small infusion will cause the central venous pressure to rise only transitorily and signs of vasodilatation will begin to appear. If there is some other cause of circulatory impairment, central venous pressure will rise sharply and remain elevated and there will be no evidence of improved flow (Sykes, 1963).

The choice of fluid depends on the nature of the fluid lost, together with serial measurements of haematocrit, plasma protein and electrolyte concentrations. Hardaway (1968) recommends the determination of red cell mass to assess the requirement for whole blood, using other fluids to continue volume repletion once the normal red cell mass has been reached, even though the haematocrit may fall as a result. However, measurements of red cell mass are not widely available, and it may in any case be wiser to maintain a normal haematocrit so that oxygen-carrying capacity is not reduced.

Plasma rather than blood will be required to correct protein loss due to inflammatory exudates. Human plasma protein fraction has similar oncotic

18/Table 4 Defects of Distribution and O_2 Utilisation

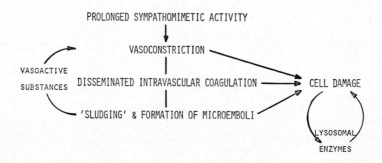

properties but the risk of serum hepatitis is virtually eliminated; fresh frozen plasma contains a high concentration of clotting factors and the risk of hepatitis is lower than with reconstituted dried plasma. The various dextran preparations also avoid the risk of hepatitis but may interfere with cross-matching and with *in vivo* coagulation if they are used in large volumes. Most dextran preparations not only expand the blood volume by the amount infused but also have a powerful osmotic effect, so causing a considerable expansion of blood volume at the expense of the extracellular fluid. Low molecular weight dextran may also have some specific action on the red cells, minimising the tendency to sludging.

Colloid-free electrolyte solutions are needed to replace deficits in extracellular fluid but only a percentage of their volume is retained in the vascular compartment. If the plasma protein concentration of blood is decreased or the capillary walls damaged, electrolyte solutions will contribute to the formation of oedema rather than restore the blood volume to normal.

When a rapid rate of transfusion is required, all solutions should be raised to body temperature and the use of calcium salts to cover massive transfusion of citrated blood is generally recommended (Royal Society of Medicine Symposium, 1968). Once a normal central venous pressure has been reached, the rate of fluid infusion should be decreased so that the venous pressure remains constant while vasodilatation occurs. If vasodilatation and evidence of improved tissue flow does not appear, some authors (Hardaway, 1968; MacLean, 1966) recommend continued transfusion to raise the central venous pressure above normal in the hope that cardiac output will rise in response to greater diastolic filling (Starling's law). However in patients with disease affecting the left side of the heart, in those with reduced levels of plasma proteins and those suffering from septicaemia, this may lead to the development of pulmonary oedema (Guyton and Lindsey, 1959; Guyton, *et al.*, 1973; MacLean *et al.*, 1967). Even monitoring the left atrial pressure does not eliminate the risk if the permeability of the pulmonary capillaries is abnormal. If, therefore, evidence of adequate tissue perfusion cannot be achieved when the central venous pressure is within the normal range, it may be wiser to consider other methods of increasing cardiac output or improving the distribution of blood flow. The only exception to this rule lies in the management of patients with known disease of the right side of the heart in whom elevation of the venous pressure above the normal range is justifiable and may well be desirable.

An inotropic agent will virtually always increase cardiac output whether this is inadequate because of a primary disorder of the heart or because myocardial impairment has developed during severe or prolonged shock. *Isoprenaline*, a powerful beta-sympathomimetic agent combining myocardial stimulation with peripheral vasodilatation, is widely used for this purpose in the treatment of all varieties of shock (MacLean *et al.*, 1965; Kardos, 1966; Elliott and Gorlin, 1966; Du Toit *et al.*, 1966; Kirklin and Rastelli, 1967). Therapy is easy to control when the drug is given intravenously (0·5–3·0 mcg/min) although its use is occasionally limited by tachycardia or dysrhythmia. In some patients, *digitalis* or drugs to control rate or rhythm may also be needed. Correction of acidosis may improve myocardial performance by permitting maximum effect of stimulating catecholamines even though evidence for direct myocardial depression by acidosis is conflicting (Weil *et al.*, 1957; Thrower *et al.*, 1961; Goodyer *et al.*, 1961; Anderson and Mouritsen, 1966).

Salbutamol.—Other sympathomimetic agents may be of greater value than isoprenaline. Salbutamol is predominantly a beta-2 stimulant; it is two to five times less potent than isoprenaline in dilating the peripheral vasculature in dogs but is one thousand times less potent as a cardiac stimulant (Cullum *et al.*, 1969; Daly *et al.*, 1971). It can therefore be given in relatively large doses (10–30 mcg/min) without alteration in heart rate or rhythm. The reduction in systemic vascular resistance permits limited myocardial work to be used to generate flow rather than pressure and, unlike beta-1 stimulants, the increase in cardiac output is not accompanied by a corresponding increase in oxygen consumption (Wyse *et al.*, 1974). The drug appears to act selectively on arteriolar resistance while leaving other components of the sympathetic nervous system intact; unlike alpha-blocking or ganglionic-blocking agents, generalised vasodilatation of both resistance and capacitance vessels does not occur. It is therefore of value in patients suffering from acute circulatory failure, particularly when there is evidence of peripheral vasoconstriction and the cardiac output is inappropriately low for systemic oxygen requirements. More recently, infusions of *sodium nitroprusside* have been advocated to promote vasodilatation and a reduction in cardiac work (Tinker and Michenfelder, 1976).

Dopamine is the precursor of noradrenaline. It is an inotropic agent and peripheral vasoconstrictor but selectively dilates the renal vascular bed (Loeb, 1971). It has been advocated for the treatment of septic shock (*Lancet*, 1974) but although elevation of the blood pressure and improvement of renal perfusion appear desirable theoretically, it is unlikely that the drug exerts a beneficial effect on the peripheral microvasculature, and survival rates in the series reported by Winslow *et al.* (1973) were disappointingly low. If dopamine *is* chosen, it is infused intravenously at a rate of 2–25 mcg/kg body weight/minute.

Alpha-adrenergic blocking agents, particularly *phenoxybenzamine*, have been advocated to relieve microcirculatory obstruction (Lillehei *et al.*, 1964). Phenoxybenzamine must be infused slowly (1 mg/kg administered over one hour) and it is essential to monitor the central venous pressure very carefully because dilatation of capacitance vessels lowers cardiac filling and further volume infusion is generally necessary. The obliteration of all peripheral vascular tone renders such patients very vulnerable to haemodynamic stress and enthusiasm for alpha-adrenergic blockade has receded with the advent of beta-sympathomimetic stimulant drugs with more selective peripheral vasodilator properties. However, there is some evidence which suggests that the beneficial actions of phenoxybenzamine are unrelated to its alpha-adrenergic blocking properties (Halmagyi, 1972), and in a few highly-selected patients monitored in units with considerable experience in the management of circulatory failure, both alpha- and beta-adrenergic blocking agents may have a useful role (Halmagyi, 1972; Berk, 1972).

If peripheral vasodilating agents of any type are used, they should be infused cautiously in patients suffering from severe vasoconstriction accompanied by hyperkalaemia and metabolic acidosis. If the peripheral vascular bed is dilated abruptly, acid metabolites are swept into the circulation and may accentuate the biochemical derangements and even precipitate cardiac arrest.

Preliminary biochemical control, using peritoneal dialysis if necessary, will minimise this risk.

Vasopressor agents are used infrequently but they may have occasional value for patients with coronary arterial disease in whom myocardial performance cannot be maintained without an adequate diastolic blood pressure (Braunwald, 1968). Noradrenaline, metaraminol, dopamine or adrenaline may be given, differences between them being related to the relative potency of their alpha- and beta-adrenergic stimulant properties.

The role of corticosteroids in the prophylaxis or treatment of acute circulatory failure remains highly controversial and was reviewed in a symposium held in 1973 (Glenn, 1974). The beneficial effects which have been claimed for high dose corticosteroid regimes include a positive inotropic action on the myocardium, peripheral and pulmonary vasodilatation, stabilisation of cell and lysosomal membranes and specific anti-endotoxic properties. Much of the controversy can be attributed to three factors:

(a) shock is not a single entity;

(b) the experimental work has been undertaken in controlled circumstances, generally using a single haemodynamic insult—haemorrhage, endotoxin administration or myocardial ischaemia;

(c) there is considerable variation in the vascular responses of different species.

It is therefore difficult to define unequivocal indications for steroid therapy and at the present time, the most convincing evidence relates to septicaemic shock (Motsay et al., 1972; Schumer, 1976) and the pulmonary sequelae of sepsis or trauma (Lozman et al., 1975; Kusajima et al., 1974). There is also controversy surrounding the choice of steroid preparation and the dosage required. Methyl prednisolone sodium succinate in a dose of 30 mg/kg given slowly intravenously over 20 to 30 minutes may be the agent of choice (Wilson, 1972b and 1974; Fuenfer et al., 1975) and a further injection of 15–30 mg/kg may be required four to six hours later. These doses are greatly in excess of even the maximum required for the anti-inflammatory actions of corticosteroids and should only be given for one or two days. It can be argued that continued steroid treatment is advisable in the treatment of adult respiratory distress syndrome to promote resolution rather than healing by fibrosis, and in these circumstances, the dosage should be reduced to the minimum considered necessary for an effective anti-inflammatory action. If corticosteroids are only indicated for the cardiovascular manifestations of septicaemia, therapy can be discontinued safely as soon as a normal haemodynamic pattern is re-established and there is no need to decrease the steroid dosage gradually because adrenal suppression does not occur so quickly.

Efforts to improve overall blood flow and its distribution will be of little value if the microcirculation is obstructed by disseminated intravascular coagulation. Anticoagulants or fibrinolysins may be of some value in resolving these changes (Hardaway and Drake, 1963; Corrigan et al., 1968) although by the time the syndrome is well-established, significant improvement can only be demonstrated very occasionally.

Therapy directed at restoring blood flow is incomplete without ensuring that the arterial oxygen content is high. A normal haemoglobin concentration and full saturation must be maintained and oxygen administration is virtually always necessary. Unless a normal arterial oxygen tension can be achieved with spontaneous ventilation through a simple face-mask, controlled ventilation is often advisable and the benefits of improved oxygenation and decreased respiratory work are generally more apparent than any deterioration caused by the effects of the raised intrathoracic pressure on cardiac output.

Sedation, muscular paralysis or cooling decrease metabolic demands and may be valuable if tissue oxygen requirements cannot be supplied, either because the cardiac output cannot be improved or because gross pulmonary pathology prevents adequate gas exchange. Mechanical support is implemented occasionally, either by aortic balloon counter-pulsation (Kantrowitz *et al.*, 1968) or by extracorporeal circulation using a membrane oxygenator (*Brit. med. J.*, 1975).

If satisfactory systemic perfusion is not restored rapidly, severe and widespread tissue damage is inevitable and may be irreversible. Renal damage is particularly likely to occur but the prophylactic use of mannitol decreases the incidence of acute renal failure (Luke and Kennedy, 1967; Dawson, 1968).

The principles governing the management of the shock syndrome are set out in Table 5. The actions listed above the horizontal line are simple to implement and are sufficient to abolish the manifestations of circulatory failure in a high proportion of patients; indications for the actions listed in the lower panels are discussed in the text. If this chart is considered in conjunction with Tables 3 and 4, it is apparent that a number of the defects which can be identified are amenable to therapeutic intervention. However, the information available about the pathology which occurs at cellular level is scanty, and until this aspect of the syndrome has been clarified, patients will continue to suffer from "irreversible shock", defining that term as acute circulatory failure which does not respond to any of the currently accepted therapeutic manoeuvres.

18/TABLE 5
MANAGEMENT OF SHOCK

1. Establish aetiology and institute appropriate therapy.
2. Measure CVP.
3. Transfuse if necessary to restore CVP to normal.
4. Correct abnormalities of oxygenation, haematocrit, electrolytes or acid-base balance.

Improve cardiac performance	Consider:	Support other systems, especially
(a) specific measures	Corticosteroids	(a) kidneys
(b) non-specific measures	Vasodilator drugs	(b) lungs
	Heparin	

REFERENCES

ANDERSON, M. N., and MOURITZEN, C. (1966). Effect of acute respiratory and metabolic acidosis on cardiac output and peripheral resistance. *Ann. Surg.*, **163**, 161.

AUSTEN, W. G., and BUCKLEY, M. J. (1967). Treatment of various forms of surgical shock. *Progr. cardiovasc. Dis.*, **10**, 97.

BAINBRIDGE, F. A., and TREVAN, J. W. (1917). Some actions of adrenalin upon the liver. *J. Physiol. (Lond.)*, **51**, 460.

BERK, J. L. (1972). Use of beta blockers in shock. In: *Shock in Low- and High-flow States*. Ed. Forscher, B. K., Lillehei, R. C. and Stubbs, S. S. Amsterdam: Excerpta Medica.

BHAGAT, B. D. (1974). Effects of methyl prednisolone on endotoxin-induced changes in adrenal catecholamine enzymes. In: *Steroids and Shock*. Ed. Glenn, T. M. Baltimore: University Park Press.

BLAISDELL, F. W. (1974). Pathophysiology of the respiratory distress syndrome. *Arch. Surg.*, **108**, 44.

BLAISDELL, F. W., LIM, R. C., and STALLONE, R. J. (1970). The mechanism of pulmonary damage following traumatic shock. *Surg. Gynec. Obstet.*, **130**, 15.

BLALOCK, A. (1930). Experimental shock: cause of low blood pressure produced by muscle injury. *Arch. Surg.*, **20**, 959.

BLOCH, J. H., DIETZMAN, R. H., PIERCE, C. H., and LILLEHEI, R. C. (1966). Theories of the production of shock. *Brit. J. Anaesth.*, **38**, 234.

BORDEN, G. W., and HALL, W. H. (1951). Fatal transfusion reactions from massive bacterial contamination of blood. *New Engl. J. Med.*, **245**, 760.

BRAND, E. C., and LEFER, A. M. (1966). Myocardial depressant factor in plasma from cats in irreversible post-oligaemic shock. *Proc. Soc. exp. Biol. (N.Y.)*, **122**, 200.

BRANTHWAITE, M. A., and BRADLEY, R. D. (1968). Measurement of cardiac output by thermal dilution in man. *J. appl. Physiol.*, **24**, 434.

BRAUNWALD, E. (1968). The pathogenesis and treatment of shock in myocardial infarction. *Bull. Johns Hopk. Hosp.*, **121**, 421.

BRILL, N. R., and SHOEMAKER, W. C. (1960). Studies on the hepatic and visceral micro-circulation during shock and after epinephrine administration: a preliminary report. *Surg. Forum*, **11**, 119.

British Medical Journal (1974). Endotoxaemia. **4**, 730.

British Medical Journal (1975). Extracorporeal oxygenation for acute respiratory failure. **3**, 340.

BURTON, A. C. (1951). On the physical equilibrium of small blood vessels. *Amer. J. Physiol.*, **164**, 319.

CAHILL, J. M., JOUASSETT-STRIDER, D., and BYRNE, J. J. (1965). Lung function in shock. *Amer. J. Surg.*, **110**, 324.

CANNON, W. B., and BAYLISS, W. M. (1919). Notes on muscle injury in relation to shock. *Med. Res. Comm.*, **81**, 19.

CORRIGAN, J. J., Jr., RAY, W. L., and MAY, N. (1968). Changes in the blood coagulation system associated with septicemia. *New Engl. J. Med.*, **279**, 851.

CRILE, G. W. (1899). *An Experimental Research into Surgical Shock*. Philadelphia: J. B. Lippincott.

CULLUM, V. A., FARMER, J. B., JACK, D., and LEVY, G. P. (1969). Salbutamol: a new, selective beta-adrenoceptive receptor stimulant. *Brit. J. Pharmacol.*, **35**, 141.

DAINTREE-JOHNSON, H. (1966). Central venous pressure and blood volume. *Lancet*, **2**, 701.

DALY, M. J., FARMER, J. B. and LEVY, G. P. (1971). Comparison of bronchodilator and cardiovascular actions of salbutamol and isoprenaline. *Brit. J. Pharmacol.*, **43**, 624.

DAWES, G. S., and COMROE, J. H., Jr. (1954). Chemoreflexes from the heart and lungs. *Physiol. Rev.*, **34**, 167.

DAWSON, J. L. (1968). The etiology and prevention of acute renal failure in surgical patients. *Proc. roy. Soc. Med.*, **61**, 1163.

DIETZMAN, R. H., and LILLEHEI, R. C. (1968). The nature and treatment of shock. *Brit. J. hosp. Med.*, **1**, 300.

DUCASTAING, R. (1919). La vaso-constriction peripherique chez les shockés. Action du nitrite d'angle. *Presse méd.*, **27**, 782.

Duff, J. H., Wright, C. J., McLean, A. P. H., and MacLean, L. D. (1972). Oxygen consumption in septic shock. In: *Shock in Low- and High-flow States*. Ed. Forscher, B. K., Lillehei, R. C. and Stubbs, S. S. Amsterdam: Excerpta Medica.

Du Toit, H. J., Dommisse J., Theron, M. S., Du Plessis, J. M. E., Rorke, M. J., and De Villiers, V. P. (1966). Treatment of endotoxic shock with isoprenaline. *Lancet*, **2**, 143.

Eley, A., Hargreaves, T., and Lambert, H. P. (1965). Jaundice in severe infections. *Brit. med. J.*, **2**, 75.

Elliott, W. C., and Gorlin, R. (1966). Isoproterenol in treatment of heart disease. *J. Amer. med. Ass.*, **197**, 315.

Erlanger, J., Gesell, R., and Gasser, H. S. (1919a). Studies in secondary traumatic shock. I: The circulation in shock after abdominal injuries. *Amer. J. Physiol.*, **49**, 151.

Erlanger, J., Gesell, R., and Gasser, H. S. (1919b). Studies in secondary traumatic shock. III: Circulatory failure due to adrenaline. *Amer. J. Physiol.*, **49**, 345.

Fine, J. (1972). Therapeutic implications of new developments in the study of refractory non-septic shock. In: *Shock in Low- and High-flow States*. Ed. Forscher, B. K., Lillehei, R. C., and Stubbs, S. S. Amsterdam: Excerpta Medica.

Freeman, J., and Nunn, J. F. (1963). Ventilation-perfusion relationships after haemorrhage. *Clin. Sci.*, **24**, 135.

Freeman, N. E., Freedman, H., and Miller, C. C. (1951). The production of shock by the prolonged continuous injection of adrenalin in unanesthetized dogs. *Amer. J. Physiol.*, **131**, 545.

Friedman, E., Grable, E., and Fine, J. (1966). Central venous pressure and direct serial measurements as guides in blood volume replacement. *Lancet*, **2**, 609.

Fuenfer, M. M., Oson, G. E., and Polk, H. C., Jr. (1975). Effect of various corticosteroids upon the phagocytic bactericidal activity of neutrophils. *Surgery*, **78**, 27.

Gelin, L. E. (1956). Studies in the anaemia of injury. *Acta chir. scand.*, Suppl. **210**, 1.

Gerst, P. H., Rattenborg, C., and Holaday, D. A. (1959). The effect of haemorrhage on pulmonary circulation and respiratory gas exchange. *J. clin. Invest.*, **38**, 524.

Glenn, T. M., Ed. (1974). *Steriods and Shock*. Baltimore: University Park Press.

Gomez, O. A., and Hamilton, W. F. (1964). Functional cardiac deterioration during development of haemorrhagic circulatory deficiency. *Circulat. Res.*, **14**, 327.

Goodyer, A. V. N., Eckhardt, W. F., Ostberg, R. H., and Goodkind, M. J. (1961). Effects of metabolic acidosis and alkalosis on coronary blood flow and myocardial metabolism in the intact dog. *Amer. J. Physiol.*, **200**, 628.

Guyton, A. C., Jones, C. E., and Coleman, T. G. (1973). *Circulatory Physiology: Cardiac Output and its Regulation*, 2nd edit. Philadelphia: W. B. Saunders.

Guyton, A. C., and Lindsey, A. W. (1959). Effect of elevated left atrial pressure and decreased plasma protein concentration on the development of pulmonary oedema. *Circulat. Res.*, **7**, 649.

Hackel, D. B., Ratliff, N. B., and Mikat, E. (1974). The heart in shock. *Circulat. Res.*, **35**, 805.

Halmagyi, D. F. J. (1972). Combined adrenergic receptor blockade in experimental post-haemorrhagic shock. In: *Shock in Low- and High-flow States*. Ed. Forscher, B. K., Lillehei, R. C., and Stubbs, S. S. Amsterdam: Excerpta Medica.

Hardaway, R. M. (1968). *Clinical Management of Shock*. Springfield, Ill.: Charles C. Thomas.

Hardaway, R. M., and Drake, D. C. (1963). Prevention of irreversible haemorrhagic shock with fibrinolysin. *Ann. Surg.*, **157**, 39.

Hardaway, R. M., James, P. M., Jr., Anderson, R. W., Bredenberg, C. E., and West, R. L. (1967). Intensive study and treatment of shock in man. *J. Amer. med. Ass.*, **199**, 779.

HAYES, M. A. (1957). The influence of shock without clinical renal failure on renal function. *Ann. Surg.*, **146**, 523.

HEATH, M. L., and VICKERS, M. D. (1968). An examination of single-tracer, semi-automated blood volume methodology. *Anaesthesia*, **23**, 659.

HINSHAW, L. B., SPINK, W. W., VICK, J. A., MALLET, E., and FINSTAD, J. (1961). Effect of endotoxin on kidney function and renal haemodynamics in the dog. *Amer. J. Physiol.*, **201**, 144.

HYMAN, A. L., PENNINGTON, D. G., KADOWITZ, P. J., and JAQUES, W. E. (1974). Studies of the mechanisms of the pulmonary vasopressor response to endotoxin: effects of corticosteroids and catecholamines. In: *Steroids and Shock*. Ed. Glenn, T. M. Baltimore: University Park Press.

INGRAM, G. I. C. (1966). The clinical investigation of a bleeding tendency. *Hosp. Med.*, **1**, 57.

JANOFF, A. (1964). Alterations in lysosomes (intracellular enzymes) during shock; effects of preconditioning (tolerance) and protective drugs. In *Shock*. Ed. Hershey, S. G. Boston: Little Brown.

JENKINS, B. S., BRADLEY, R. D., and BRANTHWAITE, M. A. (1970). Evaluation of pulmonary arterial end-diastolic pressure as an indirect estimate of left atrial mean pressure. *Circulation*, **42**, 75.

KANTROWITZ, A., TJØNNELAND, S., FREED, P. S., PHILLIPS, S. J., BUTNER, A. N., and SHERMAN, J. L., Jr. (1968). Initial clinical experience with intra-aortic balloon pumping in cardiogenic shock. *J. Amer. med. Ass.*, **203**, 113.

KARDOS, G. G. (1966). Isoproterenol in the treatment of shock due to bacteraemia with gram-negative pathogens. *New Engl. J. Med.*, **27**, 868.

KEITH, M. N. (1919). Report of shock committee. English Medical Research Committee, No. 27.

KELMAN, G. R., NUNN, J. F., PRYS-ROBERTS, C., and GREENBAUM, R. (1967). The influence of cardiac output on arterial oxygenation: a theoretical study. *Brit. J. Anaesth.*, **39**, 450.

KIRKLIN, J. W., and RASTELLI, G. C. (1967). Low cardiac output after open intracardiac operations. *Progr. cardiovasc. Dis.*, **10**, 117.

KNISELY, M. H. (1965). Intravascular erythrocyte aggregation (blood sludge). In: *Handbook of Physiology*, Section 2, Circulation, Vol. 3, 2249. Washington: Amer. Physiol. Soc.

KUIDA, H., HINSHAW, L. B., GILBERT, R. P., and VISSCHER, M. B. (1958). Effect of gram-negative endotoxin on pulmonary circulation. *Amer. J. Physiol.* **192**, 335.

KUSAJIMA, K., WAX, S. D., and WEBB, W. R. (1974). Effects of methylprednisolone on pulmonary microcirculation. *Surg. Gynec. Obstet.*, **139**, 1.

Lancet (1963). Annotation. Septic shock. **2**, 1265.

Lancet (1974). Leading Article. Bacteraemic shock. **1**, 296.

LEFER, A. M., and GLENN, T. M. (1974). Corticosteroids and the lysosomal protease-myocardial depressant factory system in shock. In: *Steroids and Shock*. Ed. Glenn, T. M. Baltimore: University Park Press.

LEVIN, J., POORE, T. W., ZAUBER, N. P., and OSER, R. S. (1970). Detection of endotoxin in blood of patients with sepsis due to Gram-negative bacteria. *New Engl. J. Med.* **283**, 1313.

LEWIS, D. H., and MELLANDER, S. (1962). Competitive effects of sympathetic control and tissue metabolites on resistance and capacitance vessels and capillary filtration in skeletal muscle. *Acta physiol. scand.*, **56**, 162.

LILLEHEI, R. C. (1957). The intestinal factor in irreversible haemorrhagic shock. *Surgery*, **42**, 1043.

LILLEHEI, R. C., LONGERBEAM, J. K., BLOCH, J. H., and MANAX, W. G. (1964). The nature of irreversible shock: experimental and clinical observations. *Ann. Surg.*, **160**, 682.

LILLEHEI, R. C., LONGERBEAM, J. K., and ROSENBERG, J. C. (1962). The nature of irreversible shock: its relationship to intestinal change. In: *Shock; Pathogenesis and Therapy* (Ciba Internat. Symp.) Ed. Bock, K. D. Berlin: Springer-Verlag.

LOEB, H. S., WINSLOW, E. B., RAHIMTOOLA, S. H., ROSEN, K. M., and GUNNAR, R. M. (1971). Acute haemodynamic effects of dopamine in patients with shock. *Circulation*, **44**, 163.

LONGERBEAM, J. K., LILLEHEI, R. C., SCOTT, W. R., and ROSENBERG, J. C. (1962). Visceral factors in shock. *J. Amer. med. Ass.*, **181**, 878.

LOZMAN, J., DUTTON, R. E., ENGLISH, M., and POWERS, S. R., Jr. (1975). Cardiopulmonary adjustments following single high dosage administration of methylprednisolone in traumatized man. *Ann. Surg.*, **181**, 317.

LOZMAN, J., POWERS, S. P., Jr., OLDER, T., DUTTON, R. E., ROY, R. J., ENGLISH, M., MARCO, D., ECKERT, C. (1974). Correlation of pulmonary wedge and left atrial pressures. A study in the patient receiving positive end-expiratory pressure ventilation. *Arch. Surg.*, **109**, 270.

LUKE, R. G., and KENNEDY, A. C. (1967). Prevention and early management of acute renal failure. *Postgrad. med. J.,* **43**, 280.

McKENZIE, G. J., TAYLOR, S. H., FLENLEY, D. C., McDONALD, A. H., STAUNTON, H. P., and DONALD, K. W. (1964). Circulatory and respiratory studies in myocardial infarction and cardiogenic shock. *Lancet*, **2**, 825.

MACLEAN, L. D. (1966). The clinical management of shock. *Brit. J. Anaesth.*, **38**, 255.

MACLEAN, L. D., DUFF, J. H., SCOTT, H. M., and PERETZ, D. I. (1965). Treatment of shock in man based on haemodynamic diagnosis. *Surg. Gynec. Obstet.*, **120**, 1.

MACLEAN, L. D., MULLIGAN, W. G., McLEAN, A. P. H., and DUFF, J. H. (1967). Patterns of septic shock in man: a detailed study of 56 patients. *Ann. Surg.*, **166**, 543.

MILLIGAN, G. F., MACDONALD, J. A. E., MELLON, A., and LEDINGHAM, I. McA. (1974). Pulmonary and hematologic disturbances during septic shock. *Surg. Gynec., Obstet.*, **138**, 43.

MOORE, F. D., LYONS, J. H., PIERCE, E. C., MORGAN, A. P., DRINKER, P. A., MACARTHUR, J. D., DAMMIN, G. J. (1969). *Post-traumatic Pulmonary Insufficiency: Pathophysiology of Respiratory Failure and Principles of Respiratory Care After Surgical Operations, Trauma, Haemorrhage, Burns and Shock*. Philadelphia: W. B. Saunders.

MOTSAY, G. J., ALHO, A. V., DIETZMAN, R. H., SCHULTZ, L. S., ROMERO, L. H., and LILLEHEI, R. C. (1974). Forelimb, small intestine and pulmonary vascular beds in canine endotoxic shock. In: *Steroids and Shock*. Ed. Glenn, T. M. Baltimore: University Park Press.

MOTSAY, G. J., DIETZMAN, R. H., SCHULTZ, L. S., ROMERO, L. H., and LILLEHEI, R. C. (1972). Effects of massive doses of corticosteroids in experimental and clinical Gram-negative septic shock. In: *Shock in Low- and High-flow States*. Ed. Forscher, B. K., Lillehei, R. C., and Stubbs, S. S. Amsterdam: Excerpta Medica.

NAIMARK, A., DUGARD, A., and RANGNOR, E. (1968). Regional pulmonary blood flow and gas exchange in haemorrhagic shock. *J. appl. Physiol.*, **25**, 301.

NICKERSON, M. (1963). Sympathetic blockade in the therapy of shock. *Amer. J. Cardiol.*, **21**, 619.

NUNN, J. F., and FREEMAN, J. (1964). Problems of oxygenation and oxygen transport in anaesthesia. *Anaesthesia*, **19**, 120.

PERLMUTER, M., GROSSMAN, S. L., ROTHENBERG, S., and DOBKIN, G. (1959). Urine-serum urea nitrogen ratio: simple test of renal function in acute azotaemia and oliguria. *J. Amer. med. Ass.*, **170**, 1533.

PONTOPPIDAN, H., GEFFIN, B., and LOWENSTEIN, E. (1972). Acute respiratory failure in the adult. *New Engl. J. Med.*, **287**, 690, 743, and 799.

RAPAPORT, S. I., TATTER, D., COEUR-BARRON, N., and HJORT, P. F. (1964). Pseudomonas septicaemia with intravascular clotting leading to the generalized Schwartzmann reaction. *New Engl. J. Med.*, **271**, 80.

REICHGOTT, M. J., and MELMON, K. L. (1972). Does bradykinin play a pathogenetic role in endotoxaemia? In: *Shock in Low- and High-flow States*. Ed. Forscher, B. K., Lillehei, R. C., and Stubbs, S. S. Amsterdam: Excerpta Medica.

RIORDAN, J. F., and WALTERS, G. (1968). Pulmonary oedema in bacterial shock. *Lancet*, **1**, 719.

ROBB, H. J. (1963). The role of microembolism in the production of irreversible shock. *Ann. Surg.*, **158**, 685.

ROE, C. F., and KINNEY, J. M. (1965). The caloric equivalent of fever. II. Influence of major trauma. *Ann. Surg.*, **161**, 140.

Royal Society of Medicine Symposium (1968). Massive blood transfusion. *Proc. roy. Soc. Med.*, **61**, 681.

SAMPSON, J. H., and HUTCHINSON, J. C. (1967). Heart failure in myocardial infarction. *Progr. cardiovasc. Dis.*, **10**, 1.

SARDESAI, V. M., and THAL, A. P. (1966). Myocardial glucose metabolism in endotoxin shock. *Fed. Proc.*, **25**, 634.

SARNOFF, S. J., CASE, R. B., WAITHE, P. E., and ISAACS, J. P. (1954). Insufficient coronary blood flow and myocardial failure as a complicating factor in late haemorrhagic shock. *Amer. J. Physiol.*, **176**, 439.

SCHUMER, W. (1972). Cellular metabolism in shock. In: *Shock in Low- and High-flow States*. Ed. Forscher, B. K., Lillehei, R. C., and Stubbs, S. S. Amsterdam: Excerpta Medica.

SCHUMER, W. (1976). Steroids in the treatment of clinical septic shock. *Ann. Surg.*, **184**, 333.

SHARPEY-SCHAFER, E. P. (1961). Venous tone. *Brit. med. J.*, **2**, 1589.

SIEGEL, J. H., GREENSPAN, M., and DEL GUERCIO, L. R. M. (1967). Abnormal vascular tone, defective oxygen transport and myocardial failure in human septic shock. *Ann. Surg.*, **165**, 504.

SPINK, W. W. (1962). Pathogenesis and therapy of shock due to infection: experimental and clinical studies. In: *Shock; Pathogenesis and Therapy* (Ciba Internat. Symp.) Ed. Bock, K. D. Berlin: Springer-Verlag.

SWAN, H. J. C., GANZ, W., FORRESTER, J., MARCUS, H., DIAMOND, G., and CHONETTE, D. (1970). Catheterization of the heart in man with use of a flow-directed balloon-tipped catheter. *New Engl. J. Med.*, **283**, 447.

SYKES, M. K. (1963). Venous pressure as a clinical indication of adequacy of transfusion. *Ann. roy. Coll. Surg. Engl.*, **33**, 185.

THAL, A. P., and KINNEY, J. M. (1967). On the definition and classification of shock. *Progr. cardiovasc. Dis.*, **9**, 527.

THAL, A. P., and WILSON, R. (1965). Shock. In: *Current Problems in Surgery*, Vol. 9. Chicago: Yearbook Publishers.

THOMAS, M., MALMCRONA, R., and SHILLINGFORD, J. P. (1965). Haemodynamic changes in patients with acute myocardial infarction. *Circulation*, **31**, 811.

THOMAS, M., MALMCRONA, R., and SHILLINGFORD, J. P. (1966). Circulatory changes associated with systemic hypotension in patients with acute myocardial infarction. *Brit. Heart J.*, **28**, 108.

THROWER, W. B., DARBY, T. D., and ALDINGER, E. E. (1961). Acid-base derangements and myocardial contractility. *Arch. Surg.*, **82**, 56.

TINKER, J. H., and MICHENFELDER, J. D. (1976). Sodium nitroprusside: pharmacology, toxicology and therapeutics. *Anesthesiology*, **45**, 340.

WEIL, M. H., HOULE, D. B., BROWN, E. B., Jr., CAMPBELL, G. S., and HEATH, C. (1957). Influence of acidosis on the effectiveness of vasopressor agents. *Circulation*, **16**, 949.

WILKINSON, S. P., ARROYO, V., GAZZARD, B. G., MOODIE, H., and Williams, R. (1974). Relation of renal impairment and haemorrhagic diathesis to endotoxaemia in fulminant hepatic failure. *Lancet*, 1, 521.

WILSON, J. W. (1972a). Pulmonary morphologic changes due to extracorporeal circulation: a model for "the shock lung" at cellular level in humans. In *Shock in Low- and High-flow States*. Ed. Forscher, B. K., Lillehei, R. C., and Stubbs, S. S. Amsterdam: Excerpta Medica.

WILSON, J. W. (1972b). Treatment or prevention of pulmonary cellular damage with pharmacologic doses of corticosteroid. *Surg. Gynec. Obstet.*, 134, 675.

WILSON, J. W. (1974). Cellular localization of ^{3}H-labeled corticosteroids by electron microscopic autoradiography after hemorrhagic shock. In: *Steroids and Shock*. E. Glenn, T. M. Baltimore: University Park Press.

WINSLOW, E. J., LOEB, H. S., RAHIMTOOLA, S. H., KAMATH, S., and GUNNAR, R. M. (1973). Hemodynamic studies and results of therapy in 50 patients with bacteremic shock. *Amer. J. Med.*, 54, 421.

WOOD, P. (1968). *Diseases of the Heart and Circulation*, 3rd edit. London: Eyre and Spottiswoode.

WYSE, S. D., GIBSON, D. G., and BRANTHWAITE, M. A. (1974). Haemodynamic effects of salbutamol in patients needing circulatory support after open-heart surgery. *Brit. med. J.*, 3, 502.

ZWEIFACH, B. W. (1958). Microcirculatory derangements as basis for lethal manifestations of experimental shock. *Brit. J. Anaesth.*, 30, 466.

ZWEIFACH, B. W. (1961). *Functional Behaviour of the Microcirculation*. Springfield, Ill.: Charles C. Thomas.

FURTHER READING

Reviews:

BRADLEY, R. D. (1977). *Studies in Acute Heart Failure*. London: Edward Arnold.

BRANTHWAITE, M. A. (1977). Adult Respiratory Distress Syndrome. In: *Advanced Medicine, 13*. Ed. G. M. Besser. Tunbridge Wells: Pitman.

Current Topics in Surgical Research. Irving, M. (1972). *Proc. roy. Soc. Med.*, 65, 1116.

Shock and Metabolism. Powers, S. R., Jr. (1975). *Surg., Gynec. Obstet.*, 140, 211.

RUSSELL, W. J. (1974). *Central Venous Pressure: Its clinical use and role in cardio vascular dynamics*. London: Butterworths.

Book:

Treatment of Shock: Principles and Practice. Schumer W., and Nyhus, L. M. (1974). Philadelphia: Lea and Febiger.

Chapter 19

PARENTERAL FLUID THERAPY

IN order to understand how present schedules for intravenous fluids for surgical patients have evolved one must go back over the last fifty years. To begin with the practice of giving such fluids largely as isotonic saline became established and a good example of this was described by Jones and Eaton (1933): their patients received about 350 mEq (mmol) of sodium daily for a week after major surgery, equivalent to $2\frac{1}{2}$ litres of saline a day, and most of them became oedematous on about the seventh day. Stewart and Rourke (1942) described a patient undergoing colporrhaphy who was given over 6 litres of isotonic saline a day for each of the first four post-operative days. Her convalescence was uneventful and she did not become oedematous. Gamble (1958), commenting on this case, was particularly impressed that there was no change whatever in the serum sodium concentration in spite of a positive sodium balance of more than 1000 mEq (mmol). From these and other studies one can deduce that surgical patients with no cardiovascular or renal disease can tolerate large volumes of isotonic sodium infusions and that individual tolerances vary widely and are quite unpredictable. All surgical patients given such therapy go into positive sodium balance, maintain normal levels of serum sodium concentration and eventually become oedematous. It is against such a background that recent developments in parenteral fluid therapy must be judged.

As the post-operative patient's propensity to retain sodium and to become oedematous became more generally recognised, solutions of isotonic dextrose (5 per cent) were given in place of the large volumes of saline. Coller and Maddock (1933, 1940) did much to influence management at this time. They assessed insensible loss as two litres daily (though they subsequently reduced this) and recommended that a urine volume of 1 to $1\frac{1}{2}$ litres a day should be aimed at from the day of surgery. It must be remembered that patients were routinely purged and given enemas before operation and received ether or chloroform with consequent likelihood of prolonged post-operative vomiting. Heat was universally regarded as beneficial for shock and there is little doubt that extrarenal losses were often appreciably higher than they are now. In this way schedules prescribing three or more litres of water a day, mostly as 5 per cent dextrose, became established. Unfortunately the inability of the kidneys to secrete solute-free water normally was not appreciated, and it was not until ten years later that a series of papers appeared drawing attention to this (Cooper et al., 1949; Ariel et al., 1950; Zimmermann and Wangensteen 1952; Moore et al., 1952). These workers provided conclusive evidence that in the post-operative period the kidneys retained water avidly. The mechanisms underlying this are discussed more fully below, but from this time on it has been known that the administration of three litres of 5 per cent dextrose a day always puts the patient into positive water balance and occasionally can result in signs and symptoms of frank water intoxication within 48 to 72 hours of surgery.

The next phase saw the application of new and more accurate methods of metabolic balance studies by numerous workers. Accurate bed scales, the flame photometer and radioisotopes all helped to unravel some of the many unanswered problems. Thus the role of the adrenal cortex in response to stress was elucidated and aldosterone was discovered. Clinical management was strongly influenced to curtail the amount of sodium given to surgical patients and so emerged the "low salt" schedule of the 1950's. This consisted of two or two and a half litres of 5 per cent dextrose together with half a litre of isotonic saline. The saline was often withheld on the day of operation and Moore and Ball (1955) recommended that no sodium should be given for five days. The greatest advance of this period was the recognition of the need to give potassium to all patients maintained on clear fluids for more than 48 hours. Such a regime was used successfully in the management of patients undergoing all types of elective surgery. The small volumes of concentrated urine passed in the first day or two after surgery became accepted as part of the normal response to trauma and were not thought to be harmful. Since then surgeons have increased the severity and length of operations and anaesthetists have accepted patients who twenty years ago would not have been considered as operative risks. Post-operative renal failure began to occur more frequently and it was inevitable that the oliguria consequent on orthodox management should be critically reappraised. It was soon recognised that considerable falls in glomerular filtration and renal blood flow occurred during surgery, and that the oxygen demands of the kidneys were closely related to renal sodium conservation.

The change in outlook emanated from Dallas in the 1960's when Shires and his colleagues challenged the accepted teaching and asserted that all major surgical trauma was accompanied by sequestration of large volumes of sodium-containing extracellular fluid and that this should be replaced (Shires et al., 1961). The measurements were made during and immediately after surgery using an isotope dilution method with sulphate and allowing 20 minutes for equilibration. These workers claimed that the "functional" extracellular fluid contracted by several litres in a three- or four-hour operation and they gave equivalent volumes of Ringer lactate ("Balanced Salt") solution. As a result anaesthetists began to give patients litres of Ringer lactate during and after surgery; the wheel had come full circle.

The present decade has seen a swing away from these very liberal infusions since cases of obvious over-infusion began to be reported (Fieber and Jones, 1966; Hutchin et al., 1969). Subsequent investigators failed to substantiate the original work (Roth et al., 1969) so that proponents of orthodox management were unwilling to abandon their well-established schedules. Nevertheless some who had done most to establish such schedules became convinced that major surgery resulted in an accumulation of sequestered fluid in the traumatised tissues, forming the so-called "Third Space". No orthopaedic surgeon would operate on a limb and enclose it within an unpadded or unsplit plaster, or on a hand without elevating it. Similarly, prolonged and vigorous retraction of the abdominal wall and the infliction of scores of small burns by diathermy is bound to result in accumulation of interstitial fluid from the freely mobilised part of the extracellular fluid which is in equilibrium with plasma. This was acknowledged to occur and to require replacement during operation by workers such as Hayes (1968) and Dudley (1968). Moore gave his support in a joint editorial with Shires (1967) but they warned against the uncritical use of the large volumes originally recommended. Irvin and his colleagues (1972) investigated patients undergoing major bowel surgery and produced evidence of a significant fall in plasma volume in the group who received no sodium and no such fall in those who received an average of 260 mEq (mmol) of sodium as Ringer lactate during surgery and a litre daily thereafter. Anaesthetists must now assess the magnitude and the nature of the operative dissection; when this involves extensive separation of tissue planes as in oesophageal or rectal resections, allowance must be made for the extracellular fluid which is translocated.

If sodium is given during operation in amounts of from 150 to 250 mEq (mmol) it will usually result in a strongly positive sodium balance in the first eight hours (Mackenzie and Donald, 1969) which may persist for three days if sodium is continued (Hutchin et al., 1969). When pre-existing disease makes this undesirable sodium may still be given provided that diuresis is assured by intravenous frusemide or ethacrynic acid. Stahl (1970) described a regime which was used successfully in patients with creatinine clearances of less than 50 ml/minute. Ringer lactate solution is often used uncritically during surgery and there are occasions when saline is more appropriate. Frusemide and ethacrynic acid both cause a greater loss of chloride than sodium in the urine and approximate sodium and water balance can be achieved if urine output is matched by intake consisting of alternate volumes of isotonic saline and 0·18 per cent saline in 5 per cent dextrose. Patients who are hypochloraemic as a result of pyloric obstruction should also receive saline rather than sodium lactate.

It is salutary to reflect that after fifty years we still do not really know the optimum sodium intake for the day of operation. Shires may have been right in selecting the 20 minute ^{35}S space and the demonstration that hours later the isotope had a larger volume of distribution may simply have meant that it had penetrated the "sequestered" pool. It is now generally agreed that moderate amounts of sodium should be given to most patients undergoing major elective surgery even if there are no external losses of body fluids. A satisfactory regime for administration of crystalloid solutions to an adult is:

During operation	500 to 1500 ml isotonic (0·9 per cent) saline or Ringer lactate
Remainder of day of operation	500 ml dextrose 5 per cent/saline 0·18 per cent six-hourly
First post-operative day	500 ml dextrose 5 per cent/saline 0·18 per cent six-hourly
Second post-operative day	500 ml dextrose 5 per cent/saline 0·18 per cent four-hourly

Potassium may be added from the first or second post-operative day (see page 689). If intravenous fluids are required after the second day consideration should be given to the requirements to provide more calories (see page 694).

THE METABOLIC RESPONSE TO TRAUMA

In the course of evolution mammals have developed a series of endocrine responses to trauma. The main target organ for effecting these responses is the kidney which regulates its excretory activity in such a way as to preserve the volume of the extracellular fluid; in practice this simply means that both water and sodium will tend to be retained when they would normally be expected to be excreted.

The anterior pituitary secretes increased amounts of ACTH in response to surgical trauma. The afferent pathways are the peripheral somatic nerves from the site of injury and also autonomic afferents arising from intravascular pressor receptors. The main effect of ACTH is to stimulate the adrenal cortex to secrete cortisol (also called Compound F or hydrocortisone), but it is now also known to produce an increase in the adrenal secretion of aldosterone. Previously the anterior pituitary had been thought not to be concerned with aldosterone release, but two types of aldosterone activity are now recognised. The first is mediated by ACTH and results in proportionally similar increases in both cortisol and aldosterone. The other is mediated by volume-sensitive receptors thought to be in the renal juxtaglomerular bodies and results in increased levels of aldosterone and has no effect on cortisol levels. Zimmermann believes that in most surgical patients aldosterone release is predominantly due to the cortico-trophin mechanism.

The Posterior Pituitary

Plasma levels of antidiuretic hormone (ADH) are consistently raised during surgery and for the first few post-operative days. During this time the normal osmoreceptor control of the hormone is overridden by other mechanisms with the result that the urine remains hypertonic whilst the plasma osmolarity tends to fall if excess water is given. Hyponatraemia is the commonest bio-chemical change post-operatively and dilution of the body sodium stores is its usual explanation (Singh and Flear, 1968). Zimmermann and his colleagues at West Virginia (Zimmermann, 1965; Moran and Zimmermann, 1967; Ukai et al., 1968) showed that ADH levels fluctuated from minute to minute during operation in response to surgical manipulations: after operation the plasma concentration of the hormone falls but remains above the pre-operative level for up to five days. This is due to pain impulses transmitted by somatic nerves and accounts for the inability of the surgical patient to excrete hypotonic fluids at this time.

MAINTENANCE OF BODY OSMOLALITY

In health the body fluids, both cellular and extracellular, are maintained at a concentration of approximately one seventh molar:* this is chiefly due to the presence of potassium in the intracellular fluid (ICF) and sodium in the extracellular fluid (ECF), each milli-equivalent (mmol) of which will hold 7 ml of water in the cells or the extracellular fluid respectively. This water "binding" is shared equally between the cations and the anions which necessarily accom-pany them, but the cations are the vital constituents which determine the rela-tive volume of the two major divisions of the body fluid. If it is known that plasma urea and sugar concentrations are within normal limits the osmolarity of the body fluids can be calculated by doubling the plasma sodium concentra-

---

* This is true for electrolytes which are completely dissociated. Strictly speaking the body fluids are about M/3·5. Thus isotonic solutions of electrolytes are M/7 and of non-electrolytes M/3·5. Both contain 286 mosmol/1.

tion and adding 10, i.e. if plasma sodium concentration is 135 mEq/l (mmol/l), the approximate plasma osmolarity will be $2 \times 135 + 10 = 285$ mosmol/l. If there is a large difference between the calculated osmolarity and the osmolality measured by freezing point depression the most likely causes are hyperlipidaemia or alcohol (ethanol). Raised triglyceride concentrations displace plasma water and depress the plasma sodium concentration when it is measured by conventional flame photometry; ethanol will raise the plasma osmolarity by 22 mosmol/l for every 100 mg/dl in the blood (Loeb, 1974). It is now generally accepted that no sustained osmolar gradient can exist between the ECF and the cells of non-secretory tissues. This has several important implications. Firstly, water will distribute itself in the two compartments in proportion to their relative volumes. As the intracellular fluid is approximately twice the volume of the extracellular fluid,[†] a positive water balance will result in twice as much water entering the cells as will remain outside them. Secondly, a rise in serum Na will cause water to shift from the cells to the ECF and a fall in the serum Na, if due to sodium loss, will cause water to pass into the cells. Thirdly, a rise and fall in intracellular K will have precisely the opposite effects. The contribution of K loss to the expansion of the ECF and therefore the production of oedema has been documented clinically and experimentally (Black and Milne, 1952). Finally, the serum Na is an indication of the intracellular as well as the extracellular osmolarity and therefore a fall in serum Na may well be due to loss of K or to an increase in total body water with no change in the external balance of Na or K.

Isotonic Solutions

Isotonic solutions are solutions in which cells neither swell nor shrink. They must therefore contain a solute such as sodium for which there is no net influx into cells. A solution of urea containing 280 mosmol/l would be iso-osmotic but not isotonic; cells suspended in it would swell as urea penetrated them accompanied by water.

Oncotic Pressure

This refers to the colloid osmotic activity of a solution and is due to molecules of molecular weight above 40,000 which do not readily escape through the capillary endothelium. Such solutions are often incorrectly described as being hypertonic; in clinical use the commonest examples are dextran 40 and 70 in which a milliosmole of each would theoretically be 40 grams and 70 grams respectively. The solutions used would therefore contain less than 3 mosmol per litre which would make them dangerously hypotonic unless they were presented in either isotonic saline or dextrose. In fact dextran solutions contain a wide range of dextran molecules of differing weights and the smaller ones render the fluid less hypotonic than the theoretical example given.

---

† Most estimates of the size of the extracellular fluid space are based on the volume of dilution of mannitol, sucrose or inulin. These substances probably underestimate the true volume of the space due to their very slow penetration into dense connective tissue (such as cartilage and ligaments), bone and gastro-intestinal luminal fluid (Edelman and Leibman, 1959). The part of the extracellular fluid concerned with rapid changes in volume is approximately half the volume of the cellular fluid.

WATER

Earlier estimates of total body water, expressed as a percentage of body weight, were higher than they are now thought to be. Edelman and Leibman (1959) give the following figures for adults of average build:

	Water content expressed as a Percentage of Body Weight	
	Ages 17–39	Age 60+
Men	60·6%	51·5%
Women	50·2%	45·5%

For practical purposes, total body water can be assessed as half the body weight in kilograms.

Fluid Balance Charts

Accurately kept balance charts are essential whenever intravenous fluids are given. One must not however expect to balance the intake and output columns like a cash account. A daily reckoning will frequently show oscillations of water balance of one or occasionally two litres which eventually balance out over a period of days. The variable rates of tissue catabolism with associated production of water in the body make the net insensible loss very difficult to compute. Balances are the result of a mixture of measurement and guesswork and one must strive for the one to be accurate and the other to be informed. In a temperate climate an afebrile patient should be managed on the basis that the net unmeasured loss (losses from skin and lungs minus water formed in the body) is 750 ml/day. If the patient is on a ventilator and inspired gases are saturated with water vapour at body temperature there is no pulmonary water loss and the allowance for unmeasured losses should be reduced to 500 ml/day.

Water Requirements

Sodium-free water is required to make good the losses from the skin and lungs; if more is given than is necessary for this it will normally be excreted in the urine which will become hypotonic due to suppression of ADH release. It has been shown above that ADH is not suppressed after surgery and therefore any excess free water will accumulate in the body. The weight of evidence now is that whereas moderate positive balances of water plus sodium are probably beneficial, there is no such evidence that a positive free-water balance is desirable and much that it is harmful in excess. Manners (1974) has shown that when intravenous fluids are stopped soon after major surgery the voluntary water intake during the first week was approximately 25 ml/kg per day. The schedule given on page 680 restricts the free-water intake to 1600 ml/day (this is the free-water content of two litres of dextrose 5 per cent/saline 0·18 per cent) and this is close to the intake selected by post-operative patients. Any clear fluids prescribed above this intake should contain sodium in isotonic concentration.

Unless unusual steps are taken to prevent it, starvation accompanies most intravenous regimes prescribed for the first 72 hours after elective surgery. More than 80 per cent of the body's energy needs have to be met by catabolism of stores of fat and protein; this not only increases the endogenous production of water but halves the solute output in the urine. Figure 1 clearly shows that the kidney's tolerance for water varies with the excretion of solutes. The daily administration of 80–100 grams of dextrose reduces protein catabolism and so reduces the solute output further; this protein-sparing effect does not operate during the operative and immediate post-operative few hours. Figure 1 also shows that when these changes are accompanied with the increased ADH activity associated with surgery the ceiling for water is little above the minimum requirements.

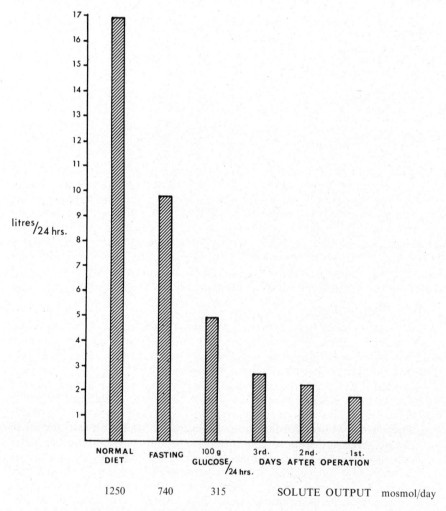

19/Fig. 1.—The ordinate shows the ceiling for water. The columns on the abscissa show how this is reduced by diminished excretion of solutes (urinary Na, K, NH$_4$ and urea). There is considerable individual variation. (After Hayes, 1968.)

Water Depletion

Water depletion without sodium depletion is uncommon in surgical patients. So effective is the sensation of thirst in its prevention that it is only likely to be seen in infants, in prolonged unconsciousness or those who are too feeble or too breathless to satisfy their need for water. Occasionally dysphagia due to lesions of the pharynx or the oesophagus can result in water depletion.

Patients suffering from prolonged unconsciousness due to head injuries or cerebrovascular accidents are more liable than most to become water depleted as they are often febrile and tend to hyperventilate. They may develop diabetes insipidus after head injuries or operations in the vicinity of the hypothalamus.

Water depletion is characterised by extreme thirst and dryness of the mouth with little or no change in cardiovascular function until its terminal stages. The rise in blood urea, if exogenous protein is not being given, is slow: its biochemical hallmark is a progressive rise in serum Na and Cl and it is the only common cause of such a finding. Man is unable to take care of himself physically or mentally when water deficits amount to 10 per cent of body weight and swallowing and talking become impossible (Schmidt-Nielsen, 1964). The approximate water deficit can be calculated from the estimated total body water and the observed serum Na. If a patient is found to have a serum Na of 160 and his normal body water is assessed to be 40 litres:

$$\text{Actual body water} \times 160 = \text{Normal body water} \times 140$$

$$\text{Actual body water} \quad = \quad \frac{40 \times 140}{160} \quad = 35 \text{ litres}$$

$$\text{Water deficit} = 40 - 35 \quad = 5 \text{ litres}$$

Treatment.—Five per cent dextrose is given to cover the normal water requirements plus the deficit. Unlike the dramatic response of extracellular depletion to appropriate treatment, the results of replacement seem disappointing in the first 12 hours. Very rapid restitution should not be aimed at: the calculated water deficit should be divided into thirds, one-third being given in the first six hours, one-third in the first 24 hours and the remainder in 48 hours. For the management of infants with hypernatraemia see page 694.

Water Excess

From the foregoing account of ADH activity in response to operation it will readily be appreciated that patients subjected to long and extensive operations are particularly liable to receive water loads in excess of their capacity to excrete them. Intakes of 3 litres of 5 per cent dextrose a day may result in a progressive accumulation of body water during the first 3–4 days after operation: when this reaches about 5 litres or the serum sodium falls below 120 mEq/l (mmol/l), the patient is likely to be confused and restless. Nocturnal disorientation and jerking movements of the limbs should arouse suspicion of water intoxication.

Treatment.—If 5 per cent saline is available, 50 to 100 ml should be given slowly intravenously. Alternatively 1·8 per cent saline can be given in volumes of half to one litre. Isotonic (0·9 per cent) saline is ineffective and should not be used.

SODIUM AND POTASSIUM

Certain aspects of the metabolism of sodium and potassium can conveniently be considered together. In an average diet the intake of both greatly exceeds the minimum requirements and both are excreted predominantly in the urine. Fruit, vegetables and meat contain up to 100 times as much potassium as sodium, nearly all the sodium in the food being added as salt in the process of cooking. Salt-free diets are therefore easy to design whereas potassium-free diets are not a practicable proposition. The kidneys, if renal function is not reduced, can retain sodium quickly and effectively so that sodium may virtually disappear from the urine. By contrast renal conservation of potassium is much less effective and potassium may be found in the urine in ten or twenty times its plasma concentration several days after intake has ceased.

If potassium is not given post-operatively the tendency for sodium to be retained is prolonged and intensified. Sodium is kept out of the cells by the energy-consuming "sodium pump". If for any reason such as hypoxia the activity of the pump is depressed, sodium and water will enter the cells and they will swell. In other circumstances, the evidence for intracellular migration of sodium is mostly inferential but Danowski's (1951) observation that potassium and sodium tend to move in opposite directions across the cell membrane has been borne out by experience.

There is a very wide range of intakes of both sodium and potassium compatible with normal health. Sodium intakes of less than five milligrams a day have been described in the highlands of New Guinea by Oomen (1961). This corresponds to less than one per cent of the intake of people accustomed to highly-seasoned food who ingest up to 200 mEq (mmol) of sodium daily. The optimum daily intakes of sodium and potassium are still not known but in the absence of abnormal losses there is general agreement that about 75 mEq (mmol) of sodium chloride and 50 to 80 mEq (mmol) of potassium chloride should be given to an adult.

Sodium and the Extracellular Fluid

The concentration of sodium in the extracellular fluid is 135 to 140 mEq/l (mmol/l) in health—figures which are well known thanks to the ease and accuracy of flame photometry. It is less well appreciated that knowledge of the sodium concentration is no sure guide to the total body stores of sodium: if the plasma sodium concentration is raised the most likely cause is water depletion. If it is lowered it may be due to loss of sodium, but it is more commonly the result of several factors of which water retention and potassium loss are important contributory causes. Moore (1960), speaking of surgical patients, states that "most hypotonicity is dilutional" and plasma sodium must be interpreted with this in mind. This is particularly likely to apply to patients who have to be re-operated upon after several days of parenteral fluid therapy. Such a patient will often be found to have a plasma sodium concentration of 125 to 130 mEq/l (mmol/l) and this should only be accepted as an indication for giving sodium if there is a likelihood of unreplaced sodium loss having occurred, or if it is associated with signs of impaired cardiovascular function.

PRE-OPERATIVE LOSSES OF EXTRACELLULAR FLUID

With the single exception of gastric juice (sodium content approximately 50 mEq/l or mmol/l) all fluids lost from the alimentary tract contain sodium in concentrations of 100 to 120 mEq/l (mmol/l). The water to sodium ratio is therefore higher than that of plasma and it follows that the plasma sodium concentration would be expected to rise as a consequence of such losses. In practice adult surgical patients usually stop all intake of electrolytes once they become acutely ill but they continue to drink water; the plasma sodium concentration is therefore often within the normal range but it tends to fall if losses are cumulative over several days.

As sodium is for practical purposes confined to the extracellular fluid, of which plasma forms a part, plasma volume will fall with the contraction of the extracellular fluid. There will be a variable loss of cell water, but the life-threatening depletion which demands urgent replacement is the loss of sodium and water from outside the cells.

Signs of Depletion of Extracellular Fluid

The term "dehydration" is too well-established to be discarded but it has been an obstacle to precision in both diagnosis and treatment. By common usage it has come to mean body fluid depletion, due either to abnormal losses or sequestration. As all such fluids are isotonic it follows that they all must contain sodium at approximately its plasma concentration. One should discipline oneself to dissect body fluid depletion into its two components and look for signs of water depletion and for signs of sodium depletion; if the signs of water depletion (see page 685) are present and cardiovascular function is good one is either dealing with mild body fluid loss or with the comparatively rare condition of true dehydration. Nearly always there will be signs of cardiovascular dysfunction. These are:

1. *Rapid pulse of poor volume*; in extreme cases the radial pulse becomes impalpable.
2. *Hypotension* and a tendency to orthostatic fainting if patient is sat up.
3. *Peripheral vasoconstriction*: coldness of the hands, feet and in extreme cases of the nose and brow. Thread-like superficial veins.
4. *Haemoconcentration*. If a venous sample is taken the blood is abnormally dark and viscous.

If cardiovascular signs are present they are accompanied by loss of normal tissue turgor which can be assessed by pinching a fold of skin over the arm or thigh. It has a dough-like feel and the fold does not immediately disappear. Retraction of the eyes is a valuable sign and one of the earliest to disappear as deficits are corrected.

Biochemical findings.—The plasma electrolyte concentrations are often unhelpful in establishing a diagnosis of body fluid loss. By contrast, the urea concentration and haemoglobin and haemotocrit may be very informative. This point is well illustrated in Table 1 which shows the average plasma sodium and urea concentrations of fifty patients. Of these twelve were assessed as being severely dehydrated and thirty-eight as being moderately dehydrated. The third column shows the percentage of each group in whom the haemoglobin concentration was over 17·5 g/100 ml (g/dl).

Note particularly the higher sodium concentration in the severely depleted group and the considerable changes in urea and haemoglobin concentrations. The highest blood urea encountered was 260 mg per cent (42·5 mmol/l) and

19/TABLE 1

THE AVERAGE PLASMA SODIUM AND UREA CONCENTRATION OF FIFTY
DEHYDRATED PATIENTS

Assessed degree of dehydration	Average plasma Na (mEq/l) (mmol/l)	Average plasma Urea mg/100ml mmol/l		Percentage of patients with Hb of 17·5 g/100ml (g/dl)
Severe (12 patients)	139	109	18	40
Moderate (38 patients)	135	78	13	10

figures of 400 mg per cent (65 mmol/l) are described and do not necessarily indicate that intrinsic renal damage has occurred. The plasma sodium concentration is therefore a very poor guide to the size of the sodium deficit.

Assessment of the Magnitude of the Loss

It is unwise to make an initial assessment of the total volume of fluid required and not be prepared to alter it as treatment is given. Cardiovascular signs thought to be solely due to dehydration are not uncommonly due in part to the presence of bacterial infections such as peritonitis or to endotoxaemia arising from non-viable bowel. In such cases the response to treatment helps to establish the diagnosis—if fluid depletion is the sole cause of the signs appropriate therapy will rapidly restore circulatory efficiency. A useful rough guide to the probable size of the fluid deficit is given by Hardy (1954):

Mild   4 per cent of body weight, i.e. 2·8 litres for a 70 kg man
Moderate   6 per cent of body weight, i.e. 4·2 litres for a 70 kg man
Severe   8 per cent of body weight, i.e. 5·6 litres for a 70 kg man

If the body weight is assessed in kilograms, these percentages are readily calculated, and in this context the weight in kilograms can be taken as half the weight in pounds. Even if the guessed weight is as much as a stone (6·5 kg) in error, it will not affect the derived therapy significantly.

The designations mild, moderate and severe depend on the signs of cardiovascular dysfunction. Mild means that they are undetectable, moderate that they are obvious and severe that the cardiovascular state is so bad that induction of anaesthesia cannot be considered until it is improved.

Replacement of Losses

An intravenous infusion should be started at once whenever there are signs of cardiovascular impairment. There is no need at this stage to spend time on central venous pressure measurement and the replacement must be with fluid that contains sodium at isotonic concentration, e.g.

1. Isotonic saline
2. Ringer lactate (Inj. Sodium Lactate Co., B.P.)
3. Dextran 70 in 0·9 per cent saline
4. Plasma protein fraction.

Patients who are critically ill as a result of body fluid loss should receive plasma or dextran 70 at first. Repletion should be rapid so that the first litre is given in about 20 minutes and half the assessed deficit is infused within an hour. A severely depleted patient might therefore receive one litre of plasma protein fraction and 1,500 ml of saline or Ringer lactate in the first hour; continuous re-assessment is essential and as soon as the circulation shows no further signs of improvement anaesthesia can be induced. The replacement of the remainder of the deficit can then be governed by the response to anaesthesia and surgery and the operative findings.

Although European practice in a temperate climate seldom requires the administration of as much as 5 litres of sodium-containing fluids in the initial replacement, much larger volumes may be required in other parts of the world. White (1961) gave up to 18 litres to Africans in the first six hours and greatly reduced the mortality of intestinal obstruction as a result. It is wise to regard five litres and 500 mEq (mmol) of sodium as the upper limit which is likely to be required during the first twelve hours of repletion and most cases will require less than this. Central venous pressure measurement should not be regarded as mandatory but it may be a helpful guide in cases suffering from both fluid loss and endotoxaemia when fluid replacement alone does not result in rapid restoration of blood pressure and tissue perfusion (see Chapter 13).

Plasma Loss in Acute Abdominal Lesions

Certain abdominal lesions, of which perforated peptic ulcers are the most common, are sometimes accompanied by large losses of plasma: this may also occur in pancreatitis, bacterial peritonitis and obstructive lesions of the mesenteric veins, e.g. volvulus. The haematocrit may rise above 60 and as Moore (1960) says "elevation of the haematocrit over 60 due to acute plasma loss alone represents a life-endangering emergency." The plasma loss is partly intraperitoneal but mostly into the wall of the bowel and therefore not obvious. The plasma volume may become seriously reduced within a few hours without any external losses occurring at all. It is in such cases that repeated estimations of haemoglobin or haematocrit can be of most help, as there is unlikely to be any significant change in the concentration of the plasma electrolytes.

Potassium and Intracellular Fluid

Potassium depletion.—Potassium is found in the cells at a concentration of approximately 150 mEq/1 (mmol/l) and in the extracellular fluid at a concentration of 3·5 to 5 mEq/l (mmol/l). The daily intake is from 60–100 mEq (mmol) and a similar amount is excreted, mostly in the urine. Intestinal juices always contain potassium at an average concentration of 10 mEq/l (mmol/l). This is very variable and when large losses occur, the potassium concentration should be measured and accurately replaced. It is important to remember that potassium excretion continues in spite of no potassium intake and an operation causes a loss of potassium of 50–100 mEq (mmol) in the first 48 hours—the loss in general varying with the severity of the operation. When protoplasm is broken down in the immediate post-operative period, each gram of nitrogen is excreted with about 2·5 mEq (mmol) of potassium. The K:N ratio is said to be 2·5. This loss occurs in starvation and is not a selective loss of potassium. If potassium is lost in excess of a K : N ratio of 2·5 the excess represents true potassium loss and this alone will affect intracellular osmolarity and accordingly be reflected by a fall in plasma sodium concentration. A patient maintained on potassium-free parenteral fluids will gradually reduce his urinary potassium loss until it stabilises at 20–30 mEq (mmol) a day—in this way deficits of 200 mEq (mmol) of potassium may readily be incurred within a few days of operation if no potassium is given. The presence of potassium deficiency is easy to infer but less easy to substantiate because the plasma potassium concentration may well be above its normal lower limit of 3·5 mEq/l (mmol/l) when there is a large overall deficit. The most reliable proof of the existence of cellular potassium depletion is provided by measuring potassium intake against urinary excretion. As long as less than 60 per cent of the intake appears in the urine, a deficit may be presumed to exist.

When potassium salts are given intravenously, they equilibrate extremely quickly with extracellular fluid if tissue circulation is normal. Equilibration is 95 per cent complete in a single transit of the circulation (Black et al., 1955) and this makes venous sampling an unreliable guide to the safety of potassium infusion. Cellular penetration is rapid when a potassium deficit exists, but occurs at different rates in different tissues—liver, lungs, heart and skeletal muscles having a rapid uptake, brain and red cells a much slower one.

If the plasma potassium concentration is below 3·5 mEq/l (mmol/l) a potassium deficit is probable and if below 3 mEq/l (mmol/l) it can be assumed with certainty. Electrocardiographic changes consist of flattening of the T wave and the occasional appearance of a small positive U wave immediately after it (see p. 524 et seq.).

Effects of potassium depletion.—Deprivation of potassium for 48 hours is harmless if intake has previously been adequate: deprivation beyond this time is associated with progressive apathy, muscular weakness and sodium retention with a tendency for oedema to form. There is experimental evidence that intestinal distension progressing to ileus results from potassium deficits (Darrow, 1950) and this may occur in man. Renal function is always affected and the kidneys lose their ability to concentrate the urine. Histological changes occur in the tubular cells and prolonged potassium depletion results in permanent renal damage. The heart is adversely affected and severe mental symptoms may appear.

Low levels of plasma potassium concentration are by no means always accompanied by obvious muscular weakness and the response to curare and other non-depolarising drugs is not necessarily altered. It is wise, if curare is to be used, to give a test dose of 5 mg and observe the effect before giving larger doses. Potassium deficiency is more likely to produce muscular weakness in acidotic patients, probably because the potassium ion and the hydrogen ion have opposite effects on neuromuscular conduction (Black and Milne, 1952).

Loss of potassium at a K : N ratio greater than 2·5 is an invariable response to water depletion and is essential if the cells are to give up their water (Elkinton and Winkler, 1944). Whenever potassium leaves the cells, it is partially replaced by sodium and hydrogen ions: this results in a fall in extracellular hydrogen ion concentration (rise in pH) which is reflected by a rise in bicarbonate concentration. If the bicarbonate is found to be raised in a surgical patient, potassium deficiency is the most likely cause.

Daily requirements.—If parenteral fluids are required for more than 48 hours after operation, potassium should be given. Ampoules containing 1 gram of potassium chloride* (13·4 mEq or mmol potassium) can be added to each half-litre bottle. Four grams daily (approximately 50 mEq or mmol) of potassium chloride is adequate to prevent progressive potassium loss and 8 grams for the treatment of established depletion.

The correction of large sodium deficits is urgent and the total amount given is aimed to restore a large part of the presumed deficit: this does not apply to potassium deficits and quantitative replacement is achieved slowly.

Potassium Toxicity

The dangers of rapid infusion of potassium salts are real and levels above 7 mEq/l (mmol/l) in the plasma are dangerous. Hypoxia and an increase in the hydrogen ion concentration (fall in pH) from whatever cause will result in potassium leaving the cells and in such circumstances potassium should not be given. Anaesthetists should beware of patients sent for surgery with infusions running: these often contain added potassium chloride and if the infusion line is used for induction there is a risk that fluid will be run in fast at the time suxamethonium is given. As a general rule potassium, in high concentrations, should never be infused during induction of anaesthesia.

Whenever potassium salts are added to plastic packs of fluids they must be thoroughly mixed. They should never be injected into the spare port of an inverted pack; if they are and the pack is left inverted the undiluted salt will pool at the bottom and enter the delivery tubing.

The accepted criteria for safety in general work are:
1. No potassium on the day of operation.
2. A urine volume of at least 500 ml in the previous 24 hours.
3. Infusion fluids should never contain more than 1·5 grams of potassium chloride per half litre pack (i.e. 40 mEq (mmol) potassium per litre).
4. Not more than 15 mEq (mmol) should be given in an hour.

These figures are well within the limits of safety and dangerous levels of plasma potassium concentration will not occur if renal and adrenal function is normal. The electrocardiograph provides the most informative evidence of potassium toxicity, the earliest changes being high, peaked T waves, followed by disappearance of P waves and widening of the QRS complex. The changes are not solely dependent upon the plasma potassium concentration and high concentrations of sodium and ionised calcium may result in a normal ECG when the plasma potassium concentration is high.

If the plasma concentration is found to be above 7 mEq/l (mmol/l) the immediate treatment is to give 10 ml of 10 per cent calcium gluconate slowly intravenously, followed by 25 grams of glucose and 15 units of soluble insulin. An infusion of 50 ml of molar (8·4 per cent) sodium bicarbonate should then be given at 1 ml per minute.

MAGNESIUM

Magnesium occurs in concentrations of 20 mg/100 ml (8·2 mmol/l) of cell

* Note that 1 g of KCl contains approximately 0·5 g of potassium.

water and the plasma range is 1·5–2·5 mg/100 ml (0·6–1·0 mmol/l). A normal diet contains 120–240 mg (5–10 mmol) a day and renal conservation is so efficient that balance can be maintained on 12 mg (0·5 mmol) per day. The excess is excreted in the urine.

The skeleton provides a large store of magnesium and even several weeks of parenteral fluid therapy with magnesium-free fluids may not cause plasma magnesium to fall significantly. Magnesium given intravenously causes vasodilatation and central nervous depression associated with some degree of myoneural block. This block is due to magnesium preventing the release of acetyl choline at the myoneural junction.

This property and the associated effect on the central nervous system led Peck and Meltzer (1916) to use intravenous magnesium sulphate to produce general anaesthesia. One of their cases received over 2·4 g (100 mmol) of magnesium in fifty minutes and this produced respiratory arrest which was treated by pharyngeal insufflation of oxygen with recovery. It is apparent that the heart must be very tolerant to great increases in plasma magnesium concentration and the small rises known to occur in hypothermia are unlikely to have any significance.

The only likely cause of significant magnesium depletion is surgical removal of most of the small intestine. Occasional cases are recorded in which hypotonia, tetany and fibrillary muscle twitching have responded to intramuscular magnesium sulphate. The surgical implications of magnesium balance have been well reviewed by Barnes (1962).

FLUID THERAPY IN INFANTS AND SMALL CHILDREN

The management of fluid and electrolyte balance in infants is very much more critical than it is in adults. Requirements vary with age and the permissible margins of error are narrow. Many of the fluid schedules prescribed for surgical causes of body fluid depletion are identical to those which are appropriate in the management of acute gastro-enteritis. This has resulted in over-generous amounts of water being given which are particularly undesirable in surgical cases. Infants with intestinal obstruction are not usually febrile and surgery corrects their lesions and induces post-operative release of antidiuretic hormone. In these circumstances too much water readily provokes water intoxication.

Infants, particularly in the first few months of life, have a greatly increased rate of turnover of water. Their body water content is greater than an adult's when related to body weight, but it is about half the adult figure if related to surface area: as surface area is more closely related to insensible loss, an infant loses water twice as fast relatively as an adult when intake ceases.

Maintenance Requirements—Infants and Children

After the first week of life and until a child weighs 25 kg (56 lb) maintenance requirements are adequately covered by doubling the adult intake expressed as a function of body weight. The daily adult intake of approximately 30 ml and 1 mEq (mmol) each of sodium and potassium per kg of body weight is therefore increased to approximately 70 ml per kg together with 2 mEq (mmol) per kg of sodium and potassium. It will be found that if the fluid is given as one-fifth normal saline in dextrose (i.e. $\frac{1}{5}$ of 0·18 per cent NaCl in 5·0 per cent dextrose) and if one gram of potassium chloride (13·4 mmol) is added to each 500 ml of fluid given, the amounts of sodium and potassium will be correct (Atwell, 1971).

Example.—A baby weighing 3 kg would receive 210 ml water: 6·2 mEq (mmol) sodium: 5·7 mEq (mmol) potassium.

This schedule can be given from the day of operation onwards, except that the potassium is omitted for 48 hours after surgery. It is easy to remember and does away with the need to refer to charts most of which are designed for medical management and necessitate various corrections to be applied to infants undergoing surgery. The only exception to the general application of this regime applies during the first week of life when the intake of fluid and electrolytes is reduced by being multiplied by

$$\frac{\text{Age in days}}{7}$$

For babies 24–48 hrs old this will result in a daily fluid intake of 50 ml or even less and it is all too easy to give far too much if explicit instructions as to rate and volume are not written down. Whenever fluids are given to babies the giving set should always incorporate a small volume-graduated burette so that large volumes of fluid cannot accidentally be infused.

Assessment of Magnitude of Body Fluid Depletion

Body fluids lost or sequestered by babies and small children all contain sodium in approximately isotonic concentration just as they do in adults. An unfortunate belief has come to be accepted that sodium should never be given to babies in a greater concentration than 30 mEq/l (mmol/l) (fifth isotonic).

In a review of the causes of death in children with appendicitis Pledger and Buchan (1969) considered that inadequate or inappropriate fluid therapy to be the commonest single cause of death. The mortality in children under 5 was eight times that of older children and this is undoubtedly related to the reluctance to treat such small children boldly. No child with peritonitis should be considered too ill for operation without an attempt being made to replenish its plasma and extracellular fluid volume.

The approximate volume of the deficit can be obtained from Table 2.

19/TABLE 2

BODY FLUIDS LOST EXPRESSED AS PERCENTAGE OF BODY WEIGHT

Age	Mild	Moderate	Severe
0–6 months	5	10	15
6 months–6 years	5	7·5	10
Older children (as for adults)	4	6	8

Note. Weight taken is observed weight. Assessment of degree depends on state of circulation. Mild implies good cardiovascular function, moderate—early, and severe—gross disturbance of circulation. (Finberg, 1967.)

Replacement

The fluid first given should contain sodium in isotonic concentration and 40 ml/kg is given in the first 40–60 minutes (Finberg, 1967). Very ill children can with advantage receive half their initial replacement (20 ml/kg) as plasma or dextran 70 in saline and the rest as either normal saline, Ringer lactate or sixth molar sodium lactate. Further replacement depends on cardiovascular signs: generally the rate may be reduced to replace the rest of the calculated deficit in 4–6 hrs and the sodium concentration reduced to 30–75 mEq/1 (mmol/l) (fifth or half isotonic saline).

Hypernatraemic Dehydration

Raised serum sodium concentrations are comparatively common in babies: they are usually the result of loss of both water and sodium, the water loss being proportionately the greater. Cardiovascular function is not usually severely affected and it is extremely important to correct this disorder very slowly with fluids containing sodium in concentrations of 50–75 mEq/1 (mmol/l) (one third to half isotonic saline). If 5 per cent dextrose alone is given convulsions due to water intoxication are readily provoked (Hughes-Davies, 1967).

Metabolic Acidosis

Normal nutrition in a healthy infant ensures that a large proportion of its food is incorporated into its growing tissues and Slater (1961) has shown that up to 50 per cent of the food protein may be used for growth and therefore impose no demand on the kidneys for excretion. This buffer provided by anabolism no longer operates and is invariably superseded by tissue catabolism in any infant requiring surgery: if extracellular fluid is lost as well, there will be a rapid development of metabolic acidosis. There is convincing evidence that correction of this with sodium lactate (which is converted into bicarbonate) or with bicarbonate itself greatly reduces the mortality (Illingworth, 1963). With the important exception of pyloric stenosis, any severely ill infant can be expected to be acidotic and should receive 1 to 2 mEq (mmol) of sodium bicarbonate per kg body weight added to the fluid given in the first hour.

PARENTERAL FEEDING

Standard regimes of parenteral fluids only provide about one fifth of a resting patient's total calories—the remainder being supplied by catabolism of tissue proteins and fat. The hundred grams of dextrose provided in the daily intake are however extremely important in reducing to a minimum the breakdown of tissue proteins to provide energy. This is often forgotten when blood has to be given, or when saline is given to replace extrarenal losses. If more than half a litre of saline is given it should be given as 0·9 per cent saline in 5 per cent dextrose, and Ringer lactate similarly should be dissolved in 5 per cent dextrose. Care must be taken to impress on the nursing staff the difference between 5 per cent dextrose in water and the same solution in saline.

If parenteral fluids are to be continued for more than five days the calorie deficit must not be allowed to progress. In the presence of severe sepsis and its associated hypercatabolic state the provision of at least 2,000 calories (8·4 MJ) a day should be aimed at within two days of surgery. Modern management of parenteral feeding involves the use of fat emulsions and amino acid preparations both of which are very expensive.

Fat Emulsions

Fat emulsions represent the most suitable source of calories as the fat is rapidly metabolised and has no osmotic activity—isotonicity is due to glycerol or sorbitol. They promote protein anabolism and do not cause thrombophlebitis (Reid and Ingram, 1967). Soya bean emulsions (Intralipid) are now preferred to emulsions of Cottonseed Oil as they can safely be given at rates of 3 g/kg/day for long periods (Lawson, 1967). Immediate reactions include nausea, headache, fever and palpitations and can be minimised by beginning the infusion very slowly. These so-called "colloid" reactions occur in about 10 per cent of patients (Hadfield, 1965). Some authorities recommend the addition of heparin to accelerate the rate of uptake of the fat but this is unnecessary (Johnston, 1969, personal communication). No drugs, vitamins or other substances should be added to the fat emulsions and the giving sets should be changed after each bottle has been run in.

Amino Acid Solutions

There are two types of amino acid solutions, those formed by enzymatic hydrolysis of casein such as Aminosol, and solutions of crystalline amino acids such as Trophysan. Both cause a high incidence of thrombophlebitis and have similar effects on nitrogen balance. The synthetic amino acids in Trophysan are a mixture of D and DL forms, whereas naturally occurring amino acids are all in the L forms. Present evidence suggests that the ideal parenteral solutions of amino acids would be one which contained synthetic amino acids in the L forms.

The solutions available are usually given with both sugar and alcohol to increase their calorie content. Fructose has some advantages over dextrose and is the hexose sugar used in Aminosol.

Administration.—There are many schemes which do not differ in essentials and the following is based on that of Peaston (1968). Half-litre bottles are given in the following sequence:

	Calories	Na	K	N
1. 20 per cent Intralipid	1,000	Nil	Nil	Nil
2. Aminosol/fructose/alcohol—1½ g KCl	435	27	20	2·1 g
3. Aminosol/fructose/alcohol—1½ g KCl	435	27	20	2·1 g
4. Either 10 per cent Aminosol or	160	80	Nil	6·4 g
5 per cent Dextrose	100	Nil	Nil	Nil
5. 20 per cent Intralipid	1,000	Nil	Nil	Nil
6. Aminosol/fructose/alcohol—1½ g KCl	435	27	20	2·1 g

N.B. 6 g Protein ≃ 2 g Urea ≃ 1 g Nitrogen.

This provides approximately 3,500 calories (14·6 MJ) and either 6·5 or 13 grams of nitrogen a day, depending on the substitution of 5 per cent dextrose for 10 per cent Aminosol. Patients with raised extrarenal losses of water are best managed with 5 per cent dextrose as the 10 per cent Aminosol represents a considerable solute load. Vitamins must be added and often repeated blood transfusions are required as haemoglobin levels invariably tend to fall.

TOTAL PARENTERAL NUTRITION

Schedules for total parenteral nutrition

Choosing a suitable mixture of nutrients depends on measuring or assessing the patient's body weight and estimating his requirement for calories. There are then essentially two decisions:

1. The choice of a nitrogen-containing preparation (Table 3).
2. The choice of the major energy-providing preparation (Table 4).

19/TABLE 3
EXAMPLES OF NITROGEN-CONTAINING PREPARATIONS

Preparation	Constituents	pH	N(g)	Cal (MJ)	Na mmol	K mmol	PO₄ mmol
Aminosol 10%	Casein hydrolysate	5·0	12·8	330 (1·4)	160	0·15	0·56
Aminosol/ fructose/ethanol	Casein hydrolysate	5·0		880 (3·7)	54	0·15	—
Trophysan 10% L	L-amino acids	6·4	6·68	573 (2·4)	6	8	—
Trophysan-L Conc.	L-amino acids	6·4	13·1	732 (3·1)	10	8	—
Vamin	L-amino acids + fructose 10%	5·2	9·4	650 (2·7)	50	20	—
Aminoplex 14	L-amino acids	7·5	13·4	340 (1·4)	35	30	—
Aminoplex 5	L-amino acids + sorbitol 10% ethanol 5%	7·5	5	1000 (4·2)	35	15	—

The column header "Contents per litre" spans the Na, K, and PO₄ columns.

Note variable sodium content: all these solutions are hypertonic and irritant to veins.

PARENTERAL NUTRITION

"In severely starved patients, if one looks to the heart, the kidneys, the liver, the readily discernible primary causes of death are not found . . . instead, in searching for the cause of death in destructive cell disease, one looks to the lungs and here finds the final mechanism of death in patients dying with rapid erosion of the body cell mass"—Moore (1962).

No field of surgical study is more active than the metabolic needs of the starving traumatised patient. For comprehensive accounts of total parenteral nutrition (TPN) the books edited by Lee (1974) and Ghadimi (1975) should be consulted. The following account attempts to relate current knowledge to its application in adults. Whenever the term "calorie" is used the kilocalorie (1 kilocalorie = 4·18 kJ) is implied.

19/TABLE 4
EXAMPLES OF ENERGY-PROVIDING PREPARATIONS

	pH	Cal/l (MJ/l)	mosmol/l
Glucose 5%	5–6	205 (0·9)	278
Glucose 50%	5–6	2000 (8·4)	3800
Intralipid 10%	7·5	1100 (4·6)	280
Intralipid 20%	7·5	2000 (8·4)	330
Aminosol/fructose ethanol	5·0	880 (3·7)	1043

(With acknowledgement to Dr. G. J. Dobb)

General Considerations

When food intake ceases, death will occur in a previously normal adult in from two to three months. Patients requiring TPN will often only survive for as many weeks due to a variety of other handicaps which beset them. It is the purpose of TPN to avert the ventilatory failure so well described by Francis Moore by preserving the proteins of the muscles.

Carbohydrate is normally the preferred energy source of the body: it is, as it were, the current account as opposed to the deposit accounts of expendable protein and fat. The metabolic response to trauma has numerous effects on the endocrine and enzyme systems which determine energy release from these body stores. As a generalisation, there is a relative intolerance of the tissue cells to glucose utilisation and enhanced breakdown and use of fat. Protein is now known to contribute only from 10 to 20 per cent of the energy requirements of surgical patients even if they are in strongly negative nitrogen balance (Kinney et al., 1970). Up to 80 per cent of the energy needs are provided by fat but certain tissues such as brain, erythrocytes, bone marrow and renal medulla normally metabolise glucose. The brain consumes more than half of the minimum daily requirement of carbohydrate, i.e. about 120 grams of glucose a day. If no carbohydrate is given the amino acids of cell proteins are mobilised and deaminated in the liver to form glucose. This gluconeogenesis from body protein is an inefficient and erosive process as it takes one kilogram of lean tissue to provide one hundred grams of glucose (Bessman, 1975). It used to be thought that muscle cells were destroyed when intracellular proteins were mobilised for the provision of energy but it is now thought that the cells simply shrink; the loss of one kilogram of lean tissue involves the movement of 750 ml of intracellular water into the extracellular fluid.

When fat provides the major contribution to energy requirements plasma ketone concentrations rise progressively to as much as ten times their normal levels. Hoover et al. (1975) found this ketonaemia to have no effect on plasma pH and in this context it should no longer be regarded as being undesirable. The brain is capable of switching from glucose to ketones as its main source of fuel thus sparing protein; other tissues such as the heart and muscles normally do so.

Fat people are often thought to have ample reserves and therefore to be in less need of TPN. In fact an average adult has the same reserves of carbohydrate, a little less protein and one-fifth the fat of an obese person twice as heavy. Because fat cannot be converted into carbohydrate, protein for gluconeogenesis determines survival and it is therefore the key fuel in prolonged starvation. Fat patients have no advantage over their slimmer brethren when they are starved.

As soon as a decision is taken to provide more than 2000 calories (8·4 MJ) a day one is faced with an alternative. One course is to provide fat in sufficient amounts to cover 75 to 80 per cent of requirements, protein to produce about 15 per cent and carbohydrate the remainder. If this is chosen it is possible to avoid hypertonic glucose and to make use of peripheral veins. The alternative is to infuse 50 per cent glucose as the main energy source and this requires the use of a central vein. Both methods have been used successfully and their relative merits are discussed under the appropriate headings.

Carbohydrate

Apart from the glucose circulating in the plasma, the only stores of carbohydrate exist as glycogen in liver and muscle. If liver glycogen stores are depleted, which happens within 12 to 18 hours of starvation, it is known that hepatocellular function is impaired. Although surgical stress interferes with glucose utilisation, the administration of some glucose on the day of operation is probably beneficial. One to one and a half grams (5·6–8·3 mmol) per kilogram of body weight is sufficient.

One to one and a half litres of fifty per cent glucose per day will provide most of the calories needed in TPN. It must be remembered that several insulin antagonists are activated by the metabolic response to trauma and of these adrenaline, glucagon, growth hormone and glucocorticosteroids are thought to be responsible. The method therefore requires the simultaneous administration of soluble insulin and frequent estimations of plasma and urinary glucose; the aim is to keep the plasma glucose below 180 mg per cent (10 mmol/l) and urinary glucose below $\frac{1}{4}$ per cent. Allison (1974) recommends the addition of 120 units of insulin and 40 mEq (mmol) of potassium chloride to each litre of 50 per cent glucose. The method is unsuitable for occasional use in general wards and should be confined to intensive care areas with adequate supervision and laboratory support. In the present state of knowledge it is the best management known for states of high catabolism due to trauma and infection, e.g. burns.

Protein

Proteins are the most complex of the three energy-producing stores. Unlike carbohydrate and fat they have essential non-nutritional functions and survival is not possible once fifty per cent of the muscle proteins have been used for gluconeogenesis. The optimum protein intake for man is still a matter of controversy (Scrimshaw, 1976; *Lancet*, 1973) and the present view is that a healthy adult requires about 50 grams a day of mixed protein if sufficient calories are provided by non-protein sources to satisfy 80 per cent of total energy requirements (Waterlow and Harper, 1975).

The daily turnover of protein is considerably greater than the daily requirement so the breakdown and re-synthesis of tissue proteins must be the result of extensive re-utilisation of amino acids. The well-recognised negative nitrogen balance and weight loss following trauma have long been assumed to indicate that there is increased breakdown of tissue proteins which form a major source of energy. Recent work has shown that neither of these beliefs is now tenable. O'Keafe and his colleagues (1974) at Cambridge have shown that the normal response to trauma is a decrease in tissue cell protein breakdown; the increased loss of nitrogen is therefore a result of failure to re-synthesise the amino acids at the normal rate.

Kinney's work (1970) established that protein only contributes about 15 per cent of the energy requirements even in the post-operative period when there is a strongly negative nitrogen balance. The reason for this apparently inconsistent finding is that tissue proteins are in solution in intracellular fluid and are probably the principal determinant of cell water (Ling and Walton, 1976). Each part by weight of protein is associated with three parts by weight of water, so when the protein is degraded the energy output per gram of tissue is only one calorie and not the four calories per gram of dry protein.

Another recent development has been the demonstration that infusion of isotonic (3 per cent) solutions of synthetic L-amino acids during and after surgery will result in re-synthesis of degraded tissue proteins and a positive nitrogen balance. Plasma levels of glucose and insulin are lower and there is enhanced utilisation of triglycerides derived from fat (Blackburn et al., 1973). This work has been confirmed by Hoover and his colleagues (1975) and it seems that in future TPN will incline to the use of amino acids and fat emulsions rather than glucose and insulin.

There is no general agreement about the best preparation of nitrogen-containing solution. The choice lies between the very costly synthetic L-amino acids which vary in the electrolyte and carbohydrate additions made to them and casein hydrolysates prepared by enzymatic hydrolysis. In spite of theoretical disadvantages of the hydrolysates they have been found to be just as effective for general use, but their high sodium content may make them unsuitable in some cases. Both are very hypertonic and tend to cause venous thrombosis in peripheral veins as a result. Whether fat or hypertonic glucose is used as the main source of calories, nitrogen must always be given and the aim should be to provide 0·2 gram of nitrogen per kilogram of body weight per day and 200 calories per day from non-nitrogenous sources for each gram of nitrogen infused.

Fat

The adipose tissues form by far the most efficient energy store on a weight basis because fat is not associated with water in the cells, so that each gram yields its full nine calories of energy when it is metabolised. Cellular fat is broken down by the enzyme triglyceride lipase and triglycerides and free fatty acids are released into the plasma. This process is accelerated by adrenaline and glucagon and strongly inhibited by insulin.

Fatty acids are oxidised directly in the tissues to provide energy. In the liver they provide the energy required by the so-called Cori cycle. Tissues such as red and white blood cells, bone marrow and renal medulla are glycolytic, i.e. they depend upon glucose which they metabolise anaerobically to lactate and pyruvate and they account for about 20 per cent of obligatory glucose utilisation. These metabolites are re-converted into glucose in the liver, making use of energy derived from fatty acids. In this way fat reduces the need for gluco-neogenesis and thus conserves tissue protein.

Preparations of fat for intravenous use are based on fractionated soya-bean oil emulsified by egg lecithin. Such emulsions have no osmotic activity and are made isotonic by the addition of 2·5 per cent glycerol which is itself metabolised: fat is therefore the only high-calorie source which can be given isotonically and it does not cause venous thrombosis (Reid and Ingram, 1967). Ten and twenty per cent emulsions are available and up to 3 grams per kilogram of body weight can be given daily. There are few disadvantages apart from rare allergy, e.g. patients with an atopy related to eggs, and a tendency to reduce adhesiveness of platelets. A new giving-set must be used for each unit of fat and changed before any other fluid is given. No drugs should ever be added to emulsions of fat, and blood for laboratory tests should be drawn at least six hours after the previous fat infusion ended; this may necessitate reducing the daily fat intake to 2 grams per kilogram.

Ethanol (Alcohol)

Ethanol can be a useful energy supplement giving 7·1 cal/g (5·6 cal/ml; 1·36 MJ/mole). It mixes well with sugars and amino acids, its metabolism being en-hanced when given at the same time as fructose or sorbitol. Coats (1972) recom-mends an upper limit of 4 per cent ethanol, though concentrations greater than 3 per cent are irritant to peripheral veins. Ethanol is rapidly metabolised by fast-ing man, its handling resembling acetate and being independent of insulin. Values for its rate of metabolism vary from 9·1 to 14 ml/hour. At an infusion rate of 1·5 g/kg/day the blood alcohol will not rise above 30 mg per cent or 6 mmol/litre (Coats, 1972) and only trivial amounts will be lost by excretion through the lungs or in urine. This will provide about one-quarter of the total energy requirements. Provided this rate of infusion is not exceeded, there are few contra-indications to the use of ethanol, although it may be better to avoid it when there is impairment of liver function (Lieber, 1966). Excessive rates of infusion may cause signs of alcohol intoxication with palpitations, excitation, torpor or nausea.

Sodium and Potassium

One millimole of sodium and potassium per kilogram of body weight is a reasonable daily intake except for those patients whose disease requires restriction of sodium intake. The contents of these elements vary considerably in the various nitrogen-containing preparations and this must be known and allowed for. Large doses of some antibiotics also must have their sodium or potassium contents included in the reckoning.

Phosphorus

Levels of plasma inorganic phosphate fall rapidly in starvation or if an insulin and carbohydrate regime is used. Sheldon and Grzyb (1975) have shown that levels of red cell 2–3 diphosphoglycerate, plasma ATP and the P50* of red cells all fall as the plasma phosphate concentration drops. If fat emulsions are

* P50—refers to the Po_2 at which the haemoglobin is 50 per cent saturated with oxygen.

not being given 20 to 25 mmol a day of potassium dihydrogen phosphate should be given from the start of parenteral feeding.

Vitamins

There is no need to add vitamins for the first week of TPN. After this the water-soluble vitamins (B and C) should be given. If TPN continues for more than two weeks the fat-soluble vitamins must also be added.

Calcium, Magnesium and Trace Elements

If TPN has to be continued for more than a month it is necessary to ensure that calcium, magnesium and trace elements are included. This is comprehensively reviewed by Wretlind (1974).

Indications for Total Parenteral Nutrition

If intravenous fluids are necessary beyond the third post-operative day one should plan to provide a gradually increasing calorie intake so that full estimated calorie needs are being given by the sixth day. Patients suffering from extensive trauma or sepsis should be given TPN from the day of surgery.

Anaemia and Colloid Oncotic Pressure

Prolonged TPN is usually associated with anaemia and requires transfusion of red cells or whole blood. Plasma albumin levels seldom fall but the administration of 500 ml of plasma protein fraction every third day is indicated in a patient suffering from states in which there is a loss of albumin, e.g. ulcerative colitis.

Precautions When Starting TPN

The casual attitude to aseptic technique which is almost universal in routine intravenous therapy has no place in TPN. When long catheters are inserted into central veins, scrupulous aseptic technique must be observed: the operator should wear gloves and have an assistant, the entry site should be effectively cleaned and the area properly draped. Giving-sets should always be changed as soon as blood or fat emulsions have gone in and at least daily in any case. The line should be broken only with the gloved hands and three-way taps should have their unused ports blocked with sterile bungs and they should only be manipulated with gloved hands. The practice of using CVP lines for both pressure measurement and TPN should be avoided if at all possible. Femoral vein lines should never be used as long as there is any possibility of access to the arm and neck veins.

Peripheral veins can be used if a deliberate policy of changing the site of administration daily is adopted and in some patients it may be possible to avoid the use of central veins altogether.

REFERENCES

ALLISON, S. P. (1974). In: *Parenteral Nutrition in Acute Metabolic Illness*, p. 293. Ed. Lee, H. A. London: Academic Press.

ARIEL, I. M., KREMEN, A. J., and WANGENSTEEN, O. H. (1950). An expanded interstitial (thiocyanate) space in surgical patients. *Surgery*, **27**, 827.

ATWELL, J. D. (1971). Personal communication.

BARNES, B. A. (1962). Current concepts relating magnesium and surgical disease. *Amer. J. Surg.*, **103**, 309.

BESSMAN, S. P. (1975). In: *Total Parenteral Nutrition*, p. 340. Ed. Ghadimi, H. New York: John Wiley.

BLACK, D. A. K., DAVIES, H. E. F., and EMERY, E. W. (1955). The disposal of radioactive potassium injected intravenously. *Lancet*, **1**, 1097.

BLACK, D. A. K., and MILNE, M. D. (1952). Experimental potassium depletion in man. *Clin. Sci.*, **11**, 397.

BLACKBURN, G. L., FLATT, J. P., CLOWES, G. H. A., and O'DONNELL, T. E. (1973). Peripheral intravenous feeding with isotonic amino acid solutions. *Amer. J. Surg.*, **125**, 447.

COATS, D. A. (1972). In: *Parenteral Nutrition*, p. 152 (Proc. Internat. Symposium in London, April 1971). Ed. W. A. Wilkinson. Edinburgh: Churchill Livingstone.

COLLER, F. A., and MADDOCK, W. G. (1933). Water requirements of surgical patients. *Ann. Surg.*, **98**, 952.

COLLER, F. A., and MADDOCK, W. G. (1940). Water and electrolyte balance. *Surg. Gynec. Obstet.*, **70**, 340.

COOPER, D. R., IOB, V., and COLLER, F. A. (1949). Response to parenteral glucose of normal kidneys and kidneys of post-operative patients. *Ann. Surg.*, **129**, 1.

DANOWSKI, T. S. (1951). Newer concepts of the role of sodium in disease. *Amer. J. Med.*, **10**, 468.

DARROW, D. C. (1950). The role of potassium in clinical disturbances of body water and electrolytes. *New Engl. J. Med.*, **242**, 978.

DUDLEY, H. A. F. (1968). Personal communication.

EDELMAN, I. S., and LEIBMAN, J. (1959). The anatomy of body water and electrolytes. *Amer. J. Med.*, **27**, 256.

ELKINTON, J. R., and WINKLER, A. W. (1944). Transfers of intracellular potassium in experimental dehydration. *J. clin. Invest.*, **23**, 93.

FIEBER, W. W., and JONES, J. R. (1966). Intraoperative fluid therapy with 5 per cent dextrose in lactated Ringer's solution. *Anesth. Analg. Curr. Res.*, **45**, 366.

FINBERG, L. (1967). Dehydration in infants and children. *New Engl. J. Med.*, **276**, 458.

GAMBLE, J. L. (1958). *Chemical Anatomy, Physiology and Pathology of Extracellular Fluid* (A Lecture Syllabus), 6th edit. Cambridge, Mass.: Harvard Univ. Press.

HARDY, J. D. (1954). *Fluid Therapy*. Philadelphia: Lea and Febiger.

HAYES, M. A. (1968). Water and electrolyte therapy after operation. *New Engl. J. Med.*, **278**, 1054.

HOOVER, H. C., GRANT, J. P., GORSCHBOTH, C., and KETCHAM, A. S. (1975). Nitrogen-sparing intravenous fluids in post-operative patients, *New Engl. J. Med.*, **293**, 172.

HUGHES-DAVIES, T. H. (1967). Hypernatraemic dehydration. *Brit. med. J.*, **2**, 737.

HUTCHIN, P., TERZI, R. G., and HOLLANDSWORTH, L. C. (1969). The influence of intravenous fluid administration on post-operative urine water and electrolyte excretion in thoracic surgical patients. *Ann. Surg.*, **170**, 813.

ILLINGWORTH, C. (1963). Bedside biochemistry in surgical care. *Lancet*, **1**, 1275.

IRVIN, T. T., MODGILL, V. K., and HAYTER, C. J. (1972). Plasma volume deficits and salt and water excretion after surgery, *Lancet*, **2**, 1159.

JONES, C. M., and EATON, F. B. (1933). Post-operative nutritional edema. *Arch. Surg.*, **27**, 159.

KINNEY, J. M., LONG, C. L., DUKE, J. H. (1970). In: *Body Fluid Replacement in the Surgical Patient*, p. 298. Ed: C. L. Fox and G. G. Nahas. New York: Grune and Stratton.

Lancet (1973). Leading article: Human energy and protein requirements, **2**, 363.

LAWSON, L. J. (1967). Parenteral nutrition in surgery. *Hosp. Med.*, **1**, 899.

LIEBER, C. S. (1966). Hepatic and metabolic effects of alcohol. *Gastroenterology*, **50**, 119.

LING, G. N., and WALTON, C. L. (1976). What retains water in living cells? *Science*, **191**, 293.

LOEB, J. N. (1974). The hyperosmolar state. *New Engl. J. Med.*, **290**, 1184.

MACKENZIE, A. I., and DONALD, J. R. (1969). Urine output and fluid therapy during anaesthesia and surgery. *Brit. med. J.*, **3**, 619.

MANNERS, J. M. (1974). Nutrition after cardiac surgery. *Anaesthesia*, **29**, 675.

MOORE, F. D. (1960). *Metabolic Care of the Surgical Patient*. Philadelphia: W. B. Saunders Co.

MOORE, F. D. (1962). Volume and tonicity in body fluids. *Surg. Gynec. Obstet.*, **114**, 276.

MOORE, F. D., and BALL, M. R. (1955). In: *The Metabolic Response to Surgery*. Springfield, Ill. Charles C. Thomas.

MOORE, F. D., HALEY, H. B., BERING, E. A., BROOKS, L., and EDELMAN, I. S. (1952). Further observations on total body water. *Surg. Gynec. Obstet.*, **95**, 181.

MOORE, F. D., and SHIRES, G. T. (1967). Editorial: Moderation. *Ann. Surg.*, **166**, 300.

MORAN, W. H., and ZIMMERMANN, B. (1967). Mechanisms of antidiuretic hormone control of importance to the surgical patient. *Surgery*, **62**, 639.

O'KEAFE, S. J. D., SENDER, P. M., and JAMES, W. P. T. (1974). "Catabolic" loss of body nitrogen in response to surgery. *Lancet*, **2**, 1035.

OOMEN, H. A. P. C. (1961). The nutrition situation in Western New Guinea. *Trop. geogr. Med.*, **13**, 321.

PEASTON, M. J. T. (1968). Parenteral nutrition in serious illness. *Hosp. Med.*, **2**, 707.

PECK, C. H., and MELTZER, S. J. (1916). Anesthesia in human beings by intravenous injections of magnesium sulphate. *J. Amer. med. Ass.*, **67**, 1131.

PLEDGER, H. G., and BUCHAN, R. (1969). Deaths in children with acute appendicitis. *Brit. med. J.*, **2**, 466.

REID, D. J., and INGRAM, G. I. C. (1967). Changes in blood coagulation during infusion of intralipid. *Clin. Sci.*, **33**, 399.

ROTH, E., LAX, L. C., and MALONEY, J. V. (1969). Ringer's lactate solution and extracellular fluid volume in the surgical patient: a critical analysis. *Ann. Surg.*, **169**, 149.

SCHMIDT-NIELSEN, K. (1964). *Desert Animals*. Oxford: Clarendon Press.

SCRIMSHAW, N. S. (1976). An analysis of past and present dietary allowances for protein in health and disease. *New Engl. J. Med.*, **294**, 198.

SHELDON, G. F., and GRZYB, S. (1975). Phosphate depletion and repletion, *Ann. Surg.*, **182**, 683.

SHIRES, T. J., WILLIAMS, J., and BROWN, F. (1961). Acute changes in extracellular fluids associated with major surgical procedures. *Ann. Surg.*, **154**, 803.

SINGH, C. M., and FLEAR, C. T. G. (1968). Why does serum sodium concentration fall postoperatively? *Brit. J. Surg.*, **55**, 858.

SLATER, J. E. (1961). Retention of nitrogen and minerals by babies 1 week old. *Brit. J. Nutr.*, **15**, 183.

STAHL, W. M. (1970). Prophylactic diuresis with ethacrynic acid for prevention of post-operative renal failure. *Ann. Surg.*, **172**, 361.

STEWART, J. D., and ROURKE, G. M. (1942). The effect of large intravenous infusions on the body fluid. *J. clin. Invest.*, **21**, 197.

UKAI, M., MORAN, W. H., and ZIMMERMANN, B. (1968). Role of visceral afferent pathways on vasopressin secretion and urinary secretory patterns during surgical stress. *Ann. Surg.*, **168**, 16.

WATERLOW, J. C., and HARPER, A. E. (1975). In: *Total Parenteral Nutrition*, p. 231. Ed: H. Ghadimi. New York: John Wiley.

WHITE, A. (1961). Intestinal obstruction in the Rhodesian African. *E. Afr. med. J.*, **38**, 525.

WRETLIND, A. (1974). In: *Parenteral Nutrition in Acute Metabolic Illness*. Ed: H. A. Lee. London: Academic Press.

ZIMMERMANN, B. (1965). Pituitary and adrenal function in relation to surgery. *Surg. Clin. N. Amer.*, **45**, 299.

ZIMMERMANN, B., and WANGENSTEEN, O. H. (1952). Observations on water intoxication in surgical patients. *Surgery*, **31**, 654.

FURTHER READING

Total Parenteral Nutrition. Editor Ghadimi, H. John Wiley, New York 1975.
Parenteral Nutrition in Acute Metabolic Illness. Editor Lee, H. A. Academic Press, London 1974.

Chapter 20

BLOOD TRANSFUSION

GENERAL CONSIDERATIONS

RECENT advances in surgery have made the transfusion of very large volumes of blood a relatively commonplace procedure. This has been made possible by a highly efficient transfusion service which, in the United Kingdom, is based on voluntary donations from over a million donors. It is likely that future developments will increase the demand for massive transfusions and that blood will become less readily available as donors become more difficult to recruit. The transfusion centres are reducing wastage by producing separate fractions of blood to meet specific needs such as antihaemophilic globulin (AHG) and platelet concentrates. This is achieved by the use of double plastic bags which make it possible to separate the red cells and plasma and re-constitute the blood after removal of the AHG or platelets. The centres will probably supply packed cells with a storage life of three weeks which is a more rational preparation for many patients who at present receive whole blood. Such economies will need to be matched by a more critical appraisal of the need for blood in operations associated with losses of up to a litre. There is an increasingly strong case to be made for the use of solutions other than blood for patients not known to be anaemic.

It is generally held that before an elective operation such as hysterectomy or prostatectomy a haemoglobin concentration of at least 10 g/100 ml (g/dl) is the minimum acceptable. Sykes (1975) points out that a drop in haemoglobin of 3 g/100 ml (g/dl) causes a 20 per cent fall in oxygen transport. This is the same change as would result from a fall in cardiac output of 1 litre/minute or from a drop of 4 volumes per cent in arterial oxygen content. Nunn and Freeman (1964) have reminded anaesthetists of the importance of thinking of the factors governing the amount of oxygen available to the tissues. These are the cardiac output, the percentage saturation of arterial blood and the oxygen carrying capacity of the blood. No surgeon can guarantee that unexpected haemorrhage will not occur, and no anaesthetist can guarantee that both cardiac output and arterial oxygen saturation will never fall during anaesthesia. It is therefore good practice to ensure that the oxygen carrying capacity of the blood is not unduly low before operation. Quite apart from its predominant role in oxygen carriage, haemoglobin constitutes the most important buffer to pH changes as a result of changes in P_{CO_2}. It should be remembered that up to ten per cent of the haemoglobin of a heavy smoker circulates as carboxyhaemoglobin. It is therefore advisable to stop smoking for 24 hours before operation (Gillies, 1974).

Figures are not available of the mortality attributable to blood transfusion. It is probably at least as great as that associated with anaesthesia for an elective operation of moderate severity and only high standards of serological control in the laboratory have made the use of stored blood as safe as it is now. Although it is in many important respects a very different tissue from circulating fresh blood, by far the commonest cause of this mortality is that a patient receives blood intended for someone else. An anaesthetist working in an unfamiliar hospital should immediately make himself aware of the methods in use for identifying patients and for checking cross-matched blood. A high "index of suspicion" should be cultivated and the patient's names alone should never be accepted as sufficient proof of identity. If a number has not been allocated, the date of birth should be used.

Good admission notes should include a record of previous transfusions and allergies, both of which may be relevant if blood is to be given. If blood is given during an operation it should be recorded in the permanent notes together with the serial numbers of the units actually given.

Pre-operative Anaemia

If anaemia is discovered immediately pre-operatively the operation should be postponed. It is essential to investigate the type of anaemia and not to assume it is due to iron deficiency. If time allows, iron should be given by mouth; intramuscular and intravenous preparations cannot produce a more rapid rise in haemoglobin synthesis and should only be prescribed by physicians if there are specific contra-indications to oral iron. If the operation cannot be postponed, packed cells should be given unless twenty-four hours can elapse between the end of the whole blood transfusion and surgery. The need for sleep on the night before operation should not be forgotten—few patients receiving blood, particularly if this involves splinting of the arm, will sleep well.

THE HAEMOSTATIC MECHANISM

The haemostatic mechanism comprises:
(a) the coagulation system
(b) the coagulation-inhibitory system
(c) the fibrinolytic system.

The Coagulation System

The coagulation factors are proteins found in the plasma in inactive precursor form (Table 1).

A much simplified scheme of the coagulation system is given in Table 2.

Apart from fibrinogen, the clotting factors exist in the plasma as inert pro-enzymes. When a factor is activated it in turn is capable of activating the next pro-enzyme in the chain of factors. Such a mechanism has been termed "an enzyme cascade" and provides a system of multiplication because each molecule of active enzyme at one stage releases many molecules of new enzyme for the pro-enzyme of the next stage. The activation of about 0·2 mg of factor VIII leads to the formation of about 250 mg of fibrin.

During blood coagulation *in vivo* both the intrinsic pathway, which is relatively slow, and the extrinsic pathway, which is faster, are activated. Thrombin formed rapidly by the extrinsic system serves two functions; it hydrolyses fibrinogen but also accelerates the intrinsic pathway by activation of factors VIII and V.

20/TABLE 1

Factor	Synonym
*I	Fibrinogen
T*II	Prothrombin
III	Thromboplastin; tissue extract
IV	Calcium
*V	Accelerator globulin; proaccelerin; labile factor
VI	Number not used
T*VII	Proconvertin; stable factor
VIII	Antihaemophilic factor; antihaemophilic globulin
T*IX	Plasma thromboplastin component (PTC); Christmas factor
T*X	Stuart-Prower factor
XI	Plasma thromboplastin antecedent (PTA)
XII	Hageman factor
*XIII	Fibrin stabilising factor

* synthesised in liver
T synthesis dependent on Vit.K
Factors V and VIII rapidly lose activity when stored as bank blood.

20/TABLE 2

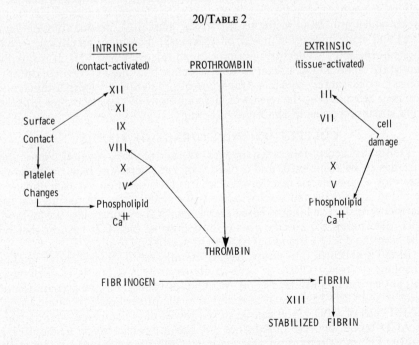

(For explanation see text)

The three tests which are most useful in the diagnosis of coagulation disorders are as follows:

i. *Prothrombin time* is an approximate measure of the extrinsic pathway. It detects deficiencies of factors V, VII, X, prothrombin (II) and fibrinogen (I).

ii. *Activated partial thromboplastin time* is the time taken for plasma which has been incubated with kaolin or some other surface active agent (to activate factors XI and XII)to clot in the presence of platelet lipid substitute and Ca^{++}. It assesses the intrinsic part of the clotting mechanism. An abnormal result is usually due to deficiency of factors VIII or IX.

iii. *Thrombin time* is the time taken for plasma to clot after the addition of thrombin. It is a measure of the formation of fibrin from fibrinogen and is prolonged if there is a deficiency of fibrinogen or if inhibitors such as heparin or fibrin breakdown products are present.

The Coagulation-inhibitory System

There is a system of inhibitors which destroy any activated factor within a few seconds of its appearance. Bleeding tendencies due to an excess of these inhibitors have been described also as having thrombotic states due to inherited deficiency.

The Fibrinolytic System

The function of this system is to digest fibrin. Plasminogen which is a β-globulin synthesised in the liver is converted to plasmin by plasminogen activators, which are found in the tissues (tissue activator), plasma (plasma activator) and urine (urinary activator or urokinase). Plasmin is an enzyme which digests fibrin and also destroys fibrinogen and factors V and VIII. It is rapidly inactivated in the blood stream by antiplasmins, but under certain conditions, such as cardiac surgery with an extracorporeal circulation, a hyperplasminaemic state may be caused by the release of large amounts of tissue activator into the blood stream resulting in abnormal bleeding.

COLLECTION AND STORAGE OF BLOOD

Donors are accepted between the ages of 18 and 65 years. A detailed questionnaire has to be completed, and a history of viral hepatitis, malaria, venereal disease or severe allergic reactions will lead to their rejection. At each donation the blood is grouped and serological tests for syphilis and a screening test for anaemia is done. The latter is based on the Van Slyke copper sulphate method, which determines the specific gravity of a drop of blood. It ensures that on collection the donor's blood has at least 12·5 g/100 ml (g/dl).

Blood is collected into plastic bags containing 65 to 75 ml of either citrate-phosphate-dextrose (CPD) or acid-citrate-dextrose (ACD). It is likely that both anticoagulants will be used as ACD has advantages in the preparation of platelets and CPD has several advantages in the preservation of whole blood. The red cells of CPD blood can be stored for 28 days compared with 21 days for ACD blood, and the blood does not become progressively acidic during storage. The most important advantage of CPD blood concerns the oxygen dissociation of the haemoglobin.

The delivery of oxygen to the tissues is governed by the tissue Po_2 and the ability of oxyhaemoglobin to dissociate from oxygen at that partial pressure. The affinity of oxyhaemoglobin for oxygen is directly related to the concentration of diphosphoglyceric acid (DPG) in the red cells. DPG is normally present in equimolar concentration with haemoglobin with which it combines to form a complex which has low oxygen affinity; thus the ability of blood to release its contained oxygen depends upon the presence of normal levels of DPG.

Stored ACD blood loses 90 per cent of its DPG after two weeks whereas CPD blood still has 80 per cent of its initial DPG preserved. An indication of the DPG level of blood is provided by determining the Po_2 (measured at 37° C, Pco_2 40 mm Hg or 5·3 kPa, pH 7·4) at which the oxyhaemoglobin is half-saturated; this is the P50 of the blood and the normal figure is 27 mm Hg (3·6 kPa). After massive transfusion of ACD blood it may fall to 18 mm Hg (2·4 kPa). The red cell DPG is restored to about 50 per cent of its normal level within 24 hours of transfusion and the significance of the lowered P50 has not been clearly determined (National Research Council Report, 1974).

Immediately after transfusion there is rapid extravascular destruction of the non-viable red cells by the cells of the reticulo-endothelial system. This is complete within a few hours and the remaining cells then behave as they would have done in the donor's circulation and therefore disappear at just under 1 per cent per day. Stored blood is based on the standard that at least 70 per cent of the red cells will remain in the recipient's circulation for more than 24 hours when transfused on the final day of storage.

Changes in Stored Blood

During storage various other changes occur which only become of importance in massive transfusions (*q.v.*) and in rare instances such as liver failure and coagulation disorders. The fall in pH of ACD blood is due to increased concentration of lactate so that after 2 weeks such blood will have a base deficit of 25 to 30 mEq/litre (mmol/l). It is quickly made good after transfusion provided that tissue perfusion and oxygenation are maintained.

Ammonium, free haemoglobin and plasma potassium all increase progressively with storage and in patients in hepatic or renal failure the freshest available blood should be used.

Prolonged Storage of Blood

Red cells mixed with a glycerol-citrate-phosphate solution under certain conditions may be stored at −20° C for several months and still show good post-transfusion survival (Mollison, 1972). Techniques such as these are still in the experimental stage and are not available for routine purposes.

Giving-Sets

Modern giving-sets have relatively small filters with a mesh of 170 μm; all the air should be squeezed out of the filter chamber in order to make use of the entire filtering surface. Giving-sets should always be changed when clear fluids follow blood and at least daily even if no blood is given.

Microfiltration of Blood

When blood is stored its components tend to coalesce to form two types of aggregate. The smaller ones consist of coalesced platelets and form "tight" aggregates of approximately 15 μm diameter. The larger "loose" aggregates range up to 50 μm in diameter and consist of clumps of white cells and platelets. Both types pass through the meshes of ordinary giving-set filters and will inevitably be trapped in the pulmonary capillaries. The presence of these aggregates can be assessed by measuring the screen filtration pressure (SFP) which is the pressure required to force the blood under standard conditions through a screen with a 20 μm mesh. Both CPD and ACD preserved blood show a progressive rise in screen filtration pressure during storage with higher values in the CPD blood.

Recently so-called "microfilters" with a pore size of 40 μm have been developed and are inserted above the giving-set. These devices will trap over 1 gram of debris from each unit of blood; although the evidence that aggregates cause detectable ventilation/perfusion inequality is conflicting, there is good reason for using microfilters whenever it is expected that 4 or more units of blood will be given to an adult or when proportionate volumes may be given to children.

By-products of Blood

Plasma

1. **Freeze dried plasma** is made from the blood of 8–10 donors. It contains everything to be found in normal blood with the exception of red cells, leucocytes and platelets. Acid–Citrate–Dextrose and a high potassium (30 mEq/l; mmol/l) which are normal constituents of stored blood, are also included. It is relatively inexpensive to produce (being made predominantly from time-expired blood) but carries the risk of transmitting viral hepatitis and is gradually being replaced by liquid plasma–protein fraction.

2. **Liquid plasma–protein fraction** costs about double that of freeze dried plasma but has the advantage that it is believed to be free of the risk of hepatitis. It is supplied in bottles of 400 ml and contains 4·5 per cent protein solution, of which 90 per cent is albumin and the remainder α- and β-globulin. The solution is stabilised with sodium caprylate and heated to 60°C for 10 hours to inactivate the causative agent for serum hepatitis. The solution contains 130–160 mEq (mmol)/l of sodium and 2 mEq (mmol)/l of potassium, but there is no fibrinogen, labile clotting factors or pseudo-cholinesterase enzyme (DHSS Report, 1973). Most important, because it is entirely free of blood group antibodies, it can therefore be safely given to people of any group.

3. **Fresh frozen plasma.**—This is prepared by centrifuging fresh ACD blood and separating the plasma which is stored at − 20° C. It contains all the clotting factors except platelets and is useful in the management of multiple clotting factor defects, e.g. after massive transfusion (*q.v.*).

Platelet Concentrates

Platelet concentrates are prepared from fresh ACD blood by centrifuging and separation of platelet-rich plasma which is again centrifuged after addition of further ACD. Twenty-five ml of concentrate contains most of the platelets from a unit of blood. Concentrates should be compatible with the recipient's ABO group.

Cryoprecipitate

If fresh plasma is frozen very rapidly some of the globulins do not re-dissolve on thawing at 4° C. In other words, the cryoprecipitate remains as a precipitate at 4° C, whereas at higher temperatures it will re-dissolve. This is the cryoprecipitate and it contains the fibrinogen and most of the antihaemophilic factor.

CORRECTION OF SOME SPECIFIC DEFICIENCIES

Haemophilia and Christmas Disease

These are rare diseases due to inherited deficiency of Factor VIII and Factor IX. They cannot be differentiated clinically and patients suffering from them will give a history of spontaneous bleeding or of prolonged bleeding after operations such as tooth extraction. It is the duration of bleeding, not its amount, which should arouse suspicion that a defect of coagulation may be responsible. Any such history demands an expert haematological investigation and admission to hospital for any surgery, however minor. In no circumstances can routine "bleeding and clotting time" tests be regarded as a substitute for this.

Haemophilia.—This is caused by deficiency of antihaemophilic factor (Factor VIII, AHG). The prothrombin time is normal however severe the disease. When Factor VIII concentration falls to 25–35 per cent of normal it becomes significant clinically, and if surgery is required the aim of management is to raise it to this level and keep it so for at least a week. This can be done by daily infusions of very large volumes of fresh frozen plasma (1½–2 litres/day) or by injection of much smaller volumes of cryoprecipitate. Factor VIII concentrates may be used but these are extremely costly and the concentrate required for a haemophiliac having a hernia repair may cost several thousand pounds.

Christmas disease.—This accounts for about 15 per cent of cases which appear to be haemophilia and is due to Factor IX deficiency. Factor IX is comparatively stable and fresh blood or plasma can be used as sources of supply. If larger amounts are required, Factor IX concentrates are now available.

Platelet Deficiency

Abnormal bleeding due to platelet deficiency is unlikely unless the count falls below 100,000/mm³. It is usually necessary to give platelet concentrates from at least five units of blood; if splenectomy is being carried out on a thrombocytopenic patient the platelets should be given after the spleen is removed.

HAZARDS OF BLOOD TRANSFUSION

Infections

Serum hepatitis, malaria and syphilis as well as some bacterial infections may all be transmitted from donor to recipient.

Serum hepatitis.—Donors are now routinely screened for surface antigen of the causative virus of hepatitis, type B. This is the "Australia" antigen and is termed HB_sAg. About one in one thousand people in the UK are positive and their rejection as donors has reduced the incidence of hepatitis due to transfusion by one quarter (*Lancet* leading article, 1975).

Mollison (1972) assesses the risk of serum hepatitis as about 0·15 per cent for each donor to whom a recipient is exposed. A three-unit transfusion would therefore carry a 1 in 200 risk of hepatitis in an average recipient. Patients whose immune responses are suppressed, e.g. those undergoing transplant surgery or being treated for leukaemia, are much more susceptible.

Precautions.—Precautions to be taken when a patient known to be Australia antigen-positive is to be anaesthetised are described in Chapter 38. In routine work, operating department staff should be trained to avoid getting blood on to their skin and to wash off any blood immediately. Anaesthetists should have a carton on their machines into which all needles etc. are discarded.

Syphilis.—*T. pallidum* is killed by storage for three to four days at 4° C. As every unit of blood is serologically screened for syphilis, the risk of transmission is small.

Malaria.—All forms of malarial parasites will survive storage for three weeks at 4° C. Donors with a history of malaria are rejected.

Bacterial infection of blood after collection.—Most common organisms are killed by storage at 4° C, but certain Gram-negative bacilli can survive and multiply at this temperature. Usually, but not invariably, the red cells are haemolysed by such organisms and the plasma becomes a mauve permanganate-like colour. Examination of the colour of the blood and evidence of the presence of haemolysis should be included in the checking routine. Blood should never be returned to the refrigerator if it has been at room temperature for more than half an hour and packed cells (if packed by hospital laboratories) should be used within six hours of preparation.

Infected blood transfused during anaesthesia is likely to manifest itself by a sudden profound fall in blood pressure and occasionally by uncontrolled bleeding.

Incompatible Transfusion

The first 100 to 200 ml of blood given to an anaesthetised patient should be considered a "test dose" and a careful watch on cardiovascular function is essential. The signs of incompatibility are the same as those of infected blood—sudden fall of blood pressure and the development of a consumption coagulation process (for example, Defibrination Syndrome) which sometimes progresses to the stage of uncontrolled pathological bleeding. Once it is known that incompatible blood has been given a sample of blood should immediately be taken from the recipient and put into a citrate container. Five to ten thousand units of heparin should then be given intravenously whether or not abnormal bleeding has occurred. Any blood deficit should at once be made good with compatible blood, and half to one litre of isotonic saline or Ringer lactate given rapidly followed by 20 g of mannitol. For further management if anuria develops see Chapter 39.

Air Embolism

Air embolism is a rare but preventible cause of death. If the atrial septum has a defect small amounts of air may pass to the left side of the heart against the pressure gradient and so reach the brain; every effort should therefore be made to ensure that no air is introduced from the giving set. Although blood is now in plastic bags, liquid plasma and dextran are only available in bottles and both may be used in haste during massive blood replacement. If roller pumps are used air should be squeezed out of both the filter and drip chambers; failure to do this has resulted in fatal air embolism (Bewes, 1961). The recognition and management of air embolism are described in Chapters 17 (p. 647) and 30 (p. 980).

Allergic Reactions

Any patient with a definite history of allergy is liable to manifest it if given blood or blood products. Piriton (chlorpheniramine maleate) 10 mg may be given intramuscularly or intravenously before starting the transfusion. As a general rule no drugs should be added to units of stored blood.

Physico-chemical Dangers of Massive Transfusion

If stored blood were to perfuse the coronary tree undiluted it would stop the heart for many reasons. The danger of cardiac arrest only arises in massive transfusions—a term which implies consideration of both rate and volume, and is most simply defined as any transfusion (in an adult) at a rate of 500 ml in five minutes or less, or replacement of half the calculated blood volume in less than an hour. The problems involved have been reviewed by Churchill-Davidson (1968) and Burton (1968). Various measures can be taken to reduce the risks.

Warming the blood.—To bring the temperature of the stored blood near to body temperature is the single most important safety measure. This is most simply done by immersion of a coil of the tubing in a water bath kept at 38–40° C. The practice of warming bottles or packs of blood in basins of water is dangerous and should never be used.

Calcium.—Although some authorities disagree (Howland et al., 1957), most now maintain that calcium should be given. Jennings et al. (1965) have provided convincing evidence that ACD is toxic in the dog, and it seems reasonable to replace an absent ionic element known to be essential to myocardial function. Apart from this consideration, calcium is the physiological antagonist to high serum potassium levels as well as protecting against the toxic effects of citrate (Mollison, 1972). Calcium salts are potentially dangerous and must be given slowly.

If calcium is to be given, 5 ml of 10 per cent calcium gluconate should be injected with every 500 ml of blood. Provided that blood is being given at rates of 100 ml/minute (and calcium should not be necessary with slower rates than this) the injection can be made into the transfusion line without causing clotting. When large masses of muscle have been injured the danger of hyperkalaemia is a very real one, and in such cases there is added reason to give calcium if massive transfusion is required.

Sodium bicarbonate.—The ultimate effect of a massive transfusion per se is to cause metabolic alkalosis as a result of the metabolism of citrate to bicarbonate. The immediate effect is a transient metabolic acidosis; this usually disappears rapidly once perfusion is restored. Sodium bicarbonate should rarely be given and then only if the patient fails to respond to rapid blood replacement. If it is necessary, 10 mEq (mmol) of bicarbonate can be given for each unit of blood up to a maximum of 60 mEq (mmol); it is best given as a slow separate injection of 4·2 per cent sodium bicarbonate, 20 ml per unit. If too much bicarbonate is given it will shift the oxygen dissociation curve of haemoglobin to the left and potentiate the effect of lowered DPG on tissue oxygenation.

Dilution.—There is both clinical and experimental support for giving isotonic sodium solutions in addition to whole blood in the management of massive bleeding. Ringer lactate is more appropriate than saline and it should be warmed to body temperature. Up to one litre may be given while blood is being cross-matched and a further $\frac{1}{2}$ to 1 litre is given for every 4 units of blood. The schedule was adopted by an Australian surgical team treating civilian battle casualties (Dudley *et al.*, 1968) and the benefits it is thought to confer are due to better tissue perfusion as a result of the fall in the viscosity of the blood and the protective effects of the induced sodium diuresis on the kidneys.

ECG monitoring.—Whenever the likelihood of massive transfusion can be foreseen, an ECG oscilloscope should be used. The changes to be looked for are usually those ascribed to hyperkalaemia—peaking of the T waves and widening of the QRS complex. If these are seen, calcium gluconate should be given slowly and the blood temporarily replaced by a potassium-free fluid such as liquid plasma or saline. The ECG should be watched for shortening of the QT interval when calcium is being injected.

DEXTRAN

Dextran 70 (Macrodex) is a suitable plasma volume expander if blood is either not available or considered to be unnecessary. It is available as a 6 per cent solution in either 0·9 per cent saline or 5 per cent dextrose and the saline preparation is the more physiological substitute for plasma. Most authorities consider 1 to 1$\frac{1}{2}$ litres as the maximum that should be given as larger amounts tend to interfere with blood clotting in ways which are not fully understood. Blood should be taken for cross-matching before dextran 70 is given.

Dextran 40 (Lomodex, Rheomacrodex) can be used as a 10 per cent solution, and according to Hardaway (1968) it will expand the plasma volume by about double the volume given. The effect is short-lived as up to 70 per cent is excreted by the kidneys within 24 hours: it should be noted that the very viscous urine which results will have an extremely high specific gravity—figures of 1050 and above are common—but there will be a negligible increase in urine osmolarity. Dextran 40 should never be given when there is any doubt about renal function and it is therefore an unsuitable fluid to use in conditions requiring very rapid blood replacement.

THE NORMAL BLOOD VOLUME

Normal blood volumes vary over a wide range if they are expressed as a function of any readily measured characteristic. The red cell volume can be shown to be closely related to total body water and to total exchangeable potassium. The most practical association relates blood volume to body weight but there is a wide variation, as shown in Table 3 by the figures quoted from three authorities.

The sex difference is due to body fat content which has about one-eighth the blood content by weight of lean tissue. In practice one can assume that 90 per cent of blood volumes will fall within the range of 5 litres $\pm \frac{1}{2}$–1 litre in adults.

20/TABLE 3
BLOOD VOLUME AS A PERCENTAGE OF BODY WEIGHT

	Men	Women
Moore	7	6·5
Mollison	7·7	6·6
Massachusetts General Hospital	9	8

Mechanisms for Control of Blood Volume

Control of plasma volume depends upon the balance between fluid uptake and fluid loss and upon the distribution of body water. Fluid intake is normally increased in response to the sensation of thirst, whereas fluid loss in the urine is reduced as a result of an increase in the output of antidiuretic hormone (ADH) from the posterior pituitary, such an increase occurring when the osmolality of the interstitial fluid of the paraventricular and supraoptic nuclei rises.

A reduction in renal blood flow causes secretion of renin by the juxta-glomerular apparatus. Renin is a proteolytic enzyme which acts on angiotensinogen, present in the plasma, to produce angiotensin.

$$\text{Angiotensinogen} \xrightarrow{\text{renin}} \underset{\text{(decapeptide)}}{\text{Angiotensin I}} \longrightarrow \underset{\text{(octapeptide)}}{\text{Angiotensin II}}$$

Angiotensin II is the most potent pressor substance known causing generalised arteriolar constriction. It stimulates secretion of aldosterone from the adrenal zona glomerulosa, so promoting renal sodium reabsorption (and potassium loss) and also causes thirst. Sodium retention and an increase in plasma volume may occur in conditions such as heart failure, cirrhosis and the nephrotic syndrome due to secondary hyperaldosteronism.

Stimulation of left atrial volume receptors inhibits ADH release, producing a consequent water diuresis, and may also influence renin release and thus sodium balance via a reflex involving the sympathetic innervation of the kidney.

The red cell component of the blood volume, in the absence of any haematological abnormality, depends upon the secretion of erythropoietin which is an α-globulin secreted mainly (but not entirely) by the kidney.

The blood volume also depends upon fluid exchange between plasma and extracellular fluid (ECF). Normally about 20 litres of fluid per day escape from the capillaries into the ECF. Of this amount, about 17 litres are reabsorbed into the capillaries and the remaining 3 litres are returned via the lymph. Factors favouring loss of fluid from the capillaries are increased permeability of the capillary wall, an increase in the hydrostatic pressure gradient across the capillary wall, and a reduction in the oncotic pressure (the osmotic pressure due to plasma proteins).

Blood Volumes in Babies and Children

The blood volume at term is high—about 85 ml/kg with a haematocrit of

60 per cent and haemoglobin concentration of 18–20 g/100 ml (g/dl). There is a rapid loss of red cells in the first three months, so that haemoglobin concentration falls to 11–12 g/100 ml (g/dl). The wide range encountered during this time must be appreciated before a baby is considered to be anaemic.

The approximate blood volume of older babies and children up to 2 years can be taken as 75 ml/kg and when anaesthetising them it is a good practice to work out their blood volume beforehand and the volume of blood which corresponds to a unit of blood in an adult.

The blood loss in infants is not easy to predict and when there is any possibility that blood may be needed intravenous access must be secured before surgery begins (see Chapter 45).

Plasma Volume

The considerable variation in blood volume in a normal subject is due to changes in plasma volume. This is mostly postural—lying down for 2 hours after prolonged standing results in expansion of the plasma volume which is reflected in a 5 per cent fall in haemoglobin concentration. This, together with the diurnal variation and small errors in measurement can produce alterations in haemoglobin concentration of 0·5–1 g/100 ml (g/dl).

The various mechanisms available for the control of plasma volume have been outlined above. Any over-expansion of the blood volume will therefore be followed by what Moore calls "plasma dispersal"—movement of water, sodium and albumin out of the intravascular compartment. Each gram of albumin takes with it nearly 20 ml of water. This is the mechanism by which a chronically anaemic patient's haemoglobin concentration is raised by the administration of whole blood, even if the haemoglobin concentration of the transfused blood is little greater than that of the recipient. The recipient, as it were, packs the red cells. This takes time and a clear 24 hours should be allowed between transfusion and surgery if it is to be complete: if time does not allow this, the cells must be packed before transfusion. In this clinical setting, and in this alone, is the clinical aphorism that a unit of blood raises the haemoglobin concentration by 1 g/100 ml (g/dl) approximately true.

If large volumes of blood are given to replace acute blood loss the resulting haemoglobin concentration in the recipient will reflect the haemoglobin concentration and haematocrit of the stored blood as it constitutes more and more of the recipient's circulating blood. After one blood volume has been given, over 60 per cent will consist of donor blood and after two blood volumes nearly 90 per cent. As a result of dilution with anticoagulant solution and rapid destruction of non-viable cells such massive transfusions will result in haemoglobin concentrations 9·5–10 g/100 ml (g/dl) and haematocrits of 35–40 per cent. This is Moore's indeterminate haematocrit of the severely injured transfused patient. "Such a haematocrit is meaningless as an indication of the circulating blood volume. It may coexist with a severe volume deficit, a normal blood volume or a dangerously overtransfused blood volume" (Moore, 1960). It follows that the more blood transfused the less reliable become the haemoglobin concentration and haematocrit as indications of the need for further transfusion.

The Response to Haemorrhage

If one or two litres of blood are lost rapidly the blood volume is made good by intravascular migration of albumin, water and electrolytes from the interstitial fluid. Fit subjects with good cardiovascular function can mobilise fluid at a maximum rate of 100 ml/hour, the rate falling progressively so that final haemodilution takes usually 36 to 48 hours. During this time the haemoglobin concentration, haematocrit and red cell count all fall progressively and such a fall should not be interpreted as an indication of further haemorrhage. Postoperative estimation of the haemoglobin concentration should therefore be deferred to the second day if operative blood loss has not been replaced. In this context (and provided that no hypertonic infusions have been given) the haemoglobin concentration, haematocrit and red cell count are all different ways of expressing the same ratio and there is nothing to be gained by measuring more than one index of this ratio.

Moore *et al.* (1966) have shown that when Ringer lactate is infused rapidly into volunteers, who have been bled approximately 10 per cent of their blood volume, more of the infused solution remains within the vascular tree than in unbled controls. It is commonly believed that saline or Ringer lactate causes albumin to be "washed out" of the intravascular compartment, but these workers showed the opposite to be true and that there was mobilisation of protein into the plasma during the time that considerable volumes of Ringer lactate were passing from the vascular to the interstitial compartment.

Acute Massive Haemorrhage

Once blood loss amounts to 20–30 per cent of blood volume the fine balance between alveolar perfusion and alveolar ventilation is seriously disturbed. The fall in both pressure and output of the right ventricle results in the uppermost parts of the lungs receiving little or no blood although they remain well ventilated. The corresponding fall in left ventricular output results in increased extraction of oxygen by the tissues so that the arteriovenous oxygen difference is greatly increased. The result of this is to increase the "shunt effect" of those alveoli which normally have a low ventilation/perfusion ratio and which are therefore critically influenced by the alveolar/arterial oxygen gradient. Freeman and Nunn (1963) have shown that both the increased dead-space effect and arterial desaturation occur in dogs and Nunn and Freeman (1964) have reviewed the clinical implications. Firstly, drugs such as morphine should be given with the greatest care and only if pain is a prominent symptom. Oxygen in concentrations of 30 per cent or more will be beneficial in some cases and finally infusion of any fluid such as dextran, plasma or saline should be given rapidly until blood becomes available.

Transfusion of Severely Anaemic Patients

Severe cases of chronic anaemia may become extremely sensitive to circulatory overload if transfused with whole blood. This is because they may be in a state of high output cardiac failure with raised central venous pressure. They are usually dyspnoeic on slight exertion and have haemoglobin levels of less than 6·0 g/100 ml (g/dl). Such patients should be given small volumes of packed cells very slowly (1 ml/kg/hr) and carefully observed. The most reliable guide is provided by a quarter-hourly pulse rate chart; incipient right heart failure and pulmonary oedema is indicated by a rising heart rate. Pulmonary oedema may develop several hours later if this warning sign is disregarded.

Sickle-cell Haemoglobin and Anaemia

Normal adult haemoglobin (Hb.A) contains two α-polypeptide chains and two β-polypeptide chains (see p. 149). If the polypeptide chains are abnormal so is the haemoglobin, most haemoglobinopathies resulting from substitution of one amino acid at a single position in either the α or β chain. In sickle-cell haemoglobin (Hb.S) glutamic acid in the 6th position of the normal β chain is replaced by valine, whereas in Hb.C it is replaced by lysine.

Alternatively, there may be defective production of qualitatively normal chains, resulting in α thalassaemia (α-chain deficiency) or β thalassaemia (β-chain deficiency). In β thalassaemia major (Cooley's anaemia or Mediterranean anaemia) the patient is homozygous for the β-thalassaemia gene and the condition is often fatal in childhood. β thalassaemia minor is the carrier state, the subject having only one normal β-polypeptide chain gene.

20/Table 4
Sickle-cell Syndromes

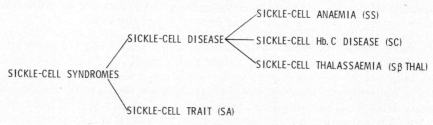

For a subject to have sickle-cell anaemia (SS) a sickle-cell β-polypeptide chain gene must have been inherited from each parent. If such a gene has only been inherited from one parent, the subject being heterozygous for Hb.S, then the other gene is usually normal. This condition is called "sickle-cell trait" (SA). Rarely the other gene is abnormal, for example Hb.C or Hb β thalassaemia, giving rise to sickle-cell haemoglobin C disease or sickle-cell thalassaemia respectively.

In equatorial Africa the incidence of sickle-cell trait (SA) is 20–30 per cent, but the overall Negro Hb.S carrier rate is probably about 10 per cent. The condition is not confined to coloured races and occurs in parts of Greece.

Sickling

When Hb.S is deoxygenated it becomes much less soluble and forms long crystals or tactoids which distort the erythrocyte, producing the sickle shape. These sickle cells tend to aggregate in the capillaries and venules obstructing the flow of blood and so causing zones of infarction. Reoxygenation of the Hb.S causes the red cells to revert to their normal form, although eventually sickling of any particular red cell may become irreversible due to damage to its membrane. Whether sickling occurs depends upon:

1. Percentage of Hb.S in the red cell.
2. Oxygen tension.
3. pH.
4. Nature of the other haemoglobins present.

Percentage of Hb.S in the red cell.—The higher the proportion of Hb.S the more likely is the cell to sickle. A simplified table of the percentages of the haemoglobins present in the various sickle-cell syndromes is given below.

20/TABLE 5
HAEMOGLOBINS IN VARIOUS SICKLE-CELL SYNDROMES

Genotype	per cent Hb.S	per cent Hb.C	per cent Hb.F (fetal)	per cent Hb.A (Normal adult)	Total Hb g/dl
SS	90–95	—	5–10	—	5–10
SA	25–45	—	—	55–75	normal
SC	50	50	—	—	10–14
S β THAL	70–100	—	—	0–30	8–14

Oxygen tension.—A red cell will sickle at a particular level of deoxygenation, the Po_2 at which this occurs depending on the position of the haemoglobin-oxygen dissociation curve. Approximate values of Po_2 at which sickling occurs are as follows:

sickle-cell anaemia (SS)   40 mm Hg (5·3 kPa)
sickle-cell Hb.C disease (SC)   30 mm Hg (4·0 kPa)
sickle-cell trait (SA)   20 mm Hg (2·7 kPa)

The oxygen tension in some vascular beds may be considerably lower than the mixed venous Po_2.

pH.—A reduction in pH causes the haemoglobin-oxygen dissociation curve to shift to the right (Bohr effect) so that for a given Po_2 the haemoglobin is more deoxygenated.

Nature of the other haemoglobins present.—Sickling is more likely to occur in the presence of Hb.C than in the presence of Hb.A or Hb.F.

Detection of Hb.S

1. *Sodium metabisulphite.* If erythrocytes which contain Hb.S are made grossly hypoxic by suspending them in a solution of the reducing agent sodium metabisulphite they will sickle.

2. *Phosphate buffer.* Reduced Hb.S precipitates in concentrated phosphate buffer, and this test can be used quantitatively to differentiate sickle-cell anaemia from the other sickle-cell syndromes (Huntsman et al., 1970). Unfortunately it cannot differentiate sickle-cell trait (SA) from sickle-cell Hb.C disease (SC) or sickle-cell thalassaemia (SβTHAL).

3. *Sickledex* (Ortho Diagnostics). This is a commercially available test which detects Hb.S by a precipitation reaction.

Anaemia with the presence of target cells in the blood film of patients with a positive test for Hb.S is suggestive of sickle-cell disease (SS, SC or SβTHAL), but whenever Hb.S is detected electrophoresis* must be carried out so that a precise diagnosis can be made.

Clinical Features

Sickle-cell trait is usually asymptomatic though sickling can occur under hypoxic conditions, e.g. flying in unpressurised aircraft, and there is an increased incidence of pyelonephritis, haematuria and renal papillary necrosis (Leading Article, *Brit. med. J.*, 1976).

In the three forms of sickle-cell disease crises may be precipitated and take several forms.

Aplastic crisis.—Marrow depression often associated with viral infection or folate deficiency causes an acute aplastic anaemia.

Haemolytic crisis.—This is due to a sudden further reduction in the red cell lifespan, possibly precipitated by infection. In patients with sickle-cell anaemia (SS) the red cell lifespan may be as little as 17 days in the absence of a haemolytic crisis.

Infarctive crisis.—Sickling causes sludging of red cells within small vessels and leads to infarction especially of lungs, spleen and bones though any organ (including the brain) may be affected. Because of the circulatory stasis produced, increasing local hypoxia and acidosis predispose to further sickling.

The treatment and prevention of infarctive crisis is controversial. Oral bicarbonate (up to 20 g/day) is strongly recommended by Huntsman and Lehmann (1974). Intravenous magnesium sulphate, which is a vasodilator and mild anticoagulant, appears to be of benefit especially in the treatment of priapism (Hugh-Jones *et al.*, 1964); cyanate (Ranney, 1972) and urea (McCurdy and Mahmood, 1971) are toxic and not very effective.

Sequestration crisis.—There is enlargement of the liver and spleen with pooling of red cells. This type of crisis mainly affects young children and infants and may necessitate immediate transfusion.

Features of sickle-cell anaemia (SS) which may be present include:
    history of bone and joint pain, osteomyelitis
    bossing of skull with overgrowth of maxilla
    leg ulcers
    lymphadenopathy
    enlarged liver (spleen usually not enlarged because of repeated infarction)
    jaundice due to haemolysis, gallstones
    haematuria
    priapism.

Anaesthesia and Sickle-cell Syndromes

This subject is well reviewed by Howells *et al.* (1972), Searle (1973), Bennett and Dalal (1975). The blood of all patients of African extraction and originating from countries bordering on the Mediterranean should be screened for Hb.S prior to anaesthesia. This is not necessary for neonates who still have a high concentration of fetal haemoglobin (Hb.F). If Hb.S is detected, electrophoresis

---

* *Electrophoresis* is a technique used for separating and identifying different proteins. Because proteins carry an electric charge they migrate in an electric field, different proteins having different electrophoretic mobilities, that is, they move at different rates.

must be carried out so that the potentially dangerous sickle-cell diseases, Hb.SS, Hb.SC and sickle-cell thalassaemia can be differentiated from sickle-cell trait (SA). If operative treatment is urgent there may not be time for conventional electrophoresis, although very rapid electrophoresis techniques are now available; as mentioned above, anaemia and the presence of target cells are indicative of one of the sickle-cell diseases rather than the trait. Abdominal pain may be caused by sickling.

1. *Sickle-cell trait.* No special precautions are needed, although gross hypoxia may cause sickling (Howells *et al.*, 1972).

2. *Sickle-cell disease.* Certain precautions should be taken in order to reduce the risk of anaesthesia to a minimum. Except for a life-saving operation, no patient should be anaesthetised during a crisis. Any infection should be treated and folate deficiency corrected if time permits.

Pre-operative transfusion is not indicated unless the haemoglobin level is less than 5–6 g/dl (Oduro and Searle, 1972; Huntsman and Lehmann, 1974); the dangers of an increased blood viscosity outweigh the advantages of increased oxygen capacity. If blood replacement is likely to be necessary during the operation fresh blood should be cross-matched. Old blood has a reduced 2:3 DPG content with a resulting shift to the left of the haemoglobin-oxygen dissociation curve; if this blood is transfused, then for a given oxygen delivery to the tissues the patient's Hb.S will be more desaturated.

The patient should be starved pre-operatively in the usual way but it is important to avoid dehydration because of the increased blood viscosity. The use of alkalis has been recommended (Gilbertson, 1967; Huntsman and Lehmann, 1974). It is difficult to achieve a significant alkalosis with oral sodium bicarbonate and its effect of shifting the haemoglobin-oxygen dissociation curve to the left is offset by a reduced production of 2:3 DPG, but it nevertheless increases the alkali reserve and so helps to prevent acidosis. The alternative is to give sodium bicarbonate intravenously at the start of anaesthesia and, if at any stage a metabolic acidosis develops, this should be corrected. Recently exchange transfusion, using a cell separator, has been used for pre-operative replacement of Hb.S by Hb.A.

During anaesthesia it is important to avoid hypoxia, hypercapnia, vasoconstriction, reduction in cardiac output and cooling (Gilbertson, 1967). Moderate hyperventilation should be used to induce a respiratory alkalosis.

Post-operatively the patient should receive a raised inspired oxygen concentration by mask for at least 24 hours, and analgesic drugs must be used cautiously so as to avoid hypercapnia due to respiratory depression. Adequate hydration has been mentioned. Chest physiotherapy is important as post-operative chest infection is a special risk in these patients. Tourniquets should be avoided whenever possible.

LIVER FAILURE AND TRANSFUSION

If anaemia is present before operation fresh packed cells should be given (Oberman, 1967). Operative blood loss should be replaced with CPD blood less than one week old. If rapid transfusion becomes necessary, calcium gluconate should be given from the start (2·5 ml of 10 per cent calcium gluconate for every 250 ml of blood).

DEFIBRINATION SYNDROME
(Consumption Coagulopathy)

This is a haemorrhagic disorder in which clotting factors and platelets are used up in a process of diffuse intravascular clotting. It is usually an acute condition caused by entry into the blood stream of factors which trigger the clotting mechanism and may occur as a complication of the conditions listed in Table 6.

20/TABLE 6
CAUSES OF ACUTE DEFIBRINATION SYNDROME

Obstetric accidents:
  (a) Abruptio placentae (premature placental separation).
  (b) Amniotic fluid embolism.
  (c) Abortion.
Surgery, especially of heart and lungs.
Haemolytic transfusion reaction.
Septicaemia.
Pulmonary embolism.
Snake bite.
Hypersensitivity reactions.

The clinical features of defibrination are bleeding, which may be generalised or localised, and the effects of organ damage due to ischaemia caused by intravascular thrombosis. After laboratory confirmation of the diagnosis, treatment should be aimed at:

1. *Elimination of the precipitating cause.* This is often not possible, but, for example, septicaemia should be treated with the appropriate antibiotics.

2. *Replacement of coagulation factors and platelets.* Fresh blood (less than 12 hours old) and platelet-rich plasma should be given. In addition, in cases with severe bleeding, fibrinogen 5–10 g in 500 ml should be infused over 2–3 hours.

3. *Inhibition of the clotting process with heparin.* Heparin should be given if the defibrination process is continuing or if intravascular thrombosis is causing organ damage. Careful laboratory monitoring is essential.

SURGERY ON PATIENTS TAKING ANTICOAGULANT DRUGS

Patients who are receiving anticoagulant treatment with one of the coumarin derivatives such as warfarin, may present for surgery. Warfarin acts as a competitive antagonist of vitamin K and so interferes with the synthesis of Factors II, VII, IX and X (Table 1).

In the case of elective surgery, normal haemostasis can be achieved by stopping the warfarin and giving vitamin K_1 (phytomenadione), 1–2 mg intravenously 48 hours in advance. Much larger doses of vitamin K_1 have previously been recommended, but are now known not to be necessary and also interfere with further anticoagulant control for several days. In the event of emergency surgery, more rapid reversal of the effect of warfarin can be achieved by giving either fresh frozen plasma or a concentrate of the vitamin-K-dependent clotting factors. The disadvantage of fresh frozen plasma is the time involved—

that is the time for it to thaw and the time taken for 500–1000 ml (the volume required which contains sufficient amounts of the clotting factors) to be infused. The alternative is to give the factor concentrate which is available either as a 3-factor concentrate (II, IX, X) or a 4-factor concentrate (II, VII, IX, X); trials comparing their efficacy are in progress, but they are probably equally effective. As with other patients whose clotting mechanism is defective, the haemostatic clot formed after clotting factor replacement may be safeguarded against physiological fibrinolysis by administration of an antifibrinolytic drug. Epsilon-aminocaproic acid should be given (5 g intravenously, 6-hourly) until oral therapy with tranexamic acid (1 g, 6-hourly) is possible, which is continued until the wound is healed. This antifibrinolytic treatment is contra-indicated if the organisation of unlysable blood clot and possible subsequent contraction of fibrous tissue at the site of operation might be dangerous, for example, after bile-duct surgery. The advantage of a factor concentrate is that normal clotting can be achieved within minutes, but against this must be set the extra risk of hepatitis due to the large plasma pools from which the factors are obtained.

REFERENCES

BENNETT, E. J., and DALAL, F. Y. (1975). Haemoglobin S and its clinical application. In: *Oxygen Measurements in Biology and Medicine.* Ed. by J. P. Payne and D. W. Hill, London: Butterworth & Co.

BEWES, P. C. (1961). Danger of air embolism in high pressure blood transfusions. *Lancet,* 1, 429.

British Medical Journal (1976). Leading Article—Sickle cell trait. 1, 1359.

BURTON, G. W. (1968). Massive blood transfusion. *Proc. roy. Soc. Med.,* 61, 682.

CHURCHILL-DAVIDSON, H. C. (1968). Massive blood transfusion. *Proc. roy. Soc. Med.,* 61, 681.

DHSS (1973). *Notes on Transfusion.* Edinburgh: H.M.S.O. Press.

DUDLEY, H. A. F., KNIGHT, R. J., McNEUR, J. C., and ROSENGARTEN, D. S. (1968). Civilian battle casualties in South Vietnam. *Brit. J. Surg.,* 55, 332.

FREEMAN, J., and NUNN, J. F. (1963). Ventilation-perfusion relationships after haemorrhage. *Clin. Sci.,* 24, 135.

GILBERTSON, A. A. (1967). The management of anaesthesia in sickle cell states. *Proc. roy. Soc. Med.,* 60, 631.

GILLIES, I. D. S. (1974). Anaemia and anaesthesia. *Brit. J. Anaesth.,* 46, 589.

HARDAWAY, R. M. (1968). In: *Clinical Management of Shock.* Springfield, Ill.: Chas. C. Thomas.

HOWELLS, T. H., HUNTSMAN, R. G., BOYS, J. E., and MAHMOOD (1972). Anaesthesia and sickle-cell haemoglobin. *Brit. J. Anaesth.,* 44, 975.

HOWLAND, W. S., BELLVILLE, J. W., ZUCKER, M. B., BOYAN, P., and CLIFFTON, E. E. (1957). Massive blood transfusion V: Failure to observe citrate intoxication. *Surg. Gynec. Obstet.,* 105, 529.

HUGH-JONES, K., LEHMAN, H., and McALISTER, J. M. (1964). Some experiences in managing sickle-cell anaemia in children and young adults, using alkalis and magnesium. *Brit. med. J.,* 2, 226.

HUNTSMAN, R. G., BARCLAY, G. P. T., CANNING, D. M., and YAWSON, G. I. (1970). A rapid whole blood solubility test to differentiate the sickle-cell trait from sickle-cell anaemia. *J. clin. Path.,* 23, 781.

HUNTSMAN, R. G., and LEHMANN, H. (1974). Treatment of sickle-cell disease. *Brit. J. Haemat.*, **28**, 437.

JENNINGS, E. R., BELAND, A. J., COPE, J. A., ELLESTAD, M. H., MONROE, C., and SHADLE, O. W. (1965). Citrate toxicity and the use of anticoagulated acid-citrate-dextrose blood for extracorporeal circulation. *Surg. Gynec. Obstet.*, **120**, 997.

Lancet (1975). Leading Article—Virus hepatitis updated. **1**, 1365.

MCCURDY, P. R., and MAHMOOD, L. (1971). Intravenous urea treatment of the painful crisis of sickle-cell disease. *New Engl. J. Med.*, **285**, 992.

MOLLISON, P. L. (1972). *Blood Transfusion in Clinical Medicine*, 5th edit. Oxford: Blackwell Scientific Publications.

MOORE, F. D. (1960). In: *Metabolic Care of the Surgical Patent*. Philadelphia: W. B. Saunders Co.

MOORE, F. D., DAGHER, F. J., BOYDEN, C. M., LEE, C. J., and LYONS, J. A. (1966). Hemorrhage in normal man. Distribution and disposal of saline infusions following acute blood loss. *Ann. Surg.*, **163**, 485.

National Research Council Report (1974). Current status of red-cell preservation in relation to the developing national blood policy. (Chaplin, H., Beutler, E., Collins, J. A., Giblett, E. R., and Ploesky, H. F.) *New Engl. J. Med.*, **291**, 68.

NUNN, J. F., and FREEMAN, J. (1964). Problems of oxygenation and oxygen transport during haemorrhage. *Anaesthesia*, **19**, 206.

OBERMAN, H. A. (1967). Indications for transfusion of freshly drawn blood. *J. Amer. med. Ass.*, **199**, 93.

ODURO, K. A., and SEARLE, J. F. (1972). Anaesthesia in sickle-cell states—a plea for simplicity. *Brit. med. J.*, **4**, 596.

RANNEY, H. M. (1972). The clinical use of cyanate in sickling. *New Engl. J. Med.*, **287**, 98.

SEARLE, J. F. (1973). Anaesthesia in sickle cell states. *Anaesthesia*, **28**, 48.

SYKES, M. K. (1975). Indications for blood transfusion. *Canad. Anaesth. Soc. J.*, **22**, 3.

Section Three

THE NERVOUS SYSTEM

Chapter 21

GENERAL PHARMACOLOGICAL PRINCIPLES

THE logical use of drugs depends on knowledge not only of what effects they exert on tissues but also of how these effects are produced and influenced by the disposal of the drugs concerned. In this chapter the general principles of drug action and disposal are discussed with special, though not exclusive, reference to drugs used in anaesthesia. No mention is made of inhalational anaesthetics in the disposal of which some special factors are involved; these are considered in Chapter 6. Stress is placed on the simple physical laws which determine the ways in which drugs reach their target cells, exert their effects, interact with substances of physiological importance or with other drugs and are then removed from their site of action and from the body. The actions of individual agents are discussed only in relation to the general principles concerned. For details of such actions the reader is referred to the special chapters dealing with particular groups of drugs.

In what follows general pharmacological principles are discussed under separate headings:

1. Drug action on receptors
2. Drug concentrations in plasma, protein binding
3. Passage of drugs across membranes
4. Drug administration
5. Drug distribution
6. Drug metabolism
7. Drug excretion
8. Variation in drug response

There is, however, much overlap in the principles involved and such a division is used only for convenience.

Drug interactions may occur clinically in a number of ways; these are considered in the appropriate sections.

DRUG ACTION ON RECEPTORS

Drugs exert many different effects on different tissues. These effects are, however, specific to a greater or lesser extent in that different drugs have different effects. Living cells must therefore possess special sites of drug action, the properties of which are to react with drugs of a specific nature and to initiate a chain of events leading to the pharmacological effect. Such sites of action are receptors. For many years no more than a useful concept for explaining in qualitative and quantitative terms how drugs act, receptors are now known to exist in fact. Recent work has revealed much about their structure, their localisation and even their number. For detailed study the reader is referred to two important symposia on the subject (Porter and O'Connor, 1970; Rang, 1973).

Drug-receptor interactions.—The attachment of drug to receptor has been the focus of much attention. Studies of the relative effects exerted by closely related drugs have shown that it involves physical bonding by a number of forces, ionic, van der Waal, hydrogen bonding and others. The extent to which each of these contributes to the drug-receptor attraction varies from one drug to another and from one receptor to another. The number of bonds involved is usually multiple and their steric arrangement critical. It is well known, for example, that L-noradrenaline exerts many times the pressor effect of D-noradrenaline, presumably because the three-point attachment of the former is more favourable than that of the latter. Bonding arrangements have been most deeply studied for cholinergic (Waser, 1961) and adrenergic (Belleau, 1963) receptors, for which optimal drug dimensions have been calculated. The relationship between receptor structure and bonding is the subject of a review (Ehrenpreis *et al.*, 1969).

Drugs which stimulate receptors are *agonists*; those which block them are *antagonists*. Drugs such as nicotine and decamethonium which have both actions are referred to as partial agonists.

Quantitative aspects of drug-receptor interaction were first studied by Clark (1937), who proposed that stimulant drugs occupied receptors and that the tissue response was proportional to the number occupied. He showed that the shape of the dose-response curve could be predicted from the law of mass action in a manner similar to that proposed by Michaelis and Menten (1913) for the behaviour of enzymes. The effect of an antagonist could be shown theoretically and in practice to modify the action of the agonist in a way which shifted the log.dose-response curve to the right without altering its shape or the size of the maximum response attainable (Fig. 1). This is competitive antagonism, seen clinically in a number of situations: atropine or tubocurarine acting against acetylcholine, phentolamine against noradrenaline, propranolol against adrenaline and naloxone against morphine or pethidine. It is so-called because agonist and antagonist compete for the same receptor.

Clark's occupation theory is not entirely satisfactory for several reasons. First, one must assume that two types of receptor occupation are possible: one for agonists which exerts an effect, another for antagonists which does not do so. Secondly, how is it possible to achieve maximal agonist responses when many receptors are occupied by antagonist molecules? In Fig. 1 the curves reach the same height even though there is antagonist present. One must assume either that the agonist displaces the antagonist from the receptor or alternatively that there is a plentiful supply of extra receptors ("spare" receptors as proposed by Stephenson, 1956) which are not needed for a maximum response. The former explanation is untrue; agonist does not displace antagonist. In anaesthetic practice, partial curarisation can be overcome by administering edrophonium, but when the edrophonium effect wears off one is left with just as much curarisation as if the edrophonium had never been given. Thirdly, how can one account for the action of partial agonists like nicotine and decamethonium which both stimulate and block receptors?

An alternative "rate" theory proposed by Paton (1960, 1961), goes some way towards overcoming these and other objections. The assumption here is that receptors are stimulated not by occupancy but momentarily by the act of combination with the drug, the rate of impact being governed by the law of mass

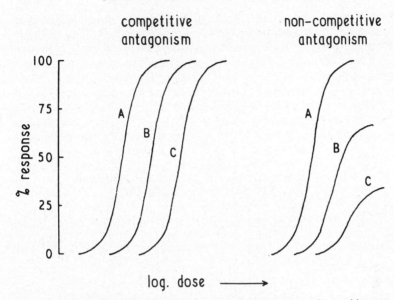

21/Fig. 1.—Theoretical log.dose-response curves for drug action. Competitive antagonists shift the curve to the right. Non-competitive antagonists alter the slope and maximal response. A = response without antagonist, B and C with increasing doses of antagonist.

action. Once occupied, the receptor is unavailable for further stimulation. On this theory the critical difference between agonists and antagonists lies in the rates of dissociation of the drug-receptor complexes. An agonist should dissociate rapidly, thus freeing the receptor for a fresh act of combination. An antagonist, on the other hand, should dissociate slowly, thus reducing the availability of receptors to agonist impacts. A partial agonist should lie between these extremes. Maximum tissue responses would be obtainable in the presence of antagonists by higher rates of impact on the reduced number of free receptors, thus obviating the need for spare receptors or for antagonist displacement. Under experimental *in vitro* conditions agonists would be rapidly, but antagonists slowly, washed out from isolated tissues, an observation which is well known and easily demonstrable.

Rate theory does not explain why some agonists are more effective than others, why different ones produce maximal effects of different sizes or why log.dose-response curves for the same receptor are not parallel for all agonists. Evidently drugs have other intrinsic properties which influence the effects they induce on the receptor containing tissue.

The action of competitive antagonists serves to verify predictions implied in drug receptor interaction theory. Other types of antagonism are also demonstrable at the tissue site. Non-competitive antagonism is shown under some conditions by phenoxybenzamine. It decreases the maximal effect of alpha adrenergic stimulants and flattens the log.dose-response curve (Fig. 1). Physiological antagonism is that which occurs when two drugs have opposite actions without real interference.

For a number of reasons it is useful to have measures of potency and specificity of drug antagonists acting on particular receptors. This is achieved by the measurement of their affinity for the receptors concerned. This function is a constant and it is usually expressed in logarithmic form (i.e. log. K) In practical terms log. K is the negative decimal logarithm of the molar concentration of antagonist required to reduce the potency of an appropriate agonist two-fold. Drugs with powerful antagonist potency therefore have high values, those with weak potency low ones. For example, against histamine's action on guinea-pig ileum mepyramine has a log. K value of 9·4, i.e. $10^{-9 \cdot 4}$ mol/l, and reduces the potency of histamine two-fold. This and other values are given in Table 1.

21/TABLE 1

LOG. AFFINITY CONSTANTS OF DRUG ANTAGONISTS ON
GUINEA-PIG ILEUM (from Schild, 1947).

Antagonist	Against histamine	Against acetylcholine
mepyramine	9·4	4·8
atropine	5·7	8·6
pethidine	6·2	5·8

Such measurements indicate the considerable specificities of mepyramine (40,000 times greater against histamine than against acetylcholine) and atropine (1,000 times vice versa) and the negligible specificity of pethidine as antagonists. One can deduce from these results the obvious clinical implications that mepyramine is a useful antihistamine but a useless anticholinergic, that atropine has the opposite properties and that pethidine is both antihistaminic and anticholinergic.

When two drugs of similar action (either agonistic or antagonistic) act together, synergistically, the resultant effect is the sum of the individual components. If the log.dose-response curves are steep this summation can result in a surprisingly large effect which is often though erroneously referred to as potentiation. It is well known, for example, that combinations of barbiturates with alcohol can produce dangerous cerebral depression, as can combinations of most central depressant drugs. The effects are the result of summation and not potentiation, the latter of which implies that the total is more than the sum of its components. Potentiation occurs almost exclusively when one drug alters the metabolism or the excretion of the other; this topic is discussed later.

Occurrences of antagonism, summation and potentiation in experimental and clinical situations are often difficult to distinguish. One useful method is the construction of isobols (Loewe, 1957), lines, analogous to isobars or isotherms on a map, joining points of equal pharmacological effect in graphs of doses of drug mixtures. Examples are shown in Fig. 2. Drug mixtures, such as barbiturates and alcohol, showing summation produce a straight-line isobol, such that combinations of two half doses produce the same effects as one whole dose (Smith and Herxheimer, 1969). In many instances, one half dose alone may have no measurable action whatsoever (reference the steepness of the log.dose-response curve above); hence the confusion with potentiation. Deviation from

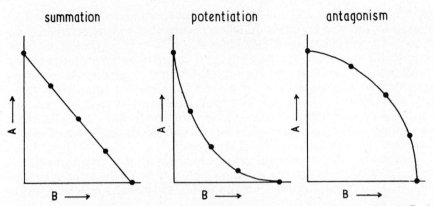

21/FIG. 2.—Theoretical isobols of drug interaction. Combined dose diagrams of equi-effective drug pairs (A and B) show summation, potentiation and antagonism.

the straight line indicates that the drugs interact so that greater or lesser doses are required to produce the defined pharmacological effect.

DRUG CONCENTRATIONS IN PLASMA

The drug concentration at its site of action is a function of its concentration in plasma. In turn the plasma concentration is influenced by the rates of drug absorption, distribution to various tissues, metabolism and excretion, and the extent to which the drug is bound to plasma protein (see below). The dynamic equilibrium established is influenced also by the extent to which the drug is ionised in each body fluid. A scheme of distribution is illustrated in Fig. 3. From measurements of drug and metabolite concentrations in plasma and urine, time courses of distribution have been simulated with the help of analogue or digital

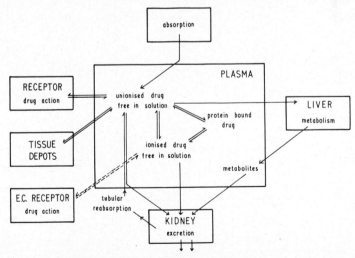

21/FIG. 3.—Distribution of drugs in the body. E.C. receptor = extracellular receptor.

computers (Wiegand and Sanders, 1964; Beckett and Tucker, 1968). Such simulations can help to predict durations of drug action under certain circumstances (e.g. for tubocurarine, Gibaldi *et al.*, 1972). In many clinical instances, however, the kinetics of drug disposition are complicated by binding to plasma protein and sequestration in tissue depots. Under such circumstances, plasma concentrations do not necessarily give direct indications of the pharmacologically active concentrations at the site of drug action and attempted correlations between plasma concentration and drug action therefore fail. Furthermore, many drugs have active metabolites whose contribution to the overall action makes such correlation too complex to evaluate.

Concentrations in plasma of drugs which are not significantly bound to plasma protein or sequestered in tissues decline by a simple exponential (first order elimination) whereby the concentration C at time t can be represented by the equation:

$$C = A.e^{-\beta t}$$

where A and β are constants. This provides a straight line on a log.concentration/time graph and gives a measure of the half-life of the drug in the plasma. For drugs administered intravenously, the decline is usually bi-exponential because disappearance from the plasma is a function of distribution to body tissues as well as elimination by metabolism or excretion. In such instances, a curve such as that for buthalitone shown in Fig. 4 results. For kinetic analysis of this and of

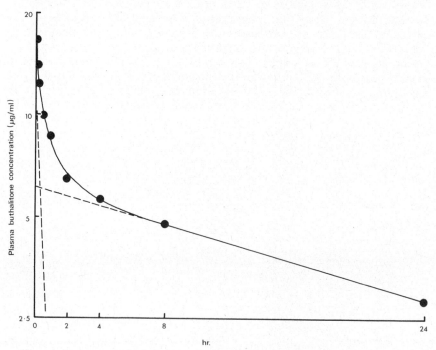

21/Fig. 4.—Plasma concentrations of buthalitone in healthy male subjects following administration of 11 mg/kg i.v. Concentrations decline bi-exponentially, as indicated by interrupted lines. (Data from Kane and Smith, 1959.)

more complex situations the reader is referred to a more specialised review (Smith and Rawlins, 1973).

Protein Binding

In the circulation many drugs are bound to plasma proteins. Acidic drugs tend to be bound to albumin and basic drugs to globulin, but there is much overlap. The extent of binding varies from one drug to another and it is dependent on the drug concentration. The subject was extensively reviewed by Goldstein in 1949. The nature of the binding process is complex and probably involves a number of binding sites of variable specificity. Some of these involve van der Waal bonding, some ionic attractions and others lipophilic affinities. The latter probably account for the binding of barbiturate molecules and explain the fact that it is the ultra-short-acting drugs in the group (the most lipid-soluble) which are most highly bound. Other sites are specific for acidic drugs such as sulphonamides and coumarin anticoagulants.

The extent to which any drug is bound is influenced by its concentration, very high concentrations tending to swamp the binding sites and lower the proportion of bound drug. A rapid increase in effect and toxicity would be expected above this level. It is difficult, however, to predict the exact behaviour because at high concentrations subsidiary binding mechanisms may come into play. For example, thiopentone may then be bound in both its ionised and non-ionised forms. At low concentrations very high proportions of circulating drugs may be bound: thiopentone about 85–90 per cent, digitoxin 95 per cent and warfarin 98 per cent. Among such drugs only a small proportion remains available for diffusion to the tissues, where the drugs exert their pharmacological actions, and some of this is metabolically degraded or filtered by the kidneys. Extensive binding therefore has the effects of limiting potency and prolonging duration of action. Bound drug is thought to be pharmacologically inactive, though the bound fraction is in a state of dynamic equilibrium with that free in solution and can therefore exert effects once it is released.

Protein binding may vary in different individuals. It is diminished by low circulating albumin levels such as occur in liver disease and malnutrition. Patients with severe liver disease are therefore intolerant of drugs which are usually highly bound because much larger proportions of the drugs circulate free in solution in plasma and are available for diffusion into the tissues. Binding of particular drugs may also be reduced by the presence of other drugs which compete for the same binding sites; this induces true potentiation. Clinically such interactions occur most obviously with acidic drugs such as sulphonamides, penicillins, salicylates, coumarin anticoagulants, sulphonylureas, phenylbutazone and methotrexate. In some instances interactions produced by concurrent administration of two or more of these drugs may be of minor importance. If they include sulphonylureas such as tolbutamide or anticoagulants such as warfarin, however, unexpected and often dangerous potentiation may occur. For further discussion of this subject the reader is referred to a survey by Prescott (1969).

Tissue proteins may also bind drugs. Barbiturates in particular are bound to homogenates of most tissues including brain (Goldbaum and Smith, 1954), the extent corresponding roughly with the distribution of these drugs *in vivo*. It is not clear how this influences the effects of such drugs at their sites of action. Some drugs have affinities for particular tissue proteins which influence their distributions in other ways. Antimony, for example, and probably other heavy metals are largely and rapidly bound by the liver because of its content of protein thiol groups (Smith, 1969). Clinically this has the effect of reducing plasma concentrations of the metals to very low levels in a short time, whereas concentrations in the liver may remain high for several weeks.

THE PASSAGE OF DRUGS ACROSS MEMBRANES

The effect of a drug at its site of action in body tissues is dependent on its presence at critical concentration at that site. To achieve this, the drug must be absorbed from its site of administration and be distributed in the body in a suitable manner, such absorption and distribution being dependent on the ability of the drug to cross cellular membrane barriers. Because the physical properties of cell membranes are similar in different parts of the body, the factors involved in absorption and distribution into different tissues are also similar.

Drugs can cross cell membranes in three ways: by diffusion, by penetration through membrane pores and by means of active transport (Christensen, 1962).

Diffusion

Many drugs used in anaesthetic and general practice are weak bases or acids which in solution are ionised to variable extents depending on the ease or difficulty with which they accept or donate protons. Conventionally this is expressed as the pK_a, the negative logarithm of the acidic dissociation constant, analogous to pH. In solution the degree of ionisation is also affected by the pH.

Thus:

$$\text{for acids—}pK_a - pH = \log\frac{Cn}{Ci}$$

$$\text{for bases—}pK_a - pH = \log\frac{Ci}{Cn}$$

where Ci and Cn are the concentrations of the ionised and non-ionised forms respectively. The pK_a values of some important compounds are illustrated in Fig. 5.

The importance of these factors to drug absorption and distribution is that in the non-ionised (undissociated) state drugs have lipid solubility and are therefore able to diffuse across cell membranes, whereas in the ionised (dissociated) form they have no lipid solubility and therefore cannot diffuse across. Drugs such as barbiturates, which have pK_a values close to physiological pH are about 50 per cent ionised in the body and, having reasonable lipid solubility, are therefore well-absorbed from the gastro-intestinal tract, cross the blood-brain and placental barriers and are reabsorbed in the renal tubule. By contrast, quaternary ammonium compounds like tubocurarine and suxamethonium which are fully ionised at physiological pH have no lipid solubility and are therefore not absorbed from the gastro-intestinal tract, do not cross the blood-brain or placental barriers and are not reabsorbed in the renal tubule. They can, however, cross capillary walls and do therefore penetrate the extracellular spaces where they act. Drug transfer across the placenta is discussed further in Chapter 44.

Transfer of a drug by diffusion across a cell membrane proceeds at a rate which is proportional to its concentration. In theory this rate is unlimited and it requires no metabolic energy. The amount of drug absorbed from the gastro-intestinal tract is therefore a direct function of the dose administered; the amount that penetrates into the brain, the fetus or any other organ is a direct function of the concentration of the drug free in solution in the plasma.

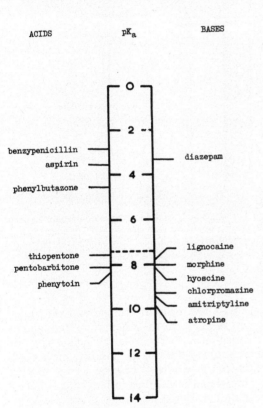

21/FIG. 5.—pK_a values of acids and bases (data from Smith and Rawlins, 1973).

Surprisingly diffusion can set up concentration gradients such that one tissue may contain much more drug than another. If there is a marked pH difference across the membrane such as exists across the gastric mucosa, total drug concentrations differ considerably because the concentrations of non-ionised drug must be the same on the two sides. The equilibrium established is illustrated in Fig. 6, which shows that a weak acid like phenylbutazone is unevenly distributed in a way which leads to its absorption from the stomach into the gastric cells. By contrast, weak bases show the opposite distribution and are therefore excreted into the stomach. Weak acids of higher pK_a than phenylbutazone are partly absorbed from and excreted into the stomach.

The same factors influence the reabsorption of weak acids and bases from the renal tubule (see below).

Penetration Through Pores

Many substances which are lipid-insoluble can enter cells and penetrate membrane barriers. Such substances as water and urea do so by filtration through pores in the cell membrane. Their movement occurs by diffusion and no energy is required, though the rate is usually slow because the pores occupy only a minute fraction of the cell surface (perhaps 0·2 per cent). Inorganic ions penetrate in the same way, though the rate of their movement is limited further by the polarisation of the membrane surface. Lipid-soluble substances may be absorbed from the gastro-intestinal tract in this manner by solution in chylomicrons.

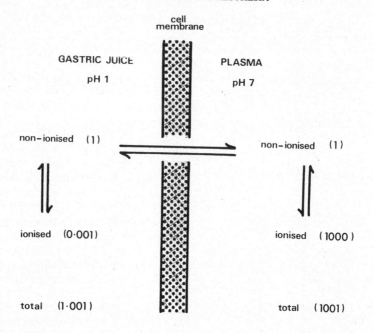

21/Fig. 6.—Theoretical distribution of a weak acid of pK_a 4·5 (e.g. phenylbutazone) between gastric juice and plasma. Differences in ionisation produce a large concentration gradient. Theoretical relative concentrations are shown in parentheses.

Active Transport

Many physiological substances and a few drugs are transferred across cell membranes by specialised transport systems. Such systems are thought to involve the use of carriers whose function is to combine reversibly with the substance at one surface of the membrane, transfer it to the opposite surface and release it there. Considerable concentration gradients may be set up and the process is energy-dependent, rate limited and susceptible to blockade by metabolic inhibitors. Special transport systems exist for sugars, amino acids, inorganic ions and neurohumoral transmitters such as noradrenaline, 5-hydroxytryptamine and gamma-aminobutyric acid. Some synthetic sympathomimetic amines are carried into nerve-endings in the same manner by use of the noradrenaline carrier.

Many drugs in common use are powerful inhibitors of these transport systems and their pharmacological actions are dependent on this property. Cocaine, for example, owes its sympathomimetic action to its ability to inhibit re-uptake of noradrenaline back into nerve-endings (Iversen, 1967). Imipramine is a powerful inhibitor of 5-hydroxytryptamine uptake by platelets (Stacey, 1961); its antidepressant effect may result from the same action in the brain. The antithyroid action of potassium perchlorate depends on its ability to antagonise thyroid iodide transport.

DRUG ADMINISTRATION

Intravenous

In anaesthetic practice many drugs are administered intravenously. Concentrations of these drugs in the plasma and indirectly in the tissues rise almost instantaneously to a maximum and the time to onset of drug effect is reduced to a minimum. Mixing of the drug solution with the whole circulating plasma volume is relatively slow, however, and is not achieved for several circulation times. Until mixing has occurred, therefore, some blood contains much more drug than the remainder, this effect being most marked immediately following the drug's administration. The difference is exaggerated further if the injection is given quickly and reduced if it is given slowly. After rapid injection, a bolus of drug solution of high concentration may travel in the circulation almost unmixed for long enough to exert a powerful drug action; if the total amount of drug administered is mixed completely by slow injection no effect may result. This "slug effect" was described by Paton (1960) and is illustrated in Fig. 7.

In clinical practice such slug effects have a profound influence on drug action. They explain, for instance, why a rapid injection of a small dose of an intravenous anaesthetic exerts a brief but powerful effect, whereas a slowly injected much larger dose has no effect at all. In patients with heart failure, of course, the time to onset of drug effect is greatly increased because of the slow circulation.

Measurements of plasma concentrations of intravenously administered drugs within 5 minutes or so of administration are therefore of doubtful value. They may produce higher or lower levels depending on the phase of mixing.

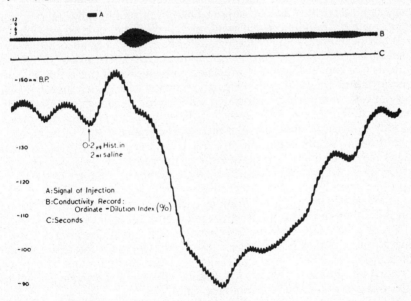

21/Fig. 7.—Slug effect of rapid i.v. administration of histamine 0·2 μg in 2 ml saline in an anaesthetised cat. Upper tracing: conductivity of carotid arterial blood gives a measure of drug concentration. Lower tracing: arterial blood pressure. The drug effect follows the slug but wanes in spite of a rising drug concentration with recirculation (Paton, 1960).

Intramuscular, Subcutaneous and Intraperitoneal

Following drug administration by these routes, absorption into the circulation occurs depending on the physico-chemical properties of the drug, the extent to which the drug solution spreads in the tissue and the state of the local circulatior Insoluble forms of drugs such as procaine penicillin and depot preparations of insulin are only slowly absorbed because solution must first occur. Given intraperitoneally, drugs are very rapidly absorbed because of rapid spread of solution over the absorptive surface and the highly vascular nature of that surface. Intramuscular and subcutaneous routes allow slower absorption because of reduced spread and blood supplies in these regions. The rates are therefore further slowed if the regional blood supply is reduced as in states of shock or by the addition of vasoconstrictors to the drug solutions. The times to peak plasma concentrations, and indirectly to drug effects elsewhere, are therefore progressively prolonged.

Oral

Absorption of drugs from the gastro-intestinal tract is influenced by the factors mentioned above and also by some special factors. Most rapid and effective absorption occurs at either end, from the oral and the rectal mucosae following local administration. Such mucosae are highly vascular and, provided the drug is lipid soluble, allow rapid transfer of the drug into the circulation. More importantly, such routes allow drug passage directly to the systemic circulation and not into the portal circulation, thus avoiding the immediate effect of the liver which in many cases inactivates drugs by metabolism. Such drugs as glyceryl trinitrate or isoprenaline, given sublingually, exert systemic actions within 2 minutes. When swallowed, these drugs have no effect at all.

When swallowed, some drugs, mostly weak acids, can be absorbed from the stomach if they are largely in the non-ionised state at the pH of the stomach contents (see above). The most important consequence of this is that high drug concentrations are built up in the gastric mucosal cells, which may explain the erosions and haemorrhage associated with the use of aspirin and phenylbutazone. Such absorption is diminished if the subject has consumed antacids in quantity sufficient to raise the intragastric pH significantly.

Although the pH conditions are not always ideal, most drug absorption occurs from the small intestine because of the enormous available absorptive surface area. Absorption is limited by the presence of food in the lumen such that some drugs taken after, rather than before, meals may hardly be absorbed at all. Meals also impede absorption by delaying gastric emptying. Malabsorption states may of course hinder absorption of drugs as they do of foodstuffs.

Drugs which interfere with intestinal function can inhibit drug absorption. Thus atropine-like drugs and drugs such as phenothiazines and antidepressants which produce atropine-like effects delay gastric emptying and thus prevent intestinal absorption of other drugs. Similar effects may be produced by shock states when gastric motility is inhibited reflexly.

Many drugs are ineffective when administered by mouth because they are inactivated in the gastro-intestinal tract. Some penicillins are acid-labile and therefore degraded by gastric juice; polypeptides are hydrolysed by gastric and intestinal enzymes; many amines such as catecholamines, histamine, and l-tyramine (e.g. cheese) are oxidised by amine oxidases in the gut wall. Drug interaction can occur within the lumen, limiting or preventing absorption. Thus, magnesium- and aluminium-containing antacids form complexes with tetracyclines and the resin cholestyramine with acidic drugs like warfarin and phenylbutazone. In each case absorption is prevented. Antibiotics may indirectly exert effects by inducing changes in bacterial flora, producing intestinal hurry and thus malabsorption. In addition, such changes can increase the effects of coumarin anticoagulants if bacterial production of vitamin K (with which the anticoagulants compete) is reduced.

DRUG DISTRIBUTION

Once a drug enters the circulation it is distributed to a variety of compartments within the body, mostly by diffusion down concentration gradients. The rate and extent of such distribution depends on several factors: the physico-chemical properties of the drug (principally its lipid solubility), the binding of the drug to plasma and/or tissue protein, the regional distribution of blood flow, and in a few instances the presence of active transport mechanisms. The total amount of drug in the body (X) and its concentration in the plasma (C) are related as follows:

$$X = C \cdot V_D$$

where V_D is the volume of distribution. In a few instances drugs are distributed into strict anatomical spaces, e.g. heparin into plasma water (0·05 1/kg), antipyrine into total body water (0·60 1/kg); the distribution volume is then a real volume which is readily envisaged. Drugs which are highly lipid-soluble or extensively bound to proteins are distributed quite differently; the distribution volume is then an apparent volume which does not conform to an anatomical space. It is merely that volume in which the drug would be dissolved were it all at the same concentration as in the plasma. It is largely independent of dosage and it is characteristic of the drug concerned. Some values of drugs which cover a wide range of distribution volume are indicated in Table 2. To the extent that drug effects must be related to drug concentrations at tissue sites and therefore indirectly to plasma concentrations, volumes of distribution are important determinants of drug action.

21/TABLE 2

DISTRIBUTION VOLUMES (V_D) AND PLASMA ELIMINATION
HALF-LIVES ($T_{\frac{1}{2}}$) OF SELECTED DRUGS IN MAN.

Drug	V_D (1/kg)	$T_{\frac{1}{2}}$ (hr)
nortriptyline	21·1	34·2
pentobarbitone	2·0*	42·0
buthalitone	1·8	21·7
thiopentone	1·2*	4·0
tubocurarine	0·14	0·8

(* approximate values)

DRUG METABOLISM

The lipid solubility of many of the drugs in common use renders them incapable of excretion by the kidney because of back diffusion in the tubules. Elimination of such drugs therefore requires hepatic biotransformation to render them more polar, less lipid-soluble and therefore more readily excretable. The metabolic processes involved are conveniently divisible into two categories: Phase I (oxidation, reduction, hydrolysis) and Phase II (conjugation). Some of the more important processes involved are summarised as follows:

Oxidation

Oxidising or hydroxylating enzymes are responsible for the degradation and inactivation of many drugs. The processes, which require triphosphopyridine nucleotide and oxygen, may involve oxidation, dealkylation, deamination, ring or side-chain hydroxylation and sulphoxide formation. Drugs which are affected by oxidative reactions include barbiturates and thiobarbiturates, ethanol, phenothiazines, sympathomimetic and other amines, analgesics and antidepressants.

Reduction

Reduction is important for only a small number of drugs and the alcoholic products which result are usually further oxidised, often quite rapidly. Adrenaline and noradrenaline are partly excreted as reduced products (phenylglycols) and chloral derivatives are reduced to yield the active metabolite trichloroethanol.

Hydrolysis

Hydrolytic splitting is responsible for the destruction of a number of compounds such as cardiac glycosides, anthracene purgatives, procaine and choline esters. Drugs such as propanidid and suxamethonium are hydrolysed by cholinesterase in the plasma as well as in the liver.

Conjugation

Synthetic processes in the liver are responsible for the formation of conjugates, particularly glucuronides and sulphates. Catecholamines, phenols, steroids, chloral derivatives and tribromethanol are all partly excreted in this form. Aromatic acids may be conjugated with glycine and some amines such as sulphonamides and histamine by acetylation.

Because of their reduced lipid solubility, most drug metabolites are not only more readily eliminated but also less potent than their parent compounds. Potency may, however, be only partly lost in any one metabolic stage and total inactivation thus often depends on more than one stage. For example, heroin (diacetylmorphine) is degraded partly to morphine which has approximately half the potency. Thiobarbiturates are converted in part to their equivalent oxybarbiturates with similar result. In some cases metabolism activates the drug with the opposite effect that the metabolite is more potent than its precursor. Thus diazepam is converted into at least three active metabolites, one of which (N-desmethyldiazepam) is so slowly eliminated that it exerts much more effect than diazepam itself.

The metabolism of drugs in the liver occurs largely by microsomal enzymes which are located in the smooth-surfaced endoplasmic reticulum. Liver damage induced by acute or chronic disease suppresses the activity of these enzymes and induces intolerance to drugs which are normally inactivated by them. Thus patients with cirrhosis or some impairment of liver function may show exaggerated and prolonged effects to compounds like ethanol, barbiturates and opiates.

Microsomal enzymes can also be affected by drugs. Administration of the experimental compound SKF 525A or of monoamine oxidase inhibitors inhibits the enzymes so that drug metabolism is slowed. Thus monoamine oxidase inhibitors render the patient intolerant not only of sympathomimetic amines which are metabolised by monoamine oxidase but also of drugs which are degraded in microsomes, amphetamine, pethidine*, ethanol, phenothiazines and most hypnotics. Drugs can also have the opposite effect.

Administration of barbiturates, phenytoin, glutethimide, dichloralphenazone and some other compounds cause enzyme induction; there is proliferation of the endoplasmic reticulum, increased enzyme formation and resultant accelerated drug metabolism. Patients under this influence become tolerant of drugs which are metabolised by these enzymes. Pharmacological aspects have been reviewed by Conney (1967) and clinical aspects by Burns and Conney (1965) and Prescott (1969).

The clinical implications of enzyme induction are still under investigation. In many instances a two- or three-fold increase in drug metabolism is probably of little consequence. In two fields, however, important interactions can result with unfortunate effects if the patient stops taking the inducing drug (e.g. a barbiturate). The two fields concern the use of coumarin anticoagulants and oral hypoglycaemic agents, most of which are inactivated by microsomal enzymes. The danger is likely to arise in patients who are stabilised on these drugs while taking enzyme-inducing agents and who stop taking the inducer at a later date while continuing on the same daily dosage of the anticoagulant or hypoglycaemic. The induction wears off in about 2–3 weeks and the original dosage of anticoagulant or hypoglycaemic agent becomes too great. Enzyme induction by phenobarbitone has recently been employed successfully to lower serum bilirubin concentrations in the newborn (Trolle, 1968).

EXCRETION

Drugs and their metabolites are excreted from the body largely by the kidney. Some compounds, however, appear in the faeces, either because they are incompletely absorbed after oral administration or because they are excreted into the intestine via the bile. The purgative phenolphthalein and many antibiotics are re-cycled in this way with resultant prolongation of their actions. Some ions such as bromides, iodides and lithium are also secreted by mucous membranes and by sweat glands.

Disposal by the kidney depends on a balance of three processes:

Glomerular Filtration

A drug free in solution in plasma enters the renal tubular lumen by filtration,

* Monoamine oxidase inhibitors are further discussed in Chapter 23.

whilst a protein-bound drug is retained unless albuminuria is present. The glomerular filtrate therefore contains drug or metabolite at the same concentration as is present free in the plasma.

Tubular Reabsorption

During its passage down the tubule, the filtrate is reduced in volume by the removal of sodium, chloride and water, so that drug or metabolite concentration increases progressively to a very high level. Under the concentration gradient thus established between tubular fluid and blood stream the drug may then diffuse passively back into the circulation, limiting its excretion. Only non-ionised drug can cross the tubular cell membrane, however, with the result that the reabsorption of weak acids and bases is strongly pH dependent. This provides the basis for alteration of the urinary pH in cases of drug poisoning. In poisoning by weak acids like barbiturates and salicylates, alkalinisation of the urine with citrates or bicarbonate increases ionisation, limits reabsorption and therefore increases their excretion in the urine; the same effect is produced in poisoning by weak bases such as amphetamines and phenothiazines by acidification of the urine with ammonium chloride. The effectiveness of such manoeuvres is dependent on effective increases in the ionised fraction of the drugs in the urine. Drugs which are totally ionised, even at the extremes of urinary pH, are not reabsorbed at all. Thus drugs such as decamethonium and neostigmine, which are quaternary ammonium compounds and fully ionised, are relatively rapidly eliminated by the kidney.

Tubular reabsorption is diminished if the flow of urine is increased because tubular fluid becomes concentrated to a lesser degree and the drug gradient across the tubular cell membrane is reduced. Thus forced diuresis increases the elimination of many drugs in proportion to the urine flow.

Tubular Secretion

A number of compounds, mostly organic acids, are actively secreted by the tubular cells into the urine. The elimination of such compounds such as penicillins and sulphonamides is thereby accelerated. A few weak bases are also secreted actively but it is doubtful whether the process is important quantitatively.

Tubular secretion is susceptible to inhibition by drugs. Thus probenecid which antagonises the secretion of organic acids has been used to delay the elimination of penicillins. Probenecid, salicylates and phenylbutazone also antagonise active tubular reabsorption of urates; hence their use in the treatment of gout.

The elimination of drugs by the kidney is retarded in renal insufficiency, largely because of the reduced glomerular filtration rate. Though this is not usually of clinical significance, with a few drugs it is important if they are liable to produce toxic effects at only moderately increased blood concentrations. Such drugs as streptomycin and kanamycin may accumulate in these circumstances to produce labyrinthine and auditory damage. Monitoring blood concentrations provides the only safeguard.

VARIATIONS IN RESPONSE

Healthy normal individuals vary in their response to drugs. This variation is quantitative and sometimes qualitative. It can occur because of differences in receptor sensitivity or because of variations in drug metabolism. It is at least partly under genetic control though how much this affects the clinical situation is not clear. Pharmacogenetics is the subject of a monograph by Kalow (1962), and variability in drug response of a recent review (Smith and Rawlins, 1973).

Some response variations due to differences in receptor sensitivity are known. Thus people with blue eyes are more sensitive to the local actions of sympathomimetic amines than are people with brown eyes. Paxson (1932) recorded similar variations in sensitivity by measuring the dose of sodium amylobarbitone needed in the presence of nitrous oxide to induce suitable anaesthetic conditions for forceps delivery. His results are illustrated as a frequency distribution of doses in Fig. 8. The subjects' requirements varied about 4-fold. A qualitative variation in response to drugs is shown by the reactions to barbiturates of patients with porphyria.

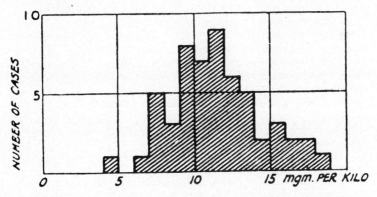

21/Fig. 8.—Frequency distribution of dose of sodium amylobarbitone needed to induce suitable anaesthetic conditions for forceps delivery in 55 subjects (Paxson, 1932).

Much interest has centred recently on genetically-determined individual variations in drug metabolism. For the anaesthetist the most important of these are the variations in suxamethonium metabolism caused by atypical varieties of plasma cholinesterase (see Chapter 26). These varieties are determined by the presence or absence of particular genes. Similar factors affect the metabolism of isoniazid and sulphadimidine by acetylation in the liver. The rate of drug metabolism is also affected by multiple genes which influence the quantity of enzyme present. Information derived from twin studies has shown that inheritance greatly influences the half-lives of dicoumarol, antipyrine and phenylbutazone (Vesell and Page, 1968) and steady-state blood concentrations of nortriptyline (Alexanderson et al., 1969). Inheritance, therefore, appears to play an important part in determining rates of drug inactivation. It remains to be seen whether receptor sensitivity is similarly affected.

REFERENCES

ALEXANDERSON, B., EVANS, D. A. P., and SJÖQVIST, F. (1969). Steady-state plasma levels of nortriptyline in twins: influence of genetic factors and drug therapy. *Brit. med. J.*, 4, 764.

ANDERSON, J., TOMLINSON, R. W. S., OSBORN, S. B., and WISE, M. E. (1967). Radio-calcium turnover in man. *Lancet*, 1, 930.

BECKETT, A. H., and TUCKER, G. T. (1968). Application of the analogue computer to pharmacokinetic and biopharmaceutical studies with amphetamine-type compounds. *J. Pharm. Pharmacol.*, 20, 174.

BELLEAU, B. (1963). An analysis of drug receptor interactions. *Proc. First International Pharmacological Meeting*, 7, 75.

BURNS, J. J., and CONNEY, A. H. (1965). Enzyme stimulation and inhibition in the metabolism of drugs. *Proc. roy. Soc. Med.*, 58, 955.

CHRISTENSEN, H. N. (1962). *Biological Transport*. New York: W. A. Benjamin.

CLARK, A. J. (1937). General pharmacology. In: *Heffter's Handbuch der experimentellen Pharmakologie*, Erg. Vol. 4. Ed. by Heubner, W. and Schüller, T. Berlin: Springer.

CONNEY, A. H. (1967). Pharmacological implications of microsomal enzyme induction. *Pharmacol. Rev.*, 19, 317.

EHRENPREIS, S., FLEISCH, J. H., and MITTAG, T. W. (1969). Approaches to the molecular nature of pharmacological receptors. *Pharmacol. Rev.*, 21, 131.

GIBALDI, M., LEVY, G., and HAYTON, W. (1972). Kinetics of the elimination and neuro-muscular blocking effect of *d*-tubocurarine in man. *Anesthesiology*, 36, 213.

GOLDBAUM, L. R., and SMITH, P. K. (1954). The interaction of barbiturates with serum albumin and its possible relation to their disposition and pharmacological actions. *J. Pharmacol. exp. Ther.*, 111, 197.

GOLDSTEIN, A. (1949). The interactions of drugs and plasma proteins. *Pharmacol. Rev.*, 1, 102.

IVERSEN, L. L. (1967). *The Uptake and Storage of Noradrenaline in Sympathetic Nerves*. London: Cambridge Univ. Press.

KALOW, W. (1962). *Pharmacogenetics: Heredity and the Response to Drugs*. Philadelphia: W. B. Saunders.

KANE, P. O., and SMITH, S. E. (1959). Thiopentone and buthalitone: the relationship between depth of anaesthesia, plasma concentration and plasma protein binding. *Brit. J. Pharmacol.*, 14, 261.

LOEWE, S. (1957). Antagonisms and antagonists. *Pharmacol. Rev.*, 9, 237.

MICHAELIS, L., and MENTEN, M. L. (1913). Die Kinetik des Invertinwirkung. *Biochem. Z.*, 49, 333.

PATON, W. D. M. (1960). The principles of drug action. *Proc. roy. Soc. Med.*, 53, 815.

PATON, W. D. M. (1961). A theory of drug action based on the rate of drug-receptor combination. *Proc. roy. Soc.*, B, 154, 21.

PAXSON, N. F. (1932). Obstetrical anesthesia and analgesia with sodium iso-amylethyl barbiturate and nitrous oxide oxygen: results in obstetrical practice. *Curr. Res. Anesth.*, 11, 116.

PORTER, R., and O'CONNOR, M., Eds. (1970). *Molecular Properties of Drug Receptors* (Ciba Foundation Symposium). London: J. & A. Churchill.

PRESCOTT, L. F. (1969). Pharmacokinetic drug interactions. *Lancet*, 2, 1239.

RANG, H. P., Ed. (1973). *Drug Receptors* (Biological Council Symposium). London: Macmillan.

SCHILD, H. O. (1947). pA, a new scale for the measurement of drug antagonism. *Brit. J. Pharmacol.*, 2, 189.

SMITH, S. E. (1969). Uptake of antimony potassium tartrate by mouse liver slices. *Brit. J. Pharmacol.*, 37, 476.

SMITH, S. E., and HERXHEIMER, A. (1969). Toxicity of ethanol-barbiturate mixtures. *J. Pharm. Pharmacol.*, **21,** 869.

SMITH, S. E., and RAWLINS, M. D. (1973). *Variability in Human Drug Response*. London: Butterworth & Co.

STACEY, R. S. (1961). Uptake of 5-hydroxytryptamine by platelets. *Brit. J. Pharmacol.*, **16,** 284.

STEPHENSON, R. P. (1956). A modification of receptor theory. *Brit. J. Pharmacol.*, **11,** 379.

TROLLE, D. (1968). Decrease of total serum-bilirubin concentration in newborn infants after phenobarbitone treatment. *Lancet*, **2,** 705.

VESELL, E. S., and PAGE, J. G. (1968). Genetic control of dicoumarol levels in man. *J. clin. Invest.*, **47,** 2657.

WASER, P. (1961). Chemistry and pharmacology of muscarine, muscarone and some related compounds. *Pharmacol. Rev.*, **13,** 465.

WIEGAND, R. G., and SANDERS, P. G. (1964). Calculation of kinetic constants from blood levels of drugs. *J. Pharmacol. exp. Ther.*, **146,** 271.

Chapter 22

SEDATIVE AND HYPNOTIC DRUGS AND INTRAVENOUS ANAESTHETICS

NORMAL SLEEP

ALTHOUGH sleep is a well-known phenomenon which is easy to define in broad terms, its scientific explanation is difficult. It is associated with a number of changes in body function: a reduction in awareness culminating in unconsciousness, progressive relaxation of body musculature, slight hypotension, bradycardia and reduction of the metabolic rate. The exact origin of sleep in the brain is not fully understood but probably arises in an integrated system involving ascending and descending pathways in the reticular formation, the cerebral cortex, intralaminary nuclei of the thalamus, caudate nucleus, posterior hypothalamus and anterior third of the pons. There appears to be no sleep centre as such, though electrical stimulation of certain parts of the reticular formation induces sleep in animals.

Different depths of sleep can be distinguished by the ease or difficulty with which the subject can be awakened and these have been correlated with electroencephalographic changes (Loomis *et al.*, 1938). Five levels were distinguished: from A (drowsiness) to E (deep sleep). The deepest level occurs only for brief periods, usually early in the night. These types of sleep are referred to as orthodox or "slow wave" sleep. The normal person spends approximately one-quarter of the night in paradoxical or "rapid eye movement" (REM) sleep, this type being characterised by fast cortical electrical activity, greater reductions in skeletal muscle tone and rapid movement of the eyes. REM sleep is associated with dreaming (Aserinsky and Kleitman, 1953). The time spent in the various depths of sleep varies with age. In older people sleep is frequently broken by periods of wakefulness (Březinová, 1975).

Total deprivation of sleep for 100 hours or more induces psychotic changes, sometimes involving hallucinations and delusions. Specific deprivation of REM sleep for much shorter periods induces anxiety and irritability, difficulties with memory and coordination and increased appetite (Dement and Fisher, 1963). Such deprivation is followed by compensatory increases of REM sleep during the following nights (Dement and Fisher, 1963).

The Effects of Drugs on Sleep

Hypnotic and anaesthetic agents induce sleep by mechanisms which are as yet poorly understood but which probably involve suppression of both cortical and subcortical activity. Progressive anaesthesia is associated with widespread inhibition, manifest by the absence of neuronal discharge. Electroencephalographic patterns change with the depth of anaesthesia (see Chapter 29). During deep anaesthesia REM periods are absent, but in light anaesthesia they are often present and dreaming is common. The content of such dreams is usually highly emotional and often of a sexual nature, the latter being one reason why a chaperone is so essential when minor operations are being performed under solely gaseous anaesthetics.

All the commonly employed hypnotic agents (barbiturates, meprobamate, methaqualone and benzodiazepines) lessen the incidence and shorten the periods of REM sleep (Oswald, 1968), thus prolonging periods of orthodox sleep. With repeated administration recovery of REM sleep occurs, after which withdrawal of the drug precipitates massive compensatory increases of REM periods. Such observations probably explain why patients so often complain of sleeping badly the first night or two after stopping treatment with hypnotics and why so many become habituated to such drugs. Antidepressant drugs and narcotics usually have similar effects but major tranquillisers like reserpine and phenothiazine derivatives may increase REM sleep and shorten the latent period before its onset. Of particular interest are some findings that these and other drugs may influence dream content as well as duration (Kramer *et al.*, 1966). In elderly subjects hot drinks last thing at night tend to improve sleep (Březinová and Oswald, 1972), an effect which is unlikely to be due entirely to suggestion (Adam *et al.*, 1976).

SEDATIVES AND HYPNOTICS

A sedative is a remedy that allays excitement, an hypnotic a drug that induces sleep: neither of these groups of drugs has any direct effect on the sensation of pain. When administered to a patient in pain they may, by depression of inhibitions, produce restlessness and make management more difficult. Pain can be controlled by the analgesics, or by the narcotics which produces sleep as well as relieving pain. Since most of these drugs have different effects depending upon dosage, it is not possible to classify them too rigidly. For instance, most hypnotic drugs will produce sedation when administered in small enough doses; but the converse does not necessarily apply, as a sedative may produce side-effects before the dose level required to produce sleep is reached.

FACTORS AFFECTING THE RESPONSE TO SEDATIVE DRUGS

The response to a given dose of a sedative drug varies within wide limits which depend in the main on the state of the patient. When prescribing a sedative an appreciation must be made of the desired effect and of the condition of the patient—this is often difficult to assess accurately. A consideration of the following points will help to obviate the risk of gross over- or under-dosage.

The degree of sedation required varies between the production of calmness and a sleep at least deep enough so that the patient has no recollection of leaving the ward or the prick of an intravenous needle. Anaesthesia may also be produced with sedative drugs.

The condition of the patient depends not only on measurable quantities such as age and weight, but also on factors such as muscularity, obesity, general fitness and previous medication with alcohol or narcotics.

There is doubt as to whether the sedatives and narcotics do actually depress the basal metabolic rate but reflex irritability varies in proportion to metabolism, so that consideration of the changes in metabolic rate is a guide to the likely effect of a given dose of sedative.

The effect of age.—The metabolic rate, which is low at birth, rises sharply until the sixth year. It then falls, and after a rise at puberty, it is back to the same value in the twentieth year as it was at the end of the first year of life. Thereafter the metabolic rate steadily declines until in old age it has returned to the same figure as in the first few weeks of life.

The effect of body weight.—Where precision of effect is required, the doses of drugs are best related to the weight of the patient, before making the necessary adjustments for the other factors. But here again allowance must be made, and the dose reduced for excess fat—or water as in patients with ascites and oedema—or increased for patients who are unusually muscular.

The effect of emotion.—The state of reflex irritability depends mainly on the emotional condition of the patient. A placid individual needs less in the way of sedatives than one in whom the nervous system is in a state of hyperactivity.

The effect of metabolic diseases.—Where the basal metabolic rate is altered by a disease such as hyperthyroidism, the action of a given dose of sedative is likely to be less evident and of briefer duration than in a normal subject. Conversely where the metabolic rate is depressed the action of sedatives is profound and prolonged.

The effect of previous medication with alcohol or narcotics.—Long-continued use of these agents produces tolerance to the psychic effects of sedatives, and larger doses may be required; but due to possible disturbances of metabolism already existing—particularly in the liver—sedatives may have a prolonged action and any depression of respiration and the circulation, which are the most important side-effects of these drugs, may be accentuated. In these circumstances a small dose given in plenty of time, so that the position can be reassessed and a further dose given if required, is the best policy.

The effect of the presence of pain.—Since drugs of this group have few if any analgesic properties, they should not be given to those who are in pain, because by removing the higher cortical functions they tend to allow the patient to over-react and produce restlessness. This may then be difficult to control with analgesics or narcotics without producing dangerous depression. The addition of a simple analgesic such as acetylsalicylic acid to a sedative will often make all the difference, and avoid the need for a narcotic. When long-acting sedatives are required pre-operatively it is important that they should be given early enough to allow most of their effect to wear off by the end of the operation, in order to avoid restlessness later.

The general fitness of the patient.—This is the most difficult factor to assess, especially for the inexperienced, and yet is the most vital because in those who are ill the margin of safety is narrow and the required dose may be extremely small. In all cases of doubt as to the fitness of the patient caution must be exercised. A dose which is thought to be too small is first given and when this has had time to act, which will vary with the drug and the route of administration, an assessment of the effect produced can be made and a further dose of the same or another drug added. Small repeated doses are safer than large doses at longer time-intervals. Patients who are ill frequently require very small quantities of a sedative to produce sleep, and these patients, who are least able to withstand any added insults, can all too easily have their respiration or circulation grossly depressed. It is often wiser not to use any pre-operative sedatives in the very ill, thus avoiding relative overdosage. Relative overdosage can cause respiratory depression which in turn allows respiratory obstruction to occur easily, and this may pass quietly into respiratory failure.

CLASSIFICATION OF SEDATIVE AND HYPNOTIC DRUGS

These drugs may be classified into four main groups:
1. Ethane derivatives.
    Paraldehyde.
    Ethyl alcohol.
    Chloral hydrate and derivatives.
    Bromethol.
2. Barbiturates.
3. Non-barbiturate hypnotics and sedatives.
4. Tranquillisers (see Chapter 23).

Many non-barbiturate hypnotics are used as tranquillisers, and some tranquillisers as hypnotics or sedatives. The distinction between the two is largely inappropriate.

ETHANE DERIVATIVES

Paraldehyde ($CH_3CHO)_3$

Paraldehyde was discovered by Wiedenbusch in 1829 and introduced into medicine by Cervello in 1882. It is a colourless, inflammable liquid, boiling point 122° C, with a pungent odour and an unpleasant burning taste. The solubility in water is only one part in eight at 25° C but it is very soluble in lipoid solvents.

Paraldehyde decomposes in the presence of light, air or acids to acetaldehyde, and should therefore be kept in dark, well-stoppered bottles.

Pharmacological actions.—Paraldehyde is a mild hypnotic, but occasionally produces excitation. Habituation may follow its use but is very infrequent.

It has a wide margin of safety and produces sleep in ten to fifteen minutes after the administration of the usual oral dose of 2 to 8 ml.

Paraldehyde produces similar changes to the barbiturates in the EEG of resting man. In therapeutic doses it does not cause cardiac or respiratory depression, but with gross overdosage it may cause death from respiratory failure and cardiovascular depression.

The metabolic fate of paraldehyde in man is not definitely known, but in patients with liver disease the duration of hypnosis is greatly prolonged, and it is thought that about 80 per cent of the paraldehyde administered is destroyed in the liver, the rest being excreted by the lungs unchanged. Soon after a dose has been given, paraldehyde can be smelt in the breath, where its continued excretion can be discerned for many hours. This smell is unnoticed by the patient. A trace is excreted by the kidneys in man, but bilateral nephrectomy in animals does not alter the duration of hypnosis.

Clinical uses.—Paraldehyde can be administered by mouth, by rectum, and by intramuscular or intravenous injection. It is rapidly absorbed and produces sleep lasting six to eight hours, within ten to fifteen minutes of its administration.

By mouth the dose is 2 to 8 ml which is administered in the proportion of 4 ml to 40 ml of water—at which strength it is completely soluble—to avoid the burning taste and gastric irritation.

By rectum it is administered in a dose of 0·5 ml/kg body weight to a maximum of 40 ml, diluted with ten times its volume of physiological saline.

By intramuscular injection the dose is 2 to 8 ml. Paraldehyde is self-sterilising so that it can be drawn straight from the bottle before injection. The dose by intravenous injection is from 2 to 8 ml. This should be given slowly to avoid a coughing spasm, but should one occur, the rate of injection must be further slowed when the spasm will soon pass. The duration of hypnosis following intravenous administration of paraldehyde is not prolonged, and there is little or no depression of respiration or of the circulation.

The advantages of paraldehyde are its safety and the absence of cardiac or respiratory depression, which make it particularly useful in the elderly. Its disadvantages are its taste, gastric irritation, and its excretion in the breath, although this is not complained of by the patient. It is particularly useful in controlling manic states and post-operatively where sleep is required without depression, as in neurosurgery.

Ethanol (Ethyl Alcohol) (C_2H_5OH)

Alcohol is a substance of more social than medical value, although a "nightcap" is a very useful hypnotic for the elderly. Its interest to the anaesthetist lies in its history and in its value for dealing with patients who are used to large quantities of it and who are therefore likely to be tolerant to the anaesthetic drugs. Alcohol was one of the first substances used to relieve pain: the giving of spirits in large quantities to patients prior to operations before 1847 is well-known. Although it may well have produced amnesia, the patients required to be restrained, since they were usually still in the so-called "excitement stage" of anaesthesia.

When a patient who is tolerant to alcohol has his normal quota withheld prior to anaesthesia, he may well be resistant, particularly when only nitrous oxide is available, as may be the case in the out-patient department. For such a person, the usual amount of alcohol, or even a little more—provided it can be given sufficiently far ahead to avoid the danger of aspiration from vomiting—may be helpful prior to anaesthesia. Induction of anaesthesia by intravenous ethanol has been reported but it is dangerous because of respiratory and circulatory depression.

Alcohol can be used as a sedative and source of calories by giving it well diluted intravenously, 1 g of alcohol liberating approximately 7 calories. Fifty ml of pure 95 per cent ethyl alcohol should be added to 1 litre of saline, or 5 per cent dextrose in water, and administered at a rate of not more than 60 drops per minute. It is oxidised at a constant rate of 10 ml per hour, so that once the required state has been produced the rate of infusion should not exceed this figure. This procedure is particularly useful in the aged (see also Chapter 19).

Chloral Hydrate ($CCl_3 . CH(OH)_2$)

Chloral hydrate was first prepared by Liebig in 1832 and introduced as a hypnotic by Liebreich in 1869. It is a colourless non-deliquescent crystalline substance with a pungent odour and a strongly bitter taste. It is freely soluble in water.

Pharmacological actions.—Chloral hydrate is a sedative and hypnotic. In the usual dosage—0·7 to 2 g—sedation occurs in ten to fifteen minutes and is followed by sleep in about half an hour. The sleep is quiet and deep, but the patient can be easily aroused, and it lasts five to eight hours. Usually there are no after-effects and "hangover" is rarely seen. The EEG in resting man is depressed in a manner similar to that produced by the barbiturates, but in a less pronounced way.

Larger doses cause a prolonged and deeper sleep and may suppress pain. With doses of 6 g or more, complete anaesthesia may occur, and with it dangerous respiratory depression.

With the usual hypnotic doses little more depression of respiration or the blood pressure occurs than in normal sleep. Cardiac depression is not seen with normal doses but does occur with large ones.

Chloral hydrate is rapidly absorbed from the gastro-intestinal tract but it is irritant to the stomach. It is mainly reduced to trichloroethanol, which is responsible for its hypnotic effect. Some of this substance is then combined in the liver with glucuronic acid to form trichloroethanol glucuronide (urochloralic acid) which is not a hypnotic. Trichloroethanol glucuronide is then excreted in the urine. In solution this reduces alkaline copper and therefore when in excess can be mistaken for glucose.

Clinical use.—Chloral hydrate is given in a dose of 0·3 to 2 g well diluted and with a suitable flavouring such as orange, to avoid gastric irritation and to mask the bitter taste. It is a non-cumulative, safe, and useful hypnotic and should be used more often than it is, especially when depression of respiration and a "hangover" effect are contra-indicated. In view of its long action, should chloral hydrate be used for premedication it must be given at least two hours before operation. Penhearow (1957) recommends the use of chloral hydrate as a pre-operative sedative for children. He gives approximately 50 mg/kg body weight.

Other preparations of chloral hydrate, its complexes or derivatives, are available. They have less gastric irritant effect and are therefore preferable for routine use (King *et al.*, 1958), particularly in elderly patients (Exton-Smith *et al.*, 1963). The most important of these are:

Approved name	Trade name	Tablet size
chloral betaine	Somilan	0·87 g
dichloralphenazone	Welldorm	0·15 g, 0·6 g
triclofos	Tricloryl	0·5 g

These and other compounds such as chloralformamide, chlorhexadol, penthrichloral and petrichloral are all metabolised in the intestine and liver to form trichloroethanol, on which their hypnotic action depends.

Bromethol (Tribromethanol; Avertin) (CBr_3CH_2OH)

Bromethol was discovered by Eicholtz in 1917 and first employed clinically by Butzengeiger (1927). It is a white crystalline powder with a slight aromatic odour and taste. It melts at 80° C. It is sparingly soluble in water (1 part in 35) but very soluble in amylene hydrate. It is unstable and is decomposed by heat, light and air to hydrobromic acid and dibromacetaldehyde. It is therefore supplied in dark bottles as a solution of 1 g bromethol in 1 ml amylene hydrate. The latter has weak hypnotic properties of its own.

Pharmacological actions.—Following the rectal administration of an adequate dose of bromethol, sleep occurs in five to fifteen minutes. Excitement is never seen. The maximal effect occurs in from twenty to thirty minutes and the patient wakes up in from one and a half to three hours when the blood concentration has fallen to 20–30 µg/ml. Skeletal muscular relaxation is only partial with safe doses.

Bromethol usually causes a fall of blood pressure varying from 15 to 40 mm Hg (2·0–5·3 kPa) lasting five to fifteen minutes, but in patients with hypertension the fall may be marked. It is caused mainly by depression of the vasomotor centre and partly by a direct action on the myocardium and blood vessels. The direct depressant action on the myocardium is negligible with normal dose levels. ECG changes are minor. Respiration is depressed, the tidal and minute volumes being decreased by about 20 per cent of normal.

The rate of absorption of bromethol from the rectum is very variable; usually 50 per cent of the dose is absorbed in the first ten minutes, and 95 per cent after 25 minutes. On reaching the liver the drug combines with glucuronic acid to form tribromethanol glucuronide (urobromalic acid). This substance is excreted by the kidneys in about 2 hours. Since bromethol may aggravate hepatic and renal disease, it is contra-indicated when they are present.

Method of administration and dosage.—Bromethol is administered by rectum. A cleansing enema should have been given the previous night and a freshly prepared solution is run in slowly, taking three to five minutes, about thirty minutes before the time of operation. The patient should be placed in a slight head-down tilt to aid retention of the fluid in the rectum. In children the buttocks should also be strapped or held firmly in apposition for a few minutes to prevent leakage.

The dose is calculated according to the patient's weight, the amount per kg being adjusted in relation to the state of the patient. The normal dose is 100 mg/kg but for a particularly robust and healthy young adult or a thyrotoxic patient 110–120 mg/kg may be required, while for the obese and sick the dose should be reduced to 60 mg/kg. Children are more tolerant of the effect of the drug and so they should be given a dose of 110–120 mg/kg. The dose so calculated is dissolved in approximately 40 times its volume of physiological saline which has been heated to 40° C—above 40° C tribromoethyl alcohol is decomposed—and shaken vigorously. The pH of the solution is tested with Congo Red; if a blue or violet colour appears the solution contains hydrobromic acid, showing that decomposition has occurred, and must not be used.

Clinical uses.—There are nowadays few indications for the administration of bromethol in clinical anaesthesia, but the drug is occasionally used for the treatment of eclampsia.

BARBITURATES

Barbituric acid was first synthesised by Conrad and Guthzeit in 1882. The 5:5′-diethyl derivative was introduced into medicine as a hypnotic by Carl Fischer and von Mering. Since this time innumerable derivatives have been synthesised and many have been introduced into medicine as hypnotics or anti-convulsants.

Structure-activity Relationships

Barbiturates are formed by three types of substitution on the parent molecule of barbituric acid. To a great extent the presence of substituents in particular parts of the molecule is associated with predictable effects on pharmacological activity. Nevertheless, there are some unexplained anomalies, such as the fact that 5 ethyl 5′ (1-3-dimethylbutyl) barbituric acid is a convulsant (Swanson, 1934) and the closely related compound 5 ethyl 5′ (1-methyl butyl) barbituric acid (pentobarbitone) is a hypnotic.

The principal variants can be enumerated as follows:

1. Substitute organic radicals for the hydrogen atoms attached to the number 5 carbon atom.

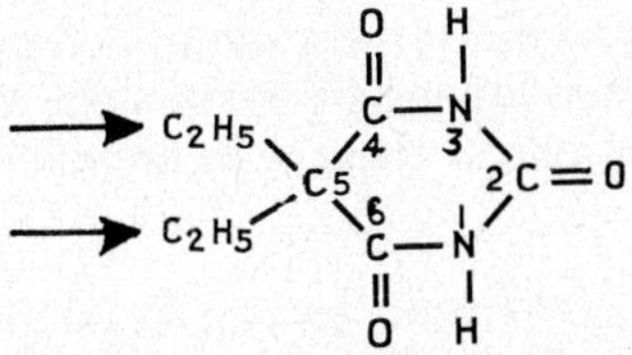

$$
\longrightarrow C_2H_5 \quad
\begin{array}{c}
O \quad H \\
\parallel \quad | \\
C-N \\
/4 \quad 3 \\
C5 \qquad 2\,C=O \\
\backslash 6 \quad | / \\
C-N \\
\parallel \quad | \\
O \quad H
\end{array}
$$

$\longrightarrow C_2H_5$

Diethyl barbituric acid

2. Substitute an alkyl radical for the hydrogen atom which is attached to the number 1 nitrogen atom, a process which makes the molecule asymmetric.

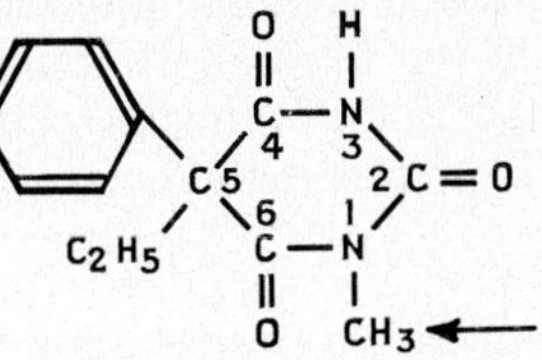

$$
\begin{array}{c}
O \quad H \\
\parallel \quad | \\
C-N \\
/4 \quad 3 \\
C5 \qquad 2\,C=O \\
\backslash 6 \quad | / \\
C-N \\
\parallel \quad | \\
O \quad CH_3
\end{array}
$$

C_2H_5 ; $CH_3 \longleftarrow$

Methyl phenobarbitone

3. Substitute a sulphur atom for the oxygen atom attached to the number 2 carbon atom.

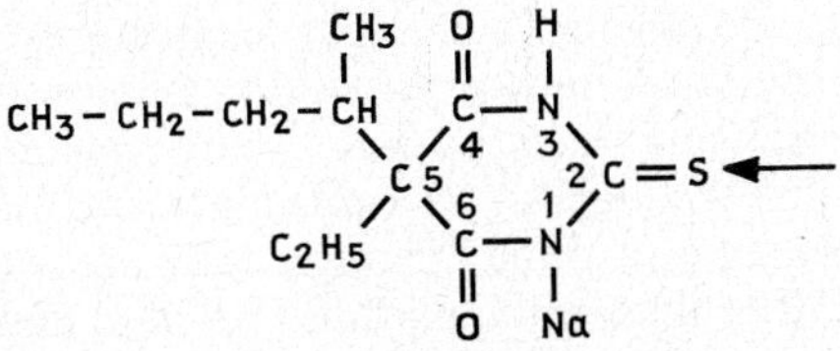

$$
CH_3-CH_2-CH_2-CH
\begin{array}{c}
CH_3 \\
| \\
\\
\end{array}
\quad
\begin{array}{c}
O \quad H \\
\parallel \quad | \\
C-N \\
/4 \quad 3 \\
C5 \qquad 2\,C=S \longleftarrow \\
\backslash 6 \quad | / \\
C-N \\
\parallel \quad | \\
O \quad N\alpha
\end{array}
$$

C_2H_5

Thiopentone

If the number of carbon atoms in the substituting groups on the number 5 position is increased, the potency is increased, and this reaches a maximum when there are seven or eight carbon atoms. Beyond this, toxicity increases out of proportion to potency. Branching or unsaturated chains lead to a further increase in potency.

The addition of certain radicals makes the derivative inactive as a hypnotic, and the presence of an aromatic nucleus in an alkyl group which is directly attached to the number 5 carbon atom produces compounds with convulsant properties. Direct substitution with a phenyl group confers anticonvulsant activity.

Substitution at the number 1 nitrogen atom by a methyl group leads to increased activity and shortened duration of action with enhanced anticonvulsant properties. Alkyl groups with more carbon atoms produce convulsant properties. Replacement of the oxygen attached to the number 2 carbon atom by a sulphur atom forms thiobarbiturates with increased solubility in lipids, and results in compounds which have a very short duration of action.

Barbituric acid and its derivatives are weak acids and therefore form salts with the alkali metals. Solutions of these salts are alkaline and decompose on keeping.

Pharmacological Actions of the Barbiturate Drugs

Traditionally, barbiturates have usually been classified according to their duration of action, but this system, originally proposed on the basis of animal experiments, does not apply in man when they are used as hypnotics and administered orally (Hinton, 1961; Parsons, 1963). Indeed the duration of action of any one drug is conditioned by the patient's reaction to it rather than by its chemical structure. Although there are individual differences between many of the barbiturate drugs, all except the ultra short-acting ones, as typified by thiopentone, are discussed together in the following sections. Thiopentone and other similar drugs are discussed in greater detail in a separate section (p. 759 *et seq.*).

Central Nervous System

All the sedative barbiturates produce a similar pattern of depression of the nervous system, the extent of which largely depends upon the level of excitability of the patient's nervous system. By choosing a suitable barbiturate, dose and route of administration, any effect can be obtained from mild sedation to deep coma.

Site and mode of action.—The cerebral cortex and the reticular activating system are most sensitive to the barbiturates, the cerebellar, vestibular and spinal systems less so, and the medullary systems least of all. The circulatory and respiratory centres are affected by high concentrations of the barbiturates, but not the vomiting centre. A number of studies using radioisotope methods indicate that the less lipid soluble barbiturates, barbitone and phenobarbitone, are uniformly distributed throughout the central nervous system (Maynert and Van Dyke, 1950; Domek *et al.*, 1960), though early after administration grey matter contains more drug than white matter. Hubbard and Goldbaum (1950) found that thiopentone tends to accumulate in the thalamus and cerebral cortex.

The mechanism of action of barbiturates is unknown and many of the biochemical effects observed may be the result rather than the cause of their general depressant action. Cerebral cell membranes are stabilised, elevation of excitatory threshold occurring. Recovery from excitation is also prolonged. Barbiturates produce metabolic effects *in vitro* (Aldridge, 1962), inhibiting oxidative phosphorylation and activating adenosine triphosphatase. The active concentrations are similar to concentrations found in the brains of barbiturate-treated animals, suggesting that these effects may be exerted *in vivo*. The link between these observations and the hypnotic action, however, remains obscure.

Hypnotic effect.—This varies from mild impairment of performance of simple tasks to sleep. Depression of the cortex produces impairment of function and with high enough dosage sleep occurs in from twenty to sixty minutes. This sleep is usually dreamless. After awakening, depression of function can still be detected for some hours and the EEG does not return to normal for up to 48 hours. Goodnow and his colleagues (1951) showed that there was altered function up to 14 hours after 100 mg pentobarbitone by mouth. Following some of the barbiturates, these effects are felt by the patient as a "hangover," but Hinton (1961) found that this also occurred after placebo medication.

Analgesic effect.—Unlike analgesic drugs such as the opium derivatives or the salicylates, the barbiturates do not have much effect on the pain threshold except in doses which affect the level of consciousness. Beecher (1951) and Keats and Beecher (1950) have shown that post-operative pain is relieved in 50 per cent of cases with an intravenous injection of 60 to 90 mg of pentobarbitone sodium, in 20 per cent by a placebo, and in 80 per cent by 8 mg of morphine. But in the presence of severe pain it is found that barbiturates have an anti-analgesic action, making the patient restless and difficult to manage, as the control exercised by the higher centres is diminished. This is seen when children who have had heavy premedication with barbiturates—so that psychic trauma is lessened—become restless and difficult to manage post-operatively. When barbiturates are combined with analgesic drugs such as salicylates or codeine, the combination is found to be more effective than the analgesic alone, but the analgesic does not enhance the hypnotic activity of the barbiturate in the absence of pain. There are many such combinations available commercially.

Anticonvulsant effect.—In anaesthetic doses all the sedative barbiturates are capable of inhibiting convulsions to some extent, such as those of tetanus, eclampsia, and epilepsy. Phenobarbitone has a specific anticonvulsant action not found in the others, which is clinically useful in treating epilepsy, particularly grand mal.

Anaesthetic effect.—If large enough doses of barbiturates are given, anaesthesia is produced, the pattern following roughly that seen with the volatile anaesthetics, but as there is no preliminary period of apparent stimulation (*cf* ether) all the vital functions are depressed. The effect on respiration is particularly marked.

The actions of the barbiturates on the brain and spinal cord differ from those produced by the volatile anaesthetics. Barbiturates inhibit spontaneous cortical activity whilst leaving the cortex accessible to afferent stimuli. Ether, however, prevents these afferent stimuli from reaching the cortex. The intrathecal injection of the barbiturates in man causes spinal anaesthesia. The motor paralysis is incomplete and there are troublesome side-effects. These drugs are therefore not suitable for this purpose. In very large doses barbiturates affect peripheral nerves, as they do nerve cells. They increase the threshold for electrical excitation, prolong the absolute and relative refractory periods, and reduce the action potential spike.

The transmission of impulses at sympathetic ganglia is depressed by small doses of barbiturates in cats (Exley, 1954). The most active drugs are butobarbitone and amylobarbitone: the least active are the thiobarbiturates.

Respiratory System

Barbiturates depress respiration by a direct action on the medullary respiratory centre. The depression is proportional to the dose of the barbiturate. The sedation and lessened muscular activity accounts for part of this fall in respiratory minute volume which is mainly brought about by a decreased amplitude of respiration. Cyclobarbitone in a dose of 600 mg does not depress the response to carbon dioxide below that which occurs in normal sleep, but does depress the response to hypoxia (Harris and Slawson, 1965). Very large doses of barbiturates produce marked respiratory depression—indeed respiratory failure is the usual cause of death from barbiturate poisoning.

Cardiovascular System

Ordinary oral hypnotic doses of the barbiturates have little effect on the circulation. The sedation they produce may cause a slight lowering of the blood pressure and/or pulse rate. Intravenous use of the barbiturates may cause a fall in blood pressure due to depression of the vasomotor centre with consequent peripheral vasodilatation. Large doses of barbiturates affect directly the small blood vessels causing dilatation and increased capillary permeability. Thiopentone is intermediate in this respect between ether and cyclopropane. Barbiturates do not appear to depress the myocardium in man, although Prime and Gray (1952) showed that thiopentone had a markedly depressant effect on the heart-lung preparation of the dog. Barbiturates do not affect cardiac rhythm or sensitise the heart to the effects of adrenaline. They may even protect the heart against dysrhythmias produced by such drugs as adrenaline or cyclopropane (Meek and Seevers, 1934; Robbins et al., 1939; Dance et al., 1956). The haemodynamic effects of short-acting barbiturates are the subject of a review (Conway and Ellis, 1969).

In dogs pentobarbitone has been shown to cause a striking leucopenia (20 per cent of the pre-anaesthetic figure) and to increase the coagulation time, while decreasing the prothrombin time (Graca and Garst, 1957). Megaloblastic anaemia has been reported in man due to the prolonged use of amylobarbitone and quinalbarbitone (Hobson et al., 1956).

Alimentary Tract

Barbiturates decrease the tone and amplitude of contractions of the gastro-intestinal tract. The mechanism is probably a direct action on the smooth muscle or on the intrinsic ganglionic plexus. Thiobarbiturates can increase intestinal tone. The gastric emptying time is little altered by hypnotic doses of the barbiturates but gastric secretion is depressed.

These findings are of little significance in clinical anaesthesia.

Kidneys

Barbiturates produce no renal damage but anaesthetic doses do temporarily alter renal function.

The urine volume is decreased owing to increased tubular reabsorption of water produced by increased secretion of the pituitary antidiuretic hormone. Any hypotension produced by the barbiturate together with renal vasoconstriction leads to a decreased glomerular filtration rate and renal plasma flow. If the hypotension is prolonged, severe oliguria or anuria may occur. An increase in the blood urea, even in the presence of normal kidneys, has been shown by Dundee and Richards (1954) to be associated with prolonged sleeping time, the extent of which can be correlated with the height of the blood urea. This may be of importance in cases of gastro-intestinal haemorrhage with a raised blood urea.

Liver

Therapeutic doses of the barbiturates have no effect on liver function. The liver is the most important organ for the destruction of the barbiturates, although other tissues such as kidney, brain and muscle also destroy the drug; therefore in cases of liver disease the action of barbiturates tends to be prolonged.

Uterus

The uterus is relatively resistant to the depressant effects of barbiturates and hypnotic doses have not been found to depress uterine contractions in labour, although full anaesthetic doses may decrease the force and frequency of the uterine contractions (Gruber, 1937). The barbiturates pass across the placental barrier easily and can produce marked respiratory depression in the fetus.

Metabolic Effects

Anderson *et al.* (1930) reported that hypnotic doses of barbitone, butobarbitone and cyclobarbitone produced some decrease in oxygen consumption, but that amylobarbitone and phenobarbitone did not do this. Anaesthetic doses of barbiturates produce a marked fall in oxygen consumption. The fall in metabolism and the peripheral vasodilatation with increased skin temperature lead to a small fall in the body temperature, depending on the environment.

The blood sugar response to the barbiturates varies from one to the other, with the previous diet, the species which is being investigated, and the dose and route of administration. In man hypnotic doses do not alter the blood sugar regularly to any degree and are therefore safe to use in the presence of diabetes mellitus.

Absorption, Metabolism and Excretion of Barbiturate Drugs

The barbiturates are readily absorbed from the intestines, the rate being slower for the longer-acting drugs. They are also easily absorbed from the rectum or from subcutaneous and intramuscular injection, but where deep anaesthesia is required it is better that they should be administered intravenously, when the rate of injection can be controlled to produce just the effect desired—remembering always the dangers of too rapid intravenous injection and the dangers of extravenous injection.

The distribution of the barbiturates and their metabolism has been reviewed by Richards and Taylor (1956). In the circulation they are adsorbed to variable extents on plasma protein. In spite of this they diffuse rapidly out of the blood stream and are taken up by all tissues. This leads to a rapid fall in blood concentration which may be below that in some of the tissues at this stage. The liver and the muscles account for most of the bulk that is withdrawn from the blood. The body fat, which has a poor blood supply, takes some time to absorb most barbiturates. Shideman and his colleagues (1953) found that in man the maximum localisation of thiopentone in fat occurs in $1\frac{1}{2}$ to $2\frac{1}{2}$ hours. Brodie and his colleagues (1950) found that fat has little affinity for pentobarbitone. When equilibration between the barbiturate in the tissues and in the blood occurs, at a varying time depending on the dose and route of administration, the fall in blood concentration is slowed and is a measure of the rate of metabolism of the drug. As the level falls in the blood and the brain, a level is reached below which waking occurs. It is the rapid removal from the blood which accounts for the brief action of the so-called "ultra-short-acting" barbiturates, and not a rapid breakdown.

Barbiturates, being lipid-soluble compounds, are largely eliminated after biotransformation in the liver to oxidised and less lipid-soluble derivatives. The rate of biotransformation is slowest with the long-acting, more polar, derivatives such as barbitone and phenobarbitone, and fastest with the ultra-short-acting ones like thiopentone. Barbitone is consequently largely excreted unchanged, phenobarbitone is about 70 per cent metabolised and 30 per cent excreted unchanged, and butobarbitone about 90 per cent metabolised and 10 per cent excreted unchanged.

Rates of drug oxidation in the liver vary greatly from one individual to another, partly from inherent variability, partly because barbiturates cause hepatic microsomal enzyme induction on repeated administration (Burns and Conney, 1965). This accelerates their breakdown and causes tolerance to the drug's actions, making the individual relatively insusceptible to its effects. Cross-tolerance appears to occur with consumption of other cerebral depressant agents, notably alcohol, though this is often in the absence of enzyme induction. The mechanisms involved are obscure.

Barbiturates cause habituation, and a true addiction with withdrawal symptoms and signs (Isbell, 1950), particularly if they are repeatedly administered intravenously. Strong political moves are currently being made to ban these drugs from use as hypnotics or sedatives.

Medium- and Long-acting Barbiturates

Individual compounds among the many available (Table 1) differ little in their pharmacological properties in that all are anticonvulsant, sedative and hypnotic according to dosage. For anticonvulsant activity, phenobarbitone (30 to 120 mg/day) is best for prophylaxis, and sodium amylobarbitone, pentobarbitone or thiopentone (see later) by intravenous injection for treatment of the fit. Barbiturates are of value in protecting against the toxic effects of local analgesics and can be given as preoperative medication for this purpose.

For controlling acute manic conditions sodium amylobarbitone or pentobarbitone can be given intramuscularly.

The disadvantages of the barbiturates are the "hangover" effect that follows the use of the longer-acting drugs, respiratory depression, and an occasional toxic skin rash.

As hypnotic agents there is little to choose between the many medium-acting drugs, amylobarbitone, butobarbitone, pentobarbitone, quinalbarbitone or the mixture Tuinal (amylobarbitone plus quinalbarbitone), all producing powerful sedation and hypnosis. Given to patients the evening before operation, any one of these drugs ensures a good night's sleep. Under the noisy conditions existing in many hospital wards, barbiturates are probably more effective than most of the alternatives presently available.

22/Table 1

Hypnotic and Anticonvulsant Barbiturates

Approved name	Proprietary and other names
allobarbitone	allobarbital, diallylbarbitone, Diadol
amylobarbitone	amobarbital, Amytal
aprobarbitone	aprobarbital, Alurate
barbitone*	barbital, Veronal
butobarbitone	butobarbital, Soneryl
cyclobarbitone	cyclobarbital, Phanadorm, Rapidal
heptabarbitone	heptabarbital, Medomin
hexobarbitone	hexobarbital
metharbitone*	metharbital
methylphenobarbitone*	mephobarbital, Prominal
nealbarbitone	alneobarbital, Censedal
pentobarbitone	ethaminal, Napental, Nembutal
phenobarbitone*	phenobarbital, Gardenal, Luminal
quinalbarbitone	secobarbital, Seconal
secbutobarbitone	Bubartal
vinbarbitone	vinbarbital, Delvinal

* Long-acting derivatives.

Some of the proprietary names given apply to the sodium salts of these drugs which, being more soluble, are more rapidly absorbed from the gastro-intestinal tract.

Tuinal is a mixture of amylobarbitone and quinalbarbitone in equal parts.

Ultra-short-acting Barbiturates

Thiopentone (Intraval, Pentothal)

Tabern and Volwiler (1935) prepared a large number of thiobarbiturates. They found that substitution by the sulphur atom shortened the period of narcosis compared with that produced by other barbiturates.

In 1934 Lundy (Lundy, 1935) at the Mayo Clinic, and Waters at Madison, Wisconsin, began clinical trials with the compound now known as thiopentone, which is the sulphur analogue of pentobarbitone. Jarman introduced thiopentone into Great Britain in 1935 (Jarman and Abel, 1936). Its property of producing peaceful sleep easily led to its rapid acceptance and the number of cases anaesthetised with thiopentone rose dramatically (Dundee, 1956).

Physical properties.—Thiopentone is a pale yellow, hygroscopic powder with a bitter taste and a slight sulphurous smell. The sodium salt of thiopentone is readily soluble in water but the acid itself much less so. In order to ensure total solution even in the presence of atmospheric carbon dioxide, commercial solutions contain 6 per cent by weight sodium carbonate. The freshly made solution has a pH of 10·6. For the formula see page 753.

Pharmacological actions.—Thiopentone rapidly crosses the blood-brain barrier and the concentration in the cerebrospinal fluid reaches a level almost as high as that of the unbound drug in the plasma. The depth of anaesthesia produced by the intravenous injection of thiopentone depends on its concentration in the blood, but the relationship is not a simple one, for the larger the initial dose the higher the brain concentration or plasma level at which the patient will awake. This has been called acute tolerance, though the fact that a patient will wake sooner from a rapid injection than from a slow one is probably accountable on the basis of the slug theory (see Chapter 21).

Thiopentone produces a progressive depression of the central nervous system. In clinical practice this is produced so rapidly that the usual signs of anaesthesia are of no value. Respiratory depression is marked, and a patient with apnoea may yet react to a surgical stimulus. The response to a surgical stimulus determines to a greater extent than with other agents the clinical signs of anaesthesia. The surgical stimulus may provide the "drive" to respiration and this may lead to fatal respiratory depression when the stimulus is removed.

Thiopentone has no analgesic properties—indeed hypersensitivity to pain and touch may be manifest.

The effect of thiopentone depends greatly on the premedication with analgesic drugs or the supplementation of thiopentone narcosis with analgesia—opiate or nitrous oxide with oxygen. These allow surgical intervention with no response at lower plasma levels of thiopentone and with less respiratory depression.

Cerebral metabolism and blood flow.—Wechsler and his colleagues (1951) showed that there was a significant depression of cerebral utilisation of oxygen in spite of a blood flow which was normal or a little increased. The blood flow is probably more affected by the carbon dioxide tension in the blood than by the thiopentone.

Respiratory system.—The usual sequence of events when a dose of thiopentone is given slowly is for a few deeper breaths to be taken just prior to the loss of consciousness. There may then be a brief period of apnoea due to the direct effect of the thiopentone on the respiratory centre coinciding with a low carbon dioxide tension from the preceding deep breaths. Respiration returns gradually and then further fades away as more thiopentone is given.

With small doses—i.e. 0·5 g given in 20 to 25 minutes—respiratory depression is not seen, but following premedication with the opiates respiratory depression is more marked (Helrich *et al.*, 1956).

The laryngeal reflexes are not depressed until the deep levels of thiopentone narcosis are reached, and stimulation, local or remote, may provoke laryngeal spasm at light levels of narcosis. If there is a predisposing cause present—such as a sensitive bronchial tree or stimulation of the larynx by mucus—thiopentone may evoke bronchospasm or laryngospasm, but does not of itself cause these conditions.

Cardiovascular system.—Under light anaesthesia there is widespread dilatation of the muscle and skin vessels but no obvious alteration in the total peripheral resistance (Fieldman *et al.*, 1955). Pauca and Hopkins (1971) showed that the forearm blood flow and vascular resistance were unchanged in unpremedicated volunteers. The increase in peripheral flow (i.e. vasodilatation) is compensated for by constriction of the splanchnic and renal blood vessels so that the blood pressure and cardiac output remain relatively unchanged. In contrast, the rapid induction of deep anaesthesia leads to a fall in cardiac output of 25 per cent or more together with a reduction in the intrathoracic blood volume (Etsten and Li, 1955; Flickinger *et al.*, 1961). These changes are thought to be due to the peripheral vasodilatation causing pooling of the blood in the extremities and a reduction of the venous return to the heart (Eckstein *et al.*, 1961). Thiopentone may also have a direct depressant action on the myocardium (Prime and Grey, 1952), but this has not been demonstrated in man.

Dysrhythmias occur in a proportion of cases, and are usually ventricular extrasystoles.

Alimentary tract.—In animals thiopentone produces some depression of intestinal motility, but this soon recovers and has returned to normal when the animal is awake.

Liver and kidneys.—Dundee (1955b) considers that doses of over 750 mg of thiopentone cause liver dysfunction in an appreciable number of patients, but Hugill (1950) notes that hypoxia is the most important factor in the causation of liver damage associated with anaesthesia. The separation of hypoxia from true hepatotoxic effects is extremely difficult in clinical practice.

The effects of thiopentone on the kidneys are secondary to its actions on the circulation, and to the liberation of antidiuretic hormone that it causes. The urine output during thiopentone anaesthesia is decreased (de Wardener, 1955).

Effect on muscles and myoneural junction.—Thiopentone, in large doses in animals, prolongs the contraction of muscle, whether stimulated directly or indirectly, and there is also evidence of a weak curare-like action at the motor end-plate, but clinically this effect is not as obvious as that caused by ether. Quilliam (1955) showed by examination of the action potential of the posterior gracilis muscle of the rat before and after the intra-arterial injection of thiopentone that its voltage was decreased, its latency increased, and duration prolonged. These facts are consistent with a decreased rate of propagation of the potential on the surface of the muscle. In man there is no evidence that thiopentone in doses up to 1·5 g affects neuromuscular transmission.

Reproductive system.—In therapeutic doses, thiopentone does not alter the tone of the gravid uterus or the motility of the Fallopian tubes. It does not influence utero-tubal spasm. McKechnie and Converse (1955) showed that when 350 mg of thiopentone was given just prior to delivery, thiopentone was present in the fetus within 45 seconds until in 2–3 minutes its concentration was equal in the maternal and fetal blood, and then fell in both synchronously. Crawford (1956), using 250 mg thiopentone, produced similar results. McKechnie and Converse could find little correlation between the level of thiopentone in the fetus and the amount of fetal depression—probably because there are so many other factors to be taken into account when considering the causes of fetal depression. Fetal respiration can be depressed by thiopentone, but the degree of depression depends upon the dose of the drug given to the mother and the duration of time that elapses between induction of anaesthesia and delivery of the baby, besides the maturity of the fetus. The available evidence suggests that unless the infant is removed from the uterus within 4 to 5 minutes of an intravenous injection of a small, sleep dose (0·15 to 0·25 g) of thiopentone, the blood level of a mature, healthy fetus will have fallen to such a degree that it is unlikely to be significant in preventing the onset of respiration (see Chapter 44).

Blood sugar.—Thiopentone has no effect on the blood sugar (Dundee and Todd, 1958).

Distribution, Metabolism and Excretion

Price (1960) traced the distribution of thiopentone in the body following a single dose administered intravenously. After one minute the blood had given up 90 per cent of the dose to the central nervous system, heart, liver and other well-perfused viscera. During the next thirty minutes other aqueous tissues acquired 80 per cent of the thiopentone leaving these viscera, and fatty tissues received the remainder. The rate at which thiopentone leaves the central nervous system depends upon the rate at which poorly perfused aqueous tissues take it up, and this depends on their blood flow. Fat is so poorly perfused that it cannot concentrate thiopentone to any great extent until the central nervous system has lost 90 per cent of its peak content. After some hours, however, fat depots may contain quite large amounts of the drug. This has a profound effect on the distribution of subsequent doses, causing a greatly increased clinical effect.

Thiopentone is practically completely metabolised in the body, only about 0·3 per cent of an administered dose being excreted in the urine unchanged (Brodie, 1952). Shideman *et al.* (1953) found in dogs that the true rate of metabolism is 6 per cent of the total dose administered per hour. Recent work suggests that in man the rate of metabolism is faster—16 to 24 per cent per hour (Rahn *et al.*, 1969).

The liver is the main site of the metabolism of thiopentone. This was demonstrated in mice and rats by Shideman and his co-workers (1947). Dundee (1952a) showed in man that the hepatic dysfunction produced by chloroform anaesthesia prolonged the recovery time from the injection of 1·0–1·5 g thiopentone.

In vitro experiments show that slices of kidney tissue inactivate thiopentone to a similar extent to liver slices. Brain slices have some activity, but muscle slices none.

Clinical use.—Thiopentone can be used for several purposes—to induce anaesthesia, as a sole anaesthetic, as the principal anaesthetic but supplemented by other drugs, in conjunction with regional analgesia, to relieve acute convulsive states of differing aetiology, and to produce simple sedation.

Thiopentone leads to a rapid and pleasant loss of consciousness that can be produced with the minimum of apparatus. Herein lie its greatest advantages and its dangers—a fatal overdose is very easily administered. The safety of thiopentone—and indeed of all intravenous anaesthetics—is largely dependent upon the skill of the administrator in assessing, both before and during anaesthesia, the requirements of the patient. Although in theory there is probably a dose that is small enough to be safe for any patient and yet produce a desired effect, there are occasions when it may be wise not to use thiopentone, or at least to give it with particular care and with special precautions. These are:

1. *General.*—Out-patients who are unaccompanied are unsuitable for thiopentone because there is frequently a stage of euphoria for some time following the return of consciousness. In this stage, the patient is in no fit state to look after himself or to take responsible action.

   Children are unsuitable for the administration of thiopentone as the sole or principal anaesthetic agent, since they need relatively large doses to produce a satisfactory depression of reflex activity. Provided venepuncture can be accomplished easily and painlessly, thiopentone is, however, an excellent induction agent for children.

2. *Respiratory disease.*—When the adequacy of the airway is in doubt, thiopentone must be used, if at all, with extreme caution (see Chapter 9). Factors which may affect the airway during induction, such as vomiting or bleeding, suggest either a special technique for the use of thiopentone or its avoidance. Thiopentone may be contra-indicated for an asthmatic patient, as it can lead to an aggravation of the condition.

3. *Cardiac and circulatory disease.*—The benefits of a smooth and pleasant induction with thiopentone must be balanced against the deleterious effects of vasomotor and respiratory depression. In fixed output cardiac diseases, such as mitral stenosis and constrictive pericarditis, vasodilatation and consequent hypotension—particularly if acute—may lead to cardiac arrest. Similarly in "shock" states, in which the blood pressure is maintained by peripheral vasoconstriction, the vasodilatation produced by even a small dose of thiopentone can prove fatal. Such conditions do not necessarily contra-indicate the use of thiopentone, unless the administrator is inexperienced and unable to assess the severity of the disease.

4. *Other diseases.*—For patients in whom coma is imminent due to diseases such as severe hepatic dysfunction, uraemia or uncontrolled diabetes, or due to over-sedation with drugs, thiopentone is either best avoided or used in minimal dosage so that recovery from its effect is rapid. Thiopentone is contra-indicated in the presence of the rare disease porphyria, since it may lead to fatal respiratory paralysis, and should be used with caution for patients with Addison's disease, in whom its action may be unduly prolonged (Dundee, 1951). Abnormal respiratory depression may follow the use of thiopentone in dystrophia myotonica (Dundee, 1952b). Untreated myxoedematous patients are sensitive to most anaesthetics, thiopentone amongst them.

Administration.—Thiopentone should not be used as a stronger solution than 2·5 per cent—i.e. 0·5 g in 20 ml. Solutions should be freshly made, although they keep for a week in a refrigerator. Bottles of solution should be shaken before use to ensure adequate mixing.

The advantages of this concentration are that it is unlikely to cause serious harm if placed extravenously or intra-arterially and it is more difficult to give a large dose rapidly.

Intravenous.—A vein should be chosen and palpated before the application of the tourniquet, which should not be applied so tightly as to occlude the arterial inflow to the arm.

When the needle is firmly in the vein and the tourniquet completely released, 2 ml of thiopentone is injected with a pause after this so that an inadvertent intra-arterial injection may become manifest. Should this have occurred, the patient will complain of a severe burning sensation in the hand (see below). The estimated dose is given at a rate and in an amount that must depend upon the state of the patient and the purpose for which the thiopentone is being given. It may range from as little as 0·05 g for the induction of anaesthesia in a severely ill patient to 1·0 g as the sole anaesthetic for a fit adult. It is best to use the smallest effective dose, and to supplement this with more flexible and potent anaesthetic agents rather than to administer large doses of thiopentone.

Rectal.—The rectal administration of thiopentone is useful in children to produce basal narcosis, particularly for such procedures as a minor operation, cardiac catheterisation and lumbar puncture. It is unsuitable when a rapid return of reflexes is required immediately after the operation. If the expected stimulation is great then supplementation should be started before the operation to prevent such reactions as laryngeal spasm.

Atropine, or other suitable anti-sialogogues, should be given 1 hour before the thiopentone and the patient should have had nothing by mouth for at least five hours. Sleep comes on within 5 to 15 minutes and the maximum effect lasts for another 20 to 30 minutes, consciousness usually beginning to return one hour after the dose has been given.

Since the volume of thiopentone solution needed for rectal instillation is small it is more likely to be retained than the larger quantities of such drugs as paraldehyde or bromethol.

The rectal injection of thiopentone by the anaesthetist provides a valuable and speedy method for inducing sleep, and has the advantage of a more limited period of action than the medium-acting barbiturates. No sterile precautions are necessary and the powder can be made up in a 5 per cent solution, the dose being assessed on the basis of 45 mg/kg body weight. When thiopentone is used some method for inflating the child's lungs with oxygen must be to hand, as central depression of the medulla may occur, particularly if the injection is made too quickly. The solution should be given over 10–20 minutes and only until the child is sleeping soundly.

Aladjemoff and her colleagues (1958) have used suppositories of sodium thiopentone in children for the induction of sleep prior to general anaesthesia. They recommend 0·25 g for children weighing from 6 kg to 12 kg, and 0·5 g for those from 12 kg to 25 kg and consider that the suppository should be given at least ten to fifteen minutes before the child leaves the ward for the operating theatre. This scaled dosage tends to be too low to produce, at best, more than a brief period of very light sleep unless the children are also sedated with morphine or pethidine—as was the case in Aladjemoff's series. A larger dose, while effective for unsedated children, is less safe.

Local complications of thiopentone injections.—Any intravenous injection carries a slight risk of introducing infection, causing a haematoma or losing the broken part of a needle. Cleanliness and efficient sterilisation of syringe and needle are essential to avoid the risk of cross-infection, particularly of infective hepatitis. The incidence of haematomata can be lessened by early release of the tourniquet and the application of pressure to the site of venepuncture while the needle is being removed and for an adequate period of time afterwards. In thin patients, particularly the elderly, pressure should be maintained for three minutes, and elevation of the arm above the level of the heart is a valuable manoeuvre.

Needles break most commonly at the junction of the shaft with the hub (Fig. 1) and they should never be inserted as far as this, so that should one unfortunately break, the shaft can be grasped and removed. To avoid trouble, the arm should be gently but firmly held so that at the slightest movement the

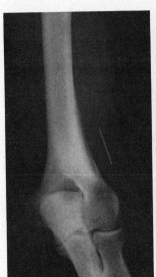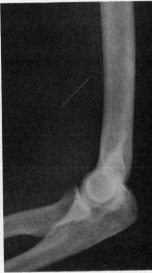

22/Fig. 1.—Broken needle following intravenous thiopentone injection.

grip can be tightened. Movement is more likely to occur in the young and in unpremedicated patients. If a needle breaks, the arm must be held still and if the shaft cannot be grasped and removed, surgical removal with X-ray localisation of the needle must be undertaken. Even with immediate fixation of the arm it is surprising how far the needle may have travelled.

Solutions of thiopentone are alkaline and therefore irritant to the tissues. If enough of the solution is placed extravenously it may cause necrosis of the subcutaneous tissue with an ulcer. If the injection is attempted on the medial side of the antecubital fossa—a site that is not recommended—damage to the median nerve may occur: this is suggested by a shooting pain down the arm and movement of the hand or wrist (Pask and Robson, 1954).

Intra-arterial injection.—The incidence of this complication, which may have extremely severe sequelae for the patient, is unknown. Cohen (1948) suggests it is 1:55,000, but Dundee (1956) considers that it is probably 1:3,500. The number of permanent sequelae that follow intra-arterial injection is also unknown. Most of the reports of permanent damage refer to those that follow the use of a 10 per cent solution, but 6 out of 16 patients in whom a 5 per cent solution had been injected had permanent sequelae (Dundee, 1956). No permanent sequelae have been reported following the use of a 2·5 per cent solution of thiopentone, and this concentration, therefore, has become the standard for clinical practice.

Intra-arterial injection occurs when insufficient attention is paid to the vessel chosen for puncture and to the initial response to a very small quantity of thiopentone. Absence of arterial pulsation may make difficult the normal differentiation between artery and vein, and this may be caused by excessive tourniquet pressure and even by bracing back the shoulders or rotating the neck in some patients. In about 10 per cent of people the ulnar artery may lie superficially beneath the skin on the medial side of the antecubital fossa, and in this position can easily be mistaken for a vein. All in all it is wisest not to select a vein in the antecubital fossa region—at least on its medial side—for the injection of thiopentone, but to choose one on the outer aspect of the forearm, and to administer a 2·5 per cent solution.

Puncture of an arterial wall is usually painless, but the injection of 2 ml of solution into the vessel nearly always causes pain of a burning character which is radiated to the hand. Following the injection, spasm of the artery occurs and the pulse at the wrist may disappear. The immediate effect is probably due to the local release of noradrenaline in or near the vessel wall (Burn and Hobbs, 1959). Waters (1966) has shown that arterial obstruction can be caused by crystallisation of the drug at the normal pH of plasma, due to the limited solubility of the non-ionised form of thiopentone. In a proportion of patients thrombosis takes place in the artery or its distal terminations. Blanching, and perhaps, cyanosis and gangrene of the distal part of the limb are therefore likely to result. Cohen (1948) suggested that thrombosis is a more dangerous factor than arterial spasm, and this view has been substantiated by the experimental work of Kinmonth and Shepard (1959). They found that intra-arterial thiopentone damaged the endothelial and subendothelial tissues of the vessels and that benign solutions buffered to the same pH (10·6) as thiopentone did not. Arterial spasm, apart from the first 30 seconds after injection, played a small part, and the damage was caused by thrombosis.

The end result depends not only on the efficacy of treatment but on many factors such as the volume and strength of the thiopentone injected and the state of the artery and circulation at the time. There is no scientific proof to support the theory that the stronger the solution the more likely are there to be permanent sequelae. But, as stated above, the facts suggest this to be the case. Cohen (1948) has shown that 4–5 ml of 35 per cent diodone can be injected intra-arterially before pain is felt in an arm in which the arterial inflow is obstructed. This volume fills the entire distal arterial tree. Four ml is also the smallest volume of 10 per cent thiopentone that has been reported as being followed by serious effects. These facts support the recommendation of Macintosh and Heyworth (1943) that the anaesthetist should inject 2 ml and then wait for a complaint of pain before proceeding with the injection. Only rarely (as in a medico-legal case reported in the *British Medical Journal* in 1951) will there be no pain.

When the accident occurs treatment must be aimed at diluting the thiopentone, overcoming the initial arterial spasm, and preventing thrombosis or extension of the clot. Operative removal of a thrombus may be necessary.

The needle must be kept in the artery—this may be difficult due to the intense pain that the patient feels—and 10 to 20 ml of 0·5 per cent procaine solution injected to dilute the thiopentone and encourage vasodilatation. When available 40–80 mg of papaverine in 10–20 ml of physiological saline is preferable. It is also advisable to inject procaine or papaverine around the artery at the site of injection, and to remove other vasoconstrictor influences by performing a brachial plexus block and putting the patient on an alpha sympathetic blocking agent and considering anticoagulant therapy. When the damage is thought to have progressed to thrombus formation, then operative removal of the clot should be undertaken within six hours of the original injection, as it is doubtful whether muscle can survive more than this period of circulatory arrest.

Stone and Donnelly (1961), reviewing the problem of accidental intraarterial injection of thiopentone, recommend the following. Light inhalational anaesthesia should be induced quickly to obtain peripheral vasodilatation and pain relief. A brachial plexus block should be performed to ensure continued vascular dilatation in the affected limb, and *anticoagulant therapy* should be started. Stone and Donnelly suggest a catheter technique for the block, so that it can be continued without the risk of bleeding from successive injections. General anaesthesia can usually be quickly induced since an anaesthetic machine is likely to be to hand, whilst a search for procaine or other vasodilator drug may take time. The surgeon must be informed at once, and a decision made whether to postpone the projected operation or not, depending upon the effectiveness of the treatment for the intra-arterial injection.

Venous thrombosis.—The incidence of venous thrombosis has rarely been reported. The belief is that it is much more common after the use of 5 per cent thiopentone than after the use of 2·5 per cent solution. Hutton and Hall (1957) reported four in a series of two hundred unselected surgical patients after the use of 5 per cent solution. Some patients seem to be predisposed to thrombosis, the complication arising on successive occasions in the same patient and despite especial care to prevent it.

Usually the thrombosis is simple, but occasionally a chemical thrombophlebitis may occur with oedema and tenderness in the neighbourhood of the injected vein and its tributaries. Rest for the affected arm is the best treatment, as the condition settles in about seven to ten days: there is no specific therapy. Dundee (1956) quotes three cases of prolonged oedema in a limb following venous thrombosis after a thiopentone injection. In two of them the blood flow from the limb was hindered and it may have been the prolonged period of the contact of the irritant with the vein wall that caused the spreading thrombosis.

Apart from the discomfort of thrombosis, there is a danger of death of tissue distal to it, but this is only inference from the fact that limbs have had to be amputated following the injection of sclerosing fluids into the deep veins of the leg (Cohen, 1948).

General complications of thiopentone administration.—These are usually due to an overdose of thiopentone having been given. This is often not a "large" dose but one too large for the patient due to an inaccurate assessment of his requirements, or attempting too much with thiopentone as the sole anaesthetic. The complications are mainly due to depression of respiration and the circulation, and have been described under the pharmacological actions of the drug. The frequency with which they lead to death is difficult to assess. Dundee (1956) has collected reports on nearly 200,000 thiopentone administrations of which 0·035 per cent (1:2,870) ended in a fatality directly attributable to the drug. Edwards and his colleagues (1956) placed 107 out of 589 deaths caused by anaesthesia in the category of immediate cardiovascular collapse following the injection of an intravenous barbiturate.

Although thiopentone ranks high amongst other anaesthetic agents and factors as a cause of anaesthetic mortality, considering its countrywide and frequent use, and, moreover, the ease with which an overdose can be given, it may be said with some reservations to be a "safe" drug.

Methohexitone Sodium (Brietal Sodium: Methohexital Sodium)

α-dl-l-methyl-5-allyl 5'-(1 methyl-2-pentynyl) barbiturate sodium salt.

Because there are two asymmetrical carbon atoms, there are four possible isomers of this substance, which can be separated into two pairs: α-dl (high melting point) and β-dl (low melting point). The α-dl pair, which is methohexitone, produce hypnosis without stimulation of skeletal muscle. The mixture of all four isomers is a potent short-acting anaesthetic agent which was found to produce excessive skeletal muscle activity and even convulsions (Taylor and Stoelting, 1960).

Physical properties.—Methohexitone sodium is a white powder. It is readily soluble in water to give a solution of pH 10–11 which is stable at room temperature for six weeks, but has been kept satisfactorily at 5° C for a year (Redish *et al.*, 1958).

Pharmacology.—Taylor and Stoelting (1960) found that methohexitone was twice as potent as thiopentone in five species of animals. In man it was three times as potent and was metabolised three times as fast. Coleman and Green (1960) found the ratio of potency to thiopentone to be 2·8:1, but Wyant and Chang (1959) had found it was only one-and-a-half times as potent as thiopentone using a 0·2 per cent intravenous infusion of methohexitone and comparing the dose per minute required to maintain satisfactory anaesthesia. The duration of action of methohexitone is shorter than that of thiopentone, therefore it is less cumulative and larger total doses are required to maintain anaesthesia for a long time. The concentration of methohexitone in the plasma is about half that of thiopentone at comparable electro-encephalographic levels of anaesthesia.

* Asymmetrical carbon atoms.

Methohexitone in the usual clinical doses produces little effect on the blood pressure. When administered during an anaesthetic, it causes a fall of blood pressure of lesser degree and shorter duration than that produced by thiopentone.

Respiratory depression occurs with methohexitone. Wyant and Chang (1959) and Taylor and Stoelting (1960) found this on occasions to be greater than that for a similar dose of thiopentone. Coleman and Green (1960) did not see any cases of apnoea in 10,142 patients.

There was no bronchospasm when methohexitone was given to a series of normal and asthmatic patients (Taylor and Stoelting, 1960). Aurup and Hougs (1963) have shown that *in vitro* methohexitone augments acetylcholine-induced bronchospasm to an extent that is midway between that of thiopentone and hexobarbitone. Extravenous injection has been found to lead to a painless erythema needing no treatment, while intra-arterial injection in animals caused gangrene similar to that produced by thiopentone in equal doses (Francis, 1964).

Some muscular twitching may be seen, which rarely is forceful. Hiccups and coughing were reported by Taylor and Stoelting (1960) but not by Coleman and Green (1960). These effects depend on the use and type of premedication. Sleep is longer-lasting in the premedicated patient and there are fewer movements if an analgesic is given (Dundee and Moore, 1961).

Administration.—Methohexitone is supplied as a powder in bottles containing 500 mg of methohexitone and 30 mg of anhydrous sodium carbonate, which should be made up as a 1 per cent solution. Solutions of methohexitone should not be mixed with acid solutions or precipitation of the sparingly soluble free acid will occur.

Methohexitone is administered intravenously. Sensations may occur at the site of injection or along the vein; these may be painful, but since they are not remembered afterwards, and thrombophlebitis does not occur, they are of no significance. The patient falls asleep peacefully but more slowly than with thiopentone. Some twitching of skeletal musculature may be observed during the initial loss of consciousness. The induction dose is approximately 1 mg/kg body weight, producing sleep lasting two or three minutes from which the patient makes a rapid recovery.

For out-patients requiring dental extractions, Coleman and Green (1960), using approximately 5 mg/stone (0·8 mg/kg approx.) of methohexitone, found that 90 per cent of patients were able to leave the dental chair within 6 minutes and 96 per cent were deemed to be safe to go home within half an hour.

Indications.—Methohexitone is recommended for any brief anaesthetic where rapid, complete recovery is required. It is especially useful for out-patients needing electro-convulsive therapy or dental extraction. It has a place in obstetrics, particularly for Caesarean section (Sliom *et al.*, 1962), and as an induction agent in paediatric anaesthesia (Miller and Stoelting, 1963). In the latter instance the dose is 0·5 mg/kg.

Other Ultra-short-acting Barbiturates

There are many of these (all thiobarbiturates), but few if any of them are now in clinical use. A list is given in Table 2.

22/TABLE 2
SOME ULTRA-SHORT-ACTING BARBITURATES

Approved name	Proprietary and other names
buthalitone	thialbutone, Transithal
hexobarbitone	sodium hexobarbital, Cyclonal, Evipan
methitural	Neraval
thialbarbitone	Kemithal
thiamylal	Surital

BARBITURATE POISONING

This may be chronic or acute. Chronic barbiturate poisoning is synonymous with barbiturate addiction. A regular daily dose of 200 mg of the powerful short-acting barbiturates can probably be taken without harm, but 800 mg per day will adversely affect performance, and after eight weeks withdrawal symptoms are likely. The average dose taken by the barbiturate addict is 1·5 g and unless this dose is exceeded severe intoxication is unusual. At any stage an overdose may be taken and then chronic poisoning becomes acute.

Acute Barbiturate Poisoning

Acute barbiturate poisoning is less common now that barbiturates themselves are less frequently prescribed. The mortality rate of patients admitted to hospital with barbiturate poisoning is less than 2 per cent with expert treatment (Clemmesen and Nilsson, 1961).

Symptoms and Signs

These reflect the degree of CNS depression. The patient may be merely lethargic with mild overdosage, inebriated in moderate overdose, or comatose in severe intoxication. Protective reflexes are impaired to an extent, related to the depth of unconsciousness. Respiration is depressed: the minute volume is decreased but the rate may be slow or rapid. Occasionally Cheyne-Stokes respiration is seen. Hypoxia and respiratory acidosis develop.

The pupils may be constricted and reacting to light or show hypoxic paralytic dilatation. The blood pressure falls, mainly due to medullary vasomotor depression but also because of a direct effect on myocardial and smooth muscle. A tachycardia is present but tissue perfusion may be impaired producing a metabolic acidosis.

Urine output is decreased because of barbiturate induced vasopressin release and poor renal blood flow. Hypothermia occurs occasionally though its presence should suggest that a phenothiazine may also have been taken.

Death, when it occurs early, is usually due to respiratory depression and obtunded laryngeal reflexes with aspiration of vomit, or to acute circulatory collapse. At a later stage bronchopneumonia, pulmonary oedema or renal failure may be responsible.

Diagnosis

This depends in part on a knowledge of the circumstances in which the patient was found. Other causes of coma must be excluded. Frequently more than one drug, including alcohol, has been taken. Circumstantial evidence in the form of empty medicine bottles may be helpful. Specimens of blood, urine and stomach contents should be obtained for analysis; they may also be required for medico-legal reasons. Physical examination alone will not differentiate between the various CNS depressants.

Management

Immediate care will depend upon an assessment of the level of consciousness and of respiratory and circulatory depression. In the fully conscious, gastric lavage may be beneficial; to be of value this should be performed soon after ingestion. Thereafter the patient is carefully observed for signs of any deepening CNS depression. In the semi-comatose and unconscious meticulous attention to the airway is essential. A patient with depressed pharyngo-laryngeal reflexes should be intubated with a plastic cuffed endotracheal tube in order to isolate the respiratory tract. Certainly no attempt at gastric lavage should be made without this precaution. In borderline cases only an oropharyngeal airway may be tolerated; such patients should be turned from side to side with a slight head down tilt and oxygen administered by a face-mask. Equipment for tracheal intubation should be readily available. In severe intoxication arterial blood gas and pH estimations are valuable. Intermittent positive-pressure ventilation may be required and concomitant metabolic acidosis needs correcting. Regular chest radiography, electrolyte, creatinine and haematocrit estimations should be performed. Prolonged intubation may necessitate tracheostomy. Analeptics have no role in the management of acute barbiturate overdose.

Circulatory collapse is a major threat in severe cases. Intravenous fluids should be infused to maintain an adequate right atrial pressure which should be monitored by a central venous pressure cannula. Plasma, dextran and crystalloid solutions may be infused, but blood should only be given if there is evidence of coincidental blood loss. Myocardial (pump) failure as shown by an inadequate cardiac output in the face of a high filling pressure is best treated with a myocardial stimulant, e.g. isoprenaline or dopamine. Shubin and Weil (1971) suggest digitalisation when diuresis does not occur with a high central venous pressure.

Hypothermia is probably best treated by passive means, and further heat loss should be avoided. Infections, especially of the respiratory tract, will require the appropriate antibiotic therapy. Corticosteroids used in the management of aspiration pneumonitis or cerebral oedema may deepen coma.

In severe intoxication methods of drug removal should be considered. These are:

(a) *Forced alkaline diuresis*

This requires normal renal function and careful, expert attention to water, electrolyte and acid-base balance. Osmotic or loop diuretics should be employed, in the presence of the high circulatory ADH to obtain a diuresis of about 10 litres/day. Sodium bicarbonate infusion is used to produce an alkaline urine. Not all barbiturates are rapidly eliminated in this way. Renal excretion plays less part in the total elimination of those barbiturates with high protein binding and lipid solubility and whose main means of elimination is metabolic (e.g.

pentobarbitone). However the elimination of longer-acting drugs such as phenobarbitone is greatly enhanced.

(b) *Haemodialysis*

This achieves rapid removal of all barbiturates. Less protein-bound drugs, e.g. long-acting barbiturates, are eliminated more quickly.

(c) *Peritoneal dialysis*

Peritoneal dialysis is far less effective than haemodialysis, and will not remove significant amounts of phenobarbitone.

NON-BARBITURATE HYPNOTICS AND INTRAVENOUS ANAESTHETICS

There is no absolute distinction between hypnotics and anaesthetic agents. The use of a particular drug for one or other purpose depends as much on its availability in particular dosage form as on its pharmacological activity. Non-barbiturate hypnotics available for oral administration are listed in Table 3.

22/TABLE 3
NON-BARBITURATE HYPNOTICS

Approved name	Proprietary names
chlormethiazole	Heminevrin
ethchlorvynol	Arvynol, Placidyl, Serenesil
ethinamate	Valmid, Valmidate
glutethimide	Doriden
methaqualone	Melsed, Melsedin
methaqualone with diphenhydramine	Mandrax
methylpentynol	Oblivon, Insomnol
methyprylone	Noludar

Their properties are similar: all produce hypnosis without marked respiratory depression (except in overdose), they summate with other cerebral depressant agents and their repeated administration may lead to dependence of the ethanol-barbiturate type. In this latter respect methaqualone is outstanding; it is now under widespread control regulations as are applied to opiates.

With the advent of benzodiazepines, discussed in Chapter 23, most of these compounds are of little importance today. For discussion of their properties the reader is referred to older textbooks. Chlormethiazole is mentioned briefly below, because it is available for intravenous administration and has been used as an anaesthetic induction agent.

Althesin (Alphadione, Alphathesin)

Althesin is a mixture of two steroids, alphaxalone (3α-hydroxy-5α-pregnane-11,20-dione) and alphadolone (3α,21-dihydroxy-5α-pregnane-11,20-dione). It is presented as a clear colourless isotonic solution of neutral pH containing alphaxalone 9 mg and alphadolone 3 mg in each ml, which also contains 20 per cent Cremophor El (polyoxyethylated castor oil) and sodium chloride. It can be diluted with any isotonic solution. Its animal pharmacology was described by Child *et al.* (1971).

It is a brief-acting intravenous anaesthetic agent which is usually non-irritant at the site of injection. Both components are bound to plasma protein to about 30–40 per cent (Child *et al.*, 1972). Following intravenous injection of 0·05 mg/kg in man sleep is induced in 30 seconds and lasts about seven minutes, whilst after 0·075 mg/kg sleep continues for around 11 minutes. Surgical anaesthesia is present for about half this time and full recovery takes 30 minutes. It appears from animal experiments that termination of its action is determined largely by rapid metabolism in the liver (Carson *et al.*, 1975; Novelli *et al.*, 1975) rather than redistribution. It should therefore not be given to patients with liver disease.

There is a fall of arterial blood pressure of 10–20 per cent due to peripheral vasodilatation, a fall in central venous pressure and an increase of 20 per cent in the pulse rate (Du Cailar, 1972; Savege, *et al.*, 1972). Apnoea may occur, particularly if the injection of Althesin is rapid, and there is a 2–3 per cent incidence of muscle tremors which is reduced by analgesic premedication (Dechene, 1976). Coughing, hiccup and laryngospasm have all been described, usually in response to stimulation during too light a plane of anaesthesia. It causes a low incidence of post-anaesthetic vomiting.

No hormonal effects due to the compounds' steroid configuration have been reported. Oyama *et al.* (1975) found that no change took place in the concentration of plasma cortisol, though it did rise at the beginning of surgery. The plasma thyroxine was decreased but there was no change in the free thyroxine index, which was raised by surgery. Mehta and Burton (1975) studied the effect of althesin on carbohydrate metabolism and showed that blood sugar rose slightly during minor surgery and more during abdominal surgery, whilst the plasma insulin and human growth hormone levels did not change. Plasma-free fatty acids increased after 15 minutes of anaesthesia and minor surgery. The hyperglycaemic response to Althesin was the same in diabetics as in non-diabetic subjects.

The most important complication associated with its use, although not occurring commonly (1 : 11,000 to 1 : 19,000, according to Clarke *et al.*, 1975) is severe bronchospasm and circulatory collapse, an anaphylactoid reaction (Hester, 1973; Horton, 1973) requiring treatment with oxygen, subcutaneous adrenaline, antihistamines, corticosteroids and plasma expanders. These reactions are probably due to the Cremophor El and have been seen following the administration of propanidid, a solution which also contains this substance.

In spite of its useful properties, Althesin cannot be recommended as a replacement for the older induction agents except where they are contra-indicated because of sensitivity reactions.

Chlormethiazole Edisylate (Heminevrin)

Chlormethiazole has sedative, hypnotic and anticonvulsant properties. Adult doses of 1 to 2 g given orally or by intravenous infusion produce unconsciousness with a tachycardia but without other cardiovascular or respiratory changes (Wilson *et al.*, 1969). It has been used to sedate elderly patients, though its repeated administration may cause dependence, and it is advocated for the management of drug- and alcohol-withdrawal states. It appears to have no certain advantage over other non-barbiturate hypnotics such as benzo-diazepines.

Etomidate

Etomidate [R-1-ethyl-1-(α-methylbenzyl)imidazole-5-carboxylate] is a newly introduced intravenous anaesthetic induction agent. Its water-soluble sulphate is available in aqueous solution at 1·5 mg/ml; the solution is of pH 3·3. In animals it has a high therapeutic index (Janssen *et al.*, 1971) and it is therefore potentially safer than many other agents.

Its effects in man have been described by Doenicke *et al.* (1973 *a* and *b*). Its rapid onset of hypnotic action coincides with the arm-brain circulation time, and within the dose range 0·1 to 0·4 mg/kg spontaneous wakening occurs in 7 to 14 min. (Kay, 1976*a*). On repeated administration there is little tendency to cumulation (Kay, 1976*b*). Anaesthesia with the larger doses is sometimes associated with apnoea of up to 45 sec duration and tachycardia of more than 20 beats per min increase (Holdcroft *et al.*, 1976). There is an increase in muscle tone and a high incidence of involuntary movement which can be decreased with opiates or diazepam premedication. The drug is without analgesic action.

Pain at the site of injection is common if the injection is made into a small vein but occurs in some patients when a large vein at the elbow is used.

The drug appears to have no great advantage over other agents and it would be of particular value only in subjects known to be sensitive to them.

Ketamine Hydrochloride (Ketalar)

2-(O-Chlorophenyl)-2-(Methylamino) cyclohexanone hydrochloride.

Physical Properties

Ketamine hydrochloride is a white crystalline solid, soluble in water to a 20 per cent clear solution that is stable at room temperature. The base component is 86·7 per cent of the salt and the solution has a pH between 3·5 and 5·5. Bensethonium chloride is added as a preservative.

Pharmacological Actions

Ketamine has unusual anaesthetic properties in that it produces un-consciousness with profound analgesia. For a brief initial period there may be a depression of respiration and a suppression of the pharyngo-laryngeal reflexes (Taylor and Towey, 1971), particularly after an intravenous injection. There is also an increase in systemic pressure and heart rate; originally this was believed to be due entirely to release of endogenous catecholamines, but other studies have suggested that ketamine produces a direct myocardial stimulant action combined with a peripheral effect (Takki *et al.*, 1972; Tweed *et al.*, 1972).

Essentially, ketamine is a cataleptic analgesic and anaesthetic with hypnotic properties which are clearly distinguishable from the barbiturates. Electro-encephalographic changes include the abolition of alpha waves and induction of theta activity. The short-lived depression of respiration and the pharyngo-laryngeal reflexes are related to a high plasma concentration following intra-venous administration.

Metabolism

Ketamine undergoes N-demethylation and hydroxylation of the cyclo-hexanone ring with the formation of conjugates which are excreted in the urine. The unconjugated N-demethylated metabolite has only one-sixth the potency of ketamine and the unconjugated cyclohexanone derivative only one-tenth.

Clinical Use

Ketamine was first introduced into clinical anaesthesia by Corssen and Domino in 1966. Since that time it has been recommended for a wide variety of anaesthetic procedures. The principal advantage of this agent is that it produces satisfactory anaesthesia lasting from about 5 to 25 minutes with a relatively stable cardiovascular situation and the maintenance of a good airway. However, as already mentioned, both the circulation and respiration and the pharyngeal reflex can be affected during the first few minutes. The main disadvantage has been the recollection of unpleasant dreams by some of the patients during the recovery period. However, not all the dreams have been described as unpleasant yet some have been classified as nightmares. Various measures can be adopted to reduce the incidence of these dreams (Johnstone, 1972) and medication with either hyoscine, droperidol or diazepam have been found useful. A quiet recovery room and minimal interference with the patient during this period can reduce the incidence of emergence phenomena.

It is difficult to assess the place of ketamine in modern anaesthesia because although it is simple to use, the services of a clinician are still of paramount importance and facilities for resuscitation must always be available. In hospital practice where an adequate supply of well-trained anaesthetists are available then it will be found that it has a useful role for repeated anaesthetic procedures in small children, e.g. change of burns dressing. It is also an invaluable agent for the treatment of the trapped casualty or even for the Mass Casualty situation, so that it should always be available for the emergency and the induction of the shocked patient (Bond and Davies, 1974). In regions where there is a dearth of anaesthetists then the satisfactory state of unconsciousness it can produce, with minimum training of the administrator, will be found useful for minor surgery but the lack of any muscular relaxation will limit this usefulness.

Dosage

Intramuscularly: 6·3–13·0 mg/kg, e.g. a dose of 10 mg/kg will usually pro-duce 12 to 25 minutes of surgical anaesthesia.

Intravenously: 1·0–4·5 mg/kg, e.g. 2·0 mg/kg will usually produce about 5 to 10 minutes of surgical anaesthesia.

N.B. It must be administered *SLOWLY* (i.e. over at least one minute) to reduce incidence of respiratory depression.

Repeated dose: Half to a full dose can be given when the patient shows the following signs.

(a) Movements in response to stimulation
(b) Nystagmus
(c) Phonation

Contra-indications

Ketamine raises both the pulse rate and the systemic pressure. Originally this was believed to be due entirely to release of catecholamines but the studies of Tweed and his co-workers (1972) have shown that ketamine has a direct stimulant action on the myocardium and peripheral vessels. In fact, they found that the myocardial minute oxygen consumption was increased and for this reason recommended that it should not be used in the presence of severe coronary or myocardial disease. Because it produces a marked rise in systemic and cerebrospinal fluid pressure, ketamine is not the drug of choice in patients with hypertension, eclampsia, raised intra-ocular and intracranial pressure.

Propanidid (Epontol)

This non-barbiturate, ultra-short-acting anaesthetic is a derivative of eugenol.

It is a pale yellow oil which, for clinical use, is dissolved in 20 per cent Cremophor El, a non-ionised, surface-active aqueous solution of ethoxylated castor oil, to give a 5 per cent solution of propanidid. This solution is highly viscous but it can be further diluted with an equal volume of physiological saline for easier administration.

It is rapidly metabolised to an anaesthetically inactive acid metabolite by enzymatic splitting of the ester bond, mainly in the liver but also in the blood by plasma-cholinesterase (Putter, 1965). This rapid breakdown determines the brief duration of anaesthesia.

When 5–6 mg/kg is administered intravenously over twenty seconds (the recommended rate) the unpremedicated patient is deeply asleep within about thirty seconds. 6 per cent of patients show involuntary muscular movements and 8 and 9 per cent a cough or hiccup. Awakening occurs in four to eight minutes and rational conversation is possible after a further two or three minutes (Wynands *et al.*, 1963). There are no "hangover" effects but phlebitis occurs in 4 per cent, and as a large needle is used for the injection greater care than usual is necessary to prevent haematoma formation.

The blood pressure falls and the pulse rate rises in most patients. The respiratory changes are characteristic (Harnik, 1964), the onset of anaesthesia being accompanied by a period of hyperventilation followed by apnoea which may last up to thirty seconds.

Propanidid prolongs the respiratory effects of suxamethonium because of their common route of metabolism, but the requirements for d-tubocurarine are increased (Clarke et al., 1967).

The brevity of its effects means that to prolong anaesthesia either the dose of propanidid must be repeated or other agents administered rapidly to achieve a smooth transition. Premedication helps this but delays recovery.

ANALEPTICS

Respiratory inadequacy has in the past been treated with a variety of analeptics, drugs which through their general nervous system stimulant properties activate medullary centres. They work either directly on the medulla or via chemoreceptor stimulation in the carotid body or both.

The management of hypoxia, whether due to respiratory disease or to overdosage with cerebral depressant drugs, is, however, not greatly helped by the use of these agents. First, their ability to increase respiration is never very good, but more importantly doses which are often only marginally greater than those needed for medullary stimulation activate cortical and other higher centres and produce convulsions. In practice, therefore, analeptic drugs are of little use and they should never be employed as substitutes for artificial ventilation if that is needed. In particular these drugs have no place in the management of drug poisoning.

Of the many agents used and available for clinical purposes, listed in Table 4, few are of more than historic interest. Ethamivan and nikethamide, both well-established drugs, and doxapram, which is the newest in the series, are discussed briefly below.

22/TABLE 4
ANALEPTICS

Approved name	Proprietary and other names
amiphenazole	Daptazole
bemegride	Megimide
doxapram	Dopram, Stimulexin
ethamivan	vanillic acid diethylamide, Vandid
flurothyl	Indoklon
leptazol	Cardiazol, Metrazol, Pentylenetetrazol
lobeline	
nikethamide	Anacardone, cardiamide, Coramine, Nikorin
picrotoxin	
prethcamide	Micoren

Doxapram (Dopram, Stimulexin)

Doxapram [1-ethyl-4-(2-morpholinoethyl)-3,3-diphenyl-2-pyrrolidone] is a general central nervous system stimulant which was introduced by Lunsford *et al.* (1962). On intravenous administration it stimulates ventilation, increases cardiac output and work, and causes arousal from anaesthesia (Noe *et al.*, 1965). This stimulant phase is not followed by reactive hypoventilation (Winnie *et al.*, 1971). The ratio of convulsant to respiratory stimulant dose in animals is 70:1, that of nikethamide is 18:1.

The drug has a brief duration of action due to rapid inactivation in the liver (Bruce *et al.*, 1965) and its ability to reverse drug-induced respiratory depression is therefore transient. Doses can be repeated hourly if necessary, or it may be given (well-diluted) in an infusion.

Doxapram has been advocated as an adjunct to opiate analgesia for it does not reverse the analgesic effect (Dundee *et al.*, 1973) and by overcoming respiratory depression may allow more opiate to be given. Gawley *et al.* (1976)

Role of Doxapram in Reducing Pulmonary Complications after Major Surgery

Treatment group	Cough	Sputum	Abnormal physical signs	Radio-logical changes	Any compli-cation
Morphine	40	52	52	44	68
Morphine + naloxone ...	48	56	52	28	72
Morphine + doxapram (single injection)	20	28	40	32	64
Morphine + doxapram (infusion)	25	25	25	45	65

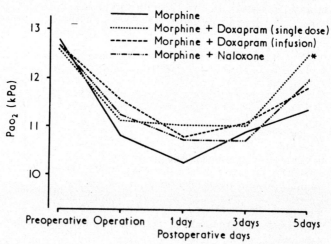

Mean PAO$_2$ values before and after operation in patients on the four treatment regimens. * = Significant difference from the control series. For clarity SE at each point is omitted.

22/Fig. 2.—Percentage incidence of cough, expectoration of purulent sputum, abnormal physical signs, and adverse radiographic signs and percentage overall complication rate in patients in the four treatment groups.

showed that doxapram 1·8–2·0 mg/kg combined with morphine following upper abdominal surgery decreased cough and sputum production by comparison with morphine alone (Fig. 2). A transient increase in ventilation at the end of operation can also be produced in order to prevent post-operative hypoxia (Winnie and Collins, 1966).

In the elderly and in patients with heart disease doxapram should be given cautiously, as ECG changes have been reported (Noe *et al.*, 1965).

Ethamivan. Vanillic Acid Diethylamide (Vandid)

Vanillic acid diethylamide is a central respiratory and circulatory stimulant. An intravenous dose of 0·6–2·0 mg per kg body weight will produce a rapid increase in the volume of respiration, followed in about a minute by an increase in respiratory and pulse rates with a moderate rise in blood pressure (Auinger *et al.*, 1952). All these effects are, however, of short duration—ten to fifteen minutes.

Nikethamide (Coramine, Anacardone)

Nikethamide is a synthetic substance which is made up as a 25 per cent solution. It stimulates respiration via the chemoreceptors of the carotid body and has a weak vasoconstrictor effect on the peripheral circulation. It has little, if any, effect on the myocardium unless large doses are given, when it raises the output slightly. The action of nikethamide is brief (10–15 minutes) and the dose is 1–2 ml of the 25 per cent solution given intravenously.

REFERENCES

ADAM, K., ADAMSON, L., BŘEZINOVÁ, V., and OSWALD, I. (1976). Do placebos alter sleep? *Brit. med. J.*, **1**, 195.

ALADJEMOFF, L., KAPLAN, I., and GETESH, T. (1958). Sodium thiopentone suppositories in paediatric anaesthesia. *Anaesthesia*, **13**, 152.

ALDRIDGE, W. N. (1962). Action of barbiturates upon respiratory enzymes. In: *Enzymes and Drug Action*, p. 155. Ed. Mongar, J. L. and de Reuck, A. V. S. London: J. & A. Churchill.

ANDERSON, H. H., CHEN, M. Y., and LEXAKE, C. D. (1930). The effects of barbituric acid hypnotics on basal metabolism in humans. *J. Pharmacol. exp. Ther.*, **40**, 215.

ASERINSKY, E., and KLEITMAN, N. (1953). Regularly occurring periods of eye motility and concomitant phenomena during sleep. *Science*, **118**, 273.

AUINGER, W., KAINDL, F., SALZMANN, F., and WEISSEL, W. (1952). Zur Atem- und Kreislauf wirkung von 3-Methoxy-4-oxy-benzoesäurediä thylamid. *Wien. Z. inn. Med.*, **33**, 23.

AURUP, R., and HOUGS, W. (1963). Effect of enallynymal natrium (Briétal), enhexymal natrium (Evipan) and thiomebumal natrium (Pentothal) on bronchial muscles. *Acta anaesth. scand.*, **7**, 83.

BEECHER, H. K. (1951). Pain and some factors which modify it. *Anesthesiology*, **12**, 633.

BOND, A. C., and DAVIES, C. K. (1974). Ketamine and pancuronium for the shocked patient. *Anaesthesia*, **29**, 59.

BŘEZINOVÁ, V. (1975). The number and duration of the episodes of the various EEG stages of sleep in young and older people. *Electroenceph. clin. Neurophysiol.*, **39**, 273.

BŘEZINOVÁ, V., and OSWALD, I. (1972). Sleep after a bedtime beverage. *Brit. med. J.*, **2**, 431.

British Medical Journal (1951). Medico-Legal Notes, **1**, 707.

BRODIE, B. B. (1952). Physiological disposition and chemical fate of thiobarbiturates in the body. *Fed. Proc.*, **11**, 632.

BRODIE, B. B., MARK, L. C., PAPPER, E. M., LIEF, P. A., BERNSTEIN, E., and ROVENSTINE, E. A. (1950). Fate of thiopental in man and a method for its estimation in biological material. *J. Pharmacol. exp. Ther.*, **98**, 85.

BRUCE, R. B., PITTS, J. E., PINCHBECK, F., and NEWMAN, J. (1965). Excretion, distribution and metabolism of doxapram hydrochloride. *J. med. pharm. Chem.*, **8**, 153.

BURN, J. H., and HOBBS, R. (1959). Mechanism of arterial spasm following intra-arterial injection of thiopentone. *Lancet*, **1**, 1112.

BURNS, J. J., and CONNEY, A. H. (1965). Enzyme stimulation and inhibition in the metabolism of drugs. *Proc. roy. Soc. Med.*, **58**, 955.

BUTZENGEIGER, O. (1927). Klinische Erfahrungen mit Avertin (E 107). *Dtsch. med. Wschr.*, **53**, 712.

CARSON, I. W., GRAHAM, J., and DUNDEE, J. W. (1975). Clinical studies of induction agents XLIII. Recovery from althesin, a comparative study with thiopentone and methohexitone. *Brit. J. Anaesth.*, **47**, 358.

CERVELLO, V. (1882). Sull 'Azione Fisiologica della Paraldeide e Contributo Allo Studio del Chloralio Idrato. Richerche. *Arch. Sci. med.*, **6**, 177.

CHILD, K. J., CURRIE, J. P., DAVIES, B., DODDS, M. G., PEARCE, D. R., and TWISSEL, D. J. (1971). The pharmacological properties in animals of CT–1341, a new steroid anaesthetic agent. *Brit. J. Anaesth.*, **43**, 2.

CHILD, K. J., GIBSON, W., HARNBY, G., and HART, J. W. (1972). Metabolism and excretion of althesin (CT–1341) in the rat. *Postgrad. med. J.*, **48** (suppl. 2), 37.

CLARKE, R. S. J., DUNDEE, J. W., GARRETT, R. T., MCARDLE, G. K., and SUTTON, J. A. (1975). Adverse reactions of intravenous anaesthetics; a survey of 100 reports. *Brit. J. Anaesth.*, **47**, 575.

CLARKE, R. S. J., DUNDEE, J. W., and HAMILTON, R. C. (1967). Interactions between induction agents and muscle relaxants. *Anaesthesia*, **22**, 235.

CLEMMESEN, C., and NILSSON, E. (1961). Therapeutic trends in the treatment of barbiturate poisoning. The Scandinavian method. *Clin. Pharmacol. Ther.*, **2**, 220.

COHEN, S. M. (1948). Accidental intra-arterial injection of drugs. *Lancet*, **2**, 361, 409.

COLEMAN, J., and GREEN, R. A. (1960). Methohexital. A short acting barbiturate. *Anaesthesia*, **15**, 411.

CONWAY, C. M., and ELLIS, D. B. (1969). The haemodynamic effects of short-acting barbiturates. *Brit. J. Anaesth.*, **41**, 534.

CORSSEN, G., and DOMINO, E. F. (1966). Dissociative anesthesia: further pharmacologic studies and first clinical experience with the phencyclidine derivative CI-581. *Anesth. Analg. Curr. Res.*, **45**, 29.

CRAWFORD, J. S. (1956). Some aspects of obstetric anaesthesia. *Brit. J. Anaesth.*, **28**, 146.

DANCE, C. L., BOOZER, J., NEWMAN, W., and BURSTEIN, C. L. (1956). Electrocardiographic studies during endotracheal intubation. *Anesthesiology*, **17**, 730.

DECHENE, J. P. (1976). Alphathesin, a new steroid anaesthetic agent. *Canad. Anaesth. Soc. J.*, **23**, 163.

DEMENT, W., and FISHER, C. (1963). Experimental interference with the sleep cycle. *Canad. psychiat. Ass. J.*, **8**, 395.

DE WARDENER, H. E. (1955). Renal circulation during anaesthesia and surgery. *Anaesthesia*, **10**, 18.

DOENICKE, A., LORENZ, W., BEIGL, R., BEZECNY, H., UHLIG, G., KALMAR, L., PRAETORIUS, B., and MANN, G. (1973a). Histamine release after intravenous application of short-acting hypnotics. *Brit. J. Anaesth.*, **45**, 1097.

DOENICKE, A., WAGNER, E., and BEETZ, K. H. (1973b). Blutgasanalysen (arteriell) nach drei kurzworkenden i.v. Hypnotica (Propanidid, Etomidate und Methohexital). *Anaesthesist*, **22**, 353.

DOMEK, N. S., BARLOW, C. F., and ROTH, L. J. (1960). An ontogenetic study of phenobarbital–C^{14} in cat brain. *J. Pharmacol. exp. Ther.*, **130**, 285.

DU CAILAR, J. (1972). The effects in man of infusions of althesin with particular regard to the cardiovascular system. *Postgrad. med. J.*, **48** (suppl. 2), 72.

DUNDEE, J. W. (1951). Thiopentone in Addison's disease. *Brit. J. Anaesth.*, **23**, 167.

DUNDEE, J. W. (1952a). Thiopentone narcosis in the presence of hepatic dysfunction. *Brit. J. Anaesth.*, **24**, 81.

DUNDEE, J. W. (1952b). Thiopentone in dystrophia myotonia. *Curr. Res. Anesth.*, **31**, 257.

DUNDEE, J. W. (1955). Thiopentone as a factor in the production of liver dysfunction. *Brit. J. Anaesth.*, **27**, 14.

DUNDEE, J. W. (1956). *Thiopentone and Other Thiobarbiturates*. Edinburgh: E. & S. Livingstone.

DUNDEE, J. W., GUPTA, P. K., and JONES, C. J. (1973). Modification of the analgesic action of pethidine and morphine by three opiate antagonists, a respiratory stimulant (doxapram) and an analeptic (nikethamide); a study using an experimental pain stimulus in man. *Brit. J. Pharmacol.*, **48**, 326P.

DUNDEE, J. W., and MOORE, J. (1961). The effects of premedication with phenothiazine derivatives on the course of methohexitone anaesthesia. *Brit. J. Anaesth.*, **33**, 382.

DUNDEE, J. W., and RICHARDS, R. K. (1954). Effect of azotaemia upon the action of intravenous barbiturate anesthesia. *Anesthesiology*, **15**, 333.

DUNDEE, J. W., and TODD, U. M. (1958). Clinical significance of the effects of thiobarbiturates and adjuvant drugs on blood sugar and glucose tolerance. *Brit. J. Anaesth.*, **30**, 77.

ECKSTEIN, J. W., HAMILTON, W. K., and McCAMMOND, J. M. (1961). The effect of thiopental on peripheral venous tone. *Anesthesiology*, **22**, 525.

EDWARDS, G., MORTON, H. J. V., PASK, E. A., and WYLIE, W. D. (1956). Deaths associated with anaesthesia. A report on 1,000 cases. *Anaesthesia*, **11**, 194.

ETSTEN, B., and LI, T. H. (1955). Haemodynamic changes during thiopental anesthesia in humans. *J. clin. Invest.*, **34**, 500.

EXLEY, K. A. (1954). Depression of autonomic ganglia by barbiturates. *Brit. J. Pharmacol.*, **9**, 170.

EXTON-SMITH, A. N., HODKINSON, H. M., and CROMIE, B. W. (1963). Controlled comparison of four sedative drugs in elderly patients. *Brit. med. J.*, **2**, 1037.

FIELDMAN, E. J., RIDLEY, R. W., and WOOD, E. H. (1955). Hemodynamic studies during thiopental sodium and nitrous oxide anesthesia in humans. *Anesthesiology*, **16**, 473.

FLICKINGER, H., FRAIMOW, W., CATHCART, R. T., and NEALON, T. F. (1961). Effect of thiopental induction on cardiac output in man. *Anesth. Analg. Curr. Res.*, **40**, 693.

FRANCIS, J. G. (1964). Intra-arterial methohexitone. *Anaesthesia*, **19**, 501.

GAWLEY, T. H., DUNDEE, J. W., GUPTA, P. K., and JONES, C. J. (1976). Role of doxapram in reducing pulmonary complications after major surgery. *Brit. med. J.*, **1**, 122.

GOODNOW, R. E., BEECHER, H. K., BRAZIER, M. A. B., MOSTELLAR, F., and TAGIURI, R. (1951). Physiological performance following a hypnotic dose of a barbiturate. *J. Pharmacol. exp. Ther.*, **102**, 55.

GRACA, J. G., and GARST, E. L. (1957). Early blood changes in dogs following intravenous pentobarbital anesthesia. *Anesthesiology*, **18**, 461.

GRUBER, C. M. (1937). On certain pharmacologic actions of newer barbituric acid compounds. *Amer. J. Obstet. Gynec.*, **33**, 729.

HARNIK, E. (1964). A study of the biphasic ventilatory effects of propanidid. *Brit. J. Anaesth.*, **36**, 655.

HARRIS, E. A., and SLAWSON, K. B. (1965). The respiratory effects of therapeutic doses of cyclobarbitone, triclofos and ethchlorvynol. *Brit. J. Pharmacol.*, **24**, 214.

HELRICH, M., ECKENHOFF, J. E., JONES, R. E., and ROLPH, W. D. (1956). Influence of opiates on the respiratory response of man to thiopental. *Anesthesiology*, **17**, 459.

HESTER, J. B. (1973). Reaction to althesin. *Brit. J. Anaesth.*, **45**, 303.

HINTON, J. M. (1961). The actions of amylobarbitone sodium, butobarbitone and quinalbarbitone sodium upon insomnia and nocturnal restlessness compared in psychiatric patients. *Brit. J. Pharmacol.*, **16**, 82.

HOBSON, Q. J. G., SELWYN, J. G., and MOLLIN, D. L. (1956). Megaloblastic anaemia due to barbiturates. *Lancet*, **2**, 1079.

HOLDCROFT, A., MORGAN, M., WHITWAM, J. G., and LUMLEY, J. (1976). Effect of dose and premedication on induction complications with etomidate. *Brit. J. Anaesth.*, **48**, 199.

HORTON, J. N. (1973). Adverse reaction to althesin. *Anaesthesia*, **28**, 182.

HUBBARD, T. F., and GOLDBAUM, L. R. (1950). Distribution of thiopental in the central nervous system. *J. Lab. clin. Med.*, **36**, 218.

HUGILL, J. T. (1950). Liver function and anesthesia. *Anesthesiology*, **11**, 567.

HUTTON, A. M., and HALL, J. M. (1957). Incidence of thrombosis following thiopentone. *Anaesthesia*, **12**, 467.

ISBELL, H. (1950). Addiction to barbiturates and the barbiturate abstinence syndrome. *Ann. intern. Med.*, **33**, 108.

JANSSEN, P. A. J., NIEMEGEERS, C. J. E., SCHELLEKENS, K. H. L., and LENAERTS, F. M. (1971). Etomidate, R-(+)-ethyl-1-(α-methylbenzyl)imidazole-5-carboxylate (R 16659). *Arzneimittel Forsch.*, **21**, 1234.

JARMAN, R., and ABEL, A. L. (1936). Intravenous anaesthesia with pentothal sodium. *Lancet*, **1**, 422.

JOHNSTONE, M. (1972). The prevention of ketamine dreams. *Anaesth. Intens. Care*, **1**, 70.

KAY, B. (1976a). A clinical assessment of the use of etomidate in children. *Brit. J. Anaesth.*, **48**, 207.

KAY, B. (1976b). A dose-response relationship for etomidate, with some observations on cumulation. *Brit. J. Anaesth.*, **48**, 213.

KEATS, A. S., and BEECHER, H. K. (1950). Pain relief with hypnotic doses of barbiturates and a hypothesis. *J. Pharmacol. exp. Ther.*, **100**, 1.

KING, R. A., BIERER, I., RICHMOND, P., and WATSON, A. J. (1958). A new form of chloral hydrate. *Lancet*, **1**, 262.

KINMONTH, J. B., and SHEPHERD, R. C. (1959). Accidental injection of thiopentone into arteries. *Brit. med. J.*, **2**, 914.

KRAMER, M., WHITMAN, R. M., BALDRIDGE, B. J., and ORNSTEIN, P. H. (1966). The pharmacology of dreaming. In: *Enzymes in Mental Health*. Ed. Martin, G. J. and Kisch, B. Philadelphia: J. B. Lippincott Co.

LEE, H. A., and AMES, A. C. (1965). Haemodialysis in severe barbiturate poisoning. *Brit. med. J.*, **1**, 1217.

LIEBREICH, O. (1869). *Das Chloralhydrat, ein neues Hypnoticum und Anästheticum.* Berlin.

LOOMIS, A. L., HARVEY, E. N., and HOBART, G. A. (1938). Distribution of disturbance-patterns in the human EEG with special reference to sleep. *J. Neurophysiol.*, **1**, 413.

LUNDY, J. S. (1935). Intravenous anesthesia: preliminary report of the use of two new thiobarbiturates. *Proc. Mayo Clin.*, **10**, 536.

LUNSFORD, C. D., CALE, A. D., and JENKINS, H. (1962). 4-(β substituted ethyl)-3,3-diphenyl-2-pyrolinones, a new series of C.N.S. stimulants. *Abstr. 141st Meeting Amer. Chem. Soc.*, 2.

MACINTOSH, R. R., and HEYWORTH, P. S. A. (1943). Intra-arterial injection of pentothal: a warning. *Lancet*, **2**, 571.

MCKECHNIE, F. B., and CONVERSE, J. G. (1955). Placental transmission of thiopental. *Amer. J. Obstet. Gynec.*, **70**, 639.

MAYNERT, E. W., and VAN DYKE, H. B. (1950). The absence of localisation of barbital in divisions of the central nervous system. *J. Pharmacol. exp. Ther.*, **98**, 184.

MEEK, W. J., and SEEVERS, M. H. (1934). Cardiac irregularities produced by ephedrine and protective action of sodium barbital. *J. Pharmacol. exp. Ther.*, **51**, 287.

MEHTA, S., and BURTON, P. (1975). Effects of althesin anaesthesia and surgery on carbohydrate and fat metabolism in man. *Brit. J. Anaesth.*, **47**, 863.

MILLER, J. R., and STOELTING, V. K. (1963). A preliminary communication on the sleep-producing effects of intramuscular methohexitone sodium in the paediatric patient. *Brit. J. Anaesth.*, **35**, 48.

NOE, F. E., BORRILLO, N., and GREIFENSTEEN, F. E. (1965). Use of a new analeptic, doxapram hydrochloride, during general anaesthesia and recovery. *Anesth. Analg. Curr. Res.*, **44**, 206.

NOVELLI, G. P., MARSILI, M., and LORENZI, P. (1975). Influence of liver metabolism on the actions of althesin and thiopentone. *Brit. J. Anaesth.*, **47**, 913.

OSWALD, I. (1968). Drugs and sleep. *Pharmacol. Rev.*, **20**, 305.

OYAMA, T., MAEDA, A., JIN, J., SALTORE, T., and KUDO, M. (1975). Effect of althesin (CT-1341) on thyroid adrenal function in man. *Brit. J. Anaesth.*, **47**, 837.

PARSONS, T. W. (1963). Clinical comparison of barbiturates as hypnotics. *Brit. med. J.*, **2**, 1035.

PASK, E. A., and ROBSON, J. G. (1954). Injury to the median nerve. *Anaesthesia*, **9**, 94.

PAUCA, A. L., and HOPKINS, A. M. (1971). Acute effects of halothane, nitrous oxide and thiopentone on the upper limb blood flow. *Brit. J. Anaesth.*, **43**, 326.

PENHEAROW, A. (1957). Paediatric anaesthesia. *Brit. med. J.*, **1**, 644.

PRICE, H. L. (1960). A dynamic concept of the distribution of the thiopental in the human body. *Anesthesiology*, **21**, 40.

PRIME, F. J., and GRAY, T. C. (1952). The effect of certain anaesthetic and relaxant agents on circulatory dynamics. *Brit. J. Anaesth.*, **24**, 101.

PUTTER, J. (1965). Uber den firmentativen Abbau des Propanidid. In: *Die intravenose Kurznarkose mit dem neuen Phenoxyersigisaurederivat Propanidid (Epontol)*, p. 61. Eds. Horatz, K., Frey, R. and Zindler, M. Berlin: Springer-Verlag.

QUILLIAM, J. P. (1955). The action of thiopentone sodium on skeletal muscle. *Brit. J. Pharmacol.*, **10**, 141.

RAHN, E., DAYTON, P. G., and FREDERICKSON, E. L. (1969). Lack of effect of halothane on the metabolism of thiopentone in man. *Brit. J. Anaesth.*, **41**, 503.

REDISH, C. H., VORE, R. E., CHERNIOSH, S. M., and GRUBER, C. M., Jnr. (1958). A comparison of thiopental sodium, methitural sodium and methohexital sodium in oral surgery patients. *Oral Surg.*, **11**, 603.

RICHARDS, R. K., and TAYLOR, J. D. (1956). Some factors influencing distribution, metabolism and action of barbiturates: a review. *Anesthesiology*, **17**, 414.

ROBBINS, B. H., BAXTER, J. H., Jr., and FITZHUGH, O. G. (1939). Studies of cyclopropane: the use of barbiturates in preventing cardiac irregularities under cyclopropane or morphia and cyclopropane anesthesia. An experimental study. *Ann. Surg.*, **110**, 84.

SAVEGE, T. M., FOLEY, E. I., ROSS, L., and MAXWELL, M. P. (1972). A comparison of the cardiorespiratory effects during induction of anaesthesia of althesin with thiopentone and methohexitone. *Postgrad. med. J.*, **48** (suppl. 2), 66.

SHIDEMAN, F. E., GOULD, T. C., WINTERS, W. D., PETERSON, R. D., and WILNER, W. K. (1953). The distribution and *in vivo* rate of metabolism of thiopental. *J. Pharmacol. exp. Ther.*, **107**, 368.

SHIDEMAN, F. E., KELLY, A. R., and ADAMS, B. J. (1947). The role of the liver in the detoxication of thiopental (pentothal) and two other thiobarbiturates. *J. Pharmacol. exp. Ther.*, **91**, 331.

SHUBIN, H., and WEIL, M. H. (1971). Shock associated with barbiturate intoxication. *J. Amer. med. Ass.*, **215**, 263.

SLIOM, C. M., FRANKEL, L., and HOLBROOK, R. A. (1962). A comparison between methohexitone and thiopentone as induction agents for Caesarean section anaesthesia. *Brit. J. Anaesth.*, **34**, 316.

STONE, H. H., and DONNELLY, C. C. (1961). The accidental intra-arterial injection of thiopental. *Anesthesiology*, **22**, 995.

SWANSON, E. E. (1934). The present status of the barbiturate problem. *Proc. Soc. exp. Biol. (N.Y.)*, **31**, 963.

TABERN, D. L., and VOLWILER, E. H. (1935). Sulfur-containing barbiturate hypnotics. *J. Amer. chem. Soc.*, **57**, 1961.

TAKKI, S., NIKKI, P., JAATTELA, A., and TAMMISTO, T. (1972). Ketamine and plasma catecholamines. *Brit. J. Anaesth.*, **44**, 1318.

TAYLOR, C., and STOELTING, V. K. (1960). Methohexital sodium—a new ultrashort-acting barbiturate. *Anesthesiology*, **21**, 29.

TAYLOR, P. A., and TOWEY, R. M. (1971). Depression of laryngeal reflexes during ketamine anaesthesia using a standard challenge technique. *Brit. J. Anaesth.*, **44**, 1163.

TWEED, W. A., MINUCK, M., and MYRNIA, D. (1972). Circulatory response to ketamine anesthesia. *Anesthesiology*, **37**, 613.

WATERS, D. J. (1966). Intra-arterial thiopentone. *Anaesthesia*, **21**, 346.

WECHSLER, R. L., DRIPPS, R. D., and KETY, S. S. (1951). Blood flow and oxygen consumption of the human brain during anesthesia produced by thiopental. *Anesthesiology*, **12**, 308.

WILSON, J., STEPHEN, G. W., and SCOTT, D. B. (1969). A study of the cardiovascular effects of chlormethiazole. *Brit. J. Anaesth.*, **41**, 840.

WINNIE, A. P., and COLLINS, V. J. (1966). The search for a pharmacologic ventilator. *Acta anaesth. scand.*, Suppl. **23**, 63.

WINNIE, A. P., GLADISH, J. T., ANGEL, J. T., RAMAMURTHY, S., and COLLINS, V. J. (1971). Chemical respirogenesis II. Reversal of postoperative hypoxaemia with the "pharmacologic sigh". *Anesth. Analg. Curr. Res.*, **50**, 1043.

WYANT, G. M., and CHANG, C. A. (1959). Sodium methohexital: a clinical study. *Canad. Anaesth. Soc. J.*, **6**, 40.

WYNANDS, J. E., and BURFOOT, M. F. (1963). A clinical study of propanidid (F.B.A. 1420). *Canad. Anaesth. Soc. J.*, **12**, 587.

Chapter 23

PSYCHOTROPIC AGENTS, ANTI-EMETICS AND ANTI-SIALOGOGUES

ANTIHISTAMINES

THE antihistamine group of drugs is important because, apart from their value in treating conditions associated with the liberation of histamine, some of the compounds have useful side-effects.

The antihistamine drugs are defined as those drugs which oppose or prevent the actions of histamine, but which do not produce the opposite pharmacological effects if they are given when no histamine has been released. This definition excludes those drugs whose pharmacological actions are opposed to those of histamine. Therefore, a drug such as adrenaline, which will relax the smooth muscle contraction produced by histamine in the intestine or bronchioles but which produces this relaxation even if there is no histamine present, is not an antihistamine.

These drugs originated from the work of Bovet and his colleagues at the Pasteur Institute in Paris, who in 1937 produced Compound No. 929F which had antihistaminic properties but was too toxic for clinical use.

To understand the value of the antihistaminics a knowledge of the pharmacological actions of histamine is essential.

$$HN\diagdown N \quad CH_2 - CH_2 - NH_2$$

Histamine

Actions of histamine.—Histamine produces (1) *contraction of smooth muscle* which is most marked in the intestines, uterus and bronchioles; (2) *a fall of blood pressure* in man due to arteriolar and capillary dilatation with increased permeability and a flushed skin (essentially the same as the triple response to stroking of Lewis); (3) *increased glandular secretion*, particularly of the stomach, where it produces maximal stimulation to the secretion of hydrochloric acid— in fact histamine acid phosphate has been used as a test to find out how much hydrochloric acid the stomach can secrete. Pepsin secretion has been found to be increased in man (Ashford *et al.*, 1949 *a* and *b*), although this has not been confirmed by other observers. Histamine may also stimulate salivary, pancreatic and intestinal secretions in man, but these effects are more pronounced and easier to study in certain animals. The headache, which occurs after the subcutaneous administration of histamine, commences when the blood pressure has returned to normal and is thought to be due to the stretching of pial and dural arteries (Pickering, 1939).

Research in recent years has shown that the actions of histamine are exerted on two populations of receptors, denoted H_1 and H_2 (Black *et al.*, 1972), which can be distinguished by the actions of histamine analogues and of antagonists. Smooth muscle and vascular effects are determined predominantly by H_1-receptors and are susceptible to blockade by H_1-antagonists. Gastric secretory effects are determined by H_2-receptors and are blocked by H_2-antagonists. There is, however, some overlap between the two and the hypotensive effect produced by histamine appears to involve both types (Black *et al.*, 1975).

H_1-antihistamines

Since the original work of Bovet, many compounds have been synthesised and much comparative work done on their relative merits. A list is given in Table 1. These compounds differ in potency and to some extent in their elimination characteristics, making some longer-acting than others, but there is no firm evidence of qualitative differences between them. Various animal tests have been used for quantitating the drugs' actions.

23/TABLE 1
H_1-ANTIHISTAMINES

Approved name	Proprietary name
brompheniramine	Dimotane
chlorpheniramine	Haynon, Piriton
clemastine	Tavegil
cyproheptadine	Periactin
dimethindene	Fenostil
dimethothiazine	Banistyl
diphenhydramine	Benadryl
diphenylpyraline	Histryl, Lergoban
embramine	Mebryl
mebhydrolin	Fabahistin
mepyramine	Anthisan
methdilazine	Dilosyn
phenindamine	Thephorin
pheniramine	Daneral
promethazine	Phenergan
trimeprazine	Vallergan
triprolidine	Actidil, Pro-Actidil

Although Hawkins and Schild (1951) using human material in the same way that Castillo and de Beer (1947) used guinea-pig tracheal rings, found that the sensitivity of this tissue to histamine and the antihistaminics was of the same order, the relationship of the potency of the different compounds varies with the tests used, and the correlation between the results in animals and those in man is uncertain.

In man using the inhibition of the histamine weal in the skin it has been shown that 25 mg of promethazine (Phenergan) was equivalent to 175 mg of mepyramine (Bain, 1949) and 2·5 mg of triprolidine.

That the histamine antagonists can prevent the increase in capillary permeability produced by histamine was shown by Last and Loew (1947), when they demonstrated that trypan blue could be kept in the circulation by diphenhydramine and mepyramine after the administration of histamine.

Concentrations of the order produced by giving promethazine in the usual doses by mouth or by injection cause a powerful contraction of the precapillary sphincters in the rat's meso-appendix and this has been suggested as the mechanism of its protective action against capillary permeability (Halpern, 1947; Haley and Harris, 1949).

Pharmacological Actions

The H_1-antihistamines show a variety of different pharmacological actions which can be summarised as follows:

1. *Antihistaminic action.*—The antagonistic action on bronchial and circulatory histamine receptors is competitive in type and depends therefore on the relative concentrations of histamine and antagonist present.

2. *Analgesia.*—Mepyramine (Dews and Graham, 1946) and promethazine (Haranath, 1954) have local anaesthetic properties. The former has also some systemic analgesic activity (Hewer and Keele, 1948).

3. *Central nervous system depression.*—Many of the anti-histamines produce depression of the central nervous system which varies from an allaying of anxiety to intense drowsiness. For this reason promethazine, which produces the greatest depression, is given by mouth or injection as a pre-operative sedative and, in the form of an elixir, as a hypnotic for children. Diethazine (Diparcol)—a closely related compound with a weak antihistaminic action—is used for its property of producing muscular relaxation in Parkinsonism. Other members of the group also have this property but to a lesser extent.

4. *Anti-emetic action.*—A particular part of the brain that is depressed by some of these compounds is the vomiting centre.

This property was discovered by chance. Dimenhydrinate (Dramamine) was given to a pregnant woman with urticaria, and she noticed that car sickness, from which she suffered regularly, was prevented by the tablets. This led to a carefully controlled trial among servicemen crossing the Atlantic (Gay and Carliner, 1949).

5. *Synergism with analgesics and anaesthetics.*—Promethazine was used in anaesthesia by Laborit and Leger (1950) in the hope that its antihistamine activity would avert certain forms of phlebitis which were thought to be due to anaphylaxis.

It was found that promethazine was a powerful hypnotic and prolonged the action of the barbiturates and opiates.

It was also postulated by Laborit (1950) that the value of promethazine during anaesthesia is due to the diminution of capillary permeability and basal metabolism.

Diethazine was used by Laborit, who found that it not only enhances anaesthesia and analgesia but also the muscular relaxation produced by gallamine.

6. *Autonomic actions.*—Most antihistamines have atropine-like actions and dry salivary secretions. They show also mild alpha-adrenoceptor blocking properties and some show quinidine-like activity on the heart (Dews and Graham, 1946).

Some individual differences in pharmacology.—Diphenhydramine produces a moderate hypnotic effect, whereas promethazine is a powerful hypnotic with a prolonged effect—its half decay time being 19½ hours. Triprolidine acts rapidly to produce an antihistamine effect which lasts for twelve hours. It produces few side-effects and has little hypnotic action. Phenindamine has little if any hypnotic action. Mepyramine has a half decay time of 5 hours.

Toxicity

H_1-antihistamines have been given continuously for periods up to two years with no signs of tolerance or toxicity. There are some reports of granulocytopenia following their use, and also of the fatal results of overdose either accidental, in children, or suicidal, when the drugs produced central nervous depression followed by convulsions—with cerebral oedema and upper nephron nephrosis discovered at autopsy.

Clinical Uses

The H_1-antihistamines are used in the treatment of urticaria and other allergic skin conditions, including drug sensitivity rashes, in the management of serum sickness, in hay fever, in vasomotor rhinitis and other respiratory diseases where there may be an allergic background. They are of little value in the treatment of an established attack of asthma but may be of value in prophylaxis. They have been used in most diseases where an antigen antibody reaction might play a part, and they have been found to be most useful in the acute stages of the allergic diseases. They are unable to influence the established disease.

Side-effects

Drowsiness is common with most of these drugs except phenindamine. Other side-effects which may occur are dizziness, headache, dry nose and mouth, with—more rarely—nausea and vomiting, intestinal colic and diarrhoea. The latter are seen most frequently with antazoline, mepyramine and tripelennamine, and can best be avoided by taking the drugs during or immediately after meals. If unpleasant side-effects are produced one of the other drugs should be used instead.

Promethazine in full doses of 25 to 50 mg daily may produce ataxia and aching limbs. It is best administered at night because of the drowsiness produced. The other antihistaminics are best administered throughout the day in repeated doses—triprolidine 2·5 mg, phenindamine 25–50 mg, diphenhydramine and tripelennamine 50 mg, mepyramine 100 mg.

Uses Associated with Anaesthesia

Promethazine has been used more in this context than the other true antihistaminics because of its marked sedative properties which are unassociated with respiratory depression. It is used as a premedicant, to supplement anaesthesia during operation, and post-operatively.

There have been many reports of its use (Lyon, 1956; Sadove, 1956; Hopkin *et al.*, 1957) and all agree that a dose of 50 mg given with pethidine 50 or 100 mg and atropine 0·6 mg before operation produces a calm patient, sleepy but rousable, and with a normal blood pressure. A dose of 25 mg is often sufficient. Less thiopentone is required for the induction of anaesthesia than after the more usual premedication of papaveretum and hyoscine; there is a rapid return of reflexes post-operatively and a decreased need for post-operative analgesics for the first twelve hours, with less post-operative nausea and vomiting.

Promethazine appears to be particularly helpful for elderly patients with bronchitis, bronchospasm or emphysema, by preventing such disturbances as bucking, coughing and spasm which often make anaesthetising these patients difficult.

When promethazine is given as premedication it is seldom necessary to give more during the operation, since it has such a long action. Combinations of promethazine, chlorpromazine and pethidine have been used as the "lytic cocktail" in premedication and for neuroleptanalgesia. The combined action of these drugs induces powerful central depression, severe hypotension from widespread vasodilatation and cholinergic blockade. When used as premedication, requirements of anaesthetic agents and post-operative analgesics are greatly reduced but recovery is slow and fluid replacement is critical.

For children there is a syrup of promethazine which is palatable and is given in a dose of 0·50 mg/kg with atropine; if the child is resistant it can be combined with an equal dose of pethidine.

H$_2$-antihistamines

To date three such compounds have appeared, *burimamide*, *metiamide* and *cimetidine*. Of these, metiamide has been subject to most testing and shown to inhibit gastric-acid secretion both at rest and provoked by histamine, pentagastrin, food and insulin hypoglycaemia. Neither burimamide nor metiamide are, however, likely to be used clinically, the former because it is poorly absorbed from the gastro-intestinal tract and the latter because of occasional bone marrow depression. This adverse effect is thought to be due to the thiourea residue present in the molecule, rather than to H$_2$-antagonism as such. If so then cimetidine, which lacks this particular residue, should prove safe. H$_2$-antagonists are the subject of a recent review (*Lancet*, 1975).

The principal clinical application of this group of drugs lies in the management of peptic ulcer. Cimetidine has already been shown to produce effective control of gastric acidity in duodenal ulceration (Pounder *et al.*, 1975) and to promote healing.

PSYCHOTROPIC DRUGS

Various terms such as "tranquillisers" or "ataractics" have been loosely applied to a whole group of drugs which have only one property in common—namely an ability to produce "peace of mind". Yet this nebulous term makes it difficult or even impossible to measure or assess their efficacy with any real degree of accuracy, especially as they have little action on normal subjects. No general agreement has yet been reached on a satisfactory classification of this diverse group of drugs, largely because each one has so many actions that it is almost impossible to place them in a select compartment. The following groups of drugs are considered here:

(*a*) Major tranquillisers.
(*b*) Minor tranquillisers.
(*c*) Antidepressants.

The distinction between major and minor tranquillisers is that the former have widespread effects on the central and peripheral autonomic nervous systems and the ability to calm grossly disturbed psychotic patients. Minor tranquillisers have only restricted central action and in practice are useful only in mild anxiety and other reactive states.

MAJOR TRANQUILLISERS

Reserpine

Reserpine is one of a large number of similar alkaloids found in *Rauwolfia serpentina* and related species of plant found in Asia. It has been used widely for its sedative and tranquillising properties and for its antihypertensive action. Its clinical use has greatly declined, except in those countries where it is indigenous, because of the occurrence of side-effects, mental depression, Parkinsonism and diarrhoea.

Reserpine and the other alkaloids induce bradycardia and hypotension (Plummer *et al.*, 1954) as a result largely of their peripheral adrenergic neurone blocking actions. These occur because of disruption of synaptic vesicles in the nerve-endings which depletes these endings of their noradrenaline stores. This is associated with supersensitivity to direct-acting, and insensitivity to indirect-acting, sympathomimetic amines in animals (Burn and Rand, 1958) and man (Gelder and Vane, 1962).

Hypotension associated with reserpine treatment is of consequence in anaesthesia. Coakley *et al.* (1956) reported that in 16 out of 40 patients severe circulatory depression occurred in association with anaesthesia and that the blood pressure did not always respond to vasopressors.

The Phenothiazine Derivatives

The phenothiazine nucleus has no antihistaminic action and little or no depressant effect upon the central nervous system; but derivatives of phenothiazine possess these as well as various other properties. Stemming from the work of Bovet and his colleagues in Paris very many have been synthesised. The first of the group to be used in medicine was promethazine, which has been discussed under the heading of the antihistamine drugs, since it is one of the most powerful antihistaminics known. The addition of a chlorine atom to the nucleus and rearrangement of the side-chain of promethazine makes chlorpromazine, the most studied of the phenothiazine derivatives.

Chlorpromazine (Largactil, Thorazine).—2-chloro-10-(3-dimethyl-amino-n-propyl) phenothiazine hydrochloride.

Physical Properties

Chlorpromazine is a greyish-white crystalline powder with a slightly pungent odour. It is very soluble in water (1 g in 2·5 ml). A 5 per cent aqueous solution has a pH of between 4 and 5. The powder and solution become discoloured in bright light, but this is not thought to impair the potency or increase the toxicity.

Pharmacological Actions

Chlorpromazine has very little antihistaminic activity but has a profound action on the central nervous system and the peripheral circulation. It has so many actions on the central nervous system that it is very difficult to elucidate the different sites and mode of production of its effects. It is said that the hypothalamus is depressed, with a decrease in the amount of secretion from the anterior pituitary. It is also stated that the mesodiencephalic alerting system, which consists of the reticular formations and the thalamic diffuse cortical projections, is depressed as well (Himwich, 1955; Rinaldi and Himwich, 1955; Moruzzi and Magoun, 1949; Jasper, 1949). These areas, which are all depressed by chlorpromazine, are involved in the control of basal metabolism, body temperature, sleep and wakefulness, vasomotor tone, vomiting and hormonal balance.

The electro-encephalogram reflects the state of consciousness after a dose of chlorpromazine but shows no special features. During the phase of "disinterestedness" there is an accentuation of the theta element but the patterns during sleep are indistinguishable from those of normal sleep (Terzian, 1952).

The mental effects noted in the conscious patient are drowsiness and loss of interest in the surroundings; euphoria sometimes occurs. If the drowsiness leads to sleep the patient can still be easily roused. The depressant action on the central nervous system is not affected by amphetamine, caffeine or nikethamide, and lasts about eight hours after 0·7 mg/kg given intravenously in man. Lehmann and Hanrahan (1954) have shown that although the sedation is greater with chlorpromazine the reaction times are longer with quinalbarbitone, and they summarise the mental effects of chlorpromazine thus: ". . . chlorpromazine is the only powerful sedative whose action is restricted to a selective inhibition of drive without producing disinhibition of effect at any level of dosage."

The depressant actions of chlorpromazine are synergistic with those of other cerebral depressants, hypnotics, analgesics, alcohol and anaesthetics. Following chlorpromazine smaller quantities of general anaesthetics are needed to produce adequate anaesthesia.

Autonomic nervous system.—Chlorpromazine is not a true ganglion-blocking agent, but since it antagonises the effects of adrenaline, and to a lesser extent those of noradrenaline and acetylcholine, it does modify some of the responses that are used as tests of ganglion-blocking ability.

Cardiovascular system.—Chlorpromazine causes dilatation of peripheral blood vessels in man by a direct action (Foster et al., 1954). This action has been demonstrated in the rabbit's ear, which also revealed an outpouring of fluid from the dilated vessels. In the isolated heart a reversible reduction of contractile force and irritability has been demonstrated with an increase in the coronary artery flow (Courvoisier et al., 1953; Melville, 1954). The centrally and peripherally produced vasodilatation leads to hypotension which is very responsive to changes in posture. The pulse rate rises, but the cardiac output changes are variable.

Respiratory system.—In spite of clinical reports of stimulation of respiration by chlorpromazine, Dobkin and his co-workers (1954) found that the tidal and minute volumes decreased in both conscious and anaesthetised patients after intramuscular or intravenous administration of 0·3–2 mg/kg. The respiratory rate was variable and the breathing frequently became irregular.

Liver and kidney function.—The prolonged use of chlorpromazine as a cause of jaundice is now well-established, but the effects of single doses, or short courses of the drug, on the liver are not clearly understood. Moyer and his co-workers (1954) found that in patients with liver dysfunction the drug appeared to be potentiated. Lehmann and Hanrahan (1954), studying 71 patients who were on daily doses of chlorpromazine, found that about half showed alteration in the cephalin-flocculation tests, that one third had changes in the total serum protein values and albumin-globulin ratios, and that three developed jaundice. Whether these effects are a primary action on the liver cells or secondary to the hypotension has not been established. Stein and Wright (1956) suggest that chlorpromazine causes increased viscosity of bile, leading to stasis and intrahepatic canalicular obstruction which is indistinguishable from other types of obstructive jaundice. It seems likely that this reaction is allergic in origin (Sherlock, 1964) as it is commoner with second than with first courses of treatment and is not associated with high dosage.

Hyperglycaemia has been noticed, and Courvoisier and her co-workers (1953) found that the hyperglycaemia produced by adrenaline was little affected by chlorpromazine. Moyer and his colleagues (1955) found no evidence of acute renal toxicity or any significant change in renal haemodynamics. Renal blood flow changes in dogs are variable but tend to increase. Sodium and water excretion are slightly increased.

Effects on metabolism.—Decourt (1953) reviews the evidence set out in his many publications, and he suggests that the fundamental activity of chlorpromazine is a reversible inhibition of cellular activity, which he terms "narcobiotic action". He has been able to demonstrate this inhibition—which with higher doses becomes irreversible—in many lower forms of life. In man, Dobkin and his co-workers (1954) were unable to demonstrate any reduction in oxygen consumption following a dose of 1–2 mg/kg but they were making sundry other measurements at the same time, which may have interfered with this observation.

Hypothermic action.—Dundee and his colleagues (1954) postulate that it is the prevention of shivering coupled with the peripheral dilatation produced by chlorpromazine that makes it such a powerful hypothermic agent. They consider it superior to the ganglion-blocking agents and the adrenolytic drugs in this respect. Decourt and his co-workers (1953) found that the central temperature of an animal under the influence of chlorpromazine falls, even if the surrounding temperature is high.

Anti-emetic action.—Chlorpromazine is a powerful anti-emetic drug especially against vomiting produced by drugs and by radiation. It appears to act by depressing the vomiting centre.

Anti-shock effect.—Courvoisier and her co-workers (1953) found that, given to a dog immediately after the haemorrhage produced by Wiggers' method, chlorpromazine in a dose of 2 mg/kg intravenously provided complete protection and a survival time of over 72 hours. Of the non-treated animals 83 per cent died within a few hours. The results in cats were less dramatic. It is postulated that the mechanism of action is its anti-adrenaline action and the maintenance of blood flow through the tissues.

Fate in the body.—Chlorpromazine, like the other phenothiazines, undergoes metabolic degradation by a number of pathways of which ring hydroxylation followed by conjugation and sulphoxide formation are the most important. These and several subsidiary pathways contribute to the formation of about 50 metabolites which appear in the urine and faeces. Some of these have modest biological activity but the extent to which their influence contributes to the action of the parent drug is unknown at present.

Miscellaneous effects.—Chlorpromazine increases the effects of both competitive and depolarising muscle relaxants. Burn (1954) found that skeletal muscle became unresponsive to direct stimulation after 3 mg/kg of chlorpromazine. This paralysis was delayed in onset and might be preceded by augmentation. Chlorpromazine is two to three times more powerful in this respect than promethazine. Su and Lee (1960) found that in high doses in rat and frog muscles this paralysis could not easily be reversed.

Chlorpromazine has a local analgesic action, but if the concentration of the solution is above 0·1 per cent necrosis of nerves may occur.

Reilly and Tournier (1953) found that chlorpromazine protected 55 per cent of mice from an otherwise fatal dose of the endotoxin of typhoid fever.

Toxicity

Animal studies show wide species variation in the amount of chlorpromazine required to kill. Large intravenous doses produce loss of tone followed by convulsions and death from respiratory arrest. Small areas of congestion may be found in the kidneys, but these are unlike the glomerulitis and lesions of the convoluted tubules, caused by toxic doses of promethazine. Burn (1954) showed that chlorpromazine slowed the rate of growth in rats. Leucopenia has been reported (Anton-Stephens, 1954), but no cases of agranulocytosis have been mentioned in the literature. Large doses of all phenothiazines accumulate with repeated administration and may cause extrapyramidal signs, Parkinsonism, dystonia, dyskinesia and akathisia. These signs disappear on stopping treatment or they can be abated by concurrent administration of anti-Parkinson drugs.

Dermatitis may occur in those who handle the drug constantly, and urticaria and other allergic manifestations have been observed in some patients, but these cleared rapidly after withdrawal of the drug. Other rare sequelae include nausea, anorexia, and epigastric distress.

Acute poisoning from chlorpromazine is rare, but Dilworth and his colleagues (1963) have reported sudden respiratory failure. As well as artificial respiration, they recommend the use of plasma expanders and vasoconstrictors. Of the latter, phenylephrine and noradrenaline are most likely to be effective.

Clinical Uses

Anaesthesia.—Chlorpromazine has been used before, during, and after anaesthesia, but because it has been given in combination with a great variety of drugs the assessment of its true worth in this field is difficult. Laborit and Huguenard in many publications from 1950 onwards described the complicated technique of "artificial hibernation". In this technique, which was described in *Pratique de l'hibernotherapie en chirurgie et en medicine* (1954), many drugs were used, but this technique is now seldom practised.

The disadvantages of chlorpromazine are that it causes postural hypotension which may last for up to four hours, and also prolonged depression of reflexes, which may be dangerous.

Administration.—Concentrated solutions of chlorpromazine—and other phenothiazines—are irritant to the tissues, and must therefore be injected intra-muscularly. Intravenous injections should be limited to diluted solutions.

Control of vomiting.—Chlorpromazine is a powerful anti-emetic and has been used successfully in vomiting due to such varied causes as carcinomatosis, labyrinthitis, disulfiram (Antabuse) and alcohol, uraemia, nitrogen mustard, digitalis, hyperemesis gravidarum, acute gastritis and radiotherapy, as well as post-anaesthesia.

The doses used vary from 25 mg daily to 50 mg four times a day, but if vomiting is not controlled by two or three injections of 25 to 50 mg of chlor-promazine it is unwise to push the dosage because of the depression that is pro-duced. A better alternative is to use another phenothiazine, such as perphena-zine (dose 5 mg). Unless the cause of vomiting is known before treatment is begun, the sedation might mask the signs and prevent the diagnosis of a condition which might be serious.

Psychiatry.—Chlorpromazine has proved of value in the symptomatic control of most types of severe psychomotor excitement. Winkelman (1954) summarises his results in 142 patients: "Chlorpromazine . . . is particularly outstanding in that it can reduce a severe anxiety, diminish phobias and obsessions, reverse or modify a paranoid psychosis, quieten manic or extremely agitated patients and make hostile, agitated senile patients quiet and easily manageable." Experimentally it antagonises the psychotomimetic effects of lysergide (LSD).

Intractable pain.—Because of its ability to increase the effectiveness of anal-gesics and its property of producing "pharmacological leucotomy"—a state where pain, although felt, does not distress the patient—chlorpromazine has found a place in the management of patients with intractable pain. Chlorpro-mazine has no analgesic properties, and therefore is of no value by itself, but in doses of 25 mg two or three times a day it is a useful adjuvant to the analgesics. It has been used extensively in the treatment of persistent hiccup.

Other Phenothiazine Compounds

Many compounds based on the phenothiazine nucleus have been synthesised in an attempt to obtain more specificity without so many or dangerous side-effects and disadvantages. The structural grouping, approved and proprietary names of these derivatives are given in Table 2.

Individual compounds in this vast collection differ from each other and from chlorpromazine itself only slightly in their properties. First, they differ in potency such that different doses are needed to produce equivalent effects. Secondly, they differ in anticholinergic activity, thioridazine being outstanding in its tendency to produce atropine-like side-effects. Thirdly, the piperidine and piperazine derivatives tend to produce antanalgesia, while the dimethyl-

23/Table 2

PHENOTHIAZINES AND RELATED DRUGS

Group	Approved name	Proprietary and other names
Dimethylamino-propyl side-chain	acepromazine	Acetylpromazine, Notensil
	chlorpromazine	Chloractil, Largactil, Thorazine
	fluopromazine	Trifluopromazine, Vespral, Vesprin
	methotrimeprazine	Levomepromazine, Levoprome, Veractil
	promazine	Sparine
	propiomazine	Indorm, Largon
	prothipendyl	Phrenotropin, Tolnate
	trimeprazine	Alimemazine, Panectyl, Temaril, Vallergan
Piperidine side-chain	mesoridazine	Lidanil, Serentil
	pecazine	Mepazine, Pacatal
	pericyazine	Neulactil, Propericiazine
	pipamazine	Mornidine
	thioridazine	Melleril
Piperazine side-chain	acetophenazine	Tindal
	butaperazine	Repoise
	carphenazine	Proketazine
	fluphenazine	Modecate, Moditen, Moditen enanthate, Permitil, Prolixin
	perphenazine	Fentazin, Trilafon
	prochlorperazine	Compazine, Prochlorpemazine, Stemetil
	thiethylperazine	Torecan
	thiopropazate	Dartalan
	thioproperazine	Majeptil
	trifluoperazine	Stelazine
Thioxanthines	chlorprothixene	Taractan, Tarasan
	clopenthixol	Sordinol
	flupenthixol	Depixol
	thiothixene	Navane

aminopropyl group tend to be analgesic (Dundee *et al.*, 1963). Fourthly, the piperazine group have exaggerated antipsychotic and anti-emetic properties and are more likely to produce extrapyramidal toxicity. The piperazine-substituted compounds have preferential use as anti-emetics.

Butyrophenone Derivatives

This group of drugs has actions which are essentially similar to those of the phenothiazines, though their structure is quite different. Important examples are:

droperidol —Droleptan
haloperidol —Serenace
trifluperidol—Triperidol

They induce mild sedation and tranquillisation in normal and neurotic patients and calm hyperactive psychotics. Their use in anaesthesia—particularly droperidol in combination with fentanyl—is becoming increasingly popular for the production of neuroleptanalgesia (see Chapter 33).

They have generalised cerebral depressant actions which are equivalent to those of the piperazine-substituted phenothiazines. They show similar anti-psychotic and anti-emetic properties and they are likely to produce extrapyramidal upsets. They do not appear to cause cross-sensitisation with phenothiazines and can safely be administered to patients who have developed jaundice after chlorpromazine.

They can cause hypotension because of both central and peripheral adrenergic blocking actions and the cerebral depressant actions summate with those of hypnotics, narcotics, analgesics and other tranquillisers. For general anaesthesia, therefore, requirements of all drugs are greatly reduced but, as with phenothiazines, recovery may be very slow.

MINOR TRANQUILLISERS

A number of mild cerebral depressant drugs have been used as sedatives and minor tranquillisers. Most of these, such as hydroxyzine, meprobamate, methylpentynol and tybamate, are largely of historic interest only. The most important of the minor tranquillisers in current use are the benzodiazepines.

Benzodiazepines

Since their introduction into clinical practice in the early 1960s, a large number of compounds in this series has been introduced. A current list of approved and proprietary names, together with their advocated uses, is given in Table 3. The distinction implied in these uses is, however, not borne out by real differences in pharmacological activity. There is therefore at present no satisfactory evidence that any of the alternatives differ significantly from diazepam, which can be regarded as the parent drug.

23/TABLE 3
BENZODIAZEPINES

Approved name	Proprietary name	Advocated use
bromazepam		tranquilliser
chlordiazepoxide	Librium	tranquilliser
clobazam		tranquilliser
clonazepam	Rivotril	anticonvulsant
clorazepic acid	Tranxene	sedative
clozapine		sedative
diazepam	Atensine, Valium	anaesthetic, anticonvulsant, tranquilliser
flunitrazepam		hypnotic
flurazepam	Dalmane	hypnotic
lofendazam		tranquilliser
lorazepam	Ativan	tranquilliser
medazepam	Nobrium	tranquilliser
nitrazepam	Mogadon	hypnotic
oxazepam	Serenid-D	tranquilliser
prazepam		muscle relaxant
temazepam		tranquilliser

Diazepam (Atensine, Valium).—7-Chloro-1,3-dihydro-1-methyl-5 phenyl-2H-1,4-benzodiazepin-2-one.

Actions.—Diazepam has general cerebral depressant properties, which make it suitable for use as anaesthetic, hypnotic, sedative or minor tranquilliser. At low dosage, it impairs concentration and the ability to perform skilled tasks. Larger doses produce amnesia, sleep or anaesthesia. Its depressant actions summate with those of all other cerebral depressant drugs, including anaesthetics. It has anticonvulsant activity (Randall *et al.*, 1961), probably supraspinal in origin, which makes it a useful agent in the management of tetanus, severe pre-eclamptic toxaemia and upper motor neurone lesions. High doses markedly reduce the EEG voltage.

Used alone, large doses do not usually depress medullary respiratory and vasomotor centres, but in combination with other depressant agents severe respiratory and cardiovascular depression may result. Given alone in doses sufficient to induce anaesthesia, airway maintenance can be difficult because of muscular relaxation brought about by inhibition of spinal reflexes.

Absorption and fate.—Diazepam is well absorbed when given by mouth and widely distributed in body tissues. It is inactivated predominantly by oxidative metabolism in the liver, but this process is slow and at least two of the metabolites formed have marked pharmacological activity (Schwartz *et al.*, 1965). Thus much of the effect produced results from N-desmethyldiazepam (which has an elimination half-life of 100 hours) as well as from diazepam itself (with a half-life of 24 hours). Nitrazepam, having a somewhat shorter half-life (12–15 hours) is possibly more suitable as a hypnotic agent than diazepam, though the difference is slight. On repeated administration diazepam accumulates in the body, and the effects of the drug and its metabolites take a long time to wear off. This is true also in cases of acute poisoning.

Uses.—Diazepam is at present one of the most commonly prescribed drugs in general and hospital practice. In mild anxiety states doses of 2 to 5 mg three times daily are used. In the management of agitated patients and in status epilepticus, as well as in premedication, larger doses may be needed.

Intravenous diazepam (5 mg/ml in propylene glycol) produces anaesthesia in healthy subjects at 1 mg/kg doses. Debilitated and elderly patients require much less. The solution is irritant and should be given only into large veins to prevent thrombosis occurring. Onset of, and recovery from, anaesthesia are slow (Brown and Dundee, 1968). Diazepam anaesthesia is the subject of a review (Dundee and Haslett, 1970). It is currently employed for endoscopy, dentistry, cardiac catheterisation and cardioversion.

ANTI-EMETICS

About one-third of all patients undergoing anaesthesia and surgery suffer nausea and vomiting afterwards. This may be peripheral or central in origin, the latter arising either from stimulation of the chemoreceptor trigger zone or by activation of labyrinthine reflexes. Anti-emetic drugs act either in the periphery or on the vomiting centre or both. Though anti-emetic drugs often reduce the incidence of post-operative nausea and vomiting, their accurate assessment is very difficult (Riding, 1963). The most useful drugs are antihistamines and phenothiazines, the anti-emetic activity of which are indicated in Table 4.

23/TABLE 4
ANTI-EMETICS

Approved name	Proprietary name
betahistine	Serc
buclizine	Equivert
cinnarizine	Stugeron
cyclizine	Marzine, Valoid
dimenhydrinate	Dramamine, Gravol
hyoscine	
meclozine	Ancoloxin
metoclopramide	Maxolon, Primperan
perphenazine	Fentazin, Trilafon
prochlorperazine	Stemetil, Vertigon
promethazine theoclate	Avomine
prothipendyl	Tolnate
thiethylperazine	Torecan
trifluoperazine	Stelazine

All writers are agreed that perphenazine is the most potent anti-emetic among the phenothiazines but it does have side-effects. The choice of an anti-emetic depends on circumstances, but Purkis and Ishii (1963) have summarised their criteria for selection of a particular drug. When minimal hypotension and rapid awakening from anaesthesia is important they recommend trifluoperazine; when only small quantities of post-operative narcotic are required they suggest fluopromazine, and when no specific contra-indications to one or other drug exist they consider perphenazine the drug of choice.

Metoclopramide (Maxolon)

This white crystalline substance, which is freely soluble in water, is an anti-emetic. In doses of 10 mg t.d.s. it is non-tranquillising. It acts by reducing the sensitivity of both the vomiting centre and the afferent nerves arising in the viscera. It is not effective in vomiting of labyrinthine origin such as travel sickness, vertigo and Mèniere's disease. Handley (1967) showed that metoclopramide (10 mg given at the end of the operation) was as effective as perphenazine 5 mg in preventing post-operative vomiting. Side-effects of prolonged administration of 60 mg per day include drowsiness, muscle dystonia, diarrhoea and headache.

Metoclopramide accelerates gastric emptying and has been advocated in the preparation of patients for obstetric anaesthesia (Howard and Sharp, 1973). The degree of emptying obtained within a reasonable time is, however, small and no reliance should be placed on its action in this situation.

ANTIDEPRESSANT DRUGS

The Monoamine Oxidase Inhibitors (MAO inhibitors)

The commonly used drugs of this group are listed in Table 5. Their beneficial effect in the treatment of reactive depression is probably related to the accumulation of brain monoamines (5-hydroxytryptamine, dopamine and noradrenaline) which they cause. Inhibition of monoamine oxidase in the periphery causes sympathetic blockade and consequent hypotension, probably due to the formation of octopamine as a false transmitter (Kopin *et al.*, 1965). Severe hypertensive episodes following ingestion of monoamine-containing foods (cheese, Marmite, wine, broad beans) should be treated by alpha-sympathetic blockade with phentolamine or chlorpromazine. Patients under treatment with MAO inhibitors should not be given sympathomimetic vasopressor agents; all will be greatly potentiated.

23/TABLE 5
MONOAMINE OXIDASE INHIBITORS

Approved name	Proprietary name
iproniazid	Marsilid
isocarboxazid	Marplan
mebanazine	Actomol
nialamide	Niamid
(pargyline	Eutonyl)
phenelzine	Nardil
tranylcypromine	Parnate
tranylcypromine with trifluoperazine	Parstelin

MAO inhibitors have inhibitory actions also on other enzyme systems, particularly those liver microsomal enzymes responsible for hydroxylation or oxidation of drugs such as barbiturates, alcohol, opiate narcotics, hypnotics and tranquillisers. These drugs are thus potentiated and should be used only in small test doses to assess their effects. Pethidine should probably be avoided altogether, for on occasion hyperpyrexia, restlessness, unconsciousness, hypotension and death have followed its use (see Perks, 1964). If pethidine administration is essential, a small intramuscular test dose of 5 mg should be given followed by 10 mg and 20 mg at hourly intervals if no untoward effect on pulse, blood pressure, respiration or state of consciousness occurs. Thereafter the dose may be increased until normal dosage is achieved without complication. Such a procedure indicates that many patients respond normally (Evans-Prosser, 1968). It is mandatory, however, that other analgesics such as pentazocine, dihydro-codeine, or even morphine should be used before resorting to pethidine in view of the known sensitivity reaction.

The reason for the interaction between pethidine and monoamine oxidase inhibitors is not absolutely clear. In the resting state, amine neurotransmitters in the brain (noradrenaline; 5-hydroxytryptamine) are stored in granules at the nerve-ending. Any unstored transmitter is rapidly inactivated by the mono-amine oxidase *enzyme* in the vicinity of the granules. On stimulation, the trans-mitter is released to act at the receptor. Thereafter some will be inactivated but the majority is *actively* taken up by the nerve-ending and re-stored in granules.

Pethidine and the tricyclic antidepressants tend to block the re-uptake pro-cess whilst the MAO inhibitors tend to build up the concentration of the neuro-transmitter. By this means the combination of an MAO inhibitor (permitting accumulation of transmitter in the nerve-ending) and pethidine (allowing accu-mulation near the receptor site) could lead to a severe reaction (convulsions, hypertension, etc.).

In animals, Gong and Rogers (1973) were able to reproduce a similar reac-tion using a combination of MAO inhibitors and pethidine but not when morphine was substituted. The finding that this sensitivity reaction is only rarely encountered in man remains a mystery but it might be explained by the hypo-thesis that patients with endogenous depression have a low output of neuro-transmitter.

There is no evidence that gaseous or volatile anaesthetic agents or neuro-muscular blockers are influenced by the administration of MAO inhibitors. The conduct of an anaesthetic may be made more difficult because of the combined hypotensive actions of the antidepressant and anaesthetic agents used. Elective operations under general anaesthesia are probably better postponed for one month, stopping MAO inhibitor treatment if the patient's psychiatric state permits. Stopping antidepressant treatment carries the risk that patients may make a suicidal attempt. This risk must be balanced against that of anaesthesia in the presence of the drugs. (See also Chapter 33.)

Tricyclic (Dibenzazepine) Antidepressants

Many compounds of this group are in common use for the treatment of depression, particularly of the endogenous or involutional type. The most important ones are listed in Table 6. These compounds have no inhibitory action against monoamine oxidase or other similar enzymes, their beneficial effect probably resulting from their action in preventing uptake of monoamines by nerve-endings (Glowinski and Axelrod, 1964). Like the MAO inhibitors, they cause mild sympathetic blockade and consequent hypotension. They have also

23/TABLE 6
TRICYCLIC AND RELATED ANTIDEPRESSANTS

Approved name	Proprietary and other names
amitriptyline	Laroxyl, Lentizol, Tryptizol
amitriptyline with perphenazine	Triptafen
butriptyline	
clomipramine	Anafranil
desipramine	Pertofran
dibenzapin	Noveril
dothiepin	Dosulepin, Prothiaden
doxepin	Sinequan
imipramine	Tofranil
iprindole	Pramindole, Prondol
nortriptyline	Allegron, Aventyl
opipramol	Ensidon, Insidon
protriptyline	Concordin
trimipramine	Surmontil, Trimeprimine

mild parasympathetic blocking (atropine-like) actions. The drugs are meta-bolised in the liver, partly by N-demethylation. Thus imipramine is converted into desipramine and amitriptyline into nortriptyline. Klerman and Cole (1965) have reviewed the clinical pharmacology of this group of compounds.

In patients taking tricyclic antidepressant drugs dangerous potentiation of the cardiovascular effects of adrenaline and noradrenaline may occur, produc-ing acute hypertension and dysrhythmias (Boakes et al., 1973). It is possible that some sudden deaths during local analgesia for dental treatment (where 1:80,000 adrenaline is commonly used) may have been caused by this inter-action. Felypressin has been recommended as a safer alternative vasoconstrictor.

ANTI-SIALOGOGUE DRUGS

The value of arresting or diminishing salivary secretions during anaesthesia is frequently questioned (Holt, 1962) and there is no doubt that an anaesthetic sequence involving no irritant inhalational agent and no intra-oral instrumenta-tion rarely causes excessive salivation. The use of atropine-like drugs may merely submit the patient to the discomfort of a dry mouth, unpleasant tachycardia and tacky bronchial secretions which are difficult to expectorate. In conventional premedicant doses, atropine does not fully block vagal activity so that it is difficult to justify the claim that it protects the heart against reflexly-induced dysrhythmias. However, instrumentation is commonly needed, albeit only an oral airway, and anti-sialogogues are therefore generally given. Hyoscine (Scopolamine) has the additional advantages of sedation and a powerful anti-emetic effect, but its ability to protect the heart from vagal stimulation is some-what less and it may cause confusion and restlessness in the elderly and very young, in whom it is better avoided.

A number of synthetic and semi-synthetic atropine-like drugs are available for anti-sialogogue or anti-spasmodic activity, the best known of which are probably propantheline and hyoscine butyl bromide. Their spectra of activity differ only slightly from that of atropine itself. Details of their potency and pharmacological profiles were studied by Herxheimer (1958).

Glycopyrrolate (Robinul) is a synthetic quaternary ammonium compound and unlike atropine (a tertiary amine) it does not cross the blood-brain barrier. Like atropine, however, it is a powerful anti-cholinergic agent which inhibits the action of acetylcholine at the peripheral cholinergic (muscarinic) receptors. Various advantages over atropine have been claimed (Ramamurthy et al., 1972; Klingenmaier et al., 1972; Gyermek, 1975), namely, it does not produce CNS stimulation, when combined with neostigmine it is slower to act on the sino-auricular node thereby producing less initial tachycardia, and it has a duration of action about three to four times that of atropine (see Chapter 27). The recommended dose is 1 µg/kg I.M. for premedication and for reversal of a non-depolarising block 0·2 mg is given along with each 1·0 mg neostigmine.

REFERENCES

ANTON-STEPHENS, D. (1954). Preliminary observations on psychiatric uses of chlorpromazine (Largactil). *J. ment. Sci.*, **100**, 543.

ASHFORD, C. A., HELLER, H., and SMART, G. A. (1949*a*). The action of histamine on hydrochloric acid and pepsin secretion in man. *Brit. J. Pharmacol.*, **4**, 153.

ASHFORD, C. A., HELLER, H., and SMART, G. A. (1949*b*). The effect of antihistamine substances on gastric secretion in man. *Brit. J. Pharmacol.*, **4**, 157.

BAIN, W. A. (1949). Discussion on antihistamine drugs. *Proc. roy. Soc. Med.*, **42**, 615.

BLACK, J. W., DUNCAN, W. A. M., DURANT, G. J., GANELLIN, C. R., and PARSONS, M. E. (1972). Definition and antagonism of histamine H_2-receptors. *Nature (Lond.)*, **236**, 385.

BLACK, J. W., OWEN, D. A. A., and PARSONS, M. E. (1975). An analysis of the depressor responses to histamine in the cat and dog: involvement of both H_1- and H_2-receptors. *Brit. J. Pharmacol.*, **54**, 319.

BOAKES, A. J., LAURENCE, D. R., TEOH, P. C., BARAR, F. S. K., BENEDIKTER, L. T., and PRICHARD, B. N. C. (1973). Interactions between sympathomimetic amines and antidepressant agents in man. *Brit. med. J.*, **1**, 311.

BOVET, D., and STAUB, A. M. (1937). Action protectrice des éthers phénoliques au cours de l'intoxication histaminique. *C.R. Soc. Biol. (Paris)*, **124**, 547.

BROWN, S. S., and DUNDEE, J. W. (1968). Clinical studies of induction agents. XXV: Diazepam. *Brit. J. Anaesth.*, **40**, 108.

BURN, J. H. (1954). The pharmacology of chlorpromazine and promethazine. *Proc. roy. Soc. Med.*, **47**, 617.

BURN, J. H., and RAND, M. J. (1958). The action of sympathomimetic amines in animals treated with reserpine. *J. Physiol. (Lond.)*, **144**, 314.

CASTILLO, J. C., and DE BEER, E. J. (1947). Tracheal chain; preparation for study of antispasmodics with particular reference to bronchodilator drugs. *J. Pharmacol. exp. Ther.*, **90**, 104.

COAKLEY, C. S., ALPERT, S., and BOLRING, J. S. (1956). Circulatory responses during anesthesia of patients on rauwolfia therapy. *J. Amer. med. Ass.*, **161**, 1143.

COURVOISIER, S., FOURNEL, J., DUCROT, R., KOLSKY, M., and KOETSCHET, P. (1953). Propértiés pharmaco-dynamiques du chlorohydrate de chloro-3(diméthylamino-3-propyl)-10 phénothiazine (4560 R.P.); étude experimentale d'un nouveau corps utilisé dans l'anesthésie potentialisée et dans l'hibernation artificielle. *Arch. int. Pharmacodyn.*, **92**, 305.

DECOURT, P. (1953). Mecanisme de l'action thérapeutique de la chlorpromazine (4560 R.P. ou Largactil). *Thérapie*, **8**, 846.

DECOURT, P. L., BRUNAUD, M., and BRUNAUD, S. (1953). Action d'un narcobiotique (chlorpromazine) sur la température centrale des animaux homéothermes soumis à des températures ambiantes supérieures, égales ou inférieures a leur température centrale normale. *C.R. Soc. Biol. (Paris)*, **147**, 1605.

DEWS, P. B., and GRAHAM, J. D. P. (1946). The antihistamine substance 2786 R.P. *Brit. J. Pharmacol.*, **1**, 278.

DILWORTH, N. M., DUGDALE, A. E., and HILTON, H. B. (1963). Acute poisoning with chlorpromazine. *Lancet*, **1**, 137.

DOBKIN, A. B., GILBERT, R. G. B., and LAMOUREUX, L. (1954). Physiological effects of chlorpromazine. *Anaesthesia*, **9**, 157.

DUNDEE, J. W., and HASLETT, W. H. K. (1970). The benzodiazepines. A review of their actions and uses relative to anaesthetic practice. *Brit. J. Anaesth.*, **42**, 217.

DUNDEE, J. W., LOVE, W. J., and MOORE, J. (1963). Alterations in response to somatic pain associated with anaesthesia. XV. Further studies with phenothiazine derivatives and similar drugs. *Brit. J. Anaesth.*, **35**, 597.

DUNDEE, J. W., MESHAM, P. R., and SCOTT, W. E. B. (1954). Chlorpromazine and the production of hypothermia. *Anaesthesia*, **9**, 296.

EVANS-PROSSER, C. D. G. (1968). The use of pethidine and morphine in the presence of monoamine oxidase inhibitors. *Brit. J. Anaesth.*, **40**, 279.

FOSTER, C. A., O'MULLANE, E. J., GASKELL, P., and CHURCHILL-DAVIDSON, H. C. (1954). Chlorpromazine. A study of its action on the circulation in man. *Lancet*, **2**, 614.

GAY, L. N., and CARLINER, P. E. (1949). The prevention and treatment of motion sickness. I. Seasickness. *Bull. Johns. Hopk. Hosp.*, **84**, 470.

GELDER, M. G., and VANE, J. R. (1962). Interaction of the effects of tyramine, amphetamine and reserpine in man. *Psychopharmacologia (Berl.)*, **3**, 231.

GLOWINSKI, J., and AXELROD, J. (1964). Inhibition of uptake of tritiated-noradrenaline in the intact rat brain by imipramine and structurally related compounds. *Nature (Lond.)*, **204**, 1318.

GYERMEK, L. (1975). Clinical studies on the reversal of the neuromuscular blockade produced by pancuronium bromide. 1. The effects of glycopyrrolate and pyridostigmine. *Curr. ther. Res.*, **18** (3), 377.

HALEY, T. J., and HARRIS, D. H. (1949). The effect of topically applied antihistaminic drugs on the mammalian capillary bed. *J. Pharmacol. exp. Ther.*, **95**, 293.

HALPERN, B. N. (1947). Recherches sur une nouvelle série chimique de corps cloués de propriétés antihistaminiques et anti-anaphylactiques: les dérivés de la thiodiphényl-amine. *Arch. int. Pharmacodyn.*, **74**, 314.

HANDLEY, A. J. (1967). Metoclopramide in the prevention of post-operative nausea and vomiting. *Brit. J. clin. Pract.*, **21**, 460.

HARANATH, P. S. R. K. (1954). Comparative study of the local and spinal anaesthetic actions of some antihistamines, mepyramine and Phenergan with procaine. *Indian J. Med. Sci.*, **8**, 547.

HAWKINS, D. F., and SCHILD, H. O. (1951). The action of drugs on isolated human bronchial chains. *Brit. J. Pharmacol.*, **6**, 682.

HERXHEIMER, A. (1958). A comparison of some atropine-like drugs in man, with particular reference to their end-organ specificity. *Brit. J. Pharmacol.*, **13**, 184.

HEWER, A. J. H., and KEELE, C. A. (1948). A method of testing analgesics in man. *Lancet*, **2**, 683.

HIMWICH, H. E. (1955). Prospects in psychopharmacology. *J. nerv. ment. Dis.*, **122**, 413.

HOLT, A. T. (1962). Premedication with atropine should not be routine. *Lancet*, **2**, 984.

HOPKIN, D. A. B., HURTER, D., and JONES, C. M. (1957). Promethazine and pethidine in anaesthesia. *Anaesthesia*, **12**, 276.

HOWARD, F. A., and SHARP, D. S. (1973). Effect of metoclopramide on gastric emptying during labour. *Brit. med. J.*, **1**, 446.

JASPER, H. H. (1949). Symposium. Thalamocortical relationships: integrative action of thalamic reticular system. *Electroenceph. clin. Neurophysiol.*, **1**, 405.

KLERMAN, G. L., and COLE, J. O. (1965). Clinical pharmacology of imipramine and related antidepressant compounds. *Pharmacol. Rev.*, **17**, 101.

KLINGENMAIER, H. C., BULLARD, R., THOMPSON, D., and WATSON, R. (1972). Reversal of neuromuscular blockade with a mixture of neostigmine and glycopyrrolate. *Anesth. Analg. Curr. Res.*, **51**, 468.

KOPIN, I. J., FISCHER, J. E., MUSACCHIO, J. M., HORST, W. D., and WEISE, V. K. (1965). "False neurochemical transmitters" and the mechanism of sympathetic blockade by monoamine oxidase inhibitors. *J. Pharmacol. exp. Ther.*, **147**, 186.

LABORIT, H. (1950). La phenothiazinyl-éthyldiéthylamine en anesthesia (2987 R.P.). *Presse. méd.*, **58**, 851.

LABORIT, H., and HUGUENARD, P. (1954). *Pratique de l'hibernothérapie en chirurgie et en médicine.* Paris: Masson.

LABORIT, H., and LEGER, L. (1950). Utilisation d'un antihistaminique de synthèse en therapeutique pré, per et post-opératoire. *Presse méd.*, **58**, 492.

Lancet (1975). Leading article: Burimamide, metiamide and cimetidine. **2**, 802.

LAST, M. R., and LOEW, E. R. (1947). Effect of antihistamine drugs on increased capillary permeability following intradermal injections of histamine, horse serum and other agents in rabbits. *J. Pharmacol. exp. Ther.*, **89**, 81.

LEHMANN, H. E., and HANRAHAN, G. E. (1954). Chlorpromazine: new inhibiting agent for psychomotor excitement and manic states. *A.M.A. Arch. Neurol. Psychiat.*, **71**, 227.

LYON, W. G. G. (1956). Promethazine in burns. *Brit. J. Anaesth.*, **28**, 126.

MELVILLE, K. I. (1954). Observations on the adrenergic blocking and anti-fibrillatory actions of chlorpromazine. *Fed. Proc.*, **13**, 386.

MORUZZI, G., and MAGOUN, H. W. (1949). Brainstem reticular formation and activation of EEG. *Electroenceph. clin. Neurophysiol.*, **1**, 455.

MOYER, J. H., KENT, B., KNIGHT, R., MORRIS, G., HUGGINS, R., and HANDLEY, C. A. (1954). Laboratory and clinical observations on chlorpromazine (SKF 2601-A): hemodynamic and toxicological studies. *Amer. J. med. Sci.*, **227**, 283.

MOYER, J. H., KINROSS-WRIGHT, V., and FINNEY, R. M. (1955). Chlorpromazine as a therapeutic agent in clinical medicine. *Arch. intern. Med.*, **95**, 202.

PERKS, E. R. (1964). Monoamine oxidase inhibitors. *Anaesthesia*, **19**, 376.

PICKERING, G. W. (1939). Experimental observations on headache. *Brit. med. J.*, **1**, 907.

PLUMMER, A. J., EARL, A., SCHNEIDER, J. A., TRAPOLD, J., and BARRETT, W. (1954). Pharmacology of rauwolfia alkaloids including reserpine. *Ann. N.Y. Acad. Sci.*, **59**, 8.

POUNDER, R. E., WILLIAMS, J. G., MILTON-THOMPSON, G. J., and MISIEWICZ, J. J. (1975). 24-hour control of intragastric acidity by cimetidine in duodenal-ulcer patients. *Lancet*, **2**, 1069.

PURKIS, I. E., and ISHII, M. (1963). The effectiveness of anti-emetic agents: comparison of the anti-emetic activity of trifluopromazine (Vesprin), perphenazine (Trilafon), and trifluoperazine (Stelazine) with that of dimenhydrinate (Gravol) in post-anaesthetic vomiting. *Canad. Anaesth. Soc. J.*, **10**, 539.

RAMAMURTHY, S., SHAKER, M. H., and WINNIE, A. P. (1972). Glycopyrrolate as a substitute for atropine in neostigmine reversal of muscle relaxant drugs. *Canad. Anaesth. Soc. J.*, **19**, 399.

RANDALL, L. O., HEISE, G. A., SCHALLEK, W., BAGDON, R. E., BANZIGER, R., BORIS, A., MOE, R. A., and ABRAMS, W. B. (1961). Pharmacological and clinical studies on Valium, a new psychotherapeutic agent of the benzodiazepine class. *Curr. ther. Res.*, **3**, 405.

REILLY, J., and TOURNIER, P. (1953). The action of chlorpromazine (4560 R.P.) on the toxin in experimental typhoid. *Presse méd.*, **61**, 1031.

RIDING, J. E. (1963). The prevention of postoperative vomiting. *Brit. J. Anaesth.*, **35**, 180.

RINALDI, F., and HIMWICH, H. E. (1955). Drugs affecting psychotic behaviour and function of mesodiencephalic activating system. *Dis. nerv. Syst.*, **16,** 133.

SADOVE, M. S. (1956). Promethazine in surgery. Preliminary report. *J. Amer. med. Ass.*, **62,** 712.

SCHWARTZ, M. A., KOECHLIM, B. A., POSTMA, E., PALMER, S., and KROL, G. (1965). Metabolism of diazepam in rat, dog and man. *J. Pharmacol. exp. Ther.*, **149,** 423.

SHERLOCK, S. (1964). Jaundice due to drugs. *Proc. roy. Soc. Med.*, **57,** 881.

STEIN, A. A., and WRIGHT, A. W. (1956). Hepatic pathology in jaundice due to chlorpromazine. *J. Amer. med. Ass.*, **161,** 508.

SU, C., and LEE, C. Y. (1960). The mode of neuromuscular blocking action of chlorpromazine. *Brit. J. Pharmacol.*, **15,** 88.

TERZIAN, H. (1952). Studio elettroencefalografico dell' azione centrale del Largactil (4560 R.P.). *Rass. Neurol. veg.*, **9,** 211.

WINKELMAN, N. W., Jnr. (1954). Chlorpromazine in the treatment of neuropsychiatric disorders. *J. Amer. med. Ass.*, **155,** 18.

Chapter 24

NORMAL NEUROMUSCULAR TRANSMISSION

THE resting cell membrane is described as being in a state of polarity. This is associated with a potential difference between the inside and outside of the cell. This electromotive force is the result of the semipermeable property of cell membranes which permits some ions to traverse the cell barrier more readily than others. The magnitude of this *transmembrane potential* is, in the resting state, proportional to the ratio of the concentrations of the most permeable ions on either side of the membrane; this follows from the Gibbs-Donnan law. In the resting state, that is before or after excitation, in nerve and muscle cells the most permeable ion is potassium. It follows that the magnitude of the resting membrane potential and therefore the excitability of nerve and muscle depends almost entirely upon the ratio of potassium ions inside the cell to those outside.

At a normal mammalian neuromuscular junction this transmembrane potential is 90 mV with the inside of the cell membrane conventionally considered to be negative relative to the outside. This is associated with a relative concentration of potassium inside the cell of about 150 mmol/l and 3·5 to 5·5 mmol/l in the extracellular fluid. Whilst potassium is the principal intracellular ion, the main extracellular ion is sodium. The concentration of sodium ions outside the cell is 30 to 60 times that inside the cell, largely as a result of the sodium pump mechanism. However, as in the resting state sodium is only one-fiftieth as permeable as potassium, it plays little part in determining the membrane potential or excitability. During electrical activity, the cell membrane becomes specifically permeable to sodium. As the membrane potential depends upon the concentration ratio of the most permeable ion, it now relates to sodium. As a result the cell membrane potential falls, and depending upon the extent of the altered permeability, it may become reversed. Provided the polarity of the cell membrane reaches a critical threshold level an *action potential* results. This is the process of *depolarisation*. It is the distribution of potassium ions between the inside and outside of the cell that determines the magnitude of the resting transmembrane potential and therefore the ease with which it is depolarised, whilst the distribution ratio of sodium ions affects the magnitude of the action potential.

In order to restore the transmembrane potential after depolarisation the sodium ions that have entered the cell during the initial depolarisation must be removed by the sodium pump and the potassium equilibrium restored. These events and their relative relationships have been analysed by Hodgkin (1951) and del Castillo and Katz (1956). It is the event of depolarisation and the restoration of ionic equilibrium that are associated with the absolute and relative refractory state of cell membranes.

Pre-junctional or Pre-synaptic Area

The arrival of an impulse or nerve action potential at the end of the nerve gives rise to a special situation. It is now almost universally accepted that the

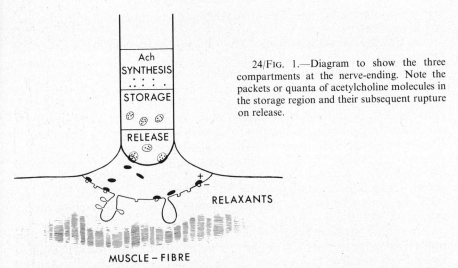

24/Fig. 1.—Diagram to show the three compartments at the nerve-ending. Note the packets or quanta of acetylcholine molecules in the storage region and their subsequent rupture on release.

conduction of an impulse from nerve to muscle is not a simple electrical response but relies on the release of acetylcholine at the nerve-ending to bridge the gap. This is the chemical theory of neuromuscular transmission as propounded by Dale *et al.* (1936). The work of Katz and Miledi (1965*a*) has produced convincing evidence to support this theory because they demonstrated that there was a measurable time-lag between the arrival of an impulse at the nerve-ending and the release of the transmitter substance (acetylcholine), the synaptic delay time.

The area of the nerve-ending is obviously very important because at this point the formation, storage and finally the liberation of acetylcholine have a very special significance. For purposes of description, therefore, these roles of acetylcholine are best considered as three separate compartments: (a) acetylcholine synthesis, (b) acetylcholine storage, (c) acetylcholine release (Fig. 1.).

(a) **Synthesis of acetylcholine.**—Acetylcholine is formed by the acetylation of choline with the help of the enzyme of choline acetylase*. In normal circumstances there is an abundance of both choline and the enzyme available at the nerve terminals because large quantities of choline can be absorbed from the extracellular space (Birks and Macintosh, 1957 and 1961). Experiments with hemicholinium have thrown further light on this matter as this compound is capable of interfering with acetylcholine synthesis. It is, therefore, experimentally possible to reduce the amount of acetylcholine formed at the nerve-ending. The result of poisoning the nerve-ending with hemicholinium is that whilst electrophysiological response to a single stimulus can be recorded, the demand of fast or tetanic rates of stimulation is too great and neuromuscular transmission fails. Under the influence of hemicholinium the supply of acetylcholine is no longer adequate, so that the phenomenon of post-tetanic exhaustion is observed following bursts of tetanic stimulation. Such a condition is observed in the experimental animal under the influence of hemicholinium, and clinically in patients with severe myasthenia gravis (Desmedt, 1966) and in the

* The enzyme aids the transfer of an acetyl group from acetyl-CoA to choline.

premature infant under the influence of a depolarising drug (Churchill-Davidson and Wise, 1964).

(b) **Storage of acetylcholine.**—The advent of electron microscopy has revealed the presence of vesicles at the nerve-ending. These packets, or quanta, are believed to contain molecules of acetylcholine. In normal circumstances they are stored after manufacture to await their final release. The number of quanta available may vary but the size of the packets remains constant. Acetylcholine is probably also formed in the neurone and transported to the presynaptic region by axonal transport. Acetylcholine is stored in two forms at the nerve-ending, as pre-packed readily available acetylcholine and as quanta of stored acetylcholine. If the rate of transfer from the stored to the *immediately available source* is slower than the demands of the nerve then the amount of acetylcholine released during stimulation of the motor nerve will fall. Drugs such as neostigmine have an important facilitatory action in speeding up this rate of transfer.

(c) **Release of acetylcholine.**—Once the packets have been formed and duly transferred to the immediately available store, all awaits the arrival of a stimulus. However, it is known that even in the resting state small quantities of acetyl-choline are being sporadically released. It is believed that this results in the miniature end-plate potentials (MEPP) due to the random contact of one of the packets of acetylcholine with a critical spot or thickening on the terminal part of the nerve opposite the secondary clefts on the post-synaptic or muscle surface. The arrival of an impulse (action potential) enlarges the reactive site and so numerous packets of acetylcholine are released. If a motor nerve is stimulated in the presence of d-tubocurarine, then acetylcholine will still be released from the nerve-ending (Krryević and Mitchell, 1961), but these molecules fail to produce a muscle response because they are prevented from reaching the post-junctional receptors on the muscle.

Magnesium and calcium have been shown to play a very important role in the *release* of acetylcholine. Either a fall in calcium ion concentration or a rise of magnesium ion concentration will greatly reduce the number of acetylcholine molecules that are liberated from the nerve-ending (del Castillo and Engbaek, 1954; Katz and Miledi, 1964 and 1965b). Other substances which are believed to interfere with the release of acetylcholine are some of the aminoglycoside group of antibiotics (for details see p. 856), botulinus toxin and possibly procaine. The pathological condition called the myasthenic syndrome (Eaton Lambert syn-drome), which is sometimes found in patients with a bronchial carcinoma, is also believed to be associated with a difficulty in release of acetylcholine. It is probable that d-tubocurare and other muscle relaxants also affect the amount of acetylcholine released as a result of a pre-synaptic stimulus; the significance of this pre-synaptic site of action of the muscle relaxants probably varies from drug to drug; it has been most clearly demonstrated with curare, it is negligible when pancuronium is used, whilst gallamine may actually facilitate acetylcholine release.

THE NEUROMUSCULAR JUNCTION

On leaving the pre-synaptic or pre-junctional area (i.e. the nerve-ending) the acetylcholine molecules traverse a minute gap before arriving at the post-junctional (post-synaptic) area on the muscle membrane. The term "neuro-muscular junction", therefore, includes both pre- and post-synaptic areas. The post-synaptic area, however, is sometimes also referred to as the *motor end-plate*. Evidence of the function of this area again outstrips a knowledge of its structure but the advent of the electron microscope has thrown new light on the possible relationship between structure and function. Much of the basic informa-tion about the micro-anatomy of this area has been provided by the remarkable studies of Couteaux (1955 and 1958), Robertson (1956) and Waser (1970).

As the myelinated motor nerve fibre approaches the muscle fibres, it divides into numerous non-myelinated terminal branches. Each of these fibres runs parallel to the axis of the muscle fibre it supplies and lies embedded in a shallow "gutter" or depression in the muscle surface. This situation is represented in diagrammatic form in Fig. 2 (Birks *et al.*, 1960).

At the myoneural junction the nerve fibre is covered by a membrane com-plex, sometimes referred to as the Schwann, axoplasmic or perineural membrane. The precise nature of this membrane is unclear; however, it forms an anatomical barrier separating the end-plate from the ECF.

At regular intervals these layers are folded inwards to make indentations towards the muscle fibre (Fig. 3a and b). These junctional folds (secondary clefts) are important because they pass close to and actually indent the muscle "basement membrane" itself. It is in this region that there is a high concentration of cholinesterase. Robertson (1956) has summarised the importance of this area as follows:

"The folds of the junction are admirably constructed to bring a very great increase in the total area of the muscle surface membrane complex in contact

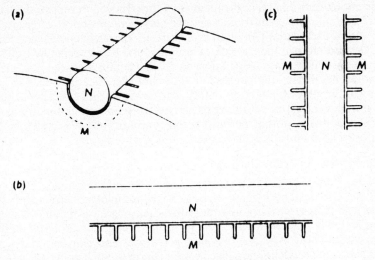

24/Fig. 2.—Diagram of Neuromuscular Junction.

(*a*) Shows a small portion of the terminal axon branch N lying in a gutter formed by the surface of the muscle fibre M. The semicircular post-junctional folds are illustrated.

(*b*) Same in longitudinal section.

(*c*) Same in tangential section.

with the nerve-ending. Since it seems likely that acetylcholine is secreted in discrete packets or quanta at the endings, one might expect to see something analogous to secretion granules of acetylcholine either in axoplasm, sarcoplasm or within the junctional membranes. It seems reasonable to speculate that the tubular or vesicular bodies of terminal axoplasm might represent such packets of acetylcholine."

Electron microscopic studies of this region demonstrate the close proximity of the vesicles (containing acetylcholine) on the one hand with these junctional folds on the other (Fig. 4a and b). On this basis, Waser (1970) has put forward the hypothesis that these junctional folds contain the sodium "pores". Each pore has a narrow neck guarded by two cholinesterase molecules, each with two curare receptor sites whilst the acetylcholine receptors are scattered around the mouth of the pore. Depolarisation occurs when sufficient acetylcholine receptors have been activated to cause deformation of the surface and open up the neck of the pore to a sufficient size to allow sodium ions to pass easily into the interior of the cell. It is envisaged that non-depolarising drugs like curare act by obstructing the neck of the pore.

Function of the Neuromuscular Junction

The arrival of sufficient acetylcholine molecules at the end-plate to cause a threshold depolarisation will trigger off a mechanism for the whole of the muscle fibre, so that a wave of depolarisation spreads outwards along its entire length, causing a mechanical contraction in its wake. The acetylcholine molecules are destroyed by a specific enzyme—cholinesterase—almost as rapidly as they are produced. Fortunately they do not have far to travel because electron-microscope studies have revealed that the distance between the nerve membrane and the motor end-plate is in the region of 1 µm. (Indeed, recent studies suggest that the synaptic cleft is an artefact and the nerve ending abuts the receptor area of the muscle end-plate.) This short range enables the acetylcholine molecules to excite the end-plate in the fraction of a millisecond before being hydrolysed by cholinesterase. The close association of cholinesterase with the post-synaptic membrane has led to the suggestion that cholinesterase is itself part of the receptor molecule (Miledi et al., 1971). The existence and function of this enzyme can be verified by inhibiting its activity with an anti-cholinesterase drug (e.g. neostigmine) and thus permitting the concentration of acetylcholine ions to multiply, with a resulting increase in muscle activity.

The Resting End-plate Potential

When a micro-electrode is inserted at random into the middle of a resting muscle fibre, a steady potential of about 60–90 millivolts (inside negative) will be recorded. If the electrode is now moved gradually towards the end-plate region a point is finally reached where small potential changes of about 0·5 millivolts are recorded. These *miniature end-plate potentials* represent the release of the small packets of acetylcholine as each vesicle ruptures. Such miniature potentials occur at fairly regular intervals (about one per second) and are only observed in the resting state. The amplitude of one of these miniature potentials is 0·5–2 mV and is insufficient to reach the threshold necessary to trigger off depolarisation of the end-plate itself.

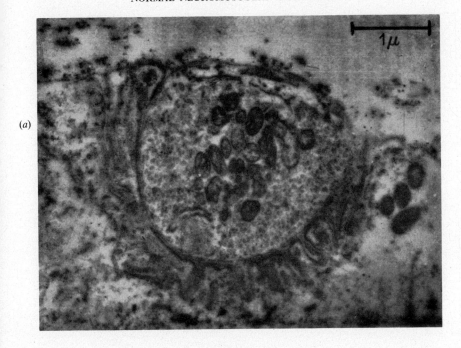

(a)

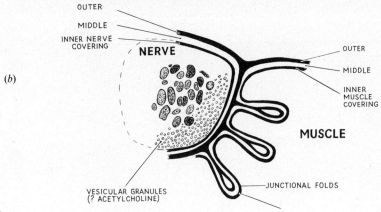

(b)

24/Fig. 3.—The Neuromuscular Junction

(a) Electron microphotograph of a reptilian neuromuscular junction.
(b) Diagrammatic representation of the neuromuscular junction.

The frequency of these miniature potentials (i.e. the rate of spontaneous rupture of vesicles) depends on the conditions prevailing in the pre-synaptic region of the nerve-ending. For example, hemicholinium interferes with the synthesis of acetylcholine whilst botulinus toxin prevents the release of the transmitter substances. Both these agents reduce the frequency of the miniature

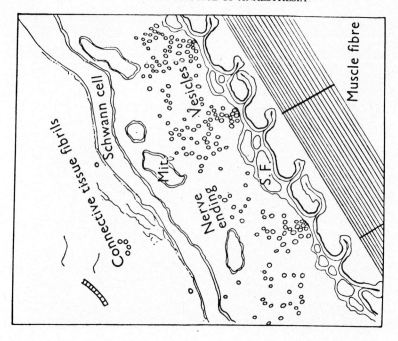

24/FIG. 4(b).—Diagram of the various structures seen in (a).

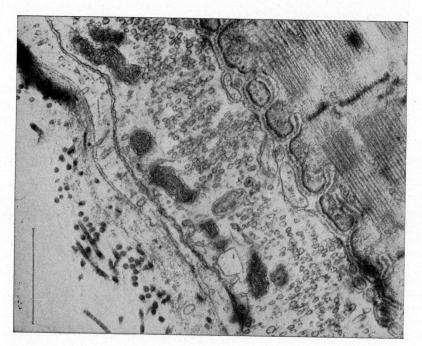

24/FIG. 4(a).—Longitudinal section through the neuromuscular junction (frog).

potentials. Calcium increases the rate of release of acetylcholine and hence the frequency of the miniature potentials.

The receptor substance is situated on the external surface of the cell membrane and is insensitive to stimulation from within the cell. For example, if a micropipette is so arranged that acetylcholine molecules are injected on to the outer surface of the end-plate region, then activity results. On the other hand, if the end of the pipette is advanced slightly so that it now lies within the muscle cell, then the acetylcholine molecules are no longer effective (del Castillo and Katz, 1955).

Margin of safety of neuromuscular transmission (*Receptor occupancy*).—In the normal patient there is a large margin of safety in neuromuscular transmission. This concept was introduced by Paton and Waud (1967) to indicate that although the neuromuscular junction was the most vulnerable part of the normal sequence of events in the indirect (nervous) excitation of muscle contraction, it was possible for the system to function in response to Faradic stimulation even though over 70 per cent of the receptors on the post-synaptic membrane were blocked by curare (Fig. 5). In other words over 70 per cent of the cholinergic receptors needed to be occupied before any signs of paresis took place.

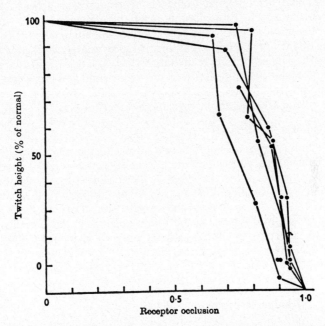

24/Fig. 5.—Receptor occupancy required to produce depression of twitch height (Paton and Waud, 1967). There is no depression of twitch response until over 70 per cent (0·7) receptors are occupied by curare.

This indicated that there was a large reserve in cholinergic transmission either because an excess of acetylcholine is normally produced or because a superfluity of receptors is normally available. In later work, Waud and Waud (1971) showed that this reserve, although still considerable, was reduced when tetanic rates of indirect stimulation were used. Some skeletal muscles require a higher percentage of receptor occupancy than others before signs of paresis are evident. For example, it has been suggested that the diaphragm (clinically a very resistant muscle) requires 90 per cent occupancy before its function starts to fail. It is evident that one cannot detect the presence of a non-depolarising muscle relaxant by Faradic stimulation unless 70 per cent or more of the receptors are occupied. It is important to realise that a patient may appear to have completely recovered from the effects of these drugs and yet have a greatly reduced margin of safety of neuromuscular transmission.

Normal muscle contraction is the result of nerve excitation at 40–50 Hz when muscle weakness would not be expected to become obvious until more than 70 per cent of the receptors were inactivated by curare, or there had been a considerable reduction in the release of acetylcholine.

The Role of the Inorganic Ions in Neuromuscular Transmission

The part played by potassium and sodium in the conduction of a nerve impulse has already been mentioned. Apart from these two ions which behave in the muscle fibre in a similar fashion to that described in the nerve fibre, both magnesium and calcium can influence neuromuscular activity. Magnesium blocks neuromuscular transmission, probably by interfering with the pre-synaptic release of acetylcholine (del Castillo and Engbaek, 1954). If given in increasing quantities magnesium finally produces complete blockade. Similarly, withdrawal of calcium produces the same effect. The role of calcium is to oppose the neuromuscular blocking action of the magnesium and these two ions appear to be antagonistic. Glucose is also necessary for the formation of acetylcholine since this is an active metabolic process (Feldberg, 1945).

Removal of Acetylcholine

Acetylcholine molecules only have a minute distance (1 μm) to travel before reaching their target. Their subsequent fate, however, is a little more obscure. The majority are certainly hydrolysed by the specific enzyme—cholinesterase—to acetic acid and choline. The molecules of choline are then available for resynthesis by the nerve terminal. Nevertheless, some of the acetylcholine molecules probably diffuse into the interstitial space and are then no longer available to take part in the resynthesis process. Evidence for this diffusion process is based on the finding that acetylcholine molecules can be collected from the perfusion fluid of a nerve-muscle preparation that has been protected from hydrolysis by an inhibitor such as eserine (Brown et al., 1936).

The Acetylcholine Receptor

The nature of this important structure is still in dispute. It is known that when a muscle is denervated specific end-plate receptors disappear and the whole of the muscle membrane becomes responsive to acetylcholine and cholinergic agonist drugs. Waser (1970), using radioactive curare, took this further and demonstrated that the curare molecules became attached to new receptors all over the muscle membrane. This led to the suggestion that the nature of the receptor material might be a mucopolysaccharide. Other authors have contended that although mucopolysaccharides have an affinity for curare they are an integral part of the basement membrane structure and not a physiological acetylcholine receptor (Chagas, 1962; Zacks and Blumberg, 1961). Undoubtedly most quaternary ammonium compounds such as d-tubocurare, gallamine and suxamethonium do have a high affinity for mucopolysaccharide.

Further suggestions have been made that the receptor must be of a phosphate nature (Nastuk, 1967), or a polypeptide or protein (Gill, 1965). More recently Changeux et al. (1972) have isolated a substance that has many of the properties of a cholinergic receptor.

The use of radioactive muscle relaxants has enabled investigators to estimate the amount of uptake of the various compounds in the vicinity of the motor end-plate. Labelled depolarising drugs such as decamethonium are taken up in far greater quantities than the non-depolarising drugs. Waser (1970) has suggested that there are twenty times as many decamethonium receptors as there are for curare. Miledi et al. (1971) have demonstrated that the cholinergic receptor of the electric organ of Torpedo fish is intimately associated with cholinesterase. Waser has suggested that the mouth of the pore permitting ionic flux (i.e. responsible for depolarisation) is guarded by two molecules of acetylcholinesterase with four active curare receptors. Under normal conditions acetylcholine combines with its own cholinergic receptor surrounding the pore: this action pulls open the mouth and allows ionic movement to take place. In the presence of d-tubocurarine, the molecule of relaxant combines with the active centres of the acetylcholinesterase molecules and effectively blocks the opening of the pore. This theory would concede that the receptors for d-tubocurarine need not be the same as those for the depolarising drug, but they must be strategically placed.

TERMINOLOGY

Much confusion has arisen over the multiplicity of terms that are in use to describe phenomena occurring at the neuromuscular junction. This is largely due to a failure to agree an international nomenclature, the use of different experimental techniques and the common practice of extrapolating from experimental results obtained in *in vitro* preparations and applying them to man. A conference was held in London in 1975 to discuss these problems and the following text is based on the recommendations.

Fatigue of normal neuromuscular transmission is known to occur when very fast rates of nerve stimulation are used. When these fast rates are employed the rate of synthesis of acetylcholine molecules is increased and likewise more molecules are liberated from the nerve-ending. However, following rapid tetanic stimulation the supply may be insufficient to cope with the demand and neuromuscular transmission will start to fail. In man, if a hand-bulb of an ergometer is squeezed maximally, fatigue occurs in 1–2 minutes. But, if the arm is ischaemic it occurs in approximately 30 seconds (Merton, 1956). When electrical stimulation of 30–50 Hz is used the first signs of failure of neuromuscular transmission occur in about 30 seconds.

Wedensky inhibition or fade.—When small doses of a non-depolarising relaxant are given in man there is a very characteristic "fade" at both slow and fast rates of nerve stimulation. Almost the whole of this failure of neuromuscular transmission takes place during the first four stimuli at both twitch and tetanic rates of stimulation (see 25/Fig. 12). This has led to the suggestion that twitch stimulation using the "train-of-four" method can be used satisfactorily for monitoring patients during relaxant anaesthesia (Ali *et al.*, 1970). In such patients the ratio of the fourth twitch height to the first is calculated by a digital computer as a quantitative measure of the amount of neuromuscular block (see Chapter 25, Fig. 14). However, other authorities claim that the "train-of-four" method does not yield as much information as the simpler twitch-tetanus-twitch sequence where not only is the fade (at both twitch and tetanic rates) evident, but the further sign of post-tetanic facilitation is revealed (see below).

Post-tetanic augmentation of contraction.—The normal response to tetanic stimulation is a small increase in muscle tension over and above that observed with the single twitch. Following cessation of tetanic stimulation, a subsequent single twitch stimulus produces a modest increase in the height of the response. This is termed *Post-tetanic Augmentation of Contraction* and is principally due to an effect on the muscle contraction.

Post-tetanic Facilitation of Transmission

Following the administration of sub-paralytic doses of non-depolarising relaxants a characteristic feature of this type of block is the "fade" of successive stimuli (described above) *and* the improvement of neuromuscular transmission immediately following a period of tetanic stimulation, i.e. *Post-tetanic Facilitation*. This is believed to be due to the release of increased quantities of acetylcholine molecules for a few seconds following the period of tetanus. There is clearly some relationship between the speed of the nerve stimulation and the amount of acetylcholine molecules produced or released. The duration of tetanic stimulation is important and clinically the best examples of post-tetanic facilitation of transmission are seen when the nerve is stimulated at 50 Hz for at least 4 to 5 seconds.

Post-tetanic facilitation (of transmission) is also seen following halothane and ether anaesthesia and in myasthenia gravis.

Post-tetanic Exhaustion

If the rate of acetylcholine production or release is depressed, as occurs after administration of hemicholinium, anoxia and hypothermia, post-tetanic exhaustion is seen. With this phenomena the initial increased response that occurs immediately after a tetanic stimulation is later followed by a period of sub-normal response. This latter aspect is believed to coincide with depleted stores of readily releasable acetylcholine. Post-tetanic exhaustion is commonly seen in patients with myasthenia gravis and also in neonatal neuromuscular transmission.

THE MOTOR UNIT

The term "motor unit" comprises the anterior horn cell in the spinal cord and its corresponding motor nerve fibre passing peripherally to divide into numerous branches, each one of which terminates at a single muscle fibre. The point of branching takes place near the skeletal muscle fibres and is an important landmark in electromyographic recordings. Stimulation below this point leads to the initial contraction of an individual muscle fibre (fibrillation potential)

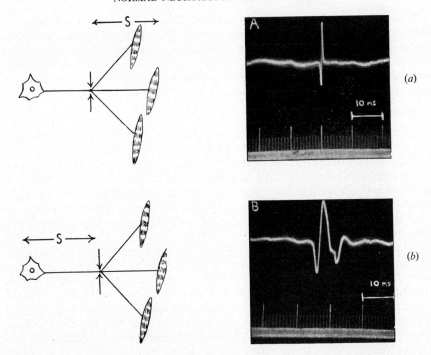

24/FIG. 6.—Electromyographic appearances from stimulation of the motor unit. (*a*) Stimulation (S) below the point of branching of the lower motor neurone produces a single fibre potential (A) or a motor unit potential. (*b*) Stimulation (S) above the point of branching of the lower motor neurone produces a motor unit potential (B).

whereas stimulation of the motor nerve above this point leads to the simultaneous contraction of all the muscle fibres in the motor unit (a motor unit action potential) (Fig. 6).

The remaining fibres of the motor unit are stimulated antidromically (Masland and Wigton, 1950) and can be recognised as the remnants of the motor unit discharge following rapidly after the single-fibre potential.

The number of muscle fibres supplied by each anterior horn cell varies widely, depending largely on the delicacy of its function. In the highly specialised skeletal muscles such as those moving the eyeball, relatively few fibres are present in each unit (5–15), whereas in the large muscles of the back or limbs the numbers are far greater (up to 300 per unit). Similarly both the height (amplitude) and the width (duration) of the action potential (as detected by the electromyograph apparatus) differ characteristically, as the electromyograph represents the summation of many action potentials. Thus:

	Number per unit	Duration	Amplitude
Eye muscles	5– 15	1 millisecond	100 microvolts or less
Large limb muscles	150–300	5–10 millisecond	300 microvolts to 1·5 millivolts

Electromyography can also be used to demonstrate lesions affecting the motor unit and it is widely employed on this basis in the diagnosis of neurological conditions. It can be used, therefore, to determine the site of action of the various drugs producing muscle relaxation and to demonstrate whether the paralysis of muscle is due to a pure central action on the spinal cord and brain or to an action at the neuromuscular junction.

Fibrillation Potential

The potential (recorded electromyographically) that occurs on the contraction of a single muscle fibre is termed a fibrillation potential. A motor unit action potential is the sum of all the fibre potentials occurring simultaneously in a single motor unit (i.e. 150–300 fibres). Ordinarily, it is not possible to stimulate a single muscle fibre, and besides this, such a contraction would be invisible to the naked eye. Nevertheless, in the presence of degeneration of the lower motor neurone, spontaneous fibrillation potentials can readily be recognised on the electromyograph.

As the depolarising drugs are believed to act like acetylcholine, theoretically their injection should create a shower of fibrillation potentials as each motor end-plate is depolarised. However, this is not the case. The muscle responds with numerous full action potentials and some of these may be seen with the naked eye as "fasciculations" occurring all over the body. The explanation of this phenomenon is probably that these agents have a pre-synaptic action on the motor nerve as well as the well-documented post-synaptic effect. The pre-synaptic action causes antidromic firing of the motor nerve (Riker et al., 1957; Galindo, 1972).

Occasionally spontaneous fasciculation potentials are observed electromyographically following the administration of a depolarising drug. Gradually, on volition, there is a progressive disintegration of the full motor unit (as the fibres drop out one after another) so that both the amplitude and the duration of its potential are diminished. Finally, when the block is established, the picture resembles a severe case of myopathy.

Contracture

Contracture is the term used to define the localised but sustained shortening of the muscle fibre that follows the intra-arterial injection of acetylcholine in birds and certain reptiles. It must be clearly differentiated from a normal *contraction* of the muscle fibre which is found in mammalian muscle. Nevertheless, if the nerve supply to mammalian muscle is cut and the nerve fibre allowed sufficient time to degenerate, then the intra-arterial injection of acetylcholine produces a typical contracture which is associated with an increased sensitivity to acetylcholine.

In some cases of upper motor neurone lesions in man, a muscle contraction unassociated with supersensitivity to acetylcholine is observed. Axelsson and Thesleff (1959) have shown that the supersensitivity to acetylcholine which develops in chronically denervated muscle is due to the whole of the muscle fibre membrane becoming as sensitive to acetylcholine as the end-plate region.

In the young chick, the intravenous injection of either acetylcholine or decamethonium produces a state of generalised contracture in which the

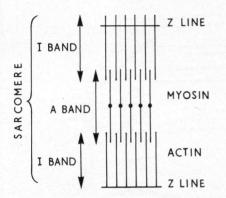

24/FIG. 7.—Diagram of a sarcomere showing the actin of the I band and the myosin of the A band.

animal assumes a position of opisthotonos. Provided the dose has not been excessive, the bird continues to breathe but the head and neck are held forcibly retracted and the spine is curved in such a manner that the tail nearly touches the back of the neck. So typical is this response that Buttle and Zaimis (1949) have used it as the basis of their test for the presence of depolarising properties in a muscle relaxant drug.

THE MUSCLE FIBRE

A striated muscle fibre possesses three principal components: (1) the myofibril which contains the contractile element; (2) the mitochondria and nuclei; and (3) the cell membrane and intercommunicating systems. These latter aqueous channels have recently assumed a much greater importance as their role in relation to function can now be partly surmised (Page, 1968).

A closer study of the myofibril reveals that it contains a series of two important overlapping bands—the A and the I bands (Fig. 7). The I bands are attached to another important structure which runs transversely round the fibre and is called the Z line. The area between two Z lines is referred to as a sarcomere. The A band, on the other hand, is darker and contains the important enzyme adenosine triphosphatase (ATPase) which is essential for the breakdown of ATP in order to release energy.

A muscle contraction takes place when two types of protein—actin of the I band and myosin of the A band—interdigitate to produce a shortening of the fibre length (Huxley and Taylor, 1958; Huxley, 1963).

A closer look at the Z line using electronmicroscopy reveals that it is really a transverse aqueous channel connecting the cell membrane with the interior of the fibre. The mouth of this system lies on the surface where it merges with the cell membrane and is open to the extracellular medium (Page, 1968). This channel is called the transverse tubular or "T" system (Fig. 8a and b). On passing to the interior it comes very close to another aqueous channel system—the sarcoplasmic reticulum.

The "T" system and the sarcoplasmic reticulum system do not actually join but in certain areas they lie in very close proximity. The sarcoplasmic reticulum is a much larger system and runs vertically between two Z bands.

Thus, when a motor end-plate becomes depolarised the excitatory disturbance is believed to spread into the interior of the fibre along the "T" system

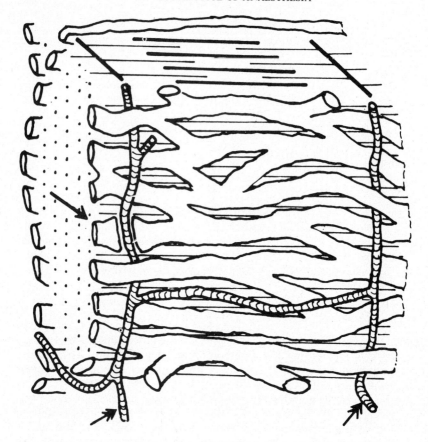

24/Fig. 8(b).—Diagram of the "T" system showing the transverse tubular system.

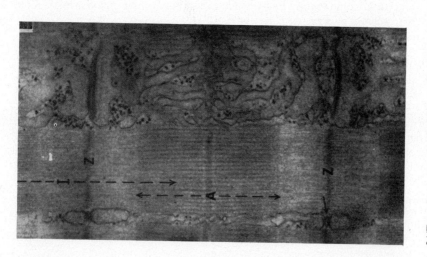

24/Fig. 8(a).—Electronmicroscopic section of frog's muscle fibre showing the A and I bands.

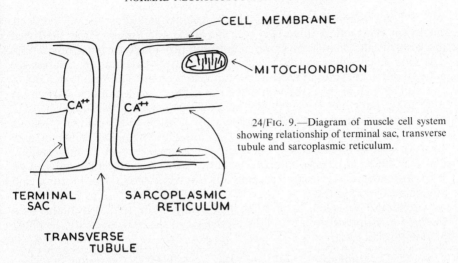

24/Fig. 9.—Diagram of muscle cell system showing relationship of terminal sac, transverse tubule and sarcoplasmic reticulum.

(Huxley and Taylor, 1958). Here it comes into contact with the terminal sacs of the sarcoplasmic reticulum (Fig. 9). There is considerable evidence to support the view that the tubules of this system act as an intracellular store for calcium ions which are released on depolarisation. The resulting rise in calcium ion concentration of the sarcoplasm triggers the activity of the enzyme ATPase, thereby initiating the breakdown of the stored adenosine triphosphate to release energy and produce a contraction (Weber *et al.*, 1964). Relaxation occurs when the calcium ions re-accumulate within the sarcoplasmic reticulum by the means of a calcium pump (Page, 1968). This process is repeated again and again as the contraction wave spreads along the length of the fibre.

Heat, Energy and Oxidative Phosphorylation in Muscle

The method of producing heat and energy in muscle is a complex one involving a series of reductions and oxidations within the respiratory chain. At each stage in the chain a certain amount of heat and energy is produced. At three stages this energy is made available for the oxidative phosphorylation of adenosine diphosphate (ADP) to form adenosine triphosphate (ATP) with the help of the enzyme adenosine triphosphatase (ATPase) which is associated with the respiratory chain of the Krebs' cycle.

The process could be presented as follows:

(*a*) *Within the mitochondrion:*

$$\text{Energy from respiratory chain} + \text{ADP} + \text{P} \xrightarrow[\text{ATPase in respiratory chain}]{} \text{ATP}$$

(*b*) *Within the cytoplasm:*

$$\text{ATP} + \text{H}_2\text{O} \xrightarrow[\substack{\text{ATPase associated} \\ \text{with myosin}}]{} \text{ADP} + \text{P} + \text{Energy of muscle contraction}$$

In muscle, adenosine triphosphate acts as the principal store of energy which can be released on contraction. As mentioned earlier calcium ions in muscle are believed to stimulate the activity of the enzyme myosin ATPase thereby releasing energy for contraction. It has also been shown (Snodgrass and Piras, 1966) that an excess of calcium ions can cause an uncoupling of oxidative phosphorylation. The most likely effect of this mechanism is that the calcium ions depress the activity of the enzyme ATPase in the respiratory chain. This results in a fall in the level of ATP in the cytoplasm and a rise in the concentration of ADP in the mitochondrion whilst the energy of the respiratory chain is released as heat. In these unusual circumstances it is theoretically possible to release vast amounts of heat very rapidly. Another interesting observation is that ATP not only acts as a store of muscle energy but it also causes relaxation of the muscle fibre. Thus, in the event of uncoupling of oxidative phosphorylation the fall in ATP level causes the muscle fibre to become stiff as is witnessed in rigor mortis and in malignant hyperpyrexia.

Creatinine phosphate is another high energy store that is available as a reserve for the production of ATP with the aid of the enzyme creatinine phosphokinase (CK), viz.

$$\text{Creatinine P} + \text{ADP} \xrightleftharpoons[\text{Creatinine phosphokinase}]{} \text{ATP} + \text{Creatinine}$$

In many myopathies, in malignant hyperpyrexia and cases of cell destruction a raised level of the creatinine kinase (CK) can be detected.

In recent years these facts have assumed particular significance to anaesthetists since the recognition of the syndrome of malignant hyperpyrexia (see p. 937).

INTERNUNCIAL CELL SYSTEM

The internuncial neurones are situated in the spinal cord between the anterior and posterior horns of the grey matter. Their function appears to be the co-ordination of impulses reaching the cord from many sources. This function allows the relaxation of one group of muscles when an opposing muscle group contracts during reflex and evoked activity. Thus they have connections with both sensory and motor fibres but are primarily influenced by impulses from the cerebellum. The role of the internuncial cell system has been likened to a telephone exchange in that it relays impulses from various sources to the appropriate cell station. A single muscle movement can no longer be regarded merely as an impulse arising in the motor cortex and passing down the appropriate pathway via the anterior horn cell in the spinal cord to the muscle fibre. The muscles themselves have a complex system of signalling the degree of their contraction (see below) and the internuncial neurones play a role in regulating this movement and passing impulses to antagonistic muscles.

Clinically, the importance of the internuncial cell system has increased since it has been found that certain drugs—notably mephenesin, diazepam and phenothiazines—can reduce or interrupt their activity and so lead to alterations in muscle tone. Nevertheless, the side-effects of mephenesin have made it unsuitable as an agent for producing muscular relaxation in clinical anaesthesia. Other members of the "tranquillising" series of drugs have been found to alter internuncial fibre activity and large doses of chlorpromazine and meprobamate have been found to be effective, but their clinical value in this respect is largely limited to the treatment of tetanus.

Muscle Spindles and the Small Fibre System

The motor pathway from the anterior horn cell down to the neuromuscular junction on the skeletal muscle fibre is now familiar to all (Fig. 10). Conduction along this route is rapid as the size of the fibre (α efferent) is large, i.e. 14 μm in diameter. Closer scrutiny of this nerve fibre reveals that besides these large fibres there are smaller ones—γ efferent fibres measuring some 4 μm in diameter —which when traced peripherally are found to end in a special structure—the *muscle spindle* (Fig. 11).

The simple act of picking up a pencil from a table not only employs the motor pathway, but afferents reach the spinal cord from the sensory endings in the skin, joints and muscles. In fact, the muscle spindles are the sensory end-organ of the skeletal muscles and are responsible for signalling the degree of shortening of the whole muscle. In this way they can provide information so that only the exact amount of muscle activity required for the task is used. Histologically, the muscle spindle is an elongated and encapsulated structure

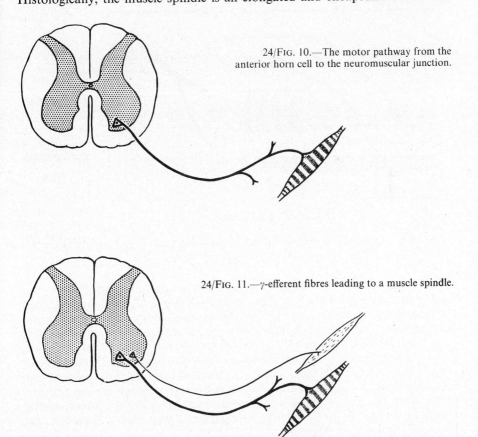

24/FIG. 10.—The motor pathway from the anterior horn cell to the neuromuscular junction.

24/FIG. 11.—γ-efferent fibres leading to a muscle spindle.

24/Fig. 12(*a*).—Intrafusal fibres.

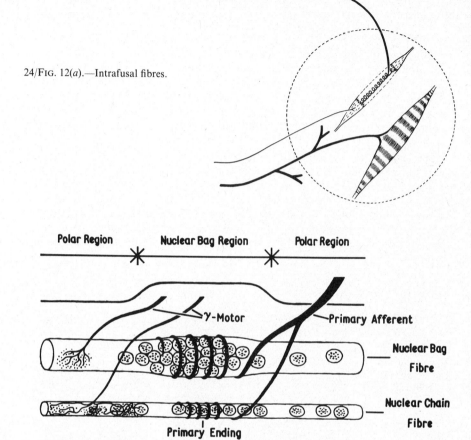

24/Fig. 12(*b*).—Diagram of central region of the muscle spindle showing innervation of nuclear bag and nuclear chain fibre (Collier, 1975).

which lies in parallel with the skeletal muscle fibres and shares its attachment. This latter point is of particular importance as its principal function is to signal the exact length of the skeletal fibre. Within the capsule small specialised (*intra-fusal*) fibres can be recognised—the *nuclear bag* fibre and the *nuclear chain* fibre (Fig. 12*b*). Because the muscle spindle receives a motor innervation from the small efferent nerve fibres, contraction of the intrafusal fibres of the spindles sends a stimulus back to the spinal cord along the large afferent sensory fibre. This fibre enters the spinal cord through the dorsal root and then traverses the grey matter, finally to synapse with the anterior horn cell of the corresponding muscle fibre (Fig. 13), or through an interneurone it may affect a motor nerve at a different spinal level (Fig. 14).

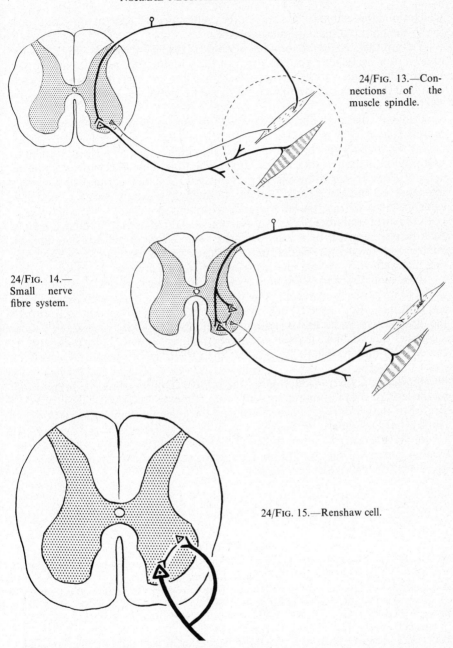

24/Fig. 13.—Connections of the muscle spindle.

24/Fig. 14.— Small nerve fibre system.

24/Fig. 15.—Renshaw cell.

The small fibre system, therefore, consists of the gamma efferent fibre, the muscle spindle, and the large afferent fibre synapsing with the anterior horn cell of the motor unit. A servo-loop or feed-back mechanism is thus created which can either enhance or dampen the contraction of skeletal muscle according to the nature of the stimulus received.

Yet another feed-back loop has been described by Renshaw (1941); as the main motor nerve fibre courses through the white matter of the spinal cord a branch loops backwards to synapse with a cell in the anterior horn (Renshaw cell), and in turn this communicates with the large anterior horn cell again (Fig. 15).

Clinically the small fibre system has three important functions in relation to muscle activity:

(a) *Volitional effort* by modulating and damping the response of muscles to motor nerve activity results in a gradual regulation of muscle changes in muscle activity necessary for co-ordinated movements. The action of the various muscle relaxants on muscle spindle activity is difficult to study but the available evidence suggests that the interference with activity occurs simultaneously at both the intrafusal fibre of the muscle spindle and the neuromuscular junction. As a result there will be a loss of muscle tone, a loss of ability accurately to control volitional movements and a decrease in the nervous input into the reticular activating system and hence an indirect effect upon the brain.

Rack and Westbury (1966) have shown that prolonged tetanic stimulation of the fibres of the muscle spindle in the cat can lead to damage to the mechanism (Fig. 12b). Both acetylcholine and suxamethonium are known to stimulate the motor and sensory nerve-endings on the muscle spindle. Collier (1975) has suggested that the muscle pains of suxamethonium could be due to damage to the delicate muscle-spindle fibre rather than the tougher skeletal muscle-fibre (see Chapter 26).

(b) *Reflex activity*—The tone of the muscle spindles in resting muscle will set the level of stimulation required to produce a reflex response. This is demonstrated by the reinforcing effect of clasping the fingers upon the knee jerk reflex (Buller and Dornhorst, 1957).

(c) *Resting muscle-tone*—Buller (1956) has described muscle tone as the level of activity of the small fibre activity. Increased muscle spindle activity is associated with a greater muscle tone.

REFERENCES

ALI, H. H., UTTING, J. E., and GRAY, C. (1970). Stimulus frequency in the detection of neuromuscular block in humans. *Brit. J. Anaesth.*, **42**, 967.

AXELSSON, J., and THESLEFF, S. (1959). A study of supersensitivity in denervated mammalian skeletal muscle. *J. Physiol. (Lond.)*, **147**, 178.

BIRKS, R., HUXLEY, H. E., and KATZ, B. (1960). The fine structure of the neuromuscular junction of the frog. *J. Physiol. (Lond.)*, **150**, 134.

BIRKS, R. I., and MACINTOSH, F. C. (1957). Acetylcholine metabolism at nerve-endings. *Brit. med. Bull.*, **13**, 157.

BIRKS, R. I., and MACINTOSH, F. C. (1961). Acetylcholine metabolism of a sympathetic ganglion. *Canad. J. Biochem.*, **39**, 787.

BROWN, G. L., DALE, H. H., and FELDBERG, W. (1936). Reactions of the normal mammalian muscle to acetylcholine and to eserine. *J. Physiol. (Lond.)*, **87**, 394.

BULLER, A. J. (1956). Muscle tone. *Physiotherapy*, **42**, 203.

BULLER, A. J., and DORNHORST, A. C. (1957). Reinforcement of tendon reflexes. *Lancet*, **2**, 1261.

BUTTLE, G. A. H., and ZAIMIS, E. J. (1949). The action of decamethonium iodide in birds. *J. Pharm. (Lond.)*, **1**, 991.

CHAGAS, C. (1962). "The fate of curare during curarisation." In: Ciba Foundat. Study Group, No. 12. *Curare and Curare-like Agents*, p. 2. Ed. De Reuck, A. V. S. London: J. & A. Churchill.

CHANGEUX, J. P., HUCHET, M., and CARTAUD, J. (1972). Reconstitution partielle d'une membrane excitable après dissolution par le deoxycholate de sodium. *C.R.Acad. Sci. (Paris)*, **274**, 122.

CHURCHILL-DAVIDSON, H. C., and WISE, R. P. (1964). The response of the newborn infant to muscle relaxants. *Canad. Anaesth. Soc. J.*, **11**, 1.

COLLIER, C. (1975). Suxamethonium pains and fasciculations. *Proc. roy. Soc. Med.*, **68**, 105.

COUTEAUX, R. (1955). Localisation of cholinesterases at neuromuscular junctions. *Int. Rev. Cytol.*, **4**, 335.

COUTEAUX, R. (1958). Morphological and cytochemical observations on the postsynaptic membrane at motor end-plates and ganglionic synapses. *Exp. Cell. Res.* Suppl., **5**, 294.

DALE, H. H., FELDBERG, W., and VOGT, M. (1936). Release of acetylcholine at voluntary motor nerve endings. *J. Physiol. (Lond.)*, **86**, 353.

DEL CASTILLO, J., and ENGBAEK, L. (1954). The nature of the neuromuscular block produced by magnesium. *J. Physiol. (Lond.)*, **124**, 370.

DEL CASTILLO, J., and KATZ, B. (1955). On the localization of acetylcholine receptors. *J. Physiol. (Lond.)*, **128**, 157.

DEL CASTILLO, J., and KATZ, B. (1956). Biophysical aspects of neuromuscular transmission. *Progr. Biophys.*, **6**, 122.

DESMEDT, J. E. (1966). Presynaptic mechanisms in myasthenia gravis. *Ann. N.Y. Acad. Sci.*, **135**, 209.

FELDBERG, W. (1945). Synthesis of acetylcholine by tissue of the central nervous system. *J. Physiol. (Lond.)*, **103**, 367.

GALINDO, A. (1972). The role of prejunctional effects in myoneural transmission. *Anesthesiology*, **36**, 598.

GILL, W. E. (1965). Drug receptor interactions. *Progr. medicinal Chem.*, **4**, 39.

HODGKIN, A. L. (1951). The ionic basis of electrical activity in nerve and muscle. *Biol. Rev.*, **26**, 339.

HUXLEY, A. F. (1963). Electron microscope studies on the structure of natural and synthetic protein filaments from striated muscle. *J. molec. Biol.*, **7**, 281.

HUXLEY, A. F., and TAYLOR, R. E. (1958). Local activation of striated muscle fibres. *J. Physiol. (Lond.)*, **144**, 426.

KATZ, B., and MILEDI, R. (1964). Localisation of calcium action at the nerve muscle junction. *J. Physiol. (Lond.)*, **171**, 10–12 PP.

KATZ, B., and MILEDI, R. (1965a). The measurement of the synaptic delay and the time course of acetylcholine release at the neuromuscular junction. *Proc. roy. Soc. B.*, **161**, 483.

KATZ, B., and MILEDI, R. (1965b). The effect of calcium on acetylcholine release from motor nerve terminals. *Proc. roy. Soc. B.*, **161**, 496.

KRRYEVIĆ, K., and MITCHELL, J. F. (1961). The release of acetylcholine in the isolated rat diaphragm. *J. Physiol. (Lond.)*, **155**, 246.

MASLAND, R. L., and WIGTON, R. S. (1950). Nerve activity accompanying fasciculation produced by prostigmin. *J. Neurophysiol.*, **3**, 269.

MERTON, P. A. (1956). Problems of muscular fatigue. *Brit. med. Bull.*, **12**, 219.

MILEDI, R., MOLINOFF, P., and POTTER, L. T. (1971). Isolation of cholinergic receptor protein of torpedo electric tissue. *Nature (Lond.)*, **229**, 554.

NASTUK, W. L. (1967). Activation and inactivation of muscle post-junctional receptors. *Fed. Proc.*, **26**, 1639.

PAGE, S. (1968). Structure of the sarcoplasmic reticulum in vertebrate muscle. *Brit. med. Bull.*, **24**, 170.

PATON, W. D. M., and WAUD, D. R. (1967). The margin of safety of neuromuscular transmission. *J. Physiol. (Lond.)*, **191**, 59.

RACK, P. M. H., and WESTBURY, D. R. (1966). The effects of suxamethonium and acetylcholine on the behaviour of cat muscle spindles during dynamic stretching, and during fusimotor stimulation. *J. Physiol. (Lond.)*, **186**, 698.

RENSHAW, B. (1941). Influence of discharge of motoneurones upon excitation of neighboring motoneurones. *J. Neurophysiol.*, **4**, 167.

RIKER, N. F., ROBERTS, J., STANDAERT, F. G., and FUJIMAN, H. (1957). The motor nerve terminal as the primary focus for drug-reduced facilitation of neuromuscular transmission. *J. Physiol. (Lond.)*, **121**, 286.

ROBERTSON, J. D. (1956). The ultrastructure of a reptilian myoneural junction. *J. biophys. biochem. Cytol.*, **2**, 381.

SNODGRASS, P. J., and PIRAS, M. M. (1966). Effects of halothane on rat liver mitochondria. *Biochemistry*, **5**, 1140.

WASER, P. G. (1960). The cholinergic receptor. *J. Pharm. Pharmacol.*, **12**, 577.

WASER, P. G. (1970). On receptors in the postsynaptic membrane of the motor endplate. *Ciba Foundation Symposium on Molecular Properties of Drug Receptors*, p. 59. Ed. Porter, R., and O'Connor, M. London: J. & A. Churchill.

WAUD, B. E., and WAUD, D. R. (1971). The relation between tetanic fade and receptor occlusion in the presence of competitive neuromuscular block. *Anesthesiology*, **35**, 456.

WEBER, A., HERZ, R., and REISS, I. (1964). The regulation of myofibrillar activity by calcium. *Proc. roy. Soc. B.*, **160**, 489.

ZACKS, S. I., and BLUMBERG, J. M. (1961). Observations on the fine structure and cytochemistry of mouse and human intercostal neuromuscular junctions. *J. biophys. biochem. Cytol.*, **10**, 517.

Chapter 25

NEUROMUSCULAR BLOCK

Non-depolarisation Block

Claude Bernard's classical experiments demonstrated that curare acted at the myoneural junction. The ability of curare to prevent muscle contraction following close intra-arterial injection of acetylcholine demonstrated that it affected the post-synaptic membrane. Initially it was considered that it acted by fitting into the cholinergic receptors by virtue of a structural similarity of its molecule to that of acetylcholine. Its molecule was likened to two molecules of acetylcholine, each centered around a quaternary ammonium group and it was believed to act like an almost perfect key to fit into the receptor site. However, as it was not hydrolysed rapidly by cholinesterase, it remained for some time occupying the receptor and preventing the access of acetylcholine. When sufficient receptors were occupied, the ability of acetylcholine to cause a threshold depolarisation of the end-plate was prevented and a "curare-like" or non-depolarising block ensued.

This concept of receptor occupancy was later modified by the introduction of the competition theory of neuromuscular blockade in which it is envisaged that the molecules of curare compete with acetylcholine for the receptor sites on the post-junctional membrane. The competition theory implies that the activity of a curare-like drug will be the result of its concentration at the end-plate, relative to the concentration of acetylcholine. As the amount of acetylcholine released in response to a series of supramaximal nerve stimuli will be relatively constant, it follows that following an injection of a curare-like drug its activity, as revealed by indirect stimulation of the motor nerve, will be proportional to its concentration. However, if an anti-cholinesterase drug is administered, the concentration of acetylcholine will be increased relative to that of the curare-like drug, reversing its activity. This theory of action of the non-depolarising muscle relaxants expresses the competition of two differing molecules for the same receptor site. It follows therefore that:

$$\text{amount of neuromuscular block} \propto \frac{\text{concentration of drug}}{\text{concentration of acetylcholine}}$$

This was recently challenged by Feldman and Tyrrell (1970) using the "isolated arm technique". This technique involves injecting the drug under study into an arm isolated from the circulation by means of an arterial tourniquet. They demonstrated that if neuromuscular block was induced using d-tubocurare or gallamine—and the blood concentration of the drug was suddenly reduced by releasing the tourniquet—neuromuscular block still continued for almost the same duration as occurs following the slow fall in blood concentration accompanying a systemic injection of the drug (Fig. 1). It has also been found that in spite of reducing the blood concentration of both

25/TABLE 1

REVISED TERMINOLOGY AS AGREED AT THE INTERNATIONAL CONFERENCE ON MUSCLE
RELAXANTS, 1975

Terminology	
Name of block	*Test for presence*
Non-depolarisation also called:— —competitive —curare-like —antagonist	Fade with *Train of 4* at 2 Hz Tetanic fade at 30 or 50 Hz Post-tetanic facilitation Reversal by anti-cholinesterase drugs
Depolarisation also called:— —Phase I —agonist	Reduced twitch height Absence of fade Weak but maintained tetanus at 30 or 50 Hz
Phase II also called:— —Dual block	Fade at both twitch and tetanic rates Sometimes reversed by anti-cholinesterase drugs Other times potentiated (see text)
Desensitisation	No response to anti-cholinesterase drugs

drugs equally rapidly the 50 per cent recovery index (time for 25–75 per cent recovery of indirectly elicited muscle twitch) reflected the relative clinical duration of action of these drugs when used in equipotent doses during anaesthesia. Thus the recovery index for curare was in the order of 12 minutes, pancuronium 10 minutes and gallamine 9 minutes. Had the competitive theory of action been correct, then the recovery of neuromuscular block should have been equally rapid for all three drugs reflecting the time required to wash the drugs out of the synaptic cleft and away from the receptor. It was therefore suggested that when a non-depolarising drug reacts with a receptor it forms a union with that receptor. The energy value of this union depends upon the molecular configuration of the drug and this will determine its duration of action.

It was further suggested that acetylcholine or other depolarising agents were capable of actively removing the drug from the receptor thus breaking the union between the non-depolarising drug and the receptor site. This is believed to be the cause of the phenomenon of post-tetanic facilitation. Any agent that reduced acetylcholine release would therefore prolong the action of the drug. An increase in acetylcholine concentration, either due to increased release (i.e. by repeated tetanic stimulation or the administration of facilitatory drugs) or by preventing its destruction (i.e. by anticholinesterase drugs) would shorten the recovery time provided that the blood concentration of the non-depolarising drug had been reduced sufficiently to allow the drug to diffuse away once it had been displaced from the receptor.

Site of action of non-depolarising drugs.—The assumption that because neuromuscular agents could be demonstrated to act upon the post-synaptic

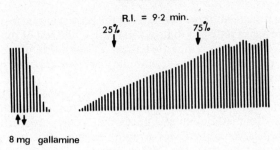

R.I. = 9·2 min.

25%   75%

8 mg gallamine

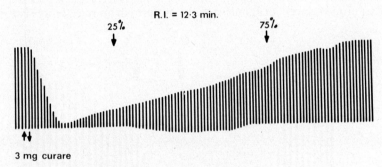

R.I. = 12·3 min.

25%   75%

3 mg curare

25/Fig. 1.— The isolated arm experiment.
Upper trace: recovery from gallamine paralysis in the absence of circulating gallamine. The recovery index (25–75 per cent recovery of twitch height) 9·2 min.
Lower trace: recovery from *d*-tubocurarine paralysis in absence of circulating curare. The recovery index (25–75 per cent of twitch height) 12·3 min.

membrane, this was the only or even the principal site of action, has been challenged in recent years (Riker and Okamoto, 1969). Indeed curare and gallamine undoubtedly do have some action upon the pre-synaptic motor nerve endings (Hubbard and Wilson, 1973). The quantitative importance of this action upon the release of acetylcholine and the development and recovery of neuromuscular block with clinical drugs is uncertain. A review of the evidence for this activity by Galindo (1972) leaves this question unresolved.

Depolarising Block

The original concept of a depolarising block was one that resulted from a lowering of the transmembrane potential of the post-synaptic membrane to a level that prevented the triggering of a propagated action potential by acetylcholine. Jenerick and Gerard (1953) suggested that once the resting membrane potential fell from −90 to −57 mV it became refractory to stimulation. It was demonstrated by del Castillo and Katz (1956) that decamethonium produced a fall in resting potential of the post-synaptic membrane thereby producing a depolarising neuromuscular block. Katz and Thesleff (1957) found, however, that the duration of the depolarisation produced was very much shorter than the duration of the loss of sensitivity of the membrane to acetylcholine. The fact that even after the transmembrane potential of the post-synaptic membrane of the muscle had once again returned to its normal value, the rest of the muscle remained unresponsive to acetylcholine, led them to term this phase of the neuromuscular block produced by decamethonium the *desensitisation phase* of depolarising neuromuscular block.

In their studies of the relationship of blood concentration to the activity of muscle relaxants, Feldman and Tyrrell demonstrated that unlike the non-depolarising relaxants, decamethonium was not bound to the receptor site and once the blood level was lowered there was a rapid recovery of neuromuscular transmission. They postulated that the determining factor as to whether a neuromuscular blocking drug acted as depolarising or non-depolarising agent was whether or not it became bound to the receptor (Fig. 2). This is in keeping with Paton's concept of agonist activity outlined in his rate theory (Paton, 1961).

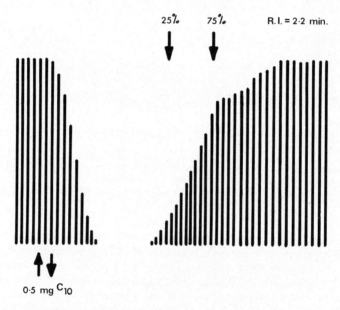

25/FIG. 2.—The isolated arm experiment. Following paralysis induced by decamethonium recovery is rapid (Recovery Index = 2·2 min.) once the blood concentration of drug falls.

Phase II Block (Dual Block)

Clinical experience has demonstrated that depolarising drugs do not always continue to exhibit the characteristics of a depolarising block if administered for prolonged periods or in excessive doses. The demonstration by Jenden *et al.* (1951) that the prolonged administration of decamethonium produced a change in the nature of the neuromuscular block to one that more closely resembled a complete failure of neuromuscular transmission suggested that other mechanisms might be involved. Zaimis *et al.* (1952) and Zaimis (1953) demonstrated that different animals responded differently to decamethonium and indeed in the dog, monkey and rabbit rapidly produced a response that had many of the characteristics of a non-depolarising neuromuscular block. When the closely related drug C_{13} (tridecamethonium) was administered to chicks, it first produced a tonic contracture and opisthotonos, typical of depolarising agents, rapidly followed by flaccid paralysis characteristic of non-depolarising drugs like curare.

Zaimis termed this phenomenon *dual block*. The demonstration of a similar change in activity of decamethonium in myasthenic patients by Churchill-Davidson and Richardson (1952) led to the concept of dual block in man. Churchill-Davidson and his colleagues (1960) demonstrated that a similar phenomenon occurred in normal man following the administration of 0·5 g of suxamethonium. Although this changing nature of the depolarising block has been termed "dual block" in man, it is now considered better to refer to the block as occurring in two stages; *Phase I*, the typical depolarising phase in which its effect is potentiated by anti-cholinesterase drugs or by tetanic stimulation; *Phase II* in which the block assumes some non-depolarising characteristics in that significant, but often short-lived, reversal occurs if an anti-cholinesterase is administered, tetanic stimulation produces some degree of post-tetanic facilitation, and tachyphylaxis to further doses of depolarising agents can be demonstrated. The term desensitisation block should be reserved for neuromuscular block associated with a complete lack of response to either acetylcholine or tetanus.

The cause of the Phase II block is unknown. It may be associated with a pre-synaptic site of action of the drug as suggested by Galindo (1971). Feldman and Tyrrell (1970) suggested that it represented an increasing proportion of the depolarising drug molecules becoming bound to the receptor so producing a significant degree of receptor occupancy and therefore a non-depolarising component to the neuromuscular block. It is probable that subclinical Phase II block develops very rapidly but that with increasing dose and increasing time of exposure, the block becomes clinically significant (Crul *et al.*, 1966).

Block Caused by Effect on Acetylcholine

Even during the resting state, small quantities of acetylcholine are released at the nerve terminals, and these ions give rise to small end-plate potentials which are insufficient to depolarise the muscle membrane. Many local analgesics—particularly procaine—are believed to suppress the release of acetylcholine directly and thus cause muscle weakness and paralysis (Harvey, 1939). Other substances which have this property are botulinus toxin (from *Clostridium botulinum*), the aminoglycoside antibiotics, severe calcium deficiency (Harvey and MacIntosh, 1940), excessive doses of phosphate (Brown and Dias, 1947) and magnesium (Paton, 1956).

The *hemicholinium* group of compounds are quaternary bases which are highly toxic. Though they are not used in clinical practice, their mode of action has excited considerable pharmacological interest. When administered to an animal they ultimately produce complete respiratory paralysis, but this is delayed in onset and can be prevented by the administration of choline. MacIntosh *et al.* (1958) have concluded that these compounds interfere with acetylcholine synthesis by impeding the transport of choline to its site of acetylation. Feldman (1973) has demonstrated that hypothermia also induces a partial neuromuscular block. This has been shown to be due to reduced release of acetylcholine (Thornton *et al.*, 1976).

Mixed Block

The muscles of respiration are normally amongst the first to recover full activity after the injection of a relaxant drug. Electromyographic recordings taken from any peripheral muscle can demonstrate that despite adequate respiratory activity a high degree of neuromuscular block still persists. If, at this point, a further relaxant drug of a different type is given, theoretically some of the motor units will be under the influence of one drug and some affected by the other. A mixed type of neuromuscular block is present.

MEASUREMENT OF NEUROMUSCULAR BLOCK

In the past the action of the various muscle relaxants has been investigated mainly in animals and these findings have often been erroneously assumed to be uniformly applicable to man. Unfortunately, there is no single species that responds to these drugs in exactly the same manner as man. This has led to considerable confusion in the literature.

The earliest attempts to study the effects of these drugs in man were based on clinical observations, grip-strength measurements in conscious volunteers, and tidal volume studies in the anaesthetised patient. None of these methods proved entirely satisfactory. The pitfalls of clinical observations are known to all, grip-strength recordings are always subject to volitional effort on the part of the individual, and most untrained volunteers have difficulty in making a maximum possible effort under the influence of these drugs. Tidal volume measurements have been widely used in anaesthetised patients; yet many other drugs, such as narcotics, hypnotics, or even inhalational anaesthetic agents, can all depress the tidal volume but are not muscle relaxants. Tidal volume measurements, therefore, can never be considered a satisfactory method of monitoring neuromuscular transmission. Clinically, it has often been wrongly assumed that the muscle relaxants were responsible for respiratory depression at the end of an operation. The danger of this assumption cannot be emphasised too strongly. Such a suggestion can only be satisfactorily upheld if it is demonstrated that neuromuscular transmission is depressed.

There is only one satisfactory method of studying neuromuscular transmission—namely, stimulation of any peripheral motor nerve and observing or measuring the response of the corresponding muscle (i.e. indirect muscle stimulation). The electric current used must be of sufficient intensity to excite all the nerve fibres in the bundle, i.e. it must be supramaximal. Once a stimulus has been propagated down a nerve fibre then, on the basis of the "all or none" law, every one of the corresponding muscle fibres must contract if there is no impairment of neuromuscular transmission.

The principal methods of measuring neuromuscular transmission are outlined below:

Volitional measurements.—It has already been mentioned above that the value of such measurements is limited. They have, however, proved useful as a guide to laboratory investigations and particularly if repeated comparative measurements are to be made in the same individual. The instrument commonly used is the *recording ergograph*. The subject squeezes a hand-bulb with a maximum effort at regular intervals. The results are displayed with a pen-recorder. The effect of a particular dose of a relaxant drug or the degree of paresis due to a pathological state can be assessed.

Involuntary measurement.—Such a technique does not require the co-operation of the patient and therefore is more suitable for use in the unconscious patient. Furthermore, as a supramaximal electrical stimulus can be used, the measurements are more reliable. The resulting contraction of the muscle fibres can be measured either mechanically or electrically. Measurement of mechanical contraction is easier but has the small disadvantage of the inertia of the apparatus, e.g. the strain-gauge. The electrical response of the contracting muscle fibres requires more complex apparatus but gives a greater degree of accuracy. Such recordings, however, are often difficult to obtain in the operating room, where electrical interference is common. Ideally both methods of study should be used.

(a) **Mechanical method.**— The commonest method employs a force transducer to measure the force of adduction of the thumb muscles following electrical stimulation of the ulnar nerve (Fig. 3). The strain-gauge used must be capable of measuring a force displacement of 50–100 g.

(b) **Electrical method.**— The technique is based on the application of a supramaximal stimulus to a motor nerve and recording the electrical potential generated by a group of muscle fibres all contracting synchronously, i.e. electromyography.

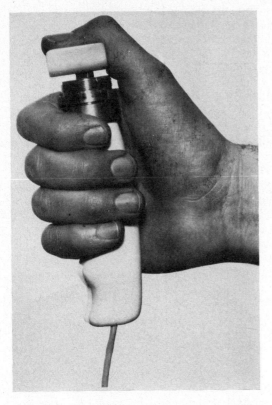

25/Fig. 3.—A Statham UC3 force transducer mounted in a bicycle handle grip to record contraction of the thumb muscle.

The upper limb is particularly useful in the anaesthetised patient because it is nearly always possible to obtain access to an extended arm in most surgical operations. For measurements the fingers and arm are bound to a splint to prevent movement and the contraction of the hypothenar muscles is recorded on the electromyograph (Fig. 4). On stimulation of the nerve fibre (i.e. ulnar), a full motor unit action potential is produced. That is to say, all the 150–300 muscle fibres supplied by that nerve fibre are compelled to contract synchronously. Each of these contractions helps to build the action potential. If the surface electrodes are correctly placed, a number of biphasic motor unit action potentials are recorded as a single large summated potential on the electromyograph.

A normal action potential of the hypothenar muscles in response to a single supramaximal twitch stimulus of the ulnar nerve is shown in Fig. 5. The stimulus artefact (represented as a small deflection prior to the action potential) represents the administration of the electrical current to the nerve. The time interval between the stimulus artefact and the beginning of the action potential represents the time taken for the stimulus to pass down the nerve fibre and across to the motor end-plate. If the stimulus is administered at two different points along a nerve fibre (e.g. at the elbow and wrist) the difference in the time interval in this case is due to transmission down the nerve between these points.

Under normal physiological conditions a subject can send stimuli down a motor nerve at a rate varying from 20 to 50 Hz, depending on the amount of effort expended (Fig. 6). It is impossible to send a single twitch stimulus or a rate as slow as 10 per second without recourse to artificial stimulation.

Regardless of the rate of stimulation (i.e. from 1 to 50 Hz), if normal neuromuscular transmission is present then the height of successive action potentials should be well sustained. That is to say, both the height and the shape of the potential will remain virtually unaltered. The size of the action potential is always slightly greater at tetanic, as opposed to twitch, rates of nerve stimulation. Furthermore, a rate of 50 Hz can be maintained in a normal adult for at least twenty seconds before the first signs of fatigue become apparent.

The height of the action potential (or more correctly, the surface area contained within its boundaries) is directly related to the number of muscle fibres that are functioning. Thus, as a muscle relaxant is administered so the height (or area) of the action potential is diminished until finally only the base-line remains when complete paralysis is present.

There are certain other features of abnormal neuromuscular transmission that have already been discussed in Chapter 24, namely post-tetanic facilitation, post-tetanic exhaustion and Wedensky inhibition.

DIFFERENTIATION OF NEUROMUSCULAR BLOCK

The various characteristics of the two principal types of neuromuscular block—depolarisation and non-depolarisation—are fortunately so different that they can easily be distinguished. This differentiation has important clinical bearings because it enables the anaesthetist to diagnose the exact type of neuromuscular block that is present, even if he does not know the agent used. Principally it is made on four counts:

1. The presence or absence of spontaneous *fasciculations*. These may be observed or recorded electromyographically from an appropriate muscle.
2. The response of the muscle fibre to both *fast* (*tetanic*) and *slow* (*twitch*) rates of nerve stimulation.
3. The presence or absence of *post-tetanic facilitation*.
4. The response to the administration of an anti-cholinesterase drug.

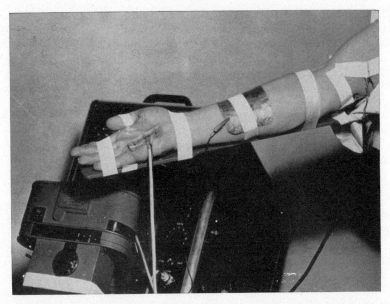

25/FIG. 4.—The electromyographic apparatus arranged for recording from the hypothenar muscles.

Depolarisation Block (Figs. 7–9)

This type of neuromuscular block follows the administration of acetylcholine (lasting a fraction of a second), suxamethonium (2–4 minutes) and decamethonium (lasting about 20 minutes or more). The four main characteristics of this type of block are:

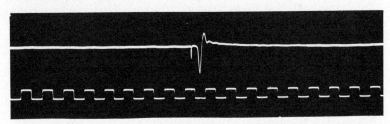

25/FIG. 5.—A normal action potential (twitch stimulus). The small downward depression before the origin of the complete action potential is the artefact caused by the electrical stimulus.

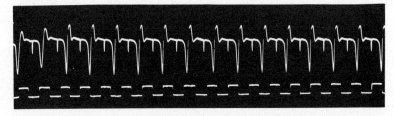

25/FIG. 6.—Normal action potentials (tetanic stimulation).

1. *Fasciculations* can be observed or recorded in muscle just prior to the onset of paralysis. They are particularly well seen after the rapid administration of suxamethonium.

2. Both *fast* (*tetanic*) and *slow* (*twitch*) rates of nerve stimulation are well *sustained*. This statement requires further clarification. Some "fade" or Wedensky inhibition can be observed during a depolarisation block. It is only seen when fast rates are used and when present will be accompanied by post-tetanic potentiation. It is almost always observed during the very early stages of recovery from complete paralysis, but by the time 50 per cent recovery has been achieved the typical signs of a well-sustained response at both twitch and tetanic rates of stimulation are present. If the patient is inhaling halothane then the "fade" at tetanic rates of stimulation is more marked (de Jong and Freund, 1967).

To observe the signs of the block correctly it is necessary to test neuro-muscular transmission in the manner demonstrated above. In other words, the sequence of events of nerve stimulation should be *twitch-tetanus-twitch*.

3. *Post-tetanic facilitation* is absent. It will be observed in Fig. 7 that the height of the muscle response to twitch or slow nerve stimulation is the same after a period of fast (tetanic) nerve stimulation as it was before.

4. *Anti-cholinesterase drugs* either produce no effect or *increase* the neuro-muscular block. These drugs have an action on the neuromuscular junction tending to potentiate a depolarisation block. Edrophonium (Tensilon) 10 mg is sometimes used as a diagnostic agent in the presence of a Phase II block (see p. 848).

The effect of first administering a depolarising drug alone and then a com-bination of a depolarising drug with an anti-cholinesterase is illustrated in Fig. 8. It will be observed that the classical signs of a depolarisation block are present. The decamethonium has produced about 95 per cent paralysis of the muscle fibres. Only a minimal change can be observed on the administration of an anti-cholinesterase, though there is some slight increase in the neuromuscular block.

Clinical significance.—These electromyographic changes can also be ob-served clinically as movements of the fingers. A simple nerve-stimulator is all that is required and there is no necessity for complex electromyographic equip-ment. If the ulnar nerve is stimulated either at the wrist or in the ulnar groove at the elbow, the fingers will be seen to take on the characteristic "main en griffe" position each time the stimulus is administered. The main deflexion appears in the 5th and 4th fingers and the hypothenar muscles, but the other muscles of the hand (particularly the thenar muscles) are also often involved.

Clinically, two features of a depolarisation block can be particularly well demonstrated provided total paralysis is not present. As previously mentioned, some "fade" and post-tetanic facilitation may be present in the early stages of recovery and during the inhalation of halothane. Once 50 per cent recovery has been achieved both twitch and tetanus are well sustained. However, in contrast with a non-depolarisation block the slow twitch rates (i.e. 2–5 Hz) are always well sustained at any stage of the recovery period. Also, in a non-depolarisation block even the twitch rates show a "fade" or Wedensky inhibition, especially marked in the first 3 or 4 twitches.

To summarise:

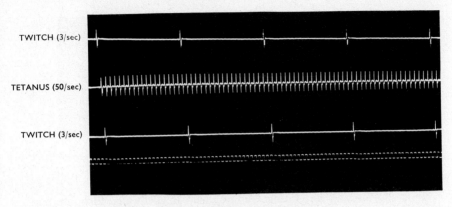

TWITCH (3/sec)

TETANUS (50/sec)

TWITCH (3/sec)

25/FIG. 7.—Depolarisation block.

1. Successive stimuli are *well-sustained* with both fast and slow rates of nerve stimulation.

2. There is *no* post-tetanic facilitation.

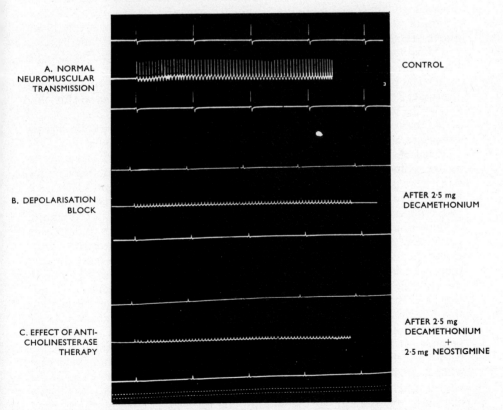

A. NORMAL NEUROMUSCULAR TRANSMISSION — CONTROL

B. DEPOLARISATION BLOCK — AFTER 2·5 mg DECAMETHONIUM

C. EFFECT OF ANTI-CHOLINESTERASE THERAPY — AFTER 2·5 mg DECAMETHONIUM + 2·5 mg NEOSTIGMINE

25/FIG. 8.—Depolarisation block and the effect of neostigmine.

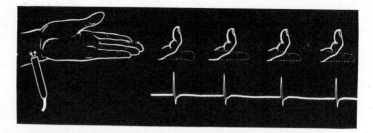

25/Fɪɢ. 9.—Depolarisation block. Movements of the fingers on peripheral nerve stimulation correlated with the electromyographic response.

If a short-acting anti-cholinesterase drug (e.g. 10 mg edrophonium) is given intravenously, a momentary increase in the paresis may be observed. Such therapy, however, is entirely unnecessary (and may even be harmful) if the other signs of a depolarisation block have already been observed.

Non-depolarisation Blocks (Figs. 10 and 11)

This type of block normally follows the administration of *d*-tubocurarine chloride, gallamine triethiodide and similar agents.

In direct contrast with the features described for a depolarisation block above, the signs of a non-depolarisation block are as follows:

1. *No fasciculations.*—There is a complete absence of muscle-fibre activity prior to the onset of paralysis.

2. The presence of "fade" of successive stimuli on both fast (tetanic) and the initial 3 or 4 responses to slow (twitch) rates of nerve stimulation (Fig. 10).

3. The presence of *post-tetanic facilitation* (see above).

4. Improvement of neuromuscular transmission by anti-cholinesterase drugs (see below).

Clinical significance.—The signs of a non-depolarisation block can easily be recognised with the aid of a peripheral nerve stimulator. Stimulation of a motor nerve reveals the characteristic *fade* and *post-tetanic facilitation*. These are best observed in the movements of the fingers. As the mechanical movements of the fingers are directly related to the electrical response, the interpretation of these results is virtually interchangeable. Sometimes it is easier to detect the presence of fade and potentiation by "feeling" the movements of the fingers rather than simply observing them. The sense of touch is often more delicate than vision in this respect. The "fade" of successive stimuli occurs maximally in the first four stimuli whether the rate be fast or slow. In a severe non-depolarisation block the initial contraction may be so short-lived during tetanic stimulation that it is unobserved by the eye yet perceived by touch. To demonstrate post-tetanic facilitation, the actual period of tetanic stimulation should be at least five seconds; at the termination about two seconds should be allowed to elapse before returning to a slow (i.e. twitch) rate of stimulation. In an average case some facilitation can be observed for about thirty seconds after the end of the tetanic stimulation, but this duration depends on many factors such as the rate of tetanus, the duration of the tetanus, and the plasma concentration of the muscle relaxant. However, it rarely persists more than one minute.

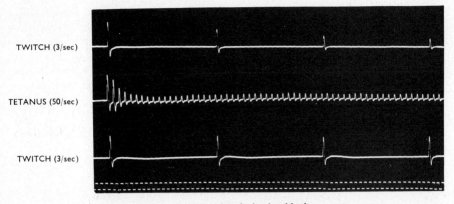

TWITCH (3/sec)

TETANUS (50/sec)

TWITCH (3/sec)

25/Fig. 10.—Non-depolarisation block.

From the clinical aspect, therefore, the anaesthetist (with the aid of a nerve-stimulator) can gauge at the end of every case in which a relaxant has been given an approximate estimate of the degree of neuromuscular block; he can also observe the effectiveness of anti-cholinesterase therapy. For example, if both "fade" and "facilitation" are present, then this is a clear indication for a further dose of anti-cholinesterase, whereas it is unnecessary if they are absent and

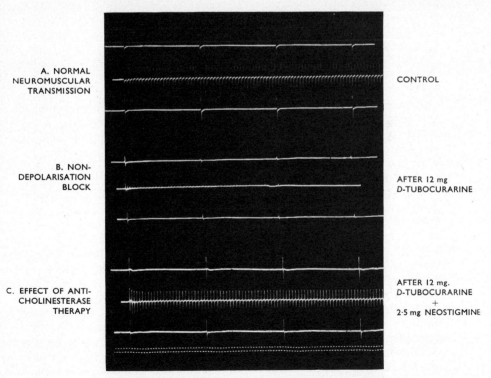

A. NORMAL NEUROMUSCULAR TRANSMISSION

CONTROL

B. NON-DEPOLARISATION BLOCK

AFTER 12 mg D-TUBOCURARINE

AFTER 12 mg. D-TUBOCURARINE + 2·5 mg NEOSTIGMINE

C. EFFECT OF ANTI-CHOLINESTERASE THERAPY

25/Fig. 11.—Non-depolarisation block and the effect of neostigmine.

neuromuscular transmission has recovered. This titration of the clinical effect is particularly useful in cardiac cases, small children, and the severely ill, where it is desired to obtain the maximum benefit to neuromuscular transmission with the minimum quantity of drugs. Finally, with careful observation of the characteristic movements of the fingers on both slow and fast nerve stimulation, then the precise type of neuromuscular block that is present can be diagnosed (Fig. 12).

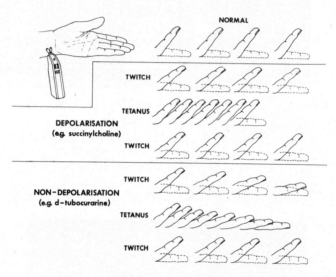

25/FIG. 12.—Finger movements with nerve stimulation.

Comment on the reversibility of *d*-tubocurarine paresis.—Electromyographically it has been observed that it is difficult completely to reverse the neuromuscular block produced by *d*-tubocurarine unless either the dose of relaxant is very low or the time interval between relaxant and antagonist is very long. In clinical practice, when a fully paralysing dose of *d*-tubocurarine has been used (i.e. 25–30 mg in an average adult) then a 100 per cent return of normal neuromuscular transmission is difficult to obtain rapidly unless sufficient time has elapsed to allow a fall in plasma level of the drug before the anti-cholinesterase is given. However such perfection is seldom required because by the time neuromuscular transmission in the hand muscles has recovered to 60 per cent of normal, the respiratory muscles have recovered sufficiently for normal ventilation. Because of this sensitivity the hand muscles act as a very useful guide in the diagnosis of residual ventilatory insufficiency.

After a period of muscle paralysis the principal aim must be to return the patient to full muscle power so that he can protect himself against any untoward respiratory obstruction and also swallow salivary secretions effectively. Various suggestions have been made as to how the clinician may gauge whether any residual paresis remains or not. The simplest and *least* efficient method is to look at the reservoir bag and estimate the tidal volume. As a normal tidal volume is 500 ml and a normal vital capacity is 5,000 ml, theoretically it is possible for the patient to be 90 per cent paralysed yet have a normal tidal volume. Some authors have advocated the ability to maintain a sustained head-lift (Dam and Guldman, 1961), but this pre-supposes that all patients are sufficiently conscious immediately after operation to perform this test effectively. Also, Walts and his co-workers (1970) have shown that sustained head-lift is not a reliable index of recovery from non-depolarising blocking agents (e.g. d-tubocurare). These authors favoured use of the response of the fingers to tetanic nerve stimulation at 30 Hz, as being the best way of monitoring complete recovery. They found that sustained muscular contraction in response to tetanic nerve stimulation was always associated with greater than 90 per cent recovery of vital capacity. These studies were made on conscious volunteers and as tetanic stimulation is a painful stimulus an axillary nerve-block was required for the study. As twitch rates of nerve stimulation are far less painful, Ali and his colleagues (1975) have suggested the use of the "*train-of-four*" stimulation. In this test the motor nerve (ulnar) is stimulated at a frequency of 2 Hz and the muscle response (adductor pollicis brevis) is recorded on a digital neuromuscular transmission analyser (Fig. 13). In the presence of a non-depolarising block the characteristic fade will be observed. The ratio of the 4th twitch to the 1st twitch is expressed in percentage terms (Fig. 14). Thus, when the 4th twitch height is 60 per cent or less of the 1st twitch height, they found that vital capacity was significantly reduced.

Clinically, it would seem unlikely that many anaesthetists will have a digital neuromuscular transmission analyser readily available for the routine case. In the anaesthetised patient or in early recovery the pain of tetanic stimulation can hardly be considered applicable because of the presence of some analgesia. If visual movement of the fingers is to be used to test for the presence of any residual paresis then the sequence of *Twitch-Tetanus-Twitch* (Fig. 12) as recommended by Churchill-Davidson and Christie (1959) is still a very effective method, because not only can the anaesthetist observe the fade of twitch rates of stimulation (as in the train-of-four) but also the fade on tetanic stimulation and the remarkable post-tetanic facilitation that accompanies it.

The skill in the administration of a relaxant drug lies in finding the optimum dose that will just produce ideal conditions for surgery yet which is easily reversible by an anti-cholinesterase drug after redistribution of the relaxant. This can only be achieved by careful monitoring with a peripheral nerve stimulator.

There still remains one important type of neuromuscular block that is commonly encountered in clinical practice—namely, Phase II or dual block.

Phase II Block (Dual Block)

One of the most interesting developments in the theory of neuromuscular transmission is the finding that the depolarising drugs, e.g. decamethonium and suxamethonium, do not always behave exactly as predicted. In order to understand the background to this new conception, it is necessary to trace the evidence in both animal and human experiments from the introduction of the methonium compounds into clinical medicine.

Investigation in animals.—By 1950 it had been firmly established that decamethonium acted by depolarising the muscle fibre in a small area in the region of the motor end-plate (Brown *et al.*, 1949). Later, this led to the assumption

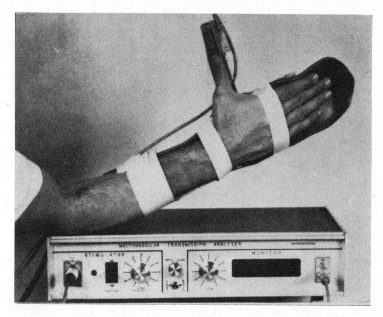

25/Fig. 13.—A view of the digital neuromuscular transmission analyser with the hand and forearm immobilised for recording from the thumb.

that both decamethonium and suxamethonium produced their neuromuscular block by pure depolarisation in all mammals (Paton and Zaimis, 1952). It had, however, been noted that the response of different muscle groups in the cat to depolarising drugs varied widely, and this difference was thought to be related to the colour of the muscle groups following exsanguination—namely red or white muscle. Thus, the soleus muscle (an example of "red" muscle) is resistant

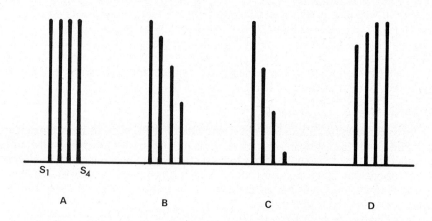

25/Fig. 14.—Train-of-four stimuli at 2 Hz.
A—control; B—5 mg d-tubocurarine; C—12 mg d-tubocurarine; D—reversal by neostigmine.

to the depolarising action of decamethonium whereas the tibialis muscle (an example of "white" muscle) is comparatively sensitive (Table 2).

25/TABLE 2

COMPARISON OF THE EFFECT OF DECAMETHONIUM ON THE TIBIALIS AND SOLEUS MUSCLES OF THE CAT

Soleus—Red muscle—Resistant to decamethonium.
Tibialis—White muscle—Sensitive to decamethonium.

At this stage it was generally believed that the depolarising drugs acted by simple depolarisation in all mammals, including man. Nearly all the discrepancies in the response to decamethonium could be explained on the basis of variations in sensitivity between the different muscle groups. This simple conception was shattered, however, when Jenden and his colleagues (1951) observed an altered response in the rabbit after the prolonged administration of decamethonium and Zaimis (1952) went on to show that a remarkable difference in the response of decamethonium existed amongst the various species.

There were two further important points about this species variation (Zaimis, 1953). First, although decamethonium produced depolarisation in the cat, if a compound with a slightly longer polymethylene chain was used (i.e. tridecamethonium, or C.13) then the response in the cat and chick was of the dual type. This suggested that simply producing a slight alteration in the molecular structure could change the type of response of the motor end-plate. A dual type of neuromuscular block could theoretically arise either from a change in the way in which the motor end-plate responded to the molecule of drug or from the drug acting at more than one receptor site.

Clinical interpretation.—A Phase II block always ultimately occurs after repeated doses of a depolarising drug in man. However, provided the dose of drug used is kept to the minimum required to produce a neuromuscular block, it seldom develops to a point where it is clinically obvious. Typically, the administration of a depolarising drug is at first followed by all the signs of a depolarisation block. With repeated doses, gradually some of the signs of a non-depolarisation block occur during the recovery phase. If suxamethonium is used this may be only for a fleeting moment at first, but then slowly the period of *fade* and *facilitation* becomes more obvious. This is coincident with the development of tachyphylaxis. Ultimately, if repeated doses continue to be given, a stage is reached where the signs of a full Phase II block are obvious and recovery of normal neuromuscular transmission is slow.

The five stages in the development of a Phase II block have been described (Churchill-Davidson *et al.*, 1960) as follows:

1. *Depolarisation stage.*—A typical depolarisation block with maintenance of both fast (tetanic) and slow (twitch) rates of nerve stimulation is present when observed at the stage of 50 per cent recovery of neuromuscular transmission. Anti-cholinesterase drugs potentiate the block.

2. *Tachyphylaxis stage.*—The same dose repeated again and again leads to a *diminishing* response. To gain the original response it is necessary to *increase* the dose. (Subclinical Phase II block.)

3. *Stage of Wedensky inhibition.*—There is a *fade* of successive potentials to fast rates of nerve stimulation only. Twitch stimulation remains unaltered.

4. *Stage of fade and facilitation.*—As the Phase II block develops, so this becomes more and more obvious. The administration of an anti-cholinesterase drug at this point will improve all those fibres exhibiting fade and facilitation.

5. *Non-depolarisation stage.*—All the classical signs of a non-depolarisation block are present. There is marked fade and facilitation and the initial twitch response is high, showing that a large percentage of the muscle fibres are now exhibiting a Phase II block. The administration of an anti-cholinesterase drug leads to a dramatic improvement in neuromuscular transmission.

An example of the first, fourth and fifth stages of Phase II block is given in Fig. 15.

A similar situation can develop if an infusion of suxamethonium is used. In Fig. 16 the twitch response following 50 mg of suxamethonium is compared with that after 1500 mg. The typical "fade" of a non-depolarisation block is clearly demonstrated.

Dose-relationship of Phase II Block

The concept of Phase II block in man, as being a changing response to a depolarising muscle-relaxant drug has not been universally accepted and it must be admitted that there is no completely satisfactory explanation of its aetiology. The possibility that it represents a prolongation of the desensitisation of the post-synaptic membrane reported by Katz and Thesleff (1957) would explain the difficulty of reversing the condition by the use of anti-cholinesterase drugs. However, the presence of curare-like characteristics of well-developed Phase II block, i.e. "fade", post-tetanic facilitation and partial—if only short-lived—response to anti-cholinesterase drugs strongly suggest that the block does involve a curare-like state of the myoneural function and is not the same as desensitisation. Galindo and Kennedy (1974) have produced evidence to suggest that this is the result of a depression of motor-nerve terminal activity leading to a decrease in acetylcholine release. They postulate three main sites of action of suxamethonium and that these may be responsible for the multi-phasic activity of this drug. The desensitisation phase demonstrated by Jenden and his colleagues in 1951, however, is likely to have been the result of a loss of intracellular potassium, a situation that is unlikely to occur in man. The possibility that a Phase II block represents a reaction of the drug at a separate receptor site, where it has antagonist effects, has been proposed by Feldman (1973). This concept receives some support from the observation that there may be two types of receptors at the end-plate, one reacting with depolarising drugs and the other with curare-type agents.

It must be remembered that due to the large margin of safety of neuro-muscular transmission, a non-depolarising type block will not be obvious until over 70 per cent of the receptors are occupied by the drug.

Treatment of Phase II Block

The fact that a fully-established Phase II block can be reversed by an anti-cholinesterase drug is now proven. However, Vickers (1963) has pointed out the difficulties that may be encountered in the indiscriminate use of anti-

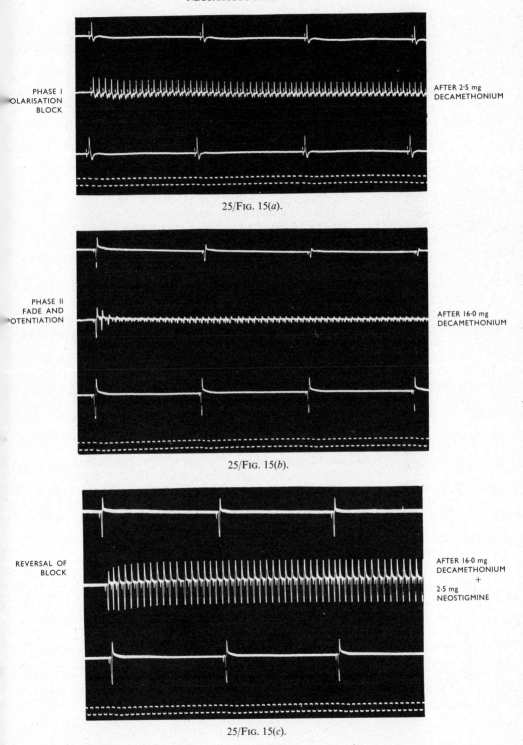

PHASE I
DEPOLARISATION
BLOCK

AFTER 2·5 mg
DECAMETHONIUM

25/FIG. 15(a).

PHASE II
FADE AND
POTENTIATION

AFTER 16·0 mg
DECAMETHONIUM

25/FIG. 15(b).

REVERSAL OF
BLOCK

AFTER 16·0 mg
DECAMETHONIUM
+
2·5 mg
NEOSTIGMINE

25/FIG. 15(c).

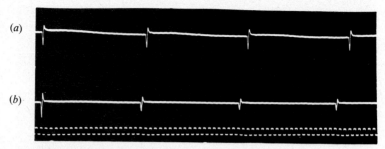

25/FIG. 16.—Effect of infusion of suxamethonium on the twitch response of the hypothenar muscles.
(*a*) After 50 mg. (*b*) After 1500 mg.

cholinesterase drugs. There are numerous clinical reports of the successful reversal of a Phase II block in clinical practice: nevertheless, there are also a number of instances when the administration of an anti-cholinesterase drug in an attempt to reverse such a block has merely increased and prolonged the paralysis (Harper, 1952; Abrams and Ginsberg, 1960; Vickers, 1963).

In considering whether or not one should use anti-cholinesterase drugs in an attempt to reverse a Phase II block there are a number of points to be taken into account. It has been demonstrated that the reversibility of an experimental Phase II block depends mainly on the concentration of the depolarising drug in the circulation (Gissen *et al.*, 1966). When the concentration is high the block cannot be reversed, whilst when it is low recovery can be achieved.

It is known that a fully established Phase II block (like a non-depolarisation block) can be reversed by an anti-cholinesterase. Equally it is known that if suxamethonium is still circulating, then the injection of an anti-cholinesterase will slow down any hydrolysis even further and may even augment the block. Unless there is well-marked and prolonged post-tetanic facilitation, it is inadvisable to give anti-cholinesterase drugs. At least thirty minutes should have elapsed since the last recorded dose of the suxamethonium and there should be some signs of improving neuromuscular transmission, thereby denoting the presence of hydrolysis. Patients exhibiting Phase II block should normally be treated symptomatically by means of artificial ventilation with 50 per cent nitrous oxide and oxygen. Normal neuromuscular conduction usually returns in 1–4 hours.

FACTORS ALTERING THE DURATION OR DEGREE OF NEUROMUSCULAR BLOCK

The use of the muscle relaxants has now become firmly established as an integral part of modern anaesthesia. It is not surprising, therefore, that their use is sometimes blamed for the failure of the patient to breathe adequately at the end of an operation. Often the muscle relaxants are unjustly convicted when the real blame lies with the administrator for failing to assess the requirements of a particular patient accurately. Occasionally, however, a number of cases are reported in which the relaxants appear to be incriminated. Each time this occurs a new theory is born, often with the minimum of experimental evidence.

The various factors which are known or believed to affect either the degree or duration of neuromuscular block are reviewed below.

It is important to appreciate the distinction between the factors that affect the degree of neuromuscular block that occurs following the administration of a given dose of drug, from those that prolong the recovery process. If a given dose of drug causes a more profound neuromuscular block, it will take longer for the recovery of normal neuromuscular transmission as this recovery will start from a lower base line (Fig. 17). The *recovery index* is the term used to denote the time taken for the twitch height to recover from 25 per cent (of control) to 75 per cent, and therefore can be useful for expressing the rate of

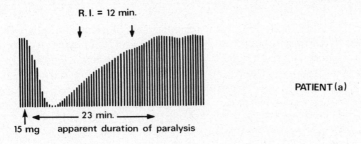

R. I. = 12 min.

23 min. ——
15 mg   apparent duration of paralysis

PATIENT (a)

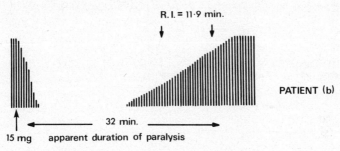

R. I. = 11·9 min.

32 min. ——
15 mg   apparent duration of paralysis

PATIENT (b)

25/FIG. 17.—In both these patients the recovery rate, as measured by the Recovery Index was similar; however, the apparent duration of paralysis in (b) was 32 min compared with 23 min in patient (a).

recovery (Feldman, 1974). The most important factors determining the amount of neuromuscular block produced are the peak plasma level of drug achieved following injection and the sensitivity of the receptors to neuromuscular block (i.e. a reduced margin of safety of neuromuscular transmission will result in less molecules of a non-depolarising agent being required to produce a neuro-muscular block). The recovery index of a drug depends upon its affinity with the receptor, the amount of acetylcholine produced and the establishment of a concentration gradient along which the drug can diffuse following displacement from the receptor site.

Blood Flow

Alterations in blood flow affect both the rate of onset and the degree of paralysis produced by a given dose of neuromuscular blocking agent (Goat *et al.*,

1976). If a drug is injected into a slow circulation it will take longer to produce neuromuscular block and the resulting effect will be less profound than if the same dose had been given into a fast circulation (Harrison, 1972). This effect may be of clinical significance as both the amount and distribution of cardiac output may vary considerably from patient to patient and may be altered by other drugs given during anaesthesia.

The effect of blood flow upon the recovery index of the drug depends upon whether the drug is depolarising or non-depolarising in nature.

(a) *Depolarising drugs* are not bound closely to the receptor and therefore recovery time depends on the rate at which the drug is washed out from the muscle. The effect of blood flow on a depolarising block can be seen in the results obtained by Churchill-Davidson and Richardson (1952) using decamethonium (Fig. 18), and Harrison (1972) using suxamethonium. Exercise or tetanic

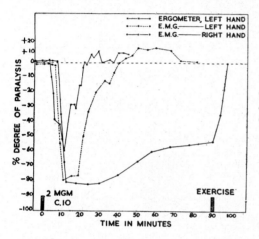

25/Fig. 18.—Comparison of the duration of paralysis from the administration of 2 mg of decamethonium in resting limb (right) and exercising limb (left).

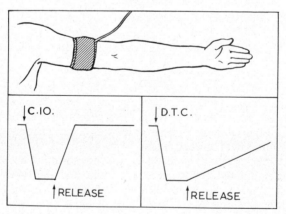

25/Fig. 19.—Diagram showing rapid recovery of decamethonium (C.10) as opposed to the slow recovery of *d*-tubocurarine after release of the cuff. An injection of a small dose of relaxant is made into the isolated limb thus ensuring that the plasma concentration in the remainder of the body is zero (Feldman and Tyrell, 1970).

stimulation of the motor nerve leads to muscle contraction, increased blood flow and improvement of neuromuscular transmission.

(b) *Non-depolarising drugs* have a high affinity for the receptor and are less susceptible to the effect of blood flow. This is well illustrated in the work of Feldman and Tyrrell (1970) (Fig. 19). Reducing the blood concentration of the non-depolarising drug to virtually zero does not appreciably affect the recovery index, and it is therefore to be anticipated that increasing the blood flow would also have little effect upon recovery from a neuromuscular block. Goat *et al.* (1976) have confirmed that in the dog an 8-fold alteration of the blood flow through a hind limb does not affect the recovery from a neuromuscular block induced by gallamine whereas it has a profound effect on the rate of onset of the block (Fig. 20*a* and *b*).

Body Temperature

(a) **Normal neuromuscular transmission.**—MacLagen and Zaimis (1957) demonstrated a depression of muscle contraction during hypothermia. In 1965, Katz and Miledi described how lowering the temperature reduced the amount of acetylcholine released at the motor nerve-ending, increased the synaptic delay time, and lessened the incidence of miniature end-plate potentials. Feldman (1973) demonstrated a reduction in the indirectly elicited twitch response in patients undergoing profound hypothermia when the muscle temperature fell to 35° C and below—this effect being partially reversed by edrophonium.

(b) **Muscle relaxants.**—The effect of hypothermia upon the action of the muscle relaxant drugs has been studied in animal preparations by Holmes *et al.* (1951) and Bigland *et al.* (1958), and in humans by Cannard and Zaimis (1959). They found that moderate hypothermia produced a mild antagonism to curare-like drugs, yet, markedly potentiated depolarising agents like decamethonium.

In contrast, Thornton *et al.* (1976) working in animals, found that cooling to temperatures below 30° C produces a more profound effect—noticeably potentiating gallamine and other curare-like drugs (Fig. 21). This effect has been confirmed by Park *et al.* (1977).

This conflict of data probably arises because there are two systems concerned with cholinergic transmission which are affected by cold—the activity of the cholinesterase enzyme and the release of acetylcholine from the nerve-ending. Moderate hypothermia, therefore, may depress the activity of the cholinesterase enzyme, thus antagonising curare-like drugs and potentiating depolarising agents. Profound cooling reduces the production of acetylcholine. This second effect becomes of overriding importance at temperatures below 32° C in humans and 30° C in dogs. At these lower temperatures non-depolarising drugs are markedly potentiated. This latter effect is likely to be of particular importance in neonates and in the elderly where body temperature can readily fall to 32° C during anaesthesia if adequate preventative measures are not taken.

Plasma Concentration

All the neuromuscular blocking drugs used are highly ionised, positively charged molecules. As a result of this property they will have little lipid solubility and will not easily diffuse across cell membranes. On theoretical grounds it would be expected that the initial rapid distribution volume of all these drugs

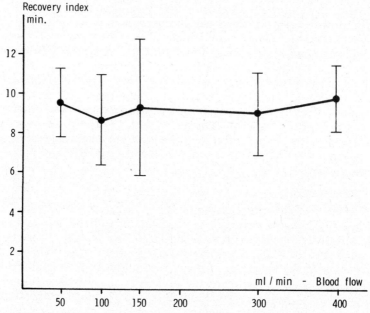

25/Fig. 20(*a*).—Alterations in blood flow on hind-limb of a dog paralysed with gallamine showing that an eight-fold increase in flow does *not* alter recovery index. (After Goat *et al.*, 1976)

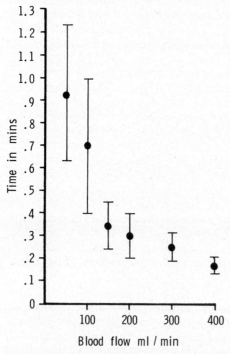

25/Fig. 20(*b*).—*Onset* of neuromuscular block by gallamine is profoundly influenced by changes in blood flow, but *no* alteration in recovery index. (After Goat *et al.*, 1976)

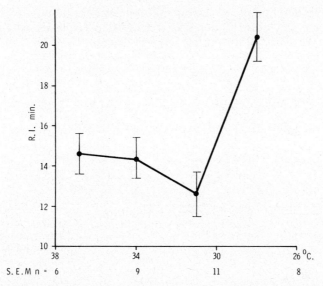

25/Fig. 21.—The effect of cold on the recovery index of gallamine in dogs demonstrating the markedly prolonged duration of action of this drug below 30° C (Thornton *et al.*, 1976).

would be restricted to the extracellular water. In a 70 kg adult the plasma volume will be about 3 litres and the total extracellular fluid (ECF) volume in the region of 15 litres. As a result it would be expected that the plasma concentration should fall rapidly to 20 per cent of the calculated value, due to rapid redistribution of the drug in the ECF. In experiments in dogs, the plasma curare and plasma gallamine levels fall rapidly to about 8–10 per cent of the calculated initial plasma values. This may be partially the result of binding of the drug to plasma protein, or on to the surface of cells, or the result of the active transfer of drug into cells of the body.

Protein binding occurs to a limited extent with most muscle relaxants. Curare binds to γ-globulin fraction of blood (Skivington, 1972), gallamine to a limited extent to albumin and pancuronium may be up to 20 per cent protein bound. Changes in plasma protein concentrations affect the peak plasma level achieved by the affected muscle relaxants and hence determine the effect produced by a given dose of drug. This relationship has been demonstrated by Stovner *et al.* (1971).

However, the quantitative effect of plasma protein must be small compared to the effect of the distribution of neuromuscular blocking drugs to the parenchymatous organs. Cohen *et al.* (1968) demonstrated that within 5 minutes of the injection of curare, gallamine and decamethonium into rats the concentration of drug in the kidneys, liver and spleen was far greater than in blood or muscle. It is likely, therefore, that alterations in the distribution of blood flow to these organs plays a major role in determining the effective peak plasma level of drug achieved following intravenous injection (Fig. 22).

As it is the peak ECF level that will determine the degree of receptor occupancy and hence the amount of neuromuscular block produced, it is evident that a consideration of the factors that influence the amount of drug reacting in these non-active distribution sites is essential to a consideration of the factors affecting the action of the muscle relaxant drugs.

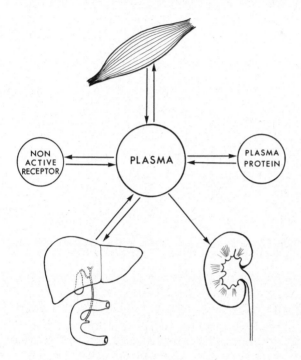

25/Fig. 22.—Diagram of the possible distribution of a relaxant drug.

Renal Excretion

All the muscle relaxants, with the exception of suxamethonium, are largely excreted unchanged in the urine. Originally, gallamine was the only relaxant believed to be excreted in entirety by the renal tract. Mushin and his colleagues (1949) recovered 30–100 per cent of the original dose from the urine of rabbits within two hours of administration.

Until recently the fate of *d*-tubocurarine was surrounded by mystery. The studies of Cohen and his colleagues (1967) have now clearly shown that the vast bulk (80 per cent of the injected dose) is excreted unchanged by the kidneys in dogs (probably only about 50 per cent is excreted in this way in humans; Miller *et al.*, 1977). A further fraction (5 per cent) passes through the biliary system to the bowels. This latter pathway plays an insignificant role when renal function is normal but it assumes great importance during renal failure because much larger proportions (up to 40 per cent) can now leave the circulation by this route (Fig. 23a and b). Gallamine does not possess this alternative pathway of excretion nor can it be metabolised. It should, therefore, not be used in the absence of renal excretion.

Clinically, a number of reports have indicated a close correlation between poor renal excretion and a prolonged response to the muscle relaxants (Fairley,

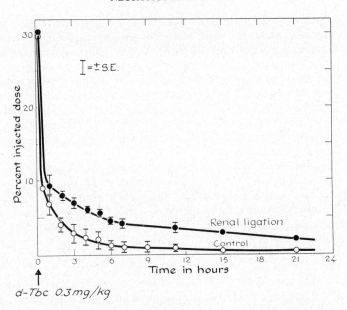

25/FIG. 23(a).—Plasma concentration of d-tubocurarine-H[3] in control dogs and in those with bilateral renal ligation. Note the raised plasma level in the presence of renal ligation.

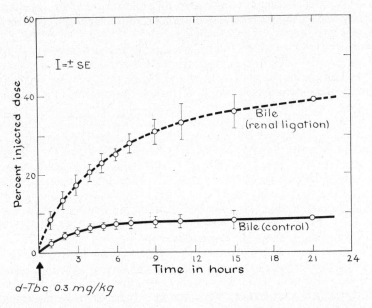

25/FIG. 23(b).—Recovery of d-tubocurarine-H[3] in the bile in control dogs and in those with bilateral renal ligation. Note the tremendous increase in biliary excretion in the presence of renal ligation.

1950; Montgomery and Bennett-Jones, 1956; Feldman and Levi, 1963). As might be expected, there are more instances involving gallamine than d-tubo-curarine. Furthermore, in a study of patients undergoing bilateral nephrectomy prior to renal transplantation, Churchill-Davidson and his associates (1967) noted the paralysis of d-tubocurarine followed a normal pattern of recovery whereas there was evidence of a very prolonged response in one patient who received gallamine. Pancuronium is usually largely excreted in the urine, but also undergoes some hepatic metabolism of the 3 and 17 acetyl radicles. The amount of non-renal excretion is variable but it is increased if the renal circulation is impaired (Agoston et al., 1973).

It is clear, therefore, that in the presence of poor renal function d-tubocurarine and pancuronium are much safer relaxant drugs than gallamine which relies entirely on the renal system for its elimination from the body. If, however, the liver and biliary system are also damaged—as is often the case in the presence of a hepato-renal syndrome—then all these relaxant drugs are best avoided or used in minimal quantities.

Antibiotics

In 1950, Molitor and Graessle studied the toxicity of streptomycin and observed that the survival rate of their animals was increased if artificial respiration was used. This evidence suggested some action of the drug at the neuromuscular junction. In 1957, Brazil and Corrado took the matter one stage further and demonstrated that streptomycin produced a neuromuscular block in both dogs and pigeons. This block was partially reversed by neostigmine but calcium chloride proved even more effective. In the following year Pittinger and Long (1958) showed that ether potentiated the neuromuscular block of neomycin and this could be antagonised by neostigmine.

It was not long before the full clinical significance of this work was appreciated. Reports were soon forthcoming of accidental deaths associated with anaesthetic and antibiotic drugs. Sabawala and Dillon (1959), using isolated muscle specimens, demonstrated that many of the antibiotic agents of the aminoglycoside group were really quite potent neuromuscular blocking drugs. Streptomycin and neomycin appeared to produce a non-depolarising block which could be potentiated by ether and d-tubocurarine and reversed by neostigmine. On the other hand kanamycin and polymyxin B appeared to be weak depolarising drugs.

Markalous (1962) analysed the clinical effect of neomycin sulphate in a group of patients and found that 1·0 g of neomycin given intraperitoneally was sufficient to reduce appreciably the minute volume. In fact, nearly one-half required artificial respiration after this dose. Nevertheless, if 1·0 g of neomycin was mixed with 20 ml of low-molecular-weight dextran sulphate this mixture did not appear to produce respiratory depression.

To summarise, from the clinical and experimental data available there is little doubt that large doses of streptomycin, kanamycin, dihydrostreptomycin, neomycin, polymyxin B, colomycin and viomycin all have significant neuromuscular blocking properties. Their action is believed to be the result of depressing acetylcholine release from the motor nerve-endings. It is quite possible that large doses of these drugs alone in children or the seriously ill patient may limit respiratory activity: in the presence of anaesthetic agents their activity becomes doubly important.

Experiments in animals suggest that in many instances neostigmine will partially antagonise this block. However, calcium chloride in small doses (200–500 mg; 5–12 mmol) appears to be the drug of choice for antagonising not only the neuromuscular blockade but also the hypotension caused by streptomycin in animals (Pandey *et al.*, 1964). The recent introduction of 4-amino pyridine, an agent that promotes calcium transport across cell membranes, appears to be the most promising specific reversal agent (Lee *et al.*, 1977).

Carbon Dioxide and the pH of Blood

The results of studies of the effect of metabolic acidosis on the degree and recovery of a non-depolarising neuromuscular block have been at variance. This may be a reflection on the method employed, the animal chosen for study, or the degree of metabolic acidosis produced.

The most pronounced effect of pH change within the clinical range is upon the action of *d*-tubocurare. There is universal agreement that respiratory acidosis in man potentiates the activity of this drug to a clinically meaningful extent and most workers accept that a similar pH change produced by a combination of metabolic and respiratory acidosis also has a similar effect. pH affects the action of suxamethonium in an opposite manner, potentiation occurring in alkalaemia and antagonism during acidaemia; however, the effect is less marked than with curare. The effect of acid-base changes upon the action of the other relaxants including dimethyl curare, alcuronium, pancuronium and decamethonium appear to be negligible. Gallamine is mildly antagonised by acidaemia and potentiated by alkalaemia and suxamethonium activity is antagonised by acidaemia.

In clinical practice the only drug whose activity is sufficiently affected by pH changes in a clinical range to produce a noticeable effect is *d*-tubocurare and the reason for this remains uncertain. Utting (1963) found that the plasma level of *d*-tubocurare varied with the pH of the blood during acidaemia, and this was confirmed in man by Baraka (1964). This could be ascribed to a reduction in plasma protein binding at a lower pH. The change in binding, however, is small and may not account for the increased blockade observed. A more likely theory is that the change in pH can alter the binding of *d*-tubocurarine to the end-plate receptor (Maclagan, 1976). An alternative theory suggested by Feldman (1973) was based upon the new structure of *d*-tubocurarine proposed by Everett *et al.* (1970). This new formula suggests that at a high pH *d*-tubocurarine is likely to be a *mono*-quaternary *mono*-tertiary compound. With this proposed structure of *d*-tubocurarine, the more acidic the media the greater will become the charge density on the second nitrogen atom and hence it will become more quaternised. As it approaches a *bis*-quaternary form it is likely to become more potent as a myoneural blocking agent. This would help to explain the unique potentiating effect of acidaemia upon the myoneural block produced by *d*-tubocarare.

Potentiation by Volatile Anaesthetics and Other Drugs

Many drugs affect the amount or duration of neuromuscular block produced by muscle relaxant drugs. Volatile anaesthetics lessen the dose requirement in clinical practice and also prolong the duration of effect of the drug. Some of this effect is due to central depression of evoked motor nerve activity causing less acetylcholine to be released at the nerve-endings but there is also some direct potentiation. Diethyl ether has been demonstrated to have a curare-like effect on the post-synaptic junction (Karis *et al.*, 1966). Halothane was found to have weak neuromuscular blocking properties (Karis *et al.*, 1967), which has been attributed to its effect on the muscle membrane raising the threshold at which an end-plate potential is propagated. A possible pre-synaptic effect of halothane causing a reduced release of acetylcholine has been described (Kennedy and Galindo, 1975). Enflurane and isoflurane have curare-like effects affecting the release of acetylcholine (Kennedy and Galindo, 1975) and depressing propagation of the end-plate potential (Waud and Waud, 1975).

In spite of this evidence of the activity of these volatile anaesthetics at the neuromuscular junction it is difficult to produce convincing experimental evidence of the effect of halothane in clinical concentration on the twitch response (Hughes, 1970). Higher concentrations of halothane will potentiate curare but as Hughes points out, in these high concentrations halothane also affects cardiac output and regional blood flow and the observed neuromuscular effect may be secondary to other changes.

From experimental work in dogs and controlled observations in man it would appear that halothane does produce some potentiation of both amount of neuromuscular block and the recovery index following the administration of pancuronium. The effect, although clinically significant, is not as great as the potentiation observed during clinical anaesthesia when mechanisms other than those at the neuromuscular junction may be involved. Nitrous oxide had no effect on neuromuscular blockage by non-depolarising relaxants, whereas a thiopentone infusion increased the neuromuscular blockade produced by curare and gallamine in cats (Hughes, 1970). Local anaesthetic agents may affect either the pre-synaptic site depressing the release of acetylcholine (Miller *et al.*, 1967), or reduce the amplitude of the end-plate response to transmitter substance by interfering with sodium conductance across the cell membrane. Wisliki and Rosenblum (1967) suggest that beta blockers may also potentiate the non-depolarising relaxant drugs by reducing acetylcholine release. Other drugs that have been demonstrated to affect the action of the non-depolarising agents administered in high concentrations include quinidine, frusemide, hexamethonium, trimetaphan, imuran (Azathioprine) and hydrocortisone.

Age

For some years past the response of the newborn infant to the relaxant drugs has always been regarded as different from that of the average adult patient. Jackson Rees (1959) went so far as to suggest that the neonate responded to the muscle relaxants like a patient with myasthenia gravis. Support for this suggestion arose from the observation that suxamethonium did not produce fasciculations in the newborn. Furthermore, neonates appeared to be "resistant" to the depolarising drug and "sensitive" to the non-depolarisers, as in myasthenia (see p. 928).

In a clinical study, Bush and Stead (1962) observed the dose of *d*-tubocurarine required to produce "adequate control of ventilation and satisfactory operating conditions" in a large series of newborn infants undergoing surgery. They concluded that only during the first ten days of life did the neonate show some "sensitivity" to *d*-tubocurarine.

Neuromuscular Transmission in the Newborn

Using an electromyographic technique, Churchill-Davidson and Wise (1963; 1964) reported that neuromuscular transmission in the newborn appeared comparable with that in the adult except for the presence of post-tetanic exhaustion (see p. 816). This is not observed in normal adults but is sometimes seen in patients with myasthenia gravis. In the newborn it occurred primarily in premature infants and during the first two weeks of life.

Using a dose based on body weight, these workers found that neonates were resistant to the depolarising drugs but they did not observe any clear-cut sensitivity to the non-depolarising drugs. Furthermore they found that neuro-muscular block produced by the depolarising drugs had some of the typical features of a Phase II block in that both fade and facilitation were observed and neuromuscular transmission was improved by an anti-cholinesterase drug (Fig. 24).

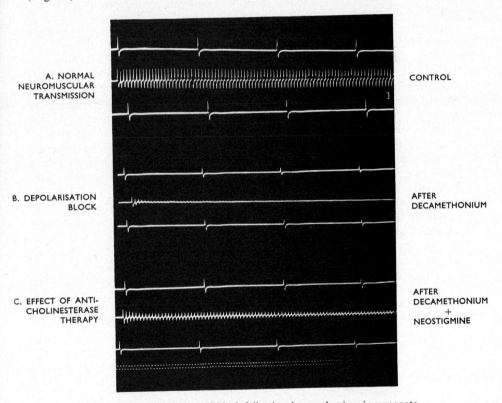

25/Fig. 24.—Signs of Phase II block following decamethonium in a neonate.

Walts and Dillon (1969) carried out a similar study with one important difference. Instead of selecting their dose on a body-weight basis, they used one determined by body surface area. Their results were significantly different. Neither neonates nor adults showed much difference in the degree or duration of action of suxamethonium, but neonates proved 2 to 3 times more sensitive to *d*-tubocurarine than adults. They pointed out, however, that had they based their selected dose on body weight rather than body surface area, the results would then have been very different. Surface area, unlike body weight, bears a close correlation with extracellular fluid volume which is the principal initial distribution volume of all the muscle relaxant drugs.

It is safe to assume that the neonate responds to a depolarising relaxant in a similar way to the adult, or may show some "resistance" if very young, but will show "sensitivity" to (i.e. will need less of) non-depolarising drugs. A dose selected by body surface area requirements is more accurate than that based on body weight.

Clinical Significance

The neonatal neuromuscular transmission possesses many features which differentiate it from that seen in the adult. Clinically, fasciculations are rarely seen with depolarising drugs. Furthermore, though these infants have a plasma cholinesterase level on the low side of normal, they require relatively large amounts of these drugs to produce paresis.

Electromyographic studies have revealed that the premature infant and the neonate respond to a depolarising drug by the easy production of a Phase II block. Under clinical conditions in operations lasting only a short time (i.e. about 1 hour), the slightly prolonged recovery time from a Phase II block as opposed to a purely depolarisation block is rarely noticed. However, if large doses are given over a long period the possibility of a delayed recovery time increases. The younger the infant, the earlier this change is likely to be observed.

With the reservations mentioned above, the non-depolarising drugs appear to act normally in the neonate. Provided an excessive dose is not used, an anti-cholinesterase drug will reverse the neuromuscular block.

Adequate dilution of the neuromuscular blocking drug is the single most important factor in the administration of relaxant drugs to the newborn. A body weight basis is often chosen for comparison, but it must be remembered that the muscle mass of an infant represents a much smaller proportion of the total body weight than in an adult. Muscle mass is about 20 per cent of body weight at birth, increasing to 33 per cent in early adolescence (Long and Bachman, 1967). The dilution chosen must be related to the fluid requirements of the patient; in clinical practice a dilution of 100 µg (0·1 mg)/ml is often found satisfactory. Although on occasions it may be necessary to use a slightly stronger solution for the initial dose, subsequent doses should always be in a very dilute concentration.

It is evident that the premature baby and the neonate have a much reduced margin of safety of neuromuscular conduction and this may easily be further reduced by hypothermia.

Nightingale and his associates (1966) studied the effects of a suxamethonium infusion on neuromuscular activity at differing age levels in infants and young children. They found that the younger the child the more suxamethonium (on a mg/kg basis) was required to achieve a comparable degree of paresis. As children grew older so this "resistance" to the paralysing action of suxamethonium became less.

Anti-cholinesterase drugs can also be used safely in this class of patients provided the same principles are applied as in adults (see p. 913). The actual injection using the intravenous route must always be given *very slowly* over a period of ten minutes. The ratio of neostigmine methyl sulphate to atropine sulphate is the same as that used for adults, namely—2·5 mg neostigmine + 1·0 mg atropine. This solution is then diluted ten or twenty times before it is used for administration. The total dose used may be calculated on a body weight basis. However, the most satisfactory method for selecting the correct dose of anti-cholinesterase in both infants and children is with the aid of a peripheral nerve stimulator. In the presence of a non-depolarising type of block there will be signs of both fade and post-tetanic facilitation: as the anti-cholinesterase drug is given these signs will disappear and neuromuscular transmission will improve. When there is no further improvement in transmission the administration of the anti-cholinesterase drug is suspended.

REFERENCES

ABRAMS, M. W., and GINSBERG, H. (1960). Prolonged apnoea following the use of suxamethonium. *Anaesthesia*, **15**, 265.

AGOSTON, S., KERSTEN, U. W., and MEIJER, D. K. (1973). The fate of pancuronium bromide in the cat. *Acta anaesth. scand.*, **17**, 129.

ALI, H. H., WILSON, R. S., SAVARESE, J. J., and KITZ, R. J. (1975). The effect of tubocurarine on indirectly elicited train-of-four muscle response and respiratory measurements in humans. *Brit. J. Anaesth.*, **47**, 570.

BARAKA, A. (1964). The influence of carbon dioxide on the neuromuscular block caused by tubocurarine chloride in the human subject. *Brit. J. Anaesth.*, **36**, 272.

BIGLAND, B., GOETZEE, B., MACLAGAN, J., and ZAIMIS, E. (1958). The effect of lowered muscle temperature on the action of neuromuscular blocking drugs. *J. Physiol. (Lond.)*, **141**, 425.

BRAZIL, O. V., and CORRADO, A. P. (1957). Curariform action of streptomycin. *J. Pharmacol. exp. Ther.*, **120**, 452.

BROWN, G. L., and DIAS, M. V. (1947). A acão do fosfato sobre a transmissão neuro-muscular na rã. *Ann. Acad. bras.*, **19**, 359.

BROWN, G. L., PATON, W. D. M., and DIAS, M. V. (1949). The depression of the demarcation potential of cat's tibialis by bistrimethylammonium decane diiodide (C.10). *J. Physiol. (Lond.)*, **109**, 15P.

BUSH, G. H., and STEAD, A. L. (1962). The use of *d*-tubocurarine in neonatal anaesthesia. *Brit. J. Anaesth.*, **34**, 721.

CANNARD, T. H., and ZAIMIS, E. J. (1959). The effect of lowered muscle temperature on the action of neuromuscular blocking drugs in man. *J. Physiol. (Lond.)*, **149**, 112.

CHURCHILL-DAVIDSON, H. C., and CHRISTIE, T. H. (1959). The diagnosis of neuromuscular block in man. *Brit. J. Anaesth.*, **31**, 290.

CHURCHILL-DAVIDSON, H. C., CHRISTIE, T. H., and WISE, R. P. (1960). Dual neuromuscular block in man. *Anesthesiology*, **21**, 144.

CHURCHILL-DAVIDSON, H. C., and RICHARDSON, A. T. (1952). Decamethonium iodide (C.10): Some observations on its action using electromyography. *Proc. roy. Soc. Med.*, **45**, 179.

CHURCHILL-DAVIDSON, H. C., WAY, W. L., and DE JONG, R. H. (1967). The muscle relaxants and renal excretion. *Anesthesiology*, **28**, 540.

CHURCHILL-DAVIDSON, H. C., and WISE, R. P. (1963). Neuromuscular transmission in the newborn infant. *Anesthesiology*, **24**, 271.

CHURCHILL-DAVIDSON, H. C., and WISE, R. P. (1964). The response of the newborn infant to muscle relaxants. *Canad. Anaesth. Soc. J.*, **11**, 1.

COHEN, E. N., BREWER, H. W., and SMITH, D. (1967). The metabolism and elimination of d-tubocurarine-H^3. *Anesthesiology*, **28**, 309.

COHEN, E. N., HOOD, N., and GOLLING, R. (1968). Use of whole-body autoradiography for the determination of uptake and distribution of labelled muscle relaxants in the rat. *Anesthesiology*, **29**, 987.

CRUL, J. F., LONG, G. J., BRUNNER, E. A., and COOLEN, J. M. W. (1966). The changing pattern of neuromuscular blockade caused by succinylcholine in man. *Anesthesiology*, **27**, 729.

DAM, W. H., and GULDMAN, N. (1961). Inadequate postanaesthetic ventilation. Curare, anaesthetic, narcotic, diffusion hypoxia. *Anesthesiology*, **22**, 699.

DE JONG, R. H., and FREUND, F. G. (1967). Characteristics of the neuromuscular block with succinylcholine and decamethonium in man. *Anesthesiology*, **28**, 583.

DEL CASTILLO, J. C., and KATZ, B. (1956). Interaction of end plate receptors between different choline derivatives. *Proc. roy. Soc. B.*, **146**, 369.

EVERETT, A. J., LOWE, L. A., and WILKINSON, S. (1970). Revision of the structure of (+)— tubocurarine chloride and (+) chondrocurarine. *Chem. Communications*, p. 1020.

FAIRLEY, H. B. (1950). Prolonged intercostal paralysis due to a relaxant. *Brit. med. J.*, **2**, 986.

FELDMAN, S. A. (1973). *Muscle Relaxants*, p. 37. London: W.B. Saunders Co.

FELDMAN, S. A. (1974). *Measurement of Neuromuscular Block in Measurement in Anaesthesia* (Boerhaave Series). Ed., Feldman, Leigh and Spierdijk. Leiden: Univ. of Leiden Press.

FELDMAN, S. A., and LEVI, J. A. (1963). Prolonged paresis following gallamine. *Brit. J. Anaesth.*, **35**, 804.

FELDMAN, S. A., and TYRRELL, M. F. (1970). A new theory of determination of action of the muscle relaxants. *Proc. roy. Soc. Med.*, **63**, 692.

GALINDO, A. (1971). Depolarising neuromuscular block. *J. Pharmacol. exp. Ther.*, **178**, 339.

GALINDO, A. (1972). The role of prejunctional effects in myoneural transmission. *Anesthesiology*, **36**, 598.

GALINDO, A., and KENNEDY, R. (1974). Further observations on depolarising neuromuscular block; the so-called Phase II block. *Brit. J. Anaesth.*, **46**, 405.

GISSEN, A. J., KATZ, R. L., KARIS, J. H., and PAPPER, E. M. (1966). Neuromuscular block in man during prolonged arterial infusion with succinylcholine. *Anesthesiology*, **27**, 242.

GOAT, V. A., YEUNG, M. L., BLAKENEY, C., and FELDMAN, S. A. (1976). Effect of blood flow upon the activity of gallamine triethiodide. *Brit. J. Anaesth.*, **48**, 69.

HARPER, J. K. (1952). Prolonged respiratory paralysis after succinylcholine (correspondence). *Brit. med. J.*, **1**, 866.

HARRISON, G. A. (1972). The cardiovascular effects and some relaxant properties of four relaxants in patients about to undergo cardiac surgery. *Brit. J. Anaesth.*, **44**, 485.

HARVEY, A. M. (1939). Action of procaine on neuromuscular transmission. *Bull. Johns Hopk. Hosp.*, **65**, 223.

HARVEY, A. M., and MACINTOSH, R. C. (1940). Calcium and synaptic transmission in a sympathetic ganglion. *J. Physiol. (Lond.)*, **97**, 408.

HOLMES, P. E. B., JENDEN, D. J., and TAYLOR, D. B. (1951). The analysis of action of curare on neuromuscular transmission: the effect of temperature changes. *J. Pharmacol. exp. Ther.*, **103**, 382.

HUBBARD, J. I., and WILSON, D. F. (1973). Neuromuscular transmission in a mammalian preparation in the absence of blocking drugs and the effect of d-tubocurarine. *J. Physiol. (Lond.)*, **228**, 307.

HUGHES, R. (1970). Effects of anaesthetics and their interactions with neuromuscular blocking agents in cats. *Brit. J. Anaesth.*, **42**, 826.

JENDEN, D. J., KAMIJO, K., TAYLOR, D. B. (1951). The action of decamethonium (C.10) on the isolated rabbit lumbrical muscle. *J. Pharmacol. exp. Ther.*, **103**, 348.

JENERICK, H. P., and GERARD, R. W. (1953). Membrane potential and threshold of single fibre *J. cell. comp. Physiol.*, **42**, 79.

KARIS, J. H., GISSEN, A. J., NASTUK, W. L. (1966). Mode of action of diethyl ether in blocking neuromuscular transmission. *Anesthesiology*, **27**, 42.

KARIS, J. H., GISSEN, A. J., and NASTUK, W. L. (1967). The effect of volatile anesthetic agents on neuromuscular transmission. *Anesthesiology*, **28**, 128.

KATZ, B., and MILEDI, R. (1965). The effect of temperature on the synaptic delay at the neuromuscular junction. *J. Physiol. (Lond.)*, **181**, 656.

KATZ, B., and THESLEFF, H. S. (1957). A study of desensitisation produced by acetylcholine at the motor end plate. *J. Physiol. (Lond.)*, **138**, 63.

KENNEDY, R. D., and GALINDO, A. D. (1975). Comparative site of action of various anaesthetic agents at the mammalian myoneural junction. *Brit. J. Anaesth.*, **47**, 533.

LEE, C., DESILVA, A. J. C., and KATZ, R. L. (1977). Reversal of Polymyxin B induced neuromuscular and cardiovascular depression by 4-aminopyridine. *Abstr. of Scientific Papers, ASA meeting*, New Orleans, p. 465.

LONG, G., and BACHMAN, L. (1967). Neuromuscular blockade by *d*-tubocurarine in children. *Anesthesiology*, **28**, 723.

MACINTOSH, F. C., BIRKS, R. I., and SASTRY, P. B. (1958). Mode of action of an inhibitor of acetylcholine synthesis. *Neurology (Minneap.)*, **8**, Suppl. I, 90.

MACLAGEN, J. (1976). Competitive neuromuscular blocking drugs. In: *Neuromuscular Junction*, p. 421. Ed. by E. Zaimis. Berlin: Springer Verlag.

MACLAGEN, J., and ZAIMIS, E. (1957). The effect of muscle temperature on twitch and tetanus in the cat. *J. Physiol. (Lond.)*, **137**, 89.

MARKALOUS, P. (1962). Respiration and the intraperitoneal application of neomycin and meolymphin. *Anaesthesia*, **17**, 427.

MILLER, R. D., MATTEO, R. S., BENET, L. Z., and SOHN, Y. J. (1977). The pharmacokinetics of *d*-tubocurarine in man with and without renal failure. *J. Pharmacol. exp. Ther.*, **202**, 1.

MILLER, R. D., WAY, W. L., and KATZUNG, B. G. (1967). The potentiation of neuromuscular blocking agents by quinidine. *Anesthesiology*, **28**, 1036.

MOLITOR, H., and GRAESSLE, O. E. (1950). Pharmacology and toxicology of antibiotics. *Pharmacol. Rev.*, **2**, 1.

MONTGOMERY, J. B., and BENNETT-JONES, N. (1956). Gallamine triethiodide and renal disease. *Lancet*, **2**, 1243.

MUSHIN, W. W., WIEN, R., MASON, D. F. J., and LANGSTON, G. T. (1949). Curare-like actions of tri(diethylaminoethoxy)benzene triethiodide. *Lancet*, **1**, 726.

NIGHTINGALE, D. A., GLASS, A. G., and BACHMAN, L. (1966). Neuromuscular blockade by succinylcholine in children. *Anesthesiology*, **27**, 736.

PANDEY, K., KUMAR, S., and BADALA, R. P. (1964). Neuromuscular blocking and hypotensive actions of streptomycin and their reversal. *Brit. J. Anaesth.*, **36**, 19.

PARK, W. Y., KIM, Y. D., and MACNAMARA, T. E. (1977). Neuromuscular block of gallamine in hypothermia. *Abstr. of Scientific Papers, ASA meeting*, New Orleans, p. 311.

PATON, W. D. M. (1956). *Proceedings of the Conference on the Myoneural Junction.* (Sponsored by Columbia University Division of Anesthesiology and Burroughs Wellcome & Co., U.S.A.) November 4th and 5th, 1955. New York City, N.Y.

PATON, W. D. M. (1961). A theory of drug action based on the rate of drug-receptor combination. *Proc. roy. Soc. B*, **54**, 21.

PATON, W. D. M., and ZAIMIS, E. J. (1952). Methonium compounds. *Pharmacol. Rev.*, **4**, 219.

PITTINGER, C. B., and LONG, J. P. (1958). Neuromuscular blocking action of neomycin sulfate. *Antibiot. & Chemother.*, **8**, 198.

REES, G. J. (1959). In: *General Anaesthesia*, Vol. 2. Eds. F. T. Evans and T. C. Gray. London: Butterworth & Co.

RIKER, W. F. J., and OKAMATO, M. (1969). Pharmacology of nerve terminals. *Ann. Rev. Pharmacol.*, **9**, 173.

SABAWALA, P. B., and DILLON, J. B. (1959). The action of some antibiotics on the human intercostal nerve-muscle complex. *Anesthesiology*, **20**, 659.

SKIVINGTON, M. A. (1972). Protein binding of three tritiated muscle relaxants. *Brit. J. Anaesth.*, **44**, 1030.

STOVNER, J., THEODORSEN, L., and BJELKE, E. (1971). Sensitivity to tubocurarine and alcuronium with special reference to plasma protein pattern. *Brit. J. Anaesth.*, **43**, 385.

THORNTON, R. J., BLAKENEY, C., and FELDMAN, S. A. (1976). Presented to the Anaesthetic Research Group, Summary. *Brit. J. Anaesth.*, **48**, 264.

UTTING, J. (1963). pH as a factor influencing plasma concentrations of *d*-tubocurarine. *Brit. J. Anaesth.*, **35**, 706.

VICKERS, M. D. A. (1963). The mismanagement of suxamethonium apnoea. *Brit. J. Anaesth.*, **35**, 260.

WALTS, L. F., and DILLON, J. B. (1969). The response of newborns to succinylcholine and *d*-tubocurarine. *Anesthesiology*, **31**, 35.

WALTS, L. F., LEVIN, N., and DILLON, J. B. (1970). Assessment of recovery from curare. *J. Amer. med. Ass.*, **213**, 1894.

WAUD, B. E., and WAUD, D. R. (1975). The effects of diethyl ether, enflurane and isoflurane at the neuromuscular junction. *Anesthesiology*, **42**, 275.

WISLICKI, L., and ROSENBLUM, I. (1967). Effects of propranolol on the action of neuro-muscular blocking drugs. *Brit. J. Anaesth.*, **39**, 939.

ZAIMIS, E. J. (1953). Motor end-plate differences as a determining factor in the mode of action of neuromuscular blocking substances. *J. Physiol. (Lond.)*, **122**, 238.

ZAIMIS, E. J., CHURCHILL-DAVIDSON, H. C., and RICHARDSON, A. T. (1952). Motor end-plate differences as a determining factor in the mode of action of neuromuscular blocking substances. *Nature (Lond.)*, **170**, 617.

Chapter 26

NEUROMUSCULAR BLOCKING DRUGS

MOST of the drugs that are active at the neuromuscular junction have certain chemical similarities that are believed to affect the specificity of their actions. Like the transmitter substance acetylcholine they possess a quaternary ammonium group:

$$R - \overset{\overset{\displaystyle R}{|}}{\underset{\underset{\displaystyle R}{|}}{N}} - CH_2 - C$$

in the most active compounds $R = CH_3$
in gallamine $R = C_2H_5$

Generally the longer the side-chain in the organic series the less reactive is the quaternary ammonium. This activity of acetylcholine-like drugs is termed "specific intrinsic activity". Acetylcholine consists of the ester of choline and acetic acid.

$$CH_3 - \overset{\overset{\displaystyle CH_3}{|}}{\underset{\underset{\displaystyle CH_3}{|}}{N}} - CH_2 - CH_3 - COO - CH_3$$

Acetylcholine

In 1935 King established a formula for d-turbocurarine in which he presented it as a bis-quaternary ammonium compound (see page 886). This formula has recently been challenged and it is now thought to be incorrect. Nevertheless it stimulated research into the special relationship between the two quaternary ammonium groups and the activity of the compound as a myoneural blocking agent (SAR—structure activity relationship).

In their classical study of the bis-quaternary polymethylene series Paton and Zaimis (1949) showed that the most active compound was decamethonium (C.10). The distance between the two quaternary ammonium groups was similar to that in the King formula of curare (14–15 Å; 1·4–1·5 nm). This led to the concept that this intermolecular distance was "ideal" for relaxant activity. Doubt has recently been thrown upon this concept since it has been demonstrated that curare is not a bis-quaternary compound and that pancuronium has a stereoisometric distance of 10–11 Å (1·0–1·1 nm) between its two quaternary ammonium groups whilst the new relaxant fazadinium (AH 8165) has only 7 Å (0·7 nm) between its two quaternary ammonium groups. Indeed, it has long been appreciated that the alkaloid erythrina extracted from the plant *Erythrina Americana* has only one onium group, yet it is an active neuromuscular blocking compound (Folkers and Major, 1937).

It is convenient to divide the muscle relaxants into two groups, the depolarising and non-depolarising relaxants, although it is appreciated these terms may not explain all activities of these drugs at the neuromuscular junction. Generally, depolarising relaxants have a high intrinsic specific activity and a low affinity constant with the receptor. They are usually small molecules compared with the non-depolarising relaxants and their two-dimensional structure depends upon the two terminal polar groups which repel each other, rather than upon molecular rigidity.

DEPOLARISING RELAXANTS

DECAMETHONIUM IODIDE

History

In the same year Barlow and Ing (1948) and Paton and Zaimis (1948) independently described the neuromuscular blocking properties of decamethonium. The latter pair of workers were methodically examining the pharmacological properties of the polymethylene-bistrimethyl ammonium compounds and they found that one member of this series, namely decamethonium (C.10), with ten CH_2 molecules in the chain, was remarkably effective as a muscle relaxant in animals. Later Organe and his colleagues (1949) reported on the effect of this drug on conscious subjects and in clinical anaesthesia.

Physical and Chemical Properties

Decamethonium is a white crystalline powder.

$$CH_3 \diagdown \atop CH_3 \diagup \!\!\!\! - \!\! N^+ \!\! - (CH_2)_{10} - N^+ \!\! - \!\!\!\! {\diagup CH_3 \atop \diagdown CH_3}$$

Decamethylene 1:10 bistrimethylammonium

It is soluble in water, neutral in solution, and relatively stable. It is odourless and non-irritant to the tissues and blood vessels, and is not destroyed by plasma cholinesterase.

Pharmacological Actions

Mode of action.—The action of decamethonium in man is believed to be similar to that of acetylcholine in that it produces depolarisation of the end-plate region. Gissen and Nastuk (1968) found that the action of decamethonium is limited to the post-synaptic membrane of the neuromuscular junction. The neural action potential recorded at the nerve-ending was unaffected by the drug and direct stimulation of the muscle fibre in the presence of neuromuscular block still elicited a contraction. On this evidence they concluded that decamethonium causes post-synaptic membrane stimulation.

Cardiovascular system.—Decamethonium has no action on the myocardium (Prime and Gray, 1952). Given intra-arterially in minute doses it leads to muscle weakness without any severe pain. There have been no reports of venous thrombosis following intravenous decamethonium.

Central nervous system.—Within the range of doses used in clinical practice there is no evidence of any action on the spinal cord, brain or autonomic ganglia.

Heavy doses in animals have been shown to produce a weak ganglion-depressant action.

Fasciculations and muscle pains.—Decamethonium may cause widespread fasciculations of muscle in man, but these are not as marked as after suxamethonium. Soon after its intravenous injection a "tight feeling" develops in the masseter muscles of the jaw and in the posterior muscles of the calf. This is an aching type of pain which may persist for several hours.

Histamine release.—Decamethonium liberates only small quantities of histamine and has about half the activity in this respect of *d*-tubocurarine (Sniper, 1952).

Placental barrier.—Decamethonium has been demonstrated not to cross the placental barrier in the guinea-pig and rabbit (Young, 1949), but there is no evidence available for man.

Distribution

The distribution of decamethonium throughout the body following an intravenous injection has been beautifully demonstrated by the autoradiograph technique of Cohen and his collaborators (1968). They showed that decamethonium does not cross either the blood-brain barrier or the placental barrier to reach the fetus (Fig. 1). Considerable quantities, however, could be observed

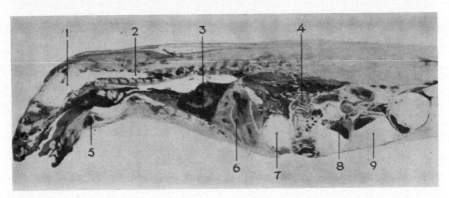

26/Fig. 1.—Autoradiograph of rat sacrificed 15 minutes after intravenous injection of 0·15 mg/kg decamethonium. 1, brain; 2, spinal cord; 3, heart; 4, intestine; 5, salivary gland; 6, liver; 7, stomach; 8, placenta; 9, fetus.

in the cardiac muscle though (as mentioned above) no cardiac action has so far been demonstrated. The concentration in the liver (although higher than in muscle or blood) was less than with all non-depolarising drugs. There is no doubt that this whole-body autoradiograph technique offers an excellent manner of comparing the distribution of the various relaxant drugs. Nevertheless, the presence of a drug at a particular receptor site does not necessarily indicate that it produces any activity in this area as there are numerous non-active receptor sites in the body.

Decamethonium, unlike the non-depolarising muscle relaxants, readily passes into the muscle around the end-plate area. However, it has not been demonstrated to exert any action once it has penetrated the muscle membrane.

Detoxication and Excretion

There is no evidence available either in animals or man that decamethonium undergoes any form of breakdown *in vivo*. The excretion rate in animals is slow and persists for many hours after a complete recovery of muscle power has been attained; 80–90 per cent of the total dose injected has been recovered unchanged in the urine over a 24-hour period (Paton and Zaimis, 1952). In man, 40 per cent has been recovered unchanged over a three-hour period following a single injection (Churchill-Davidson and Richardson, 1953). As the renal tract is the principal, and possibly the only, route of excretion, severe renal damage or hypotension could theoretically produce a prolonged action of the drug. Clinically, however, there is no evidence available to suggest that the duration of action of decamethonium is related to renal function.

Waser (1962) supports the view that some decamethonium is metabolised *in vivo* from a quaternary to a tertiary compound. However, following a single dose, it is probable that redistribution within the body and slow renal excretion, result in a lowering of the blood drug concentration, below that necessary for clinical activity.

Administration

The intravenous route is the only satisfactory method of giving decamethonium in clinical practice. Thirty to forty seconds after the initial injection the conscious patient notices a difficulty or blurring of vision followed gradually by a generalised weakness which spreads to involve the trunk and limb muscles. In the anaesthetised patient, perfect conditions for endotracheal intubation may not arise until two to three minutes have elapsed.

Dosage.—A dose of 2·25 to 2·50 mg of decamethonium will produce almost complete paralysis of the limb musculature in the average patient. A dose of 3·0 to 4·0 mg is necessary for intubation. Phase II block occurs readily following repeated doses of this drug.

Duration of action.—The time taken to return to complete recovery after 95 per cent paresis of the grip-strength is approximately 15–20 minutes in the conscious subject. The conditions of measurement, however, are not comparable to those in the anaesthetised subject, for electromyographic recordings have shown that the duration of action bears a close relationship to the muscle blood flow (see "Factors altering the duration or degree of neuromuscular block," p. 849). Decamethonium produces excellent relaxation for operations lasting up to 40 minutes. It is unsuitable for prolonged procedures, as it readily produces Phase II block.

SUXAMETHONIUM (SUCCINYLDICHOLINE; ANECTINE)

History

In 1906 Reid Hunt and Taveau first described the pharmacological action of suxamethonium, but though they studied its effect on blood pressure they failed to observe that it caused neuromuscular block, because they were using a previously curarised animal. Glick (1941) demonstrated that the hydrolysis rate was high and that it was broken down by cholinesterase in horse serum. Bovet and his colleagues (1949) in Italy, and Phillips (1949) in the United States, both independently described the neuromuscular blocking properties of suxamethonium. In the same year Bovet-Nitti showed that this substance was broken down by cholinesterases and this hydrolysis could be inhibited by eserine. In the following year Castillo and de Beer (1950) confirmed these findings in animal experiments. The drug was first used in man as a neuromuscular blocking agent by Thesleff at the Karolinska Institute in Stockholm (1951), and by Brucke and his associates (1951) and Mayrhofer and Hassfurther (1951) in Austria. Scurr (1951) and Bourne and his colleagues (1952) described its use in Great Britain, and Foldes and his associates (1952) introduced it in the United States.

Physical and Chemical Properties

Suxamethonium is a synthetic bis-quaternary ammonium compound. It is a

$$CH_3-\overset{+}{\underset{\underset{Cl^-}{CH_3}}{N}}(CH_3)-CH_2-CH_2-OOC-CH_2-CH_2-COO-CH_2-CH_2-\overset{+}{N}(CH_3)(CH_3)CH_3 \quad Cl^-$$

Suxamethonium chloride

white crystalline substance with a melting point of 150° C. It is relatively unstable and may deteriorate in solution if kept in a warm cupboard. It has shown to be unstable in alkaline solution (pH 9·3) and can lose 50 per cent of its activity in 3 hours under such conditions. Owing to its instability it was originally marketed combined with various halogens as the chloride, iodide and bromide. Some manufacturers preferred only to produce it in powder form, but later experience has shown that provided it is not kept for too long in a warm atmosphere the chloride solution is satisfactory for clinical use.

Pharmacological Actions

Mode of action.—Suxamethonium is believed to act like acetylcholine in man and to bring about a depolarisation type of neuromuscular block. If repeated doses are used the block gradually undergoes a change from one of depolarisation to one showing many of the signs of non-depolarisation (see Phase II Block p. 843).

Cardiovascular system.—The ability of suxamethonium to produce bradycardia was described by Leigh and his colleagues (1957). In view of the chemical similarity between suxamethonium and acetylcholine, it is hardly surprising that the drug exerts an acetylcholine-like action. In the isolated perfused heart the action of suxamethonium cannot be distinguished from acetylcholine (Goat and Feldman, 1972b). The action is dose-related and is blocked by atropine. The finding that severe bradycardia and asystole occurred most frequently after the second injection of suxamethonium (Bullough, 1959; Martin, 1958; Lupprian and Churchill-Davidson, 1960) is more difficult to explain. It would appear that a critical period of 5 minutes following the first dose of suxamethonium renders the heart most sensitive to the effect of the second injection (Mathias and Evans Prossar, 1970) (Fig. 2). It is possible that the first dose sensitises the cardiac vagal receptors to the effect of the second dose.

Suxamethonium and potassium-induced cardiac dysrhythmias.—Berlin and

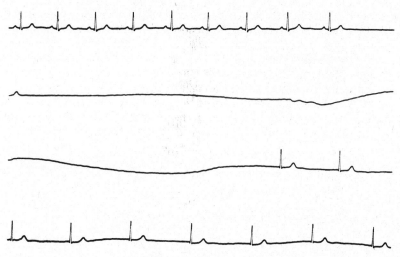

26/Fig. 2.—Example of the bradycardia seen on the administration of a second dose of suxamethonium.

Karlin (1966) noted cardiac dysrhythmias in patients receiving suxamethonium for dressings of burns some weeks after their injury. Birch *et al.* (1969) suggested that this was due to a shift in potassium ions in these patients consequent upon the depolarisation (Fig. 3). Since that time the dangers of potassium leaking out of damaged and denervated muscle cells has been appreciated as a cause of dangerous and potentially fatal ventricular dysrhythmias.

Denervation of muscle has been demonstrated to cause a loss of specificity of the end plate to acetylcholine and suxamethonium; as a result the whole muscle membrane becomes permeable and the resulting potassium shift becomes dangerous. The effect is also found in some forms of upper motor neurone disease due to the loss of the ill-understood trophic effect upon the muscle. In an excellent review of this subject Gronert and Theye (1975) have drawn attention to the increase in oxygen consumption and potassium flux that occurs after denervation, upper motor neurone lesions and following thermal and traumatic injuries to muscle (Fig. 4). These changes do not occur following simple immobilisation of the muscle.

In view of these findings and the case reports of cardiac arrest following suxamethonium, the drug should be avoided after major muscle injury, denervation of muscle (lower motor neurone lesions, motor nerve disease and spinal injury). It should be used cautiously, if at all, in patients with widespread muscular disturbance, following upper motor neurone and central nervous system disease. This risk appears to be maximal at 10 days to 3 weeks following denervation, but is still present up to 6 months after injury.

The danger of suxamethonium administration in renal disease has probably been exaggerated. It is probable that in the absence of renal neuropathy and with a normal potassium distribution, the risks are minimal (Miller *et al.*, 1972).

d-Tubocurarine in small doses (5–6 mg) and gallamine (8–10 mg) given 60 seconds before the suxamethonium will modify but not prevent the release of

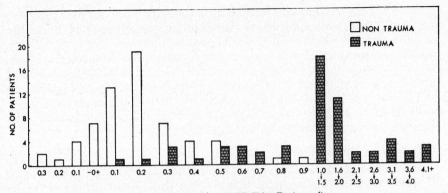

26/Fig. 3.—The changes in serum potassium in two groups of patients (normal and traumatised) receiving suxamethonium.

potassium. The prior use of a small dose of non-depolarising relaxant does however increase the dose requirements of suxamethonium from 1 mg/kg to 1·5 mg/kg (Miller and Way, 1971).

Central nervous system.—There is very little evidence either in animals or in man to suggest that suxamethonium has any direct action on the spinal cord or brain. Like both decamethonium and *d*-tubocurarine, suxamethonium has been

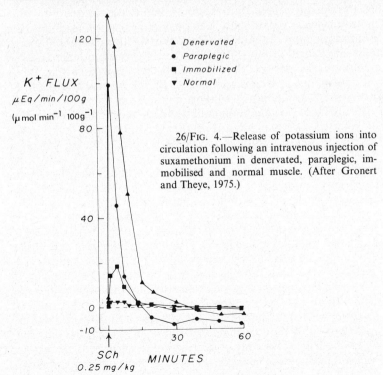

26/Fig. 4.—Release of potassium ions into circulation following an intravenous injection of suxamethonium in denervated, paraplegic, immobilised and normal muscle. (After Gronert and Theye, 1975.)

found to depress the spontaneous activity of the respiratory centre in cats (Ellis *et al.*, 1952). Suxamethonium has an initial stimulating action on the autonomic ganglion, but large doses will finally depress conductivity and bring about a block in transmission. However, the doses required are enormous and are some 700 times greater than that needed to produce paralysis of skeletal muscle. This compares favourably with *d*-tubocurarine in similar circumstances where only double the muscle-paralysing dose is required to block autonomic activity. Nevertheless, the effect of these drugs on autonomic activity in patients with autonomic irritability has yet to be fully determined.

Route of Administration

Walts and Dillon (1967) compared the intravenous and intramuscular route of administration of suxamethonium on the duration of paralysis. Using comparable doses they found the paresis lasted approximately twice as long when the intramuscular route was used. The intramuscular route is sometimes used in infants because of the simplicity of administration but it allows less immediate control over the paralysis. Also, it must be remembered that the formation of a Phase II block is both dose- and time-dependent, so that for a given dose of suxamethonium this change is more likely to be observed when the intramuscular, as opposed to the intravenous, route is used.

Fasciculations and muscle pains.—Suxamethonium causes marked fasciculations of the muscles. These contractions frequently lead to muscle pains which are usually noticed by the patient on the day after the operation—particularly when the operative procedure is minor, and therefore does not keep the patient in bed or produce pain itself. The precise mechanism leading to the production of muscle pain is obscure, but Rack and Westbury (1966) observed a high incidence of changes in the muscle spindles of cats when large doses of suxamethonium were used. It is possible, therefore, that these pains may be due to mechanical damage to these muscle spindles. Muscle fasciculations can be severe and may cause clinically obvious myoglobinuria due to excessive muscle destruction. The ability of suxamethonium to stimulate the motor nerve-ending has been demonstrated. This may produce antidromic firing either in the motor nerve or in the muscle spindle leading to and possibly causing muscle pains (see also Chapter 24, p. 817).

In ambulant patients the incidence of these pains is about 60–70 per cent, whereas if the patient is confined to bed after the injection the incidence drops to 10 to 14 per cent or less (Churchill-Davidson, 1954; Morris and Dunn, 1957; Foster, 1960; Lamoreaux and Urbach, 1960). These muscle pains are only rarely observed in young children and the aged. Bush and Roth (1961) have pointed out that in children aged 5–14 years the incidence is only 10 per cent, whereas it falls to 3 per cent if the age group of 5–9 years is studied.

Various methods have been tried to eliminate or modify the incidence of these pains. The only satisfactory methods are to administer a small dose of a non-depolarising drug (i.e. 3–5 mg *d*-tubocurarine or 10 mg gallamine) at least sixty seconds before the suxamethonium is given. As the two types of block are antagonistic, however, this reduces the effectiveness of the suxamethonium. An alternative method is to give 8 mg of suxamethonium followed, 60 seconds later, by the full paralysing dose (Baraka, 1977), but the results are unknown.

Action on the eye.—The action of suxamethonium on the extra- and intra-ocular muscles is both interesting and complex. The matter has assumed some importance because the anaesthetist frequently uses this drug in anaesthesia for ophthalmic surgery.

Early reports suggested that the rise in intra-ocular tension brought about by suxamethonium is capable of expelling vitreous from the inner chamber of the open eye (Dillon *et al.*, 1957; Lincoff *et al.*, 1957). Katz and Eakins (1969) reviewed all the evidence and in the light of their own work concluded that suxamethonium was capable of increasing intra-ocular tension not only by a contraction of the extra-orbital musculature but also by contracting the intra-orbital smooth muscle. They also pointed out that if suxamethonium produced a rise in systemic pressure then this also would tend to increase intra-ocular tension.

Hess and Pilar (1963) drew attention to two distinct systems of neuromuscular transmission that can be found in the extra-ocular muscles. First, there is the *twitch* system characterised by muscle fibres with small, well-defined fibrils and supplied by the large efferent nerve fibres. These respond with action potentials similar to those found at other mammalian neuromuscular junctions. Secondly, there is the *tonic* system characterised by muscle fibres with poorly defined fibrils and supplied by small efferent nerve fibres. Stimulation of this system leads to a slow summating contraction—a contracture—as occurs in amphibian and avian muscle.

Katz and Eakins (1969) concluded that the varied response to suxamethonium could be explained on the basis of this double neuromuscular system. They postulated that suxamethonium (like other depolarising drugs) stimulates the tonic system, thereby increasing intra-ocular tension. At the same time it depresses the twitch system, though this plays no part in the overall result. *d*-Tubocurarine, on the other hand, depresses both systems and blocks the stimulating effect of suxamethonium not only on the tonic system of the extra-ocular muscles but also on intra-ocular smooth muscle.

Comment.—It is now fully recognised that suxamethonium can produce a rise in intra-ocular pressure. This might prove harmful in cases of penetrating injury to the eye, in glaucoma (where there is already increased tension) or in cases of detached retina (where a further rise in pressure might increase the damage) or by expelling vitreous humour during open eye surgery. In such instances the use of suxamethonium alone is obviously contra-indicated. The alternative is to use a non-depolarising drug which does not raise intra-ocular pressure, or a small dose of *d*-tubocurarine (3 mg) or gallamine (10 mg) given 1–2 minutes before the suxamethonium will block this effect of suxamethonium on the orbital musculature (Miller *et al.*, 1968). The increase in intra-ocular pressure is of 3–10 minutes duration.

Alimentary system.—In animals no deleterious effect on the contraction of the intestine has been noted, even with large doses. If massive quantities are given which are a long way outside the therapeutic range in man there is some evidence that irregular contractions and a decreased sensitivity to acetylcholine may be produced (Thesleff, 1952). It should be remembered that plasma cholinesterase is formed in the liver, and this enzyme is responsible for the breakdown of suxamethonium. In the event of severe liver damage, cachexia, or malnutrition, therefore, an increased duration of action of suxamethonium should be anticipated.

Histamine release.—The release of histamine by suxamethonium is believed to be about one hundredth of the activity of *d*-tubocurarine (Bourne *et al.*, 1952; Davies, 1956). However, Laurie Smith (1957) has drawn attention to the fact that patients can be found in whom the intradermal injection of small doses of suxamethonium (10 mg) produces a weal and flare of almost identical proportion with that of a small dose of *d*-tubocurarine (2 mg). Certainly cases of possible bronchospasm have been reported (Fellini *et al.*, 1963), and Jerum and his colleagues (1967) described a case of anaphylaxis with the onset of tachycardia, hypotension, bronchospasm, and pharyngeal and facial oedema in a 26-year-old woman.

Placental transmission.—A method for the study of small concentrations of suxamethonium in serum has been described (Kvisselgaard and Moya, 1961). This technique has been used to study the possible transmission of suxamethonium across the placental barrier in women. It has been established that the placental tissue itself (in homogenous suspension) does not significantly contribute to the hydrolysis of suxamethonium (Moya and Margolies, 1961).

Drabkova *et al.* (1973) using radioactive tagged suxamethonium demonstrated that provided the concentration of drug in the uterine artery was sufficient, it would pass readily through the placental barrier to fetal monkeys, and also if injected into the fetal animal, suxamethonium would pass back to the mother. These workers demonstrated that the placenta at term is not an anatomical barrier even to quaternary ions. The lack of effect on the fetus during human Caesarean section and parturition is mainly due to the low concentration of drug in the uterine artery.

Distribution

The distribution of suxamethonium is well illustrated in Fig. 5 which is based on whole body autoradiography in a monkey fetus.

Detoxication and Excretion

Suxamethonium has held a leading role in clinical anaesthesia principally because of its very short duration of action. Thus, following an intravenous dose it is believed that nearly all the suxamethonium in the plasma has been hydrolysed within one minute of the injection (Pantuck, 1967). This is brought about by rapid enzymatic hydrolysis with (plasma) cholinesterase. However, redistribution, alkaline hydrolysis and renal excretion may play an important role if enzymatic hydrolysis is impaired.

(*a*) **Enzymatic hydrolysis.**—Plasma cholinesterase is a glycoprotein that is synthesised in the liver and abounds in the plasma. The purpose of its presence in man (other than to destroy suxamethonium) is not yet clear. It must be readily distinguished from another enzyme, true (specific) cholinesterase, which is present in red blood cells and at the neuromuscular junction. This latter enzyme is responsible for the rapid hydrolysis of acetylcholine at the nerve-ending.

The breakdown of suxamethonium takes place in two stages—one rapid and the other slow (Table 1).

1. *Succinyldicholine to succinylmonocholine and choline.*—Within seconds of

Whole Body Autoradiography; Monkey Fetus (Macaca Mulatta)
SUXAMETHONIUM
Intracordal Injection *in situ*

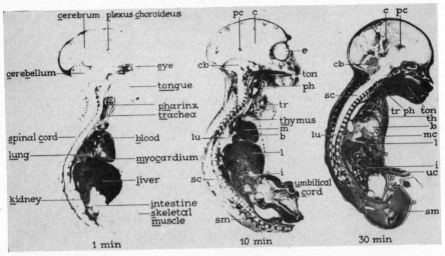

26/FIG. 5.—The distribution of suxamethonium in the monkey fetus (by courtesy of Prof. J. F. Crul).

entering the plasma this process has begun, and is so effective in the normal case that probably not more than 5 per cent of the injected dose reaches the muscles in the periphery. Less than 2 per cent appears in the urine (Foldes and Norton, 1954). The administration of suxamethonium brings about a depression of the plasma cholinesterase level, for Doenicke and his colleagues (1968) have been able to demonstrate that this inhibition bears a direct relationship to the duration of apnoea. As soon as no further enzyme inhibition was measurable spontaneous respiration returned.

26/TABLE 1
THE BREAKDOWN OF SUXAMETHONIUM (SUCCINYLDICHOLINE)

1st stage:

$$\text{Suxamethonium} \xrightarrow[\text{Plasma cholinesterase}]{\text{(Rapid)}} \text{Succinylmonocholine} + \text{Choline}$$

2nd stage:

$$\text{Succinylmonocholine} \xrightarrow[\substack{\text{Specific liver enzyme and} \\ \text{Plasma cholinesterase}}]{\text{(Slow)}} \text{Succinic acid} + \text{Choline}$$

2. *Succinylmonocholine to succinic acid and choline.*—This stage is slow and though plasma cholinesterase does play some role there is a specific enzyme for hydrolysis of succinylmonocholine found in the liver (Greenway and Quastel, 1955). Though the monocholine derivative is theoretically capable of producing a neuromuscular block in its own right, as it only has one-twentieth

to one-eightieth the activity of suxamethonium, paresis is unlikely to occur unless large doses of the parent drug have been used (i.e. over 500 mg of suxamethonium). Foldes and his associates (1954) demonstrated that 5–7 mg/kg of succinylmonocholine produced good relaxation in an anaesthetised subject lasting 8–12 minutes. This observation was also confirmed by Brennan (1956). The monocholine is largely excreted in the urine (Dal Santo, 1968).

(b) **Alkaline hydrolysis.**—This is a non-enzymatic process which in normal circumstances plays only a very small role in the metabolism of suxamethonium. Even in the absence of an enzymatic process it can only play a minor role in shortening the period of paresis, as less than 5 per cent per hour is destroyed by this method (Kalow, 1959). In other words, less than 50 per cent of the injected dose would have been broken down in ten hours.

(c) **Re-distribution.**—The uptake of suxamethonium at receptor sites (active and non-active) clearly has an important role to play in reducing the concentration in the plasma. The extent to which suxamethonium is bound to protein has yet to be elucidated. Autoradiographic studies suggest that the liver, kidney, spleen, muscle and mucopolysaccharide are major sites for the re-distribution of suxamethonium and succinylmonocholine (Fig. 5).

(d) **Excretion.**—It has already been mentioned that less than 2 per cent of suxamethonium is excreted unchanged in the urine, but in the absence of enzymatic hydrolysis this percentage might prove to be very much higher. No data is available on this subject.

Plasma Cholinesterase

The enzymatic hydrolysis of suxamethonium in man is now well understood. Nevertheless, patients are occasionally encountered who exhibit a prolonged response to this drug. Originally it was believed that all these could be accounted for on the basis of a diminished production of plasma cholinesterase enzyme by the liver. However, not all these cases appeared to be suffering from malnutrition or liver damage; in fact, some of the apnoeas occurred in very fit, healthy young patients with apparently normal levels of plasma cholinesterase. The puzzle was resolved when Kalow and Davies (1958) discovered that in man there were at least two types of plasma cholinesterase enzyme—a normal and an atypical one. Apparently individuals could lead perfectly normal lives with either one of these enzymes and it was only when they received an injection of suxamethonium that any differentiation could be made. A fit person with the normal plasma cholinesterase enzyme could hydrolyse suxamethonium rapidly, whereas one with the atypical enzyme could not do it at all. The only difference between these two enzymes is one of degree. Both are capable of hydrolysing suxamethonium *in vitro* but only the normal enzyme can do it in clinical conditions where the concentration of suxamethonium is low. Thus, if a patient with the atypical enzyme receives a dose of suxamethonium, the dilution caused by the blood volume rapidly causes a drop in its concentration below the effective level for the atypical esterase. In these circumstances the patient remains paralysed for a prolonged period of time.

(a) *Normal plasma cholinesterase.*—The enzyme level is normally determined by the Warburg apparatus but this estimation is both difficult and tedious. In clinical practice a simple test paper (incorporating the same principle) has been

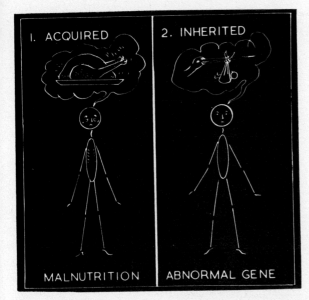

26/Fig. 6.—Illustration of the two causes of reduced plasma cholinesterase enzyme activity.

found satisfactory and reasonably accurate (Churchill-Davidson and Griffiths, 1961). Such methods will give an estimation of the total *amount* of enzyme in the blood but they will not differentiate the *type* of enzyme, i.e. between the normal and the atypical. Fortunately, the patients with only the atypical enzyme in their blood give low values for these tests, but there are a number of patients who have a mixture of some normal esterase and some atypical who merely give values on the low side of normal. For this reason, a low value for plasma

26/Fig. 7.

THE GENES
OF PLASMA CHOLINESTERASE ——

SYMBOL

HOMOZYGOTE
(SIMILAR GENES) or

HETEROZYGOTE
(DISSIMILAR GENES)

Pear Banana

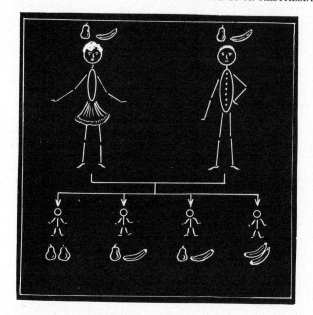

26/Fig. 8.—Diagram of genetic response in the offspring when two heterozygotes marry.

cholinesterase may be due to two causes (Fig. 6). One is liver damage due to disease and malnutrition; the other is genetically determined.

Kalow and Genest (1957) demonstrated that the presence of an abnormal plasma cholinesterase could be detected as it behaves differently when a local analgesic agent (dibucaine) is added to the plasma.

(*b*) *Atypical cholinesterase enzyme.*—The presence of this enzyme is due to the inheritance of an abnormal gene. An understanding of this process is most easily achieved if the genes for the cholinesterase enzyme are expressed as symbols (Fig. 7).

On the basis of Kalow's studies (1959) the vast majority of the population (96·2 per cent) are normal (i.e. homozygotes or similar genes). These two genes are normal (2 pears). Such people can destroy suxamethonium very rapidly. A small percentage of the population (3·8 per cent) have a mixture, i.e. one normal and one atypical gene. They are described as heterozygotes (dissimilar genes) which are represented above as one pear and one banana. Such persons destroy suxamethonium, but far less efficiently, so that its duration of action may be prolonged to 5–10 minutes. Very rarely (1:2800 people) someone is encountered who has only two atypical genes—i.e. an abnormal homozygote (2 bananas). In clinical practice it is estimated that an abnormally prolonged response to suxamethonium is encountered in 1 out of 2400 cases (Churchill-Davidson, 1961), so that it is probable that the great bulk of "apnoeas" which are met with are due to the presence of an atypical gene.

The manner in which two heterozygotes happen to marry and produce a child with the atypical homozygotic enzyme is illustrated above (Fig. 8).

The dibucaine test.—The basis for this test is to examine the amount of inhibition of a particular plasma cholinesterase activity by dibucaine. If a specimen has a high normal enzyme content then it will be inhibited to a large extent by the dibucaine. This percentage is usually expressed as a number—the dibucaine number (Table 2).

26/TABLE 2
DIBUCAINE NUMBERS FOR VARIOUS TYPES OF SERA

	Dibucaine Number
A. Normal homozygote (two normal genes) NN	70–85
B. Heterozygote (one normal and one atypical gene) DN	50–65
C. Abnormal homozygote (two abnormal genes) DD	16–25

Significance of plasma cholinesterase and dibucaine test.—Patients with a low dibucaine number also have a low plasma cholinesterase, but the converse is not necessarily true. For example, a patient with malnutrition may have a low plasma cholinesterase value yet have a normal dibucaine number. In this manner, it is now possible to distinguish between those patients who have a prolonged apnoea due to malnutrition and liver failure and those who have simply inherited an atypical gene. The clinical importance of making this differentiation may seem small but if the process is traced through a family it is possible to forewarn a certain member(s) of that family that a prolonged response to suxamethonium may be anticipated.

The possible results of these two tests (when combined), along with the diagnosis of the result, are presented in Table 3 (Lehmann, 1962).

26/TABLE 3
POSSIBLE RESULTS OF THE COMBINATION OF THE PLASMA CHOLINESTERASE
ESTIMATION (NORMAL = 60 – 120 UNITS) AND THE DIBUCAINE NUMBER

Ps. ch. esterase in units	Dibucaine Number % inhibition	Diagnosis	Genes
60–120	70–85	Normal homozygote	2 normal
8–59	70–85	Normal homozygote with liver damage	2 normal
26–90	50–65	Heterozygote	1 normal 1 atypical
8–40	50–65	Heterozygote with liver damage	1 normal 1 atypical
8–35	16–25	Atypical homozygote	2 atypical

Other genetic variants.—Further studies on the serum of patients who had a prolonged response to suxamethonium soon revealed certain interesting variations.

1. *Fluoride-resistant variant.*—Harris and Whittaker (1961; 1962a and b) found that sodium fluoride could be used in place of dibucaine. However, they noticed in comparing the results of the two methods that a few patients had a normal-looking dibucaine number yet an abnormally low fluoride number (Table 4). They suggested that here was yet another gene for plasma cholinester-

ase. The homozygote of this fluoride gene was known to give a moderately prolonged response to suxamethonium (Kalow, 1964).

2. *Silent gene.*—Liddell and his colleagues (1962), using the dibucaine test, found evidence for yet another gene. These patients have complete absence of all plasma cholinesterase activity. The clinical importance for such patients is that they have a *very* prolonged response to suxamethonium.

3. C_5 *variant*, described by Harris *et al.* in 1963, is another rare variety of genetic disturbance of normal plasma cholinesterase. This produces a very rapid hydrolysis of suxamethonium.

Comment.—There would appear to be at least five genes for plasma cholinesterase—the normal, the dibucaine resistant, the fluoride resistant, the

26/TABLE 4

THE VALUES QUOTED BY HARRIS AND WHITTAKER (1961) FOR THE DIBUCAINE AND FLUORIDE NUMBERS IN A STUDY OF 285 PATIENTS

Phenotype		Dibucaine No.		Fluoride No.	
		Mean	Standard Deviation	Mean	Standard Deviation
Normal Homozygote	"Usual"	80·06	1·56	61·35	3·21
Heterozygote	"Intermediate"	61·93	21·17	47·79	4·48
Abnormal Homozygote	"Atypical"	21·82	2·92	23·14	2·23

26/TABLE 5

HEREDITARY VARIANTS OF PLASMA CHOLINESTERASE IN MAN
(adapted from Pantuck, 1967)

Genotype	Incidence	Response to suxamethonium	Av. Dibucaine No.	Av. Fluoride No.
N–N	96 per cent	Normal	80	60
D–D	1:2,500	Prolonged + +	20	20
S–S	1:100,000	Prolonged + + +	0	0
F–F	Rare	Prolonged +	70	30
N–D	1:25	Prolonged	60	45
N–F	?	Prolonged	75	50
N–S	1:200	Prolonged	80	60
D–F	?	Prolonged +	45	35
D–S	1:800	Prolonged + +	20	20
F–S*	?	Prolonged	70	20

N = gene for normal plasma cholinesterase
D = gene for dibucaine-resistant variant
F = fluoride-resistant variant
S = silent gene
* Not yet observed

C_5 variant and the silent gene. These can combine to form ten genotypes (Table 5), of which six are associated with markedly increased sensitivity to suxamethonium (Pantuck, 1967). It is estimated that one of these six will appear in every 1500 patients (Kalow, 1964).

Administration

Suxamethonium is usually administered intravenously, but it can be given intramuscularly or even by the subcutaneous route if the dose is sufficient. If either of the latter routes is used then there is a considerable delay in the onset of paresis and once established it lasts much longer than normal. An increase of 50 per cent in dose is required to produce paralysis by these routes. With the intravenous route the arrival in any group of muscle fibres is heralded by brief but visible twitches or fasciculations, and these are usually first observed in the eyebrow and eyelid muscles, passing later to the shoulder girdle and abdominal musculature, and finally to the hands and feet. Muscle fasciculations are more obvious in patients who are lightly anaesthetised.

Dosage.—The average single dose in man is 1 mg/kg, but when administered by continuous infusion as a 0·1 per cent solution a dose of 20–40 µg/kg/min will give relaxation of most skeletal musculature, but some assistance to respiration is required. Doses of 50–60 µg/kg/min and above usually result in complete respiratory paralysis. If total paralysis is produced by continuous infusion there is a considerable danger of administering an overdose, as there are no signs of muscle activity available. It is essential to monitor neuromuscular transmission continuously whenever an infusion of suxamethonium is used, as this will remove the risk of overdosage.

Duration of action.—A single injection of suxamethonium (50–75 mg) produces, on average, respiratory paralysis for 2–4 minutes. Doubling the dose does not necessarily double the duration of cessation of respiration. A period of apnoea (in the presence of adequate manual ventilation) lasting longer than ten minutes must be considered as an abnormal response. Electromyography, however, has shown that the recovery of the limb muscles lags far behind that of the respiratory muscles.

Antagonists

Like that of decamethonium, the action of suxamethonium can be opposed by the previous administration of a non-depolarising drug such as d-tubocurarine or gallamine; similarly, it can be potentiated by anti-cholinesterase or depolarising drugs whether given before or after the suxamethonium. In clinical practice both hexafluorenium bromide (Foldes *et al.*, 1960) and tetrahydroaminoacridine (tacrine) (Gordh and Wahlin, 1961; MacCaul and Robinson, 1962; Benveniste and Dyrberg, 1962) have been used to potentiate the duration of action of suxamethonium. Both are inhibitors of plasma cholinesterase with only weak or absent muscarinic effects, e.g. salivation and bradycardia. The advantage of this combination is claimed to be that it reduces the total amount of suxamethonium required and therefore lowers the incidence of Phase II block.

PROLONGED RESPONSE

As has been previously stated, the duration of action of a single dose of

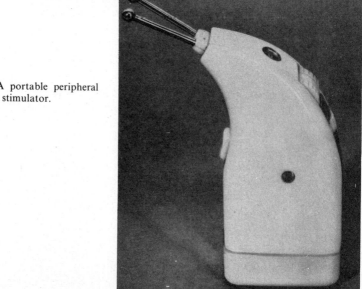

26/Fɪɢ. 9(*a*).—A portable peripheral nerve stimulator.

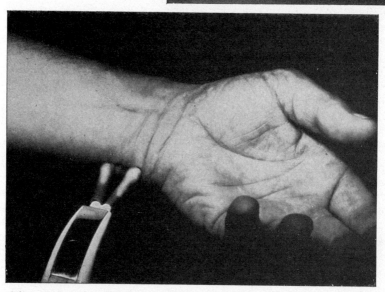

26/Fɪɢ. 9(*b*).—Method of applying the peripheral nerve stimulator to the ulnar nerve at the wrist.

suxamethonium (e.g. 50–75 mg) is 2–4 minutes in adults, and apnoea lasting longer than ten minutes must be considered abnormal. Often the cause of failure of return of respiration is not related to the relaxant at all but to the sedation, the depression of the respiratory centre or the hyperventilation. The diagnosis of a prolonged response to suxamethonium, therefore, must be made with a peripheral nerve-stimulator (Fig. 9). This instrument, when applied to a peripheral nerve, will indicate first the amount of neuromuscular block that is present, and secondly the characteristics of this block—i.e. depolarisation or non-depolarisation. If, after ten minutes of apnoea, the hand muscles are still completely paralysed, then it is safe to assume that this is an abnormal response to suxamethonium. For routine continuous monitoring it is necessary to place needle electrodes under the skin in the vicinity of the ulnar nerve either at the wrist or elbow. Care must be exercised to ensure that the needle point does not impinge on the nerve causing a high local charge density and that there is no possibility of this needle acting as an earth for an inadequately earthed diathermy machine. Some peripheral nerve-stimulators are so arranged that they automatically deliver a single twitch stimulus every 3–5 seconds, thereby enabling the anaesthetist to gauge the depth of paresis and to regulate the suxamethonium infusion. For diagnostic purposes a single application using external electrodes will usually reveal all the information required. Peripheral nerve-stimulators are useful for monitoring the degree of neuromuscular block produced during a continuous suxamethonium infusion and for differentiating between apnoea caused by central nervous system depression and one resulting from residual effect of a neuromuscular blocking agent. A well-maintained twitch response and an absence of post-tetanic facilitation indicates that neuromuscular conduction is unimpaired.

A prolonged response to suxamethonium may occur for three reasons:

1. *Low or atypical plasma-cholinesterase enzyme activity.*—Patients with a low enzyme activity are most often encountered in severe liver disease, starvation —as in carcinoma of the oesophagus—or in women in late pregnancy (Shnider, 1965; Robertson, 1966). The duration of paralysis in this type of case rarely exceeds $\frac{1}{2}$–1 hour. Similarly, a patient with a heterozygous type of enzyme activity will take longer than usual to complete the breakdown of the relaxant. However, it is those patients with the atypical homozygous enzyme who cannot hydrolyse any of the suxamethonium *in vivo* who exhibit the longest periods of paralysis. During the prolonged period of recovery many of these patients will show evidence of a Phase II block which may increase the recovery time.

2. *Overdose of suxamethonium.*—This may arise when an intravenous infusion is used to produce relaxation for abdominal surgery without a nerve stimulator being used to monitor the degree of neuromuscular blockade. Added to this the situation may be further confused by the development of Phase II block (Fig. 10). These signs can often be demonstrated briefly after a dose of only 200 mg suxamethonium (White, 1963; Katz *et al.*, 1963). Nevertheless, this early Phase II block rarely poses a problem in clinical practice because the recovery time is not unduly increased.

3. *Long-term anti-cholinesterase therapy.*—The increasing use of anti-cholinesterase drugs in medicine has increased this danger. Such agents are frequently used to lower intra-ocular tension in cases of glaucoma with ecothiopate iodine (Phospholine). Certain of the cytotoxic agents used in the treatment of cancer and some anti-bilharzia drugs also have some anti-cholinesterase action (Wang and Ross, 1963). Propanidid also has moderate anti-cholinesterase activity, although it is transient.

Treatment of prolonged response to suxamethonium.—The development of a Phase II block following prolonged exposure to suxamethonium presents the anaesthetist with a great temptation to try to expedite natural recovery by the administration of drugs. The dangers of this have been reviewed by Vickers (1963) and Hunter (1966). Anti-cholinesterase agents may initially improve neuromuscular conduction but the results are seldom prolonged and unless the plasma level of drug is very low it will result in prolonging the action of suxamethonium in the depolarising phase. The use of cholase (purified human serum esterase) may effectively reduce the duration of the depolarising block (Doenick *et al.*, 1968; Stovner, 1976), but the shelf life of the enzyme is short. Many patients do not recover normal neuromuscular function after cholase, possibly due to the residual Phase II effect. Most anaesthetists are agreed that should there be a very prolonged effect from suxamethonium then the patient should be ventilated with 50 per cent nitrous oxide and oxygen until neuromuscular recovery occurs. Fluid infusions may assist recovery by increasing the distribution volume and promoting a diuresis and thus lowering the plasma concentration of drug.

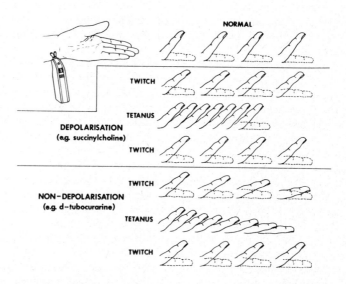

26/Fig. 10.—Diagram of the characteristic movement of the fingers on stimulation of the ulnar nerve in the presence of both depolarisation and non-depolarisation block.

Every patient who demonstrates a prolonged response to suxamethonium (over 30 min apnoea) should be investigated to determine if they have a reduction of plasma cholinesterase or an abnormal genotype. If an abnormal genotype is revealed then the immediate relatives of the patient should have their blood examined to determine the familial pattern. All patients with either the homozygous or heterozygous abnormality should carry warning cards to be given to the anaesthetist should an operation be necessary.

d-TUBOCURARINE CHLORIDE

History

The early history of the white explorers and their hunt for the secret of the arrow poison used by the South American Indians is a fascinating one, and the reader is strongly advised to consult two excellent monographs on this subject, one by McIntyre (1947) and the other by Bryn Thomas (1964). McIntyre suggests that the conception that Sir Walter Raleigh introduced curare to Europe is wrong. Many Spanish and English explorers of the sixteenth century wrote accounts of this interesting arrow poison, however, and it can reasonably be assumed that small quantities of it reached Europe.

The first authentic account of its preparation with all the native ritual did not come until Humboldt travelled to South America in 1805 to satisfy his curiosity. About that time, this remarkable man was also working with Gay-Lussac on the composition of various gases.

One of the earliest accounts of the experimental use of curare comes from the work of Sir Benjamin Brodie. In 1851 he published a book describing some early experiments and in one of these (circa 1814) curare was administered to an ass belonging to the famed naturalist and explorer Charles Waterton. This was the first time the value of artificial respiration in the treatment of curare paralysis was appreciated. In fact, the animal was paralysed for two hours but was kept alive by artificial respiration, so that in time a complete recovery was made.

The history of curare can never be told without paying faithful tribute to the phenomenal experiments of that great physiologist Claude Bernard. About 1850 he was studying various poisons and noted that curare, when injected into a frog, brought about paralysis of skeletal muscle; yet skeletal muscle, when stimulated directly, responded. With a series of simple yet lucid experiments he was able to show that neither the muscle itself nor the nerves were affected by the drug, but that somewhere between these two a block in neuromuscular transmission occurred. It is to Kuhne (1862), a former pupil of Bernard's, that the credit goes for concentrating interest on the neuromuscular junction, as we know it today.

Towards the end of the nineteenth century (1886–1897), Boehm published a series of articles which greatly clarified the position of curare. Up to that time the preparation of this poison had been surrounded with weird native superstition and no two samples were identical in their constituents. Boehm pointed out that these "concoctions" contained three main types of curare depending on the method of preparation used. Thus there was calabash (gourd) curare, pot curare, and finally tube curare, each prefix signifying the vessel that had been used in its preparation. Boehm's curarine, which was a potent quaternary ammonium compound obtained from calabash curare, was never found in a crystalline form. It is generally believed that this drug, which was used in a great many pharmacological and physiological experiments, contained a high proportion of toxiferae. One of the most notable of these is toxiferine-I which was isolated from the bark of the Strychnos Toxifera by King (1949) and found to possess potent neuromuscular blocking properties (Paton and Perry, 1951).

In 1928, Späth, Leithe and Ladeck examined a sample of Boehm's original crystalline "curarine" and were able to show that this was merely the laevo-

26/Fig. 11(a).—Original formula of d-tubocurarine chloride (after King, 1935).

26/Fig. 11(b).—New structure of d-tubocurarine chloride (after Everett et al., 1970).

modification of d-bebeerine. This latter drug was known to be an alkaloid found in the dried roots of a small bush plant, the *chondodendron tomentosum*. This valuable piece of information was sufficient to excite King (1935) who proceeded to isolate the pure alkaloid—d-tubocurarine—from the same plant. His method of extraction was complex, using first ether and then chloroform.

A similar alkaloid, d-chondocurarine, can also be isolated from this plant root, and this also has neuromuscular blocking properties. As it has about four times the potency of its sister alkaloid, Dutcher (1951) has suggested that the presence of small amounts of this substance might account for some of the variations in potency that are sometimes found during manufacture.

In 1940, Bennet and his associates first described the administration of d-tubocurarine in man. They used it to soften the effects of electroconvulsion therapy and from that day onwards the muscle relaxants have played an important part in this treatment. In 1942, Griffith and Johnson in Montreal introduced curare into anaesthesia, and together they contributed to one of the most spectacular advances in modern surgery. In 1946, Gray and Halton in England presented a series of cases describing the use of d-tubocurarine in anaesthesia.

Standardisation

d-Tubocurarine chloride is a purified extract of *chondodendron tomentosum* (Wintersteiner and Dutcher, 1943); 1 ml of the solution contains 10 mg of the active principle in the U.K. and 3 mg in the U.S.A. This substance has now been universally adopted in clinical anaesthesia.

Physical and Chemical Properties

Chemical analysis of d-tubocurarine is very difficult. A spectrophotometric method described by Elert (1956) was revised by Elert and Cohen (1962) and Utting (1963). Some workers have used biological assay but most have utilised the specific radioactivity of tritium-labelled drug (Cohen *et al.* 1967). More recently, Horowitz and Spector (1973) have described a radioimmune assay technique for estimating the quantity of drug in blood.

The original formula of *d*-tubocurarine chloride (Fig. 11*a*) is now thought to be incorrect and the new formula that is gaining acceptance was elucidated by Everett *et al.* (1970) at the Burroughs Wellcome laboratories in London (Fig. 11*b*). In this form *d*-tubocurarine is not a di-methyl substituted bis-quaternary ammonium compound. As a result it has only one stable quaternary ammonium group. The structure of the other nitrogen ion will vary according to the pH of the media behaving more like a tertiary ammonium compound at an alkaline pH.

Pharmacological Actions

Mode of action.—*d*-Tubocurarine was the first of a long line of neuromuscular blocking drugs. It acts by non-depolarisation block of the neuromuscular junction. The curare molecule combines with the end-plate receptor and this denies the acetylcholine molecule access to its normal destination. The characteristics of this type of neuromuscular block have already been discussed in detail (Chapter 25). Briefly, they can be summarised as follows:

1. "Fade" of successive response to both slow (twitch) and fast (tetanic) rates of nerve stimulation.
2. The presence of post-tetanic facilitation.
3. The above signs are reversed by anti-cholinesterase drugs.

An example of a non-depolarisation block is illustrated (Fig. 12).

Other features of a non-depolarisation block that may sometimes be observed are:

(*a*) Antagonism or reversal of the block by depolarising drugs. This is more theoretical than practical in clinical anaesthesia as it requires a perfect balance of dosage that can seldom be attained.

(*b*) The absence of fasciculations or muscle pains either during or after the injection.

In animal experiments great importance has been attached to the presence of Wedensky inhibition (i.e. the passage of slower rates of nerve stimulation even when the faster rates are blocked). In clinical practice, when full paralysing doses are used this discrepancy between fast and slow rates of nerve stimulation is not so obvious. Whether the rate be fast or slow, the decrement of successive responses occurs mainly with the first four stimuli. Following this, continued stimulation leads to a slight waxing and waning of neuromuscular transmission.

Cardiovascular system.—Until a few years ago it was generally believed that *d*-tubocurarine had virtually no effect on myocardial activity. However, Dowdy and her associates (1965) found that 15–30 mg of *d*-tubocurarine "corrected ventricular fibrillation in patients in whom all other conventional means had failed". This observation suggested that the relaxant drug had a direct anti-dysrhythmic action on the myocardium. These authors also found that *d*-tubocurarine (when injected into the isolated rabbit heart) led to a reduction of contractile tension which resembled quinidine. This effect may have been due

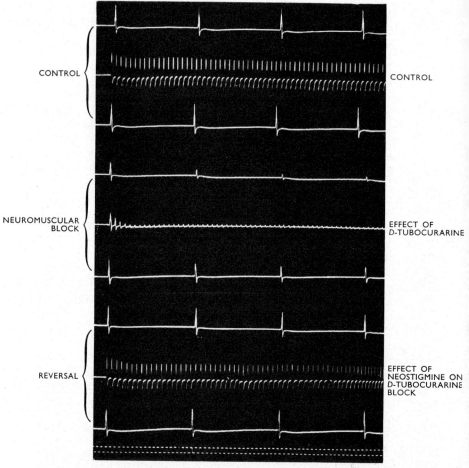

CONTROL

NEUROMUSCULAR
BLOCK

REVERSAL

CONTROL

EFFECT OF
D-TUBOCURARINE

EFFECT OF
NEOSTIGMINE ON
D-TUBOCURARINE
BLOCK

26/Fig. 12.—Electromyograph of classical *d*-tubocurarine neuromuscular block.

to a preservative which is present in the U.S.P. preparation but not in the B.P. curare. It cannot be reproduced using "pure" *d*-tubocurarine.

Support for the thesis that *d*-tubocurarine may have a direct myocardial action is also given by the work of Cohen and his colleagues with their auto-radiographic studies in rats. They observed that, unlike gallamine, a large part of the injected dose could be found in heart muscle (Fig. 13).

Apart from a possible direct negative inotropic effect on the myocardium, *d*-tubocurarine is often referred to as a ganglion-blocking drug. This arose largely from the observation that some patients developed hypotension following the injection of the relaxant (Thomas, 1957; Bono and Mapelli, 1960; McDowall and Clarke, 1969). The evidence for actual ganglionic blockade rests with animal experiments and it is extremely effective as such in the cat. In man, all known ganglion-blocking drugs produce a tachycardia yet *d*-tubocurarine causes either no change or a fall in pulse rate. A possible explanation of this dilemma is that the hypotension is due to the release of histamine. Iwatsuki and his associates (1965), working with dogs, demonstrated that d-tubocurarine produced a marked decrease in ventricular contractile force which they believed to be due to histamine release. Contrary to the results of earlier workers (Mongar and Whelan, 1953) it now seems more certain that d-tubocurarine is capable of raising the blood level of histamine in man (Westgate and Van Bergen, 1962; Salem et al., 1968; Crul, 1970; McDowall and Clarke, 1969) and this could account for the fall in blood pressure observed in some patients, an effect, however, that cannot be prevented by the prior administration of an antihistamine.

Finally, Mathias and Evans-Prosser (1970), in a far-ranging study of the bradycardia and dysrhythmia produced by suxamethonium, have drawn attention to the fact that only very small doses of d-tubocurarine are required to protect the patient against an alteration in either cardiac rate or rhythm. As many other drugs, such as atropine and the ganglion-blockers, are also capable of affording this protection, they have suggested that the most likely site of action for d-tubocurarine is on the vagal afferent system. In this way the relaxant is able to protect the heart from afferent stimulation arising in other parts of the body and which otherwise would lead to vagal slowing and possible dysrhythmias. In concentrations about twice that found in patients d-tubocurarine does prevent the bradycardia produced by acetylcholine on the isolated rabbit heart (Goat and Feldman, 1972a). However, d-tubocurarine also reduces the response of the isolated perfused adrenal medulla to sympathetic nerve stimulation.

Paton (1959) reviewed much of the evidence for the possible passage of d-tubocurarine across the blood-brain barrier and concluded that "although there is little likelihood that these (muscle relaxants) should be able to penetrate the central nervous system . . . a number of conditions such as asphyxia, anaesthesia, dehydration or haemorrhage may weaken the selectiveness of the entry from the blood to the brain." Using radioimmunoassay Matteo et al. (1977) have detected small concentrations of d-tubocurarine in the cerebrospinal fluid of nine patients during anaesthesia. They comment that the quantities of d-tubocurarine found were unlikely to produce any pharmacologic effect in man.

Neostigmine-resistant curarisation was a term used by Hunter (1956) to describe cases in which an electrolyte imbalance (often associated with acute intestinal obstruction) was believed to be responsible for a prolonged neuromuscular block that could not be reversed by neostigmine. Despite the passing of nearly fifteen years, evidence is still lacking that a neuromuscular block with the classical signs of a non-depolarisation block was present and that neostigmine failed to improve neuromuscular transmission. Brooks and Feldman (1962) drew attention to the similarities in the syndrome described by Hunter, and that produced by metabolic acidaemia. In both conditions there is depression of consciousness, hypotension that is unresponsive to catecholamine infusion and gasping respiration. With the recognition and early treatment of metabolic acidosis in patients with obstructive gut lesions the incidence of neostigmine-resistant curarisation has greatly diminished.

Skeletal muscle.—The order of paralysis of muscles following the intravenous injection of d-tubocurarine is similar to that with any other muscle relaxant. The eye muscles are the first to be affected and the weakness then rapidly spreads to involve the face and limb musculature before finally reaching the trunk muscles. Fortunately, the bulbar muscles are the last to be affected and for this reason it always is possible to select a dose of d-tubocurarine in clinical anaesthesia which will produce complete paralysis of the limb musculature without reducing the respiratory tidal volume. It is not possible, however, to paralyse the abdominal musculature without seriously impairing the function of the respiratory muscles.

Exceptions to this order of muscle paralysis sometimes do occur, but only in rare instances. First, in the presence of generalised myasthenia gravis, where the respiratory muscles are affected by the disease, the administration of d-tubocurarine may produce a state of affairs where the patient is apnoeic yet able to signal his distress with his arms. Secondly, in the anaesthetised patient, after large doses of d-tubocurarine the muscles of the eyebrow and forehead can be seen to move occasionally, although the other muscles in the body still appear to be completely paralysed. The explanation may lie in the theory that the levator palpebrae superioris muscles have a double innervation and that they contain some smooth muscle fibres with a nerve supply from the autonomic system. They would thus remain unaffected by the dose of d-tubocurarine used. Some support for this suggestion is given by the occurrence of ptosis after a stellate ganglion block. Thirdly, following the rapid injection of a massive (bolus) dose, the sequence of muscle paralysis follows the pattern of distribution of the cardiac output to the periphery.

Interaction with volatile anaesthetic agents.—In the presence of halothane anaesthesia less d-tubocurarine is required to produce the same degree of neuromuscular block (Katz and Gissen, 1967). In other words halothane potentiates the neuromuscular block of a non-depolarising relaxant. The two drugs, however, do not have the same mechanism of action. Halothane interferes with neuromuscular transmission principally by desensitising the post-junctional membrane (Gissen et al., 1966).

In an interesting study in man Katz (1966) has demonstrated that ether has a weak neuromuscular blocking action. Nevertheless, he observed that ether depressed the motor activity of the abdominal muscles *before* there was any evidence of paresis in the limb musculature. From this he concluded that under normal clinical conditions the muscle relaxation of ether is mainly attributable to depression of the conduction mechanism in the spinal cord rather than an action at the neuromuscular junction.

Liver and kidneys.—There is no evidence that d-tubocurarine has any action on the liver or kidney cells. The kidneys provide the principal route of elimination, with the biliary system in the liver offering an alternative (Cohen et al., 1967). In the event of renal failure the amount excreted through the biliary system is greatly increased. In liver disease larger doses of d-tubocurarine than normal may be required (Dundee and Gray, 1953). A possible explanation of the phenomenon is a change in the albumin and globulin content of plasma. In severe liver disease the plasma albumin level falls, but the globulin level rises since this protein is formed in other places than the liver. As a result, protein binding of tubocurarine may be increased.

Uterus and placental barrier.—d-Tubocurarine has no detectable action on the smooth muscle of the uterus (Harroun and Fisher, 1949).

Clinically, d-tubocurarine does not appear to cross the placental barrier because infants born of curarised mothers do not show any obvious signs of paresis. This clinical impression has been confirmed in animal studies by Harroun and his colleagues (1947) and Buller and Young (1949). In an investigation of six human patients, Crawford and Gardiner (1956) found that the concentrations of *d*-tubocurarine in the cord blood at delivery were imperceptible, even following a maternal dose as high as 20 mg. Furthermore, Cohen and his co-workers (1953) in a comparative study between the maternal and fetal circulations in patients undergoing Caesarean section, found that although thiopentone crossed the placental barrier *d*-tubocurarine did not. Later studies (Cohen *et al.*, 1968), using autoradiographic techniques in the curarised rat, have confirmed that *d*-tubocurarine does not reach the fetus (Fig. 13). This evidence justifies the use of modest doses of *d*-tubocurarine in parturient patients. However, large doses or the continuous administration (as in the treatment of tetanus) to a mother during pregnancy may cause arthrogryposis multiplex congenita, possibly indicating intra-uterine action of *d*-tubocurarine upon the fetus (Drachman and Coulombre, 1962)—see Chapter 44.

Distribution

This is illustrated in Fig. 13 (Cohen *et al.*, 1968).

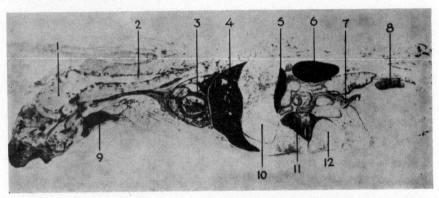

26/Fig. 13.—Autoradiograph of rat sacrificed 15 minutes after intravenous injection of 0·6 mg/kg *d*-tubocurarine. 1, brain; 2, spinal cord; 3, heart; 4, liver; 5, spleen; 6, kidney; 7, intestine; 8, bladder; 9, salivary gland; 10, stomach; 11, placenta; 12, fetus.

Detoxication and Excretion

Contrary to earlier reports, it is now generally accepted that *d*-tubocurarine is not broken down *in vivo* but is excreted unchanged. The principal route of elimination is the kidney, with the biliary system offering an alternative pathway (Cohen *et al.*, 1968). In the presence of normal renal function, 85 per cent of an injected dose can be recovered in dogs, and of this only 5 per cent leaves the circulation via the biliary tract. In patients, rather less curare appears to be excreted by the kidney. On the other hand, in renal failure as much as 38 per cent of the injected dose may leave the body by biliary excretion (see Chapter 25).

Recovery of spontaneous respiration cannot occur unless the plasma concentration of drug falls below a critical threshold level. This occurs, not only due to urinary and biliary elimination but, more importantly, by redistribution. *d*-Tubocurarine is taken up by active and non-active receptors; the active receptors are those found at the neuromuscular junction whilst the non-active ones are spread throughout the body. The widespread distribution is well illustrated in Fig. 13. The most important redistribution sites include the kidneys, liver and spleen.

Administration

Method of administration.—(*a*) *Intravenously.*—This route is most commonly used as it produces maximum relaxation within two to three minutes. Provided the pH of the solution has been suitably adjusted, *d*-tubocurarine can be mixed in the same syringe with thiopentone.

(*b*) *Intramuscularly.*—In the presence of hyaluronidase the paralysing action of intramuscular *d*-tubocurarine is apparent within 2–5 minutes and reaches a maximum in about 5–8 minutes. There is, however, a wide margin of variation in response with this route; consequently the relaxant effect is difficult to control. Clinically, an intramuscular injection is only used in exceptional circumstances when the intravenous route is impracticable.

(*c*) *Orally.*—This route has proved unfavourable as doses at least 50 times greater than those used intravenously are required. Absorption takes place slowly through all mucous surfaces and the gastric juices do not appear to interfere with the passage of the drug, but the main area of absorption is in the small intestine.

(*d*) *Dissolved in oil.*—*d*-Tubocurarine can be dissolved in oil and administered by deep intramuscular injection, so that its duration of action is prolonged. Although used in the past in the treatment of some spastic states, this route is rarely if ever used nowadays. The theory underlying the use of "curare in oil" for patients with spastic paralysis, and also in the treatment of poliomyelitis, lay in the belief that though some muscles were weak or paralysed there were others that were antagonistic to the affected muscles but which remained in a state of spasm; thus weak muscles were hindered in their movements by spasm in their antagonists. Some of this antagonism was believed to be reflex in origin. Theoretically it was argued that *d*-tubocurarine could reduce the spasm of the antagonistic muscles yet leave the already weak muscles unaffected. This is not the case, and the initial benefits claimed were not borne out in clinical practice.

Dosage.—Many attempts have been made to assess the dose of *d*-tubocurarine required on a body-weight basis. There is such a wide variability in the response that this is not possible. For this reason it is better to test each patient individually once he is anaesthetised. This can be done by giving incremental doses until the signs of impending respiratory inadequacy occur. This dose (when combined with controlled respiration) is usually sufficient for abdominal relaxation, though it is inadequate for endotracheal intubation. In the average adult (70 kg) a dose of 0·1 to 0·2 mg/kg is required to produce paresis of limb musculature, 0·4 to 0·5 mg/kg for abdominal relaxation, and 0·5 to 0·6 mg/kg for endotracheal intubation. General anaesthesia (depending on depth) reduces the dose required.

Reversal of *d*-Tubocurarine Paresis (see Chapter 27)

Neostigmine methylsulphate is the anti-cholinesterase of choice for the reversal of *d*-tubocurarine paresis because it is long-acting and therefore avoids the dangers of recurarisation. It must be combined with atropine to prevent the unpleasant muscarinic side-effects such as salivation, sweating, bradycardia and colic. An important point to remember is that provided the dose of *d*-tubocurarine is not excessive (i.e. paresis is less than 100 per cent) then neostigmine can be administered at any time interval after *d*-tubocurarine and it will be an effective antagonist (Bridenbaugh and Churchill-Davidson, 1968). In other words, a further dose of *d*-tubocurarine can be used to close the peritoneum and it is not necessary to wait another 20–30 minutes before reversal with neostigmine. These authors have also pointed out that often it is necessary to use a dose of neostigmine of more than 2·5 mg and they recommend a dose of up to 5·0 mg neostigmine (with 2·0 mg atropine) for all cases that have received large doses of *d*-tubocurarine (40–50 µg/kg body weight). Any increase in dosage above 5·0 mg is valueless. Pyridostigmine (Mestinon) which has about one-quarter the potency of neostigmine has also been recommended.

Recurarisation

Although neostigmine may produce an apparent complete reversal of neuromuscular blockade it does not necessarily completely remove all the curare molecules from the receptors. As a result, in stressful situations where a high degree of receptor response may be required, residual paresis may be evident. This can often be demonstrated as weakness of the eye muscles (Hannington-Kiff, 1970). True recurarisation is fortunately exceedingly rare and may follow a massive shift in K^+ ions altering the sensitivity of the receptors or following a shift of sequestrated drug from a non-active receptor site such as the liver or kidneys, into the blood.

Tests of the reversal of non-depolarising block vary in sensitivity. The ability to maintain sustained contraction in response to a 30–50 Hz stimulation is usually considered evidence of adequate reversal as it coincides with return of a normal ventilatory capacity. The train-of-four stimuli, each given at 2 Hz, will show a fall in the twitch height of the fourth stimulus that exceeds 20 per cent of the first twitch height if reversal of curarisation is incomplete and ventilatory power remains affected (Ali *et al.*, 1975). Lesser degrees of residual receptor occupancy by non-depolarising drugs can be demonstrated by using fast tetanic stimulation (100 Hz) but such fast rates are outside the physiological range and the problem of muscle fatigue becomes important.

Duration of action.—The time taken to recover from complete paralysis of the limb musculature is about 30–50 minutes. In clinical practice it is often unnecessary to give a further dose of relaxant following the original paralysing dose until some 40–60 minutes have elapsed. This interval will be influenced by the amount of paralysis produced by the first dose—thus if the first dose produced only 90 per cent depression of twitch height, the second dose will be required earlier than if all the receptors had been saturated—and other factors, such as the depth of anaesthesia, the carbon dioxide level of the blood, and the degree of surgical stimulation will determine the duration of action of the original dose of drug. When a second dose is required it is rarely necessary to exceed one-fifth of the original amount in order to restore paralysis, as a considerable proportion of the receptors will still be occupied by the curare in spite of apparent complete recovery of neuromuscular transmission.

GALLAMINE TRIETHIODIDE (FLAXEDIL)

History

Following the introduction of *d*-tubocurarine into clinical anaesthesia, pharmacologists throughout the world sought for synthetic drugs with a similar action. In 1947, Bovet and his co-workers described the muscle relaxant properties of a synthetic product—gallamine triethiodide. The effects of this relaxant in man were first described by Huguenard and Boué (1948) in France and by Mushin and his colleagues (1949) in England.

Physical and Chemical Properties

Gallamine triethiodide is chemically tri-(β-diethylaminoethoxy)-benzene triethiodide with the following structural formula:

$$I^-$$

$$O-CH_2-CH_2-N^+-(C_2H_5)_3$$
$$I^-$$
$$O-CH_2-CH_2-N^+(C_2H_5)_3$$
$$I^-$$
$$O-CH_2-CH_2-N^+-(C_2H_5)_3$$

It is a white amorphous powder with a melting point of 145–150° C and a molecular weight of 891. It is non-irritant. Gallamine is prepared synthetically in the laboratory and supplied commercially in a 4 per cent solution containing 40 mg/ml. Ampoules of 80 mg (2 ml) and 120 mg (3 ml) are available. It is relatively stable and can be mixed with thiopentone.

Pharmacological Actions

Mode of action.—Gallamine triethiodide acts at the neuromuscular junction by non-depolarisation in a similar manner to *d*-tubocurarine.

Cardiovascular system.—Gallamine does not appear to have any direct action on the myocardium although it has been suggested that it reduces the incidence of cardiac dysrhythmias under cyclopropane anaesthesia (Riker and Wescoe, 1951). It has a very marked vagal-blocking activity in the doses used in clinical anaesthesia and this factor is particularly useful in combination with halothane, a drug which tends to stimulate this nerve. The action of gallamine on the parasympathetic system was not recognised in the early animal experiments using cats, but was described in man by Doughty and Wylie (1951). These authors noted that it occurred within 1–1½ minutes of an intravenous injection of the drug and was particularly marked in young people. The degree of tachycardia varied widely but, in over half the patients studied, showed an increase of 20–60 per cent over the control value. The rise in pulse rate is some-times accompanied by an increase in the systemic blood pressure and cardiac output (Kennedy and Farman, 1968). The tachycardia can be abolished by both cyclopropane and halothane.

Central nervous system.—Like *d*-tubocurarine, there is no clear evidence available to suggest that gallamine has any action on the central nervous system in man. In animals, however, its intrathecal injection can lead to convulsions.

Liver and kidneys.—Gallamine has no direct action on either the liver or kidney. Indirectly, however, it has a weak inhibitory effect on the plasma cholinesterase produced by the liver (Vincent and Parant, 1954). Like *d*-tubocurarine it is believed to be excreted in the urine. Mushin and his colleagues (1949) recovered 30 to 100 per cent of the original dose from the urine of rabbits in the two hours following its administration. Feldman *et al.* (1969) found up to 82 per cent of the initial dose was excreted in the urine of dogs in 24 hours.

A number of reports have appeared in the literature suggesting that a pro-longed paresis may follow the use of gallamine in cases with poor renal function (Fairley, 1950; Montgomery and Bennett-Jones, 1956; Feldman and Levi, 1963). This is partly due to loss of redistribution sites in the kidney and also to the lack of alternative pathways of excretion for the drug (Feldman *et al.*, 1969) (Fig. 14).

Some support for the suggestion that the duration of action of gallamine triethiodide can be modified by the presence or absence of renal function has

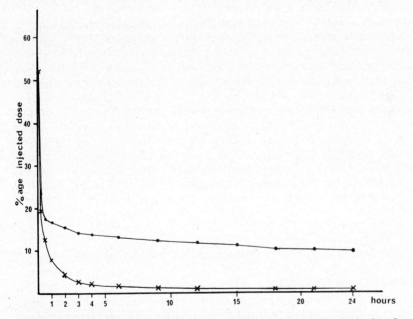

26/Fig. 14.—Blood level of gallamine following intravenous injection in the dog. *Lower trace*: in presence of normal kidneys. *Upper trace*: after bilateral renal pedicle ligation.

N.B. In the absence of renal distribution sites the blood level does not fall below 18 per cent of the original concentration and that level is then maintained due to lack of an excretory pathway.

been observed (Churchill-Davidson *et al.*, 1967). A patient undergoing bilateral nephrectomy (i.e. with complete absence of renal function) received a paralysing dose of the relaxant drug. Although reversal was achieved with an anticholinesterase drug, the signs of recurarisation were clearly visible many hours after the operation.

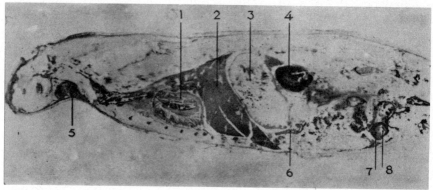

26/Fig. 15.—Autoradiograph of rat sacrificed 15 minutes after intravenous injection of 2·4 mg/kg gallamine. 1, heart; 2, liver; 3, stomach; 4, kidney; 5, salivary gland; 6, intestine; 7, placenta; 8, fetus (Cohen *et al.*, 1968).

On the basis of the available evidence it would appear unwise to use gallamine as the relaxant agent in the presence of poor renal function.

Histamine release.—Courvoisier and Ducrot (1948) failed to find any evidence of histamine release in dogs. Mushin and his colleagues (1949), working with the rat diaphragm preparation, found that gallamine liberated 1/5th–1/2 the quantity of histamine as compared with *d*-tubocurarine. Sniper (1952), using the intradermal weal test in human subjects, found that the activity of gallamine in liberating histamine was considerably less than that of *d*-tubocurarine.

Uterus and placental barrier.—There is no evidence available to suggest that gallamine influences the contractions of the pregnant uterus. Crawford (1956) found direct evidence in patients undergoing forceps delivery or Caesarean section that gallamine crossed the placenta "in appreciable concentrations". Although he failed to notice any signs of paresis in the infants, gallamine was easily detectable in the cord serum. Nevertheless, Crawford was unable to find a simple relationship between the concentration of gallamine in the maternal and fetal bloods.

Distribution

The distribution of gallamine throughout the body is illustrated in Fig. 15.

Detoxication and Excretion

Gallamine is not detoxicated *in vivo* but is excreted unchanged in the urine. In the cat, 30–100 per cent of the total dose injected can be recovered from the urine within two hours (Mushin *et al.*, 1949). In the dog, 82 per cent of the total dose can be recovered from the urine in 24 hours, the majority being excreted in the first 5 hours (Feldman *et al.*, 1969).

Method of Administration

The intravenous route is the only method that has gained widespread popularity in clinical anaesthesia. When injected subcutaneously the activity is about one-quarter that of an intravenous injection (Bovet, 1951).

Dosage.—In the average adult subject 50 mg is sufficient to produce almost complete paralysis of the limb musculature, yet leaving the respiratory tidal excursion unimpeded. In comparison, 8–9 mg of d-tubocurarine and 2·25–2·5 mg of decamethonium are required to produce the same effect. A dose of 100–140 mg of gallamine leads to total cessation of respiration.

Duration of action.—This is between 20 and 35 minutes and therefore on a comparative basis is slightly shorter than that of d-tubocurarine (30–50 minutes).

Antagonists

Both neostigmine and edrophonium oppose the action of gallamine triethiodide in a similar manner to that described for d-tubocurarine.

PANCURONIUM BROMIDE (PAVULON)

History

Whilst investigating a series of amino-steroids, Hewitt and Savage in 1964 observed that when two acetylcholine-like groups were added to the steroid ring neuromuscular blocking agents were obtained. One such compound—pancuronium bromide—appeared to be a very effective neuromuscular blocking agent without evidence of steroid activity, and the pharmacology has been extensively studied in animals (Buckett and Bonta, 1966; Buckett et al., 1968). It was introduced into clinical anaesthesia by Baird and Reid in 1967, and is now widely used throughout Europe and the U.S.A.

Physical and Chemical Properties

Pancuronium bromide is chemically 3β, 16β-dipiperidine-5α-androstane-3α, 17β-diol diacetate dimethobromide with the following structural formula:

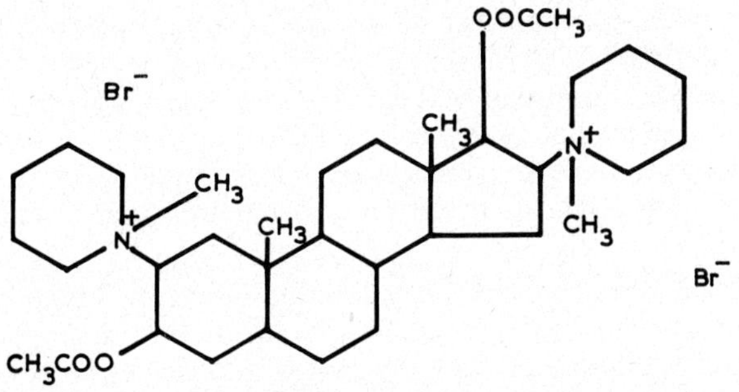

It is an odourless, white crystalline powder with a bitter taste, which melts at 215° C with decomposition. Pancuronium is a bis-quaternary ammonium salt which is relatively stable and is supplied for clinical purposes in 2 ml ampoules containing 2 mg/ml.

Pharmacological Action

Mode of action.—Pancuronium acts at the neuromuscular junction in man by non-depolarisation (Baird and Reid, 1967) and has no steroidal activity.

Cardiovascular system.—Pancuronium has little effect on the cardiovascular system. There is little change in pulse rate in doses less than 0·06 mg/kg although some vagolytic activity occurs at higher dose levels. The absence of hypotension (compared with *d*-tubocurarine) is particularly noticeable (Baird, 1968; Crul, 1970; Sellick, 1970; McDowall and Clarke, 1969). It has even been suggested that pancuronium may tend to produce an increase in blood pressure by sympathetic stimulation, especially in the presence of autonomic irritability. Seed (1976) has produced evidence of a direct but short-lived inotropic effect of pancuronium upon the intact heart. Evidence has been presented that indicates some increase in peripheral resistance following the administration of pancuronium. Because of the absence of hypotension this drug is preferred by many anaesthetists for patients with cardiovascular instability and in those with possible low output states. Pancuronium (like *d*-tubocurarine) prevents the bradycardia and dysrhythmias produced by the second dose of suxamethonium in man (Mathias and Evans-Prosser, 1970).

Central nervous system.—Although there is no evidence available in man it is not believed to cross the blood-brain barrier. Like all the muscle relaxants it is a highly charged ion and is therefore unlikely to pass vital membranes easily. It possesses very little fat-solubility.

Liver and kidneys.—Pancuronium is principally excreted unchanged by the kidneys. Agoston *et al.* (1973) have demonstrated that in the cat about 20 per cent of a normal dose is taken up by the liver and excreted in the bile. The liver is capable of metabolising up to 30 per cent of the drug in experimental animals in whom the renal pedicles are ligated. Although there are quantitative differences in the way the human liver and kidney handle pancuronium, there is little doubt that significant but very variable amounts can be metabolised and excreted by extrarenal processes in the presence of anuria.

Histamine release.—A particular advantage claimed for pancuronium is the lack of histamine release. This is believed to account for the absence of both hypotension and bronchospasm following its use; however allergic reactions have been recorded.

Uterus and placental barrier.—No evidence is available in man but animal experiments suggest that in clinically effective amounts it does not cross the placental barrier. Wide experience with this drug in patients undergoing Caesarean section confirms that it has no apparent deleterious effect on the fetus.

Metabolism.—Pancuronium is believed to be excreted mainly unchanged in the urine but can be biodegraded to less active and inactive compounds by metabolism of the 3 and 17 acetyl groups of the parent compound (Agoston, 1975). Up to 15 per cent of an injected dose of pancuronium may be recovered from the urine as the 3-hydroxy derivative. In the absence of renal excretion large amounts of the drug can be recovered from the bile much in the form of steroids in which the 3 and/or 17 acetyl group has been hydrolysed to either the hydrogen or hydroxy derivative.

Method of Administration

The intravenous route is used although the drug is active following intramuscular injection.

Dosage.—Pancuronium has about five times the potency of d-tubocurarine. Therefore to produce apnoea a dose of 0·04 to 0·08 mg/kg will be required in the adult, and if it is used for endotracheal intubation then doses of 6–10 mg will be required to provide good conditions.

Duration of action.—The paresis produced by pancuronium lasts for about 25–40 minutes and a satisfactory "topping-up dose" is about $\frac{1}{5}$ to $\frac{1}{10}$ of the original paralysing dose. For simplicity, the duration of action of pancuronium could be described as lying midway between the shorter action of gallamine and the longer duration of d-tubocurarine.

Antagonists.—Pancuronium can be easily reversed by neostigmine in the usual manner. Pancuronium is a weak inhibitor of plasma cholinesterase, but some of its metabolic derivatives are more active in this respect. Caution should be exercised if suxamethonium were to be used for the closing stages of an operation in which pancuronium has been used.

MISCELLANEOUS GROUP OF MUSCLE RELAXANTS

The muscle relaxants in common clinical use are suxamethonium, d-tubocurarine, gallamine and pancuronium. There are others, apart from decamethonium, which enjoy popularity on a limited scale, and many more which have never seen the light of day outside the laboratory. For the latter the reader must search in a textbook of pharmacology. It is proposed here to describe briefly some of the principal points about a miscellaneous selection of relaxants which have been or still are being used in clinical practice.

Dimethyl Ether of d-Tubocurarine (DME; Metocurine)

History.—This preparation was first described as a methylated derivative of d-tubocurarine by King in 1935. It was not until several years later, however, that Collier (1950) described its pharmacological actions in animals. Soon afterwards Wilson and his associates (1950) reported on its use in man.

DME is a substance with a melting point of 236° C. It is commercially available as the chloride or iodide salt and can be mixed with thiopentone. It has recently been reintroduced commercially in the U.S.A.

Mode of action.—This is similar to that of d-tubocurarine.

General properties.—Dimethyl tubocurarine is administered intravenously, and as it is 2–2$\frac{1}{2}$ times as potent as d-tubocurarine, 4 mg of it are sufficient to produce relaxation of the limb muscles. A dose of 8–10 mg leads to total paralysis of all muscles including those of respiration. The duration of action is believed to be slightly shorter than that of d-tubocurarine, and it is also claimed to have less effect on the autonomic ganglia and to release less histamine (Collier, 1950). Its neuromuscular blocking activity is rapidly reversed by neostigmine and edrophonium. It has less effect upon the cardiovascular system in cats than d-tubocurarine (Hughes, 1974). However, it can cause hypotension in patients with quite moderate doses of the drug, and it has been demonstrated to reduce myocardial contractility in patients with cardiac disease.

Despite these possible advantages dimethyl tubocurarine has never gained wide popularity in clinical practice (it has recently been reintroduced under the trade name, Metocurine). The principal reason for this is that it possesses no obvious advantages over *d*-tubocurarine. Moreover, Mogey and Trevan (1950) have pointed out that its molecule is so complex that it is difficult to be certain that all batches of the drug possess identical activity.

OTHER STEROID RELAXANTS

By modifying the side chains of the steroid nucleus a series of muscle relaxants of different properties have been produced. Two of these, NB. 68 and ORG 6368, have been tested in man.

NB. 68 (Dacuronium)

This has an hydroxyl group replacing the 17-acetyl group of pancuronium. It is one of the naturally occurring breakdown products of that drug. NB. 68 is a non-depolarising neuromuscular blocking agent that resembles gallamine both in potency and duration of action. It also shares gallamine's vagolytic activity in clinical doses (Feldman and Tyrrell, 1970).

ORG 6368

This is a non-depolarising relaxant that is of slightly shorter duration of action than pancuronium. Its potency is about 40 per cent that of pancuronium and it only produces tachycardia in large doses. It has the interesting and potentially useful property of having 40 per cent of an injected dose cleared from the blood during its passage through the liver in animals (Agoston, 1975). This should reduce the cumulative effect and make reversal of the drug by an anticholinesterase, much easier and safer.

Fazadinium Bromide (Fazadon; AH 8165)

Fazadinium bromide is an azo bis-arylimidazo-pyridinium compound of yellow colouration. It produces a non-depolarising neuromuscular block in man of about 30 minutes duration. It is claimed to be particularly rapid in onset (Simpson *et al.*, 1972). However, the speed of onset appears to be related to the dose administered. The dose requirements vary between 0·5 mg/kg and 0·8 mg/kg. Fazadinium does not cause hypotension, indeed it may reverse the fall in cardiac output produced by halothane (Savege *et al.*, 1973). In clinical doses it produces marked vagal blockade. In cats, almost complete vagal blockade occurs at a dose of drug that induces 80 per cent inhibition of twitch height, an effect even more marked than that observed with gallamine (Hughes, 1974). The inability of neostigmine to completely reverse the activity of fazadinium in the rat-phrenic nerve diaphragm preparation and its tonic effect upon the chick neck muscle have led Hiser *et al.* (1975) to suggest that fazadinium may have some depolarising action, prior to onset of non-depolarising block. In this respect it is interesting to note that the distance between the quaternary ammonium groups in fazadinium is about 7Å (0·7 nm), making it structurally more like acetylcholine than curare.

Diallyl-nor-Toxiferine; Alcuronium (Alloferin)

This compound is a derivation of C-Toxiferine I and was introduced into clinical anaesthesia by Hugin and Kissling (1961). It has twice the potency of *d*-tubocurarine and the same duration of action. The original claim that it did not produce a fall in systemic pressure has been discounted, although the degree of sympathetic block produced by an effective dose of alcuronium is less than with curare. The drug has been widely used for some ten years, 10–15 mg producing complete paralysis in most patients.

CLINICAL USE OF THE NEUROMUSCULAR BLOCKING DRUGS

Indications for a Relaxant

The specific indications for a muscle relaxant in anaesthesia fall into three categories:

1. To relax the muscles for surgical access, and for anaesthetic and investigational procedures.
2. To facilitate the control of respiration.
3. To limit the amount of general anaesthetic when relaxation itself is not the prime requisite.

The first two of these are self-explanatory and, together with suggestions for the choice of relaxant, they receive more detailed discussion in the various clinical sections of the text where anaesthetic procedure is mentioned. The third, although to some extent part of the other two, needs amplification. By dividing anaesthesia into the three components of narcosis, analgesia and muscle relaxation (Gray, 1954), an attempt can be made to control reflex activity on a more specific basis than can be done with a single anaesthetic agent, and particular drugs chosen to block each subdivision. But—haemorrhage and chemical depression apart—our knowledge of the basic cause of deterioration in the condition of a patient during surgery is so incomplete that such a simple division is no more than a suggested guide. Indeed clinical opinion is divided between those anaesthetists who consider that provided the patient is unconscious, and all motor response to surgical stimuli abolished by adequate paralysis, nothing is to be gained by adding other agents, and those who argue that in such a state, deeper anaesthesia or analgesia may be needed to suppress sensory or autonomic activity. Few anaesthetists, however, doubt that the judicious use of a muscle relaxant can avoid most of the detrimental effects of excessive chemical depression by diminishing the need for deep anaesthesia.

However, the "purist" school of nitrous oxide, oxygen and relaxant anaesthesia has lost ground in recent years as it has become increasingly apparent that judicious supplements of narcotics or volatile anaesthetics can greatly lessen the dose requirements of muscle relaxants making reversal of their actions complete and safe at the end of the operation. Opinion still remains divided, however, between those who use very small doses of muscle relaxants to supplement full general anaesthesia, as in some centres in the USA, and the European method of using fully paralytic doses of muscle relaxants together with relatively light planes of general anaesthesia. Theoretical considerations of the two techniques are discussed by Feldman (1973).

Choice of Relaxant

Pancuronium has become the most widely used muscle relaxant in the

United Kingdom in the past five years. Suxamethonium and curare are still widely used whilst gallamine, alcuronium and decamethonium have become less popular. Personal preference, suitably modified by experience and a knowledge of the pharmacology of each drug, must be the final arbiter when making a choice. However, as a general rule a short-acting relaxant is used for short procedures and a long-acting one for those lasting more than 30 minutes. For this reason suxamethonium is principally used for intubation of the trachea, endoscopies, electro-convulsive therapy, and the setting of fractures. In more prolonged operations the choice will very often depend on whether halothane is to be the principal anaesthetic agent or not. If it is, then the vagal-blocking activity of gallamine makes this drug a particularly suitable choice. On the other hand, if bleeding during the operation is a major consideration then the mild hypotension produced by the combination of halothane and d-tubocurarine may make this selection preferable. In cardiac surgery, renal disease and poor-risk cases pancuronium is very often selected because it is the drug least likely to lower the blood pressure or change cardiac rate.

In recent years, d-tubocurarine has largely replaced suxamethonium in paediatric anaesthesia because it has been found reliable, easily reversible, and avoids the complications of possibly overloading the circulation with a continuous infusion or obtaining a Phase II block (see p. 843).

Suxamethonium has certain well-known disadvantages, namely potassium ion shift causing cardiac dysrhythmias or arrest, severe muscle pains in ambulant patients, the raising of intra-ocular pressure and the alteration of cardiac rate and rhythm in hypertensive patients or in those receiving multiple doses. All these disadvantages can be modified or minimised if a small dose of a non-depolarising drug (e.g. 3 mg d-tubocurarine) is given 1–2 minutes before the suxamethonium. Because these two drugs are antagonistic, it is necessary to increase the dose of suxamethonium slightly (e.g. 1·5 mg/kg instead of 1 mg/kg) in order to achieve the same degree and duration of paralysis.

Although the search for the ideal relaxant continues, and in spite of the very real dangers and disadvantages of suxamethonium, it is extremely rare for a patient's life to be jeopardised by the use of these agents as their therapeutic ratio is very large provided adequate artificial ventilation is maintained. It would seem that anaesthetists need to be more flexible in the choice of relaxant and the way in which it is used, so as to select the drug therapy best suited to the requirements of the surgery and the safety of the patient.

Mixing of Relaxants

Theoretical considerations suggest that it is unwise to use drugs of differing actions at the neuromuscular junction on the same patient on the same occasion, and there is some practical support for this view as evidenced in the number of bizarre and occasionally long-lasting sequelae following the practice reported in the literature. Yet accumulated clinical experience lends support to the contention that with a proper appreciation of the risks involved and avoidance of certain pitfalls (see below), drugs such as suxamethonium and d-tubocurarine can be given with safety to the same patient for a single operation. Needless to say, this practice should not be adopted unless it has a sound clinical indication. For example, it may be desirable to produce total paralysis with suxamethonium, so that the best possible conditions are achieved for intubation of the trachea, and yet to obtain relaxation throughout the subsequent operation with *d*-tubo-curarine. Provided the effects of the suxamethonium—as judged clinically from respiratory activity or as demonstrated with a peripheral nerve stimulator—have worn off, there does not seem to be any good reason for supposing that the administration of *d*-tubocurarine will now lead to an abnormal response. The theoretical argument that following a single dose of suxamethonium the neuromuscular junction remains abnormal for a far longer period than is suggested by the clinical state of the patient, does not in our view prejudice this practice. The use of suxamethonium at the termination of an operation to secure full relaxation, say for peritoneal closure, and following a non-depolarising agent, is more problematical. The precise manner in which the motor end-plate responds to suxamethonium under these conditions is unknown. To some extent it may act as an antidote to the residue of the non-depolarising drug, and this action would be helpful. On the other hand, it is equally possible that it might enhance the underlying non-depolarisation block if an excessive dose is administered. A danger arises later when the operation is completed and evidence of muscle paralysis remains. Neostigmine can now only be adminis-tered with safety provided the suxamethonium and its breakdown products are ineffective; if they are not, there will be a real risk of prolonged paralysis or paresis.

Complications Following the Use of Relaxants

Major complications caused by muscle relaxants are more often than not due to their misuse rather than to any peculiarity in their action. The side-effects of both *d*-tubocurarine and gallamine, however, must be remembered since these may be responsible for some complications in unduly sensitive or physically handicapped patients. Inadequate ventilation, residual paralysis sufficient to enhance or cause difficulty with the airway, and the removal or depression of protective glottic reflexes in the presence of foreign material are the principal causes of mortality and morbidity. The bizarre and occasionally prolonged periods of apnoea that follow the use of relaxants, or injudicious mixtures of them with or without an antidote, should not of themselves lead to death unless artificial respiration is inadequately carried out, or the patient is already moribund.

Patients who have received a relative overdose of muscle relaxant may benefit from the expansion of their extracellular fluid (the drug distribution volume) and also from the promotion of a diuresis. The rationale behind this treatment is that it lowers the plasma drug concentration and promotes excretion by the kidney.

Regional Use of Muscle Relaxants

In selected cases requiring limb surgery, muscle paresis has been achieved by injecting the relaxant intravenously after a tourniquet has been applied (Torda and Klonymus, 1966). The recommended doses and dilutions are given below:

	Volume of Diluent (ml)	Dose (mg) d-Tubocurarine	Gallamine	Suxamethonium
Upper limb	30	1·5	10·0	4·0
Lower limb	50	3·0	20·0	6·0

A similar technique using smaller doses has been advocated as a test for myasthenia gravis (Foldes, 1970).

REFERENCES

AGOSTON, S. (1975). Pharmakokinetics of the steroid muscle relaxants. In: *Anaesthesia and Pharmacology* (Proc. Boerhaave Course). Leiden: Univ. of Leiden Press.

AGOSTON, S., KERSTEN, U. W., and MEIJER, D. F. K. (1973). The fate of pancuronium in the cat. *Acta anaesth. scand.*, **17,** 129.

ALI, H. H., WILSON, R. S., SAVARESE, J. J., and KITZ, R. J. (1975). The effect of tubocurarine on indirectly elicited train-of-four muscle response and respiratory measurements in humans. *Brit. J. Anaesth.*, **47,** 570.

BAIRD, W. L. M. (1968). Some clinical experiences with a new neuromuscular blocking drug—pancuronium bromide (Pavulon NA97). *Irish J. Med.*, 7th series, **1.** 559.

BAIRD, W. L. M., and REID, A. M. (1967). The neuromuscular blocking properties of a new steroid compound, pancuronium bromide. *Brit. J. Anaesth.*, **39,** 775.

BARAKA, A. (1977). Self-taming of succinylcholine-induced fasciculations. *Anesthesiology*, **46,** 292.

BARLOW, R. B., and ING, H. R. (1948). Curare-like action of polymethylene bis quaternary ammonium salts. *Nature (Lond.)*, **161,** 718.

BELIN, R. P., and KARLEEN, C. I. (1966). Cardiac arrest in the burned patient following succinyldicholine administration. *Anesthesiology*, **27,** 516.

BENNET, A. E., MCINTYRE, A. R., and BENNETT, A. L. (1940). Pharmacologic and clinical investigations with crude curare. *J. Amer. med. Ass.*, **114,,** 1791.

BENVENISTE, D., and DYRBERG, V. (1962). Tetrahydroaminoacridine. Clinical use of a cholinesterase inhibitor in conjunction with succinylcholine. *Acta anaesth. scand.*, **6,** 1.

BIRCH, A. A., MITCHELL, G. D., PLAYFORD, G. A., and LANG, C. A. (1969). Changes in serum potassium response to succinylcholine following trauma. *J. Amer. med. Ass.*, **210,** 490.

BOEHM, R. (1886). *Chemische Studien über das Curare.* Leipzig.

BOEHM, R. (1895). Das sudamerikanische Pfeilgift. *Abhandl. d. kgl. sachs. Gesselsch. d. Wiss.*, **22,** 199.

BOEHM, R. (1897). Ueber Curare und Curare Alkaloide. *Arch. d. Pharmakol.*, **235,** 660.

BONO, F., and MAPELLI, A. (1960). The effect of d-tubocurarine chloride on arterial pressure during general anaesthesia. *Minerva anest.*, **26,** 29.

BOURNE, J. G., COLLIER, H. O. J., and SOMERS, G. F. (1952). Succinylcholine (succinoylcholine) muscle-relaxant of short action. *Lancet*, **1,** 1225.

BOVET, D. (1951). Some aspects of the relationship between chemical constitution and curare-like activity. *Ann. N.Y. Acad. Sci.*, **54,** 407.

BOVET, D., BOVET-NITTI, F., GUARINO, S., LONGO, V. G., and MAROTTA, M. (1949). Proprieta farmacodinamiche di alcuni derivati della succinilcolina dotati di azione curarica. *R.C. Ist. sup. Sanità*, **12,** 106.

BOVET, D., DEPIERRE, F., and DE LESTRANGE, Y. (1947). Propriétés curarisantes des éthers phénoliques à fonctions ammonium quaternaires. *C.R. Acad. Sci. (Paris)*, **225,** 74.

BOVET-NITTI, F. (1949). Degradazione di Alcune sostanze curanzzanti per Azione di Colinesterasi. *R.C. Ist. sup. Sanità*, **12,** 138.

BRENNAN, H. J. (1956). Dual action of suxamethonium chloride. *Brit. J. Anaesth.*, **28**, 159.

BRIDENBAUGH, P. O., and CHURCHILL-DAVIDSON, H. C. (1968). Response to tubocurarine chloride and its reversal by neostigmine methylsulfate in man. *J. Amer. med. Ass.*, **203**, 541.

BRODIE, B. C. (1851). "Physiological Researches". Note C. p. 142. Quoted in: *Curare: Its History and Usage*, p. 34, by K. Bryn Thomas. London: Pitman Medical Publishing Co.

BROOKS, D. K., and FELDMAN, S. A. (1962). Metabolic acidosis—a new approach to neostigmine resistant curarisation. *Anaesthesia*, **17**, 161.

BRÜCKE, H., GINZEL, K. H., KLUPP, H., PFAFFENSCHLAGER, F., and WERNER, G. (1951). Bis-cholinester von Dicarbonsäuren als Muskelrelaxantien in der Narkose. *Wien. klin. Wschr.*, **63**, 464.

BUCKETT, W. R., and BONTA, I. L. (1966). Pharmacological studies with NA97 (2β, 16β Dipiperidine-5α-androstane-3α, 17β-diol diecetate dimethobromide). *Fed. Proc.*, **25**, 718.

BUCKETT, W. R., MARJORIBANKS, C. E. B., MARWICK, F. A., and MORTON, M. B. (1968). The pharmacology of pancuronium bromide (Org. NA–97), a new potent steroidal neuromuscular blocking agent. *Brit. J. Pharmacol.*, **32**, 671.

BULLER, A. J., and YOUNG, I. M. (1949). The action of *d*-tubocurarine chloride on foetal neuromuscular transmission and the placental transfer of this drug in the rabbit. *J. Physiol. (Lond.)*, **109**, 412.

BULLOUGH, J. (1959). Intermittent suxamethonium injections. *Brit. med. J.*, **1**, 786.

BUSH, G. H., and ROTH, F. (1961). Muscle pains after suxamethonium chloride in children. *Brit. J. Anaesth.*, **33**, 151.

CASTILLO, J. C., and DE BEER, E. J. (1950). Neuromuscular blocking action of succinylcholine (Diacetylcholine). *J. Pharmacol. exp. Ther.*, **97**, 458.

CHURCHILL-DAVIDSON, H. C. (1954). Suxamethonium (succinylcholine) and muscle pains. *Brit. med. J.*, **1**, 74.

CHURCHILL-DAVIDSON, H. C. (1961). The changing pattern of neuromuscular block. *Canad. Anaesth. Soc. J.*, **8**, 91.

CHURCHILL-DAVIDSON, H. C., and GRIFFITHS, W. J. (1961). Simple test-paper method for for the clinical determination of plasma pseudocholinesterase. *Brit. med. J.*, **2**, 994.

CHURCHILL-DAVIDSON, H. C., and RICHARDSON, A. T. (1953). Neuromuscular transmission in myasthenia gravis. *J. Physiol. (Lond.)*, **122**, 252.

CHURCHILL-DAVIDSON, H. C., WAY, W. L., and DE JONG, R. H. (1967). The muscle relaxants and renal excretion. *Anesthesiology*, **28**, 540.

COHEN, E. N., BREWER, H. W., and SMITH, D. (1967). The metabolism and elimination of *d*-tubocurarine-H[3]. *Anesthesiology*, **28**, 309.

COHEN, E. N., HOOD, N., and GOLLING, R. (1968). Use of whole-body autoradiography for determination of uptake and distribution of labeled muscle relaxants in the rat. *Anesthesiology*, **29**, 987.

COHEN, E. N., PAULSON, W. J., WALL, J., and ELERT, B. (1953). Thiopental, curare, and nitrous oxide anesthesia for Cesarian section with studies on placental transmission. *Surg. Gynec. Obstet.*, **97**, 456.

COLLIER, H. O. J. (1950). Pharmacology of D-O, O-Dimethyl tubocurarine iodide in relation to its clinical use. *Brit. med. J.*, **1**, 1293.

COURVOISIER, S., and DUCROT, R. (1948). Sur l'effet histaminoide de la *d*-tubocurarine et des curares de synthèse. *C.R. Soc. Biol. (Paris)*, **142**, 1209.

CRAWFORD, J. S. (1956). Some aspects of obstetric anaesthesia. *Brit. J. Anaesth*, **28**, 146.

CRAWFORD, J. S., and GARDINER, J. E. (1956). Some aspects of obstetric anaesthesia. The use of relaxant drugs. *Brit. J. Anaesth.*, **28**, 154.

CRUL, J. F. (1970). Studies on new steroid relaxants. *Progress in Anaesthesiology* (Proc. 4th World Congr. Anaesthesiol., Sept. 1968). Amsterdam: Excerpta Medica.

DAL SANTO, G. (1968). Kinetics of distribution of radio-active labelled relaxants III. *Anesthesiology*, **29**, 435.

DAVIES, J. I. (1956). Untoward reactions to succinylcholine. *Canad. Anaesth. Soc. J.*, **3**, 11.

DILLON, J. B., SABAWALA, P., TAYLOR, D. B., and GUNTER, R. (1957). Action of succinyl-choline on extra-ocular muscles and intra-ocular pressure. *Anesthesiology*, **18**, 44.

DOENICKE, A., SCHMIDINGER, ST., and KRUMEY, I. (1968). Suxamethonium and serum cholinesterase. Comparative studies *in vitro* and *in vivo* on the catabolism of suxa-methonium. *Brit. J. Anaesth.*, **40**, 834.

DOUGHTY, A. G., and WYLIE, W. D. (1951). An assessment of Flaxedil (gallamine tri-ethiodide, B.P.). *Proc. roy. Soc. Med.*, **44**, 375.

DOWDY, E. G., DUGGAR, P. N., and FABIAN, L. W. (1965). Effect of neuromuscular block-ing agents on isolated digitalised mammalian hearts. *Anesth. Analg. Curr. Res.*, **44**, 608.

DOWDY, E. G., and FABIAN, L. W. (1963). Ventricular arrhythmias induced by succinyl-choline in digitalised patients. *Anesth. Analg. Curr. Res.*, **42**, 501.

DRABKOVA, J., CRUL, J. K., and VAN DER KLEIJN, E. (1973). Placental transfer of C_{14}-labelled succinylcholine in near-term Macaca Mulatta monkeys. *Brit. J. Anaesth.*, **45**, 1087.

DRACHMAN, D. B., and COULOMBRE, A. J. (1962). Experimental clubfoot and arthrogryposis multiplex congenita. *Lancet*, **2**, 523.

DUNDEE, J. W., and GRAY, T. C. (1953). Resistance to *d*-tubocurarine chloride in the presence of liver damage. *Lancet*, **2**, 16.

DUTCHER, J. (1951). Curare and anti-curare drugs. *Ann. N.Y. Acad. Sci.*, **54**, 326.

ELERT, B. (1956). A new ultraviolet spectrophotometric method for the determination of *d*-tubocurarine chloride in plasma. *Amer. J. med. Technol.*, **22**, 331.

ELERT, B. T., and COHEN, E. N. (1962). A micro spectrophotometric method for the analysis of minute concentrations of *d*-tubocurarine chloride in plasma. *Amer. J. med. Technol.*, **28**, 125.

ELLIS, C. H., NORTON, S., and MORGAN, W. V. (1952). Central depression by drugs which block neuromuscular transmission. *Fed. Proc.*, **11**, 42.

EVERETT, A. J., LOWE, L. A., and WILKINSON, S. (1970). Revision of the structure of (+) tubocurarine and (+) chondrocurarine. *Chem. Communications*, **16**, 1020.

FAIRLEY, H. B. (1950). Prolonged intercostal paralysis due to a relaxant. *Brit. med. J.*, **2**, 986.

FELDMAN, S. A. (1973). *Muscle Relaxants*, p. 150. London: W. B. Saunders Co.

FELDMAN, S. A., COHEN, E. N., and GOLLING, R. C. (1969). The excretion of gallamine in the dog. *Anesthesiology*, **30**, 593.

FELDMAN, S. A., and LEVI, J. A. (1963). Prolonged paresis following gallamine. *Brit. J. Anaesth.*, **35**, 804.

FELDMAN, S. A., and TYRRELL, M. F. (1970). N.B. 68. A new steroid muscle relaxant. *Anaesthesia*, **25**, 349.

FELLINI, A. A., BERNSTEIN, R. L., and ZAUDER, H. L. (1963). Bronchospasm due to suxa-methonium. *Brit. J. Anaesth.*, **35**, 657.

FOLDES, F. F. (1970). Regional intravenous neuromuscular block: a new diagnostic and experimental tool. *Progress in Anaesthesiology* (Proc. 4th World Congr. Anaesthesiol., Sept. 1968). Amsterdam: Excerpta Medica.

FOLDES, F. F., MCNALL, P. G., and BIRCH, J. H. (1954). The neuromuscular activity of succinylmonocholine iodide in anaesthetized man. *Brit. med. J.*, **1**, 967.

FOLDES, F. F., MCNALL, P. G., and BORREGO-HINOJOSA, J. M. (1952). Succinylcholine: a new approach to muscular relaxation in anesthesiology. *New Engl. J. Med.*, **247**, 596.

FOLDES, F. F., MOLLOY, R. E., ZSIGMOND, E. K., and ZWARTZ, J. A. (1960). Hexafluore-nium: its anti-cholinesterase and neuromuscular activity. *J. Pharmacol. exp. Ther.*, **129**, 400.

FOLDES, F. F., and NORTON, S. (1954). The urinary excretion of succinyldicholine and succinylmonocholine in man. *Brit. J. Pharmacol.*, **9**, 385.

FOLKERS, K., and MAJOR, R. T. (1937). Isolation of erythroidine, an alkaloid of curare action. *J. Amer. chem. Soc.*, **59**, 1580.

FOSTER, C. A. (1960). Muscle pains that follow administration of suxamethonium. *Brit. med. J.*, **2**, 24.

GISSEN, A. J., KATZ, R. L., KARIS, J. H., and PAPPER, E. M. (1966). Neuromuscular block in man during prolonged arterial infusion with succinylcholine. *Anesthesiology*, **27**, 242.

GISSEN, A. J., and NASTUK, W. L. (1968). The mechanism of action of decamethonium. *Anesthesiology*, **29**, 197.

GLICK, D. (1941). Some additional observations on specificity of cholinesterase. *J. biol. Chem.*, **137**, 357.

GOAT, V. A., and FELDMAN, S. A. (1972a). The effect of non-depolarising muscle relaxants on cholinergic mechanisms in the isolated rabbit heart. *Anaesthesia*, **27**, 143.

GOAT, V. A., and FELDMAN, S. A. (1972b). The dual action of suxamethonium on the isolated rabbit heart. *Anaesthesia*, **27**, 149.

GORDH, T., and WAHLIN, A. (1961). Potentiation of the neuromuscular effect of succinylcholine by tetrahydro-amino-acridine. *Acta anaesth. scand.*, **5**, 55.

GRAY, T. C. (1954). Disintegration of the nervous system. *Ann. roy. Coll. Surg. Engl.*, **15**, 402.

GRAY, T. C., and HALTON, J. (1946). A milestone in anaesthesia? (*d*-tubocurarine chloride). *Proc. roy. Soc. Med.*, **39**, 400.

GREENWAY, R. M., and QUASTEL, J. H. (1955). Hydrolysis of succinylmonocholine by liver esterase. *Proc. Soc. exp. Biol.* (*N.Y.*), **90**, 72.

GRIFFITH, H. R., and JOHNSON, G. E. (1942). The use of curare in general anesthesia. *Anesthesiology*, **3**, 418.

GRONERT, G. A., and THEYE, R. A. (1975). Pathophysiology of hyperkalemia induced by succinylcholine. *Anesthesiology*, **43**, 89.

HANNINGTON-KIFF, J. G. (1970). Residual post-operative paralysis. *Proc. roy. Soc. Med.*, **63**, 73.

HARRIS, H., HOPKINSON, D. A., ROBSON, E. B., and WHITTAKER, M. (1963). Genetical studies on a new variant of serum cholinesterase detected by electrophoresis. *Ann. hum. Genet.*, **26**, 359.

HARRIS, H., and WHITTAKER, M. (1961). Differential inhibition of human serum cholinesterase with fluoride: recognition of two new phenotypes. *Nature* (*Lond.*), **191**, 496.

HARRIS, H., and WHITTAKER, M. (1962a). The serum cholinesterase variants. A study of 22 families selected via the intermediate phenotype. *Ann. hum. Genet.*, **26**, 59.

HARRIS, H., and WHITTAKER, M. (1962b). Differential inhibition of the serum cholinesterase phenotypes by solanine and solanidine. *Ann. hum. Genet.*, **26**, 73.

HARROUN, P., BECKERT, F., and FISHER, C. W. (1947). The physiologic effects of curare and its use as adjunct to anesthesia. *Surg. Gynec. Obstet.*, **84**, 491.

HARROUN, P., and FISHER, C. W. (1949). The physiological effects of curare, its failure to pass the placental membrane or inhibit uterine contractions. *Surg. Gynec. Obstet.*, **89**, 73.

HESS, A., and PILAR, G. (1963). Slow fibres in the extraocular muscles of the cat. *J. Physiol.* (*Lond.*), **169**, 780.

HEWETT, C. L., SAVAGE, D. S., LEWIS, J. J., and SUGRUE, M. F. (1964). Anticonvulsant and interneuronal blocking activity in some synthetic amino-steroids. *J. Pharm., Pharmacol.*, **16**, 765.

HISER, P. T., DRETCHEN, K. L., and KUGER, G. O. (1975). *In-vitro* investigation of a new neuromuscular relaxant AH.8165. *Anesthesiology*, **42**, 245.

HOROWITZ, P. E., and SPECTOR, S. (1973). Determination of serum *d*-tubocurarine concentration by radio-immunoassay. *J. Pharmacol. exp. Ther.*, **185**, 94.

HUGHES, R. (1974). Pharmacological concepts. Paper presented at *Symposium on Muscle Relaxants at IV European Congress, Madrid*, 1974.

HUGIN, W., and KISSLING, P. (1961). Preliminary reports on a new short-acting relaxant of the depolarisation-inhibiting type, Ro 4–38161. *Schweiz. med. Wschr.*, **91**, 445.

HUGUENARD, P., and BOUÉ, A. (1948). Un nouvel ortho-curare français de synthèse, le 3697 R.P. *Rapport à la Soc. d'Anesthésie de Paris*, Seance du 17.

HUNT, R., and TAVEAU, R. (1906), On physiological action of certain choline derivatives and new methods for detecting choline. *Brit. med. J.*, **2**, 1788.

HUNTER, A. R. (1956). Neostigmine resistant curarization. *Brit. med. J.*, **2**, 919.

HUNTER, A. R. (1966). Suxamethonium apnoea. *Anaesthesia*, **21**, 325.

IWATSUKI, K., YUAS, T., and KATAOKA, Y. (1965). Effects of muscle relaxants on ventricular contractile force in dogs. *Tohoku J. exp. Med.*, **86**, 93.

JERUM, G., WHITTINGHAM, S., and WILSON, P. (1967). Anaphylaxis to suxamethonium. *Brit. J. Anaesth.*, **39**, 73.

KALOW, W. (1959). The distribution, destruction and elimination of muscle relaxants. *Anesthesiology*, **20**, 505.

KALOW, W. (1964). Pharmacogenetics and anesthesia. *Anesthesiology*, **25**, 377.

KALOW, W., and DAVIES, R. O. (1958). The activity of various esterase inhibitors towards atypical human serum cholinesterase. *Biochem. Pharmacol.*, **1**, 183.

KALOW, W., and GENEST, K. (1957). A method for the detection of atypical forms of human serum cholinesterase; determination of dibucaine numbers. *Canad. J. Biochem.*, **35**, 339.

KATZ, R. L. (1966). Neuromuscular effects of diethyl ether and its interaction with succinylcholine and *d*-tubocurarine. *Anesthesiology*, **27**, 52.

KATZ, R. L., and EAKINS, K. E. (1969). The actions of neuromuscular blocking agents on extraocular muscle and intraocular pressure. *Proc. roy. Soc. Med.*, **62**, 1217.

KATZ, R. L., and GISSEN, A. J. (1967). Neuromuscular and electromyographic effects of halothane and its interaction with *d*-tubocurarine in man. *Anesthesiology*, **28**, 564.

KATZ, R. L., WOLF, C. E., and PAPPER, E. M. (1963). The nondepolarizing neuromuscular blocking action of succinylcholine in man. *Anesthesiology*, **24**, 784.

KENNEDY, B. R., and FARMAN, J. V. (1968). Cardiovascular effects of gallamine triethiodide in man. *Brit. J. Anaesth.* **40**, 773.

KING, H. (1935). Curare. *Nature (Lond.)*, **135**, 469.

KING, K. (1949). Curare alkaloids. X. Some alkaloids of *strychnos toxifera*. *J. chem. Soc.*, **4**, 3263.

KUHNE, W. (1862). *Uber die peripherischen Endergon der motorischen Nerven*. Leipzig: Engelmann.

KVISSELGAARD, N., and MOYA, F. (1961). Estimation of succinylcholine blood levels. *Acta anaesth. scand.*, **5**, 1.

LAMOREAUX, L. R., and URBACH, K. F. (1960). Incidence and prevention of muscle pain following the administration of succinylcholine. *Anesthesiology*, **21**, 394.

LEHMANN, H. (1962). Personal communication.

LEIGH, M. D., McCOY, D. D., BELTON, M. K., and LEWIS, G. B. (1957). Bradycardia following intravenous administration of succinylcholine chloride to infants and children. *Anesthesiology*, **18**, 698.

LIDDELL, J., LEHMANN, H., and SILK, E. (1962). A silent pseudocholinesterase gene. *Nature (Lond.)*, **193**, 561.

LINCOFF, H. A., BREININ, G. M., and DE VOE, A. G. (1957). The effect of succinylcholine on the extraocular muscles. *Amer. J. Ophthal.*, **43**, 440.

LUPPRIAN, K. G., and CHURCHILL-DAVIDSON, H. C. (1960). Effect of suxamethonium on cardiac rhythm. *Brit. med. J.*, **2**, 1774.

McCaul, K., and Robinson, G. D. (1962). Suxamethonium "extension" by tetrahydro-aminoacrine. *Brit. J. Anaesth.*, **34,** 536.

McDowall, S. A., and Clarke, R. S. J. (1969). A clinical comparison of pancuronium with *d*-tubocurarine. *Anaesthesia*, **24,** 581.

Martin, H. V. (1958). Paper read at an International Symposium in Venice on Curare and Curare-like Drugs.

Mathias, J. A., and Evans-Prosser, C. D. G. (1970). An investigation into the site of action of suxamethonium on cardiac rhythm. *Progress in Anaesthesiology* (Proc. 4th World Congr. Anaesthesiol., Sept. 1968). Amsterdam: Excerpta Medica.

Mattes, R. S., Pua, E. K., Khambatta, H. J., and Spector, S. (1977). Cerebrospinal fluid levels of *d*-tubocurarine in man. *Anesthesiology*, **46,** 396.

Mayrhofer, O., and Hassfurther, M. (1951). Kurzwirkende Muskelerschlaffungsmittel. *Wien. klin. Wschr.*, **47,** 885.

Miller, R. D., and Way, W. L. (1971). The interaction between succinylcholine and sub-paralyzing doses of *d*-tubocurarine and gallamine in man. *Anesthesiology*, **35,** 567.

Miller, R. D., Way, W. L., Hamilton, W. K., and Layzer, R. B. (1972). Succinylcholine induced hyperkalaemia in patients with renal failure? *Anesthesiology*, **36,** 138.

Miller, R. D., Way, W. L., and Hickey, R. F. (1968). Inhibition of succinylcholine-induced increased intra-ocular pressure by non-depolarising muscle relaxants. *Anesthesiology*, **29,** 123.

Mogey, G. A., and Trevan, D. W. (1950). *D*-tubocurarine salts and derivatives. *Brit. med. J.*, **2,** 216.

Mongar, J. L., and Whelan, R. F. (1953). Histamine release by adrenaline and *d*-tubocurarine in the human subject. *J. Physiol. (Lond.)*, **120,** 146.

Montgomery, J. B., and Bennett-Jones, N. (1956). Gallamine triethiodide and renal disease. *Lancet*, **2,** 1243.

Morris, D. D. B., and Dunn, C. H. (1957). Suxamethonium chloride administration and post-operative muscle pain. *Brit. med. J.*, **1,** 383.

Moya, F., and Margolies, A. B. (1961). Hydrolysis of succinylcholine by placental homogenates. *Anesthesiology*, **22,** 11.

Mushin, W. W., Wien, R., Mason, D. F. J., and Langston, G. T. (1949). Curare-like actions of tri-(diethylaminoethoxy)-benzine triethyliodide. *Lancet*, **1,** 726.

Organe, G. S. W., Paton, W. D. M., and Zaimis, E. J. (1949). Preliminary trial of bistri-methylammonium decane and pentane di-iodide (C.10 and C.5) in man. *Lancet*, **1,** 21.

Pantuck, E. J. (1967). Genetic aspect of neuromuscular blockade. In: *Advances in Anesthesiology: Muscle Relaxants*, Chap. 5, p. 63. New York: Hoeber.

Paton, W. D. M. (1959). The effects of muscle relaxants other than muscular relaxation. *Anesthesiology*, **20,** 453.

Paton, W. D. M., and Perry, W. L. M. (1951). The pharmacology of the toxiferenes. *Brit. J. Pharmacol.*, **6,** 299.

Paton, W. D. M., and Zaimis, E. J. (1948). Clinical potentialities of certain bisquaternary salts causing neuromuscular and ganglionic block. *Nature (Lond.)*, **162,** 810.

Paton, W. D. M., and Zaimis, E. J. (1949). The pharmacological actions of polymethylene bistrimethylammonium salts. *Brit. J. Pharmacol.*, **4,** 381.

Paton, W. D. M., and Zaimis, E. J. (1952). Methonium compounds. *Pharmacol. Rev.*, **4,** 219.

Phillips, A. P. (1949). Synthetic curare substitutes from aliphatic dicarboxylic acid amino-ethyl esters. *J. Amer. chem. Soc.*, **71,** 3264.

Prime, F. J., and Gray, T. C. (1952). The effect of certain anaesthetic and relaxant agents on circulatory dynamics. *Brit. J. Anaesth.*, **24,** 101.

Rack, P. M. H., and Westbury, D. R. (1966). The effect of suxamethonium and acetyl-choline on the behaviour of cat muscle spindles during dynamic stretching and during fusimotor stimulation. *J. Physiol (Lond.)*, **186,** 698.

RIKER, W. F., Jnr., and WESCOE, W. C. (1951). Pharmacology of Flaxedil, with observations on certain analogs. *Ann. N.Y. Acad. Sci.*, **54**, 373.

ROBERTSON, G. S. (1966). Serum cholinesterase deficiency. II. Pregnancy. *Brit. J. Anaesth.*, **38**, 361.

SALEM, M. R., KIM, Y., and EL ETR, A. A. (1968). Histamine release following intravenous injection of *d*-tubocurarine. *Anesthesiology*, **29**, 380.

SAVEGE, T. M., BLOGG, C. E., ROSS, L., LANG, M., and SIMPSON, B. R. (1973). The cardio-vascular effects of AH 8165. *Anaesthesia*, **28**, 253.

SCURR, C. F. (1951). A relaxant of very brief action. *Brit. med. J.*, **2**, 831.

SEED, R. (1976). Communication to the *VI World Congress of Anesthesiologists*, Mexico.

SELLICK, B. A. (1970). Clinical experience of a new muscle relaxant—pancuronium bromide. *Progress in Anaesthesiology* (Proc. 4th World Congr. Anaesthesiol., Sept. 1968). Amsterdam: Excerpta Medica.

SHNIDER, S. M. (1965). Serum cholinesterase activity during pregnancy, labour and the puerperium. *Anesthesiology*, **26**, 335.

SIMPSON, B. R., SAVEGE, T. M., and FOLEY, E. I. (1972). An azobis-arylimidazopyridinium derivative; a rapidly acting non-depolarizing muscle relaxant. *Lancet*, **1**, 516.

SMITH, N. L. (1957). Histamine release by suxamethonium. *Anaesthesia*, **12**, 293.

SNIPER, W. (1952). The estimation and comparison of histamine release by muscle relaxants in man. *Brit. J. Anaesth.*, **24**, 232.

SPÄTH, E., LEITHE, W., and LADECK, F. (1928). Curare alkaloids. I. Constitution of curine. *Ber. dtsch. chem. Ges.*, **61**, 1698.

STOVNER, J. (1976). Newer aspects of reversing neuromuscular block. *VI World Congress of Anesthesiologists, Mexico.*

THESLEFF, S. (1951). Pharmacologic and clinical experiments with o.o. succinylcholine iodide. *Nord. med.*, **46**, 1045.

THESLEFF, S. (1952). The pharmacological properties of succinylcholine iodide. *Acta physiol. scand.*, **26**, 103.

THOMAS, E. T. (1957). The effect of *d*-tubocurarine chloride on the blood pressure of anaesthetised patients. *Lancet*, **2**, 772.

TORDA, T. A. G., and KLONYMUS, D. H. (1966). The regional use of muscle relaxants. *Anesthesiology*, **27**, 689.

UTTING, J. (1963). pH as a factor determining plasma concentration of *d*-tubocurarine. *Brit. J. Anaesth.*, **35**, 706.

VICKERS, M. D. A. (1963). The mismanagement of suxamethonium apnoea. *Brit. J. Anaesth.*, **35**, 260.

VINCENT, D., and PARANT, M. (1954). Action des alcoloides des curares sur les cholin-estérases. *Bull. Soc. Chim. biol. (Paris)*, **36**, 405.

WALTS, L. F., and DILLON, J. B. (1967). Clinical studies on succinylcholine chloride. *Anesthesiology*, **28**, 372.

WANG, R. I. H., and ROSS, C. A. (1963). Prolonged apnoea following succinylcholine in cancer patients receiving AB-132. *Anesthesiology*, **24**, 363.

WASER, P. G. (1962). In: *Curare and Curare-like Agents.* (Ciba Foundation Study Group No. 12). Ed. de Reuck, A. V. S. London: J. & A. Churchill.

WESTGATE, H. D., and VAN BERGEN, F. H. (1962). Changes in histamine blood levels following *d*-tubocurarine administration. *Canad. Anaesth. Soc. J.*, **9**, 497.

WHITE, D. C. (1963). Dual block after intermittent succinylcholine. *Brit. J. Anaesth.*, **35**, 305.

WILSON, H. B., GORDON, H. E., and RAFFAN, A. W. (1950). Dimethyl ether of *d*-tubocurarine iodide as a curarising agent in anaesthesia for thoracic surgery. *Brit. med. J.*, **1**, 1296.

WINTERSTEINER, O., and DUTCHER, J. D. (1943). Curare alkaloids *chondodendron tomento-sum*. *Science*, **97**, 467.

YOUNG, I. M. (1949). The action of decamethonium iodide (C. 10) on foetal neuromuscular transmission and its transfer across the placenta. *J. Physiol. (Lond.)*, **109**, 31P.

FURTHER READING

BRYN THOMAS, K. (1964). *Curare. Its History and Usage*. London: Pitman Medical Publishing Co.

FELDMAN, S. A. (1973). Major Problems in Anaesthesia. In: *Muscle Relaxants*. London: W. B. Saunders Co.

KATZ, R. L. (1975). *Muscle Relaxants*. Amsterdam: Excerpta Medica.

McINTYRE, A. R. (1947). *Curare, its History, Nature and Clinical Use*. Chicago: Univ. Chicago Press.

Chapter 27

CHOLINESTERASES AND ANTI-CHOLINESTERASES

CHOLINESTERASES

IT is generally agreed that the cholinesterases play a very important part in normal neuromuscular transmission, for there is clear evidence that this enzyme is responsible for the rapid breakdown of acetylcholine to choline and acetic acid. Some observers question whether the speed of activity in tetanic nerve stimulation could ever be accounted for on a purely molecular basis. However, the distance that the acetylcholine molecule has to travel is extremely short (1 μm) and the speed at which it is broken down by cholinesterase is phenomenal (1/500th of a second). This time may be compared with the apparently slower process of repolarising the muscle membrane after a contraction has taken place—namely 1/250th of a second. In consequence any objection to the chemical theory of neuromuscular transmission on these grounds is unjustified.

During a period of quiescence the enzymes of the *choline acetylase* system (present inside the nerve fibre) are responsible for the synthesis of acetylcholine. Acetylcholine molecules are then sorted in the matrix of the nerve-ending as freely revolving packets or "quanta". Outside the nerve fibre in the surrounding tissue fluids are found the cholinesterase enzymes. These are distributed widely throughout the body but the highest concentrations are to be found in brain, nerve and muscle. The experiments of Marnay and Nachmansohn (1938), however, have shown that the concentration of cholinesterase enzyme at the myoneural junction is many thousand times greater than that to be found in other parts of the muscle.

Essentially, there are two distinct types of cholinesterase enzymes and the difference is largely based on their site of origin. *Pseudo* or *plasma* cholinesterase is to be found in the serum and in the pancreatic tissue. The normal values in the plasma vary from 40 to 100 units* depending on the method of estimation used. *True* or *specific* cholinesterase is found mainly in the red blood corpuscles, the neuromuscular junction, and the brain. The distinction between these two enzymes is not clear except that plasma cholinesterase is capable of hydrolising certain non-choline esters (e.g. tributyrin) whereas the activity of true cholinesterase is confined to the choline esters only. Plasma cholinesterase is also relatively insensitive to eserine and responds readily to di-fluorophosphate

---

* *Electrometric Method of Michel* (1949).

An indirect method of measuring cholinesterase based on the fall in pH of a barbitone/phosphate buffered system due to the acid produced.

Normal Values:	Lower Limit	Upper Limit
Red Blood Corpuscles .	51	100
Plasma . . .	40	100
Whole Blood . .	80	129

Aldridge and Davies (1952).

(DFP), but its action in destroying acetylcholine is at its best when the concentration of acetylcholine is high. True cholinesterase is also inhibited by DFP but in contrast the hydrolytic activity of the true esterase is greatest when the concentration of acetylcholine is low.

ANTI-CHOLINESTERASES

As their name implies, all these compounds block the activity of both types of cholinesterase enzyme in varying degrees.

Mode of action.—The principal activity of anti-cholinesterase drugs is to depress the cholinesterase enzyme—both the plasma and true—thus permitting the local concentration of acetylcholine molecules to rise. There are, however, other effects of these drugs that must be mentioned. They are capable of acting in their own right to produce depolarisation if sufficiently large doses are used. This effect may be seen as a fibrillation of small muscles which may proceed to paresis in man if doses of more than 5·0 mg of neostigmine are given intravenously in the absence of any d-tubocurarine. The presence of even the smallest quantity of the latter drug will normally prevent this in clinical practice. These drugs may also have an action on the nerve-ending causing repetitive firing and increasing release of acetylcholine directly (Katz, 1967). Indeed, there is considerable evidence to suggest that this facilitatory effect on acetylcholine mobilisation may be the primary mode of action of the anti-cholinesterase drugs (Riker, 1960; Riker and Standaert, 1966).

Acetylcholine has a very widespread activity in the body, affecting not only peripheral autonomic ganglia, smooth muscle (including myocardium) and secretory glands, but also skeletal muscle. So various are these actions that they are usually sub-divided into two main groups. First, the *nicotine-like* activity accounting for the action at the neuromuscular junction and also at the autonomic ganglia. Secondly, the *muscarine-like* action which accounts for the effect on the myocardium, bowel, bladder, pupil, and secretory glands (Table 1).

27/TABLE 1

ACTIONS OF ACETYLCHOLINE

Muscarinic effects	*Nicotinic effects*
1. Myocardium = bradycardia. 2. Gut = contraction. 3. Bronchioles = constriction. 4. Pupil = contraction. 5. Salivary glands = mucus + +. 6. Sweat glands = stimulated. 7. Bladder = contracted.	1. Autonomic ganglia stimulated. 2. Skeletal muscle stimulated.
Opposed by atropine sulphate.	

Atropine sulphate opposes the muscarinic actions of acetylcholine and therefore is the drug of choice in the treatment of nerve-gas casualties where the most important lesion is usually spasm of the smooth muscle of the bronchioles. The anti-cholinesterases stimulate both the muscarinic and the nicotinic actions of acetylcholine. If, however, they are combined with a large dose of atropine (1–2 mg) then only the nicotinic action is revealed and the muscarinic side-effects are reduced or prevented.

Blaber and Bowman (1963) have investigated the action of the anti-cholinesterase drugs and conclude that three distinct sites of activity can be illustrated. These are:—

1. *Depression of acetylcholinesterase activity.*—This increases the amount of acetylcholine available at the motor end-plate.

2. *Action on the pre-junctional nerve-ending.*—The anti-cholinesterase drugs hasten the release of acetylcholine from the nerve-ending. Thus when high rates of nerve stimulation are used, the stores of acetylcholine are rapidly exhausted and neuromuscular transmission fails. However, these stores are sufficient for slow rates of nerve stimulation.

3. *Action on the post-junctional motor end-plate.*—This is one of simple depolarisation due to the presence of a greater quantity of acetylcholine for longer than the normal fraction of a millisecond.

Neostigmine Methyl Sulphate (Prostigmin)

This is a white crystalline powder, odourless and soluble in water. The formula is:

The fate of neostigmine in the body is interesting, for though a large proportion of the injected material can be accounted for by direct contact with the enzyme cholinesterase, a small proportion is excreted by glomerular filtration in the kidneys and a similar proportion destroyed by the liver. When taken orally the gastro-intestinal tract appears to possess powerful destructive properties for neostigmine, as none survives long enough to reach the faeces, yet only one-thirtieth of the ingested material ever reaches the general circulation (Goldstein et al., 1949).

Fasciculations.—When neostigmine is given intravenously to a conscious subject, fasciculations may be seen or experienced by the individual. These are activations of motor units brought about partly by the accumulation of the packets or quanta of acetylcholine at the end-plate, but also by the direct action of the neostigmine on the motor nerve-ending causing repetitive firing with anti-dromic excitation of the motor unit. Massive doses of neostigmine cause severe and widespread fasciculations which on some occasions may involve a whole limb in a vigorous unco-ordinated twitch. This type of response is usually the prelude to neuromuscular block with failure of respiration. Coupled with the muscarinic symptoms (see below) the whole goes to make up a condition sometimes described as a *cholinergic crisis*. It is rarely seen in normal subjects except after the ingestion of large quantities of anti-cholinesterase drugs. It may follow poisoning with organophosphatides and other compounds sometimes used in the chemical industry. It is most commonly seen in patients with myasthenia gravis who have received excessive parenteral dosage of neostigmine.

Neostigmine and the heart rate.—Neostigmine produces a vagotonic effect causing bradycardia. For this reason it has always been advocated that it should be preceded by atropine. A number of isolated cases of cardiac arrest following the use of neostigmine have been reported but most of these date back to the early days of the use of the muscle relaxants combined with the belief that neostigmine should not be administered until after the return of spontaneous respiration. This resulted in high levels of CO_2 at the time of its administration and consequently frequent cardiac dysrhythmias (Macintosh, 1949; Clutton Brock, 1949; Lawson, 1956; Riding and Robinson, 1961). Other observations suggest that the atropine may have been responsible. In fact, Eger (1962) states that "the injection of atropine intravenously in the presence of cyclopropane or halothane anaesthesia may produce disastrous arrhythmias."

In the past it has been common practice to administer atropine sulphate (1·0 mg) at least two minutes before the commencement of neostigmine therapy. Atropine leads to a rapid rise in the heart rate which is followed a few minutes later by a gradual reduction in the rate as the effect of the neostigmine becomes apparent. At that time, based on the work of Bain and Broadbent (1949), it was believed that the combination of atropine and neostigmine was dangerous because the initial bradycardia due to the so-called "central effect" of atropine might summate with that of neostigmine to provide a fatal cardiac arrest. Later it was realised that the slowing of the heart rate produced by atropine was dependent on both the size of the dose and the mode of administration. If atropine is given subcutaneously the slow rate of absorption produces a low blood level and therefore a slowing before the onset of an increase in the pulse rate. On the other hand, if 0·5 mg or more is injected intravenously then no preliminary bradycardia can be observed since a high blood level is quickly achieved (Morton and Thomas, 1958).

Kemp and Morton (1962) took the matter one stage further and demonstrated that if the atropine and neostigmine were administered together intravenously then no initial slowing of the heart rate was observed. With this combination the action of atropine speeding up the pulse rate was evident in about 25 seconds and reached its peak in 45 seconds. The effect of neostigmine came on much later and the heart rate did not begin to be reduced until at least 100 seconds had passed. The conclusion was reached, therefore, that if atropine and neostigmine are combined together the action of the atropine on the heart rate will always precede that of the neostigmine.

Clinical comment.—Experience has shown that neostigmine in a dose of 40–45 μg/kg and atropine 20 μg/kg can be used with safety to reverse a non-depolarising block in man, and that neostigmine and atropine may be combined because the action of the atropine always precedes that of the neostigmine. In clinical practice a ratio of 1·0 mg of atropine sulphate to 2·5 mg neostigmine methylsulphate has been found satisfactory. The optimum time to administer this mixture is whilst the patient is still being hyperventilated and the carbon dioxide level of the blood is low. It should, however, never be administered in the presence of a high concentration of halothane or cyclopropane.

Though almost every case that has received a paralysing dose of a non-depolarising drug will probably require reversal of the neuromuscular block, it is now possible to demonstrate the degree of this block with a peripheral nerve-stimulator (see p. 882). If, for example, the hand muscles show adequate recovery of transmission then it can safely be concluded that the respiratory muscles are no longer under the influence of the relaxant drug. Recovery of the respiratory muscles always precedes that of the peripheral hand muscles. The only exception to this rule is when a pathological state exists at the motor end-plate, e.g. myasthenia gravis.

In small children, cardiac cases, and severely ill patients it is advisable to titrate the exact dose of neostigmine and atropine required with the nerve-stimulator. Also, in those patients who have received very large doses of a non-depolarising relaxant over a long period of time, then it is often necessary to exceed a total dose of 2·5 mg of neostigmine and 1·0 mg of atropine. How-ever, before further therapy is attempted it is important to verify with the stimu-lator that the signs of a non-depolarising neuromuscular block are still present.

If a dose of *d*-tubocurarine has been used which is much greater than the blocking dose (i.e. 100 per cent paralysis) then neostigmine will be unable to bring about complete reversal until the plasma level of relaxant has fallen below the critical threshold (Baraka, 1967). In clinical practice it is never advisable to exceed a total dose of 2·0 mg atropine and 5·0 mg neostigmine, as this is sufficient to depress all cholinesterase enzyme activity severely. Reports have varied on the time of activity of neostigmine but this largely depends on whether the heart rate or skeletal muscle activity is being studied (Gravenstein and Perkins, 1966; Katz and Katz, 1967). Nevertheless, it is generally agreed that an interval of about 1–2 minutes elapses before the first signs are present. The maximum effect at the neuromuscular junction is not reached until about twenty minutes later and it persists for more than one hour. Generally, the larger the dose adminis-tered, the more rapid is the onset of its action. Blitt and his co-workers (1976) using a technique of giving neostigmine *before* the administration of *d*-tubo-curare have suggested that the duration of action of neostigmine may be as long as 2–3 hours.

Though the combination of atropine and neostigmine is now considered safe it is perhaps wiser not to administer the mixture in the presence of a brady-cardia. In such an instance atropine alone in dilute solution is sometimes used to raise the pulse rate to around 80 per minute before mixing the remainder of the atropine with 2·5 mg of neostigmine.

Edrophonium Chloride (Tensilon)

In a study of the quaternary ammonium compounds analogous to neo-stigmine the pharmacological activity of edrophonium was revealed. The com-pound is 3-hydroxy-phenyldimethylethylammonium chloride, a white, odour-less and crystalline powder which is readily soluble in water but not in alkali.

The mode of action of edrophonium has aroused considerable interest, since it was originally believed that it acted mainly by a direct action on the neuro-muscular junction similar to that of acetylcholine. Its anti-cholinesterase activity was considered to be very weak (Randall, 1950; Riker and Wescoe, 1950). Subsequently, however, Hobbiger (1952) attacked this concept, and it is now generally accepted that the main action of the drug is an anti-cholinesterase one and that the direct depolarising activity is of secondary importance. The principal reason for this difference of opinion was based on the mode of experi-mentation. In the early stage *in vitro* experiments suggested that edrophonium had only 1/100–1/400 the anti-cholinesterase activity of neostigmine. However, the use of *in vivo* experiments showed that in fact the anti-cholinesterase activity was in the order of 1/5–1/15 that of neostigmine.

Following the intravenous injection of 10 mg of edrophonium in a patient partially paralysed with *d*-tubocurarine, a rapid improvement in muscle power occurs between 30–45 seconds after it has been given. The return of muscle power, however, is not maintained, and after a further two to three minutes the original paresis begins to return. The degree of secondary paralysis is rarely as severe as that before the administration of edrophonium. Nevertheless, the fact that the improved muscle power is not maintained is sufficient to prohibit the therapeutic use of this drug. It should be used for diagnostic measures only. In this respect it will be found most useful to diagnose the presence or absence of Phase II block in a patient suffering from prolonged apnoea following the use of muscle relaxants, or to differentiate between a myasthenic or cholinergic crisis in a patient with myasthenia gravis (see Chapter 28, p. 932).

Pyridostigmine (Mestinon).—This compound (i.e. the dimethylcarbamic ester of 1-methyl-3-hydroxy-pyridinium bromide) is an analogue of neostigmine and was introduced into medicine for the treatment of cases of myasthenia gravis. Pyridostigmine has about one-quarter the potency of neostigmine so that 10 mg given intravenously are equivalent to 2·5 mg neostigmine by the same route, but the action of pyridostigmine on the myocardium and the bowel are far less marked.

Brown (1954) investigated the use of this drug in anaesthesia and verified that the muscarinic side-effects are less than with an equivalent dose of neostig-mine. He found, however, that about four minutes elapsed before the action at the neuromuscular junction became evident, and also that the drug was generally less reliable than neostigmine.

OTHER DRUGS AFFECTING NEUROMUSCULAR FUNCTION

Galanthamine hydrobromide (Nivalin).—This compound is an alkaloid which is extracted from the snowdrop bulb. It was widely used in Bulgaria as an antagonist to non-depolarising relaxants. Galanthamine has about one-tenth the anti-cholinesterase activity of neostigmine but the side-effects on heart rate and salivation are less (Wislicki, 1967). The use of atropine is recommended.

Germine acetate.—Germine mono- and di-acetate are derivatives of the semi-synthetic ester alkaloids of the veratrum family. They are an interesting group of drugs because their principal site of action is on the muscle fibre itself. Germine diacetate is capable of improving neuromuscular transmission in the presence of both a depolarisation and a non-depolarisation block. This is achieved by converting a single muscle action potential into a brief period of tetanic firing by a direct effect on the fibre itself. However, it can have no effect at all if all neuromuscular transmission is blocked by complete paralysis. It would appear to be of possible value in the treatment of myasthenia gravis.

Hexafluorenium.—This is a drug with a variety of interesting actions. It achieved some notoriety in clinical anaesthesia when combined with suxamethonium because it prolonged the latter drug's action, reduced the dose required and therefore lessened the risk of Phase II block (Foldes *et al.*, 1960). The main action is one of inhibition of plasma cholinesterase activity but it also has a specific action on the post-junctional membrane (Nastuk and Karis, 1964). Apart from these actions, it also inhibits true cholinesterase and is a weak non-depolarising agent. It often causes disconcerting salivation in patients.

To those accustomed to using suxamethonium for short procedures and *d*-tubocurarine for long procedures, the value of combining hexafluorenium with suxamethonium has never seemed obvious. The combination lacked an adequate antidote. Added to this, there were reports of tachycardia, hypertension, cardiac dysrhythmias and fatal bronchospasm (Katz, 1967), so it is hardly surprising that it failed to gain universal popularity.

Tetrahydroaminacrine (THA).—This drug has also been advocated for combination with suxamethonium. It is a weak anti-cholinesterase but a powerful direct stimulant of the respiratory centre.

Quinidine.—This agent potentiates the neuromuscular block of both the depolarising and the non-depolarising relaxants. In fact, the combination of quinidine and a muscle relaxant has resulted in a case of prolonged apnoea lasting six hours (Way *et al.*, 1967). The most likely explanation of this enhancement of the activity of the muscle relaxants is that the cinchona alkaloids (like the local analgesic agents) depress the release of acetylcholine at the nerve-ending. However, Usubiaga (1968) attacks this thesis and argues that the most likely explanation is a depressant action on the muscle fibre itself.

4-Aminopyridine.—This drug has been used to reverse the non-depolarising muscle relaxants at the end of operations, to reverse the effect of the aminoglycoside antibiotics at the myoneural junction (Lee *et al.*, 1977) and to treat the Eaton-Lambert syndrome (myasthenic syndrome) (Agoston, personal communication, 1977). The drug is not an anti-cholinesterase but is believed to act by increasing the rate of calcium transport across membranes, thereby increasing the rate of acetylcholine release and the force of muscle contraction.

Clinical Comment on the Indications for the use of an Antidote to the Muscle Relaxants

Most anaesthetists today give an anti-cholinesterase drug at the end of all operations in which a non-depolarising muscle relaxant has been administered. This practice is usually commendable as it will lower the drug receptor occupancy to a safe level, but this can only be safely achieved if the blood level of the relaxant has been suitably reduced to a non-paralytic level. However, anti-cholinesterase therapy is not without complications and may cause disruption of intestinal anastomosis by promoting gut activity (Bell and Lewis, 1968). The more proximal the gut involved the more active is the resulting peristalsis caused by the neostigmine. But clinically all patients must be adequately reversed.

REFERENCES

ALDRIDGE, W. N., and DAVIES, D. R. (1952). Determination of cholinesterase activity in human blood. *Brit. med. J.*, **1**, 945.

BAIN, W. A., and BROADBENT, J. L. (1949). Death following neostigmine. *Brit. med. J.*, **1**, 1137.

BARAKA, A. (1967). Irreversible tubocurarine neuromuscular block in the human. *Brit. J. Anaesth.*, **39**, 891.

BELL, C. M. A., and LEWIS, C. B. (1968) Effect of neostigmine on integrity of iliorectal anastomosis. *Brit. med. J.*, **3**, 587.

BLABER, L. C., and BOWMAN, W. C. (1963). Studies on the repetitive discharges evoked in motor-nerve and skeletal muscle after injection of anti-cholinesterase drugs. *Brit. J. Pharmacol.*, **20**, 326.

BLITT, C. D., MOON, B. J., and KARTCHNER, C. D. (1976). Duration of action of neostigmine in man. *Canad. Anaesth. Soc. J.*, **23**, 80.

BROWN, A. K. (1954). Pyridostigmin. *Anaesthesia*, **9**, 92.

CLUTTON BROCK, J. (1949). Death following neostigmine. *Brit. med. J.*, **1**, 1007.

EGER, E. I. (1962). Atropine, scopolamine and related compounds. *Anesthesiology*, **23**, 365.

FOLDES, F. F., HILLMER, N. R., MOLLOY, R. E., and MONTE, A. P. (1960). Potentiation of the neuromuscular effect of succinylcholine by hexafluorenium. *Anesthesiology*, **21**, 50.

GOLDSTEIN, A., KRAYER, O., ROOT, M. A., ACHESON, G. H., and DOHERTY, M. E. (1949). Plasma neostigmine levels and cholinesterase inhibition in dogs and myasthenic patients. *J. Pharmacol. exp. Ther.*, **96**, 56.

GRAVENSTEIN, J. S., and PERKINS, H. M. (1966). The effect of neostigmine, atropine and ephedrine on heart rate in man. *Anesthesiology*, **27**, 298.

HOBBIGER, F. (1952). The mechanism of anticurare action of certain neostigmine analogues. *Brit. J. Pharmacol.*, **7**, 223.

KATZ, R. L. (1967). Neuromuscular effects of *d*-tubocurarine, edrophonium and neostigmine in man. *Anesthesiology*, **28**, 327.

KATZ, R. L., and KATZ, G. J. (1967). Clinical use of muscle relaxants. In: *Advances in Anesthesiology—Muscle Relaxants*, Chap. 6. Ed. by L. C. Mark and E. M. Papper. New York; Hoeber.

KEMP, S. W., and MORTON, H. J. V. (1962). The effect of atropine and neostigmine on the pulse rates of anaesthetised patients. *Anaesthesia*, **17**, 170.

LAWSON, J. I. (1956). Cardiac arrest following the administration of neostigmine. *Brit. J. Anaesth.*, **28**, 336.

LEE, C., DESILVA, A. J. C., and KATZ, R. L. (1977). Reversal of Polymyxin B induced neuromuscular and cardiovascular depression by 4-aminopyridine. *Abstr. of Scientific Papers, ASA Meeting*, New Orleans, p. 445.

MACINTOSH, R. R. (1949). Death following injection of neostigmine. *Brit. med. J.*, **1**, 852.

MARNAY, A., and NACHMANSOHN, D. (1938). Choline esterase in voluntary muscle. *J. Physiol. (Lond.)*, **92**, 37.

MICHEL, H. O. (1949). Electrometric method for determination of RBC's and plasma cholinesterase activity. *J. Lab. clin. Med.*, **34**, 1564.

MORTON, H. J. V., and THOMAS, E. T. (1958). Effect of atropine on the heart rate. *Lancet*, **2**, 1313.

NASTUK, W. L., and KARIS, J. H. (1964). The blocking action of hexafluorenium on neuromuscular transmission and its interaction with succinylcholine. *J. Pharmacol. exp. Ther.*, **144**, 236.

RANDALL, L. O. (1950). Anticurare action of phenolin quaternary ammonium salts. *J. Pharmacol. exp. Ther.*, **100**, 83.

RIDING, J. E., and ROBINSON, J. S. (1961). The safety of neostigmine. *Anaesthesia*, **16**, 346.

RIKER, W. F., Jr. (1960). Pharmacological considerations in a re-evaluation of the neuro-muscular synapse. *Arch. Neurol. (Chic.)*, **3**, 488.

RIKER, W. F., Jr., and STANDAERT, F. G. (1966). The action of facilitory drugs on neuro-muscular transmission. *Ann. N.Y. Acad. Sci.*, **135**, 163.

RIKER, W. F., Jr., and WESCOE, W. C. (1950). Studies on the inter-relationship of certain cholinergic compounds. V. The significance of the actions of the 3-hydroxy phenyl-trimethylammonium ion on neuromuscular function. *J. Pharmacol. exp. Ther.*, **100**, 454.

USUBIAGA, J. E. (1968). Potentiation of muscle relaxants by quinidine. *Anesthesiology*, **29**, 1068.

WAY, W. L., KATZUNG, B. G., and LARSON, C. P. (1967). Recurarisation with quinidine. *J. Amer. med. Ass.*, **200**, 153.

WISLICKI, L. (1967). Nivalin (galanthamine hydrobromide), an additional decurarizing agent: some introductory observations. *Brit. J. Anaesth.*, **39**, 963.

Chapter 28

NEUROLOGICAL DISEASE
IN RELATION TO ANAESTHESIA

THE mode of action of various anaesthetic drugs at the motor end-plate and on the spinal cord is gradually being elucidated. Nevertheless, at the present time the theories underlying the response of people to these drugs are constantly undergoing change, so that it is hardly surprising that the subject becomes even more confusing when the pathological states of neurological disease are considered. Frequently the anaesthetist is confronted with such a patient undergoing some surgical operation unrelated to his neurological condition. In the majority of patients the response to anaesthetic drugs does not differ from that found in normal subjects; unhappily an abnormal response, particularly to one of the muscle relaxants, is sometimes encountered. This complication most often arises in the presence of undiagnosed myasthenia gravis and, therefore, this disease is considered in detail.

MYASTHENIA GRAVIS

Myasthenia gravis is a chronic disease characterised by variable fatigue and weakness of voluntary muscles which gradually recover with rest. Although loss of reflex activity is not commonly observed, in long-standing cases some wasting of the muscle fibres may be present. The site of this fatigue has long been known to be in the peripheral neuromuscular system and the results of modern research have led to a general acceptance that the abnormality is at the neuromuscular junction.

History

In 1684, Thomas Willis first suggested the existence of such a disease in his book entitled *A Practice of Physick*; he went on to describe in detail the signs in a young woman affected with the disease. Nearly two hundred years later the syndrome again excited great interest when it became known as Erb-Goldflam's disease (Erb, 1879; Goldflam, 1893) and finally received the name of myasthenia gravis pseudo-paralytica from Jolly in 1895; in 1900 this name was modified to myasthenia gravis by Campbell and Bromwell.

Pathological Changes

In early myasthenia gravis the motor end-plates are morphologically normal but as the condition becomes established so sprouting and branching of the terminal fibres is observed. The end-plates become elongated and show widening of the synaptic clefts and folds (Santa *et al.*, 1972). Infiltration with lymphorrhages is common. Atrophic end-plates are most frequently associated with neostigmine-resistant myasthenia gravis.

Two types of thymic enlargement have been described in patients with this disease. The commonest is simple hypertrophy of the gland in which lymphorrhages and germ centres are often seen. The second type is a tumour—a thymoma. This may be benign and encapsulated or it may be locally malignant within the thoracic cage. There is a close association between both thymic hyperplasia or tumour and the symptoms of myasthenia gravis, but their presence is by no means certain in every case.

Clinical Features

(a) *Neonatal myasthenia* occurs in 1 out of 8 infants born to myasthenic mothers and a previous thymectomy performed on the mother is believed to reduce this incidence. The symptoms develop within three days of birth and the weakness persists for about six weeks after which it usually resolves. The condition responds well to the anti-cholinesterase drugs and may be related either to maternal anti-cholinesterase therapy or to maternal antibodies.

(b) *Juvenile type.*—In the condition before the age of two years it is usually confined to the bulbar musculature and consists of ptosis and ophthalmoplegia. It is usually mild or slowly progressive. In older children the pattern is similar to that found in the adult.

(c) *Adult type.*— Little can be added by modern physicians to the early description by Willis and others. Most cases occur in adults of either sex between the ages of 20 and 50, but it has been described in all the various age groups.

The onset of muscle fatigue is often so insidious that its significance may be missed by both doctor and patient. Occasionally it is precipitated by a severe illness or emotional disturbance. Fatigue of the eyelid muscles (on staring upwards) or of the limb girdle muscles (with elevation of the arms) are sometimes useful in eliciting the early signs of myasthenia. Though the bulbar muscles (i.e. eyelid, facial and swallowing) are the most commonly affected, the signs of the disease can appear in any skeletal muscle throughout the body. Typically, the patient gives a history of fatigue increasing throughout the day with some recovery on awakening in the morning. In long-standing cases some wasting of the muscle fibres can be observed. The progress of the disease fluctuates but often reaches a certain level and then remains static for many years. In the early stages a remission may occur but these are rarely permanent. Abnormalities of thyroid function are present in a high proportion of patients with myasthenia gravis.

Electromyographic Changes

At the end of the last century Jolly was able to demonstrate a difference with electrical stimulation between normal and myasthenic muscle. Classically, the severe myasthenic cannot maintain tetanic stimulation of a motor nerve. The "fade" and post-tetanic facilitation observed are similar to those already described for *d*-tubocurarine, viz. Fig. 1 *a* and *b*.

After a period of post-tetanic facilitation (lasting about 30 seconds) in cases of myasthenia there is a secondary period of post-tetanic exhaustion (see p. 816) which lasts for 20 minutes or more (Desmedt, 1957). This latter phenomenon is not observed in a paralysis due to *d*-tubocurarine chloride.

Unfortunately the classical electromyographic findings cannot be demonstrated in every case of myasthenia. This is probably because they are only

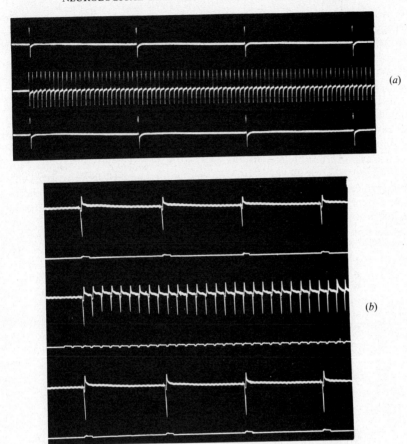

28/Fig. 1.—A comparison of the effects of electrical stimulation in a normal and myasthenic patient.

    (*a*) Normal neuromuscular transmission.

    (*b*) Myasthenia gravis. Note the "fade" of the twitch and tetanic response, and also the presence of post-tetanic facilitation.

observed when the muscles under test are actually showing clinical evidence of myasthenic weakness.

Aetiology of Myasthenia Gravis

The aetiology of myasthenia gravis has fascinated physicians for many years but still remains unknown. The superficial resemblance of this condition to the paresis of curare is known to all, but in the light of present knowledge the old theory of a circulating curare-like substance can no longer be entertained. The three current theories are based on the results of investigations:—

    (*a*) *Diminished synthesis or release of acetylcholine.*—This is a pre-junctional theory. It is based on electromyographic recordings made from myasthenic muscle (Desmedt, 1961). The presence of fade of successive responses, post-tetanic facilitation, and post-tetanic exhaustion have been described above.

Desmedt pointed out that though post-tetanic exhaustion did not occur in the presence of *d*-tubocurarine in normal muscle, a very similar pattern was observed in the muscle of cats treated with hemicholinium. This drug is believed to inhibit either the synthesis or the release of acetylcholine (see p. 811). On this basis he postulated that myasthenia was primarily a failure of the synthesis or release of acetylcholine at the nerve-ending.

Further support for this theory is given by the finding of Dahlback and his colleagues (1961) who investigated isolated specimens (*in vitro*) of both normal and myasthenic muscle with an intracellular micro-electrode. They measured the output of miniature end-plate potentials in both types of muscle and found that it was considerably reduced in cases of myasthenia gravis. Elmquist and his co-workers (1964) took the matter one stage further and demonstrated that the miniature end-plate potentials were diminished to one-fifth of normal (Fig. 2). From further analysis they concluded that the primary fault in myasthenia was a reduction not in the total number of quanta but in the number of *molecules* in each packet.

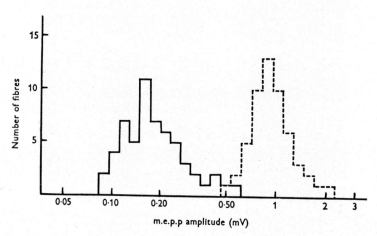

28/Fig. 2.—Distribution of mean miniature end-plate potential amplitudes from 57 myasthenic (solid line) and 54 normal (dotted line) human muscle fibres. All amplitudes corrected to a membrane potential of 85 mv. (From Elmqvist *et al.*, 1964.)

The interpretation of this work has recently been challenged (Engel *et al.*, 1974; Newsom Davis, 1974). A snake venom α-Bungarotoxin is believed to bind specifically (and irreversibly) with the nicotinic cholinergic receptor on the end-plate. Studies using this labelled agent have shown that in myasthenia gravis the number of receptors is reduced (Fambrough *et al.*, 1973). On this basis, it is argued that the widening of the synaptic cleft (a typical feature of myasthenia) could cause a volumetric dilution of each quanta of acetylcholine and thereby explain the diminution in the size of the miniature end-plate potentials.

(*b*) *Altered response of the motor end-plate.*—This is a post-junctional theory which is based largely on a pharmacological and electromyographic study of neuromuscular transmission. Churchill-Davidson and Richardson (1953) observed that myasthenic patients were resistant to the depolarising action of decamethonium iodide. This resistance can be demonstrated in every muscle of the body even though there are no signs of clinical weakness in the muscles under study. If repeated doses are given this resistance is overcome and a dual response at the motor end-plate is observed. As decamethonium is believed to act like acetylcholine on the post-junctional neuromuscular junction the basic fault in myasthenia was believed to be an alteration in the response of the motor end-plate. In this context it is particularly important to remember two things about the action of decamethonium in a myasthenic patient. First, the finding that all the motor end-plates in the body (whether clinically affected or not) are *resistant* to decamethonium demonstrates clearly that myasthenia gravis is a generalised condition. Some myasthenic patients can receive double or even quadruple the dose of decamethonium which is sufficient to paralyse a normal subject. Secondly, this *resistance* is best demonstrated in the very early or mild case and does not disappear either during a remission or after thymectomy. As it is such an early sign of myasthenia it could well be postulated that amongst the general population there is someone with a marked resistance to decamethonium who at some future date will develop the clinical signs of myasthenia gravis. Such a case has not been described.

The resistance of the myasthenic patient to depolarising drugs is not easily explicable on the basis of a primary pre-junctional lesion. If a gradual reduction of either acetylcholine production or liberation was the principal cause then one might presuppose that the motor end-plate would become more, rather than less, sensitive to acetylcholine in an attempt to compensate for the changing circumstances.

The post-junctional concept is supported by the work of Grob and his colleagues (1955) who used injections of intra-arterial acetylcholine and found that myasthenic muscle reacted differently from the normal subject. Thus, when injected into the brachial artery of a normal patient there was a brief contraction followed by a rapid recovery. But in cases of myasthenia gravis a secondary period of paresis developed which was not so severe but lasted about twenty minutes or more (Fig. 3). This secondary effect alone could be reproduced by the injection of choline, which is a breakdown product of acetylcholine. On this basis they postulated that myasthenia was an alteration of the response of the motor end-plate to either acetylcholine or to the choline formed from its hydrolysis. Engel *et al.* (1977) have clearly demonstrated a destructive auto-immune reaction involving the post-synaptic membrane in myasthenia gravis. Electron micrographs revealed that immune complexes (absent in the controls) were more abundant in the less severely affected myasthenic patients. They attributed this finding of fewer immune complexes in the severely affected patients to a smaller quantity of acetylcholine receptor (AChR) remaining at their end-plates.

(c) *Auto-immune response.*—It has been suggested that the physiological function of the thymus is essential for the proper development of lymphoid structures throughout the body. The maximum activity probably occurs during the development of the embryo but it also functions for some time after birth. The principal purpose of the gland is believed to be to ensure that the body can distinguish its own cells from other cells and antigens. This is the basis of the

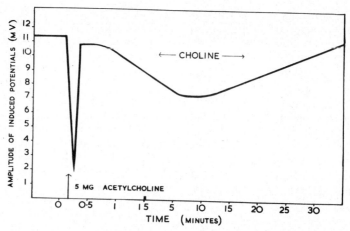

28/Fig. 3.—The intra-arterial injection of acetylcholine in a patient with myasthenia gravis. Note the primary paralysis due to acetylcholine with almost complete recovery, followed rapidly by a secondary phase of prolonged paralysis due to the choline. The second phase of paralysis is reversible by neostigmine, and is not seen in normal neuromuscular transmission.

antigen-antibody response and is one of the body's principal protective mechanisms. However, sometimes it functions to the individual's disadvantage as in the case of organ grafting; it is well-known that skin cells can be transplanted from one area to another on the same patient but that this same person cannot normally receive a graft of cells from another donor unless they are identical twins.

The development of the auto-immune response is believed to be associated with the thymus gland. On Burnet's hypothesis (1962 *a* and *b*) various mutations occur during early development in the blood cells; it is the responsibility of the thymus gland to destroy or disable these mutations. Once this has been accomplished it no longer has a function to perform so that it gradually atrophies. In myasthenia gravis the body is presumed to lose this ability to be able to distinguish between the different cells, so that antibodies are formed which react with both skeletal and cardiac muscle.

Support for this hypothesis is given by the finding of Nastuk and his associates (1959) who observed an abnormally wide fluctuation in the serum complement activity of myasthenic patients. The level fell with the active phases of the disease and rose during remission. They believed that in myasthenia gravis the muscle fibre itself becomes antigenic and sets up an antibody reaction. An autoimmune concept of this disease could account for the alteration in structure of this region that is observed on histological examination of the area and also for the defect of neuromuscular transmission. Myasthenic symptoms are occasionally associated with other autoimmune diseases, i.e. polyarteritis nodosa, disseminated lupus, etc. An increased level of muscle A antibody is commonly found in myasthenic patients. It is probably a true antibody and is highly characteristic of myasthenia, being found in 30 per cent of patients with symptoms and 100 per cent of those with a thymoma. However, this antibody is found elsewhere and has not been demonstrated to fix only to the A band of striated muscle (Osserman *et al.*, 1966) and is not thought to be responsible for muscle weakness (Engel *et al.*, 1974).

Summary.—There is now general agreement that the defect in myasthenia gravis is located at the neuromuscular junction. Both the pre- and post-junctional sites would appear to be involved. Current opinion favours the acceptance of a theory based on the auto-immune response but the reason why this phenomenon should suddenly or slowly develop still remains a mystery. It is possible that some infection is responsible (Simpson, 1960).

TESTS FOR MYASTHENIA GRAVIS

Mild cases of myasthenia gravis present a difficult problem of diagnosis. It is hardly surprising, therefore, that many drugs have been used at one time or another as tests for the presence of this condition. The anaesthetist is often called upon to carry out these tests and must be familiar with their anticipated result.

1. **Anti-cholinesterase tests.**—Both neostigmine and edrophonium have been widely used as tests for myasthenia. In fact, without a positive response to either of these drugs the physician is powerless to make a diagnosis on physical grounds alone. Both drugs inhibit the action of cholinesterase thus enabling the concentration of acetylcholine at the motor end-plate to undergo a temporary rise. These drugs also cause repetitive motor nerve discharge in response to a single stimulus thus increasing the output of transmitter substance and an increase in the twitch tension developed following indirect stimulation.

(*a*) *Edrophonium*, by virtue of its short duration of action (2–5 minutes) and minimal side-effects, can be given intravenously (dose 10 mg). It has now largely replaced neostigmine as a diagnostic agent. Although atropine is usually omitted in this test there may be some slowing of the heart rate and increased salivation. In normal subjects fine fascicular tremors may be observed in the eyelids 30–45 seconds after the injection. These are absent in cases of myasthenia gravis.

(*b*) *Neostigmine* can be used intramuscularly in a dose of 1·0–2·0 mg (combined with 0·5–1·0 mg atropine to reduce the side-effects). Some improvement in muscle power should be observed within 10–15 minutes.

For accurate assessment of any increase in muscle strength the ergograph can be used both before and after the drug. A false positive must be avoided by repeating the procedure with a placebo or atropine.

2. *d*-**Tubocurarine test.**—Before attempting any test with a muscle relaxant it is imperative that adequate measures for artificial ventilation are at hand.

Foldes and McNall (1962) recommend the administration of 0·5–1·0 mg of *d*-tubocurarine chloride at 3-minute intervals up to a total of 4·0 mg. They conclude that when this drug is combined with the ergograph the maximum dose should produce a marked reduction in grip strength or vital capacity in cases of myasthenia gravis. This test has now been replaced by the isolated arm test with curare (Foldes, 1970).

Rowland and his associates (1961) are more conservative and suggest a maximum dose of 0·016 mg/kg of *d*-tubocurarine chloride. They found that 84 per cent of myasthenia gravis patients exhibited "sensitivity."

Foldes (1970) has described the value of the isolated arm test using 0·2 mg of *d*-tubocurarine in the diagnosis of myasthenia gravis. In normal patients this dose produced a decrease in grip strength of 10 ± 4 per cent, whereas in myasthenic patients the fall was 67.9 ± 7 per cent.

Details of technique.—The patient lies on a couch and the muscle-power in the upper limbs is measured by dynamometry, ergography or electromyography. After control measurements a needle is inserted into a vein in each arm. Both limbs are then raised for 1 minute in order to empty the venous channels, after which tourniquets are applied and inflated to 40 mm Hg (5·3 kPa) above the systolic pressure. 0·2 mg *d*-tubocurarine diluted in 40 ml of 0·9 per cent sodium chloride is injected into one arm and the diluent only into the other. The cuffs are kept inflated for five minutes. Two minutes after their release the arms are tested for muscle-power.

Decamethonium.—This drug is believed to act in a similar manner to acetyl-choline but has the advantage that it is not destroyed by cholinesterase (Zaimis, 1951; Burns *et al.*, 1949; Burns and Paton, 1951). Its action in myasthenia gravis is, therefore, of particular importance and has been fully described by Churchill-Davidson and Richardson (1953 and 1955).

Essentially, in normal subjects the injection of decamethonium produces a neuromuscular block with all the signs of depolarisation; in cases of myasthenia gravis it shows evidence of resistance leading finally to a dual block. Thus fibrillary twitching of fasciculations are common in normal subjects but are rarely observed in cases of myasthenia. The combination of electromyographic techniques with decamethonium and edrophonium has enabled three stages in the development of myasthenia to be identified (Fig. 4).

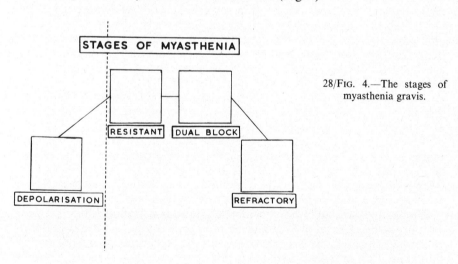

28/Fig. 4.—The stages of myasthenia gravis.

1. *Stage of resistance.*—In this stage the patient's muscles show no evidence of clinical weakness yet the motor end-plate shows a remarkable resistance to the paralysing action of decamethonium. Whereas in normal subjects a dose of 2·5 to 3·0 mg is capable of producing profound paralysis, myasthenic muscle in the stage of resistance can tolerate doses three to four times as great without

showing evidence of any weakness. The muscles of myasthenic patients which do not show clinical weakness and function normally are classified as in this stage. The fact that this resistance is so clearly evident in very mild cases of myasthenia makes decamethonium useful as a test in the diagnosis of this condition.

2. *Stage of dual block*.—The onset of this stage is heralded by the appearance of clinical weakness. Decamethonium, acting like a large dose of acetylcholine, produces a dual block which is partially reversible by the injection of an anti-cholinesterase substance (edrophonium). In contrast, decamethonium in normal subjects leads to a depolarisation type of neuromuscular block; if at this point an anti-cholinesterase drug is given the block either exhibits no change or shows a dramatic increase.

3. *Stage of myopathy (or refractoriness)*.—After prolonged periods in which the muscle fibre has not contracted due to the persistence of a neuromuscular block, the fibre finally atrophies from disuse. At this point the signs of a myopathy are evident. If a diligent electromyographic search is made, such signs can be found in at least one sixth of all cases of myasthenia gravis: they are more common in long-standing cases.

The evidence available suggests that the natural history of the development of myasthenia goes through the stages in the order that they have been enumerated above. The severity of the disease depends on the number of muscle fibres that are in the dual block and myopathic stages. If most of the fibres are merely in the resistant phase then the condition is mild.

The development of dual block in myasthenics receiving decamethonium can be demonstrated using the isolated arm technique described above, replacing curare with 0·5 mg of decamethonium (Feldman, 1973).

Suxamethonium.—Though this relaxant drug acts in a similar manner to decamethonium, its short duration of action coupled with the high initial dosage make it difficult to demonstrate the resistance stage before the onset of a dual neuromuscular block. Thus in myasthenia, suxamethonium brings about a paralysis of muscles through the medium of a dual response, but as it is rapidly destroyed by the enzyme cholinesterase (normal level in myasthenia) the duration of the weakness is only a few minutes. Nevertheless, the recovery does not appear to be either so rapid or so complete as in normal subjects, though the time taken may be shortened by administering an anti-cholinesterase drug.

Summary

In the majority of cases of myasthenia gravis the edrophonium test reveals a dramatic improvement in neuromuscular transmission. The patient's diagnosis is then finally confirmed by the improvement of muscle strength with anti-cholinesterase therapy. There are some cases, however, in which the response to both the test and therapy are equivocal and it is in these cases that further evidence is sometimes required. If there is generalised weakness then the *d*-tubocurarine test will reveal "sensitivity". On the other hand, if the weakness is limited to one group of muscles (e.g. the eye muscles) then *d*-tubocurarine is of little value because the "sensitivity" reaction is confined largely to those muscles that are already showing evidence of clinical weakness. As the "resistance" to decamethonium is universal throughout the body, this test is the most specific for cases of myasthenia gravis (Churchill-Davidson and Richardson, 1961), but nevertheless is the most complex. It is particularly useful in differentiating an ocular myopathy from ocular myasthenia gravis.

TREATMENT OF MYASTHENIA GRAVIS

The anaesthetist may encounter the myasthenic patient unwittingly, in the labour ward, in the course of routine surgery, or for the operation of thymectomy. He may also be called in to advise with the problem of ventilation in a myasthenic or cholinergic crisis; therefore some knowledge of the treatment of myasthenia is essential.

Medical Treatment

General care.—Any concomitant disease (i.e. thyroid or other autoimmune condition) should be actively treated. Anaemia should be corrected and the plasma potassium should be well-maintained and any deficiency treated vigorously.

There are two principal approaches to medical treatment: first, to enhance function at the neuromuscular junction with anti-cholinesterase drugs and alternatively, to suppress the supposed immune response with corticosteroid therapy (chiefly prednisone).

The anaesthetist encounters the myasthenic patient under medical care in two particular emergencies.

1. *Myasthenic crisis.*—Often the patient will give a history of a recent pulmonary infection associated with some difficulty in breathing. In a true myasthenic crisis there is dramatic improvement following the administration of an intravenous anti-cholinesterase such as edrophonium (10 mg). However, in most instances the patient has already increased his normal intake of anti-cholinesterase drugs so that often he is unresponsive to further therapy. The treatment of this condition is control of the airway, suction and adequate artificial ventilation.

2. *Cholinergic crisis.*—This produces very similar symptoms and signs to a myasthenic crisis and although the two are theoretically distinguishable, in practice both myasthenic and cholinergic elements are often present in each case. The diagnosis is made by either no improvement or increased paresis following the injection of 10 mg edrophonium intravenously. This condition is believed to be due to excessive anti-cholinesterase therapy. However, as both the patient's requirements and the response to an anti-cholinesterase drug may change rapidly in the presence of infection the management becomes extremely complex. Furthermore, whereas some patients may remain stable for years others may become increasingly unresponsive to anti-cholinesterase therapy. Refractoriness to these drugs is one of the basic problems in the treatment of myasthenia patients. It can only be overcome if all such therapy is withdrawn for a period of time. This is the basis for the use of *d*-tubocurarine therapy. The treatment of this condition is the same as for a myasthenic crisis with the exception that no anti-cholinesterase drugs should be used.

With both myasthenic and cholinergic crises adequate artificial ventilation must be maintained. ACTH therapy has proved useful in the treatment of myasthenic crisis but it not infrequently causes an initial increase in the muscle weakness (presumably as a result of a shift of K^+ ions, or antagonism with the anti-cholinesterase drugs) before producing any symptomatic relief. It is preferable therefore to combine this form of treatment with artificial ventilation.

A. *Anti-cholinesterase therapy*

Many myasthenic patients are adequately controlled with anti-cholinesterase drugs given by mouth in tablet form. Those most commonly used are:

Neostigmine bromide as a 15 mg tablet is sometimes used. The duration of action rarely exceeds four hours so that from 1–3 tablets are needed at intervals varying from every 2 to 6 hours depending on the severity of the myasthenia. The objective of all therapy is to achieve the maximum benefit of muscle strength pertinent to the patient's requirements with the minimum number of tablets. As the symptoms may vary during the day, the maximum dose should be timed to coincide with the occurrence of the most troublesome symptoms.

Pyridostigmine (Mestinon) is less potent than neostigmine and the 60 mg tablet corresponds approximately in activity to 15 mg of neostigmine. In some patients it is better tolerated than neostigmine with less gastro-intestinal disturbance and a slightly longer duration of action. For this reason it is often used at night.

Ambenonium chloride (Mytalase) is used as a 6 mg tablet which is roughly equivalent to 15 mg of neostigmine. It is believed to be more rapid in onset, longer acting and with less gastro-intestinal disturbance.

Other factors and drugs improving function.—*Ephedrine* is often combined with these drugs but its value is doubtful. Atropine in the form of tincture of belladonna (5–15 minims) is sometimes used for the treatment of colic. Steroid therapy may exacerbate the myasthenia gravis and therefore should be used with caution in such patients (see below).

Guanidine hydrochloride (20–40 mg four times a day). This is believed to benefit some patients by increasing the rate of release of acetylcholine following motor nerve stimulation.

Germine diacetate.—Originally the veratrum alkaloids were tried and abandoned due to their marked cardiovascular and emetic side-effects. This compound is a synthetic relative without side-effects. It leads to repetitive firing in the motor axon after a single normal action potential.

Cold.—The application of local hypothermia has been beneficial in some patients. This is especially useful for facial weakness and in improving swallowing in myasthenic patients. Cold is believed to have mild anti-cholinesterase effects.

B. *Corticosteroid therapy*

A short course of ACTH at high dosage has sometimes been followed by remarkable improvement in muscle power. However, during the early part of the treatment there is sometimes a marked increase in myasthenic weakness and ventilatory failure. Recent work has suggested that this is principally due to the steroid therapy antagonising the beneficial effect of the anti-cholinesterase drugs. Therefore, the new approach is first to reduce the anti-cholinesterase drugs to zero over a 3–5 day period and then to substitute high dose prednisone therapy, particularly after a thymectomy operation.

C. *Alternate day prednisone therapy*

Very good results have been described for maintenance treatment with prednisone following an initial high dose (Brunner *et al.*, 1972; Engel *et al.*, 1974). 100 mg prednisone is given daily for two weeks followed by continued treatment with the alternate day regime on a reduced dosage. The best results have been obtained in the elderly male and this therapy is often used following thymectomy. In all severe cases the vital capacity should be monitored regularly with a Wright respirometer. A reduction to 1·2–1·0 litre indicates that respiratory failure is imminent.

D. *Plasma exchange*

The technique is designed to remove the patient's plasma together with any immune complexes and antibodies and replace with fresh frozen plasma from various donors, as well as the patient's own red cells. It has been claimed to be of value in the treatment of severe cases of myasthenia and systemic lupus erythematosus, particularly where there is extensive involvement of the cardio-respiratory or renal systems. The process may cause a reduction in coagulation factors and also possibly a fall in plasma cholinesterase levels.

Surgical Treatment

A patient with myasthenia gravis may require anaesthesia on a variety of occasions. The principles of management, however, remain the same whatever the operation.

Principles of management.—If possible the patient should be stabilised on oral anti-cholinesterase therapy pre-operatively. The dose selected should not be the same as that used when leading an active life at home but rather should be the amount required by a subject lying at rest in bed. In the past most of the problems in the management of the myasthenia patient for surgery have been created by over-enthusiastic therapy. Anti-cholinesterase drugs may temporarily increase muscle strength but at the same time the production of secretions is also increased. Once stabilised on an oral dose of a suitable drug the patient usually ceases to be affected by the side-effects of colic and increased salivary secretions. Yet, a sudden increase in the dosage will initiate the return of these symptoms. Whenever possible, therefore, the dose of anti-cholinesterase both before and after operation should be administered by mouth and it should be reduced to as small as possible a dose to enable the patient to reach the operating room in comfort. On some occasions with complete bed rest pre-operatively it is possible to withdraw all anti-cholinesterase therapy.

Specific instances in which the myasthenia patient requires anaesthesia for operation may be considered under three different headings.

(*a*) *Incidental general surgery.*—Whenever possible anti-cholinesterase drugs should be administered orally, if necessary through a naso-gastric tube, rather than parenterally. Anaesthesia can be obtained satisfactorily with most agents but halothane has proved particularly useful. If muscle relaxation is not adequate, it can be produced by a local analgesic technique. (It is preferable to use a technique requiring a low total dose of local anaesthetic as most local anaesthetics depress neuromuscular transmission by interfering with membrane depolarisation). If the patient requires bowel surgery then control must be by parenteral therapy but this will probably lead to an increase in the secretions in the respiratory tract. In the presence of severe generalised myasthenia and a large abdominal or thoracic incision then the use of prolonged endotracheal intubation or a prophylactic tracheostomy should be seriously considered.

(b) *Obstetrics.*—The course of myasthenia gravis in relation to pregnancy is variable. Some patients improve remarkably whilst others become much weaker. Myasthenia gravis, however, is not an indication for Caesarean section unless there are associated obstetrical reasons. These patients tolerate analgesic drugs well but it should be remembered that the anti-cholinesterase drugs may enhance the effect of the opiates and their analogues (Slaughter *et al.*, 1940). A regional analgesic technique such as pudendal nerve block, epidural or subarachnoid block will provide very satisfactory conditions for delivery. If general anaesthesia is required then ether or cyclopropane are preferable to halothane since at comparable depths of anaesthesia there is less reduction in uterine tone.

(c) *Thymectomy.*—The value of this operation in the treatment of myasthenia gravis is more widely accepted and although the most successful results have been obtained in females under 40 years of age (Keynes, 1954; Eaton and Claggett, 1955), it is now recommended for most younger patients with the disease. The particular risks of this operation centre around the problem of the control of secretions due to anti-cholinesterase drugs, the pain in the post-operative period caused by splitting the sternum, the possible complication of bilateral pneumothorax, and the depression of ventilation by analgesic drugs.

Halothane anaesthesia in the presence of controlled respiration (to rest the respiratory muscles during surgery) has proved the most satisfactory agent for general anaesthesia.

In the presence of a severe myasthenia in the pre-operative period then it is advisable to perform an elective tracheostomy at the end of the operation. In this manner the high mortality previously associated with the operation of thymectomy can be eliminated provided adequate means of suction and ventilation are available. Unless the symptoms are very mild, it is better to ventilate all patients electively for 2 to 10 days after the operation so as to avoid the need for anti-cholinesterase therapy and obviate the production of thick sputum which is difficult for the patient to "cough up" following a thoracotomy. During this period the end-plates can be resensitised to anti-cholinesterase therapy. With a better understanding of the problems associated with surgery in these patients, thymectomy is now a far safer operation and the indications have been extended to include all patients with rapidly progressive disease and those with disabling symptoms.

CARCINOMATOUS NEUROPATHY

Henson and his colleagues (1954) drew attention to the relationship between carcinoma (particularly of the bronchus) and a motor neuropathy. In most cases of advanced carcinoma the cachexia, anaemia and loss of weight are sufficient to produce severe peripheral weakness. However, in true carcinomatous neuropathy the fatiguability is out of all proportion to the severity of the disease. Microscopic examination discloses demyelination of nerve fibres and atrophy of muscle fibres. The response to anti-cholinesterase therapy is poor.

The relationship of this condition to the myasthenic syndrome is not clear but carcinomatous neuropathy is much commoner than the myasthenic syndrome and lacks the characteristic electromyographic "growth" of successive tetanic response which is so essential for diagnosis of the later condition.

MYASTHENIC SYNDROME

In recent years a number of cases have been described suggesting an association between a condition resembling myasthenia gravis and bronchial carcinoma. This relationship was first pointed out by Anderson and his associates (1953) but it was not until four years later that Eaton and Lambert (1957) detailed the specific condition which they termed "myasthenic syndrome".

Although superficially many of the features of the myasthenic syndrome resemble myasthenia gravis, a closer investigation has revealed a wide margin of differentiation. These have been fully described by Wise and Wylie (1964) and are tabulated in Table 1.

The myasthenic syndrome is essentially a condition of peripheral muscle weakness developing in a patient with a bronchial carcinoma. This association is so common that the finding of the characteristic electromyographic response in the absence of obvious evidence of a neoplasm should be sufficient to stimulate an intensive search for its presence.

The specific electromyographic features are illustrated in Fig. 5.

They can be summarised as follows:

1. Low-voltage potential on twitch stimulation (Fig. 6).
2. The "fade" of successive responses on twitch stimulation.
3. The "growth" of successive responses on tetanic stimulation.
4. The presence of post-tetanic facilitation.

In a clinical assessment of the effect of relaxant drugs on patients with the myasthenic syndrome Wise (1962) pointed out that these patients were highly sensitive to both the depolarising and the non-depolarising drugs. The presence

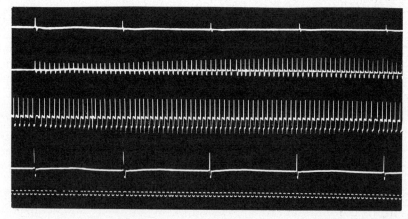

28/Fig. 5.—Electromyographic pattern of myasthenic syndrome. This patient has a proven carcinoma of bronchus.

28/Table 1

	Myasthenia gravis	Myasthenic syndrome
Sex	Twice as common in women.	Almost entirely men.
Age of onset	Commonly 20–40 years.	Commonly 50–70 years.
Presenting signs	Weakness of external ocular, bulbar and facial muscles.	Weakness and fatiguability of proximal limb muscles (legs > arms).
Other signs	Weakness of limbs, usually proximal, is a later sign (arms > legs).	Weakness of ocular and bulbar muscles is infrequent.
Other clinical features	Fatigue on activity.	Transient increase in strength on activity precedes fatigue.
	Muscle pains uncommon.	Muscle pains common.
	Tendon reflexes normal.	Tendon reflexes reduced or absent.
Response to muscle relaxants	Good response to neostigmine.	Poor response to neostigmine.
	Increased sensitivity to non-depolarising relaxants in clinically weak muscles.	Marked sensitivity to non-depolarising relaxants even in muscles relatively un-affected.
	Resistance to depolarising relaxants.	Sensitivity to depolarising relaxants.
Electromyographic features	Normal or slightly reduced amplitude of action potentials at slow rates of stimulation.	Very low voltage action potentials at slow rates of stimulation with fade.
	Fade of successive potentials especially on tetanic stimulation.	Marked growth of potentials on tetanic stimulation.
	Post-tetanic potentiation and post-tetanic exhaustion present.	Post-tetanic potentiation present.
Pathologic states	Thymoma in 25 per cent of patients.	Small-celled carcinoma of bronchus usually present.
	Motor end-plates abnormally elongated and distal nerves unusually branched.	Non-specific degenerative process of nerve fibres and end-plates.
Prognosis	Often good.	Rapid deterioration and death.

of the peripheral weakness is always demonstrable in these cases if actually sought by the anaesthetist. However, if the patient has been confined to bed or is suffering from some incapacitating lesion then the presence of a myasthenic syndrome may be missed. The possible presence of this condition should always be borne in mind during the pre-operative examination of the patient for bronchoscopy under general anaesthesia or a thoracotomy for carcinoma of lung. If this condition is suspected then the diagnosis can easily be confirmed by electromyography. The use of all the muscle relaxants is contra-indicated in the presence of the myasthenic syndrome. Improvement of neuromuscular conduction following the administration of 4-aminopyridine has been described (Agoston, personal communication, 1977).

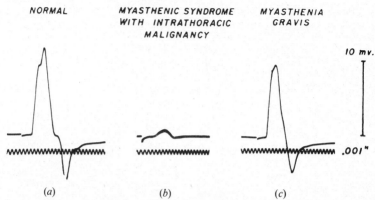

28/Fig. 6.—Illustrates the different height (i.e. voltage) of the action potential in response to a single twitch stimulus in (a) normal, (b) myasthenic syndrome, (c) myasthenia gravis (Lambert *et al.*, 1961).

DYSTROPHIA MYOTONICA

Dystrophia myotonica is a familial disease, usually occurring in adult life, characterised by muscle wasting, fatigue, and an inability to relax the muscles after a contraction (myotonia). The myotonia may precede the muscle wasting by many years or may occur independently. The condition is commonly associated with cataract, baldness and testicular atrophy. Occasionally the anaesthetist may be privileged to diagnose the presence of myotonia when the patient "opens and squeezes" his hand before the induction of intravenous anaesthesia.

The abnormality in dystrophia myotonica is believed to be an increase in the sensitivity of the muscle fibre. Brown and Harvey (1939) working with myotonic goats found that the myotonia persisted even after nerve-section and curarisation. Later Geschwind and Simpson (1955) showed in man that neither *d*-tubocurarine nor decamethonium will abolish the myotonia. MacDermot (1961), however, has demonstrated histologically that not only is the muscle fibre itself involved but there is also a defect of the nerve-ending.

Kaufman (1960) investigated the effect of anaesthetic drugs, including the relaxants and thiopentone, in patients with dystrophia myotonica. He observed that thiopentone did not influence neuromuscular transmission. The intense depression of respiration, therefore, that may follow the use of barbiturate or narcotic drugs is probably related to central depression of the respiratory centre in a patient with a limited respiratory reserve.

Both neostigmine and the depolarising drugs (Thiel, 1967) may increase the degree of myotonia whereas *d*-tubocurarine will block neuromuscular transmission without necessarily overcoming the myotonia. Thiel (1967) described a case in which the myotonic episodes were directly attributable to the action of suxamethonium.

Patients with dystrophia myotonica may also have some cardiac or endocrine dysfunction. Regional analgesic techniques are well tolerated. The use of respiratory depressant drugs should be strictly limited. If general anaesthesia is required halothane (which is rapidly eliminated) is most useful.

MALIGNANT HYPERPYREXIA

This syndrome represents one of the most interesting yet baffling conditions associated with anaesthesia. Originally described in North America (Saidman et al., 1964; Stephen, 1967; Relton et al., 1966; Wilson et al., 1967) it has now been recognised in reports from all over the world.

The paradox of the situation is that in ordinary circumstances the onset of general anaesthesia reduces the ability of a patient to make heat, so that (unless he can shiver) his body temperature gradually falls to that of his environment (i.e. he becomes poikilothermic). In modern operating theatres with air-conditioning, therefore, it is often difficult to prevent the onset of insidious hypothermia. Yet, in the rare instance of malignant hyperpyrexia, it is possible for the anaesthetised patient to raise his body temperature at the phenomenal rate of 1° C every 5–10 minutes. Once the body-core temperature exceeds 42° C recovery is unusual.

Clinical Features

Often the patient is young and healthy, undergoing some relatively minor procedure, and in most cases suxamethonium has been used for intubation. In many of these case reports, the anaesthetist has observed a stiffness or rigidity of the jaw muscles and occasional tonic contractions of the skeletal muscles. Intubation is difficult which is usually attributed to an inadequate effect of the muscle relaxant. In malignant hyperpyrexia this rigidity persists and is not abolished by d-tubocurarine. In other cases—particularly those who have not received suxamethonium—the induction of anaesthesia is normal, the skeletal musculature is flaccid and the first untoward signs do not develop until about 30–45 minutes from the start. The anaesthetist may observe a tachycardia, a rise in blood pressure, and an increase in ventilation. A particular feature is a hot, dry skin with flushed facies and ultimately, when the body temperature rises rapidly, peripheral cyanosis occurs.

All these signs indicate a greatly increased metabolism. This rise in metabolic rate is so great that the normal inspired oxygen concentration is outstripped and the patient gradually becomes hypoxic and acidaemic. Simultaneously, the enormously increased carbon dioxide concentration during expiration often leads to exhaustion of the soda-lime canister. If untreated, the body temperature will continue to rise, the pupils become fixed and dilated, and death ensues due either to cardiac failure or cerebral damage.

Investigations made during the pyrexia have revealed a raised serum potassium level, high carbon dioxide tension, a grossly acidic pH of the blood and a raised serum CPK (Saidman et al., 1964; Thut and Davenport, 1966; Davies et al., 1969).

Aetiology

As stated above, the cause of this condition is unknown. However, it appears to be genetically determined and distinct from the neuropathies and myopathies. **Hereditary metabolic defect.**—In a study of various family histories certain interesting observations have been made. For example, Britt and her colleagues (1969) found a family of 115 people in the Wisconsin area. Twenty of this family received a general anaesthetic whilst in good health, yet eight of them died. Again, Denborough and his associates (1962) reported another family of 116 people in Australia. Thirty-seven of them received general anaesthesia and ten died. Furthermore, Relton and his co-workers examined four sisters and found that one had died under anaesthesia. The remaining three sisters produced twenty-two children between them, and one half of this number died under general anaesthesia—eight with known hyperpyrexia.

Such figures are so alarming that it is impossible to believe that a hereditary defect is not in some way responsible. Isaacs and Barlow (1970) took the matter a stage further and investigated ninety-nine relatives of a patient who had developed malignant hyperpyrexia. They found that the resting levels of serum creatin phosphokinase and aldolase were raised in a significantly high proportion of their patients. They concluded that the high level of these muscle enzymes was evidence of a subclinical myopathy and that pre-operative estimations might reveal potential sufferers. Further support for the hereditary metabolic defect is given by the observations of Furniss (1971) that hyperpyrexia in association with muscle rigidity occurred predominantly in those patients under the age of twenty. It was argued that a congenital defect would be most likely to be revealed by the young rather than the old.

Support for the hereditary defect theory is also given by the finding that hyperpyrexia occurring during anaesthesia is occasionally observed in certain strains of pigs. Hall et al. (1966) found three pigs from the same litter of the Landrace-Wessex strain who developed hyperpyrexia after an injection of suxamethonium. An even more interesting finding was that of Harrison and his associates (1969) who were working on the problem of liver transplantation in the pig. By chance, they came across the fact that one in every four pigs of the pure Landrace strain would develop rigidity and hyperpyrexia if given an injection of suxamethonium. Furthermore, other anaesthetic agents such as halothane and chloroform could also produce this response, though ether, thiopentone and trichloroethylene would not do so.

Subsequently other varieties of pigs have been demonstrated to show some of the characteristics of malignant hyperthermia, including the Poland, China and Pietrain strains. It would seem that suxamethonium and the combination of suxamethonium and halothane is most effective in provoking hyperpyrexia although most anaesthetic drugs including nitrous oxide have now been incriminated as triggering mechanisms. It is possible that the stress associated with the fear of anaesthesia may also be a contributing factor. Once the condition is established anaerobic glycolysis takes place with an enormous increase in plasma potassium, magnesium and phosphate. A twenty-fold increase in the circulating catecholamines has also been noted (Lucke et al., 1976).

The problems associated with screening relatives of patients who may exhibit this lethal syndrome has led to the study of muscle biopsy specimens and their response to suxamethonium and to halothane. Ellis and his colleagues in 1971 (and Ellis and Harriman, 1973) demonstrated that exposure of the muscle biopsy specimens from susceptible individuals to halothane caused contracture of the muscle. Histological examination of the muscles from these patients demonstrated degenerative lesions suggestive of a myopathy. This halothane-induced contracture can be prevented by pretreating the muscle preparation with procaine, but not lignocaine (Keaney and Ellis, 1971). Harrison (1971) has demonstrated a reduced mortality in Landrace pigs by pretreatment with procaine. The rationale of the use of procaine is that is is known to accelerate the uptake of calcium by the sarcoplasmic reticulum. Both in this effect and in its ability to block the leak of calcium from the sarcoplasmic reticulum caused by certain chemicals it is superior to lignocaine. It is of interest that procaine and procainamide have been used in patients with this condition (Kalow et al., 1970; Maisel et al., 1973; Barrett, 1973); however it has not always prevented a fatal outcome. It has been suggested that there are funda-mental differences between the halothane-induced malignant hyperpyrexia in the pig and the clinical condition in man, although there appears to be a common defect of calcium transport in the muscle.

Britt and Kalow (1970) reviewed the possible aetiology of this condition and concluded that "the malignant hyperthermia which occurs on the basis of a genetic defect in Landrace pigs is not only clinically identical with the human syndrome but also identical in many of the biochemical features". In a later investigation they reported on the study of muscle biopsy specimens of two patients who had previously undergone an episode of malignant hyperpyrexia accompanied by muscle rigidity. They found that in each instance the calcium uptake in the sarcoplasmic reticulum was low after exposure to halothane. They concluded that the lesion in the rigid type of the condition was due to an inability of the sarcoplasmic reticulum to store calcium. This meant that the concentra-tion of calcium in the cytoplasm remained constant and the enzyme myosina-deno triphosphatase was not activated in the usual manner. The result was that the myofibrils remained locked together in a persistent contraction. They were unable to suggest the aetiology of those cases in which hyperpyrexia occurred in the absence of muscle rigidity.

Treatment

It must be emphasised that this is an exceedingly rare complication of anaesthesia but because of the high mortality anaesthetists must be wary of warning signs such as a family history suggesting an unexplained anaesthetic death, a failure of the patient to relax following suxamethonium or the develop-ment of muscle rigidity. The hot, vasodilated patient producing excessive respiratory drive suggests the onset of acidaemia. Treatment recommended includes termination of the anaesthetic, administration of 100 per cent oxygen, hyperventilation, infusion of sodium bicarbonate, immersion of patient in ice-cold water, extracorporeal cooling, massive doses of corticosteroids and procaine or procainamide. In spite of these treatments, the mortality of the condition remains high. Dantrolene has been recommended to treat the hyper-pyrexia (Harrison, 1975).

The relatives of any patient demonstrating this condition, or those who react to anaesthetic drugs, especially halothane and suxamethonium in a manner suggestive of this condition, should be subjected to muscle screening. A per-sistently raised creatinine phosphokinase level is suggestive of muscle disease but a normal CPK does not exclude the condition. Muscle biopsies should be carried out and halothane screening of the biopsy specimen performed in conditions that allow a quantitative measurement of any contracture. Histological evidence of cellular infiltration in the muscle specimen should be sought. Any patient at risk must be warned so that general anaesthesia can be avoided unless it is for a life-threatening condition.

FAMILIAL PERIODIC PARALYSIS

This is a hereditary condition characterised by recurrent attacks of flaccid paralysis. It is associated with an abnormality of potassium and is of two types:

(a) *Hypokalaemic form.*—The attacks of paresis are generally associated with a fall in the serum potassium concentration, but there is no critical level for the onset of muscular weakness. These attacks can be induced by the administration of glucose, insulin and epinephrine. During the paresis the muscles will no longer respond to electrical stimulation. Nevertheless, the volume of the muscle fibre increases, suggesting that not only potassium but water enters the fibre during the period of paralysis.

There is no data available on the response of these patients to anaesthetic drugs, but it is reasonable to assume that during an attack the patient will have an increased sensitivity to non-depolarising agents.

(b) *Hyperkalaemic form.*—This is a much rarer form of this condition and is associated with a high serum potassium producing an intermittent depolarising type of neuromuscular block.

PORPHYRIA

Porphyrins are tetrapyrrolic pigments produced mainly in the liver and bone marrow as intermediates in the synthesis of haem. The porphyrias are disorders of porphyrin metabolism causing excessive production of porphyrins or their precursors and are classified according to the major site of abnormal porphyrin production, the hepatic porphyrias being more common than the erythropoietic. The reader is referred to Goldberg *et al.* (1975) for further details of the porphyrias in general; the only variety which will be mentioned below is acute intermittent porphyria.

Acute Intermittent Porphyria

This is the commonest and most severe form of hepatic porphyria and usually presents in young adults. It is inherited as an autosomal dominant, but in 30 per cent of cases there is no family history. Typically there is an acute onset of colicky central abdominal pain with vomiting and constipation, although diarrhoea occurs in 10 per cent of cases. There is usually evidence of peripheral neuropathy which gives rise to paraesthesiae, numbness and cramp-like pains as well as weakness of limb and girdle muscles; weakness of trunk muscles is less common but can lead to respiratory embarrassment. The cardiovascular system is involved in about 70 per cent of attacks of acute intermittent porphyria; sinus tachycardia and hypertension are common and may be associated with left ventricular failure. It is important to remember that many of these patients present with psychiatric disturbances which include depression.

The diagnosis is confirmed initially by examination of the urine which turns dark on standing and has a very high (during an attack) porphobilinogen content.*

A large number of drugs may precipitate or exacerbate an attack of acute porphyria. Barbiturates, especially thiopentone sodium, are most frequently involved and can produce severe porphyric neuropathy and coma. Other drugs, including those containing oestrogens, may precipitate an attack of the disease. If anaesthesia is needed for a patient suffering from porphyria, induction is best achieved with Althesin or an inhalational agent; there is no contra-indication to the use of opiate analgesics, diazepam or promazine and all these drugs may be needed in the treatment of an attack of porphyria itself. Most anaesthetists would be reluctant to use a local anaesthetic technique in a patient with (or at risk of) peripheral neuropathy.

DERMATOMYOSITIS

Certain patients with this disease show a profound peripheral weakness and in some this is associated with an improvement on the administration of an anti-cholinesterase drug. There is also a close relationship between carcinoma and dermatomyositis.

In an investigation of ten patients with dermatomyositis, Churchill-Davidson and Richardson (1958) found positive evidence of a myasthenic response (using decamethonium) in two: in one of these a neoplasm of bronchus was present. The muscle relaxants, therefore, must be used with caution when anaesthetising patients with dermatomyositis.

SUMMARY OF ANAESTHESIA AND NEUROLOGICAL DISEASE

In general, patients with some neurological impairment of muscle function are extremely susceptible to respiratory depressant or relaxant drugs; a fact which could safely be predicted, for in normal subjects the respiratory reserve is such that a considerable number of muscle fibres can be inactive yet the minute volume is well maintained. This is emphasised by the statement, "tidal volume is only 10 per cent of vital capacity in a normal patient," signifying that theoretically it is possible to lose 90 per cent of the fibre activity before diminished ventilation is apparent. In the presence of neurological disease the requirements for anaesthetic drugs are drastically reduced and the dose of any agent used should be selected accordingly.

TETANUS

This disease is characterised by muscle stiffness and paroxysmal spasms which, unless suitably treated, often prove fatal. The causative organism is *Clostridium tetani*, a spore-bearing anaerobe, which enters a wound or small

---

* To test for porphobilinogen in the urine:
—mix equal parts of fresh urine and Ehrlich's reagent.
—red colour develops if porphobilinogen is present.
—add 3 ml n-butanol, shake, allow to separate.
—if red colour does not enter butanol (upper layer) it is porphobilinogen.

abrasion from infected material—typically soil. Sometimes the site of entry is small and almost insignificant, but from the moment that the bacilli reach the wound the incubation period of the disease begins. This may be as brief as two or three days or as long as three weeks, but the longer the duration of time between infection and the onset of the first symptoms, the more favourable is the ultimate prognosis.

Route of Infection

The bacilli produce an extremely potent toxin which is absorbed by the motor end-plate and gradually passes centripetally to affect the motor nerve cells in the anterior horn of the spinal cord. From the spinal cord the toxin ascends to the bulbar nuclei (Wright, 1954). It has also been suggested from experimental evidence in animals that the brain stem may be affected by circulating toxin (Lawrence and Webster, 1963).

Symptoms and Signs

The earliest sign of the onset of tetanus is usually stiffness in the muscles of the jaw which progresses to trismus—hence the name "lockjaw". The masseter muscles are thus the first to become involved but very soon other muscles of the face are affected so that "risus sardonicus" results. The tendon jerks throughout the body become exaggerated as a general increase in muscle tone becomes apparent, until on a sudden stimulation muscle spasm everywhere becomes accentuated resulting in a full scale paroxysm. At this stage there is generally marked opisthotonos, and breathing is hampered. Death may occur suddenly from anoxia due to respiratory difficulties from the toxic effects of heat, or after several days as a result of exhaustion.

The spasms of tetanus are very similar to those found in patients with strychnine poisoning but the essential difference lies in their constancy. The muscles of patients with tetanus are in a state of continuous contraction which is accentuated during a paroxysm. Parsons and Hofman (1966) have demonstrated that tetanus toxin lowers the pre-synaptic membrane potential. In strychnine poisoning the muscles are completely relaxed in the intervals between paroxysms.

Patients with severe tetanus may also show signs which are thought to be caused by overactivity of the sympathetic nervous system (Kerr et al., 1968). There is profuse sweating with an increased metabolic rate, extreme peripheral vasoconstriction with a glove-and-stocking distribution and sharp line of demarcation between warm and cold skin, hyperpyrexia, sinus tachycardia with multifocal ventricular ectopics and hypertension leading terminally to hypotension which does not respond to pressor agents. Treatment with β-blockers has been recommended if sympathetic overactivity occurs (Prys-Roberts et al., 1969).

Prophylaxis

The following prophylactic measures are available to a patient with a contaminated wound (Editorial, 1974):
(a) Surgical treatment
(b) Active immunisation
(c) Passive immunisation
(d) Antibiotic therapy

(a) *Surgery.*—*Clostridium tetani* thrives in a wound where the oxygen tension is low. The aim of surgery is to remove dirt, foreign bodies and any necrotic tissue or blood clot and to restore the blood supply to the part. Antibiotics can be directly applied.

(b) *Active immunisation.*—This is obviously the prophylactic measure of choice and can be instituted at any age by giving two doses of adsorbed toxoid at an interval of 4 to 6 weeks followed by a third dose 6 to 12 months later. Tetanus toxoid is often combined with diphtheria and pertussis toxoids in a triple vaccine. Maintenance reinforcing doses are given every 5 to 10 years. It is important to remember that clinical tetanus provides no significant immunity to the patient who must therefore receive active immunisation to protect him from a second episode.

(c) *Passive immunisation.*—A patient presenting with a contaminated wound who has not been immunised against tetanus should be given antitoxin. The best preparation is human antitetanus immunoglobulin (homologous antitoxin) which is given intramuscularly in a dose of 250–500 I.U., a first dose of adsorbed toxoid is given at the same time. The availability of this preparation is limited, and in its absence the use of refined horse serum antitoxin (heterologous antitoxin) should be considered. However, since this carries a high risk of causing allergic reactions and is less effective than homologous antitoxin, it is usually safer to rely on surgical treatment and antibiotic therapy.

(d) *Antibiotic therapy.*—The drug of choice is penicillin which should be given as soon after the injury as possible and continued for five days. In penicillin-sensitive patients, tetracycline or erythromycin can be used.

Treatment

In recent years anaesthetists have been able to give practical help in the treatment of many patients with tetanus, particularly when the muscles of respiration have been involved. But the many papers in the literature on the subject of treatment testify to the variety of opinions that exists on this subject. Mild cases of tetanus are seldom a problem and can be adequately treated by careful nursing and simple sedation using diazepam. The onset of paroxysms of muscle spasm calls for more radical treatment. Here the muscle relaxants used to produce total paralysis, combined with artificial respiration, some sedation and careful control of nourishment and the electrolyte balance offer great possibilities (Woolmer and Cates, 1952; Shackleton, 1954; Lassen *et al.*, 1954; Smith *et al.*, 1956; Wilton *et al.*, 1958). Smythe and Bull (1961) have added weight to the argument in favour of the more liberal use of complete paralysis and controlled ventilation. They report that in the years 1951–57 there were 55 cases of tetanus neonatorum which were primarily treated by sedation. The mortality was about 50 per cent. When they adopted tracheostomy and IPPR in the more serious cases the death rate fell to 11 per cent in the next twenty-five cases. Smythe (1963) has emphasised the importance of total muscle paralysis, regular tracheal suction, and adequate ventilation with regular monitoring of the carbon dioxide level of the blood.

General measures.—Careful and devoted nursing in a quiet and darkened room is essential, and every effort must be made to avoid triggering off paroxysmal spasms. The value of anti-tetanus serum once the disease has become apparent is still debated, but nevertheless it should be given as soon as possible. Provided there is no reaction to a test dose, an intravenous dose of 100,000 units has been recommended. Patel and his colleagues (1963), however, in a series of 3,295 cases of tetanus, found that there was no significant difference in the overall mortality provided a minimum dose of 10,000 units was used. Increasing the dose did not improve the results. Then the wound should be attended to surgically under general anaesthesia. Penicillin should be administered prophylactically to control secondary infection both in the wound and in the lungs, and other antibiotics prescribed should a particular organism suggest their use.

Sedation.—The drugs of choice are diazepam, chlorpromazine and the barbiturates, so there is little indication for mephenesin which needs to be given via a nasogastric tube in order to avoid the haemoglobinuria which may follow intravenous administration, or the potentially dangerous local analgesia of the pharynx following oral administration.

Chlorpromazine has a number of actions of specific value in the treatment of tetanus. It depresses the internuncial neurones of the spinal cord when given in large doses and has an effect on the basal ganglia in the brain. It will abolish the muscle spasm of experimental tetanus in rabbits (Hougs and Andersen, 1954; Kelly and Laurence, 1956). Webster (1962) concludes that chlorpromazine reduces the muscle spasms of tetanus by an action on the reticular system with the aid of the tranquillising effect also reducing the impact of afferent stimuli. Chlorpromazine can be used clinically to control tetanus with some sedative effect but without loss of consciousness and without any clinical impairment of respiratory activity. Laurence and his colleagues (1958) used 100 to 150 mg of chlorpromazine intramuscularly four- to six-hourly for adult patients and seldom exceeded a total of 1 g in 24 hours. An intravenous dose of the same size was occasionally used when a spasm urgently needed controlling. For neonates Laurence gave 20–25 mg approximately four-hourly, using a total of about 220 mg in 24 hours. These same workers compared a series of patients treated with chlorpromazine with a series treated with barbiturates—adults, phenobarbitone 200 mg intramuscularly three- to six-hourly or amylobarbitone intramuscularly or intravenously 0·25–1·0 g for urgent control, neonates phenobarbitone 60 mg six- to eight-hourly at first and at longer intervals after the first two or three days —and found no statistically significant difference in the outcome of the tetanus. They commented, however, that chlorpromazine is easier to manage than barbiturates since it does not cause loss of consciousness nor noticeable respiratory depression. On the other hand, there is increasing evidence that chlorpromazine alone does not produce sufficient mental sedation to make the patient entirely comfortable, even though it may be controlling the muscle spasm very satisfactorily. It is thus best combined with a small dose of a barbiturate.

Diazepam like mephenesin depresses the internuncial neurones in the spinal cord. It has now become the most useful drug in the treatment of muscle spasms that do not necessitate complete paralysis. It is less toxic than mephenesin or chlorpromazine and its central sedative properties make it a suitable drug for this distressing condition.

Muscle relaxation.—If sedation fails to prevent widespread spasms, full paralysis of the body, including the muscles of respiration, must be produced and maintained. For details of the care of patients during long-continued artificial respiration see Chapter 10. Once tracheostomy has been performed under general anaesthesia, full narcosis is no longer necessary; indeed the maintenance of anaesthesia with nitrous oxide throughout the period of treatment—a matter of weeks for many patients—may be dangerous. Bone marrow depression with an acute aplastic anaemia has been recorded during such treatment (Lassen *et al.*, 1956).

Nutrition and fluid balance.—In a severe case of tetanus the treatment is likely to continue for at least two weeks. It is important, therefore, to ensure that an adequate fluid and caloric intake is maintained during this period. Intragastric feeding is both easier and preferable to intravenous infusion but carries with it the risk of regurgitation and inhalation of stomach contents. If, however, tracheostomy has been necessary, a cuffed tube will avoid such a complication.

The daily caloric intake should be not less than 2,000 (preferably 2,500) and the total fluid intake should aim at 3·5 litres/24 hours with a urinary output of not less than 2 litres/24 hours. If intravenous therapy is used it is advisable to insert either a cannula or a polythene tube into a central vein to allow full mobility while nursing the patient.

Discussion

In practice it is the assessment of the progress of the disease that suggests the form of treatment. The clinical picture may change in a matter of hours, let alone days. At the earliest stage, as soon as a tentative diagnosis is made, the administration of drugs such as chlorpromazine and diazepam would seem reasonable. The dosage must be large and fully adequate to control and prevent paroxysms. In certain cases it may be justifiable to combine this treatment with tracheostomy to avoid laryngeal crises in a patient particularly sensitive to such a complication. At the first sign that full control with drugs is not possible without producing respiratory depression, a change to muscle relaxants and full paralysis must be made. To delay and risk death from respiratory inadequacy during a paroxysm is dangerous and unnecessary. Although radical treatment has undoubtedly led to a reduction in the mortality from severe tetanus, it is also unfortunately true that some cases die despite adequate control of their muscle spasms. The report from Ellis (1963) of 36 consecutive patients treated successfully would indicate that many of the deaths which result from tetanus are avoidable.

REFERENCES

ANDERSON, H. J., CHURCHILL-DAVIDSON, H. C., and RICHARDSON, A. T. (1953). Bronchial neoplasm with myasthenia. Prolonged apnoea after administration of succinylcholine. *Lancet*, **2**, 1291.

BARRETT, J. T. (1973). Recovery from malignant hyperthermia; a case report. *N.Z. med. J.*, **77**, 84.

BRITT, B. A., and KALOW, W. (1970). Malignant hyperpyrexia: aetiology unknown. *Canad. Anaesth. Soc. J.*, **17**, 316.

BRITT, B. A., LOCHER, W. G., and KALOW, W. (1969). Hereditary aspects of malignant hyperthermia. *Canad. Anaesth. Soc. J.*, **16**, 89.

BROWN, G. L., and HARVEY, A. M. (1939). Congenital myotonia in the goat. *Brain*, **62**, 341.

BRUNNER, N. G., NAMBA, T., and GROB, D. (1972). Corticosteroids in management of severe, generalized myasthenia gravis. Effectiveness and comparison with corticotropin therapy. *Neurology (Minneap.)*, **22,** 603.

BURNET, F. M. (1962*a*). Auto-immune disease—experimental and clinical. *Proc. roy. Soc. Med.,* **55,** 619.

BURNET, F. M. (1962*b*). Role of the thymus and related organs in immunity. *Brit. med. J.,* **2,** 807.

BURNS, B. D., and PATON, W. D. M. (1951). Depolarization of the motor end-plate by decamethonium and acetylcholine. *J. Physiol. (Lond.),* **115,** 41.

BURNS, B. D., PATON, W. D. M., and DIAS, M. V. (1949) Action of decamethonium iodide (C.10) on the demarcation potential of cats' muscle. *Arch. Sci. physiol.,* **3,** 609.

CAMPBELL, H., and BROMWELL, E. (1900). Myasthenia gravis. *Brain,* **23,** 277.

CHURCHILL-DAVIDSON, H. C., and RICHARDSON, A. T. (1953). Neuromuscular transmission in myasthenia gravis. *J. Physiol. (Lond.),* **122,** 252.

CHURCHILL-DAVIDSON, H. C., and RICHARDSON, A. T. (1955). Mestinon in myasthenia gravis. *Lancet,* **1,** 1123.

CHURCHILL-DAVIDSON, H. C., and RICHARDSON, A. T. (1958). Personal communication.

CHURCHILL-DAVIDSON, H. C., and RICHARDSON, A. T. (1961). A study of neuromuscular transmission in one hundred cases of myasthenia gravis. *Proceedings 2nd International Symposium on Myasthenia Gravis.* Ed. H. R. Viets. Springfield, Ill.: Charles C. Thomas.

DAHLBACK, O. ELMQVIST, D., JOHNS, T. R., RADNER, S., and THESLEFF, S. (1961). An electrophysiologic study of the neuromuscular junction in myasthenia gravis. *J. Physiol. (Lond.),* **156,** 336.

DAU, P. C., LINDSTROM, J. M., CASSEL, C. K., DENYS, E. H., SHEV, E. E., and SPITLER, L. E. (1977). Plasmapheresis and immunosuppressive drug therapy in myasthenia gravis. *New Engl. J. Med.,* **297,** 21.1134.

DAVIES, R. M., PACKER, K. J., TITEL, J., and WHITMARSH, V. (1969). Case report: malignant hyperpyrexia. *Brit. J. Anaesth.,* **41,** 703.

DENBOROUGH, M. A., FORSTER, J. F. A., LOVELL, R. R. H., MAPLESTONE, P. A., and VILLIERS, J. D. (1962). Anaesthetic deaths in a family. *Brit. J. Anaesth.,* **34,** 395.

DESMEDT, J. E. (1957). Nature of the defect of neuromuscular transmission in myasthenic patients; post-tetanic exhaustion. *Nature (Lond.),* **179,** 156.

DESMEDT, J. E. (1961). Neuromuscular defect in myasthenia gravis. *Proceedings 2nd International Symposium on Myasthenia Gravis.* Ed. H. R. Viets. Springfield, Ill.: Charles C. Thomas.

EATON, L. M., and CLAGGETT, O. T. (1955). Present status of thymectomy in the treatment of myasthenia gravis. *Amer. J. Med.,* **19,** 703.

EATON, L. M., and LAMBERT, E. H. (1957). Electromyography and electric stimulation of nerves in diseases of motor unit. Observations on myasthenic syndromes associated with malignant tumours. *J. Amer. med. Ass.,* **163,** 1117.

EDITORIAL (1974). Human antitoxin for tetanus prophylaxis. *Lancet,* **1,** 51.

ELLIS, F. R., and HARRIMAN, D. G. F. (1973). A new screening test for susceptibility to malignant hyperpyrexia. *Brit. J. Anaesth.,* **45,** 638.

ELLIS, F. R., HARRIMAN, D. G. F., KEANEY, N. P., KYEI-MENSAH, K., and TYRRELL, J. H. (1971). Halothane-induced muscle contracture as a cause of hyperpyrexia. *Brit. J. Anaesth.,* **43,** 721.

ELLIS, M. (1963). Human antitetanus serum in the treatment of tetanus. *Brit. med. J.,* **1,** 1123.

ELMQUIST, D., HOFMANN, W. W., KUGELBERG, J., and QUASTEL, D. M. J. (1964). An electrophysiological investigation of neuromuscular transmission in myasthenia gravis. *J. Physiol. (Lond.),* **174,** 417.

ENGEL, A. G., LAMBERT, E. H., and HOWARD, F. M., Jr. (1977). Immune complexes (IgG and C3) at the motor end-plate in myasthenia gravis: ultra-structural and light microscopic localization and electrophysiologic correlations. *Proc. Mayo Clin.*, **52/5**, 267.

ENGEL, W. K., FESTOFF, B. W., PATTEN, B. M. *et al.* (1974). Myasthenia gravis. *Ann. intern. Med.*, **81**, 225.

ERB, W. (1879). Ueber einen neuen, wahrscheinlich bulbären Symptomencomplex. *Arch. Psychiat. Nervenkr.*, **9**, 336.

FAMBROUGH, D. M., DRACHMAN, D. B., and SATYAMURI, S. (1973). Neuromuscular junction in myasthenia gravis: decreased acetylcholine receptors. *Science*, **182**, 293.

FELDMAN, S. A. (1973). *Muscle Relaxants—major problems in anaesthesia*, p. 101. London: W. B. Saunders.

FOLDES, F. F. (1970). Regional intravenous neuromuscular block: a new diagnostic and experimental tool. In: *Progress in Anaesthesiology*, p. 425 (Proc. 4th World Congr. Anaesthesiol.). Amsterdam: Excerpta Medica.

FOLDES, F. F., and MCNALL, P. G. (1962). Myasthenia gravis. A guide for anesthesiologists. *Anesthesiology*, **23**, 837.

FURNISS, P. (1971). The aetiology of malignant hyperpyrexia. *Proc. roy. Soc. Med.*, **64**, 216.

GESCHWIND, N., and SIMPSON, J. A. (1955). Procaine amide in the treatment of myotonia. *Brain*, **78**, 81.

GOLDBERG, A., BEATTIE, A., and CAMPBELL, B. (1975). The porphyrias and heavy metal intoxication. *Medicine (Baltimore)*, Series 2, 600.

GOLDFLAM, S. (1893). Ueber einen scheinbar heilbaren bulbärparalytischen Symptomencomplex mit Betheiligung der Extremitäten. *Dtsch. Z. Nervenheilk.*, **4**, 312.

GROB, D., JOHNS, R. J., and HARVEY, A. M. (1955). Alterations in neuromuscular transmissions in myasthenia gravis as determined by studies of drug action. *Amer. J. Med.*, **19**, 684.

HALL, L. W., WOOLF, N., BRADLEY, J. W. P., and JOLLY, D. W. (1966). Unusual reaction to succinylcholine. *Brit. med. J.*, **2**, 1305.

HARRISON, G. G. (1971). Anaesthetic induced malignant hyperpyrexia a suggested method of treatment. *Brit. med. J.*, **3**, 454.

HARRISON, G. G. (1975). Control of the malignant hyperpyrexia syndrome in malignant-hyperpyrexia-susceptible swine by dantrolene sodium. *Brit. J. Anaesth.*, **47**, 62.

HARRISON, G. G., SAUNDERS, S. J., BIEBUYEK, J. F., HICKMAN, R., DENT, D. M., WEAVER, F., and TERBLANCHE, J. (1969). Anaesthetic-induced malignant hyperpyrexia and a method for its prediction. *Brit. J. Anaesth.*, **41**, 844.

HENSON, R. A., RUSSELL, D. S., and WILKINSON, M. (1954). Carcinomatous neuropathy and myopathy. A clinical and pathological study. *Brain*, **77**, 82.

HOUGS, W., and ANDERSEN, E. W. (1954). The action of atropine, promethazine and chlorpromazine on experimental local tetanus in cats and rabbits. *Acta pharmacol. (Kbh.)*, **10**, 227.

ISAACS, H., and BARLOW, M. B. (1970). The genetic background to malignant hyperpyrexia revealed by serum creatine phosphokinase estimations in asymptomatic relatives. *Brit. J. Anaesth.*, **42**, 1077.

JOLLY, F. (1895). Ueber Myasthenia gravis pseudoparalytica. *Berl. klin. Wschr.*, **32**, 1.

KALOW, W., BRITT, B. A., TERREAU, M. E., and HAIST, C. (1970). Metabolic error of muscle metabolism after recovery from malignant hyperthermia. *Lancet*, **2**, 895.

KAUFMAN, L. (1960). Anaesthesia in dystrophia myotonica—a review of the hazards of anaesthesia. *Proc. roy. Soc. Med.*, **53**, 183.

KEANEY, N. P., and ELLIS, F. R. (1971). Malignant hyperpyrexia. *Brit. med. J.*, **4**, 49.

KELLY, R. E., and LAURENCE, D. R. (1956). Effect of chlorpromazine on convulsions of experimental and clinical tetanus. *Lancet*, **1**, 118.

KERR, J. H., CORBETT, J. L., PRYS-ROBERTS, C., SMITH, A. C., and SPALDING, J. M. K. (1968). Involvement of the sympathetic nervous system in tetanus. *Lancet*, **2**, 236.

KEYNES, G. (1954). Surgery of the thymus gland. Second (and third) thoughts. *Lancet*, **1**, 1197.

LAMBERT, F. H., ROOKE, E. D., EATON, L. M., and HODGSON, C. H. (1961). Myasthenic syndrome occasionally associated with bronchial neoplasm: neurophysiologic studies. *Proceedings 2nd International Symposium on Myasthenia Gravis*, p. 368. Ed. H. R. Viets, Springfield, Ill.: Charles C. Thomas.

LASSEN, H. C. A., BJØRNEBOE, M., IBSEN, B., and NEUKIRCH, F. (1954). Treatment of tetanus with curarisation, general anaesthesia, and intratracheal positive pressure ventilation. *Lancet*, **2**, 1040.

LASSEN, H. C. A., HENRIKSEN, E., NEUKIRCH, F., and KRISTENSEN, H. S. (1956). Treatment of tetanus. Severe bone marrow depression after prolonged nitrous oxide anaesthesia. *Lancet*, **1**, 527.

LAURENCE, D. R., BERMAN, E., SCRAGG, J. N., and ADAMS, E. B. (1958). A clinical trial of chlorpromazine against barbiturates in tetanus. *Lancet*, **1**, 987.

LAWRENCE, D. R., and WEBSTER, R. A. (1963). Pathologic physiology, pharmacology and therapeutics of tetanus. *Clin. Pharmacol. Ther.*, **4**, 36.

LUCKE, J. N., HALL, G. M., and LISTER, D. (1976). Porcine malignant hyperthermia—metabolic and physiological changes. *Brit. J. Anaesth.*, **48**, 297.

MACDERMOT, V. (1961). The histology of the neuromuscular junction in dystrophia myotonica. *Brain*, **84**, 75.

MAISEL, R. H., SESSIONS, D. G., and MILLER, R. N. (1973). Malignant hyperpyrexia during general anaesthesia—successful management of a case. *Ann. Otol. (St. Louis)*, **82**, 729.

NASTUK, W. L., PLESCIA, O. J., and OSSERMAN, K. E. (1959). Search for a neuromuscular blocking agent in the blood of patients with myasthenia gravis. *Amer. J. Med.*, **26**, 394.

NEWSOM DAVIS, J. (1974). Myasthenia. *Brit. J. hosp. Med.*, **2**, 933.

OSSERMAN, K. E., TSAIRIS, P., and WEINER, L. B. (1966). Myasthenia gravis and thyroid disease: clinical and immunological correlations. *Fed. Proc.*, **25**, 309.

PARSONS, R. L., and HOFMAN, W. W. (1966). Mode of action of tetanus toxin on the neuromuscular junction. *Amer. J. Physiol.*, **210**, 84.

PATEL, J. C., MEHTA, B. C., NANAVATI, B. H., HAZRA, A. K., RAO, S. S., and SWAMINATHAN, C. S. (1963). Role of serum therapy in tetanus. *Lancet*, **1**, 740.

PRYS-ROBERTS, C., CORBETT, J. L., KERR, J. H., and CRAMPTON SMITH, A. (1969). Treatment of sympathetic overactivity in tetanus. *Lancet*, **1**, 542.

RELTON, J. E. S., CREIGHTON, R. E., JOHNSTON, A. G., PELTON, D. A., and CONN, A. W. (1966). Hyperpyrexia in association with anaesthesia in children. *Canad. Anaesth. Soc. J.*, **13**, 419.

ROWLAND, L. P., ARANOW, H., and HOEFER, P. F. A. (1961). "Observations on the curare test in the differential diagnosis of myasthenia gravis". *Proceedings 2nd International Symposium on Myasthenia Gravis*. Ed. H. R. Viets. Springfield, Ill.: Charles C. Thomas.

SAIDMAN, L. J., HAVARD, S. E., and EGER, E. I., II. (1964). Hyperthermia during anesthesia. *J. Amer. med. Ass.*, **190**, 1029.

SANTA, T., ENGEL, A. G., and LAMBERT, E. H. (1972). Histiometric study of neuromuscular junction ultrastructure. *Neurology (Minneap.)*, **22**, 71.

SHACKLETON, P. (1954). The treatment of tetanus. Role of the anaesthetist. *Lancet*, **2**, 155.

SIMPSON, J. A. (1960). Myasthenia gravis. A new hypothesis. *Scot. med. J.*, **5**, 419.

SLAUGHTER, D., PARSONS, J. C., and MUNAL, H. D. (1940). New clinical aspects of the analgesic action of morphine. *J. Amer. med. Ass.*, **115**, 2058.

SMITH, A. C., HILL, E. E., and HOPSON, J. A. (1956). Treatment of severe tetanus with *d*-tubocurarine chloride and intermittent positive pressure respiration. *Lancet*, **2**, 550.

SMYTHE, P. M. (1963). Studies on neonatal tetanus and on pulmonary compliance of the totally relaxed infant. *Brit. med. J.*, **1**, 565.

SMYTHE, P. M., and BULL, A. B. (1961). Treatment of tetanus, with special reference to tracheotomy. *Brit. med. J.*, **2**, 732.

STEPHEN, C. R. (1967). Fulminant hyperthermia during anesthesia and surgery. *J. Amer. med. Ass.*, **202**, 221.

THIEL, R. E. (1967). The myotonic response to suxamethonium. *Brit. J. Anaesth.*, **39**, 815.

THUT, W. H., and DAVENPORT, H. T. (1966). Hyperpyrexia associated with succinylcholine induced muscle rigidity: a case report. *Canad. Anaesth. Soc. J.*, **13**, 425.

WEBSTER, R. A. (1962). Site of action of chlorpromazine and mephenesin in experimental tetanus. *Brit. J. Pharmacol.*, **18**, 150.

WILLIS, T. (1684). *A Practice of Physick*, p. 167. London.

WILSON, R. D., DENT, T. E., TRABER, D. L., McCOY, N. R., and ALLEN, C. R. (1967). Malignant hyperpyrexia with anesthesia. *J. Amer. med. Ass.*, **202**, 183.

WILTON, T. N. P., SLEIGH, B. E., and CHANDLER, C. C. D. (1958). Tetanus. *Lancet*, **1**, 940.

WISE, R. P. (1962). A myasthenic syndrome complicating bronchial carcinoma. *Anaesthesia*, **17**, 488.

WISE, R. P., and WYLIE, W. D. (1964). "The thymus gland. Its implications in clinical anesthetic practice." *Clinical Anesthesia: Anesthesia for Patients with Endocrine Disease*, Chapter II. Ed. M. T. Jenkins. Philadelphia: Davis & Co.

WOOLMER, R., and CATES, J. E. (1952). Succinylcholine in the treatment of tetanus. *Lancet*, **2**, 808.

WRIGHT, G. P. (1954). Tetanus. *Brit. med. Bull.*, **10**, 59.

ZAIMIS, E. J. (1951). The action of decamethonium on normal and denervated mammalian muscle. *J. Physiol. (Lond.)*, **112**, 176.

FURTHER READING

LAWRENCE, D. R., and WEBSTER, R. A. (1963). Pathologic physiology, pharmacology and therapeutics of tetanus. *Clin. Pharmacol. Ther.*, **4**, 36.

OSSERMAN, K. E., FOLDES, F. F., and GENKINS, G. (1972). *Myasthenia Gravis. International Encyclopedia of Pharmacology and Therapeutics*, Section 14. Oxford: Pergamon Press.

Chapter 29

CEREBRAL CIRCULATION AND BRAIN METABOLISM

THE importance of the blood supply to the brain is well known and is emphasised by the frequency with which neurological damage is the factor limiting full recovery after an episode of circulatory arrest.

ANATOMY

The arterial supply to the brain is derived from the internal carotid and vertebral arteries on each side, two-thirds of the supply coming from the carotid vessels. The left common carotid artery arises directly from the aorta, whereas the right is a branch of the innominate artery. The vertebral vessels arise from the subclavian artery on their respective sides and join together at the lower border of the pons to form the basilar artery. The circle of Willis (Fig. 1) is formed by an anastomoses between the terminal branches of the basilar and two internal carotid arteries.

Kramer (1912) using a methylene blue technique, first suggested that the streams of blood passing to the circle of Willis do not normally mix but are distributed to sharply demarcated areas of brain on the same side, and work with cerebral angiography (McDonald and Potter, 1951) has confirmed this. Flow across the anastomotic communications does occur though, and the importance of the circle of Willis was underlined by Brain (1957) who stated "the purpose served by the circle of Willis is to guarantee that whatever the

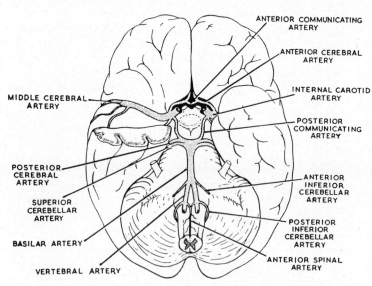

29/Fig. 1.—The circle of Willis.

position of the head in relation to gravity and to the trunk, and however from one moment to another the relative flow through either carotid or vertebral artery may vary as a result, these variations are always compensated for distal to those vessels, and within the cranial cavity, by the freest possible anastomosis before the brain is reached." The efficiency of the circle of Willis in equalising pressures has been demonstrated in animal studies by Symon (1967) who showed that complete occlusion of one internal carotid artery reduced pressure in both ipsilateral and contralateral middle cerebral arteries by about 14 per cent. Bilateral internal carotid occlusion caused a 50 per cent fall in middle cerebral artery pressure. Whilst in young subjects unilateral internal carotid occlusion does not affect total cerebral blood flow, a similar occlusion in the elderly often produces evidence of cerebral ischaemia. Individual anatomical variations, generalised arterial disease or acute reductions in systemic arterial pressure may all affect the efficiency of the circle of Willis.

Cerebral venous drainage, even in health, does not follow the unilateral pattern of the arterial supply (Batson, 1944). About two-thirds of the blood in the superior jugular bulb comes from the ipsilateral side and there is also a small (approximately 3 per cent) extracerebral contribution at this level (Shenkin et al., 1948). This may be important when a sample from one jugular bulb is taken as representative of the entire cerebral venous drainage. Kety and Schmidt (1948) concluded that for most purposes, unilateral sampling is adequately representative, although Munck and Lassen (1957) recommend bilateral sampling for greatest accuracy.

PHYSIOLOGY

Methods of Measurement

A variety of methods have been used for the study of cerebral blood flow in man (Ingvar and Lassen, 1965). All feasible methods are based on the Fick principle, which states that the uptake or clearance of a suitable indicator from an organ is a function of the blood flow through that organ and the concentration gradient of indicator between blood supplying and draining the organ. The methods in general, use either diffusible indicators which are inhaled or suitable isotopes injected intra-arterially.

Inhalation techniques.—The best known application of inhaled indicators to perfusion measurement is the Kety-Schmidt method of using nitrous oxide to measure cerebral blood flow (Kety and Schmidt, 1948). A mixture of 15 per cent nitrous oxide and 21 per cent oxygen in nitrogen is inhaled for ten minutes whilst arterial and cerebral venous blood is sampled either intermittently or continuously. At the end of this time brain uptake is usually complete and is given by the product of the final cerebral venous indicator concentration and the blood-brain partition coefficient of nitrous oxide (which is approximately unity). Cerebral blood flow per unit weight of brain is obtained by dividing this uptake figure by the integrated arteriovenous nitrous oxide difference during the uptake period. Whilst simple in theory the Kety-Schmidt method is beset with practical difficulties. Estimation of blood nitrous oxide concentration is tedious. This problem can be overcome by using ^{85}Kr as the inhaled indicator and employing standard counting techniques to blood sample analysis (Lassen and Munck, 1955). If flow is slow equilibrium will not be reached in ten minutes, and inhalation may have to be extended to 15–30 minutes, or arteriovenous differences extrapolated to infinite time. Simultaneous arterial and venous blood samples are needed and venous blood must be drawn from the jugular bulb. The method gives no indication of regional blood flow.

Lassen and Klee (1965) suggest that for accurate results under low flow conditions subjects should inhale low concentrations (1 mCu/litre) of ^{85}Kr, and arteriovenous differences measured during the desaturation period following inhalation.

Intra-arterial injection technique.—When a bolus of ^{85}Kr or ^{133}Xe is injected into an internal carotid artery, entry of indicator into and its subsequent exit from brain tissue will depend upon blood flow, diffusion and solubility. As these two indicators have a very low blood solubility, pulmonary excretion will be virtually complete in one circulation and there will be no effective arterial recirculation. In practice clearance of the indicator is detected by an array of externally placed scintillation crystals. Cerebral blood flow per unit weight of brain is calculated from the height of the clearance curve, the area underneath it and the tissue blood partition coefficient of indicator (Lassen and Ingvar, 1963; Veall and Mallett, 1963). An array of scintillation crystals allows some regional discrimination of flow. As a further refinement each clearance curve can be treated as the sum of two exponential components, an initial fast component representing flow through grey matter and a slow component reflecting white-matter flow.

Other methods.—Heat clearance from the surface of the cortex has been described by Carlyle and Grayson (1956) as a method of measuring cerebral blood flow, whilst Meyer and Gotoh (1964) have used a thermovelocity method to estimate internal jugular flow. These and other thermal methods suffer from severe calibration problems. Other indicators which have been used include Evans Blue (Gibbs *et al.*, 1947*b*) and labelled red cells (Nylin *et al.*, 1960). Impedance plethysmography (Jenkner, 1962) and direct measurements on exposed vessels (Kristiansen and Krog, 1962) have also been employed.

NORMAL VALUES AND PHYSIOLOGICAL VARIATION IN CEREBRAL BLOOD FLOW

Cerebral blood flow measured by the nitrous oxide technique is 50–55 ml/ 100 g/minute in normal adults, indicating a total cerebral flow of approximately 750 ml/minute (Kety and Schmidt, 1948). The flow rate is greater in the first decade of life, falling at puberty towards the adult values (Kennedy and Sokoloff, 1957). Although most evidence suggests that cerebral blood flow tends to fall from middle age onwards (Shenkin *et al.*, 1953), this does not necessarily occur (Sokoloff, 1959*a*). There are direct relationships between cerebral metabolic activity and cerebral blood flow. Flow is reduced during barbiturate anaesthesia, and is increased when analeptic and convulsant drugs are given. Risberg and Ingvar (1968) have shown that this also holds on a regional basis, photic stimulation for instance producing increased flow in the occipital lobes. Blood flow rises markedly during rapid eye movement sleep but is only slightly raised in slow-wave sleep.

FACTORS CONTROLLING CEREBRAL BLOOD FLOW

The Munro-Kellie doctrine of 1783 postulated that because the nearly incompressible brain is housed within a rigid cranium, the quantity of blood in the cerebral circulation will remain constant and flow through it will respond passively to changes in arterial pressure. In 1890, Roy and Sherrington suggested that in addition to the effects of the systemic arterial pressure, the calibre of the cerebral vessels could vary in response to chemical changes in their environment, and it is now accepted that intrinsic regulation of the cerebrovascular resistance is the most important determinant of cerebral blood flow under normal conditions (Sokoloff and Kety, 1960). The many factors which can influence cerebral blood flow do so either by altering the pressure gradient across the vessels, or by changing the resistance within them.

1. Factors Affecting the Pressure Gradient Across the Cerebral Vessels

(a) **Arterial blood pressure.**—In the absence of hypotension, the systemic blood pressure is believed to play little part in the regulation of the cerebral blood flow, and until the mean blood pressure is less than 40 mm Hg (5 kPa) the cerebral blood flow is maintained (Finnerty et al., 1954). This autoregulation of cerebral flow in response to changes in arterial pressure has been demonstrated by a variety of techniques and over a wide range of both high and low abnormal pressures, spontaneous and induced (Lassen, 1959). However, the autoregulatory response is abolished by elevation of the arterial carbon dioxide tension (Harper and Glass, 1965) and by deep anaesthesia, extensive surgery, arterial hypoxaemia and circulatory arrest (*Lancet*, 1968). A transitory failure of autoregulation can also follow sudden changes in pressure (Schneider, 1963), and is common in the presence of cerebral tumours and with infarcted areas of brain.

The mechanism of autoregulatory control of the cerebral vessels is obscure —Bayliss (1902) postulated a direct effect of pressure on the musculature of the blood vessels whereas Lassen (1959) suggests that the tissue carbon dioxide tension is the regulating factor. The existence of conditions under which the mechanism fails may explain the discrepancy between some reports of the effect of arterial pressure on cerebral blood flow, and also provides a warning that even moderate hypotension occurring during some of the circumstances met in clinical anaesthesia may endanger cerebral perfusion. In addition, it is important to recall that the critical pressure at which autoregulation begins to fail even in the conscious subject may well be higher in the elderly and arteriosclerotic, and Bromage (1953) has produced electroencephalographic evidence in support of this. When autoregulation fails a passive pressure-flow relationship governs cerebral perfusion.

(b) **Venous pressure.**—The effect of the pressure in the great veins is normally insignificant even in heart failure (Novak et al., 1953) but when coughing or straining or during occlusion of the great veins, much higher pressures may be reached. Moyer et al. (1954) demonstrated no change in cerebral blood flow when the internal jugular venous pressure of man was elevated to 23 cm of water (2·3 kPa), and Jacobson et al. (1963a) have produced evidence to suggest that autoregulation of cerebral blood flow can occur in response to changes in venous pressure. These authors also showed that moderate increases in cerebral venous pressure, by limiting vessel collapse, may improve cerebral blood flow. Alternatively, a very high right atrial pressure may occasionally be encountered during by-pass heart surgery due to distortion of the vessels—this can compromise cerebral blood flow.

2. Factors Affecting the Cerebrovascular Resistance

(a) **Chemical control.**—Arterial carbon dioxide tension is the most important single factor controlling cerebral blood flow. Increasing arterial CO_2 tension increases flow whilst reduction in arterial CO_2 tension reduces cerebral blood flow. Harper (1965) showed that in dogs cerebral blood flows changed by about 2·5 per cent for every 1 mm Hg (0·1 kPa) change in P_{CO_2}, that sensitivity was greatest around the normal P_{CO_2} of 40 mm Hg (5·3 kPa), and that the relationship between P_{CO_2} and cerebral blood flow was virtually linear between 30 and 60 mm Hg (4–8 kPa). At P_{CO_2} levels over 150 mm Hg (20 kPa) no further increase in cerebral blood flow occurs, presumably because maximum cerebral vascular dilatation has then occurred. Similarly cerebral blood flow reaches a level of about 45 per cent of normal at a P_{CO_2} of 15 mm Hg (2 kPa), and further reduction of P_{CO_2} does not cause a further decrease in flow. This limitation is probably due to local hypoxia, produced by vasoconstriction, exerting a local vasodilator effect which counters the effects of further hypocapnia.

Harper and Glass (1965) showed that this response to CO_2 is diminished in the presence of hypotension and abolished when systemic blood pressure reaches 50 mm Hg (6·7 kPa). Similarly Lennox and Gibbs (1932) showed that the response of cerebral blood flow to carbon dioxide is diminished in the presence of arterial hypoxaemia.

Whilst acute changes in CO_2 tension cause the above changes, prolonged maintenance of arterial CO_2 at abnormal levels is associated with a return of cerebral blood flow to normal levels. After six to twelve hours of hyperventilation during acclimatisation to high altitude, Severinghaus and his colleagues (1966) found cerebral blood flow to be unchanged from normal levels. Chronic hypercapnia, as seen in chronic respiratory failure, is usually associated with a normal cerebral blood flow.

The effect of carbon dioxide on cerebral blood flow is almost certainly due to a direct action on the smooth muscle of cerebral arterioles, mediated by local tissue pH changes (Lassen, 1966). If arterial carbon dioxide tension is kept constant marked changes in arterial pH produced by infusing acids or alkalis do not affect cerebral blood flow (Harper and Bell, 1963). Thus the blood-brain barrier protects cerebral blood flow from the effects of metabolic acidosis and alkalosis.

The effects of changes in arterial oxygenation on cerebral blood flow are opposite to those produced by carbon dioxide. However, the cerebral circulation does not respond to Pa_{O_2} changes around the normal value. When Pa_{O_2} falls below 60 mm Hg (8 kPa) cerebral blood flow increases, and is doubled at a Pa_{O_2} of about 35 mm Hg (4·7 kPa). The cerebral vasodilatation produced by hypoxia may be due to local tissue acidosis causing a fall in tissue pH and affecting smooth muscle of cerebral arterioles.

Higher than normal oxygen tensions cause a diminution in cerebral blood flow, 100 per cent oxygen inhalation reducing cerebral blood flow by 10 per cent, whilst a similar oxygen concentration at 2 atmospheres pressure causes a

20 per cent fall in cerebral blood flow. Whilst part of this response may be due to hypocapnia accompanying hyperoxia, oxygen also appears to have a direct constrictor effect on cerebral vessels. The fall in cerebral blood flow due to hyperoxia is not associated with fall in cerebral available oxygen (Jacobson et al., 1963). Harper, McDowall and Ledingham (1965) showed that cerebral vasoconstriction did not occur with hyperbaric oxygenation in dogs suffering from haemorrhagic hypotension, and Holbach and Gött (1970) have shown a similar lack of effect of hyperbaric oxygenation on regional cerebral blood flow in areas of cerebral oedema following head injury.

(b) **Neurogenic control.**—The cerebral circulation is less subject to auto-nomic control than other vascular beds in the body. Limited effects of the autonomic nervous system on cerebral vascular reactivity have been demon-strated (James et al., 1968; Harper et al., 1972; Lassen, 1968). Harper and his associates (1972), on the basis of their own results, have recommended that the cerebral circulation should be considered in two parts. First, the *extraparen-chymal* arteries and veins which are mainly under neurogenic control, and secondly, the *intraparenchymal* small arteries which are controlled by local metabolites. It has also been demonstrated that denervation of the systemic baroreceptors and chemoreceptors probably reduces the effects of carbon di-oxide on cerebral blood flow, whilst reactivity to carbon dioxide is increased following cervical sympathectomy. This evidence suggests that sympathetic tone normally has an opposing action on the cerebrovascular dilator effects of carbon dioxide.

(c) **Intracranial pressure.**—At pressures up to about 50 cm H_2O (4·9 kPa) increases of intracranial pressure do not reduce cerebral perfusion pressure (arterial—CSF pressure difference) below the lower limit at which autoregula-tion occurs and cerebral blood flow is unaffected. Above this level there is a considerable fall in cerebral blood flow (Kety et al., 1948a).

(d) **Viscosity.**—Cerebral blood flow was found by Kety (1950) to be less than half normal in polycythaemia and it can be significantly increased in severe anaemia (Robin and Gardner, 1953).

EFFECTS OF DRUGS ON THE CEREBRAL CIRCULATION

Many of the conflicting reports on the effects of drugs on cerebrovascular resistance and some of the variations in response are attributable to choice of species or the dose and route of administration. Thus aminophylline in man causes cerebral vasoconstriction, the effect of the falling carbon dioxide tension predominating over the direct vasodilator effect seen in other species (Wechsler et al., 1950; Shenkin, 1951). Adrenaline given intravenously in doses which raise the mean arterial pressure by 20 per cent causes an increase in cerebral blood flow, whereas with noradrenaline the vasoconstrictor effect predominates and the cerebral blood flow falls in spite of the rise in blood pressure (King et al., 1952). A review of the effects of drugs on the cerebral circulation is given by Sokoloff (1959b) and of the effects of anaesthetic drugs by McDowall (1965, 1971)—see Table 1. McDowall points out the many ways in which changes induced by anaesthetic drugs may affect the cerebral circulation, and emphasises the difficulty of attributing observed changes in cerebral blood flow to the direct action of the anaesthetic drugs.

29/Table 1.

EFFECTS OF GENERAL ANAESTHETIC DRUGS ON CEREBRAL BLOOD FLOW

AGENT	CEREBRAL BLOOD FLOW	CEREBRAL METABOLIC RATE	CEREBROVASCULAR RESPONSE TO CO_2
Barbiturates	↓	↓↓	unchanged
Narcotic analgesics	o,↓	↓	unchanged
Nitrous oxide	o	↓	unchanged
Cyclopropane	↓,↑	↓	unchanged
Halothane	↑	↓	unchanged
Trichloroethylene	↑	↓	unchanged
Methoxyflurane	↑	↓	unchanged
Chloroform	↑	↓	unchanged
Diethyl ether	↑	↓	unchanged
Enflurane	↑	↓(↑)	unchanged
Isoflurane	↑	↓	unchanged

Barbiturates.—Marked falls in cerebral blood flow can occur when barbiturates are given in doses sufficient to produce general anaesthesia. The reduction in blood flow is proportional to the related reduction in cerebral metabolic activity, mediated by a reduced local production of carbon dioxide.

Narcotic analgesics.—These agents have little effect on cerebral blood flow if arterial CO_2 levels are controlled. If respiratory depression occurs the increase in P_{CO_2} markedly increases cerebral blood flow. Large doses of potent analgesics such as fentanyl and phenoperidine cause some reduction in cerebral metabolic activity and a concomitant fall in cerebral blood flow (Fitch et al., 1969).

Inhalational anaesthetics.—All the volatile anaesthetic agents increase cerebral blood flow by producing cerebral vasodilatation. The increase in general is proportional to the concentration of drug administered. In deep general anaesthesia blood pressure may fall below the lower limit of auto-regulation and cerebral blood flow may return to normal levels or be reduced below normal. Inhalational anaesthetics also produce a dose-related reduction in cerebral metabolic activity. The combination of raised blood flow and reduced metabolism leads to an increase in cerebral venous oxygen content. Nitrous oxide has little effect on cerebral blood flow but clinical concentrations reduce cerebral metabolic activity by about 25 per cent (Alexander et al., 1965). Low concentrations of cyclopropane reduce both cerebral blood flow and cerebral metabolic activity, but high concentrations of this gas behave like other agents in increasing cerebral blood flow (Alexander et al., 1968).

GENERAL ANAESTHETICS AND INTRACRANIAL PRESSURE

The inhalational anaesthetics (which raise cerebral blood flow by vaso-dilatation) lead to an increase in cerebral blood volume which, in turn, causes a rise in intracranial pressure. Usually the rises in CSF pressure are slight and readily controlled by hyperventilation. Large changes in intracranial pressure can occur in patients with space-occupying brain lesions (Jennett *et al.*, 1969). Rapid fluctuations in cerebral blood volume can in these patients lead to dangerous pressure gradients being developed between different brain compartments. These effects of volatile anaesthetics can be reduced by a period of hyperventilation before their administration (Adams *et al.*, 1972; Misfeldt *et al.*, 1975).

Effects of Hypothermia

Both cerebral blood flow and cerebral metabolic rate fall in dogs with decrease in body temperature (Rosomoff and Holaday, 1954; Kleinerman and Hopkins, 1955). Rosomoff (1956) showed a diminution in cerebral blood flow in dogs of 6–7 per cent for each degree centigrade fall in temperature. At a temperature of 28° C, a fall in cerebral blood flow of 50 per cent was recorded and Kleinerman and Hopkins reported that at temperatures between 22 and 27° C the reduction in cerebral blood flow exceeded the diminution of cerebral oxygen consumption. Albert and Fazekas (1956) reported five cases of induced hypothermia in man; in two of these the diminution in cerebral blood flow exceeded the decrease in cerebral metabolic rate. However, Rosomoff and Holaday reported a parallel reduction in both metabolic rate and blood flow in dogs cooled to 26° C and in clinical practice the technique is widely and successfully used to prevent cerebral damage during procedures which may jeopardise cerebral blood flow.

Regional Variations in the Cerebral Circulation

The development of measurement techniques to measure regional cerebral blood flow has produced evidence that marked abnormalities in the distribution of cerebral blood flow may occur when brain damage is present.

Luxury perfusion.—This is the name given by Lassen (1966) to a localised over-abundant cerebral blood flow relative to metabolic needs, and is commonly seen round areas of damaged brain. It is due to local tissue acidosis caused by tissue damage.

Steal syndrome.—The blood supply to damaged areas of brain may not react to changes in arterial CO_2 tension, but have a circulation which varies passively with perfusion pressure. Hypercarbia under these conditions will cause vasodilatation in normal cerebral vessels and divert blood from diseased to healthy areas (Brock *et al.*, 1969).

Robin Hood (Inverse Steal) syndrome.—The opposite phenomenon to the Steal syndrome can occur during hypocapnia where vasoconstriction in normal areas of brain causes an increased blood flow to the diseased area.

Hyperventilation and Anaesthesia

Hyperventilation raises the pain threshold in conscious volunteers and appears to reduce requirements for central depressant drugs during anaesthesia. It has been shown that hypocapnia does not alter anaesthetic requirements in man (Bridges and Eger, 1966) and greater depth of anaesthesia during hyperventilation may be due to the higher alveolar tension of anaesthetic agent which develops when increased ventilation occurs at constant inspired concentration (Eger *et al.*, 1965). There is conflicting evidence on the possible occurrence of cerebral hypoxia secondary to cerebral vasoconstriction and shift of the oxygen dissociation curve due to a low arterial carbon dioxide tension (Sugioka and Davis, 1960; Robinson and Gray, 1961; Pierce et al., 1962; Bollen, 1962; Wollman et al., 1965). Many of these authors support the view that mild degrees of cerebral hypoxia can be produced by hyperventilation, but despite this theoretical disadvantage there is no clinical evidence that moderate hyperventilation of the anaesthetised patient to a Pco_2 of 30–35 mm Hg (4·0–4·7 kPa) produces cerebral damage and the benefits of controlled respiration, circulatory stability and minimal central depression, have made the technique widely popular. Full arterial saturation throughout is obviously essential to minimise any possible hypoxic hazard.

Value of Hyperventilation in Neurosurgery

Although it is sometimes claimed that hyperventilation can "shrink" the normal brain, Rosomoff (1963) showed in dogs that hyperventilation does not reduce the volume of the brain tissue and that intracranial pressure is unaffected provided the carbon dioxide tension is normal before the onset of increased ventilation. The spontaneously breathing, anaesthetised patient is almost always hypoventilating to some extent so that controlled ventilation is likely to provide better and safer operating conditions. Likewise in head injuries or patients with cerebral oedema, controlled ventilation with a guaranteed airway may be more satisfactory than possibly inadequate spontaneous respiration and an airway jeopardised by coma. Because of the factors associated with regional variations in cerebral blood flow hyperventilation may be of therapeutic value where localised areas of brain damage occur. By inducing an inverse steal syndrome blood flow to damaged areas will be increased and tissue damage may be minimised (Alexander and Lassen, 1970).

CEREBRAL METABOLISM

Measurements of overall cerebral metabolism depend on the determination of cerebral arteriovenous differences and total blood flow. The venous sample is drawn from the superior jugular bulb in man (Myerson et al., 1927) and this provides blood which is almost exclusively representative of cerebral activity.

The brain is unique in that it relies entirely upon carbohydrate utilisation to provide its energy requirements. Under normal circumstances glucose is oxidised aerobically to produce carbon dioxide and water. The initial stage in this process is the production of pyruvate. In the absence of an adequate oxygen supply pyruvate can be converted to lactate. Anaerobic metabolism results in the liberation of a far lesser amount of energy-providing ATP than does the aerobic oxidation of pyruvate. The supply of oxygen determines which of the two metabolic pathways will be used (Wollman et al., 1968).

Oxygen consumption of the brain is normally high (3·5 ml/100 g/min) and is independent of cerebral blood flow, there being no diminution in oxygen consumption until cerebral flow has fallen to 60 per cent by hypotension (Finnerty et al., 1954). Available stores of oxygen in the brain are so small that an uninterrupted circulatory supply is essential. Oxygen deprivation by total circulatory arrest causes loss of consciousness in 10 seconds (Rossen et al., 1943). Hypoglycaemia, by reducing the amount of substrate, produces all degrees of functional disturbance progressing to coma, the degree of hypo-glycaemia correlating well with the level of impairment.

Relationship to Functional Activity

Physiological variations of cerebral activity produce no change in the overall metabolic rate or cerebral blood flow (Mangold *et al.*, 1955; Sokoloff *et al.*, 1955), but regional variations in flow induced by changes in cerebral activity may well account for this (Landau *et al.*, 1955; Sokoloff, 1957). It is also possible to correlate depression of mental activity in a variety of pathological conditions affecting consciousness with cerebral metabolic rate (Fazekas and Bessman, 1953; Kety, 1950; Freyhan *et al.*, 1951).

Marked reductions in cerebral oxygen supply, as occur during severe hypocapnia with a Pco_2 of about 20 mm Hg (2·7 kPa), have been shown to affect the EEG (Cohen *et al.*, 1966), and following anaesthesia with such a level of hypocapnia alterations in critical flicker fusion and reaction time have been shown to occur (Allen and Morris, 1962; Wollman and Orken, 1968).

Changes in Pathological Conditions

Circulatory deficiency rapidly causes irreversible metabolic changes as witnessed by prolonged unconsciousness and a lowered cerebral oxygen consumption even after cerebral blood flow has been restored (Fazekas and Bessman, 1953). Lesser degrees of anoxia cause an increase in glycolysis and depletion of energy-rich phosphate compounds together with an increased production of lactic acid (Gurdjian *et al.*, 1944). Young animals have a greater capacity for withstanding cerebral anoxia without harm because of prolonged retention of the fetal ability to metabolise anaerobically (Himwich, 1951).

During hypoglycaemic coma, a persistent low level of oxygen consumption together with a respiratory quotient which is still unity suggests that other carbohydrate stores can be utilised slowly (Kety *et al.*, 1948*b*). When these are exhausted, hypoglycaemic coma becomes irreversible and as with prolonged anoxic damage, coma and a low oxygen consumption persist even when higher than normal blood sugar levels have been restored (Fazekas *et al.*, 1951).

THEORIES OF ANAESTHESIA

Anaesthesia may be defined as a progressive reversible depression of nervous tissue, or more simply as the controlled production of unconsciousness.

There is no simple theory explaining the production of the unconscious state. The many theories of anaesthesia which have been advanced depend either on physical properties of anaesthetics or the localisation of a site of action of anaesthetics.

PHYSICAL PROPERTIES OF ANAESTHETICS

A vast number of compounds have been shown to be capable of producing anaesthesia, and they lack any common chemical features. No theories have been advanced relating anaesthetic action to overall chemical structure. The anaesthetic agents in general use have however several common physical features. They are all substances of comparatively low molecular weight, chemically unreactive and uncharged. A fruitful source of theories of anaesthesia has been to correlate some physical property of anaesthetics with anaesthetic potency.

Lipid Solubility

Meyer and Overton were the first workers to correlate narcotic potency with lipid solubility, expressed as an oil-water partition coefficient (Meyer, 1899; Overton, 1901). There is general agreement that all anaesthetics are lipophylic, and the greater the lipid solubility the lower the concentration of anaesthetic required to produce its effects. It is more conventional to correlate potency with an oil/gas partition coefficient rather than differential solubility in oil and water. The minimum anaesthetic concentration (MAC) of any agent multiplied by its oil-gas partition coefficient tends towards a constant value of 140 (Eger *et al.*, 1969). Lipid solubility does not lead to any explanation of how anaesthetics act but strongly suggests that they are acting in lipid regions of cells.

Water Solubility

The majority of anaesthetics are poorly soluble in water. Miller (1961) and Pauling (1961) independently showed that many anaesthetic molecules were capable of forming hydrates in the form of clathrates. In these compounds a cage of water molecules surrounds a central anaesthetic molecule. The presence of such "microcrystals" was believed to produce anaesthesia by affecting membrane permeability or altering the electrical properties of cells. Whilst there is a correlation between anaesthetic potency and its hydrate dissociation pressure, it is a far poorer correlation than was originally thought. Moreover whilst clathrates of many anaesthetic compounds can be formed, their formulation often requires extremes of pressure at body temperature.

Thermodynamic Activity

Ferguson (1939) pointed out that many of the correlations invoked in theories of anaesthesia were concerned with partition of an anaesthetic between different phases. At equilibrium in such a partition the thermodynamic potential—the partial molal free energy—will be the same in all phases. Ferguson showed that equipotent concentrations of anaesthetics had equal thermodynamic activities, assessed as the ratio of anaesthetic tension to saturated vapour tension. This finding, like that of lipid solubility, does not explain how anaesthetics act. It does explain why many different physical properties of anaesthetics can be to a greater or lesser extent correlated with narcotic potency.

Anaesthetic Sites of Action

Synaptic action of anaesthetics.—There is general agreement that anaesthetics are capable of depressing synaptic transmission (De Jong *et al.*, 1968; Larrabee and Posternak, 1952). The effects of anaesthetics on central transmission have been shown to be greater on the polysynaptic pathways through the reticular-activating substance than on more direct pathways (French *et al.*, 1953). However as anaesthetics can act at many sites in the central nervous system no single site can be pinpointed as a primary site of action.

Anaesthetics and cell membranes.—In searching for a hydrophobic area of cells where anaesthetics may exert their effects much attention has been centred on the possible effects of anaesthetics on cell membranes. Seeman (1966) showed that red cell membranes could be stabilised against lysis by exposure to optimal concentrations of anaesthetics. The effect is related to an increased membrane bulk caused partly by insertion of anaesthetic molecules into the membrane. It has been suggested, though supportive evidence is slight, that swelling of membranes due to anaesthetic action reduces membrane permeability to sodium and other ions. Reduced permeability at pre- and post-synaptic membranes could considerably affect synaptic transmission. Pressure reversal of anaesthesia—the reversal of the anaesthetic state produced by pressures above 150 atmospheres—has been explained as being due to a compression of an expanded membrane to its normal state with a restoration of normal permeability. The evidence supporting these various theories of altered permeability is of the most indirect variety, based mainly on the effects of anaesthetics on models such as artificial membranes (Bangham *et al.*, 1965).

Biochemical theories.—As a result of *in vitro* studies on cortical brain slices Quastel (1952) suggested that depression of oxidation is the mechanism by which the anaesthetic state is produced. The sensitive stage in carbohydrate metabolism was suggested as being the oxidation of NADH to NAD and therefore ATP production (Quastel, 1965). *In vivo* studies by Michenfelder and his colleagues (1970) have shown that brain ATP concentration is unchanged during anaesthesia. Although biochemical effects of anaesthetics can be demonstrated it is very possible that these effects are the result of rather than the cause of anaesthesia.

ELECTROENCEPHALOGRAPHY

The electroencephalogram (EEG) is conveniently recorded from multiple symmetrically paired electrodes placed on the skull, although monitoring during anaesthesia is commonly performed with only two electrodes (frontal and occipital). A number of extraneous signals may interfere with the recording of these very small potentials (tens of microvolts only); excessive sweating, eye movements and contraction of scalp or limb muscles can all produce artefacts, and arterial or venous pulses, respiratory changes and the electrocardiogram can be superimposed on the EEG, particularly if the electrodes or earth lead are poorly applied or incorrectly sited. Proximity to other apparatus frequently causes interference and it may be necessary to perform the recording in a screened room.

Normal Activity

A wide variety of patterns may be recorded from normal individuals and the following wave forms have been recognised.

Delta waves, 0·5–3·5 Hz, occur in infants and sleeping adults with an amplitude of about 100 microvolts. They are largest in the frontal lobes, symmetrical but asynchronous.

Theta waves, 4–7 Hz, occur in children with an amplitude of 50 microvolts and in adults with an amplitude of 10 microvolts. They are diffuse in children but become localised to the parietal and temporal regions in adults.

Alpha waves, 8–13 Hz, occur in infants with an amplitude of 20 microvolts, in children with an amplitude of 75 microvolts and in adults with an amplitude of 50 microvolts. These, like the theta rhythms, are diffuse in children but become localised to the parietal and occipital areas in adults. They are symmetrical and synchronous. The alpha waves are augmented by closing the eyes and during mental repose, and are reduced by visual and mental activity, sometimes to the extent of total removal or "blocking".

Beta waves, 14–15 Hz, of about 20 microvolts, usually occur in the fronto-central areas in children and are symmetrical and asychronous.

Gamma waves, 26 or more Hz, usually have an amplitude of 10 microvolts and are rare in normal subjects.

Some Abnormal Patterns

It is very rare to obtain a record of a major convulsive seizure free from artefact but minor seizures are frequently well recorded, especially when a stimulus such as over-breathing is used (Fig. 2–*4*). Seizures produced in this way are often less severe than those usually suffered by the patient and are called "larval". About 50 per cent of people subject to "fits" have an "abnormal" EEG record between attacks—that is they show patterns which are never seen in normal subjects (Fig. 2–*5*). Hysterical fits do not affect the EEG.

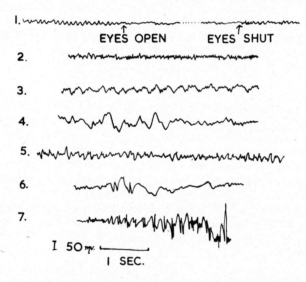

29/FIG. 2.—SOME ELECTROENCEPHALOGRAPHIC PATTERNS

1. Normal *alpha* rhythm showing effect of opening the eyes; 2. Normal fast activity; 3. Normal slow activity; 4. Slow activity in a child of 10 produced by hyperventilation; 5. Typical inter-seizure record; 6. Wave and spike activity; 7. Pre-convulsion trace.

As the disturbances arise in differing parts of the brain, the pattern of the electroencephalogram will vary from lead to lead. A minor seizure pattern is characterised by "wave and spike" activity containing a very large component up to 1 millivolt at a frequency from 1·5 to 3·5 Hz (Fig. 2–*6*). The spike component lasts from 0·02 second up to 0·1 second. In organic diseases the relationship between the spike and wave varies from moment to moment.

The pattern of a major convulsion appears to be an all-or-none phenomenon and it is not much altered by drugs. The pattern depends on the site of onset and route of spread of the electrical disturbance but is symmetrical and synchronous when it is fully developed. It starts to alter thirty seconds or so before the onset of the convulsion is manifest, as shown by rhythms of 2–7 Hz which increase in amplitude and are most prominent in the pre-motor regions (Fig. 2–7). The tonic stage of the convulsion is characterised by the abrupt onset of spikes of moderate amplitude. The spikes then become "grouped" and there is a slow component at 1·5–3 Hz which bears a constant time relationship to the groups of spikes. Towards the end of the convulsion, the spikes occur only in synchronised groups on the crest of a rhythmic slow wave. The frequency of this wave slows to 1 Hz with no decline in amplitude, and then it suddenly ceases. After the convulsion there is random slow activity with an occasional spike which is followed by the gradual reappearance of the normal pattern.

The Effect of Anaesthetic Drugs on the Electroencephalogram

It is difficult to correlate the classical Guedel signs of anaesthesia with changes in the EEG and there is some variation in the changes which are produced by different anaesthetic agents. Sadove and his colleagues (1967) state as a broad outline that the following changes occur. "When there is only slight mental impairment with mild analgesia and amnesia, low-voltage fast activity is increased and the record resembles the normal 'attention' trace. With the onset of light anaesthesia, fast activity of high voltage predominates. Slowing of the electrical activity occurs with deepening of the anaesthetic, followed by brief periods of inactivity and finally, total electrical silence. The stage of brief periods of inactivity may be reached transitorily after a rapid intravenous induction."

Common sedatives (barbiturates, chloral hydrate and paraldehyde) can produce variable changes in the EEG but there is no correlation with the clinical effect of the drug. All sedatives producing sleep, even those used clinically as anticonvulsants, tend to activate seizure discharges in epileptic or predisposed persons (Gibbs *et al.*, 1947a). Atropine, pethidine and morphine used in conventional doses produce no change in the EEG and curare likewise has no effect provided respiration is controlled (Kiersey *et al.*, 1951). Spinal anaesthesia produces no change in the EEG although coincidental sleep or sedation may have some effect on the record.

Effects of Hypoxia

Slowing of the wave frequency of the EEG is the most characteristic change associated with hypoxia, but cerebral venous oxygen tensions of 18 mm Hg (2·4 kPa) may be reached before there is any alteration of the record. An initial increase of frequency and amplitude lasting 1 to 2 seconds occurs sometimes with the onset of sudden and complete anoxia. By ten seconds there is slow cortical activity of 1 to 3 Hz which becomes slower and of greater amplitude. When it reaches 1 Hz the amplitude decreases so that by 18 to 20 seconds after complete anoxia, the EEG becomes a straight line. If hypoxia is rapidly relieved the EEG returns to normal in the reverse order, but changes may persist long after the oxygen tension has been restored to normal if the period of hypoxia was prolonged. Following a long period of hypoxia, a flat trace with superimposed low-voltage (5 microvolts), fast (50 Hz), spiky activity may occur (Gronquist *et al.*, 1952). This is known as "file pattern" and carries a poor prognosis.

It has been suggested that the EEG may be used to identify "cerebral death" in patients requiring support of cardiorespiratory function, and Hockaday *et al.* (1965) were able to predict with considerable accuracy from the EEG whether anoxic damage following cardiac or respiratory arrest would prove fatal or non-fatal. However Haider *et al.* (1968) have reported survival with complete normality in patients with a persistently flat EEG for many hours after barbiturate intoxication and it must therefore be realised that the EEG alone is insufficient evidence on which to decide whether supportive therapy should be continued or withdrawn from a patient with severe cerebral damage. Serial recordings, considered in conjunction with clinical assessment of the function of the central nervous and other systems and the aetiology of the condition, may be of some value in making these individual and difficult decisions.

Effects of Hypercapnia

Moderate increases in carbon dioxide tension (5 per cent inspired CO_2) cause an increase in frequency of cortical activity. Greater increases (more than 10 per cent CO_2) reverse this acceleration and slow waves appear (Sadove *et al.*, 1967). High carbon dioxide tensions also potentiate the effects of barbiturates and other anaesthetic drugs (Clowes *et al.*, 1953).

Effects of Hypocapnia

Voluntary hyperventilation in man produces high-voltage slow waves in the EEG which Brazier (1943) concluded are due to the direct effect of a low Pco_2 and are not secondary to hypoxia due to cerebral vasoconstriction. Holmberg (1953) however found that voluntary hyperventilation with oxygen produced less alteration in brain potentials than voluntary hyperventilation with air, and Bollen (1962) considered that the slow wave activity and accompanying analgesia of hyperventilation were indicative of mild cerebral hypoxia. The relevance of this clinical practice is discussed in the section on hyperventilation and anaesthesia.

Effects of Hypotension

The electroencephalographic pattern during hypotension depends not only on the level of blood pressure but also on the rate of fall to that level. At a rate of under 10 mm Hg (1·3 kPa)/minute, a fall of 100 mm Hg (13·3 kPa) in a hypertensive patient produced no electroencephalographic change (Bromage, 1953), whereas a rapid but smaller decrease in blood pressure can produce slow, high-amplitude waves or even temporary cessation of cortical activity (Fig. 3). These effects may be due to delay in the response of the cerebral blood vessels to sudden changes in blood pressure.

Effects of Hypothermia

Little change occurs in the EEG until the temperature has fallen to 35–31° C when some decrease in amplitude and frequency takes place. At 25° C the amplitude is further decreased and at 20° C there is no appreciable activity in either

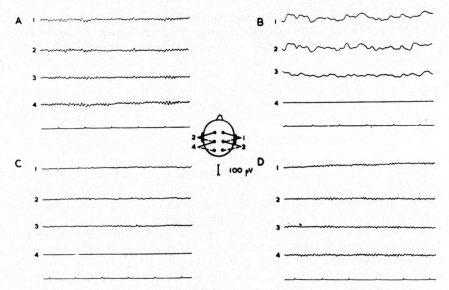

29/FIG. 3.—THE EFFECTS OF HYPOTENSION ON THE ELECTROENCEPHALOGRAM

EEG records of normal man, aged 38.
Time marker: 1 second intervals.
A—Normal resting rhythm of 9 Hz B.P. 130/80.
B—During acute fall of B.P. to unrecordable levels, after 100 mg C5 and 45 degrees foot-down tilt. Subject unconscious.
C—One minute after B, 10 degrees head-down. B.P. 40/? Consciousness returning.
D—Four minutes after C. B.P. 105/70. Conscious. Normal α-rhythm.

parietal or occipital regions, and only a very low-amplitude wave remains at 2 cycles per second in the frontal regions. Prolonged maintenance at low temperatures produces no further alterations. With rewarming the changes occur in the reverse order but at one or two degrees higher than on cooling and there are no permanent changes (Wilson, 1957).

The effect of circulatory arrest in the hypothermic patient is to produce a flat record but this appears more slowly than would be the case at normal temperatures. "File pattern" low-voltage fast activity may be seen in these circumstances, but it is not of grave significance (Pearcy and Virtue, 1959).

Effects of Surgery and Cardiopulmonary By-pass

Studies before and after major surgery show that in a high percentage of cases, changes are produced which generally last for two or three days but which can persist for up to two weeks (Sadove *et al.*, 1967). During cardiopulmonary by-pass, transitory slowing of the EEG may occur with the onset of perfusion, possibly due to differences in temperature, chemistry or drug content of the blood in the apparatus, but subsequently the EEG may be used to monitor the adequacy of cerebral perfusion.

Interpretation of EEG Data

The availability of analogue and digital computers has led to many refinements in EEG presentation and interpretation. Sophisticated methods of power spectral analysis have been used to assess depth of anaesthesia from the EEG (Berezowskyj *et al.*, 1976). Simple methods of interpreting the EEG have also been investigated. The "Cerebral Function Monitor" described by Maynard, Prior and Scott (1969) filters a single EEG signal to accept that portion with frequencies between 2 and 15 Hz. Branthwaite (1973) has shown the value of this simple monitor in differentiating cerebral changes occurring during open heart surgery.

TEMPERATURE REGULATION AND SWEATING

Man, like birds and other mammals, maintains a relatively constant body temperature over a wide range of climatic and environmental conditions. The deep body or "core" temperature is controlled within narrow limits whilst superficial tissues act as a variable insulator. Temperature control consists of a balance between heat production and heat transfer to the environment. The hypothalamus contains centres which respond to impulses from cutaneous cold and warm receptors. The hypothalamus also responds to local changes in blood temperature.

Heat is produced in the body mainly by metabolic activity. Heat production can be increased by increased muscle activity—shivering. Under most circumstances heat production is relatively constant and body temperature is controlled by variations in heat loss. Heat is lost by processes of conduction, convection, radiation and evaporation. Increasing skin blood flow is the primary mechanism by which heat loss is increased, the loss being mainly due to convection and radiation. Above a certain threshold the sweating rate markedly rises to increase heat loss by evaporation. The sweat glands are innervated by cholinergic sympathetic fibres. Sweating provoked by anxiety, anoxia and other non-thermal stimuli merely reflects increased sympathetic activity.

Current theories of temperature regulation suggest that the anterior hypothalamus acts as a biological thermostat with a built-in "set point" (Benzinger, 1970; Hammel, 1972). Variations in this set point account for diurnal temperature variations, temperature changes during the menstrual cycle and changes during exercise. Fever is an example of a gross disturbance in the set point.

The anaesthetised patient tends to become poikilothermic. Depression of metabolism reduces heat production, whilst central depression and loss of vascular control impair the regulation of heat loss. Body temperature tends to fall, especially in children and when visceral cavities are opened. Alternatively, it should be remembered that atropine in children can block the activity of the sweat glands thereby sometimes leading to pyrexia in the presence of inflammatory conditions. A hot environment, theatre lights and impermeable drapes can cause an increase in body temperature. Unless central depression is profound this will produce sweating. Sweating during anaesthesia is more usually indicative of increased sympathetic activity due to too light an anaesthetic plane, hypoxia or hypercapnia. Extreme hyperpyrexia during general anaesthesia—malignant hyperthermia—is due to a massive increase in heat production, and is discussed in some detail in Chapter 28, p. 937.

Appendix to Chapter 29

DIAGNOSIS OF BRAIN DEATH

THE code of practice agreed by the Conference of Medical Royal Colleges and Faculties of the United Kingdom (1976). (Reproduced in full by kind permission of the Editor, *British Medical Journal*).

With the development of intensive care techniques and their wide availability in the United Kingdom it has become commonplace for hospitals to have deeply comatose and unresponsive patients with severe brain damage who are maintained on artificial respiration by means of mechanical ventilators.

This state has been recognised for many years and it has been the concern of the medical profession to establish diagnostic criteria of such rigour that on their fulfilment the mechanical ventilator can be switched off, in the secure knowledge that there is no possible chance of recovery.

There has been much philosophical argument about the diagnosis of death, which has throughout history been accepted as having occurred when the vital functions of respiration and circulation have ceased. With the technical ability to maintain these functions artificially, however, the dilemma of when to switch off the ventilator has been the subject of much public interest. It is agreed that permanent functional death of the brain stem constitutes brain death and that once this has occurred further artificial support is fruitless and should be withdrawn. It is good medical practice to recognise when brain death has occurred and to act accordingly, sparing relatives from the further emotional trauma of sterile hope.

Codes of practice, such as the Harvard criteria (1968), have been devised to guide medical practitioners in the diagnosis of brain death. These have provided considerable help with the problem and they have been refined as the knowledge gained from experience has been collated. More recently Forrester has written on established practice in Scotland (1976) and Jennett has made useful observations (1975).

The diagnostic criteria presented for brain death here have been written with the advice of the subcommittee of the Transplant Advisory Panel, the working party of the Royal College of Physicians, and the working party of the Faculty of Anaesthetists and the Royal College of Surgeons and have been approved by the Conference of Medical Royal Colleges and their Faculties in the United Kingdom. They are accepted as being sufficient to distinguish between those patients who retain the functional capacity to have a chance of even partial recovery from those in whom no such possibility exists.

Conditions for considering diagnosis of brain death

All of the following should coexist.

1. *The patient is deeply comatose.*

(*a*) There should be no suspicion that this state is due to depressant drugs. Narcotics, hypnotics, and tranquillisers may have prolonged durations of action, particularly when some hypothermia exists. The benzodiazepines act cumulatively and their effects persist, and they are commonly used as anti-convulsants or to assist synchronisation with mechanical ventilators. It is therefore recommended that the drug history should be carefully reviewed and adequate intervals allowed for the persistence of drug effects to be excluded. This is of particular importance in patients whose primary cause of coma lies in the toxic effects of drugs followed by anoxic cerebral damage.

(b) Primary hypothermia as a cause of coma should have been excluded.

(c) Metabolic and endocrine disturbances that can cause or contribute to coma should have been excluded. Metabolic and endocrine factors contributing to the persistence of coma must be carefully assessed. There should be no profound abnormality of the serum electrolytes, acid base balance, or blood glucose concentrations.

2. *The patient is being maintained on a ventilator because spontaneous respiration had previously become inadequate or had ceased altogether.*

Relaxants (neuromuscular blocking agents) and other drugs should have been excluded as a cause of respiratory inadequacy or failure. Immobility, unresponsiveness, and lack of spontaneous respiration may be due to the use of neuromuscular blocking drugs, and the persistence of their effects should be excluded by eliciting spinal reflexes (flexion or stretch) or by showing adequate neuromuscular conduction with a conventional nerve stimulator. Equally, persistent effects of hypnotics and narcotics should be excluded as the cause of respiratory failure.

3. *There should be no doubt that the patient's condition is due to irremediable structural brain damage. The diagnosis of a disorder which can lead to brain death should have been fully established.*

It may be obvious within hours of a primary intracranial event such as severe head injury, spontaneous intracranial haemorrhage, or after neuro-surgery that the condition is irremediable. But when a patient has suffered primarily from cardiac arrest, hypoxia, or severe circulatory insufficiency with an indefinite period of cerebral anoxia or is suspected of having cerebral air or fat embolism then it may take much longer to establish the diagnosis and to be confident of the prognosis. In some patients the primary condition may be a matter of doubt and a confident diagnosis may be reached only by continuous clinical observation and investigation.

Tests for confirming brain death

All brain-stem reflexes should be absent.

(a) The pupils are fixed in diameter and do not respond to sharp changes in the intensity of incident light.

(b) There is no corneal reflex.

(c) The vestibulo-ocular reflexes are absent. These are absent when no eye movement occurs during or after the slow injection of 20 ml of ice-cold water into each external auditory meatus in turn, clear access to the tympanic membrane having been established by direct inspection. This test may be contra-indicated on one or other side by local trauma.

(d) No motor responses within the cranial nerve distribution can be elicited by adequate stimulation of any somatic area.

(e) There is no gag reflex or reflex response to bronchial stimulation by a suction catheter passed down the trachea.

(f) No respiratory movements occur when the patient is disconnected from the mechanical ventilator for long enough to ensure that the arterial carbon dioxide tension rises above the threshold for stimulating respiration— that is the $Paco_2$ must normally reach 50 mm Hg (6·7 kPa). This is best achieved by measuring the blood gases; if this facility is available the patient should be disconnected when the $Paco_2$ reaches 40–45 mm Hg (5·3–6·0 kPa) after administration of 5 per cent CO_2 in oxygen through the ventilator. This starting level has been chosen because patients may be moderately hypothermic (35° C to 37° C), flaccid, and with a depressed metabolic rate, so that $Paco_2$ rises only slowly in apnoea (about 2 mm Hg/min; 0·27 kPa/min). (Hypoxia during disconnection should be prevented by delivering oxygen at 6 l/min through a catheter into the trachea.)

If blood gas analysis is not available to measure the $Paco_2$ and Pao_2 the alternative procedure is to supply the ventilator with pure oxygen for 10 minutes (preoxygenation), then with 5 per cent CO_2 in oxygen for five minutes, and to disconnect the ventilator for 10 minutes while delivering oxygen at 6 l/min by catheter into the trachea. This establishes diffusion oxygenation and ensures that during apnoea hypoxia will not occur even in 10 or more minutes of respiratory arrest.

Those patients with pre-existing chronic respiratory insufficiency, who may be unresponsive to raised levels of carbon dioxide and who normally exist on a hypoxic drive, are special cases and should be expertly investigated with careful blood gas monitoring.

Other Considerations

Repetition of testing.—It is customary to repeat the tests to ensure that there has been no observer error. The interval between tests must depend on the primary condition and the clinical course of the disease. Some conditions in which it would be unnecessary to repeat tests since a prognosis of imminent brain death can be accepted as being obvious are listed under the third criteria for considering a diagnosis of brain death (see above). In some conditions the outcome is not so clear-cut and in these the tests should be repeated. The interval between tests depends on the progress of the patient and might be as long as 24 hours. This is a matter for medical judgment, and repetition time must be related to the signs of improvement, stability, or deterioration that present themselves.

Integrity of spinal reflexes.—It is well established that spinal cord function can persist after insults that irretrievably destroy brain-stem function. Reflexes of spinal origin may persist or return after an initial absence in brain-dead patients (Ivan, 1973).

Confirmatory investigations.—It is now widely accepted that electro-encephalography is not necessary for diagnosing brain death (Walker, 1976; Mohandas and Chou, 1971; *Lancet*, 1974; *British Medical Journal*, 1975; MacGillivray, 1973).

Indeed, this view was expressed from Harvard in 1969 by Beecher, only a year after the original Harvard criteria were published. Electroencephalography has its principal value at earlier stages in the care of patients, when the original diagnosis is in doubt. When electroencephalography is used the strict criteria recommended by the Federation of EEG Societies (1974 and 1975) must be followed. Other investigations such as cerebral angiography or cerebral blood flow measurements are not required for diagnosing brain death.

Body temperature.—The body temperature in these patients may be low because of depression of central temperature regulation by drugs or by brain-stem damage and it is recommended that it should be not less than 35° C before the diagnostic tests are carried out. A low-reading thermometer should be used.

Specialist opinion and status of doctors concerned.—Experienced clinicians in intensive care units, acute medical wards, and accident and emergency departments should not normally require specialist advice. Only when the primary diagnosis is in doubt is it necessary to consult with a neurologist or neurosurgeon. The decision to withdraw artificial support should be made after all the criteria presented above have been fulfilled and can be made by any one of the following combinations of doctors. (*a*) A consultant who is in charge of the case and one other doctor; (*b*) in the absence of a consultant, his deputy, who should have been registered for five years or more and who should have had adequate experience in the case of such cases, and one other doctor.

REFERENCES

ADAMS, R. W., GRONERT, G. A., SUNDT, T. M., and MICHENFELDER, J. D. (1972). Halothane, hypocapnia and cerebrospinal fluid pressure in neurosurgery. *Anesthesiology*, **37**, 510.

ALBERT, F. N., and FAZEKAS, J. F. (1956). Cerebral haemodynamics and metabolism during induced hypothermia. *Curr. Res. Anesth.*, **35**, 381.

ALEXANDER, S. C., COHEN, P. J., WOLLMAN, H., SMITH, T. C., REIVICH, M., and VAN DER MOLEN, R. A. (1965). Cerebral carbohydrate metabolism during hypocarbia in man. *Anesthesiology*, **26**, 624.

ALEXANDER, S. C., and LASSEN, N. A. (1970). Cerebral circulatory response to acute brain disease. *Anesthesiology*, **32**, 60.

ALEXANDER, S. C., MARSHALL, B. E., and AGNOLI, A. (1968). Cerebral blood flow in the goat with sustained hypocarbia. *Scand. J. clin. lab. Invest.*, Suppl. 102.

ALLEN, C. D., and MORRIS, L. E. (1962). Central nervous system effects of hyperventilation during anaesthesia. *Brit. J. Anaesth.*, **34**, 296.

BANGHAM, A. D., STANDISH, M. M., and MILLER, N. (1965). Cation permeability of phospholipid model membranes—effects of narcotics. *Nature (Lond.)*, **208**, 1295.

BATSON, O. V. (1944). Anatomical problems concerned in the study of cerebral blood flow. *Fed. Proc.*, **3**, 139.

BAYLISS, W. M. (1902). On the local reaction of the arterial wall to changes of internal pressure. *J. Physiol. (Lond.)*, **28**, 220.

BEECHER, H. K. (1969). After the "definition of irreversible coma". *New Engl. J. Med.*, **281**, 1070.

BENZINGER, T. H. (1970). *Physiological and Behavioural Temperature Regulation*, p. 831. Edited by J. D. Hardy, A. P. Gagge and J. A. J. Stolwijk. Springfield, Ill.: Chas. C. Thomas.

BEREZOWSKYJ, J. L., McEWEN, J. A., ANDERSON, G. B., and JENKINS, L. C. (1976). A study of anaesthesia depth by power spectral analysis of the electroencephalogram (EEG). *Canad. Anaesth. Soc. J.*, **23**, 1.

BOLLEN, A. R. (1962). The electroencephalogram in anaesthesia; some aspects of hyperventilation. *Brit. J. Anaesth.*, **34**, 890.

BRAIN, R. (1957). Order and disorder in the cerebral circulation. (*Harvey Tercentenary Lecture*). *Lancet*, **2**, 857.

BRANTHWAITE, M. A. (1973). Factors affecting cerebral activity during open heart surgery. *Anaesthesia*, **28**, 619.

BRAZIER, M. A. B. (1943). The physiological effects of carbon dioxide on the activity of the central nervous system in man. *Medicine (Baltimore)*, **22**, 205.

BRIDGES, B. E., and EGER, E. I., II (1966). The effect of hypocapnia on the level of halothane anesthesia in man. *Anesthesiology*, **27**, 634.

British Medical Journal (1975). Brain death. **1**, 356.

BROCK, M., FIESCHI, C., INGVAR, D. H., LASSEN, N. A., and SCHÜRMANN, K. (Eds) (1969). *Cerebral Blood Flow: Clinical and Experimental Results*. Berlin; Springer.

BROMAGE, P. R. (1953). Some electro-encephalographic changes associated with induced vascular hypotension. *Proc. roy. Soc. Med.*, **46**, 919.

CARLYLE, A., and GRAYSON, J. (1956). Factors involved in the control of cerebral blood flow. *J. Physiol. (Lond.)*, **133**, 10.

CLOWES, G. H. A., KRETCHMER, H. E., McBURNEY, R. W., and SIMEONE, F. A. (1953). Electroencephalogram in evaluation of effects of anaesthetic agents and carbon dioxide accumulation during surgery. *Ann. Surg.*, **138**, 558.

COHEN, P. J., REIVICH, M., and GREENBAUM, L. J. (1966). Electroencephalographic changes induced by 100% oxygen breathing at 3 ata in awake man. In: *Proc. 3rd Internat. Conf. on Hyperbaric Medicine*. Ed. by I. W. Brown & B. G. Cox. Washington D.C.: National Academy of Sciences.

DE JONG, R. H., ROBLES, R., and CORBIN, R. W. (1968). Effect of inhalational anesthetics on monosynaptic and polysynaptic transmission in the spinal cord. *J. Pharmacol. exp. Ther.*, **162**, 326.

EEG SOCIETIES (1974). The International Federation of EEG Societies. Report. *Electroenceph. clin. Neurophysiol.*, **37**, 430.

EEG SOCIETIES (1975). The International Federation of EEG Societies. Report. *Electroenceph. clin. Neurophysiol.*, **38**, 536.

EGER, E. I. (II), SAIDMAN, L. J., and BRANDSTATER, B. (1965). Minimum alveolar anesthetic concentration: a standard of anesthetic potency. *Anesthesiology*, **26**, 756.

FAZEKAS, J. F., ALMAN, R. W., and PARRISH, A. E. (1951). Irreversible post-hypoglycaemic coma. *Amer. J. med. Sci.*, **222**, 640.

FAZEKAS, J. F., and BESSMAN, A. N. (1953). Coma mechanisms. *Amer. J. Med.*, **15**, 804.

FERGUSON, J. (1939). The use of chemical potentials as indices of toxicity. *Proc. roy. Soc. B.*, **127**, 387.

FINNERTY, F. A., WITKIN, L., and FAZEKAS, J. F. (1954). Cerebral haemodynamics during cerebral ischaemia induced by acute hypotension. *J. clin. Invest.*, **33**, 1227.

FITCH, W., BARKER, J., JENNETT, W. B., and MCDOWALL, D. G. (1969). The influence of neuroleptanalgesic drugs on cerebrospinal fluid pressure. *Brit. J. Anaesth.*, **41**, 800.

FORRESTER, A. C. (1976). Brain death and the donation of cadaver kidneys. *Hlth. Bull. (Edinb.)*, **34**, 199.

FRENCH, J. D., VERZEANO, M., and MAGOUN, H. W. (1953). A neural basis of the anesthetic state. *Arch. Neurol. Psychiat. (Chic.)*, **69**, 519.

FREYHAN, F. A., WOODFORD, R. B., and KETY, S. S. (1951). Cerebral blood flow and metabolism in psychoses of senility. *J. nerv. ment. Dis.*, **113**, 449.

GIBBS, F. A., GIBBS, E. L., and FUSTER, B. (1947a). Anterior temporal localisation of sleep-induced seizure discharges of the psychomotor type. *Trans. Amer. neurol. Ass.*, **72**, 180.

GIBBS, F. A., MAXWELL, H., and GIBBS, E. L. (1947b). Volume flow of blood through the human brain. *Arch. Neurol. Psychiat. (Chic.)*, **57**, 137.

GRONQUIST, Y. K. J., SELDON, T. H., and FAULCONER, J., Jr. (1952). Cerebral anoxia during anaesthesia. Prognostic significance of electroencephalographic changes. *Ann. Chir. Gynaec. Fenn.*, **41**, 149.

GURDJIAN, E. S., STONE, W. E., and WEBSTER, J. E. (1944). Cerebral metabolism in hypoxia. *Arch. Neurol. Psychiat. (Chic.)*, **51**, 472.

HAIDER, I., OSWALD, I., and MATTHEW, H. (1968). EEG signs of death. *Brit. med. J.*, **3**, 314.

HAMMEL, H. T. (1972). *Essays on Temperature Regulation*, p. 121. Edited by J. Bligh and R. Moore. Amsterdam: North-Holland.

HARPER, A. M. (1965). Physiology of the cerebral blood flow. *Brit. J. Anaesth.*, **37**, 225.

HARPER, A. M., and BELL, R. A. (1963). The effect of metabolic acidosis and alkalosis on the blood flow through the cerebral cortex. *J. Neurol. Neurosurg. Psychiat.*, **26**, 341.

HARPER, A. M., DESHMUKH, U. D., ROWAN, J. O., and JENNETT, W. B. (1972). The influence of sympathetic nervous activity on cerebral blood flow. *Arch. Neurol. (Chic.)*, **27**, 1.

HARPER, A. M., and GLASS, H. I. (1965). The effect of alterations in the arterial carbon dioxide tension on the blood flow through the cerebral cortex at normal and low arterial blood pressure. *J. Neurol. Neurosurg. Psychiat.*, **28**, 449.

HARPER, A. M., MCDOWALL, D. G., and LEDINGHAM, I. (1965). The influence of hyperbaric oxygen on the blood flow and oxygen uptake of the cerebral cortex in hypovolaemic shock. *Proc. 2nd Internat. Conf. on Hyperbaric Oxygen*, Vol. 2.

HARVARD (1968). Report of the Ad Hoc Committee of Harvard Medical School to examine the definition of brain death. Definition of irreversible coma. *J. Amer. med. Ass.*, **205**, 337.

HIMWICH, H. E. (1951). *Brain Metabolism and Cerebral Disorders*. Baltimore: Williams and Wilkins.

HOCKADAY, J. M., POTTS, F., EPSTEIN, E., BONAZZI, A., and SCHWAB, R. S. (1965). Electroencephalographic changes in acute cerebral anoxia from cardiac or respiratory arrest. *Electroenceph. clin. Neurophysiol.*, **18**, 575.

HOLBACH, K. H., and GÖTT, U. (1970). Effects of hyperbaric oxygen therapy on neurosurgical patients. In: *Proc. 4th Internat. Congr. on Hyperbaric Medicine*. Washington D.C.: National Academy of Sciences.

HOLMBERG, G. (1953). The electroencephalogram during hypoxia and hyperventilation. *Electroenceph. clin. Neurophysiol.*, **5**, 371.

INGVAR, D. H., and LASSEN, N. A. (1965). Methods for cerebral blood flow measurements in man. *Brit. J. Anaesth.*, **37**, 216.

IVAN, L. P. (1973). Spinal reflexes in cerebral death. *Neurology (Minneap.)*, **23**, 650.

JACOBSON, I., HARPER, A. M., and McDOWALL, D. G. (1963). Relationship between venous pressure and cortical blood flow. *Nature (Lond.)*, **200**, 173.

JAMES, I. M., MILLAR, R. A., and PURVES, M. J. (1968). Neural pathways involved in the control of cerebral blood flow in the baboon. *J. Physiol. (Lond.)*, **196**, 34P.

JENKNER, F. L. (1962). *Rheoencephalography*. Springfield, Ill.: Charles C. Thomas.

JENNETT, B. (1975). The donor doctor's dilemma: observations on the recognition and management of brain death. *J. med. Ethics*, **1**, 63.

JENNETT, W. B., BARKER, J., FITCH, W., and McDOWALL, D. G. (1969). Effect of anaesthesia on intracranial pressure in patients with space-occupying lesions. *Lancet*, **1**, 61.

KENNEDY, C., and SOKOLOFF, L. (1957). An adaptation of the nitrous oxide method to the study of the cerebral circulation in children; normal values for cerebral blood flow and cerebral metabolic rate in childhood. *J. clin. Invest.*, **36**, 1130.

KETY, S. S. (1950). Circulation and metabolism of human brain in health and disease. *Amer. J. Med.*, **8**, 205.

KETY, S. S., and SCHMIDT, C. F. (1948). The nitrous oxide method for quantitative determination of cerebral blood flow in man: theory, procedure and normal values. *J. clin. Invest.*, **27**, 476.

KETY, S. S., SHENKIN, H. A., and SCHMIDT, C. F. (1948a). The effects of increased intracranial pressure on cerebral circulatory functions in man. *J. clin. Invest.*, **27**, 493.

KETY, S. S., WOODFORD, R. B., HARMEL, M. H., FREYHAN, F. A., APPEL, K. E., and SCHMIDT, C. F. (1948b). Cerebral blood flow and metabolism in schizophrenia; effects of barbiturates, semi-narcosis, insulin coma and electroshock. *Amer. J. Psychiat.*, **104**, 765.

KIERSEY, D. K., BICKFORD, R. G., and FAULCONER, A., Jr. (1951). Electroencephalographic patterns produced by thiopentone sodium during surgical operations. Description and classification. *Brit. J. Anaesth.*, **23**, 141.

KING, B. D., SOKOLOFF, L., and WECHSLER, R. L. (1952). The effects of l-epinephrine and l-nor-epinephrine upon cerebral circulation and metabolism in man. *J. clin. Invest.*, **31**, 273.

KLEINERMAN, G., and HOPKINS, A. L. (1955). The effects of hypothermia on cerebral blood flow and metabolism in dogs. *Fed. Proc.*, **14**, 410.

KRAMER, S. (1912). On the function of the circle of Willis. *J. exp. Med.*, **15**, 348.

KRISTIANSEN, K., and KROG, J. (1962). Electromagnetic studies on the blood flow through the carotid system in man. *Neurology (Minneap.)*, **12**, 20.

Lancet (1968). Annotation. Cerebral blood flow and cerebrospinal fluid. **2**, 206.

Lancet (1974). Brain damage and brain death, **1**, 341.

LANDAU, W. M., FREYGANG, W. H., ROWLAND, L. P., SOKOLOFF, L., and KETY, S. S. (1955). The local circulation of the living brain; values in unanaesthetised and anaesthetised cats. *Trans. Amer. neurol. Ass.*, **80**, 125.

LARRABEE, M. G., and POSTERNAK, J. M. (1952). Selective action of anaesthetics on synapses and axons in mammalian sympathetic ganglia. *J. Neurophysiol.*, **15**, 91.

LASSEN, N. A. (1959). Cerebral blood flow and oxygen consumption in man. *Physiol. Rev.*, **39**, 183.

LASSEN, N. A. (1966). The luxury perfusion syndrome and its possible relation to acute metabolic acidosis localised within the brain. *Lancet*, **2**, 1113.

LASSEN, N. A. (1968). Neurogenic control of cerebral blood flow. *Scand. J. clin. lab Invest.*, Suppl. 102, VI, F.

LASSEN, N. A., and INGVAR, D. H. (1963). Regional cerebral blood flow measurement in man. *Arch. Neurol. (Chic.)*, **9**, 615.

LASSEN, N. A., and KLEE, A. (1965). Cerebral blood flow determined by saturation and desaturation with Krypton 85. *Circulat. Res.*, **16**, 26.

LASSEN, N. A., and MUNCK, O. (1955). The cerebral blood flow in man determined by the use of radioactive Krypton. *Acta physiol. scand.*, **33**, 30.

LENNOX, W. G., and GIBBS, E. L. (1932). The blood flow in the brain and the leg of man and the changes induced by alteration of blood gases. *J. clin. Invest.*, **11**, 1155.

McDONALD, D. A., and POTTER, J. M. (1951). The distribution of blood to the brain. *J. Physiol. (Lond.)*, **114**, 356.

McDOWALL, D. G. (1965). The effects of general anaesthetics on cerebral blood flow and cerebral metabolism. *Brit. J. Anaesth.*, **37**, 236.

McDOWALL, D. G. (1971). The cerebral circulation. In *General Anaesthesia*, Vol. I, p. 284. Eds. T. C. Gray and J. F. Nunn. London: Butterworth & Co.

MacGILLIVRAY, B. (1973). The diagnosis of cerebral death. In: *Proc. 10th Congr. European Dialysis and Transplant Assn*. Ed. by J. F. Moorhead. London: Pitman Medical.

MANGOLD, R., SOKOLOFF, L., CONNER, E. L., KLEINERMAN, J., THERMAN, P. G., and KETY, S. S. (1955). The effects of sleep and lack of sleep on the cerebral circulation and metabolism of normal young men. *J. clin. Invest.*, **34**, 1092.

MAYNARD, D., PRIOR, P. F., and SCOTT, D. F. (1969). Device for continuous monitoring of cerebral activity in resuscitated patients. *Brit. med. J.*, **4**, 545.

MEYER, H. H. (1899). Zur Theorie der Alkoholnarcose I mitt Welche Eigenschaft der Anesthetika bedingt ihre narkotische Wirkung? *Naunyn-Schmiedeberg's Arch. exp. Path. Pharmak.*, **42**, 109.

MEYER, J. S., and GOTOH, F. (1964). Continuous recording of cerebral metabolism, internal jugular flow and E.E.G. in man. *Trans. Amer. neurol. Ass.*, **89**, 151.

MICHENFELDER, J. D., VAN DYKE, R. A., and THEYE, R. A. (1970). The effects of anesthetic agents and techniques on canine cerebral ATP and lactate levels. *Anesthesiology*, **33**, 315.

MILLER, S. L. (1961). A theory of gaseous anesthetics. *Proc. nat. Acad. Sci. (Wash.)*, **47**, 1515.

MISFELDT, B. B., JÖRGENSEN, P. B., and RISHOJ, M. (1975). The effect of nitrous oxide and halothane upon the intracranial pressure in hypocapnic patients with intracranial disorders. *Brit. J. Anaesth.*, **46**, 853.

MOHANDAS, A., and CHOU, S. N. (1971). Brain death. A clinical and pathological study. *J. Neurosurg.*, **35**, 211.

MOYER, J. H., MILLER, S. I., and SNYDER, H. (1954). Effect of increased jugular venous pressure on cerebral haemodynamics. *J. appl. Physiol.*, **1**, 245.

MUNCK, O., and LASSEN, N. A. (1957). Bilateral cerebral blood flow and oxygen consumption in man by use of Krypton 85. *Circulat. Res.*, **5**, 163.

MYERSON, A., HALLORAN, R. C., and HIRSCH, H. L. (1927). Technique for obtaining blood from internal jugular vein and internal carotid artery. *Arch. Neurol. Psychiat. (Chic.)*, **17**, 807.

NOVAK, P., GOLUBOFF, B., BORTIN, L., SOFFE, A., and SHENKIN, H. A. (1953). Studies of the cerebral circulation and metabolism in congestive heart failure. *Circulation*, **7**, 724.

NYLIN, G., SILVERSKIÖLD, B. P., LÖFSTEDT, S., REGNSTRÖM, O., and HEDLUND, S. (1960). Studies on cerebral blood flow in man, using radioactive labelled erythrocytes. *Brain*, **83**, 293.

OVERTON, E. (1901). *Studien uber die Narkose.* Jena: Fischer.

PAULING, L. (1961). A molecular theory of general anaesthesia. *Science,* **134,** 15.

PEARCY, W. C., and VIRTUE, R. W. (1959). The electroencephalogram in hypothermia and circulatory occlusion. *Anesthesiology,* **20,** 34.

PIERCE, E. C., LAMBERTSEN, C. J., DEUTSCH, S., CHASE, P. E., LINDE, H. W., DRIPPS, R. D., and PRICE, H. L. (1962). Cerebral circulation and metabolism during thiopental anesthesia and hyperventilation in man. *J. clin. Invest.,* **41,** 1664.

QUASTEL, J. H. (1952). Biochemical aspects of narcosis. *Curr. Res. Anesth.,* **31,** 151.

QUASTEL, J. H. (1965). Effects of drugs on metabolism of the brain *in vitro. Brit. med. Bull.,* **21,** 49.

RISBERG, J., and INGVAR, D. H. (1968). Regional changes in cerebral blood volume during mental activity. *Exp. Brain Res.,* **5,** 72.

ROBIN, E. C., and GARDNER, F. H. (1953). Cerebral metabolism and haemodynamics in pernicious anaemia. *J. clin. Invest.,* **32,** 598.

ROBINSON, J. S., and GRAY, T. D. (1961). Observations on the cerebral effects of passive hyperventilation. *Brit. J. Anaesth.,* **33,** 62.

ROSOMOFF, H. L. (1956). Some effects of hypothermia on the normal and abnormal physiology of the nervous system. *Proc. roy. Soc. Med.,* **49,** 358.

ROSOMOFF, H. L. (1963). Distribution of intracranial contents with controlled hyperventilation: implications for neuro-anesthesia. *Anesthesiology,* **24,** 640.

ROSOMOFF, H. L., and HOLADAY, D. A. (1954). Cerebral blood flow and cerebral oxygen consumption during hypothermia. *Amer. J. Physiol.,* **179,** 85.

ROSSEN, R., KABAT, H., and ANDERSON, J. P. (1943). Acute arrest of cerebral circulation in man. *Arch. Neurol. Psychiat. (Chic.),* **50,** 510.

ROY, C. S., and SHERINGTON, C. S. (1890). On regulation of blood supply of brain. *J. Physiol. (Lond.),* **11,** 85.

SADOVE, M. S., BECKA, D., and GIBBS, F. A. (1967). *Electroencephalography for Anaesthesiologists and Surgeons.* Philadelphia: J. B. Lippincott Co.

SCHNEIDER, M. (1963). Critical blood pressure in the cerebral circulation. In: *Selective Vulnerability of the Brain in Hypoxaemia.* Eds. Schade, J. P. and McMenemy, W. H. Oxford: Blackwell Scientific Publications.

SEEMAN, P. M. (1966). Membrane stabilization by drugs: tranquillizers, steroids and anaesthetics. *Int. Rev. Neurobiol.,* **9,** 145.

SEVERINGHAUS, J. W., CHIODI, H., EGER, E. I. (II), BRANDSTATER, B., and HORNBEIN, T. F. (1966). Cerebral blood flow in man at high altitude. *Circulat. Res.,* **19,** 274.

SHENKIN, H. A. (1951). Effects of various drugs upon cerebral circulation and metabolism of man. *J. appl. Physiol.,* **3,** 465.

SHENKIN, H. A., HARMEL, M. H., and KETY, S. S. (1948). Dynamic anatomy of the cerebral circulation. *Arch. Neurol. Psychiat. (Chic.),* **60,** 240.

SHENKIN, H. A., NOVAK, P., GOLUBOFF, B., SOFFE, A. M., and BORTIN, L. (1953). The effects of aging, arteriosclerosis and hypertension upon the cerebral circulation. *J. clin. Invest.,* **32,** 459.

SOKOLOFF, L. (1957). In: *New Research Techniques of Neuroanatomy.* Ed. Windle, W. F. Springfield, Ill.: Charles C. Thomas.

SOKOLOFF, L. (1959a). *Proc. Conference on the Process of Aging in the Nervous System.* Springfield, Ill.: Charles C. Thomas.

SOKOLOFF, L. (1959b). The action of drugs on the cerebral circulation. *Pharmacol. Rev.,* **11,** 1.

SOKOLOFF, L., and KETY, S. S. (1960). Regulation of cerebral circulation. *Physiol. Rev.,* **40,** 38.

SOKOLOFF, L., MANGOLD, R., WECHSLER, R. L., KENNEDY, C., and KETY, S. S. (1955). The effect of mental arithmetic on cerebral circulation and metabolism. *J. clin. Invest.,* **34,** 1101.

SUGIOKA, K., and DAVIS, D. A. (1960). Hyperventilation with oxygen: a possible cause of cerebral hypoxia. *Anesthesiology*, **21**, 135.

SYMON, L. (1967). A comparative study of middle cerebral pressure in dogs and macaques. *J. Physiol. (Lond.)*, **191**, 449.

VEALL, N., and MALLETT, B. L. (1963). Measurement of cerebral blood flow. *Lancet*, **1**, 1081.

WALKER, A. E. (1976). The neurosurgeon's responsibility for organ procurement. *J. Neurosurg.*, **44**, 1.

WECHSLER, R. L., KLEISS, L. M., and KETY, S. S. (1950). The effects of intravenously administered aminophylline on cerebral circulation and metabolism in man. *J. clin. Invest.*, **29**, 28.

WILSON, S. M. (1957). Electro-encephalography in relation to anaesthesia. *Proc. roy. Soc. Med.*, **50**, 105.

WOLLMAN, H., ALEXANDER, S. C., and COHEN, P. J. (1968). Cerebral circulation and metabolism in anesthetized man. In: *Clinical Anaesthesia* (3). *Neurologic Considerations*, Ed. Harmel, M. H. Oxford: Blackwell Scientific Publications.

WOLLMAN, H., ALEXANDER, S. C., COHEN, P. J., SMITH, T. C., CHASE, P. E., and VAN DER MOLEN, R. A. (1965). Cerebral circulation during general anesthesia and hyperventilation in man. *Anesthesiology*, **26**, 329.

WOLLMAN, S. B., and ORKEN, L. R. (1968). Postoperative human reaction time and hypocarbia during anaesthesia. *Brit. J. Anaesth.*, **40**, 920.

Chapter 30

NEUROLOGICAL ANAESTHESIA

CEREBROSPINAL FLUID

ANAESTHESIA for intracranial surgery involves above all other considerations a constant awareness of the intracranial pressure. All space-occupying lesions, including even small aneurysms, may interfere with cerebrospinal fluid circulation and absorption. Drugs and techniques used by the anaesthetist can by direct or indirect mechanisms cause catastrophic changes in cerebrospinal fluid pressure which threaten the viability of the brain.

Formation of Cerebrospinal Fluid

Cerebrospinal fluid is secreted by the villous projections of the choroid plexuses in the lateral ventricles. It passes through the interventricular foramina into the third ventricle, cerebral aqueduct and fourth ventricle, and thence through the foramina of Magendie and Luschka into the subarachnoid space. The major portion passes upwards through the posterior fossa and over the surface of the cerebral hemispheres, whilst the remainder flows through the foramen magnum to surround the spinal cord. Absorption of cerebrospinal fluid occurs mainly through the arachnoid villi into the dural sinuses and spinal veins. A small amount passes out along the dural sheaths of cranial and spinal nerves to be absorbed into lymphatics. The volume of cerebrospinal fluid in adults is 100–150 ml, and with the subject in the lateral position this exerts a pressure of 50–150 mm (0·5–1·5 kPa) of cerebrospinal fluid.

Raised Intracranial Pressure

The classical signs of raised intracranial pressure are headache, vomiting and papilloedema. Detectable papilloedema may take up to two weeks to develop. A dangerous rise in pressure occurring due to a supratentorial lesion is marked by drowsiness, clouding of consciousness, a loss of the ability to look upwards and dilatation and loss of response to light, firstly of the pupil on the side of the lesion and finally of both pupils. Raised pressure in the posterior fossa causes bradycardia, bradypnoea and hypertension. Some drowsiness may be present. As pressure in the posterior fossa rises medullary coning occurs, when the cerebellar tonsils are pushed down behind the cervical spinal cord through the foramen magnum blocking this foramen and also the foramina of Magendie and Luschka. Increasing medullary pressure leads to respiratory failure. Developing medullary coning usually produces neck stiffness and head retraction.

Evidence of raised intracranial pressure may be seen on X-rays of the skull as enlargement of the pituitary fossa, erosion of the posterior clinoid processes and in slowly developing cases a beaten silver appearance of the vault (Fig. 1). In children the sutures may be forced apart.

Diagnostic lumbar puncture, anaesthesia, posturing the patient, and neuroradiological and neurosurgical interference can all precipitate a medullary conus in a patient already suffering from severe hydrocephalus.

A knowledge of the presence and degree of hydrocephalus is of greater importance to the anaesthetist than a diagnosis of the specific disease, while an understanding of normal cerebrospinal fluid physiology and the effects on it of anaesthetic drugs and procedures, is an essential prerequisite to the selection and administration of successful anaesthesia.

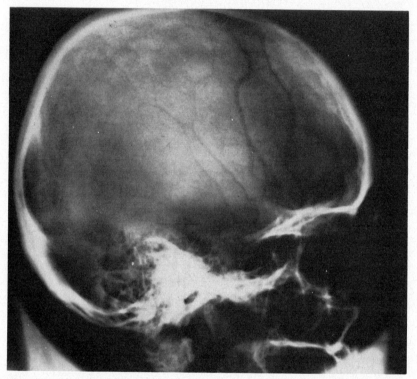

30/FIG. 1.—Raised intracranial pressure. Lateral skull radiograph of a 52-year-old woman with a malignant astrocytoma, showing a "smudged-out" appearance of the pituitary fossa typical of generalised raised intracranial pressure.

Cerebral Perfusion Pressure

Because the cerebral venous sinuses have a pressure in them which approximates to the intracranial pressure (Sosterholm, 1970), blood flow through the brain is determined by the mean arterial to intracranial pressure gradient. This cerebral perfusion pressure is normally 80–90 mm Hg (10·5–12 kPa) (Fitch *et al.*, 1969). Work by McDowall and his colleagues (1966) has drawn attention to the potentially damaging falls in cerebral perfusion pressure which can occur when volatile anaesthetic agents are given to patients with raised intracranial pressure. Such falls have been shown to occur when commonly used anaesthetic concentrations of halothane, trichloroethylene and other volatile anaesthetic agents are administered (McDowall *et al.*, 1966; Jennett *et al.*, 1969; Fitch *et al.*, 1969). All these agents cause an immediate but variable rise in cerebrospinal fluid pressure which is dose-dependent. The rise reaches a peak in 10 to 15 minutes and then declines. In the presence of an already raised intracranial pressure the rise caused by volatile anaesthetics may be very marked and intracranial pressure may continue to rise even after withdrawing the volatile agent. A high intracranial pressure, especially if associated with a reduced mean arterial pressure, may reduce cerebral perfusion pressure to near zero levels and cause hypoxic brain damage. The rise in cerebrospinal fluid pressure is due to increased cerebral blood flow and a raised cerebral blood volume and it is most evident when P_{CO_2} is either normal or raised. The practical importance of this is that when patients with raised intracranial pressure are to be anaesthetised, these agents should be avoided unless other measures to reduce intracranial pressure have been taken before they are exhibited. This is particularly applicable to investigations such as carotid angiography and in the management of patients having extracranial operations, usually for fractures, who also have recent head injuries. Relaxant drugs and moderate hyperventilation are to be preferred to spontaneous breathing and volatile agents.

POSTURE

The posture of the patient has a pronounced effect on venous drainage. Unfortunately the ideal position for the anaesthetist is not always compatible with that needed by the surgeon, and although venous congestion may mitigate against a dry operation field, other more important factors sometimes decide the ultimate choice. Whenever possible the patient should be placed in a position so that venous drainage away from the operation site is encouraged, obstruction to major veins is avoided, and respiration is not impeded. There are four classical positions commonly used in neurosurgery—the supine, prone, sitting, and lateral.

1. *Supine Position*

The supine position is used to approach the anterior fossa, and with the patient lying on his back and his head slightly raised and fixed in a special horseshoe rest, venous drainage and respiration are not embarrassed. The addition of a foot down tilt is an advantage, but since it may lead to a very low pressure in the veins above the level of the heart there is a risk of air embolus occurring during the operation. This risk is at its highest when the sitting position is used.

2. *Prone Position*

The prone position is used for laminectomies, and to approach the posterior fossa. It often leads to marked venous congestion, particularly if the operation area is dependent. Moreover, unless the patient is properly supported, undue abdominal compression may embarrass ventilation and obstruct the inferior vena cava. This last effect can seriously reduce blood pressure and also increase pressure in the vertebral veins. On the credit side, there is no risk of air embolus occurring.

The vertebral venous system consists of an extensive network of veins which drain into and communicate freely with the vena cavae (Batson, 1940). Increased abdominal or thoracic pressure will be reflected in vertebral venous pressure and may reverse the normal direction of flow. Pearce (1957) has shown that in patients in the prone position abdominal pressure sufficient to obstruct the inferior vena cava can cause caval pressure to rise by more than 30 cm of water (2·8 kPa), whilst even slight abdominal compression leads to a rapid increase in caval pressure of 3–4 cm of water (0·3–0·4 kPa). To produce minimal venous pressure Pearce recommended supporting the fully relaxed and ventilated patient so that the abdominal wall hangs free. A wedge-shaped pillow under the thorax with its broad edge just below the level of the acromion effectively maintains the patient in the correct position and gives reasonable freedom for diaphragmatic movement. Further help can be gained by raising the pelvis on supports. This position opens up the intervertebral spaces of the upper part of the spine but tends to close the lumbar intervertebral spaces. For this reason the jack-knife position with the patient flexed in the prone position over pillows or a "broken" operation table is often used for lumbar laminectomies, although respiratory embarrassment and venous congestion are more likely in this position. A modified jack-knife position with the patient raised at the pelvis to free the abdomen has been described (Taylor et al., 1956).

3. *Lateral Position*

Another approach to the problem of venous bleeding during laminectomy is to use the lateral position, which enables the patient to be postured with the back flexed. There is little, if any, venous engorgement in this position, provided the surgeon does not need excessive flexion to open up the intervertebral spaces. This can only be achieved by drawing up the thighs with full flexion at the hips, and results in some abdominal compression.

4. *Sitting Position*

The sitting or upright position is undoubtedly the most effective method for producing an uncongested operating field for a cervical laminectomy or posterior fossa craniotomy. The patient is placed in a special chair with the head supported anteriorly in a cushioned horse-shoe. An alternative method is to place the patient supine on the operating table, but with the head well over the end and held forward and supported by a wire and caliper which is fixed to the head. The table is set with a pronounced foot-down tilt.

Some Dangers of Posture

Air embolus and severe hypotension are the two dangers associated with these upright positions, although any degree of anti-Trendelenburg tilt is conducive to such potential hazards.

Air embolus.—The incidence of air embolus is difficult to assess and published figures are not available, but it undoubtedly bears a relation to the competence of the surgeon. Furthermore, prompt diagnosis and treatment by both surgeon and anaesthetist sometimes prove surprisingly successful (see Chapter 17). In neurosurgical practice the quantity of air sucked into a vein may be comparatively small, but the site of entry may not be apparent at once. A tear in a venous sinus during the removal of bone is a likely site. Other vulnerable vessels are the suboccipital venous plexus and the mastoid emissaries (Hunter, 1975). Deep breathing or one or two deep respirations following a cough add to the hazard, as they increase the subatmospheric pressure which already exists in these veins. Hunter (1960) considers that air embolism is very likely to occur when muscle relaxants and intermittent positive-pressure ventilation are used for a posterior fossa operation in the sitting position and he considers the method unacceptable because effective ventilation, even without a negative phase, reduces the venous pressure above the heart to a dangerously low level. However, Millar (1972) could find no evidence of a special danger of controlled ventilation during posterior fossa surgery. The risk of air embolism can be minimised by deliberately increasing venous pressure during the danger periods when the skull is being opened and closed by intermittent compression of the jugular veins (Hunter, 1975), by providing an expiratory resistance (Hewer and Logue, 1962), or by use of a G-suit. The early signs of air embolism are an unexplained fall in blood pressure, a rise in pulse rate and (in the spontaneously breathing patient) the occurrence of a deep breath (McComish and Thompson, 1968). Useful adjuvants to diagnosis are an oesophageal stethoscope, electrocardiogram, right atrial pressure line and a continuous monitor of end-tidal carbon dioxide concentration. A Doppler ultrasonic detector can readily detect the presence of air in the venous system (Edmonds-Seal and Maroon, 1969) but the extreme sensitivity of this apparatus to the smallest quantities of air limits its clinical application. At the first signs of air embolus treatment must be instituted at once. The ingress of more air into the circulation must be prevented by identifying and closing the open vein. The patient should be given 100 per cent oxygen, for in the presence of nitrous oxide an air bubble within the circulation will greatly increase in size. The ideal position for the patient is to be flat and on his left side, to minimise the danger of air entering the right ventricular outflow tract. It may not be easy to change posture rapidly during neurosurgery in the sitting position. If a right atrial catheter is in place air can be aspirated from the right heart (Michenfelder et al., 1966). Large air emboli cause a marked reduction in cardiac output and cardiovascular supportive measures may be necessary.

Hypotension.—Adoption of the sitting position can impose a considerable disability on the circulatory system. This is most likely to occur in the thirty minutes after the patient has been placed in an upright position. The falls in blood pressure that occur in this position are usually due to impaired vasomotor stability produced by drugs given before and during anaesthesia. Although autoregulation maintains a normal cerebral blood flow in spite of falls in blood pressure there is a lower limit of arterial pressure below which this mechanism fails. It is unwise to allow the systolic pressure of a patient who has a normal circulation to fall below 70–80 mm Hg (9·3–10·7 kPa), and even this level may be unsafe in the presence of raised intracranial tension. To minimise falls in blood pressure the sitting position should be adopted gradually. Falls in blood pressure should initially be treated by a rapid infusion of bland fluid. If this is not effective a small dose of a pressor agent such as methoxamine (5–10 mg) may be necessary. Atropine may also be useful if bradycardia is present. The most effective form of therapy is to lower the patient to a more supine position. Some help towards the prevention of undue hypotension can be gained by firm bandaging of the legs from toes to groins, flexing the thighs and raising the legs (Cheatle and MacKenzie, 1953) or by placing the lower part of the patient's body in a G-suit (Hewer and Logue, 1962).

The changes in the brain that can be caused by sub-oxygenation have been described elsewhere (see Chapter 29). Here it only needs to be stressed that specific histological changes in the cells are not visible if death takes place within 30 to 36 hours of the period of sub-oxygenation. Post-mortem diagnosis of the cause of sudden death in the operating theatre is rarely satisfactory, and depends far more upon clinical evidence of the sequence of events than upon abnormal pathology.

Discussion

The choice between the upright and prone position usually depends upon the inclinations of the surgeon. Theoretically, better access to a particular part of the brain due to an uncongested and relatively bloodless operation wound enables delicate surgery to be performed with less risk of trauma to surrounding tissue. This is an important factor in neurosurgical work where morbidity and mortality tend anyway to be high when the operation is in an area of the brain which abounds with vital functions. Yet there is insufficient practical evidence that the end results of series of similar operations differ greatly, if at all, when performed in either position by competent surgeons. For this reason it is as well to be certain that the complications specific to a particular position do not mar the ultimate result, and to select a posture which not only suits the surgeon but also the patient.

ANAESTHESIA

The basis of good anaesthesia for neurosurgery has been well summarised by Bozza Marrubini (1965) as a perfect airway, adequate ventilation, low venous pressure, a slack brain, minimal bleeding, the absence of coughing or straining and a rapid return to consciousness. Intracranial work does not require deep anaesthesia, and indeed the greatest and most frequent stimulus of an entire operation is usually the presence of an endotracheal tube in the trachea. The diathermy is an essential and constant part of neurosurgical technique, so that inflammable anaesthetic agents must not be used. Some surgeons may take upwards of six hours for an operation which is performed by others in under two. To satisfy these several requirements special techniques have been developed, but the differences between them only illustrate the importance that one anaesthetist attaches to some particular aspect of the problem and stress the value of the personal touch. There are few, if any, drugs or techniques which do not in some way adversely affect intracranial or intraspinal mechanics. Such factors can be minimised by careful selection and attention to detail.

Local or General

No single drug or combination of drugs can be considered ideal in the circumstances of neurosurgical anaesthesia. Apart from the skin, fascia, temporal muscle, periosteum and bone of the skull, and certain parts of the basal dura where it is attached to bone, cranial surgery is carried out in an area which is entirely insensitive to pain. The nerves to the skin and fascia also supply the periosteum and bone. They pass through the fascia beneath the skin on a line encircling the skull and drawn approximately from the occipital protuberance to the eyebrows (Pitkin, 1953). Thus local subcutaneous infiltration with a solution of 1 per cent lignocaine produces satisfactory analgesia for burr holes and minor operations. If the incision impinges on the temporal muscle then a deeper infiltration must be made. In terms of pain relief this form of local analgesia is also effective for major craniotomies, and has the advantage of having no adverse effects on intracranial mechanics. Why, then, general anaesthesia?

Local Analgesia

Local analgesia leaves much to be desired in terms of sedation and comfort for the patient, and does nothing to aid the surgeon should the patient be unco-operative or unable to keep perfectly still. Although the mental state of many patients with intracranial disease is confused, the majority are conscious enough to dislike the discomforts of major surgery under local analgesia. The position on the operating table and the need to remain in it, and in a motionless state, for perhaps several hours are effective deterrents. There is a good deal of mental stress associated in the minds of many patients with an operation on the brain, and surgical manipulations in this area, even though painless, evoke indirect sensations, particularly during bone work. Stimulation of brain substance sometimes produces spontaneous motor or sensory activities for the patient, and though these may be valuable under certain circumstances as a guide to the localisation of the surgeon's work, they are unpleasant if repetitive or gross. A patient who is difficult to control because of his disease, or more simply because he or she is unco-operative, cannot be adequately sedated with complete safety, and certainly not as effectively as with a good general anaesthetic. Finally, the duration of action of all known local analgesic drugs is insufficient to cover the length of time that some surgeons take to complete certain operations.

General anaesthesia supplies an answer to all these disadvantages of local analgesia, but it does so at some slight cost. The dangers and disadvantages of general anaesthesia in the hands of inexperienced administrators must be appreciated before criticising those clinics where local methods of analgesia still find favour. So far as the operation of laminectomy is concerned, local infiltration analgesia is far from satisfactory, and either a more complete form, such as an epidural or spinal, must be used, or general anaesthesia preferred.

General Anaesthesia

The airway.—There must be an adequate airway at all times. This can be assured by using a flexible but unkinkable oral endotracheal tube. Armoured tubes whose walls are reinforced with a nylon spiral fulfil these requirements. The Oxford pattern of endotracheal tube is also very satisfactory for neurosurgery (Duckworth, 1962). It is essential to cut a hole in the anterior wall of Oxford tubes close to the bevel or to cut the bevel itself square across to avoid obstruction of the outlet of the tube by the posterior tracheal wall when the neck is acutely flexed. A curved or right-angled wide-bore connector must be firmly fixed to any tube used. Because access to the face may be impossible once an operation has started any tube and its connectors must be firmly mounted and well strapped into position. In some neurosurgical operations, especially posterior fossa operations in children, there is a very real danger of accidental endobronchial intubation occurring when the neck is acutely flexed. Hunter (1975) recommends marking the distance on the tube from mouth to supra-sternal notch before intubation, and not introducing a tube further than this distance.

Ventilation.—The importance of adequate ventilation during anaesthesia for all branches of surgery is well known but is of especial relevance during neuro-surgery. Carbon dioxide retention can play havoc with the neurosurgeon's operating field, while a raised expiratory resistance from obstruction, coughing or straining is even more disastrous. The mechanisms at work have been re-viewed by Ballantyne and Jackson (1954). Expiratory resistance increases intrathoracic pressure and this is reflected in a raised pressure in the cerebral and vertebral veins. Increased intra-abdominal pressure from the work of the abdominal muscles during forced expiration contributes by compression on the inferior vena cava to the rise of pressure in the latter. Raised venous pressure causes a rise in cerebrospinal fluid pressure. Oxygen lack and carbon dioxide retention act directly to cause cerebral vascular engorgement and enlargement in the size of the brain substance (Kety and Schmidt, 1948). Hypoxia leads to an increase in capillary permeability and probably to an increase in the fluid content of brain cells.

For most operations, particularly when deep anaesthesia is neither neces-sary nor desirable, muscle paralysis and efficient controlled ventilation supply the answer to these problems and this method is now generally recommended for supratentorial intracranial surgery. There is less agreement on the place of controlled ventilation in posterior fossa surgery. Spontaneous ventilation in these circumstances can provide an indication of the integrity of vital functions and changes in spontaneous breathing may warn of impending surgical danger. Many authorities however feel that equally good indications of surgical invasion of the vital centres can be obtained by monitoring the circulation during con-trolled ventilation (Hunter, 1975). Nevertheless, it is not difficult with care and attention to detail, to maintain satisfactory spontaneous ventilation even throughout very lengthy operations. If for any reason spontaneous ventilation is unsatisfactory and seems likely to remain so, then it is wiser to take over and control ventilation properly, making use of muscle relaxants for this purpose.

There are special advantages in using controlled respiration with muscle relaxants for some neurosurgical operations. The anatomical build of an occasional patient, the state of the lungs of another, or the posture required for the operation may individually or collectively suggest that the best con-ditions will only be obtained by taking over the patient's ventilation. Irrespective of such indications, brain tension can be reduced when ventilation is controlled. Furness (1957) described how effective controlled respiration can be, and con-sidered that a negative phase has a considerable effect on brain tension. Her views have been confirmed by others (Galloon, 1959; Mortimer, 1959), though it is now generally thought that a negative expiratory phase contributes little to the reduced brain tension (Brown, 1959; Bozza Marrubini et al., 1961; Hunter, 1975). Controlled hyperventilation is widely advocated as a method of further reducing brain tension. Whilst cerebral blood volume and brain bulk is reduced as Pco_2 falls, marked hyperventilation usually requires a higher mean intrathoracic pressure and the effects of this on cerebral venous pressure may offset its other benefits. Hyperventilation to a PCO_2 of 30 mm Hg (4 kPa) seems to provide the optimal balance (Hayes and Slocum, 1962; Shenkin et al., 1965). Rosomoff (1963) considers that although hyperventilation may lower cerebrospinal fluid pressure it never reduces brain volume. The major advantage of hyperventilation may be in offsetting some of the drawbacks of spontaneous ventilation and adverse posture (Rosomoff, 1962), avoiding the need for a volatile anaesthetic and preventing straining (Hunter, 1960).

Anaesthetic system.—The type of anaesthetic system is of only slight importance, but it must be designed to avoid rebreathing and to exclude any undue resistance to expiration. It is also convenient to have the anaesthetic trolley some distance from the operation site, and to be able to institute controlled ventilation easily and efficiently. Often it is necessary to double the length of the corrugated breathing tubes in which case gas compression and tube expansion make it necessary to increase the minute volume considerably to achieve a given PCO_2 (Bushman and Collis, 1967). All methods—semi-closed, non-rebreathing, "T"-piece, and closed with absorption—have their advocates, and each offers advantages and disadvantages. Personal preference must ultimately decide.

Premedication.—The potential danger of those drugs which cause respiratory depression when given to patients with a raised intracranial pressure is well known. Opiates and their analogues must therefore be prescribed with caution, if at all. Even when there is no apparent contra-indication to using them preoperatively it must be borne in mind that their action may persist into the postoperative period, particularly when the operation is of relatively short duration. They may reduce reflex activity and the level of consciousness in the postoperative period, while the small and unreactive pupil which follows the administration of opiates is a disadvantage when assessing the state of the patient. Pre-operative sedation is an important factor in the preparation of the patient for any type of anaesthetic, but for intracranial surgery this benefit may have to be foregone. In the positive absence of any evidence of raised intracranial tension small doses of morphine (up to 10 mg) can be given. Tranquillisers such as diazepam which have little cardiovascular or respiratory effect may have advantages over opiates (Bozza Marrubini and Tretola, 1965). If a neuroleptanaesthetic technique is to be employed it is useful to premedicate the patient with small doses of droperidol (10 mg) and fentanyl (0·1 mg) thirty minutes preoperatively. During maintenance of anaesthesia there is a practical advantage in having an undepressed patient as this allows greater freedom in the use of intravenous drugs. An adequate dose of atropine sulphate should be given subcutaneously about an hour before the induction of anaesthesia.

These arguments do not apply in the case of operations on the spine—indeed opiates are of considerable value in controlling post-operative pain after a laminectomy. However, undue respiratory depression can be a marked disadvantage even during a laminectomy, and this may be accentuated by the position of the patient.

Choice of anaesthetic.—Although adequate anaesthesia can be produced with a single powerful agent such as ether, a combination of drugs has some advantages in overcoming with minimal sequelae the few sensory reflexes that neurosurgical operations and the presence of an endotracheal tube initiate.

There has been a general swing away from spontaneous breathing for supratentorial surgery and this has been given added impetus by the work of McDowall and Jennett already referred to. Most neurosurgical anaesthetists give relaxant drugs and use mechanical ventilators to produce moderate reductions in Pco_2. The omission of sedative premedication and the concern for perfect oxygenation inevitably mean that the anaesthetic is conducted close to the level of consciousness. It is therefore often necessary to take other measures to ensure that this level is never reached. Small increments of intravenous analgesics are appropriate, or volatile agents may be used. Trichloroethylene or halothane in low concentrations are the drugs which have been most commonly used to supplement nitrous oxide. Experience has shown that provided the introduction of these volatile supplements is preceded by a few minutes of hyperventilation and the use—when indicated—of mannitol, the rise in intracranial pressure which they cause need not be taken into account. If grossly raised intracranial pressure is known to be present it is unlikely that any supplement to nitrous oxide will be necessary and volatile anaesthetics should not be introduced until the dura is opened and the brain tension can be assessed.

In posterior fossa surgery a similar technique can be used if the patient is prone, but in the sitting position there may be a case for retaining spontaneous breathing.

Intravenous induction of anaesthesia is a blessing to the patient—particularly to those who are unsedated—and if the dose is moderate, less upsetting to intracranial mechanics than a stormy inhalational induction. There may be assets, it is true, in maintaining adequate spontaneous respiration throughout induction and intubation, but they hardly outweigh the intrinsic advantage of a brief period of perfect relaxation from suxamethonium during which laryngoscopy and intubation can be easily performed. Following induction with thiopentone (3–4 mg/kg) and paralysis with suxamethonium (1 mg/kg) the patient should be ventilated with oxygen for 30 seconds before thoroughly spraying the vocal cords and trachea with a suitable local anaesthetic and inserting an endotracheal tube. Ventilation is then continued with nitrous oxide and oxygen until spontaneous ventilatory activity returns. It may sometimes be advisable to allow spontaneous ventilation to continue until the patient has been positioned and the incision marked out. To prevent reactions to the presence of an endotracheal tube small doses of pethidine, thiopentone or methohexitone may be necessary at this stage.

When controlled ventilation is instituted following the administration of tubocurarine or a similar muscle relaxant nitrous oxide anaesthesia can be supplemented with a volatile agent, intravenous barbiturates or intravenous analgesics. The potentially dangerous effects of volatile anaesthetic agents on intracranial tension have already been mentioned. Thiopentone and other intravenous barbiturates will reduce intracranial tension. The cumulative effects of these drugs and their depressant cardiovascular actions are important and they must be used cautiously and in minimal doses. Pethidine has been the most widely used of the intravenous analgesics. Its anti-cholinergic, antispasmodic and sedative actions can be useful advantages in neurosurgical anaesthesia (Wylie, 1951). Neuroleptanalgesic drugs have many advantages during intracranial surgery. Circulatory stability is usually greater than with other agents and a combination of droperidol and fentanyl reduces cerebral blood flow (Miller and Barker, 1969) and therefore brain volume. These drugs may be given following induction with thiopentone or used from the outset for pre-medication and induction. In spite of the profound respiratory depression these drugs produce their use must be accompanied by complete curarisation. The occasional rigidity of abdominal and chest wall muscles which fentanyl may produce will otherwise cause a rise in cerebral venous pressure and increase brain volume and bleeding.

REDUCTION OF INTRACRANIAL TENSION

Prevention of a rise in intracranial tension is a cardinal rule of safe neuro-surgical anaesthesia. In this context the prevention of carbon dioxide retention, avoidance of venous congestion and cautious use of volatile inhalational agents are all of importance. Occasionally, in spite of all precautions, intracranial tension may rise to a dangerous level. Such rises may be due to the presence of an intracranial space-occupying lesion, or related to brain oedema caused by severe hypoxia or brain trauma. In some patients intracranial tension may be of a severity which warrants its reduction before induction of anaesthesia. Reduction of a high intracranial pressure may be produced by employing one or more of the following methods.

Removal of CSF.—The simplest method of removing CSF is by lumbar puncture, followed if necessary by continuous drainage through a malleable needle (Vourc'h, 1963). The problems associated with this method are the severe headaches that may follow removal of the large volumes of fluid which this approach entails, and the danger of precipitation of medullary coning in patients with unsuspected supratentorial lesions. Fluid can be removed from the ventricles by tapping either through burr holes or following craniotomy and may greatly assist exposure of intracranial lesions in the presence of hydrocephalus. Mechanical drainage of CSF has in the main been rendered unnecessary by the advent of powerful intravenous hypertonic solutions.

Cerebral dehydration.—Increases of plasma osmolality will cause a transfer of fluid from the brain to plasma. Many substances have been used in the past to so reduce brain bulk, including 50 per cent glucose, 50 per cent sucrose, 40 per cent fructose, hypertonic dextran and double- or quadruple-strength plasma. None of these agents was markedly efficient in shrinking a swollen brain.

Urea as a 30 per cent solution lyophilised in 10 per cent invert sugar was shown in 1956 to have a useful dehydrating effect on the brain (Javid and Settlage, 1956) when given in a dose of 1–1·5 g/kg body weight with a maximum dose of 90 g. Urea is a potent osmotic diuretic and has a more prolonged action than substances which merely increase plasma osmolality. Urea is contra-indicated in the presence of renal disease and is a profound local irritant. Its main disadvantage is that it may cause a rebound rise in brain tension (Clark and Einspruch, 1962) due to a late diffusion of urea into the brain substance and a subsequent rise of brain osmolality.

Mannitol has replaced urea for the purposes of cerebral dehydration. It too increases plasma osmolality to withdraw fluid from the brain and acts as a potent diuretic. Rebound of brain swelling is much less marked with mannitol than with urea. Mannitol is used as a 20 per cent solution and a dose of $1-1.5$ g/kg is usually given over 15–20 minutes.

It is wise when osmotic diuretics are being used to catheterise the patient and monitor urine flow. When mannitol fails to produce a diuresis the uncompensated increase in plasma volume produced may increase venous bleeding during craniotomy and can precipitate pulmonary oedema.

Other measures.—The use of hyperventilation and the resultant hypocapnia in the control of vascular volume has already been emphasised. Other measures which have been used to reduce brain swelling include hypothermia and induced hypotension. These two methods are discussed below.

Oral glycerol has been used to lower intracranial tension (Cantore *et al.*, 1964). Its advantages are simplicity of administration, lack of rebound phenomena and lack of toxicity. The oral dose is $0.5-2$ g per kg body weight, and as much as 5 g per day has been given to a single patient over several days without troublesome effects. In spite of its safety glycerol has not achieved great popularity.

Frusemide, either alone or in combination with mannitol, has also been used to produce cerebral dehydration (Fossa *et al.*, 1968). Frusemide is a powerful diuretic and can produce considerable electrolyte loss. It differs as a diuretic from mannitol, which promotes a loss of water with little electrolyte content. The use of frusemide to reduce brain bulk would seem to have a doubtful basis.

Steroids such as dexamethasone can produce dramatic reductions in intracranial pressure when the rise is due to cerebral oedema. Dexamethasone is given intravenously in a dose of 10 mg and followed by 4 mg every 6 hours intramuscularly. Its effects are most pronounced if cerebral oedema is due to a tumour.

CONTROLLED HYPOTENSION

There are few branches of surgery in which so strong a case can be made for induced hypotension, and in which the risks of the ancillary technique can be set against the advantages. At the outset, however, it is important to remember that most intracranial and spinal operations can be performed satisfactorily without it, provided due attention is paid to the essentials of good anaesthesia and posture. However, the presence of a tumour may cause congestion during surgery so that induced hypotension, by reducing swelling, may lessen the risks of some operations on the brain. Increased meningeal vascularity may lead to major haemorrhage during craniotomy which cannot be controlled until the skull is opened. Hypotension may reduce such blood loss to manageable levels. Minimal arterial bleeding with no venous ooze materially assists the surgeon to delineate the limits of the disease process and thus to remove it with less risk of damage to normal tissue. Control of haemorrhage may make possible operations which could not otherwise be attempted (Anderson and McKissock, 1953). A raised intracranial pressure makes exposure at the operation site difficult, since the distended brain tends to bulge out when the dura is opened, and aggravates venous bleeding. A distended brain also necessitates considerable retraction which in turn leads to bruising of tissue. A marked reduction in arterial pressure will help to control these factors.

There are two situations in which hypotension during intracranial surgery may be particularly indicated. During the removal of vascular tumours such as meningiomata reduction of systolic pressure to levels of 60–70 mm Hg (8·0–9·3 kPa) can be of great use. A more profound hypotension may be necessary during the control of aneurysms or angiomata to reduce the risk of vessel rupture. Hypotension during the removal of vascular tumours may have to be maintained for several hours. An adequate reduction of bleeding may be obtained by moderate hyperventilation and the use of low concentrations of halothane. Greater control of blood pressure can be obtained by the use of trimetaphan. This and other ganglion-blocking agents can produce a post-operative cycloplegia of several hours duration which may complicate neuro-logical assessment. The brief and profound hypotension necessary during aneurysmal surgery is best obtained by sodium nitroprusside (Siegel et al., 1971).

The dangers of induced hypotension are well-recognised (see Chapter 15) and there are some problems associated with this technique of specific relevance to neurosurgical anaesthesia. Aserman (1953) has described how hypotension produces a dough-like consistency of brain tissue, when it is easily compressed, slow to regain its normal conformity and equally slowly replenished with blood. In these circumstances pressure from a brain retractor may lead to "retractor anaemia". Aserman's advice that induced hypotension should only be used for those operations in which retraction is made on brain substance that is ultimately to be excised is however far too sweeping. If measures to keep brain bulk to a minimum are employed (which may necessitate ventricular tap) only minimum retraction is needed to expose even deep seated lesions. A more important problem than retractor anaemia is the possibility of brain damage due to a low blood pressure. Abnormalities of the blood-brain barrier have been demonstra-ted after lowering mean arterial pressure of experimental animals to 30 mm Hg (4 kPa) (Roth et al., 1969). The loss of autoregulation which occurs at low arterial pressures may persist for some time after restoration of perfusing pressure. The cerebral circulation may be more vulnerable to the effects of hypotension during neurosurgery. With an open skull the siphon effect of the cerebral venous drainage in potentiating cerebral perfusion is lost (Hunter, 1975).

Sodium nitroprusside has become increasingly popular for use during neurosurgery because of the ease with which its effects can be controlled and its lack of a direct myocardial action. A dangerous accumulation of cyanide may occur if large doses of nitroprusside are given or rapid rates of administra-tion used (McDowall et al., 1974; Vesey and Cole, 1975). If the use of nitro-prusside in neurosurgical anaesthesia is restricted to the production of profound hypotension as an aneurysm is about to be attacked, minimal doses are required and adverse effects of its metabolic breakdown are unlikely. Administration of hydroxocobalamin during or following nitroprusside infusion acts as an effective antagonist to any cyanide that may be produced (Vesey et al., 1974).

HYPOTHERMIA

Hypothermia leads to a fall in cerebral blood flow and cerebrospinal fluid pressure, and to a reduction in brain volume (Rosomoff and Holaday, 1954; Rosomoff and Gilbert, 1955). Access to various parts of the brain is improved, and the surgeon can temporarily occlude a major end-artery. At rectal temperatures of about 30° C Burrows and his colleagues (1956) have been able to clamp the middle cerebral artery for from $4\frac{1}{2}$ to $12\frac{3}{4}$ minutes without evidence of permanent cerebral damage. The induction of hypothermia will lead to some fall in systemic blood pressure, but not necessarily to very much. The reduction in metabolism that the fall in temperature causes will, however, offer some protection against the potential dangers of induced hypotension. It will also play an important part in reducing or preventing cerebral oedema, which in some neurosurgical procedures is often the ultimate factor leading to death. Hellings (1958) describing her experiences with surface cooling for a large series of patients with ruptured intracranial aneurysms and angiomata, reports that the technique may be used with small risks (no deaths due to it in over 100 patients), when compared with the use of a general anaesthetic alone. She considers that hypothermia can reasonably be used for other intracranial procedures, such as removal of a meningioma, when the improved operating conditions may be of value. It is difficult to be certain of the overall advantages of hypothermia for neurosurgical operations unless there is a specific indication, such as the temporary occlusion of an important vessel. Most of its advantages can be achieved by simpler means, such as controlled respiration with hyperventilation. There is a strong case for hypothermia when vascular occlusion is likely to be required, but the use of hypothermia to lower intracranial pressure *per se* or to assist in the production of induced hypotension has been rendered unnecessary by modern techniques. The popularity of hypothermia during neurosurgery seems to be waning. McDowall (1971) in a survey of many neurosurgical centres found wide variations in the use of the technique but a general tendency to reduce the indications for its employment.

NEURORADIOLOGICAL INVESTIGATION PROCEDURES

The special neuroradiological investigation procedures fall into three groups —air replacement of the cerebrospinal fluid to outline the ventricular system, intraventricular or spinal subarachnoid injection of a radio-opaque dye to outline a tumour or other obstruction to the flow of cerebrospinal fluid, and arterial and venous angiography. All these investigations can be, and indeed frequently are, performed under local analgesia with or without sedation, but some of them—particularly the air-replacement techniques—are often so unpleasant as to warrant complete loss of consciousness. Nevertheless, with the development of the new E.M.I. brain "scanner" it is hoped that the technique of computerised tomography (McDowall, 1976) will make many of these potentially dangerous anaesthetics unnecessary. Children and unco-operative adults apart, there is still little unanimity of opinion amongst the doctors concerned about the indications for general anaesthesia for these investigational procedures, and some discussion of its merits and demerits is therefore worth while.

The dangers of the anaesthetic are those common to all anaesthetics and primarily dependent on the competence of the administrator. However, anaesthesia for neurological investigations carries special risks by virtue of the varied postures the patient will need to be placed in, and the effects of the disease on the vital centres. An experienced anaesthetist is essential, and with this assumption and some selection of cases, there is little evidence that general anaesthesia increases the mortality or morbidity associated with these procedures. Indeed Brown (1955) considers that light general anaesthesia is to be preferred to local analgesia for angiography, because it enables the patient's response to the injection of dye to be more simply and quickly assessed. This facilitates quicker treatment of any complications that may occur. However, loss of consciousness does necessitate manhandling the patient at intervals during the investigation to get the correct positions for radiography, which is a distinct disadvantage if staff is very limited. Paradoxically, anaesthesia enables the radiologist concerned to get on with the procedure without undue worry about the personal feelings of the patient—an important advantage when the symptoms caused by the investigation are barely tolerable—and the head can be kept perfectly still while the pictures are taken.

In the final event pleasantness for the patient must be the object of the anaesthetist, and provided this can be achieved without increasing the hazards of the investigation or adding special risks of its own, there are no legitimate reasons for refusing full anaesthesia. Nevertheless an accurate appreciation of the true nature of the symptoms produced by each investigation is essential before recommending general anaesthesia routinely, besides cognisance of the mental state of the patient concerned when the investigation is known to be relatively simple and devoid of unpleasant sequelae.

Most neurological investigations cause only slight discomfort to the average patient, but many patients—particularly if the progress of their suspected disease has not dulled the intellect—are extremely apprehensive.

Sedation and Analgesia in Neuroradiology

The fundamental consideration in management is the presence or absence of raised intracranial pressure. A drowsy patient with papilloedema is not a suitable candidate for any form of sedation.

If apprehension and the unpleasantness of the positioning rather than pain are the main considerations then diazepam 5 to 10 mg or droperidol 5 mg intravenously are unlikely to have any unwanted effects on cardiovascular or respiratory function. They are best given by slow intravenous injection immediately before the investigation. If pain is also to be taken into account, phenoperidine may be diluted and given intravenously, 0·25 mg at a time, while its effect on respiration is very carefully watched. The use of these drugs has very much increased the versatility of sedation and the choice between them and general anaesthesia depends on many factors and is often difficult to make. A consideration of the individual procedures will enable these factors to be better understood.

Ventriculography and Air-encephalography

Ventriculography is the replacement of cerebrospinal fluid in the ventricular system from above and can be likened to the injection of air into a bottle full of fluid after the cork has been removed. Air-encephalography is replacement from below through a lumbar puncture, and by a similar analogy is injection into a bottle with the cork still in place. Thus, potentially, air-encephalography is a more dangerous procedure than ventriculography, as the passage of air into the ventricles may lead to or accentuate cerebral oedema and displace the medulla downwards. For many years the feeling that this sequence of events might occur limited the practice of air-encephalography, and the prospect of danger is still sometimes used as an argument against the production of general anaesthesia during the investigation. Indeed, if the circumstances of the patient's disease are so dire that general anaesthesia—by raising carbon dioxide tension or causing some sub-oxygenation—might accentuate the existing oedema sufficiently to produce a pressure cone, then general anaesthesia should not be induced, but, even more important, air-encephalography should not be performed at all. In such circumstances the injection of air by this method is as likely as general anaesthesia to be fatal. This type of patient is best investigated by ventriculography, and a drainage tube left in one or other lateral ventricle so that cerebrospinal fluid can be taken off at intervals. But even ventriculography may be followed by a central reaction in the brain leading to oedema and rising pressure.

At the present time air-encephalography is more frequently performed than ventriculography because it is a simple non-surgical procedure and the risks referred to are only likely in exceptional cases. These exceptional cases constitute the majority of patients who are submitted to ventriculography.

Ventriculography.—The investigation consists of making two burr holes in the posterior part of the skull, passing a canula into each lateral ventricle, and replacing part of the cerebrospinal fluid in them with air or oxygen. The outlines of the ventricular system are then defined on X-rays taken subsequently.

The patient is placed on the operating table in the supine position with head supported at a high level in a horse-shoe rest so that the occipital protuberance is well displayed.

The whole procedure can be carried out with minimal discomfort in co-operative adults under local infiltration analgesia. Premedication is neither desirable nor usually necessary, and to be effective is often more depressant than full general anaesthesia. The skin and deep tissues of the scalp down to the periosteum are infiltrated in the line of the incision with 1 per cent lignocaine. The dura and brain substance are painless, but the injection of air or oxygen into the lateral ventricles may cause some headache. There are no absolute contraindications to general anaesthesia for ventriculography—indeed the presence of a burr hole and ventricular drainage is a factor for safety in those patients who have a high intracranial pressure—but in practice the procedure is well tolerated under local analgesia.

Oxygen is best for injection since it is more rapidly absorbed from the ventricular system than air. It is also less likely to cause any reaction and is cleaner than atmospheric air. Oxygen is drawn off from a medical gas cylinder through a sterile connecting rubber tube into a 10 ml syringe and injected directly from the syringe into the canulae. Oxygen is always preferable to air, although there may be a case for using the latter when prolonged radiographic studies over a day or two are contemplated.

The patient must be carefully observed for some hours after ventriculography is completed. Removal of fluid from the ventricle relieves undue intracranial pressure but leaves room for cerebral oedema to accumulate. Even oxygen replacement causes some degree of reaction of this type and this may ultimately be sufficient to produce a rise in both systolic and diastolic blood pressures and respiratory difficulties. Further judicious drainage from the lateral ventricle will then be indicated.

Air (or oxygen) encephalography.—The patient is placed in the sitting position, preferably in a special chair which supports the front of the body and the head, which must be angled forward, and leaves the back free. A lumbar puncture is performed, about 10 ml of fluid are withdrawn and an equivalent quantity of air or oxygen replaced. Lateral X-rays of the skull are then taken to check that the gas is in the subarachnoid space and able to pass up into the ventricular system. This is sometimes difficult to achieve, particularly if a diagnostic lumbar puncture has been performed within the past week or two, since the oxygen then tends to track up in the epidural space.

Once the gas has passed into the ventricles a further 20 to 30 ml of cerebrospinal fluid are withdrawn in 10 ml quantities and replaced at once by equivalent amounts of gas. The X-rays are then taken (Fig. 2). This period may be protracted for as long as one or two hours. It will require movement of the patient, both to the supine and prone positions, to facilitate filling of the entire ventricular system and to ensure adequate pictures from different angles.

For an unanaesthetised patient lumbar encephalography is tedious and unpleasant. Nevertheless the difficulties of positioning are less if the patient can co-operate, and provided that he is carefully and skilfully managed the procedure can be made more tolerable.

Management without general anaesthesia.—The legs may be bandaged with crêpe bandages as for posterior fossa surgery: an indwelling intravenous needle is inserted and a blood-pressure cuff applied. Vasovagal fainting with its attendant nausea can be prevented by injecting 0·6 mg atropine intravenously immediately the patient is sat up. Diazepam 2·5–7·5 mg has been used as a sedative during the procedure.

General anaesthesia.—General anaesthesia is essential for children and for adults unable

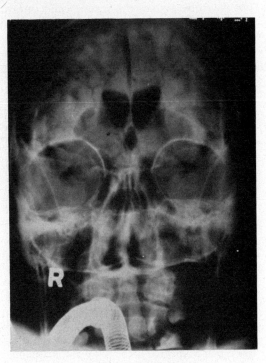

30/FIG. 2.—Normal air-encephalogram.

to co-operate. If there is any doubt about tolerance of the procedure under sedation it is better to choose general anaesthesia. The problems are similar to those of posterior fossa surgery and a marked fall of pressure must be looked for and guarded against, particularly after sudden movements or the intravenous injection of anaesthetic drugs. A cuffed non-kinkable endotracheal tube is mandatory. Spontaneous ventilation can be retained, but controlled ventilation will reduce the liability of raised intracranial pressure.

There are special problems associated with gas injections into a closed body cavity during nitrous oxide anaesthesia. If the cavity is filled with air nitrous oxide will diffuse into the cavity much faster than nitrogen leaves it and pressure within the cavity will rise (Saidman and Eger, 1965). As air encephalography should only be performed in patients with normal or near normal intracranial pressures the rise in pressure produced by nitrous oxide should not be dangerous. Oxygen as the contrast medium has some advantages over air. Although nitrous oxide will diffuse just as readily into an oxygen-containing cavity, oxygen diffuses out from such a cavity more rapidly than does nitrogen. Using nitrous oxide as the contrast medium prevents this rise of pressure during the procedure, but the rapid post-operative absorption of nitrous oxide can lead to severe intracranial hypotension which may itself produce dangerous complications (Collan and Ivanainen, 1969).

General anaesthesia not only eliminates the unpleasantness of the procedure but may also reduce the severity and duration of the headache that follows. Analgesia and sedation should be maintained in the post-anaesthetic stage by suitable drugs, provided they are compatible with the patient's neurological and general condition. The intermittent inhalation of oxygen may be of some benefit in the treatment of the headache when air has been injected (Macintosh et al., 1958).

Myelography and Ventricular Dye Injection

Myelography consists of the injection of a radio-opaque dye into the sub-arachnoid space, either at the lumbar or the cisternal level, and posturing the patient to allow it to run towards the tumour. Spinal myelography with lumbar injection of the dye should only be managed by general anaesthesia when the patient is unable to co-operate. There is often no objection to the use of sedation, if necessary with opiates, and the very steep head-down tilt in the prone position in a darkened room makes general anaesthesia hazardous. No patient should be managed in total darkness and it is essential that the oxygen rotameter and the reservoir bag are continuously watched.

For ventricular dye injection the same considerations apply as to gas ventriculography and general anaesthesia is usually strongly contra-indicated. Myodil, which is used as the contrast medium, is an iodinated lipoid with a low specific gravity, more fluid than iodised poppy-seed oil (Lipiodol) and relatively non-irritant. Injection of a dye to outline the ventricular system necessitates one or two burr holes and the passage of a rubber catheter into one or other lateral ventricle. Although the operation is done in the theatre, the dye is better injected in the X-ray department.

Cerebral Angiography

Carotid arteriography stems from the work of Moniz who in 1926 attempted puncture of this vessel under local analgesia (Moniz, 1940). Percutaneous injection of diodone into the carotid or vertebral artery on one or other side is now commonly performed to delineate the arterial tree of the brain. Aneurysms,

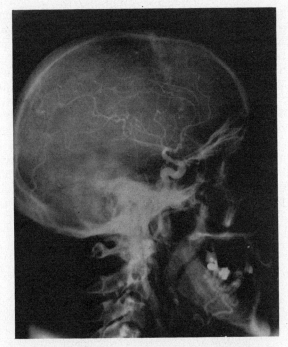

30/Fig. 3.—Normal carotid arteriogram, lateral view.

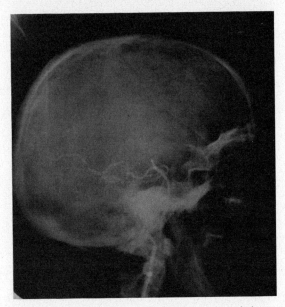

30/Fig. 4.—Normal vertebral arteriogram, lateral view.

vascular tumours or arterial displacement by other tumours may be depicted. Carotid injection will outline most of the vessels above the tentorium, while vertebral injection depicts those below this structure as well as the posterior cerebral artery (Figs. 3–6).

The internal carotid or the vertebral artery is punctured in the neck with the patient lying supine. The needle is kept clear by the continuous slow injection of normal saline, while the patient's head is angled correctly in the X-ray apparatus. The opaque dye is then injected and the pictures are taken. Although the procedure is uncomfortable it is not unbearable with simple local infiltration of the skin, and, provided the operator is adept at the technique and the patient co-operative, general anaesthesia is not essential. Recent work however has caused a re-appraisal of the role of general anaesthesia in this investigation because it has shown that lowering of the carbon dioxide tension results in much improved angiograms, particularly in patients with tumours (Samuel *et al.*, 1968; Dallas and Moxon, 1969).

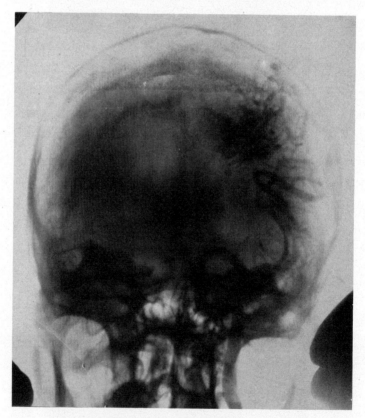

30/Fig. 5(*a*).—Carotid arteriogram—haemangioma (anteroposterior view).

The older technique involving spontaneous breathing and the use of volatile agents has definitely been shown to be much less satisfactory, and relaxation with curare or pancuronium is now the method of choice. Patients with grossly raised intracranial pressure are better managed without anaesthesia, but if this is not possible relaxation and hyperventilation is preferable to the further increase in intracranial pressure which volatile agents and a rise in arterial carbon dioxide tension inevitably cause.

Certain dangers must be noted both in relation to the technique of arterial puncture and to the results of the injection of the radio-opaque dye. In arteriosclerotic patients, particularly if firm pressure is not applied to the site of arterial puncture for some time after withdrawal of the needle, a haematoma may develop in the neck. When this lies behind the trachea it may cause respiratory embarrassment and necessitate the passage of an endotracheal tube (Fig. 7). Repeated attempts at arterial puncture may cause spasm of the vessel, and this can be offset to some extent by a liberal infiltration of local analgesic solution to which has been added a small quantity of 5 per cent papaverine solution.

The actual injection of dye may lead to various disturbances, but all are

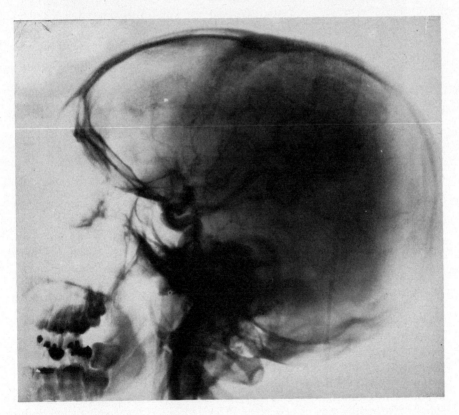

30/Fig. 5(*b*).—Carotid arteriogram—haemangioma (lateral view).

fortunately rare. Vomiting and coughing may occur, and marked hypotension may follow generalised vasodilatation (Duncalf and Thompson, 1956). The

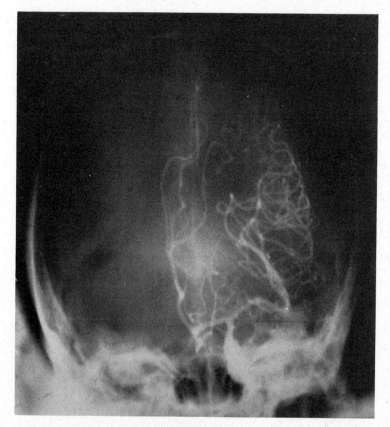

30/Fig. 6.—Subdural haematoma. Antero-posterior carotid arteriogram of a 60-year-old male with a severe head injury, showing lentiform avascular area over the cerebral hemisphere.

neurological sequelae recorded include hemiplegia, death from haemorrhage into a tumour or from an intracranial aneurysm, and transient blindness (Geddes, 1952). Temporary hypotension plays a part in the production of some palsies, but an element of vascular spasm and subsequent thrombosis is probably more dangerous. Extravasation of the dye into the neck can cause injury to the cervical sympathetic chain (Dunsmore *et al.*, 1951).

Brown (1955) has recorded a detailed description and discussion of the circulatory disturbance that may occur during or following cerebral angiography under general anaesthesia. When cases of recent spontaneous subarachnoid haemorrhage are submitted to the procedure, an immediate fall of blood pressure sometimes occurs. If the fall is slight, a return to normal usually occurs in a matter of minutes, but if it is severe recovery may take several hours, and supportive therapy may be necessary. Brown considers that hypotension of this type is due to the irritant effect of the dye on vessels which are already hypersensitive because of injury from haemorrhage in their vicinity. The degree of hypotension bears some relation to the site of the haemorrhage, its severity, and the time between its onset and the angiography.

BACKGROUND TO ANAESTHETIC PRACTICE
IN NEUROSURGERY

If the anaesthetist is to do more than satisfy the immediate aim of technical proficiency in neurosurgical anaesthesia he must have some background knowledge of the patient's disease, the neurosurgical procedure—its aims and the major steps in its performance—and the complications specific to the operation. Technical skill must not, however, be unduly denigrated, for there are few practical sides of anaesthesia in which obsessional attention to detail can be so effective in the final result, and in which a minor disruption can so quickly upset

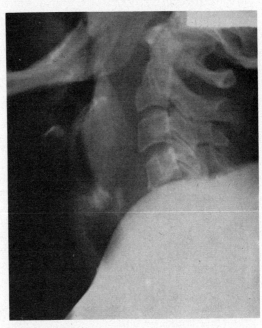

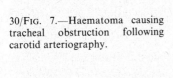

30/FIG. 7.—Haematoma causing tracheal obstruction following carotid arteriography.

the operation field, and perhaps jeopardise the patient's life. Despite the intricate formation of the brain and its connections, surprisingly extensive operations can be performed in its substance without permanent damage to important tissues, and without evoking any localised or generalised response on the part of a lightly anaesthetised patient. There are, however, exceptions, and the implications of these may be of importance.

Not every anaesthetist has the opportunity to work in a neurosurgical unit, so that some amplification of the subject is felt to be justified, even though it often represents an anaesthetist's view of the problem, largely consists of generalisation, and is far from exhaustive.

Circulatory and Respiratory Changes caused by Neurosurgical Operations

Observation of the pulse rate and blood pressure may enable the anaesthetist to warn the surgeon that he is disturbing the vital centres. Those centres which are likely to be damaged or stimulated lie in the floor of the third ventricle and hypothalamus or in the floor of the fourth ventricle near the dorsal portion of the pons and the medulla oblongata (Hunter, 1952). Interference with the hypo-thalamic centres may take place during an operation on the pituitary, or ones for a suprasellar cyst or for an olfactory groove meningioma—all of which abut on the vital area. Hypotension results and is an indication for the surgeon to stop at once. If the pressure then returns to normal in all probability all will be well, but persistent or severe hypotension suggests a bad prognosis. After irreversible hypothalamic damage the patient does not recover consciousness, but gradually succumbs over twenty-four to forty-eight hours with a rising pulse rate, hypotension and hyperpyrexia.

The centres in the floor of the fourth ventricle are sometimes affected during operations on the brain stem or in its vicinity. The damage may be direct, parti-cularly when a tumour extends into that area, but may also be due to inter-ference with the blood supply from thrombosis or the tearing of small vessels. The centres may also be indirectly affected if the brain stem is rotated during retraction. The alterations in pulse rate and blood pressure which these factors cause are variable, but usually take the form of temporary hypertension and bradycardia. The occurrence of either is an indication that all is not well. A sudden and marked hypertension, even though of brief duration, often portends permanent damage.

Bradycardia and temporary respiratory arrest have been noticed to follow deliberate or accidental stimulation of the uncal gyrus of a temporal lobe (Howland and Papper, 1952). These variations, like the tachycardia and respira-tory irregularities which follow stimulation in light anaesthesia of those few intracranial structures with a sensory nerve supply, are not of grave significance, although the anaesthetist must seek for their cause. Persistent and increasing tachycardia usually heralds a rise in intracranial pressure due to obstruction to the flow of cerebrospinal fluid, and is most commonly seen in patients with sub-tentorial lesions. It is the earliest sign that pressure is building up and a warning that worse may follow in the form of a medullary coning, unless the ventricular pressure is quickly released.

Respiratory arrest may occur during intracranial surgery as a result of in-direct interference with the vital centres—usually when tumours are growing in their vicinity—but it is usually temporary. It also occurs as the late result of medullary coning, and may momentarily follow the sudden release of a high intracranial pressure.

Cervical laminectomy for tumour removal may result in injury to the phrenic nerve roots with respiratory embarrassment. Laminectomies are sometimes associated with autonomic reflex activity. The mass reflex which may occur in patients with high spinal traumatic injuries is associated with sweating, brady-cardia, and a very high blood pressure and has been noted under anaesthesia (Ciliberti et al., 1954).

Tumours of the Cerebello-pontine Angle

The commonest tumour found in this vicinity is the acoustic neuroma, which arises from the eighth nerve within the internal auditory meatus. Although benign in nature, this tumour is in such close proximity to many cranial nerves and the vital centres of the brain that operative removal is associated with a high mortality and morbidity. Surgical treatment can be roughly divided into two groups. First, total removal, and secondly, intracapsular removal—though in fact part of the capsule is usually removed—but to appreciate the significance of each method certain factors must be considered.

The tumour is solid but usually has a quantity of fluid encapsulated in arachnoid mater around it. Within the internal meatus it is in close contact with the seventh cranial nerve, and, as it grows in size, it encroaches on the fifth, ninth, tenth, eleventh and twelfth cranial nerves, as well as the pons and cerebellum. Therefore total removal of the tumour and capsule may well result in permanent damage to the seventh nerve and enhances the risk of damage to the other nerves. Swallowing is very likely to be unco-ordinated in the post-operative period and a plastic naso-gastric tube should be passed at induction. Retraction and operation in that area may also produce effects on the vital centres which lie in the floor of the fourth ventricle either directly or as a result of damage to the blood supply (see above). If the patient survives, total removal constitutes a cure, and a facial palsy can be improved by anastomosing this nerve to the hypoglossal nerve in the neck at a later operation, or by a sling operation designed to support the facial muscles. Neither of these plastic operations is very satisfactory, but the former improves the contour and movement of the face and helps to control a watery eye and mouth dribbling. On the other hand, it leads to hemiatrophy of the tongue. Intracapsular removal, although incomplete, and therefore likely to be followed by recurrence in a matter of years, is less likely to produce damage to adjacent structures, though it can and does do so on occasion. It can be argued, certainly so far as elderly patients are concerned, and particularly if they have coexisting disease in other systems, that an intracapsular removal is perfectly satisfactory treatment and likely to suit the normal expectation of life for such a patient. Choice of operation can also be made to justify a particular posture, since there can be no doubt that perfect access to the cerebello-pontine angle materially assists the surgeon to locate and avoid these important structures. Thus the upright or sitting position is nearly always routinely used by the advocates of total removal, though this in itself probably plays a part in the death of some patients either from air embolus or severe hypotension.

Subarachnoid Haemorrhage

The commonest cause of spontaneous subarachnoid haemorrhage is rupture of an intracranial aneurysm. Other causes are intracranial angiomata, spreading haemorrhage from a burst atheromatous vessel in the brain and, very rarely, certain blood diseases. Although there may be severe hypertension, spontaneous subarachnoid haemorrhage may also occur without evidence of local disease. McKissock (1956) has summarised the position by referring to the results of carotid angiography. On a statistical basis 50–60 of 100 patients admitted to hospital with spontaneous subarachnoid haemorrhage will be found to have an intracranial aneurysm either upon the circle of Willis or one of its major branches, about 10 patients will have an intracranial angioma, and in the remaining patients no vascular lesion will be demonstrated. The distribution and incidence of the major groups of intracranial aneurysms is illustrated in Fig. 8.

Speedy diagnosis is essential, and once cerebral arteriosclerosis and essential hypertension and other systemic diseases have been excluded by clinical methods, cerebral angiography should be carried out. The risk of this investigation causing a further bleed or enhancing the generalised spasm of the cerebral vessels that the original haemorrhage causes, is probably very small, and is in any event

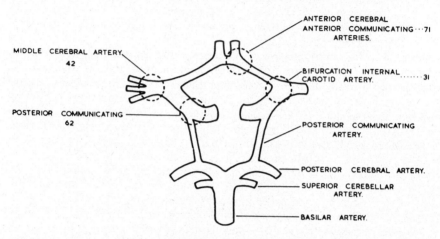

30/FIG. 8.—Diagram of the circle of Willis, showing distribution of major groups of aneurysm in a series of 206 patients.

usually accepted nowadays. Diagnosis is an urgent matter, since the choice of treatment affects the prognosis. Once more the position has been concisely summarised by McKissock (1956). With medical treatment 50 per cent of patients shown to have an aneurysm will die during the first eight weeks after the first bleed and another 20 per cent will die from recurrent haemorrhage later. With surgical treatment 33·3 per cent of patients with a proven aneurysm will die in the first eight weeks. These figures are for intracranial aneurysms in all situations, and a more impressive case for active therapy can be made when the results of medical and surgical treatment of aneurysms at particular sites are analysed. Even in the most awkward situations surgical treatment more often offers a favourable result than the natural course of the disease (McKissock and Walsh, 1956). Although early operation is, therefore, usually recommended when the site of the aneurysm suggests that surgical treatment will be possible, picking the exact time to operate needs consideration. Immediate operation after establishment of the diagnosis is common practice, though this hardly leaves time for any associated vascular spasm in the neighbourhood of the haemorrhage to settle. In any event operation must not be delayed for more than a week as a second bleed commonly occurs on or about the tenth day.

Angiomata have a different natural history. They bleed at longer intervals than aneurysms and a second bleed, even when soon after the first, is not necessarily fatal. On the other hand, they are more often than not amenable to surgical treatment.

Some of the probable changes that take place after rupture of an intracranial aneurysm have been described by Logue (1956). Immediately following the rupture, the vessels in continuity with the aneurysm and near by it go into intense spasm. The spasm has the beneficial effect of reducing the tension of blood in the sac so that the tear shrinks in size and becomes sealed with clot. The spasm has the detrimental effect of producing ischaemia in the area of the brain supplied by the vessels and in about 15 per cent of cases the consequent cerebral oedema raises the intracranial pressure. It seems probable that spasm with its associated cerebral ischaemia and swelling is the cause of death or neurological damage in many cases, although destruction of brain substance plays a major part in some. Logue also stresses the importance of spasm in the small perforating vessels, particularly following rupture of an aneurysm of the anterior cerebral artery. Here the result will be ischaemia in the hypothalamus, basal ganglia and internal capsule, and the retraction necessary for the exposure of the aneurysm at operation is very likely to accentuate the damage.

It is consideration of factors such as these which illustrates the dangers of dogmatising on the virtues of induced hypotension or hypothermia. It is now established that the major advance in the improvement of operating conditions has been the use of controlled ventilation with moderate lowering of the P_{CO_2} so that neither induced hypotension nor hypothermia is routinely used. Induced hypotension can undoubtedly make a valuable contribution to the surgical access to intracranial aneurysms, and will help to control any sudden bleed that may occur from the sac during operation. The abnormally low pressure in the presence of intense vascular spasm could, however, equally contribute to thrombosis of the small perforating vessels and enhance the dangers of retraction. Although it is commonplace to suggest that induced hypotension has made operation on these intracranial aneurysms a practical possibility, this is not the strict truth. Many have been successfully treated without it. It is, however, an undoubted aid, though not without its own dangers, which in the present state of our knowledge must be accepted.

The value of hypothermia is equally problematical but there is increasing evidence that it does not prevent the ischaemic damage to the brain consequent upon rupture of an intracranial aneurysm, and that it does not therefore improve the survival rate following surgical treatment of this condition (Hamby, 1963). McKissock and his colleagues (1965), in a study of aneurysms of the anterior communicating artery, substantiate this view. Good arguments in favour of hypothermia are that it enables the surgeon to occlude temporarily a major end-artery, leads to a reduction in brain bulk, and helps to prevent the onset of cerebral oedema. However, the disadvantages and dangers of hypothermia *per se* must not be overlooked. When it is indicated a body temperature of not less than 30° C is satisfactory, but deep hypothermia with the aid of an artificial circulation to 20° C or less has been used for the surgical repair of intracranial aneurysms (Uihlein *et al.*, 1960; Michenfelder *et al.*, 1963).

Stereotactic Operations

Localised lesions can be produced in the depths of the brain by thermocoagulation or by freezing with liquid nitrogen. Stereotaxis is the method by which the region to be treated is determined and localised. The technique is commonly used for making lesions of the globus pallidus in patients suffering from Parkinsonism. It is also valuable for the treatment of intractable pain and has recently been used for frontal leucotomy. Local analgesia will suffice but it is not always pleasant for the patient. When general anaesthesia is used it must be so chosen that at certain times during the operative procedure the patient will regain consciousness and co-operate fully with the surgeon. This is particularly important during the stage of stimulation when the area of the brain to be treated is being localised, and while the lesion is being made. Coleman and De Villiers (1964) describe a technique for anaesthesia consisting simply of the continuous intravenous infusion of a 0·1 per cent solution of methohexitone. When tremor or abnormal movements are severe they also use small paretic doses of gallamine triethiodide to induce some reduction in muscle power. No premedication is used, and all sedative drugs are stopped for 24 hours before the operation. By stopping or slowing the drip it is possible to effect a rapid return of full consciousness, or, in an unduly apprehensive subject, a co-operative but sedated patient. An alternative technique is to make use of neuroleptanalgesia which provides sedation and suppression of mental and physical discomfort, but leaves the patient co-operative (Brown, 1964), (see p. 1090). Because controlled lesions are best produced in the presence of tremor an alternative approach is to define the area to be treated under general anaesthesia, but delay the production of lesions until a later occasion and do this in a fully conscious patient.

Cordotomy (Tractotomy) and Rhizotomy

Cordotomy is a gross but effective method of treating severe pain on either or both sides of the body. It is usually performed for those patients in whom neoplastic disease is the cause of the pain and in whom a reasonable expectation of life seems likely. A successful result enables more general treatment, such as that by opiates, to be stopped, or at least diminished. It is worth noting that patients who have been treated by large doses of opiates prior to a successful cordotomy do not always crave for these drugs when they are stopped. The therapy of genuine pain by large doses of opiates does not apparently invariably lead to addiction.

Cordotomy is always done at the cervical level so that the sense of touch is undisturbed, and a bilateral cut is rarely performed at the same operation, in order to avoid sphincter disturbances. If a bilateral cordotomy is needed then an interval of 6–8 weeks is usually allowed between the two. The approach is as for a laminectomy and the actual cord division is gross enough to be performed under general anaesthesia, although a more accurate assessment of the extent of section can be made if the patient is awake and co-operative. Simple infiltration is a not very successful method of ensuring good pain relief for laminectomy, though it can be used in combination with light enough anaesthesia to ensure sufficient return of consciousness at the crucial time. Segmental epidural analgesia will provide complete analgesia in the operation site without disturbing the area of pain and thus allowing adequate testing during the operation (Krumperman et al., 1957).

In recent years stereotactic percutaneous cordotomy has become an established procedure (Mullan et al., 1963; Lipton, 1968). Radiofrequency, direct current or strontium are used to produce a localised spinothalamic lesion. This operation carries a lower mortality and morbidity than surgical cordotomy and can more readily be repeated if pain returns.

Rhizotomy, or root section, is a precise method of treating pain which can be localised. With the exception of the cranial nerves, it is usual also to cut the nerve roots above and below the one supplying the affected segment, since there is an overlap in the sensory supply from the spinal nerves.

NEUROSURGERY IN CHILDREN

Infants and small children may require neurosurgery for a variety of reasons, the commonest of which is probably the relief of congenital hydrocephalus. The other common reasons for paediatric neurosurgery are tumours such as astrocytomata and haemangioblastomata, and following severe head injury. Children with advanced intracranial tumours or head injuries may be in a critical state when they present for surgery, with a dangerously raised intracranial pressure. Management of these patients requires attention to all the basic demands of neurosurgical anaesthesia plus the problems particular to small and sick children. In general best results are attained by anaesthesia with controlled ventilation. Premedication should consist of atropine 0·02 mg/kg, with a minimum dose of 0·2 mg. Anaesthesia is best induced with intravenous thiopentone. If no suitable vein can be found an inhalation induction may be needed. As soon as consciousness is lost an intravenous line is established. Suxamethonium (1 mg/kg) is used before intubation, and may be preceded by a small dose of thiopentone to limit any rise in intracranial tension that may result from intubation. Anaesthesia is continued after intubation with nitrous oxide and oxygen, tubocurarine (0·4 mg/kg) and controlled ventilation. Volatile anaesthetics are best avoided if intracranial tension is raised. Nitrous oxide can be supplemented with fentanyl in doses of up to 3 µg/kg. A minute volume in the order of 150 ml/kg/minute will usually produce a P_{CO_2} of 30–35 mm Hg (4–4·7 kPa). Severe brain swelling during craniotomy may require mannitol (0·5–1 g/kg) for its control. At the end of the operation atropine (0·02 mg/kg) and neostigmine (0·05 mg/kg) are given to reverse the relaxant. During surgery monitoring of the cardiovascular and respiratory systems and of body temperature are important. A precordial or oesophageal stethoscope should be positioned before surgery commences, as should ECG leads. Accurate blood-pressure monitoring may require intra-arterial pressure measurements. A thermocouple or thermistor lead should be inserted in the oesophagus. Monitoring of tidal carbon dioxide concentration with a suitable infra-red analyser gives information on both respiration and cardiovascular function. Blood loss must be meticulously replaced as it occurs during surgery.

Anaesthetised infants are specially prone to hypothermia during surgery. A water blanket kept at 37° C or wrapping the infant in kitchen foil are useful methods to limit heat loss. Baum and Scopes (1968) have described a polyester sheet laminated on both surfaces with aluminium as an effective "swaddler" during major paediatric surgery.

POST-OPERATIVE CARE OF THE NEUROSURGICAL PATIENT

The immediate post-operative period is of considerable importance in neurosurgical practice. After cranial operations it may be difficult to distinguish between the effects of surgery and of anaesthesia—both may make common ground in the production of unconsciousness. In this respect anaesthesia can only be considered perfect when it ceases as soon as the surgeon completes the operation, for then the level of consciousness and the state of reflex activity are true guides to the condition of the patient. Unfortunately neither anaesthesia nor surgery is invariably perfect, and their combined or individual effects sometimes create problems which make the immediate post-operative period of considerable importance.

The sensitive intracranial mechanisms, already disturbed by the surgical procedure, may easily become unbalanced by apparently trivial complications of anaesthesia, and it is no exaggeration to suggest that a brief anoxic episode or a momentary rise in the level of carbon dioxide in the blood might even affect the patient's chance of survival. Either accentuates the element of cerebral oedema that follows all cerebral surgery. Oxygen should be given at this time for the first few hours and if there is any doubt about the adequacy of ventilation the endotracheal tube should be left in place and mechanical ventilation continued. Even successful surgery—successful that is, by the standard of removing a tumour completely—may be followed by nerve palsies, or more bizarre complications such as vasomotor collapse, hyperpyrexia, and respiratory disorders, all of which cause exceptional difficulties.

Thus the normal hazards of the post-anaesthetic period and the special requirements of the neurosurgical patient are a strong indication for the provision of recovery room space next to the operating theatre, so that both anaesthetist and surgeon can be within sight and sound of the patient at this potentially critical time.

ROUTINE POST-OPERATIVE CARE

Apart from the patient, the most important person in the recovery room is the nurse. The institution of continuous and skilled nursing care after surgery plays a vital part in the reduction of overall morbidity for many cranial operations. This is particularly so when cranial nerve palsies are present, since the dangers associated with partial respiratory obstruction and tracheal aspiration are very real. An adequate airway must be kept at all times, and in doubtful cases it is wiser to leave the endotracheal tube in position until the situation has clarified.

Observation

The nurse must observe and record all essential clinical data at regular intervals—every ten minutes for the first hour or so. Pulse and respiration rates, blood pressure level, the level of consciousness, response to stimuli, fluid intake, drugs given and any other points likely to be of value must be written down. These observations are of paramount importance in assessing the progress of intracranial complications, while differentiation of the effects of anaesthesia from those of surgery is possible only if a record is available to show the general trend of events. Thus the earliest signs of reactionary haemorrhage may be the onset of sleep in a previously sleepy but conscious patient, or a rise in blood pressure in a semi-conscious one.

Posture

As soon as consciousness is regained, and provided the systolic blood pressure is over 100 mm Hg (13·3 kPa), patients who have had cranial operations should be brought to a sitting position. Even before this, if the danger of vomiting can be circumvented or appears unlikely—patients can be reflexly normal but cerebrally unconscious—it may be advisable to have the head raised on pillows. The prime object of posture at this early stage is to reduce the twin risks of cerebral oedema and reactionary haemorrhage. However, in the exceptional case it may be wiser to wait several hours before sitting the patient up at all. Occasions of this type occur after removal of a large tumour from the posterior fossa, when the adjacent compressed tissues cannot be expected to fill up the resulting hole straight away. In these circumstances a sudden change in posture could lead to marked movement of the brain stem, due to inadequate compensation for the change in blood pressure, and consequent disturbance of function.

Patients who have had a laminectomy are nursed flat for several days.

At a later stage in the post-operative period posture must also be adjusted to encourage lung drainage, and reduce incidence of ischaemic sores, particularly for those patients who remain semiconscious or suffer from respiratory dysfunctions.

Changes in posture are facilitated by nursing all neurosurgical patients in special beds designed to tilt or rise in various ways with minimal inconvenience to the patient or nursing staff.

Sedation and Analgesia

Patients who have had cranial operations do not usually suffer from acute pain as a result of surgery. They are often restless and occasionally nauseated, particularly after operations in the posterior fossa, but rarely uncomfortable except from headache. The reason for this presumably lies in the insensitiveness of the structures involved, the skin being a notable exception, and the fact that movement of the patient is not, as in most other operative sites, reflected in increased tension in the wound. Laminectomy wounds, however, are very painful and usually require full doses of a potent analgesic such as an opiate or analogue. These agents are never necessary after cranial surgery, and indeed their potency, accentuated by the lack of acute pain, coupled with their well-known side-effects—particularly respiratory depression and pupillary contraction—contra-indicate their use.

The restlessness and headache can be adequately controlled by codeine phosphate in a dosage of from 32 to 65 mg, combined if necessary with phenobarbitone 100 to 200 mg and given intramuscularly. The effectiveness of codeine as an analgesic is open to doubt, but as a mild sedative without marked side-effects it is useful in these circumstances. Occasional patients may be so seriously disturbed by the surgery as to become vociferous and in need of restraint. For these, paraldehyde intramuscularly (2–3 ml) is very effective.

Intravenous Fluids

There is still no general agreement about the exact distribution of water between the cells and the extracellular fluid in the brain. It is however agreed that cerebral oedema, unlike oedema in its more usual manifestations, is due to intracellular accumulation of water particularly in the white matter (Aldridge, 1965). Equilibration of water between blood and brain is very rapid and occurs within a few minutes (Bering, 1952), and it is extremely important not to overhydrate neurosurgical patients in the immediate post-operative period.

Many patients are able to take fluids by mouth in a matter of hours and if the intravenous infusion has been left running it is very easy to give them more fluid than is desirable. It is wise to restrict the total fluid intake by all routes to $1\frac{1}{2}$–2 litres on the day of operation and on the following day. Temporary diabetes insipidus is not uncommon after operations near the hypothalamus and if a catheter has been passed can be recognised during operation by a sudden increase in urine volume—usually to between 7 and 12 ml/minute. In such cases dextrose/saline (4·3 per cent dextrose in 0·18 per cent saline) should be given 3-hourly in amounts equivalent to the previous 3-hourly urine volume if the patient in unable to drink.

Cerebral Oedema

Apart from posture, the most effective method of reducing raised intracranial pressure is intravenous mannitol. Its use at induction is described on page 987. When used post-operatively 500 ml of 10 per cent mannitol is given in the course of an hour and repeated 12-hourly. During this time the total fluid intake (including the volume of the mannitol solution) is restricted to 2 litres in 24 hours. Such a regime cannot usually be continued safely for more than 48 hours as it will cause progressive depletion of body water. This is indicated by a rise in serum sodium concentration which should not be allowed to exceed 155–160 mEq/l (mmol/l). Uncontrollable post-operative cerebral oedema may necessitate surgical decompression.

Reactionary Haemorrhage

Bleeding into the operation site leads to a rise in intracranial pressure which will be manifested by the signs already described, but specific localising signs, such as nerve palsies, which can be accounted for by the pressure of the accumulating blood clot, may also be present.

Treatment is essentially operative to remove the blood and stop the bleeding. Anaesthesia is often not required but an endotracheal tube should be passed with the aid of a relaxant, and adequate ventilation ensured. Once the compression has been relieved, however, anaesthesia will be needed, since consciousness often rapidly returns.

Particular note must be taken of the quantity of blood lost when a craniotomy wound is re-opened, and immediate replacement made should it appear necessary. Despite the constricted space in which the bleeding takes place, a surprisingly large quantity of blood can be lost while re-opening the wound since such an emergency allows no time for meticulous haemostasis until after the clot has been evacuated. Circulatory collapse during reactionary haemorrhage or while re-opening is in part due to central factors, but undoubtedly owes something to blood loss. This simple fact must not be forgotten.

SPECIAL POST-OPERATIVE CARE

Operations in the posterior fossa, particularly those for total extirpation of an acoustic neuroma, may be followed by cranial nerve palsies. Following removal of an acoustic tumour, a seventh nerve palsy is not uncommon, but more dangerous in the immediate post-operative period are palsies of the glossopharyngeal and vagus nerves. These may be only temporary and incomplete, but while present swallowing lacks co-ordination, and with laryngeal and glottic sensitivity diminished normal feeding may lead to aspiration into the respiratory tract. For this reason it is a good plan to have a plastic tube of 4 to 6 mm diameter passed through the nose into the stomach before the operation is started. During the post-operative period all feeds should be given down this tube and great care taken to avoid vomiting or regurgitation, either of which may lead to aspiration. A suction apparatus should be next to the bed at all times. After 48 hours, a small quantity of water should be given to the patient by mouth to test whether swallowing is normal; if it is, the tube should be removed. When there is any likelihood of fifth nerve damage, a tarsorrhaphy should be performed to protect the affected eye.

Patients who remain unconscious or semi-conscious for more than an hour or so after operation should be treated generally in a similar manner, and when they seem likely to remain in such a condition for several days—yet with a prospect of ultimate recovery—endotracheal intubation or a temporary tracheostomy must be considered. Certain complications—pulmonary aspiration lesions or inadequate ventilation—may be considered as indications for intubation or tracheostomy, but unconsciousness alone is not, provided competent nursing staff is available.

When gross aspiration of stomach contents into the lungs occurs during a bout of vomiting or regurgitation—a rare complication with adequate supervision and posturing—immediate bronchoscopy with lavage offers a reasonable prospect of removing the material and preventing infection. There are rarely, if ever, any other indications for bronchoscopy in the post-operative treatment of neurosurgical patients, or even for suction through an endotracheal tube. Simple pulmonary complications are best treated by posture and encouragement of normal drainage. If these fail, and the essential cause—such as unconsciousness or semiconsciousness—persists, then a tracheostomy enables efficient suction to be carried out simply and at regular intervals.

Respiratory Failure

This may be the terminal result of a rising intracranial pressure—in which case the essential treatment is that of the cause—of surgical interference, or of the direct effect of the disease process.

Operations on the cervical cord may be attended by bilateral phrenic paralysis, and although intercostal activity may be complete it is unlikely to be sufficient to maintain adequate ventilation, particularly during the immediate post-operative period. In cases of this type assisted or controlled respiration, preferably by a mechanical respirator, should be carried out, and a tracheostomy considered.

Vasomotor Failure

Hypotension is more often central than peripheral in origin. A peculiar type of circulatory collapse, characterised by a low blood pressure, with a slow pulse and dilated peripheral vessels, sometimes occurs after operations in the region of the fourth ventricle. The degree of hypotension is often sufficient to cause unconsciousness. Repeated intramuscular or intravenous doses of methoxamine, 5–10 mg, may be successful in restoring the blood pressure to normal, but more often than not the initial cause is incurable and the condition fatal.

Hyperpyrexia

So often in cranial surgery the post-operative complications are indicative of irreversible lesions in the brain itself, so that treatment, however effective in controlling the measurable signs or symptoms, only very rarely cures the cause. This is particularly true of severe hyperpyrexia, which is more often than not due to thrombosis in the region of the brain stem or thalamus. For such cases the production of hypothermia or the use of drugs such as chlorpromazine is unlikely to be successful—a more simple procedure, such as tepid sponging, is usually just as effective. If, however, the hyperpyrexia is likely to be due to cerebral oedema, then the more active measures may be found helpful.

Pulmonary Oedema

Certain operations in the region of the mid-brain, typically for tumours in the floor of the fourth ventricle, may be followed by pulmonary oedema. A rapid reduction in the circulating blood volume can be achieved with the use of diuretics (see Chapter 14, p. 546). Intubation followed by positive-pressure respiration with a mechanical ventilator should be commenced if diuretics alone do not quickly control the situation.

Post-operative problems peculiar to operations on the pituitary are discussed in Chapter 40.

HEAD INJURIES

Trauma is responsible for more deaths in all age groups under the age of 45 years than any other single cause, and head injury is the single most important factor in deaths due to trauma (Horton, 1975). In the care of head injuries attention has to be paid not only to the direct effects of brain trauma but also to the profound effects that disturbances in other bodily systems, especially the respiratory system, can have on intracranial mechanics.

Head injuries commonly occur in association with other trauma. The potentially lethal nature of even mild head injuries should never be overlooked in the treatment of associated injuries. Patients who have been concussed with only a transient loss of consciousness should be regarded as suffering from a potential major intracranial lesion until it is proved otherwise.

Initial treatment.—Because the commonest cause of deterioration after a head injury is due to respiratory obstruction the establishment of a clear airway is the first and major priority in the first aid treatment of these cases. The patient should be nursed on his side and blood or other foreign matter removed from the mouth. If obstruction occurs due to trismus or from soft tissues of the throat an airway can be inserted. If the cough and swallowing reflexes are depressed an endotracheal tube should be passed at an early stage. When the airway is secured haemorrhage can be controlled and steps taken to provide and maintain an adequate circulation. The extent of the patient's injuries can then be assessed and any necessary definitive treatment commenced.

Assessment.—This consists of an initial assessment to provide baseline measurements and subsequent observations to detect change in the patient's condition. A careful assessment of the level of consciousness is performed and neurological localising signs sought. Because a high proportion of head injuries have other injuries the whole patient must be carefully examined.

In the assessment of head injuries early signs which portend a rising intracranial pressure are a deteriorating level of consciousness, hypertension and bradycardia, and alterations in the respiratory pattern.

Treatment of cerebral oedema.—Cerebral oedema commonly occurs in severe head injury cases due initially to brain damage, but often greatly worsened by hypercapnia and hypoxia. The raised intracranial pressure that ensues from cerebral oedema must be controlled to prevent a vicious circle of increasing brain damage and further oedema. Prevention of hypoxia and hypercapnia and avoidance of the straining and venous engorgement which result from any degree of respiratory obstruction are important factors in the prevention of cerebral oedema. Dexamethasone in an initial intravenous dose of 10 mg followed by 4 mg six-hourly can dramatically reduce a raised intracranial pressure. Mannitol (1·5 g/kg) may also produce dramatic reduction in brain bulk, though if the blood-brain barrier is impaired its effects will be diminished. Because the rapid shrinking of the brain produced by mannitol may worsen intracranial bleeding this drug should not be given indiscriminately. The role of controlled hyperventilation in the reduction of intracranial pressure is discussed below.

Other methods of treating a raised intracranial pressure include hypothermia and drainage of cerebrospinal fluid. Whilst in theory induced hypothermia should be a valuable method of treatment the practical difficulties it entails are considerable. Of greater importance is the avoidance of hyperthermia by controlling rigidity, spasms or shivering. If intracranial pressure is being monitored through a ventricular catheter it can be reduced by removal of cerebrospinal fluid.

Respiratory management.—An endotracheal tube should be passed in any head injury case in whom an adequate airway cannot be guaranteed by use of simple methods to combat obstruction. Where prolonged coma is anticipated or in the presence of severe associated trauma early tracheostomy should be considered. Prolonged endotracheal intubation can cause severe damage of the larynx and trachea. More importantly secretions and foreign matter can be removed more efficiently through a tracheostomy than through an endotracheal tube.

Artificial ventilation may be indicated at an early stage in the treatment of head injuries. It may be needed to remedy apnoea or severe hypoventilation. Conversely pontine damage may cause marked hyperventilation which is best controlled. Decerebrate rigidity and spasms lead to hypoxia and hyperpyrexia which should be treated with muscle relaxants and controlled ventilation. The virtues of controlled ventilation are that it prevents carbon dioxide retention, reduces the increased oxygen consumption produced by hyperventilation, fits and decerebrate spasms, and usually assures an adequate degree of cerebral oxygenation. Moderate hyperventilation to a P_{CO_2} of about 25 mm Hg (3·3 kPa) will usually reduce intracranial pressure. Gordon (1971) has reported a significant reduction in mortality when controlled hyperventilation was used as a routine measure in severe head injury cases. He has ascribed this in part to a reduction in cerebral tissue acidosis and a restoration of a more appropriate cerebral perfusion consequent upon a low P_{CO_2}.

The long-term care of an unconscious patient necessitates continuous, devoted nursing and special attention to diet, sedation and the prevention of infection. Feeding should whenever possible be by naso-oesophageal tube, the only exception being when intestinal disturbances make an adequate fluid and food intake by this route impracticable. Particular care must be taken to ensure a proper fluid and electrolyte balance and to limit muscle-wasting by providing the correct amount of protein.

ANAESTHESIA FOR OPHTHALMIC SURGERY

Just as during neurosurgical anaesthesia raised intracranial pressure may damage the brain, a raised intra-ocular pressure during ophthalmic surgery may damage the contents of the orbit. In the past local anaesthetic techniques have been widely used to avoid or minimise this problem. There has been in the last few decades an increasing use of general anaesthesia as problems of the control of intra-ocular pressure have been defined and methods to overcome these problems evolved.

Local analgesia has much to recommend it for this branch of surgery, for the operations performed are usually limited in extent and complete loss of pain can be accomplished fairly easily. But local analgesia has disadvantages and hazards. It is unsatisfactory for unco-operative patients, for children and for those people with diseases of the eye which might be accentuated by local analgesia. Rosen (1962) lists three principal hazards. An incomplete block may lead to compression of the globe. If this occurs when the eye is open there will be expulsion of the intra-ocular contents. A retrobulbar haemorrhage produced during local block will cause a tense orbit and compression of the globe, prolapse of the iris, expulsion of the lens and loss of vitreous may all follow. Direct penetration of the optic nerve meninges may involve the optic nerve in trauma.

The main disadvantages of general anaesthesia are the potential complications of coughing and straining and these, though easily prevented by a skilled anaesthetist during anaesthesia, may occur in the post-operative period: there is also perhaps an increased incidence of nausea and vomiting. However these disadvantages can usually be avoided whilst on the positive side a properly selected and well-managed general anaesthetic has much to offer to both patient and surgeon. Apart from the patient's personal views, many surgeons prefer general anaesthesia provided the local conditions in the eye can match those of local analgesia, as an unconscious patient makes the whole procedure much easier.

Intra-ocular Tension

Intra-ocular tension depends on the balance between the production of aqueous humour by the ciliary body and its removal by drainage through the canal of Schlemm. Pressure in the anterior chamber of the eye is usually 10–22 mm Hg (1·3–2·6 kPa). The important disease process in which intra-ocular tension is raised is glaucoma, where drainage of aqueous humour is obstructed. Intra-ocular tension may be acutely changed by many drugs and by various physiological events. An acute rise in intra-ocular tension may be catastrophic if it occurs when the globe is open and leads to expulsion of contents.

Factors raising intra-ocular tension.—The only drugs commonly used in anaesthetic practice which may raise intra-ocular tension are atropine and suxamethonium. Because of its powerful mydriatic action atropine may cause the iris root to occlude the drainage meshwork in the angle of the anterior chamber. Considerable rises in pressure may occur when atropine is instilled topically into eyes predisposed to closed-angle glaucoma. Parenteral doses of atropine do not appear to cause serious rises of pressure even in the susceptible eye. Ketamine also produces a slight increase in intra-ocular pressure.

Suxamethonium causes a rise in intra-ocular tension due to contracture (a sustained contraction) of the extra-ocular muscles and compression of the globe (Dillon *et al.*, 1957). Contraction of orbital smooth muscle (Katz *et al.*, 1968) and a vascular element in the raised intra-ocular pressure produced by suxamethonium have also been suggested (Adams and Barnett, 1966). This effect of suxamethonium is transient, and pressure returns to normal within five minutes.

Venous engorgement due to coughing, retching or straining on an endo-tracheal tube raises intra-ocular tension by increasing the volume of blood present in the eye. In the same way acute rises in arterial pressure cause transient increases in intra-ocular tension. Hypercapnia and hypoxia also increase intra-ocular tension by affecting intra-ocular blood volume.

Increased pressure on the globe can be produced by screwing up of the eye. This can occur under light general anaesthesia and also during the immediate post-operative period. Squeezing can be eliminated if the facial nerve is blocked.

Factors decreasing intra-ocular tension.—Reduction in intra-ocular blood volume will tend to reduce intra-ocular tension. Arterial blood pressure has to be reduced to below 90 mm Hg (12 kPa) before any appreciable fall in intra-ocular tension occurs (Adams and Barnett, 1966). Hypocapnia and hyperoxia also tend to reduce pressure in the eye.

Intra-ocular tension is reduced by most general anaesthetics, narcotic analgesics and intravenous barbiturates. These effects are in most cases of no clinical importance.

Local Anaesthesia

Topical.—The instillation of 2 per cent cocaine provides satisfactory surface analgesia lasting about half an hour. Cocaine dilates the pupil and is thus contra-indicated in glaucoma. It also produces vasoconstriction and slightly damages the corneal epithelium and the haziness it produces may impede the surgeon's view of intra-capsular structures. Amethocaine 0·5 per cent or lignocaine 4 per cent are equally effective, last longer and neither damage the cornea nor dilate the pupil. These agents cause vasodilatation and mild con-junctival hyperaemia.

Infiltration and nerve block.—Simple infiltration with 0·5–2 per cent ligno-caine combined with 1 in 250,000 adrenaline provides satisfactory conditions for operations on the eyelids. A retro-ocular injection of 1–2 ml of this local anaesthetic solution within the cone formed by the ocular muscles will block the ciliary nerve and ganglion through which the sensory supply from the eye is carried. Retro-ocular block is usually combined with a block of the terminal branches of the facial nerve superficial to the neck of the mandible to prevent intra-ocular pressure increasing by the action of orbicularis oculi. These techniques are well reviewed by Burn and Knight (1969). A potential danger of retro-ocular block is haemorrhage leading to proptosis. On the other hand, successful block is associated with a decrease in intra-ocular pressure.

Patients who are to undergo major ophthalmic surgery under local analgesia should receive adequate sedation pre-operatively. A number of techniques of sedation are available. Phenothiazines such as chlorpromazine and promethazine may be given together with pethidine in divided doses. Postural hypotension is common when this drug combination is used, and difficulty may be experienced in maintaining an airway. Neuroleptanalgesia produced by a combination of droperidol and fentanyl is probably safer than phenothiazine sedation, but cardiovascular and respiratory depression can still be troublesome. Diazepam and other minor tranquillisers are becoming more widely used as judiciously administered doses produce good sedation with minimal side-effects.

General Anaesthesia

The principles and techniques of anaesthesia described for neurosurgical operations are equally important in ophthalmic practice.

Premedication.—The allaying of anxiety and drying of secretions are of obvious importance but special attention should be directed to the prevention of nausea and vomiting so that the inclusion of anti-emetic drugs such as promethazine or prochlorperazine may help considerably. The use of opiates and related compounds unfortunately increases the risk of post-operative nausea and as a post-operative tranquil state is desirable and sometimes imperative, their omission may be advisable and their use best reserved for patients in pain. Barbiturates provide an alternative. The addition of atropine dries secretions and there is no worthwhile evidence to substantiate the theoretical view that parenteral injections of atropine increase the risk of acute glaucoma in a predisposed patient. The quantity of atropine reaching the eye after such an injection is so small it can be ignored (Rosen, 1962). Alternatively, hyoscine is not only an effective antisialogogue but is also anti-emetic.

Oculo-cardiac reflex.—Traction on the extrinsic muscles of the eye may produce an oculo-cardiac reflex which is associated with bradycardia, dysrhythmia or even cardiac arrest. The afferent stimulus travels in the ciliary branches of the ophthalmic division of the trigeminal nerve—possibly in parasympathetic nerve fibres—and the efferent arises in the cardio-inhibitory centre of the brain stem reaching the heart through the vagus nerve. Retro-orbital injection of local analgesic solution may prevent the reflex but is not invariably successful. Premedication with atropine will diminish the incidence of bradycardia but does not prevent it entirely unless the dose of atropine is sufficient to block the vagus completely—given subcutaneously this might be in the region of 2 mg for an adult. An intravenous injection of atropine (1 mg for an adult) shortly before the operation begins is satisfactory. With repeated handling of the extrinsic muscles of the eye, bradycardia is less likely to occur, presumably because of fatigue of the oculo-cardiac reflex at the level of the cardio-inhibitory centre (Mooney et al., 1964).

Anaesthesia.—No special problems, other than those already described under oculo-cardiac reflex, are related to extra-ocular operations, but the anaesthesia must be sufficient to keep the eye stationary. For intra-ocular operations the degree of tension within the eye is a factor of considerable importance. Normally it is the concern of the anaesthetist to ensure that this is at least within normal limits and certainly not increased. Increases in tension are directly related to rises in venous pressure and to increasing tone in the ocular muscles. Technically good anaesthesia will circumvent these problems and if it is associated with loss of muscle tone and adequate ventilation, tend to lessen intra-ocular pressure. Suxamethonium leads to a rise in intra-ocular tension as mentioned above. The rise in intra-ocular tension is short-lived and does not contra-indicate the use of suxamethonium for intubation, but it suggests that this relaxant should not be used during an intra-ocular operation when the eye is open. The administration of 3 mg of *d*-tubocurarine or 20 mg of gallamine intravenously three minutes prior to the use of suxamethonium has been shown to prevent an increase in intra-ocular tension both in normal and glaucomatous patients (Miller *et al.*, 1968). The use of hypotensive agents is rarely necessary in practice but a head-up tilt will help reduce intra-ocular tension.

A prolonged response to suxamethonium has been reported following the use of ecothiopate iodide eye drops (Pantuck, 1966) and is due to inhibition of cholinesterase activity.

The precise technique of general anaesthesia is a matter of choice. Intubation which should be preceded by topical spraying of the larynx with 4 per cent lignocaine, may be followed by spontaneous breathing or controlled ventilation with relaxants. Both give excellent airway control but carry disadvantages of possible coughing or spasm on extubation. On the other hand, although an unintubated patient obviates the need for relaxants, meticulous attention must be paid to ensuring a good airway by keeping a hand under the angle of the jaw throughout the procedure—a task which may not only be tiring but difficult. General anaesthesia may be combined with local analgesia both of the eye and facial nerve; this latter technique permits the lightest possible general anaesthetic but it still suffers from the same disadvantage of a need to support the jaw throughout the operation.

When general anaesthesia alone is used the depth of anaesthesia must be sufficient to prevent coughing and straining. Explosive coughing must be avoided on extubation, especially following cataract surgery. For this reason anaesthesia is usually deepened prior to extubation.

ELECTRO-CONVULSION THERAPY

The precise mechanism by which the passage of an electric current through the brain should be able to bring about a therapeutic effect in cases of endogenous depression is still unknown. A simple explanation is that the current stimulates the mood centre in the hypothalamus, but in attempting to reach this innermost area of the brain it must also excite other centres such as the motor cortex. Before the introduction of anaesthesia and muscle paralysis into electro-convulsive therapy, the severity of the convulsions would put the patient at risk not only from compression fractures of the spine but from myocardial failure. An unmodified fit in a conscious subject comprises an immediate loss of consciousness with the passage of the electric current. This is followed by a tonic convulsion of about five seconds duration leading into a clonic convulsion with regular muscle movements lasting from about 10–50 seconds. Immediately after the passage of the current, signs of autonomic stimulation—"goose-pimples", dilatation of the pupil and flushing of the facial skin can be observed. Contraction of the jaw muscles is probably due to direct stimulation of the muscle fibres by the electric current as this takes place even in the completely paralysed patient. For this reason it is mandatory to protect the patient's teeth with some suitable mouth prop.

Cerletti and Bini (1938) first described this method of treatment and since that time the clinical successes in many thousands of patients throughout the world bear witness to its value. The introduction of general anaesthesia and muscle paralysis has transformed the technique into one which can be conducted either as an out-patient or an in-patient with minimal risk. Mental depression increases in frequency with advancing age, so that a considerable number of patients will be encountered with hypertension and cardiac disease. Great care must therefore be used in selecting the sleep-dose of either thiopentone or methohexitone for each patient, but these doses need only be minimal as the passage of the electric current also produces unconsciousness.

In the majority of cases the electric current is applied to both temporal areas. In 1957, unilateral ECT to the non-dominant hemisphere was first proposed. It reduces the incidence and severity of memory disturbances associated with the bilateral technique (Zinkin and Birtchnell, 1968), but there is not general agreement that the therapeutic results are identical.

Technique of General Anaesthesia

Sedative premedication is usually unnecessary but there is no objection to its use when specially indicated. A short-acting oral barbiturate is the most satisfactory method for such cases. Dobkin (1958) considers that ECT may occasionally produce a period of cardiac asystole which is normally brief, but could lead to cardiac arrest, and which can only be prevented by a large dose of atropine prior to treatment. To avoid the risk of vagal asystole, 1·0 mg of atropine sulphate should be given intravenously (either separately or mixed with the induction agent). Subcutaneous atropine in small doses given half-an-hour before treatment merely gives the patient an unpleasant dry-mouth feeling without influencing vagal activity.

Anaesthesia may be induced with any suitable intravenous induction agent. Thiopentone and methohexitone are the most widely used agents, but both propanidid and Althesin have been employed. Induction of anaesthesia is followed immediately by suxamethonium, 0·5–0·75 mg/kg. The doses of induction agent and suxamethonium and the patient's response to them are recorded so that any necessary adjustments may be made on subsequent occasions. Successful anaesthesia should allow slight twitching of the face and limbs, but little more. If no movements occur—because the dose of suxamethonium has been excessive—two signs may be useful as suggestive evidence of the successful passage of a current. The first is the presence of goose-flesh (Edridge, 1952) and the second, dilatation of the pupils and their failure to react when inspected immediately after the stimulus (Thomas and Honan, 1953).

As soon as the patient is paralysed the lungs must be adequately inflated with oxygen. A mouth prop is then inserted to protect the teeth and the electrodes applied. Great care must be used in selecting and fitting the mouth prop to protect the patient's own teeth. In rare instances it may be beneficial for the patient to retain a denture in position to give maximum support to his few remaining teeth.

Immediately after passage of the current the patient should again be gently ventilated with oxygen until adequate spontaneous respiration returns. The patient can then be turned on to his side and allowed to rest until fully conscious and orientated, when he can safely be allowed to return home provided he is accompanied.

The return to consciousness is usually quiet if the patients have been properly selected for treatment, but unsuspected neurotics or hysterics may be difficult to control for a short period. The commonest complications are headache and retrograde amnesia.

REFERENCES

ADAMS, A. K., and BARNETT, K. C. (1966). Anaesthesia and intraocular pressure. *Anaesthesia*, **21**, 202.

ALDRIDGE, W. N. (1965). The pathology and chemistry of experimental oedema in the brain. *Proc. roy. Soc. Med.*, **58**, 599.

ANDERSON, S., and MCKISSOCK, W. (1953). Controlled hypotension with Arfonad in neurosurgery. *Lancet*, **2**, 754.

ASERMAN, D. (1953). Controlled hypotension in neurosurgery with hexamethonium bromide and procaine amide. *Brit. med. J.*, **1**, 961.

BALLANTYNE, R. I. W., and JACKSON, I. (1954). Anaesthesia for neurosurgical operations. *Anaesthesia*, **9**, 4.

BATSON, O. V. (1940). The function of the vertebral veins and their role in the spread of metastases. *Ann Surg.*, **112**, 138.

BAUM, J. D., and SCOPES, J. W. (1968). The silver swaddler. *Lancet*, **1**, 672.

BERING, E. A. (1952). Water exchange of central nervous system and cerebrospinal fluid. *J. Neurosurg.*, **9**, 275.

BOZZA MARRUBINI, M. L. (1965). General anaesthesia for intracranial surgery. *Brit. J. Anaesth.*, **37**, 268.

BOZZA MARRUBINI, M. L., MASPES, P. E., and ROSSANDA, M. (1961). The control of brain volume and tension during intracranial operations. *Brit. J. Anaesth.*, **33**, 132.

BOZZA MARRUBINI, M. L., and TRETOLA, L. (1965). Diazepam as a preoperative tranquillizer in neuro-anaesthesia. *Brit. J. Anaesth.*, **37**, 934.

BROWN, A. S. (1955). Circulatory disturbances during cerebral angiography. *Anaesthesia*, **10**, 346.

BROWN, A. S. (1959). Controlled respiration in neurosurgical anaesthesia. *Anaesthesia*, **14**, 207.

BROWN, A. S. (1964). Neuroleptanalgesia for the surgical treatment of Parkinsonism. *Anaesthesia*, **19**, 70.

BURN, R. A., and KNIGHT, P. (1969). Anaesthesia in ophthalmic surgery. *Brit. J. hosp. Med.*, **2**, 1527.

BURROWS, M. MC., DUNDEE, J. W., FRANCIS, I. Ll., LIPTON, S., and SEDZIMIR, C. B. (1956). Hypothermia for neurological operations. *Anaesthesia*, **11**, 4.

BUSHMAN, J. A., and COLLIS, J. M. (1967). The estimation of gas losses in ventilator tubing. *Anaesthesia*, **22**, 664.

CANTORE, G., GUIDETTI, B., and VIRNO, M. (1964). Oral glycerol for the reduction of intracranial pressure. *J. Neurosurg.*, **21,** 278.

CERLETTI, V., and BINI, L. (1938). L'ettroshock. *Arch. gen. Neurol. Psichiat.*, **19,** 266.

CHEATLE, C. A., and MACKENZIE, R. M. (1953). Anaesthesia for cranial surgery in the sitting position. *Anaesthesia*, **8,** 182.

CILIBERTI, B. J., GOLDFEIN, J., and ROVENSTINE, E. A. (1954). Hypertension during anesthesia in patients with spinal cord injuries. *Anesthesiology*, **15,** 273.

CLARK, K., and EINSPRUCH, B. C. (1962). Osmotic rebound phenomena associated with agents used to lower intracranial pressure with emphasis on urea. *Arch. Neurol. (Chic.)*, **6,** 414.

COLEMAN, D. J., and DE VILLIERS, J. C. (1964). Anaesthesia and stereotactic surgery. *Anaesthesia*, **19,** 60.

COLLAN, R., and IVANAINEN, M. (1969). Cardiac arrest caused by rapid elimination of nitrous oxide from cerebral ventricles after encephalography. *Canad. Anaesth. Soc. J.*, **16,** 519.

DALLAS, S. H., and MOXON, C. P. (1969). Controlled ventilation for cerebral angiography. *Brit. J. Anaesth.*, **41,** 597.

DILLON, J. B., SABAWALA, P., TAYLOR, D. B., and GUNTER, R. (1957). Depolarising neuromuscular blocking agents and intraocular pressure "in vivo". *Anesthesiology*, **18,** 439.

DOBKIN, A. B. (1958). Cardiac arrest following electroplexy. *Lancet*, **1,** 640.

DUCKWORTH, S. I. (1962). The Oxford non-kinking endotracheal tube. *Anaesthesia*, **17,** 208.

DUNCALF, D., and THOMPSON, P. W. (1956). Anaesthesia for cardiovascular and neurosurgical radiological investigations. *Brit. J. Anaesth.*, **2,** 450.

DUNSMORE, R., SCOVILLE, W. B., and WHITCOMB, B. B. (1951). Complications of angiography. *J. Neurosurg.*, **8,** 110.

EDMONDS-SEAL, J., and MAROON, J. C. (1969). Air embolism diagnosed with ultrasound. *Anaesthesia*, **24,** 438.

EDRIDGE, A. (1952). Discussion on new muscle relaxants in electric convulsion therapy. *Proc. roy. Soc. Med.*, **45,** 869.

FITCH, W., BARKER, J., MCDOWALL, D. G., and JENNETT, W. B. (1969). The effect of methoxyflurane on cerebrospinal fluid pressure in patients with and without intracranial space-occupying lesions. *Brit. J. Anaesth.*, **41,** 564.

FOSSA, S., BATTISTIN, N., MARINO, C., and PALLECCHI, A. E. (1968). The use of a combination of mannitol and frusemide in endocrine operations. *Acta anaesth. (Padova)*, **19,** 1159.

FURNESS, D. N. (1957). Controlled respiration in neurosurgery. *Brit. J. Anaesth.*, **29,** 415.

GALLOON, S. (1959). Controlled respiration in neurosurgical anaesthesia. *Anaesthesia*, **14,** 223.

GEDDES, I. C. (1952). Anaesthesia for cerebral angiography. *Brit. J. Anaesth.*, **24,** 252.

GORDON, E. (1971). Controlled respiration in the management of patients with traumatic brain injuries. *Acta anaesth. scand.*, **15,** 193.

HAMBY, W. B. (1963). Intracranial surgery for aneurysm. *J. Neurosurg.*, **20,** 41.

HAYES, G. J., and SLOCUM, H. C. (1962). The achievement of optimal brain relaxation by hyperventilation technics of anesthesia. *J. Neurosurg.*, **19,** 65.

HELLINGS, P. M. (1958). Controlled hypothermia: recent developments in the use of hypothermia in neurosurgery. *Brit. med. J..*, **2,** 346.

HEWER, A. J. H., and LOGUE, V. (1962). Methods of increasing the safety of neuroanaesthesia in the sitting position. *Anaesthesia*, **17,** 476.

HORTON, J. M. (1975). The immediate care of head injuries. *Anaesthesia*, **30,** 212.

HOWLAND, W. S., and PAPPER, E. M. (1952). Circulatory changes during anesthesia for neurosurgical operations. *Anesthesiology*, **13,** 343.

HUNTER, A. R. (1952). The present position of anaesthesia for neurosurgery. *Proc. roy. Soc. Med.*, **45,** 427.

HUNTER, A. R. (1960). Discussion on the value of controlled respiration in neurosurgery. *Proc. roy. Soc. Med.*, **53**, 365.

HUNTER, A. R. (1975). *Neurosurgical Anaesthesia*. Oxford: Blackwell Scientific Publications.

JAVID, M., and SETTLAGE, P. (1956). Effect of urea on cerebrospinal fluid pressure in human subjects. Preliminary report. *J. Amer. med. Ass.*, **160**, 943.

JENNETT, W. B., BARKER, J., FITCH, W., and McDOWALL, D. G. (1969). Effect of anaesthesia on intracranial pressure in patients with space-occupying lesions. *Lancet*, **1**, 61.

KATZ, R. L., EAKINS, K. E., and LORD, C. O. (1968). The effects of hexafluorenium in preventing the increase in intraocular pressure produced by succinylcholine. *Anesthesiology*, **29**, 70.

KETY, S. S., and SCHMIDT, C. F. (1948). Effects of altered arterial tensions of carbon dioxide and oxygen on cerebral blood flow and cerebral oxygen consumption of normal young men. *J. clin. Invest.*, **27**, 484.

KRUMPERMAN, L. W., MURTAGH, F., and WESTER, M. R. (1957). Epidural block anesthesia for cordotomy. *Anesthesiology*, **18**, 316.

LIPTON, S. (1968). Percutaneous electrical cordotomy in relief of intractable pain. *Brit. med. J.*, **2**, 210.

LOGUE, V. (1956). Surgery in spontaneous subarachnoid haemorrhage due to intracranial aneurysms. *Brit. med. J.*, **1**, 473.

McCOMISH, P. B., and THOMPSON, D. E. A. (1968). Respiratory disturbances in air embolism. *Anaesthesia*, **23**, 259.

McDOWALL, D. G. (1971). The current usage of hypothermia in British neurosurgery. *Brit. J. Anaesth.*, **43**, 1084.

McDOWALL, D. G. (1976). Neurosurgical anaesthesia and intensive care. In: *Recent Advances in Anaesthesia and Analgesia*, 12th edit., Chapter 2, p. 38. Ed. by Langton Hewer, C., and Atkinson, R. S. Edinburgh: Churchill Livingstone.

McDOWALL, D. G., BARKER, J., and JENNETT, W. B. (1966). Cerebrospinal fluid pressure measurements during anaesthesia. *Anaesthesia*, **21**, 189.

McDOWALL, D. G., KEANEY, N. P., TURNER, J. M., LANE, J. R., and OKUDA, Y. (1974). Circulatory effects of sodium nitroprusside. *Brit. J. Anaesth.*, **46**, 323.

MACINTOSH, R. R., MUSHIN, W. W., and EPSTEIN, H. G. (1958). *Physics for the Anaesthetist*, 2nd edit. Oxford: Blackwell Scientific Publications.

McKISSOCK, W. (1956). Subarachnoid haemorrhage. *Ann. roy. Coll. Surg. Engl.*, **19**, 361.

McKISSOCK, W., RICHARDSON, A., and WALSH, L. (1965). Anterior communicating aneurysms. *Lancet*, **1**, 873.

McKISSOCK, W., and WALSH, L. (1956). Subarachnoid haemorrhage due to intracranial aneurysms. *Brit. med. J.*, **2**, 559.

MICHENFELDER, J. D., TERRY, H. R., DAW, E. F., MacCARTY, C. S., and UIHLEIN, A. (1963). Profound hypothermia in neurosurgery: open-chest versus closed-chest techniques. *Anesthesiology*, **24**, 177.

MICHENFELDER, J. D., TERRY, H. R., DAW, E. F., and MILLER, R. H. (1966). Air embolism during neurosurgery. *Anesth. Analg. Curr. Res.*, **45**, 390.

MILLAR, R. A. (1972). Neurosurgical anaesthesia in the sitting position. *Brit. J. Anaesth.*, **44**, 495.

MILLER, J. D., and BARKER, J. (1969). The effect of neuroleptanalgesic drugs on cerebral blood flow and metabolism. *Brit. J. Anaesth.*, **41**, 554.

MILLER, R. D., WAY, W. L., and HICKEY, R. F. (1968). Inhibition of succinylcholine-induced increased intraocular pressure by non-depolarizing muscle relaxants. *Anesthesiology*, **29**, 70.

MONIZ, E. (1940). *Die Cerebrale Arteriographie und Phlebographie*. Berlin.

MOONEY, G. T., REES, D. L., and ELTON, D. (1964). The oculo-cardiac reflex during strabismus surgery. *Canad. Anaesth. Soc. J.*, **11**, 621.

MORTIMER, P. L. F. (1959). Controlled respiration in neurosurgical anaesthesia. *Anaesthesia*, **14**, 205.

MULLAN, S., HARPER, P. V., HEKMATPANAH, J., TORRES, H., and DOBBIN, G. (1963). Percutaneous interruption of spinal pain tracts by means of Strontium 90 needle. *J. Neurosurg.*, **20**, 931.

PANTUCK, E. J. (1966). Ecothiopate iodide eye drops and prolonged response to suxamethonium. *Brit. J. Anaesth.*, **38**, 406.

PATTERSON, A. S., and KING, D. W. (1957). Electric convulsion fractures. *Brit. med. J.*, **1**, 1118.

PEARCE, D. J. (1957). The role of posture in laminectomy. *Proc. roy. Soc. Med.*, **50**, 109.

PITKIN, G. P. (1953). *Conduction Anesthesia*, 2nd edit. Philadelphia: J. B. Lippincott Co.

ROSEN, D. A. (1962). Anaesthesia in ophthalmology. *Canad. Anaesth. Soc. J.*, **9**, 545.

ROSOMOFF, H. L. (1962). Distribution of intracranial contents after hypertonic urea. *J. Neurosurg.*, **19**, 859.

ROSOMOFF, H. L. (1963). Distribution of intracranial contents with controlled hyperventilation: implications for neuroanesthesia. *Anesthesiology*, **24**, 640.

ROSOMOFF, H. L., and GILBERT, R. (1955). Brain volume and cerebrospinal fluid pressure during hypothermia. *Amer. J. Physiol.*, **183**, 19.

ROSOMOFF, H. L., and HOLADAY, D. A. (1954). Cerebral blood flow and cerebral oxygen consumption during hypothermia. *Amer. J. Physiol.*, **179**, 85.

ROTH, D. A., YANEZ, R., ANDREW, N. W., and MARK, V. H. (1969). The combined effects of hyperventilation and hypotension on the blood-brain barrier. *Anesth. Analg. Curr. Res.*, **48**, 755.

SAIDMAN, L. J., and EGER, E. I. (1965). Changes in cerebrospinal fluid pressure during pneumoencephalography under nitrous oxide anesthesia. *Anesthesiology*, **26**, 67.

SAMUEL, J. R., GRANGE, R., and HAWKINS, T. D. (1968). Anaesthetic technique for carotid angiography. *Anaesthesia*, **23**, 543.

SHENKIN, H. A., GOLUBOFF, B., and SOMACH, F. M. (1965). Control of intracranial pressure at operation. *Anesth. Analg. Curr. Res.*, **44**, 440.

SIEGEL, P., MORACA, P. P., and GREEN, J. R. (1971). Sodium nitroprusside in the surgical treatment of cerebral aneurysms and arteriovenous malformations. *Brit. J. Anaesth.*, **43**, 790.

SOSTERHOLM, J. L. (1970). Reaction of the cerebral venous sinus system to acute intracranial hypertension. *J. Neurosurg.*, **32**, 652.

TAYLOR, A. R., GLEADHILL, C. A., BILSLAND, W. L., and MURRAY, P. F. (1956). Posture and anaesthesia for spinal operations with special reference to intervertebral disc surgery. *Brit. J. Anaesth.*, **28**, 213.

THOMAS, E., and HONAN, B. F. (1953). Electro-convulsive therapy. *Brit. med. J.*, **2**, 97.

UIHLEIN, A., THEYE, R. A., DAWSON, B., TERRY, H. R., McGOON, D. C., DAW, E. F., and KIRKLIN, J. W. (1960). The use of profound hypothermia, extracorporeal circulation and total circulatory arrest for an intracranial aneurysm. *Proc. Mayo Clin.*, **35**, 567.

VESEY, C. J., and COLE, P. V. (1975). Nitroprusside and cyanide. *Brit. J. Anaesth.*, **47**, 1115.

VESEY, C. J., COLE, P. V., LINNELL, J. C., and WILSON, J. (1974). Some metabolic effects of sodium nitroprusside in man. *Brit. med. J.*, **2**, 140.

VOURC'H, G. M. (1963). Continuous cerebral spinal fluid drainage by indwelling spinal catheter. *Brit. J. Anaesth.*, **35**, 118.

WYLIE, W. D. (1951). Some aspects of anaesthesia for neurosurgery, with special reference to pethidine hydrochloride. *G. ital. Anest.*, **17**, 305.

ZINKIN, S., and BIRTCHNELL, J. (1968). Unilateral electro-convulsive therapy: its effect on memory and its therapeutic efficacy. *Brit. J. Psychiat.*, **14**, 973.

Chapter 31

NEUROLOGICAL AND OPHTHALMIC COMPLICATIONS OF ANAESTHESIA

Hypoxia and the Central Nervous System

Whatever the cause of hypoxia, the end results in the central nervous system appear to be the same, differing only in extent, which is in direct relation to the degree and duration of the period of sub-oxygenation. An acute anoxic episode caused by a period of cardiac arrest is dramatic enough to draw attention to any sequelae should the patient survive. Equally important are the equivalent degrees of acute hypoxia that can occur without cardiac arrest in some anaesthetic mishaps and certain disease states. Less obvious but just as potentially detrimental to the patient are the effects of prolonged but subacute hypoxia. Ancillary factors are the state of the brain prior to sub-oxygenation and repeated bouts of hypoxia. The normal brain will tolerate a moderate degree of oxygen lack for quite long periods without apparently being harmed, but the presence of disease, or even the ordinary changes associated with ageing, markedly increase its vulnerability. On the other hand, young babies have more resistance than adults. Repetitive bouts of moderate hypoxia may be cumulative (Lucas and Strangeways, 1952), while once hypoxia of any degree has produced changes in the brain, a vicious-circle effect leads to further sub-oxygenation. Ischaemic hypoxia is more dangerous than that associated with a normal flow of blood.

Clinical Picture

The clinical results are immensely variable, depending, as would be expected, on the severity and duration of the episode. Bedford (1955) describes the occurrence of adverse cerebral effects in old people following operations under general anaesthesia. These may vary from extreme dementia, through personality changes, to lesser degrees of incapacity which are only noticeable to the patient and his relatives, and range from inability to concentrate to simple impairment of memory. Here the sub-oxygenation, whatever its primary cause, is likely to have been slight though protracted. Acute and total anoxia may be followed by coma and death, although a period of decerebrate rigidity often intervenes. Cope (1960) emphasises that following an anoxic or hypoxic episode a patient may recover consciousness completely, only to lapse into coma soon afterwards. But far short of this, a whole series of clinical pictures, sometimes singly and sometimes together, may be portrayed. Convulsions, various paralyses—spastic and flaccid—Parkinsonism, total or partial blindness, dysphonia and multiple defects of intellectual function have been recorded (Allison, 1956). Finally, any period of hypoxia occurring during anaesthesia, although not marked enough to cause objective neurological sequelae, may result in a delayed post-operative recovery of consciousness and a prolonged period of nausea associated with severe headache.

Physiopathology

The higher centres are more vulnerable than the lower. Nerve cells have a much higher metabolism than nerve fibres so that reflex excitability is abolished if the centres are deprived of oxygen for even short periods.

Lesions due to general brain anoxia are commonly widely distributed but may vary according to the cause—hypotension, hypoxaemia, circulatory arrest, etc. Measurements of regional cerebral blood flow in patients with focal occlusive (anoxic) lesions have demonstrated a vasomotor paralysis of the blood vessels supplying the anoxic area giving rise to a "luxury perfusion syndrome" in which the rate of flow is increased above the post-anoxically lowered metabolic demands (Ingvar, 1968). This hyperaemia may lead to oedema. The same sequence of events may occur in generalised cerebral anoxia. Post-anoxic hyperaemia occurs within minutes and its duration is probably dependent on the duration and severity of the tissue hypoxia. Should generalised cerebral anoxia occur, this may set up a vicious circle which leads to raised intracranial pressure which ultimately diminishes the perfusion pressure gradient giving rise to generalised ischaemia and in severe cases to global brain ischaemia and necrosis.

Lindenberg (1963) has emphasised that the effects of acute hypoxia on the brain are influenced by the rate at which a critical level of hypoxia develops. Acute hypoxia following cardiac arrest leads to a rapid accumulation of toxic metabolites which cause destructive changes in nerve cells and irreversible cell death, and may produce cerebral oedema. Critical hypoxia of a slower onset will be preceded by a period of hypoxaemia associated with a maintained circulation. There will be a lesser build up of toxic metabolic products, few histological changes in nerve cells and no tendency to cerebral oedema.

Preventive Treatment

Although it may be considered elementary to write of prevention in relation to a complication of anaesthesia such as hypoxia, which is generally regarded as obvious in its clinical manifestation, the work of Bedford (1955 and 1957) has drawn attention to the innumerable occasions during and following anaesthesia when a mild but insidious degree of sub-oxygenation of the patient may take place. Such occasions occur with moderate hypotension due to the effects of anaesthetic drugs or techniques. Arterial oxygenation is known to be impaired during anaesthesia (Marshall and Wyche, 1972) and failure to enrich the inspired atmosphere with oxygen can lead to mild cerebral hypoxia. Virtually all patients subjected to anaesthesia and surgery undergo a period of post-operative hypoxaemia (Nunn and Payne, 1962; Conway and Payne, 1963). Whilst in itself of little consequence, moderate post-operative hypoxaemia occurring in a patient with a low haemoglobin and a reduced cardiac output may lead to a dangerous lowering of the supply of oxygen to the brain. Consideration and avoidance of adverse factors and repeated appraisal of each patient with respect to the adequacy of oxygenation is the duty of the anaesthetist. This is particularly important in patients who are to be submitted to techniques such as induced hypotension.

Active Treatment

Active treatment may save a patient who remains unconscious after an acute hypoxic episode. A complete neurological examination should be made at the earliest convenient time.

Ventilation.—Whether a patient should be allowed to breathe spontaneously or should have intermittent positive-pressure respiration instituted must depend on the degree of unconsciousness and on the adequacy of spontaneous ventilation assessed clinically and by acid-base measurements. An enriched oxygen mixture is essential. The presence of hypercarbia increases the risk of cerebral oedema, and intubation followed by moderate controlled passive hyperventilation will reduce intracranial pressure caused by hypercarbia. It remains to be proved that this technique is of value in the presence of a normal Pa_{CO_2} (Rosomoff, 1963). Secretions are more easily removed in an intubated patient. Tracheostomy may be necessary at a later stage.

Dehydrating agents.—These should be administered as soon as possible on the basis that if cerebral oedema or brain swelling occur, a reduction in brain volume, even if only temporary, is likely to be of benefit. Mannitol can be given in a dose of 1 g/kg body weight administered over 20–30 minutes. Whilst osmotic diuretics are contra-indicated in the presence of severe renal disease, it is perhaps wise in the presence of such a complication to err on the side of treatment by giving a small intravenous dose of mannitol such as 12·5 g, to assess the effect on the patient, rather than do nothing and risk the onset of a vicious circle of anoxia. For long-term administration, glycerol may be given by a gastric tube in a 50 per cent solution 1–2 g/kg body weight and may be repeated 6–8-hourly even up to a week; its use is contra-indicated where there is a suspicion of a peptic ulcer.

Steroids.—Steroid therapy has been used increasingly in recent years both for the prevention and treatment of cerebral oedema. The steroid of choice is dexamethasone for this drug has minimal sodium-retaining activity (Taylor *et al.*, 1965; French, 1966). An initial dose of up to 10 mg intravenously or intramuscularly can be followed by subsequent doses of 4 mg 6-hourly for 2–3 days.

Hypothermia.—Advantages claimed for its use include a decrease in cerebral blood flow, a corresponding reduction in cerebral metabolism, induced hypotension, decrease in brain volume and a fall in intracranial pressure. Rosomoff (1968) advocates lowering the temperature to 30–32° C for up to three weeks. Shivering is controlled by using an infusion of pethidine 100 mg, promethazine 100 mg and phenobarbitone 100 mg in 5 per cent dextrose in 0·2 per cent saline. Whilst induced hypothermia undoubtedly modifies the immediate reaction of the brain to injury, it has not yet been clearly shown that the ultimate degree of injury can be modified by lowering the body temperature (Strong and Keats, 1967). It is quite possible that the major benefit is derived from the prevention of hyperpyrexia rather than from the institution of hypothermia. Whatever method of cooling is used, it is essential that shivering be prevented.

Fluid balance.—This is best maintained by the use of intravenous Ringer lactate solution or 5 per cent dextrose in 0·2 per cent saline. The use of 5 per cent dextrose in water, although isotonic, is potentially dangerous if it is given faster than water is lost (normally 1000–1200 ml/sq metre/24 hours). This is because it is initially distributed throughout the total body water which includes the brain and cerebrospinal fluid. Subsequently the fall in blood glucose is more rapid than that in the brain and this leads to a movement of water from a relatively hypotonic plasma into a hypertonic brain and cerebrospinal fluid, thereby increasing cerebrospinal fluid pressure and possibly the cerebral oedema. These changes are exaggerated in the presence of water retention (Fishman, 1953).

Posture.—Keeping the head raised will lessen the cerebral venous pressure but hypotension may ensue.

Sedation.—There is evidence that barbiturates exert a protective action against the effects of hypoxia (Secher and Wilhjelm, 1968). Anticonvulsants may be needed if convulsions are present or anticipated.

General.—Other measures such as the passing of a nasogastric tube to avoid gastric distension or for feeding should follow those for the management of unconscious patients.

Prognosis

Although the immediate prognosis for life after a severe and protracted bout of cerebral hypoxia is undoubtedly poor, that for morbidity in patients who survive is very difficult to assess. It has long been known that the duration of cerebral anoxia or hypoxia is the most important factor determining the outcome but in clinical situations this is often unknown and the causes may be complex. Even when the period of cardiac arrest is known, it may have been preceded by an unknown period of circulatory insufficiency. Prognosis in the early post-anoxic period can be very difficult and in an unconscious patient anything other than a gross alteration in the level of the central nervous system function may not be detectable.

Pampiglione and Harden (1968) consider that the electro-encephalograph may be helpful at a very early stage in assessing the chances of survival, possible severity, occurrence of complicating factors and impending seizures, as well as "death of the brain". These workers made a prognostic evaluation of early EEG findings following resuscitation after cardiovascular arrest. They found that the best timing for EEG studies for early prognosis was between 2–12 hours after resuscitation and that these should be repeated at 2–3-hourly intervals. They emphasised that before any prognostic evaluation was attempted, the EEG should be recognised as only one physical sign to be interpreted in the context of the patient's history and other physical signs. They warned against misleading information where inadequate EEG studies were performed and suggested that at least four different areas of each hemisphere should be simultaneously studied with appropriate leads.

PERIPHERAL NERVE PALSIES

Peripheral nerve palsies occurring during general anaesthesia are usually due to the effects, singly or combined, of pressure upon, or stretching, a nerve at some vulnerable point along its course. Occasionally such complications may result from the injection of an irritant substance into or near the nerve, or more simply from the trauma of a needle point. Evidence has accumulated to show that special conditions, such as induced hypothermia or hypotension, may themselves cause a neuropathy—while they will certainly aggravate any of the more common causes.

Stephens and Appleby (1956) and Swan and his co-workers (1955) describe the onset of nerve palsies following the use of hypothermia for cardiac operations. They were able to measure temperatures of 4° C in the gastrocnemius muscle of a patient who had a rectal temperature of 28° C. Exposure to cold in an ice water bath for periods of longer than thirty minutes led to peripheral nerve palsies in a number of patients.

In the assessment of any post-operative nerve palsy, a knowledge of the pre-operative neurological condition is of considerable importance. Not only is a diseased nerve more susceptible to trauma but the debilitating effects of both surgery and anaesthesia, even without any localised factor in the nerve itself, may accentuate pre-existing neurological disease. Diabetes mellitus, periarteritis nodosa and alcoholism are known predisposing causes.

Compression and Stretching

Brachial plexus palsy.—A combination of factors is most commonly the cause of trouble. Clausen (1942) described a case of brachial plexus palsy due to the effects of pressure alone, when a patient was maintained in the Trendelenburg position with inadequately padded shoulder supports. Presumably the supports were also badly positioned, because direct pressure upon the roots of the plexus is impossible if they are placed opposite the acromion processes.

The principal factors are weight bearing through the shoulder girdle in the Trendelenburg position, stretching of the plexus by moving the arm away from the side of the body, and abnormal relaxation of the muscles in this area. Weight bearing through the shoulder girdle leads to compression of the plexus between the first rib and the clavicle. When the arm is abducted from the side it is usually extended with some external rotation so that the plexus is put on the stretch. This may easily be accentuated to more than 90° by the unintentional and unnoticed movements of the surgeon, his assistants, or bystanders during the course of the operation. A further aggravating factor consists in placing the abducted arm at a lower horizontal level than the rest of the body (Jackson and Keats, 1965). This may occur if the arm drops away from the side of the body. Moreover the ill effects of this manoeuvre, which pushes the head of the humerus up into the already tightened plexus, are increased by raising the body still higher with a gall-bladder rest. The importance of the position of the arm, and hence of stretching as the principal cause of brachial plexus palsy, is illustrated by Kiloh's (1950) description of four cases, all of which occurred during gallbladder operations. Kiloh also stresses the fact that individual variations of anatomy and idiosyncrasy, such as cervical ribs, the size of the cervico-axillary canal, the shape of the first rib and the slope of the shoulder may all play a part sometimes in rendering the brachial plexus more vulnerable. Brachial plexus palsy as a result of faulty posturing during surgery was described long before relaxant drugs were introduced into anaesthetic practice, but there is little doubt that the extreme degrees of muscle relaxation they induce renders this complication much more likely in certain circumstances than with general anaesthesia alone.

Compression

Facial nerve palsy.—The buccal branch of the facial nerve normally arises from the main stem in the substance of the parotid gland and emerges at the anterior edge of this gland to supply the lateral part of the orbicularis oris muscle. Occasionally this branch may arise more proximally and run superficial to the gland, in which case it is susceptible to pressure. Paresis of it may then be caused by compression when the jaw of an unconscious patient is held forward, or due to a firmly fitted head harness (Morris, 1959).

Radial nerve palsy.—The nerve is vulnerable as it winds round the mid-part of the inner surface of the humerus. In the lateral position—particularly with the arm placed away from the side of the body—it can easily be subjected to pressure.

Ulnar nerve palsy.—The ulnar nerve is unprotected as it passes superficially and inferior to the medial epicondyle of the humerus. Typically it may be compressed between the bone and the edge of the operating table should the arm not be placed close to the side of the body in the horizontal position. The surgeon, or his assistant, is likely to add further pressure during the operation as he stands up against the table.

Common peroneal nerve palsy.—This nerve, in a similar manner to the ulnar, may easily be compressed against the head of the fibula when the patient lies in the lateral position or from compression against the stirrups in the lithotomy position.

Saphenous nerve.—This nerve may be compressed against the stirrups on the medial side of the knee when the patient is in the lithotomy position (Schmidt and Lincoln, 1966).

Injection

Median nerve palsy.—The median nerve lies in close deep relationship to the basilic and median cubital veins at the medial side of the antecubital fossa. An extravenous injection of thiopentone in this area can easily reach the nerve. Pask and Robson (1954) have drawn attention to the difficulty of appreciating the injection of very small quantities of fluid from a 10 ml syringe, and have shown that 0·2 ml of 1 per cent lignocaine can affect the median nerve significantly. Should the patient move after the needle of a syringe containing thiopentone has been successfully placed in the basilic vein, the point might easily advance sufficiently for some of the irritant fluid to reach the nerve.

Lateral and median cutaneous nerves of the forearm.—Either of these nerves may inadvertently come into contact with thiopentone solution should an attempted intravenous injection lead to some extravasation outside the vein, or the nerve itself be pricked.

Radial nerve palsy.—The radial vein, and its tributaries lying about one to one and a half inches above the wrist on the radial side of the forearm, are popular not only for intravenous injection but also for intravenous infusion. Injudicious attempts at either of these procedures may lead to trauma of the radial nerve as it lies deep to but not far from the veins.

Sciatic nerve palsy.—Intramuscular injection into the buttock is always fraught with the potential hazard of traumatising the sciatic nerve, especially in infants. The upper and outer quadrant of the buttock should be used, but an alternative and safe site for injection is the antero-lateral aspect of the mid-thigh.

Prevention

General awareness of these dangers on the part of anaesthetists, surgeons, nurses, and all who care for unconscious patients is the best safeguard against their occurrence. Special precautions must be taken in particular instances where the risk of a certain posture must be accepted in the general interest of the patient. Thus it may be essential to use shoulder supports to maintain a patient in the Trendelenburg position, with the legs in the lithotomy position at the same time, during the operation of synchronous combined abdomino-perineal resection of the rectum. In such an instance well-padded supports placed at the acromion processes are essential, and the arms should be placed by the side of the body. In all other inclined planes the body is more safely prevented from sliding by the use of a non-slip mattress (Fig. 1; Hewer, 1953).

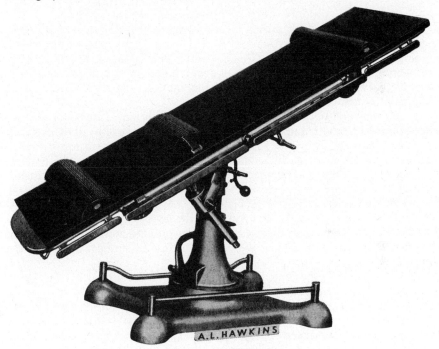

31/Fig. 1.—Non-slip mattress.

If an arm is to be abducted from the body for the purpose of intravenous injections or infusions during an operation—and this is frequently essential—it should be maintained at a higher horizontal plane from the body, and the use of a right-angle lock will help to ensure it is never abducted beyond this. In the "hands up" position, elevation of the upper arm 6 inches off the table prevents injury (Jackson and Keats, 1965).

Treatment

This should consist of splinting to prevent deformities, and active exercises. Analgesics may be needed for a day or two after the onset of paresis.

Prognosis

The greater the pressure and the longer it is applied, the more severe is the injury. Provided there is no pre-existing neurological disease the prognosis for peripheral nerve palsies of the types described is good. They may be slow to recover completely but the majority will clear within six months. The only notable exceptions are those due to hypothermia, which may take considerably longer. As a rule power returns quickest in large muscles and more slowly in those concerned with fine movements. Thus patients who rely upon their fingers for everyday work and pleasure are more handicapped than manual workers.

The **neurological sequelae of spinal analgesia** are discussed in Chapter 36.

CONVULSIONS DURING ANAESTHESIA

Convulsions may occur during local or general anaesthesia. Those due to local anaesthetic drugs are discussed in Chapter 34. Convulsions during the administration of general anaesthesia have often been associated with ether but are by no means limited to the use of this agent; indeed, accumulated experience suggests that they may be the result of a combination of factors. These may be divided into three groups:

1. *Physical predisposition.*—Children undoubtedly have a greater propensity to convulse than adults, and this is presumably due to the lability of their central nervous systems. A fit may be induced in a true epileptic by various stimuli—such as hypoxia or hypercarbia—but the evidence for believing that all patients who convulse during general anaesthesia have an epileptic tendency is inconclusive.

2. *Disease.*—Sepsis with its associated high temperature and increased basal metabolism leads to some tissue hypoxia of the histotoxic type and frequently to dehydration. An excessively high body temperature may be produced by an overheated operating theatre or the injudicious use of surgical drapes on the patient.

3. *Anaesthesia.*—The contribution of anaesthesia lies primarily in its ability to accentuate the other factors. Hence excessive premedication with atropine raises the patient's temperature by increasing both metabolism and dehydration, while deep inhalational anaesthesia adds to the tissue hypoxia. Moreover, unless respiration is at least assisted at this stage, some carbon dioxide retention occurs. Convulsions in children following premedication with "Pamergan SP100", a proprietary name for a combination of promethazine 50 mg, pethidine 100 mg and hyoscine 0·4 mg, have been recorded (Waterhouse, 1967) and an idiosyncratic reaction to the promethazine element has been postulated. Convulsions have also followed premedication in children with papaveretum and hyoscine (Holmes 1968), and the opiate held responsible.

"Malignant hyperthermia", well documented in recent years, may be a cause of convulsions (Britt and Gordon, 1969). Its features and treatment are described elsewhere (Chapter 28).

Prevention of convulsions should consist of a reasoned appraisal of the risk in likely subjects and the avoidance of all controllable and predisposing factors. The immediate treatment should be to ensure oxygenation; this is best achieved by paralysing the patient with a muscle relaxant and performing intermittent positive-pressure respiration with 100 per cent oxygen. Particular care must be taken to ensure that the carbon dioxide tension of the blood is kept within normal limits, and steps should be taken to lower the patient's body temperature. Prolonged treatment on the lines suggested on p. 1023 may be needed should a period of acute hypoxia occur before the convulsion can be controlled.

Ophthalmic Complications

Most ophthalmic complications follow direct trauma or the irritant effect of anaesthetic vapours, soda-lime dust, or sterilising solutions. Conjunctivitis, corneal abrasion and ulcers may also be caused in this fashion, and it is particularly important to ensure that the eyelids are closed, thus covering the eye at all times. In certain postures, such as the prone position in neurosurgery, and when the eyes are especially vulnerable, as in exophthalmos, it is a wise precaution temporarily to strap the eyelids together with adhesive plaster. Indeed, in the latter case it is occasionally necessary to perform a tarsorrhaphy.

Less common complications affecting the eye as a result of anaesthesia and surgery are thrombosis of the central artery of the retina, acute glaucoma and pain in the region of the supra-orbital nerve. Thrombosis of the retinal artery, which causes blindness, is only likely to occur in those patients with pre-existing disease. Shock states, and excessive induced hypotension, could be a contributory cause. Post-operative blindness may also be part of a general syndrome caused by acute or sub-acute hypoxia (see p. 1021). Givner and Jaffe (1950) suggest that compression of the eye by an anaesthetic mask may cause indirect pressure on the central artery of the retina. If the patient suffers from arterial disease then ischaemic changes in the retina may be produced. Difficulties of accommodation are not uncommon immediately after anaesthesia and can usually be related to the varying effects of the drugs used—including pre- and post-operative medicants and the relaxants—upon the ciliary and ocular muscles. Any agents which produce dilatation of the pupil and impede the circulation of the aqueous humour will accentuate a tendency towards glaucoma. Acute glaucoma, precipitated in a myopic patient, is a well-recognised post-operative complication, but its direct connection with either operation or anaesthetic is not always apparent. It has been suggested that the pressure of a face mask on the eye, and its subsequent release, is an important factor, but cases occur in which a mask has not been used. Certainly atropine and scopolamine should be used with caution for known cases of glaucoma, but the occasional acute case that occurs is more likely to be related to the general metabolic disturbance than to any single and specific factor.

Supra-orbital pain—a very rare complication—is almost certainly related to undue pressure in the area of the nerve.

The ocular complications of spinal analgesia are discussed in Chapter 36.

REFERENCES

ALLISON, R. S. (1956). Clinical consequence of cerebral anoxia. *Proc. roy. Soc. Med.*, **49,** 609.

BEDFORD, P. D. (1955). Adverse cerebral effects of anaesthesia on old people. *Lancet*, **2**, 259.

BEDFORD, P. D. (1957). Cerebral damage from shock due to disease in aged people with special reference to cardiac infarction, pneumonia and severe diarrhoea. *Lancet*, **2**, 505.

BRITT, B. A., and GORDON, R. A. (1969). Three cases of malignant hyperthermia with special consideration of management. *Canad. Anaesth. Soc. J.*, **16**, 99.

CLAUSEN, E. G. (1942). Post-operative ("anaesthetic") paralysis of brachial plexus; review of literature and report of nine cases. *Surgery*, **12**, 933.

CONWAY, C. M., and PAYNE, J. P. (1963). Postoperative hypoxaemia and oxygen therapy. *Brit. med. J.*, **1**, 844.

COPE, D. H. P. (1960). Dehydration therapy in cerebral hypoxia. *Proc. roy. Soc. Med.*, **52**, 678.

FISHMAN, R. A. (1953). Effects of isotonic intravenous solutions on normal and increased intracranial pressure. *Arch. Neurol. (Chic.)*, **70**, 350.

FRENCH, L. A. (1966). The use of steroids in the treatment of cerebral oedema. *Bull. N.Y. Acad. Med.*, **42**, 301.

GIVNER, I., and JAFFE, N. (1950). Occlusion of the central retinal artery following anaesthesia. *Arch. Ophthal.*, **43**, 197.

HEWER, C. L. (1953). Maintenance of the Trendelenburg position by skin friction. *Lancet*, **1**, 522.

HOLMES, R. P. (1968). Convulsions following pre-operative medication. *Brit. J. Anaesth.*, **40**, 633.

INGVAR, D. H. (1968). The pathophysiology of cerebral anoxia. *Acta anaesth. scand.*, Suppl. **29**, 47.

JACKSON, L., and KEATS, A. S. (1965). Mechanism of brachial plexus palsy following anesthesia. *Anesthesiology*, **26**, 190.

KILOH, L. G. (1950). Brachial plexus lesions after cholecystectomy. *Lancet*, **1**, 103.

LINDENBERG, R. (1963). Patterns of CNS vulnerability in acute hypoxaemia including anaesthesia accidents. In: *Selective Vulnerability of the Brain in Hypoxaemia*. Ed. J. P. Schade and W. H. McMenemy. Oxford: Blackwell Scientific Publications.

LUCAS, B. G. B., and STRANGEWAYS, D. H. (1952). The effects of intermittent anoxia on the brain. *J. Path. Bact.*, **64**, 265.

MARSHALL, B. E., and WYCHE, M. Q. (1972). Hypoxaemia during and after anesthesia. *Anesthesiology*, **37**, 178.

MORRIS, P. M. (1959). Personal communication.

NUNN, J. F., and PAYNE, J. P. (1962). Hypoxaemia after general anaesthesia. *Lancet*, **2**, 631.

PAMPIGLIONE, G., and HARDEN, A. (1968). Resuscitation after cardiovascular arrest. Prognostic evaluation of early electroencephalographic findings. *Lancet*, **1**, 1261.

PASK, E. A., and ROBSON, J. G. (1954). Injury to the median nerve. *Anaesthesia*, **9**, 94.

ROSOMOFF, H. L. (1963). Distribution of intracranial contents with controlled hyperventilation: implications for neuro-anesthesia. *Anesthesiology*, **24**, 640.

ROSOMOFF, H. L. (1968). Cerebral oedema and brain swelling. *Acta anaesth. scand.*, Suppl. **29**, 75.

SCHMIDT, C. R., and LINCOLN, J. R. (1966). Peripheral nerve injuries with anesthesia: a review and report of three cases. *Anesth. Analg. Curr. Res.*, **45**, 748.

SECHER, O., and WILHJELM, B. (1968). The protective action of anaesthetics against hypoxia. *Canad. Anaesth. Soc. J.*, **15**, 423.

STEPHENS, J., and APPLEBY, S. (1956). Polyneuropathy following induced hypothermia. *Trans. Amer. neurol. Ass.*, p. 102 (80th Meeting, 1955).

STRONG, M. J., and KEATS, A. S. (1967). Induced hypothermia following cerebral anoxia. *Anesthesiology*, **28**, 920.

SWAN, H., VIRTUE, R., BLOUNT, S. G., Jnr., and KIRCHER, L. T., Jnr. (1955). Hypothermia in surgery: analysis of 100 clinical cases. *Ann. Surg.*, **142**, 382.

TAYLOR, J. M., LEVY, W. A., HERZOG, I., and SCHEINBERG, L. C. (1965). Prevention of experimental cerebral oedema by corticosteroids. *Neurology* (*Minneap.*), **15,** 667.

WATERHOUSE, R. G. (1967). Epileptiform convulsions in children following premedication with Pamergan SP100. *Brit. J. Anaesth.*, **39,** 268.

Chapter 32

PAIN AND THE
ANALGESIC DRUGS

INTRODUCTION

PAIN is one of man's most compelling experiences. It is an unpleasant sensation which only the individual himself can appraise and as such is incapable of a satisfactory objective definition. It is frequently associated, by the patient, with physical damage and hence his description is often couched in terms connected with injury (Merskey and Spear, 1967). Sherrington (1906), in his classic work on the central nervous system, has defined pain as "the psychical adjunct to an imperative protective reflex". This concept certainly draws attention to the protective aspect of pain in preventing body injury by noxious stimuli. The burnt fingers of a patient with syringomyelia, or corneal ulceration after division of the fifth cranial nerve, bear testimony to the usefulness of pain.

This defensive function of pain extends also to disease. The natural inclination to rest an inflamed part not only relieves the pain but also has a beneficial effect on the body's efforts to combat the infection. Similarly, angina pectoris protects the diseased heart from acute myocardial insufficiency due to over-exertion.

Leriche (1949) has stressed that on many occasions pain seems pointless and quite often the warning which it affords is inadequate. As he points out, many of the gravest illnesses, such as cancer and heart disease, develop silently and pain only arises when the disease is far advanced, merely making sadder and harder a situation long since lost.

That the ability to experience pain is not essential for the satisfactory adaptation of man to his surroundings is evident from reports on patients with a congenital absence of pain sensation (Ford and Wilkins, 1938; Kunkle and Chapman 1943). As a symptom, pain demands instant relief and is present in two out of every three patients seeking medical advice (Devine and Merskey, 1965). Not only is it a distressing experience but if continued it may have a harmful effect on vital organs, leading to impairment of function or even tissue damage (Wolff and Wolf, 1958).

The relief of pain during surgery is the *raison d'être* of anaesthesia. Many anaesthetists have extended the scope of their activities by setting up pain clinics to help alleviate the chronic pain from which some patients suffer.

NATURE OF PAIN SENSATION (THEORIES OF PAIN)

Although the sensory nature of pain was recognised by the great Greek philosophers, it was conceived more broadly as a moral force with pain and unpleasantness as the natural opposites of virtue and pleasure.

The theory that pain could be produced by intensive stimulation of any sensory organ has been frequently discussed, although by many authors it is accepted as a separate and specific form of sensation. The neuro-anatomical basis of pain sensibility has been unfolded in the past one hundred years, following the discovery of the sensory function of the posterior spinal nerve roots and of the existence of medullary pathways comparatively specialised for pain. The doctrine of specific nerve energies was formulated by Müller in 1840 and implies that the sensation evoked by a stimulus is determined by the particular nerve fibres stimulated and not by the nature of the stimulus. As well as signalling temperature changes, heat and cold may cause pain if the relevant pathways are excited simultaneously. The discovery of separate nerve pathways for specific forms of sensation followed transection experiments on the spinal cord by Schiff (1848) and others. With the introduction by Adrian (1931) of electro-physiological techniques to the study of sensory nerve physiology, a new field was opened for studying the electrical responses in single nerve fibres following their stimulation.

The receptor organs for pain are distributed throughout the body but it is convenient from the clinical aspect to consider pain under different headings. The following classification of pain will be adopted:

Superficial or cutaneous pain. } Somatic pain.
Deep pain (muscles, bones, ligaments, joints, fascia }
Visceral pain.
Referred pain.
Psychogenic or functional pain.

Superficial or Cutaneous Pain

The description of superficial pain will be expanded to include a more general discussion on the physiological mechanisms and neural pathways underlying the reception, conduction and appreciation of painful stimuli.

(i) **Reception of painful stimuli.**—Painful stimuli are carried by a network of non-myelinated or poorly myelinated nerve fibres which ramify in the superficial, deep or visceral tissues. Pain nerve endings react to a variety of excessive stimuli, all of which pose a threat of tissue damage. Several forms of energy, thermal, mechanical and electrical, as well as chemical stimuli, are all capable of evoking pain.

It is not certain whether these forces cause a direct excitation of the bare nerve endings or whether they produce tissue damage with the secondary release of a pain-producing substance. Hardy and others (1951) found with thermal energy that the onset of pain coincided with the temperature at which alterations of tissue protein began to take place. A release of chemical substances would be anticipated under these conditions. Beecher (1956) rejects this thesis and points out that in man, wounds, widespread lacerations and extensive tissue injury can be produced without pain being experienced. He concludes that the level of anxiety is of considerable importance in determining the occurrence of pain.

Wolff and Wolf (1958) consider that in such extensive injuries coagulated serum, oedema and devitalised tissue may shield the pain endings from noxious stimuli. Moreover, damage to nerve terminals and fibres may desensitise traumatised tissue.

A pain-producing substance—probably a polypeptide—has been detected by Armstrong and his co-workers (1957) in inflammatory exudates, and there are several substances capable of producing pain on subcutaneous injection or when applied to a blister base (Armstrong *et al.*, 1953). These include histamine, acetylcholine, angiotonin, bradykinin, adenosine triphosphate, serotonin, hydrogen and potassium ions and 5-hydroxytryptamine. Recent evidence (Ferreira, 1972) suggests that prostaglandin E sensitises the pain receptors to stimuli such as pressure and also to the action of the chemical mediators. Aspirin may relieve pain by inhibiting the production of prostaglandin E peripherally and so preventing the sensitisation of the pain receptors (Vane, 1971).

(ii) **Pain pathways.**—Gasser (1943) has classified nerve fibres by correlating their diameter with the conduction velocity of nerve impulses. The myelinated somatic or A fibres are subdivided into 5 groups.

		Terminology	*Fibre diameter*	*Conduction speed metres per sec.*
		Alpha	20µm	120
		Beta		
Myelinated somatic fibres	A	Gamma		
		Delta	↓ (3–4µm)	↓ (6–30)→pain
		Epsilon	2µm	5 fibres
Myelinated visceral fibres (preganglionic autonomic))	B		< 3µm	3–15
Unmyelinated somatic fibres	C		<2µm	0·5–2→pain fibres

Two groups of fibres are responsible for the perception of pain in the epidermis and superficial layers of the dermis. These are the myelinated A-delta fibres and the more slowly conducting unmyelinated C fibres. These latter fibres are the first to be blocked by cocaine but the last to be blocked by asphyxia.

The existence of both a fast and a slow neural pathway for conducting pain impulses to the central nervous system is suggested by the occurrence of double pain sensation or echo pain. This term applies to the twin peaks of pain which may follow a brief painful stimulus to the skin. The more distally the stimulus is applied, the greater the temporal separation of the two pain waves.

From experimental work Landau and Bishop (1953) concluded that C fibre pain had a delayed, burning and persistent character as typified by that associated with inflammation. They considered that sharp, pricking pain produced by mechanical or electrical stimulation was transmitted by the delta fibres.

(iii) **Spinothalamic pathway.**—The cell bodies of the nerve fibres carrying pain impulses are located in the posterior root ganglia. On entering the spinal cord the pain fibres deviate laterally to form the ascending and descending branches of the tract of Lissauer at the tip of the posterior horn. After ascending one to three segments, these fibres synapse in the substantia gelatinosa on the tip of the posterior horn. The axons of the second neurone cross the mid-line in the anterior commissure to form the lateral spinothalamic tract, which ascends and terminates in the lateral nucleus of the thalamus (Fig. 1). The fibres which arise in the lower parts of the body are displaced laterally by fibres from the upper segments, which thus occupy a medial position in the spinothalamic tract. This laminar arrangement of the fibres in the tract ensures their precise topo-

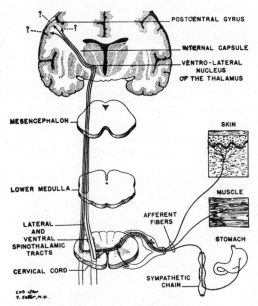

32/FIG. 1.—Pain pathways.

graphical distribution which is related to body dermatomes and is probably continued to the sensory cortex.

From the thalamus, the third neurone passes through the posterior limb of the internal capsule and is projected to the post-central gyrus of the cerebral cortex.

Pain fibres from the neck and the occipital region of the scalp pass through the 2nd and 3rd cervical nerves. Fibres supplying the face and front of the scalp arise in the cells of the trigeminal ganglion and synapse in the nucleus of the spinal tract of the trigeminal nerve.

(iv) **Reticular system.**— In addition to this classical pain pathway, it has been suggested (Gellhorn, 1953) that collaterals from it are distributed to the ascending reticular system. This multisynaptic pathway relays in the reticular formation of the brain stem and provides an alternative route for pain impulses to bombard a large area of the cerebral cortex. It is believed that stimuli following this pathway activate the cortex and help to maintain consciousness. It is probably a non-specific arousal mechanism, while localisation is a function of the thalamic radiation to the post-central gyrus.

(v) **Dermatomes.**—The cutaneous area supplied by a single posterior nerve root is termed a "dermatome." Knowledge of these is important in determining the nerve roots it is necessary to block when treating superficial pain by local anaesthetics or when relieving persistent pain with alcohol, phenol or root section. A dermatome chart of the whole body is shown in Fig. 2, every spinal root being represented except C1. The dermatomes are in fact more extensive than those shown on such a chart as there is considerable overlap in the areas supplied by adjacent roots.

(vi) **Thalamus and sensory cortex.**—The dermatomal arrangement of the sensory fibres is maintained in the cortical projection to the post-central gyrus and it is possible to map out a distorted image of the body upon the cortex itself.

The relative importance of the thalamus and the cortex in the perception of pain is still disputed. Head (1920) believed that pain is experienced when nerve impulses arrive in the appropriate part of the thalamus which he regarded as the centre of consciousness for pain. It is known that cortical lesions produce only transient and minimal disturbances of pain appreciation, whereas destruction of the thalamus abolishes pain sensibility.

Thalamic sensation is crude and poorly localised and the sensory cortex is essential for localising and detecting variations in the intensity of pain. To ascribe sensation to the thalamus and perception to the cortex is to take too narrow a view of a complex functional interrelationship.

A therapeutic problem is sometimes posed by patients with a persistent pain following some lesion which has long since disappeared or as a sequel to certain conditions affecting the spinal nerve roots or peripheral nerves. The explanation probably lies in the establishment of abnormal activity in the thalamocortical pathways which may persist despite attempts to block the afferent pain pathway at a lower level (Brain, 1962). Although cordotomy or the destruction of peripheral nerves or spinal roots may be completely ineffective in such patients, the symptoms may be relieved by a localised ablation of the sensory cortex.

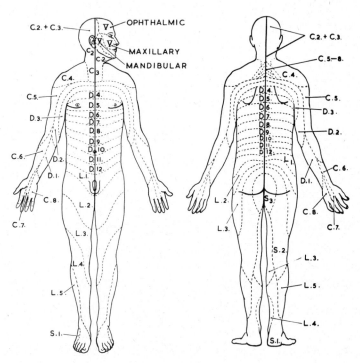

32/Fig. 2.—The dermatomes of the body.

The unpleasant affective reaction accompanying painful stimuli is determined by the prefrontal cortex and the multisynaptic pathways of the reticular formation. By performing a prefrontal leucotomy or stereotactic ablation of the thalamic nuclei, when a patient's emotional reaction to pain is severe, the thalamic influence on these areas is removed. This leads to the disappearance of the mental tension and the unpleasant affective connotation of pain. Such patients still feel pain but they no longer suffer. This may be the only procedure capable of helping patients with the persistent type of pain described above.

The conscious appreciation of pain appears to depend upon the widespread activity of the entire intact cortex, so enabling the individual to interpret and formulate his own personal reaction to a particular painful experience. The complex and diverse cortical connections which subserve this process are laid down largely on the basis of previous experience, and the intensity of pain suffered varies enormously with the personality, intelligence and culture of the individual. Uncivilised people often display a stoic disregard for pain. As a generalisation, pain is felt more intensely by artistic and cultured persons than by those of the same race or family who lack these attributes.

Emotional stress and anxiety adversely affect the pain response, while other factors which enhance the severity of pain are debility and fatigue. Pain often becomes worse during the night when the distractions of everyday life are absent and the patient has time to brood on his symptoms. The combined use of hypnotic and analgesic drugs is often necessary to prevent sleepless nights. Protracted severe pain becomes the dominant factor in a patient's life and leads eventually to both physical and psychological exhaustion.

Descending Pathways

Impulses descending from the higher centres of the central nervous system, primarily the cerebral cortex and thalamus, are able to modulate the perception of pain at spinal cord level. The transmission of pain impulses through the substantia gelatinosa is either enhanced or inhibited by such a mechanism utilising mainly the descending cortico-spinal and reticulo-spinal pathways, with additional contributions from the limbic circuit and its associated emotional influences.

Deep (Non-visceral) Pain

Pain impulses from joints, tendons, muscle and fascia arise in a network of fine fibres similar to those in the skin and travel by the same nervous pathways. The sensitivity of these tissues appears to vary with the richness of the innervation. Thus the low pain threshold of the periosteum is associated with dense innervation as compared with the relatively insensitive and sparsely supplied fibrous muscle septa (Ruch and Fulton, 1960).

The deep tissue area supplied by a single posterior nerve root is termed a sclerotome and it must be stressed that it is not directly related to the overlying dermatome. As the extent of the sclerotomes has not been worked out as accurately as the dermatomes, it is often difficult to decide which roots are involved in patients with deep pain. For this reason the therapeutic blocking of spinal nerve roots to alleviate deep pain must be more extensive than that for superficial pain.

Deep pain usually has a dull aching character, and it may be accompanied by an unpleasant sickening sensation due to an autonomic response. It is poorly localised and tends to spread to other areas utilising both superficial and deep pathways. Both myelinated and non-myelinated fibres, which travel to the posterior root ganglia by way of the sympathetic chains, may also transmit aching pains from viscera, bones and muscles (Wolff and Wolf, 1958). This pain pathway has an important clinical application when using neurolytic agents intrathecally to alleviate intractable pain.

The occurrence of pain at some point distant from the site of stimulation is termed "referred pain" and it will be discussed in a later section. Although it is associated more commonly with visceral pain, it can occur with deep non-visceral structures, as in the case of a diseased hip, when pain may be felt in the knee. Moreover, deep pain may be referred to the dermatome of the same posterior nerve root through which the impulses from the deep structures enter the spinal cord.

Deep pain endings can be stimulated by chemical substances or mechanical forces such as the stretching of muscle fibres. The receptors are especially sensitive in the presence of trauma or infection. Ischaemic muscle pain, as in intermittent claudication, and also the muscle pain provoked by excessive or sustained contractions, are probably due to stimulation of the nerve endings by various metabolic products. Sustained contraction is the likely cause of a large number of muscle pains, including many cases of backache and the neck stiffness associated with headaches. These may have an organic basis, as in meningitis, or may be due to the emotional tension accompanying an anxiety state (Holmes and Wolff, 1950).

Visceral Pain

This is transmitted mainly in the sympathetic nerves via the sympathetic chain and the white rami communicantes to the posterior root ganglia, where the cell bodies are situated. The fibres essentially are components of spinal nerves utilising but not relaying in the sympathetic system. The modern tendency is to speak of them as autonomic or visceral afferents. Although the fibres connect with the spinothalamic tract, they are distributed more widely than somatic pain fibres within the cord. This explains why a more extensive cordotomy is generally required for visceral pain. The pain innervation of the viscera is shown in Fig. 3.

Not all visceral pain impulses are conducted by sympathetic nerves. Those from certain pelvic organs such as the bladder neck, prostate, uterine cervix and lower colon travel by the parasympathetic pelvic nerves to the cord. It has also been suggested that some pain fibres from the trachea and oesophagus travel in the vagus nerve.

Viscera have evolved quite different effective stimuli from those which activate cutaneous receptors. It is possible, for example, to handle and even cut and burn viscera under local anaesthesia without producing pain, although mesenteric traction usually causes discomfort. Pain-producing stimuli include chemical irritants, as in peritonitis, sudden distension of organs and excessive contractions and spasms, especially when associated with changes in the blood supply, as in intestinal obstruction. Normal activity of smooth muscle is painless except when the blood supply is impaired.

Compared with somatic pain, visceral pain is diffuse, less easily localised and often referred. It has a dull, aching character and is often accompanied by a fall in pulse and blood pressure, whereas these usually rise with somatic pain. Muscular rigidity and hyperaesthesia are commonly associated with visceral pain.

Referred Pain

Deep pain, whether visceral or somatic in origin, may be misinterpreted so that it is felt in some part of the body other than the site of stimulation. The reference of cardiac pain to the left arm and diaphragmatic pain to the shoulder are well-known examples of this phenomenon.

Harman (1948) considers that sensation cannot be localised in deep parts of the body that are unperceived by the individual and the existence of which, as in the case of a viscus, he may not be aware. The inability to visualise the site of stimulation creates the need to project the pain to some part of the body where

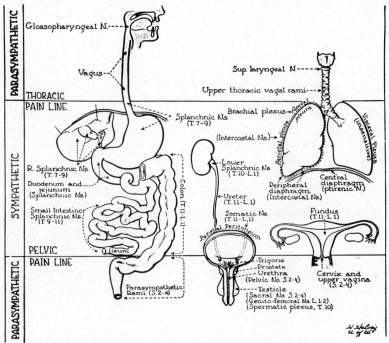

32/Fig. 3.—Pain innervation of the viscera.

perception is possible. This results in pain being referred to the dermatomes having the same or adjacent segmental innervation as the painful focus itself.

Visceral pain tends to have a characteristic localisation for each organ and it is referred to part rather than the whole of a segment. Pain from abdominal organs, for example, is usually felt anteriorly and not in the dorsal part of the segment. The neurophysiological basis of referred pain probably depends on the convergence of several cutaneous and visceral afferent fibres on the same secondary neurone at some point in the pain pathway. Although this may occur in the thalamus or cortex, it is known that the fibres in the spinothalamic tract are outnumbered by the pain fibres in the dorsal root, indicating a convergence of fibres at the spinal level (Ruch and Fulton, 1960).

On the basis of previous experience, impulses travelling by a certain tract are interpreted by the brain as arising in a particular cutaneous site. This projection will occur whether the impulses are initiated by cutaneous or visceral receptors. The mechanism is analogous to a shared "party" telephone line. Certain tracts remain "private" and transmit unreferred visceral pain impulses. The muscular rigidity and hyperaesthesia associated with conditions like acute appendicitis are due to the central spread of excitation with the evoking of somatic reflexes and the facilitation of cutaneous impulses which normally would be incapable of producing pain. This facet of referred pain can be removed and the patient's discomfort reduced by infiltrating the hyperaesthetic area with a local anaesthetic.

The therapeutic action of counter-irritants in relieving visceral pain may be in the ability of a strong cutaneous stimulus to crowd out or inhibit visceral impulses from entering the cord in the same segment. The vasodilatation which may be produced in the viscera when a rubefacient is applied to the skin of the corresponding spinal segments is unlikely to produce rapid pain relief.

Anginal pain has been reported in a phantom limb (Cohen and Jones, 1943) so that it is unnecessary for the part actually to exist in order to have pain projected to it by the cerebral cortex. Harman (1951) showed that anginal pain referred to the arm was abolished by a complete brachial plexus block. This made the patient unaware of his arm. The pain persisted, however, with a selective block which achieved analgesia without the loss of touch, position sense and motor power.

The inference from these reports is that the perception of a structure by the cortex is a fundamental requisite for referred pain.

CURRENT CONCEPT OF THE NATURE OF PAIN

In recent years the specificity of sensory perception has been questioned increasingly, especially the psychological assumption that stimulation of pain receptors results in the direct transmission to the brain of impulses which are interpreted as pain. Such a concept has the implication that the sifting of information about a stimulus occurs entirely at the peripheral receptors. Soulairac (1968) considers pain as an affective reaction, dependent not on the nature of the sensory receptors but on the intensity of the impulses transmitted to the central nervous system and on the manner in which they are utilised there.

Pain sensation is one manifestation of a more general reaction or "algic" behaviour and it is often impossible to correlate the sensory phenomenon of pain with the unpleasant affective state that occurs.

The assimilation of sensory pain at the level of consciousness depends on its integration in the central nervous system at different levels of vigilance and on its modification by other sensory information. The first level of vigilance is situated in the mesencephalic (mid-brain) reticular substance (Charpentier, 1968). It does not produce affective awareness but rather an abrupt awakening of the central nervous system and activation of protective homeostatic responses like the startle and flight reactions. The state of alert activates the higher centres, especially the frontal cortex. This first centre of integration is essentially adrenergic in nature. The second level of vigilance is in the rhinencephalon and thalamic reticular formation and is responsible for the more specific and affective reactions to pain. This system is activated by strong stimuli and is essentially cholinergic in nature. The potent narcotic analgesics such as morphine and pethidine exert their effect at this level. The third level of integration of pain sensation determines its tempero-spatial analysis and evaluation in regard to the external environment and is located in the frontal cortex. It achieves a co-ordinated response by the animal to the painful stimulus having regard to its cause, strength and its surroundings. The progress of a painful stimulus through the levels of integration is set out in the following scheme (after Charpentier):

Sensory nerve→Medulla→Brain stem→Rhinencephalon→Cortex

↓	↓	↓	↓
Reflex	Diffuse	Affective	Intellectual
	alertness	alertness	alertness

It is only in the two superior levels of integration, where affective regulation is manifest, that pain is transformed to the state of suffering.

Gate Control Theory of Pain

Melzack and Wall (1965 and 1968) have recently proposed a new theory of pain mechanisms, in which it is suggested that the sensory input from the skin is modulated by a gate control system before its eventual perception as pain. The sensory impulses from the skin are distributed to three systems in the spinal cord: the tracts of the dorsal columns for onward transmission to the brain, the cells of the substantia gelatinosa, and the first central transmission (T) cells in the dorsal horn which transmit sensory information to higher centres.

These authors suggest that the substantia gelatinosa acts as a gate control mechanism (see Fig. 4), as it has been shown (Wall, 1962; Mendell and Wall, 1964) that although impulses in large fibres are at first very potent in activating the T cells, their effect is later diminished by an inhibitory process. Impulses transmitted by the small fibres, on the other hand, bring into play an excitory mechanism, which enhances the effect of impulses arriving from the periphery. The nerve impulses which travel continuously to the spinal cord, even when there is no apparent stimulation, are transmitted primarily by the small fibres, and Melzack and Wall propose that they maintain the gate in a comparatively open position. Stimulation of the skin evokes a burst of impulses, in which large fibre activity predominates over that in the small fibres. The T cells are triggered off, but at the same time, due to the inhibitory mechanism, the gate is partly closed. During sustained stimulation, adaptation in the large fibres swings the balance in favour of the small fibre system, so opening the gate and increasing the outflow of impulses from the T cells.

It is also suggested that central influences engendered by emotion or previous experience can influence sensory input by means of the gate control mechanism (Hagbarth and Kerr, 1954; Wall, 1967). This effect may be generalised or selective and restricted to a particular part of the body, as for example has been reported in soldiers wounded in battle (Beecher, 1959), who may suffer little pain from their wound but complain vehemently about a careless venepuncture.

This process has been termed the "central control trigger", and it is suggested that it is mediated by the dorsal column system. This carries exact information on the type and location of the stimulus, so altering selective brain mechanisms and also influencing the gate control mechanism by central efferent fibres.

The onward transmission of impulses by the cord cells in response to a pain-producing stimulus depends, therefore, on the intensity of the incoming stream of impulses and the state of excitability of the T cells, under the combined inhibi-

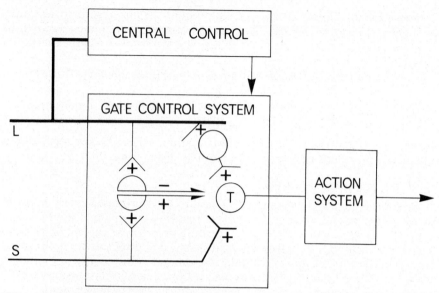

32/Fig. 4.—Diagram to illustrate the gate control theory of pain. L is the large diameter fibres; S is the small diameter fibres; T represents the first central transmission cells.

tory and excitatory balance of the afferent impulses, together with the influence of the descending control messages, sent by the brain.

This theory can explain many phenomena of pain, such as that which occurs in alcoholic and diabetic neuropathy and other neuralgias, where there is a selective degeneration of the large fibres. The impaired functioning of the inhibitory mechanism in these circumstances allows the unopposed activity of the small fibres to hold the gate open and so produce severe pain. Trigeminal neuralgia may be explained by such a process, as degenerative changes have been described (Kerr and Miller, 1966) in the large fibres in this condition.

Reservations have been expressed about this theory by Schmidt (1972) and Iggo (1972) who have doubted the evidence for constant afferent activity in the small fibres and the conflicting evidence on the potentials produced in dorsal roots by small fibre stimulation.

Psychogenic Aspects of Pain

A psychogenic basis for pain can be inferred when no satisfactory organic cause for it can be found, and its distribution does not accord with a known anatomical pattern. These symptoms, which are a manifestation of a psychological disorder, are often described in a characteristic way. A feeling of pressure or of a tight band constricting the head are well-known examples of such a pain. Pains of psychological origin are usually continuous from day to day and involve more than one part of the body but they do not tend to disturb sleep (Merskey, 1968). These patients are prone to self-pity and have an easily aroused resentment, especially concerning previous treatment. The pain may enable the patient to escape some particular situation or duty and may be heralded by symptoms suggestive of an emotional disturbance.

Protracted organic pain frequently leads to exhaustion, while psychogenic pain is often preceded by a phase of exhaustion. Symptoms may occur at the site of previous trauma or infection, the pain persisting and growing in significance as it becomes the focus of the patient's preoccupation and apprehension. Sciatic pain from a prolapsed intervertebral disc may follow this pattern even when there is no question of impending litigation.

From the practical aspect it is important for the anaesthetist to realise that there is a psychological element to a greater or lesser extent in every patient, which can not only cause pain but can also increase its severity. Simple explanation and kindliness can do much to allay the anxiety of an apprehensive patient during a pre-operative ward visit. The relief of post-operative pain by a placebo exemplifies the power of suggestion. Narcotics and sedatives are invaluable during the post-operative period but they are often given too freely when reassurance and skilled nursing could do much to relieve the patient's anxiety and over-reaction to pain.

Certain patients have an abnormal and heightened reaction to pain, so that they suffer more intensely than normal individuals. The hospital atmosphere, together with an attitude of sympathy and firmness from both medical and nursing staff, can do much to help such people. In severe cases psychotherapy may be as important as conventional pain-relieving measures. In any patient suffering from pain, both the somatic and the psychic aspects must be evaluated including the patient's personality and reaction to the present illness.

The anaesthetist should be well-versed in the pharmacological and physical means of relieving pain but will probably need expert psychiatric assistance when dealing with predominantly psychogenic pain. This would involve the use of antidepressant drugs or ECT for endogenous depression and psychotherapy and sedation in neurotic illnesses. There is no doubt that these patients can suffer as acutely as those with a clear-cut physical cause for their pain and are equally deserving of sympathy and compassion. The acceptance of pain at its face value and the institution of the appropriate treatment should be the underlying principle in cases of doubt, rather than the premature diagnosis of a psychogenic disorder.

ASSESSMENT OF PAIN AND ANALGESIC DRUGS

Assessment of pain is extremely difficult because it is so entirely a subjective sensation. Nevertheless it is essential to have some means of measuring pain if one is to assess the value of analgesic drugs or techniques.

The *type* of pain (i.e. whether burning, aching, stabbing, whether acute or chronic and whether visceral, superficial, or musculo-skeletal) must be assessed, in order to select the analgesic agents most suited to its treatment. For example, morphine-like drugs are indicated for aching, visceral pains; anti-inflammatory drugs for arthritic pains; only local anaesthesia can truly alleviate intermittent, sharp and stabbing pains. A potential addictive drug may be used for a short-lived severe pain, but should be avoided for chronic pain unless it is terminal.

The *intensity* of pain must be assessed in any analgesic clinical trial, as in many cases analgesia may only be partial. Methods of measuring pain intensity are described later.

Clinical trials of analgesic drugs and techniques are beset with difficulties, and anyone contemplating one should read at least some of the vast library that has been written on the subject of evaluating pain and analgesia (Beecher, 1957; Gruber, 1962; Frazer and Harris, 1967; Lasagna, 1964; Lasagna, 1970; Joyce *et al.*, 1975) and should turn to the *Index Medicus* for recent publications.

The effects of analgesics may be tested on:
1. Experimental pain in animals and man;
2. Clinical pain.

Experimental Pain in Animals

Techniques involving experimental pain generally measure the pain *threshold* and the effect on it of analgesic techniques. In animals a reflex response usually measures the end-point, yet this appears to be related fairly satisfactorily to the pain threshold. The response to pin-prick by twitching of the skin in guinea-pigs can measure local anaesthetic activity. The use of heat (radiant heat causing rat tail-flicking (Bonnycastle, 1962), or rats and mice jumping from hot plates) has the advantage that it can be accurately measured, and the pain it produces is more susceptible to systemic analgesics.

Animals make better experimental subjects in this field than man because they are not subject to bias, and unlikely to be placebo reactors, and to them experimental pain is just as worrying as pathological pain.

Experimental Pain in Man

Although experimental pain is useful for testing local anaesthetics in man (see Chapter 34) it is more difficult to devise experimental pain which is susceptible to systemic analgesic drugs in man. Moreover, nowadays, ethical considerations generally preclude giving potentially addictive agents to volunteers. However, unlike in animals, not only pain *threshold* but also pain *intensity* can be assessed in man.

Pain may be produced by pressure on a bony surface, by radiant heat or a faradic current to the skin, or by exercising a limb rendered ischaemic with a sphygmomanometer. In all these cases the stimulus *applied* can be measured (temperature, current, duration of exercise). The degree of pain *experienced* can then be assessed after various doses and various drugs.

The disadvantage of experimental pain in assessing systemic analgesics is that both mild analgesics and morphine-like drugs appear to have much less effect on it than on pathological pain. This is because some mild analgesics have an anti-inflammatory effect while morphine-like drugs are said to have less effect upon pain threshold than upon *response* to pain. Frazer and Harris (1967) found that morphine only reduced the perception of pain in anxiety-ridden situations, which nevertheless they did manage to reproduce in the laboratory. Morphine has, however, been found to alleviate experimentally ischaemic pain without added psychological trauma (Smith *et al.*, 1966).

Clinical Assessment

Clinical pain has the advantage that it is the real thing and is often accompanied and aggravated by a substantial element of anxiety and a psychological reaction unlike that to experimental pain. The anxiety and psychological response are more susceptible to treatment by morphine-like drugs than is the pain itself. However clinical pain has the disadvantage that it waxes and wanes spontaneously and can only be evaluated subjectively.

A clinical trial of an analgesic should be limited to one particular field, for example: post-operative, obstetric, rheumatic or terminal pain. At least two dose levels of the test drug should be compared with a standard reference drug and a placebo, that is at least four treatments. A placebo is essential in this context to ensure that the method of assessment is sufficiently sensitive to distinguish between the effect of the drug and the placebo response (Loan and Dundee, 1967). But once the technique has been validated, a placebo can be omitted, if necessary, on ethical grounds. If the pain is of sufficient duration, a patient may act to an extent as his own control, that is to say he may receive in sequence two, three or more of the different treatments being studied. If pain is too brief or variable, patients must be randomly allocated into different treatment groups, or else be matched with others for age, sex, weight, degree of pain or disability, etc., which may be wasteful of clinical material. With random allocation, groups must be checked at the end of the trial for comparability.

The possibility that a drug may have a different effect if given in a single dose or repeatedly should be remembered. It should be tested in the way that it is intended to be used. The timing and route of administration should be standardised as much as possible and doses given on a weight basis. The use of a double-blind technique need not preclude this.

Evaluation of pain.—The actual *assessment* is the most difficult part. A double-blind technique is essential as the assessment by both patient and observer is subjective and therefore open to bias. Occasionally objective methods, such as vital capacity and peak flow measurement after abdominal surgery, may reinforce evaluation of pain (Parkhouse and Holmes, 1963). Assessment should be sufficiently frequent to measure both peak effect and duration of the different treatments, otherwise variations in time course between treatments may falsify results. The patient may be asked to assess the pain as absent/slight/ moderate or severe and the response to pain may be assessed by the observer as for example none/slight/marked or excessive. This technique has been used to assess intermittent pains such as labour (Major *et al.*, 1966). Fixed interval scales as in the above example have now been superseded by the visual analogue scale, which has been found to be more sensitive, accurate and consistent (Joyce *et al.*, 1975). By this technique the patient is shown a line which he is told represents at one end 'no pain at all' and at the other 'pain as bad as he could possibly imagine', and is asked to mark the point on the line where his pain lies. This scale has the added advantage that, unlike the fixed interval scale, the pain can be given a numerical value.

Finally, *side-effects* must be assessed. Appropriate signs such as vomiting, and alterations in blood pressure or respiration should be noted regularly. When seeking symptoms, the use of a check list is often advocated, but Huskisson and Wojtulewski (1974) suggested that the incidence of side-effects may be more accurately recorded without a questionnaire, since the influence of suggestion is removed, and symptoms that might have been omitted from the check list are more likely to be volunteered.

Because the disease state may contribute to what appear to be side-effects, their incidence may be more accurately recorded in healthy volunteers, but such a technique would be acceptable only with non-addictive drugs.

ANALGESIC DRUGS

Analgesic drugs relieve pain in doses which do not impair consciousness. Some drugs relieve pain by a direct effect on its cause: thus glyceryl trinitrate relieves anginal pain by reducing venous return and so reducing heart work; migraine may be relieved by ergotamine, which constricts meningeal vessels; colchicine relieves the pain of acute gout by virtue of an anti-inflammatory effect specific for this condition. None of these drugs is classed as an analgesic, which classically has its primary effect upon the central nervous system. Such a definition, however, ignores the fact that anti-inflammatory analgesics, typified by aspirin, owe a variable but large component of their analgesic effect to a peripheral anti-inflammatory action.

Analgesics may be divided into two main groups:—
1. Mild, antipyretic and anti-inflammatory analgesics.
2. Narcotic analgesics: morphine and related drugs.

MILD ANALGESICS

Mild analgesics also possess either an antipyretic effect (e.g. paracetamol) or an anti-inflammatory effect (e.g. indomethacin), or both, as in the case of aspirin. There is increasing evidence that they act by inhibiting prostaglandin synthesases, enzymes concerned with prostaglandin synthesis, and that paracetamol affects only the central nervous system enzymes while anti-inflammatory drugs depress only the peripheral enzymes, and aspirin inhibits both.

These drugs are non-addictive and many are readily available across the counter. Many are incorporated in various BP and proprietary combination tablets, which may also contain other ingredients such as caffeine. The value of such mixtures probably lies simply in their additive effects. The cumulative self-administration over a few years of several kilograms of such combination tablets, principally those containing phenacetin, can cause renal papillary necrosis, an important cause of chronic renal failure.

Aspirin (Acetylsalicylic Acid)

This is the oldest and probably the most effective of the mild analgesics. It possesses analgesic, antipyretic and anti-inflammatory actions and although its analgesic effect is in part due to an action on the central nervous system, the peripheral, anti-inflammatory action probably accounts for its remarkable effectiveness in relieving pain associated with inflammation. Although inferior to morphine and allied drugs in relieving visceral pain and that due to severe injury, it is superior in relieving headache, toothache, arthritic pain, dysmenorrhoea (probably because of the involvement of prostaglandins in uterine contraction) and that due to skin sepsis.

Aspirin has an antipyretic action mediated via the heat-regulating centre which is set at a lower level, so increasing the heat loss in febrile patients. This is achieved by cutaneous vasodilatation and sweating; aspirin is of especial value in relieving the aching pains associated with pyrexial illnesses such as influenza. When used at night, the antipyretic effect is a useful aid to inducing sleep in febrile patients. It has no effect upon the normal temperature, but since it is a metabolic stimulant it may cause hyperpyrexia in large or toxic doses, especially if there is absence of sweating, as there may be in dehydration and electrolyte depletion.

Aspirin has no effect on mood or consciousness, except when toxic doses cause severe pH and electrolyte disturbances, when coma ensues.

The only important side-effect of a normal dose of aspirin is gastric mucosal irritation with erosion and bleeding. This reaction depends upon a high concentration of non-ionised aspirin produced by stomach contents of a very low pH. Non-ionised aspirin is readily absorbed into the mucosal cells, whose interior pH is much higher. The aspirin will therefore ionise within the cells; it cannot easily diffuse out again once ionised and so accumulates to produce concentrations which are highly irritant to the mucosal cells. Such an adverse reaction cannot occur therefore in the absence of a very low luminal pH, which explains the great differences in sensitivity between individuals. Its occurrence can be minimised by taking aspirin well crushed in a lot of water, with sodium bicarbonate or as soluble aspirin.

Hypersensitivity occasionally occurs producing skin rashes. The precipitation of an asthmatic attack in asthmatic subjects is probably not due to hypersensitivity to aspirin but rather due to a disturbance in prostaglandin balance in the lungs.

Other adverse reactions to aspirin in general occur only after excessive dosage. It produces respiratory alkalosis due to direct stimulation of the respiratory centre, and metabolic acidosis due to uncoupling oxidative phosphorylation and disturbances of intermediary metabolism. Metabolic acidosis is especially prominent in children, and can occur when they are given large doses in the treatment of rheumatic fever.

Large doses may also prolong the prothrombin time, but the value of aspirin in preventing post-operative deep vein thrombosis and other coagulative disorders is not established.

Symptoms of excessive doses typically are tinnitus and dizziness.

Administration and dosage.—Tablets contain 300 mg, and one to three tablets may be taken by adults up to four times a day. The dose commonly prescribed in adult rheumatoid arthritis is 900 mg four-hourly (5 times a day). Aspirin soluble tablets BP or Disprin, or one of many sustained release or combined preparations (*vide infra*) may be preferred to reduce gastric irritation. Children should be given aspirin paediatric preparations, or Junior Aspirin tablets, which contain 75 mg of aspirin. The dose is approximately 10 mg/kg, three to four times a day. Aspirin is contra-indicated in the presence of peptic ulceration and in those taking steroids or oral anticoagulants.

Acute salicylate poisoning represents about 15 per cent of all acute poisonings that are admitted to hospital (Matthew and Lawson, 1970). The mortality in adults is 1–2 per cent while in children it is around 7 per cent.

Direct stimulation of the respiratory centre leads initially to a respiratory alkalosis. This feature is not prominent in children. Metabolic stimulation leads to increased CO_2 production (which later overcomes the early reduction in Pa_{CO_2}), increased O_2 demand, accumulation of fixed acids and hyperpyrexia from increased heat production. The consequent metabolic acidosis becomes increasingly severe with time, and may be marked from the start in children. Dehydration, because of sweating, hyperventilation and hyperpyrexia, is a prominent and serious complication. Consciousness is maintained unless the biochemical abnormality is severe. Ultimately, as in all forms of overdose, respiration is depressed.

Treatment.—Therapeutic measures include gastric lavage and intravenous fluid therapy to correct dehydration, electrolyte losses and acid-base disturbances. These changes can best be managed if repeated blood pH and P_{CO_2} or standard bicarbonate measurements are carried out. Intravenous sodium bicarbonate is especially valuable both to correct the metabolic acidosis and to alkalinise the urine, which promotes salicylate excretion. Diuretics are not usually indicated and may actually be harmful, especially in children, as they may add to the fluid and electrolyte disturbances.

Rehydration is effected with 5 per cent dextrose solution with the addition of sodium bicarbonate and potassium chloride to correct acidosis and hypokalaemia. Sodium bicarbonate is indicated if the arterial blood pH is less than 7·5 and urinary pH less than 7·6. In severe intoxication accompanied by renal failure, haemodialysis is required, while in children in the presence of coma and hyperpyrexia, artificial ventilation may be indicated.

Paracetamol (Acetaminophen USP, Panadol)

Paracetamol is an antipyretic analgesic which has no anti-inflammatory action. Most individuals find it to be a less effective analgesic than aspirin, but it is very popular and widely used, both by prescription and across the counter, owing to its freedom from side-effects in normal doses and lack of drug interactions. It does not cause gastric irritation or bleeding and may be taken with oral anticoagulants and steroids. There are thus no contra-indications to its use. Unlike aspirin it is of no value in the treatment of rheumatoid arthritis, though both aspirin and paracetamol may be used to treat post-operative pain once the worst is over and medication can be taken by mouth. Paracetamol tablets contain 0·5 g and two tablets may be taken four times a day.

The one serious disadvantage of paracetamol is its toxicity in acute overdose. In recent years it became increasingly popular among those making suicide bids and now more than 1000 cases of paracetamol poisoning are admitted to hospital annually in England and Wales, of which at least 3 per cent die (Douglas et al., 1976). The major and notable danger of acute paracetamol overdose is hepatotoxicity which may occur after as few as 12 to 14 tablets. This is caused by toxic products of intermediary metabolism which accumulate in the liver when the normal metabolic pathways are saturated. After the overdose has been taken consciousness is not lost, and no effect is normally observed for the first few days, after which liver damage may become apparent and occasionally leads to hepatic coma and death. Treatment is extremely difficult and cannot be successful once severe liver damage has occurred. It is aimed at (i) limiting the absorption of paracetamol from the gastro-intestinal tract in the early stages with oral cholestyramine or activated charcoal, (ii) removing it from the blood by charcoal haemoperfusion, haemodialysis or diuresis, and (iii) reducing hepatotoxicity with steroids or cysteamine. Few of these procedures have proved to be of value though the use of cysteamine, itself a rather toxic substance, appears to be very successful provided it is given within 10 hours of the ingestion of paracetamol (Prescott *et al.*, 1974). More recently Douglas *et al.* (1976) recommended the usual supportive measures and in particular 5 per cent dextrose intravenously and nothing by mouth.

Phenacetin

Phenacetin used to be present in many compound analgesic tablets and was rarely used alone. Compound tablets containing phenacetin have now been withdrawn because of the danger of renal damage with continued use.

Compound Analgesic Preparations

Numerous preparations are available which contain combinations of two or more analgesics and other odds and ends, and may include aspirin, paracetamol, codeine, dextropropoxyphene (*vide infra*) and other analgesics and caffeine. Their analgesic effects summate and in some instances preparations are formulated to reduce gastric irritation from aspirin. For example Safapryn contains paracetamol in the outer layer and aspirin in the core, while benorylate is a chemical combination of aspirin with paracetamol, which is only broken down after absorption. This preparation is in a liquid form and fairly well tolerated by many, though liable to give symptoms of aspirin toxicity (Aylward, 1973).

Anti-inflammatory Agents

There is a large number of drugs of little use as analgesics except in the treatment of inflammatory conditions such as rheumatoid arthritis. All produce gastric irritation in proportion to their efficacy as anti-inflammatory agents. Phenylbutazone is one of the oldest and produces a surfeit of side-effects the most dangerous of which is hypersensitivity-type bone marrow depression. It may also produce rashes, diarrhoea and fluid retention. Indomethacin is now more commonly used since hypersensitivity to it is rare. Other preparations include ibuprofen, alclofenac, mefenamic acid, oxyphenbutazone.

NARCOTIC ANALGESICS

The second group of analgesics includes a collection of drugs related to morphine either chemically, in their effects or both.

They have certain chemical similarities, for example all are tertiary amines. They may be classified chemically into the following groups.

1. Natural alkaloids, the opiates (phenanthrene derivatives)	morphine codeine
2. Semi-synthetic derivatives:	heroin dihydrocodeine oxymorphone
3. Synthetic compounds: a. morphinans	levorphanol
b. benzmorphans	phenazocine pentazocine

  c. phenylpiperidine derivatives   pethidine
                                                       phenoperidine
                                                       fentanyl

  d. diphenyl compounds   methadone
                                                       dextromoramide
                                                       dextropropoxyphene

They vary in their efficacy as analgesics: while some such as codeine and dextropropoxyphene have a low ceiling effect, and can relieve only mild pain even in maximally effective dosage, others typified by morphine are capable of much greater analgesia and may be used to treat severe pain due to injury, operation, childbirth or burns. Morphine is generally taken as the standard with which the others are compared. It produces a number of side-effects, which are possessed by the rest to a greater or lesser degree. They may induce drug dependence to an extent related to their euphoriant effect, and also, regrettably, to their efficacy as analgesics. The maximum respiratory depressant effect tends to be related to the maximum degree of analgesia of which each is capable; thus with codeine maximum respiratory depression and analgesia are mild while with fentanyl, at the other end of the scale, both are profound. There is some variation in the sedative effect, but this may depend as much upon the individual as upon the drug. There is variation in absorption from the gastro-intestinal tract. Some such as heroin and methadone are well absorbed by mouth. Others such as morphine may be conjugated in the gut wall and little is absorbed unchanged. Those that are less well absorbed are more likely to produce constipation. Finally they vary in their duration of action, morphine, lasting about 4 hours, being intermediate in duration.

A number of N-allyl derivatives of narcotic antagonists are in use. These have *narcotic antagonist* and *partial agonist* activity and are described later (p. 1057). The actions of morphine will be described first, and the remainder compared with it.

Morphine

Morphine is the principal alkaloid contained in opium, of which it forms 10 per cent by weight. Opium is the dried powder derived from the milky exudate of the seed capsule of the poppy *Papaver somniferum*.

Morphine produces its major effects on the central nervous system and the bowel. It is believed to act on specific opiate receptors to produce its characteristic pattern of effects. It is probable that such functions are normally subserved by pentapeptides known as enkephalins, which occur in the brain and produce a similar spectrum of effects (Snyder, 1975).

Analgesia.—It produces analgesia without impairing consciousness, although as the name narcotic implies it may induce drowsiness in many individuals. It is especially effective in combating dull, aching pain and less effective in sharp, intermittent pain. Unlike the mild analgesics it relieves visceral pain. It can elevate the pain threshold experimentally but it is much more effective when an element of fear is also present (Beecher, 1957). The concomitant rise in Pa_{CO_2} also raises the pain threshold. The powerful effect of morphine upon mood is probably much more important than its effect on the pain threshold. It reduces the response to pain in reducing anxiety and dulling attention while inducing relaxation.

Mood.—Morphine reduces worry, fear, hunger and fatigue and generally induces a drowsy and detached tranquillity. Accompanying this in most individuals is quite marked euphoria and associated with it a liability to produce dependence. While a very few individuals may be "hooked" after a single dose, physical dependence can be produced in all after a large number of doses. The sedative effect is species-dependent: cats and a few humans are stimulated by morphine. *The respiratory centre* is depressed, leading to a reduction in the respiratory rate and minute volume. In therapeutic doses, the tidal volume is not necessarily decreased and may even be increased. The sensitivity of the respiratory centre to CO_2 is decreased and though the minute volume may appear to be within normal limits it will be found to be associated with a raised Pa_{CO_2}. Respiratory depression is progressive with increasing doses and is the principal toxic effect of overdose, after which the respiratory rate may fall to three per minute. *Cough* is also markedly depressed.

Other brain-stem effects.—Morphine produces pin-point pupils because it stimulates the Edinger-Westphal nucleus—the parasympathetic nucleus of the oculo-motor nerve. The chemoreceptor emetic trigger zone is stimulated, often producing nausea and vomiting, but because the vomiting centre is later depressed, this effect does not usually occur beyond the first dose. Vomiting is commoner in women than in men and in ambulant than in resting patients. Morphine should only be given therefore to those confined to bed. The vaso-motor centre is only slightly depressed except in the presence of severe respiratory depression with brain-stem hypoxia.

Cardiovascular system.—Morphine releases histamine which may produce peripheral vasodilatation and a warm itching skin. This property, coupled with mild vasomotor centre depression, may occasionally produce postural hypotension, and hypotension after haemorrhage. In the normal recumbent subject, blood pressure is not reduced unless severe respiratory depression produces medullary hypoxia. Dilatation of capacitance vessels may contribute to the beneficial effect of morphine in acute left ventricular failure.

Gastro-intestinal tract.—Visceral muscle tone is increased, especially at the pyloric and ileo-caecal sphincters. Furthermore, peristalsis throughout the gastro-intestinal tract is reduced, so causing delay in gastric emptying and constipation. The muscle tone of the biliary ducts is increased and the sphincter of Oddi is contracted, effects which may aggravate the pain of biliary colic. Powerful peristaltic waves may be generated in segments of colon affected by diverticulosis, under the influence of morphine, and the high intrasigmoid pressures so created may cause pronounced distension of the diverticula and an increased risk of perforation (Painter *et al.*, 1965).

Overdose.—After an overdose of morphine the respiratory rate is extremely slow and the patient may become comatose, hypotensive and cyanosed. The respiratory depression, coupled with pin-point pupils, is usually diagnostic of narcotic overdose, though *in extremis* the pupils may dilate. A reduced tolerance to morphine is the most usual cause of such toxicity. Intense pain may antagonise the side-effects of morphine and the patient may require increasing doses of the drug. With a reduction in pain, tolerance is diminished and the patient may show signs of overdose. In acute coronary thrombosis such a collapse may be ascribed to the disease rather than to morphine, and similarly in the post-operative period surgical shock and blood loss may be incorrectly blamed. An addict becomes tolerant of narcotics, and may require vastly increasing doses. After a period of abstinence, sensitivity is restored, and if the addict then gives himself his previous dose, acute toxicity ensues.

Narcotic overdose should be treated with a narcotic antagonist (*vide infra*) as well as with the usual supportive measures.

Absorption, distribution and fate.—Morphine is poorly absorbed from the gastro-intestinal tract because it is conjugated in the gut wall (Brunk and Delle, 1974). For an analgesic effect therefore it must be given by injection. As a basic drug, it is quite extensively taken up in the tissues, readily crosses the blood-brain barrier though not as rapidly as heroin, and crosses the placenta to the fetus, who is highly susceptible to its respiratory depressant effects. Having free −OH groups, morphine is conjugated in the liver and the conjugated metabolites are rapidly excreted by the kidneys.

Uses.—The tranquillising effect of morphine makes it an excellent premedicant; moreover its analgesic property is a useful adjunct to anaesthesia. Probably its greatest value is in the treatment of severe pain due for example to myocardial infarction, injury, surgery and terminal cancer. It is little used in obstetrics, in which pethidine is the preferred narcotic in most centres. It is an effective cough suppressant, but other related drugs such as codeine or pholcodine, with more specific antitussive effects and less addiction liability, are to be preferred. It is sometimes used in the treatment of dyspnoea associated with acute left ventricular failure and pulmonary oedema, in which both the reduced respiratory drive and the cardiovascular effect described above are valuable. It may be used to facilitate controlled respiration, as depressing the respiratory centre may help to stop the patient fighting the ventilator, when prolonged mechanical ventilation is required in intensive care. Finally, morphine is an excellent remedy for diarrhoea, for which purpose it is taken orally in kaolin and morphine mixture or in Chlorodyne, which cause minimal systemic effects.

Contra-indications and dangers.—Narcotics should not be used in the control of chronic pain in non-terminal conditions, such as various musculo-skeletal disorders, because the risk of producing dependence is too great. In such conditions aspirin, indomethacin or even steroids are to be preferred.

In subjects receiving morphine regularly the risk of addiction must be constantly borne in mind. The onset of tolerance gives warning that addiction is developing. When satisfactory relief cannot be obtained with other analgesics the risk of addiction must be accepted, especially in the terminal stages of cancer when a fatal outcome is inevitable in a matter of months.

Narcotics should be avoided in acute asthmatic attacks and acute or chronic bronchitis and emphysema, not because of any effect upon the airways but because in such patients respiratory drive must be preserved otherwise carbon dioxide narcosis may be precipitated. Moreover obese and scoliotic patients may be quite disastrously sensitive to the respiratory depressant effects of even small doses of narcotics.

Morphine and all allied drugs are contra-indicated in head injury in the absence of controlled ventilation, because the CO_2 retention they produce causes cerebral vasodilatation and so increases the intracranial pressure. Exactly the same danger exists in eclampsia.

So long as the dose is administered on a body-weight basis, age makes little difference to narcotic sensitivity. Those with adrenocortical and thyroid deficiencies require reduced doses, which should probably also be used in renal failure, to avoid accumulation of conjugates. Patients with hepatic disease may require a reduced frequency of dosage, but hepatic disease does not always impair drug inactivation.

Dosage.—The usual dose of morphine is 0·1–0·2 mg/kg though more than this may be required in resistant individuals. It may be given 4-hourly by intramuscular or subcutaneous injection, though in the presence of severe vasoconstriction absorption from subcutaneous tissues may be very slow and small divided intravenous doses are preferred. One-ml ampoules may contain 10, 15, 20, or 30 mg of morphine sulphate. Morphine sulphate contains 75 per cent of anhydrous morphine base.

Other Morphine Preparations

Papaveretum (Omnopon, Opoidine).—This consists of all the water-soluble alkaloids of opium (morphine, codeine, papaverine, thebaine, narcotine, etc.) in the same proportions as they are in opium, and is standardised to contain 50 per cent of anhydrous morphine. The contribution of the other constituents to the overall effect of papaveretum is minimal. The adult dose of papaveretum is 10–20 mg, and that for a child 0·25 mg/kg. For premedication 10 mg of papaveretum combined with hyoscine 0·4 mg gives good sedation for the average adult and a lower incidence of nausea and oversedation than when 20 mg of papaveretum is used.

Nepenthe.—Nepenthe is a liquid preparation of the opium alkaloids with added morphine such that one ml of nepenthe contains 8·4 mg of anhydrous morphine. It is thus slightly stronger than the ordinary preparation of morphine sulphate 10 mg/ml and has no advantage over it for paediatric administration.

Codeine

Codeine, or methyl morphine, is a homologue of morphine in which the −OH group on the benzene ring is replaced with −OCH$_3$.

The analgesic effect of codeine is very weak and resides in part in the very small proportion of codeine which is converted to morphine in the liver. Codeine does not normally produce sedation, euphoria, addiction or marked respiratory depression though it is an effective cough suppressant and usually causes constipation.

The analgesic dose of 60 mg of codeine phosphate serves no useful purpose for pain relief though it may help to suppress diarrhoea. 8–10 mg of codeine, present in various proprietory compound analgesic tablets, can have little analgesic effect. Codeine linctus, for cough suppression, contains 15 mg codeine phosphate per 5 ml dose.

Heroin (Diamorphine Hydrochloride)

Heroin is available legally in few western countries outside Great Britain but several differences from morphine make it valuable in certain fields of medicine.

In heroin, the two hydroxyl groups of morphine are replaced by acetyl (CH_3 COO$-$) groups. This chemical alteration makes heroin more lipid-soluble, more readily and completely absorbed from the gastro-intestinal tract (until de-acetylated it cannot be conjugated) and more rapid in its passage across the blood-brain barrier. It has a high ceiling for analgesia and produces less vomiting, constipation and sedation than morphine, but a very marked degree of euphoria. It is active as the unchanged drug and also as monoacetyl morphine and morphine to which it is broken down.

Its rapid onset of action and high-ceiling effect undoubtedly contribute to its worldwide popularity as a drug of abuse. However its oral effectiveness and relative freedom from side-effects make it of special value in the treatment of pain in terminal malignant disease, and in combination with cocaine it is of remarkable benefit. It is also used in a few centres in Great Britain for obstetric pain relief.

It is of similar potency to morphine.

Dihydrocodeine (DF 118)

This is a semisynthetic derivative of codeine with superior analgesic activity. It is therefore an analgesic of intermediate activity producing little respiratory depression and dependence liability. Although useful for the latter reason in chronic pain, constipation can be a problem. It may be taken orally or by injection in a dose of 30–60 mg.

Oxymorphone

This is a very potent morphine analogue with a high ceiling for analgesia and side-effects. It is little used clinically but its N-allyl derivative, naloxone (*vide infra*) is the first pure antagonist in therapeutic use.

Levorphanol

The properties of levorphanol are similar to those of phenazocine and methadone (*vide infra*) and because it is older it is less used nowadays. Its N-allyl derivative levallorphan, however, is in clinical use as an antagonist.

Phenazocine (Narphen)

Phenazocine is of similar efficacy as an analgesic to morphine but is effective orally, produces less sedation and has a longer duration of action. The incidence of other side-effects is similar. Two mg are equivalent to 10 mg of morphine by injection and the oral dose is usually 5 mg.

Pentazocine (Fortral)

Pentazocine was first tested in animals as a narcotic antagonist but was found in man to be a partial agonist with useful analgesic activity. It was originally hoped that it would be as effective an analgesic as morphine but with less risk of addiction and severe respiratory depression. In practice it is intermediate in its efficacy as an analgesic: less effective than morphine and similar to or slightly better than dihydrocodeine. It also produces only slight respiratory depression and neither of these effects is augmented by increasing the dose. Hypertension rather than hypotension may be produced (Keats and Telford, 1964). It produces little or no euphoria, but quite substantial dysphoria in a few individuals. Addiction is rare and typical physical dependence is not seen.

Unlike pure narcotic agonists, its effects cannot be reversed by nalorphine or levallorphan, but naloxone is effective.

It is indicated in the treatment of chronic pain of intermediate severity when dependence must be avoided. It is also used in obstetrics. It produces less effective pain relief than pethidine, but fewer side-effects, and crosses the placenta less (see Chapter 44). It is of briefer duration than pethidine and less cumulative.

Because of its flat dose response curve, 20–60 mg may be equivalent to 10 mg of morphine by injection, while the oral dose is 25–100 mg. Because of its extremely brief duration it is rarely given with sufficient frequency.

Pethidine (Meperidine USP, Demerol)

The effects of pethidine are very similar to those of morphine, the principal difference being that both analgesia and side-effects are of briefer duration. The sedative and tranquillising effects are almost as good, and though the incidence of nausea, vomiting, dry mouth, hypotension and dizziness is transiently higher than after morphine, the duration of these side-effects is briefer (Dundee et al., 1965). Respiratory depression, though as profound, is of shorter duration than with morphine, and pethidine cannot usefully suppress the cough reflex. Euphoria cannot be as reliably produced by pethidine as by morphine and heroin, nevertheless pethidine is widely used.

Pethidine does not cause gastro-intestinal tract spasm as does morphine; it is less likely to produce constipation and cannot be used to treat diarrhoea. It has no spasmolytic action in therapeutic doses, and cannot relax the sphincter of Oddi, though it is probably preferable to morphine for biliary colic. It does not produce meiosis. One serious disadvantage of pethidine is its dangerous interaction with monoamine oxidase inhibitors. Pethidine given to patients taking this type of antidepressant may produce coma, convulsions, hypertension, hyperpyrexia and occasionally hypotension and respiratory depression. The mechanism is probably an interaction occurring within the brain where pethidine inhibits neuronal 5-HT re-uptake, an action not shared by opiates or pentazocine (Gong and Rogers, 1973). Although monoamine oxidase inhibitors may slightly retard the metabolism of all narcotics, they do not contra-indicate the cautious use of any except pethidine and dextromethorphan, a cough suppressant.

Pethidine, having no −OH groups, cannot be directly conjugated by the liver, though it is fairly rapidly broken down by this organ. A principal product of its metabolism, nor-pethidine, is itself a convulsant, and may contribute to the apparent stimulant effect of pethidine in overdose.

Pethidine may be used for analgesia in all the situations in which morphine is used, though for most patients it has no advantages over morphine, except in the case of biliary colic. It has been found useful in combating the tachypnoea that may develop during trichloroethylene anaesthesia. The important place it has in obstetric analgesia is hallowed by tradition. The effects it may have upon the fetus and neonate are far-reaching (see Chapter 42) but it is the preferred narcotic in this field if only because experience with it is so extensive.

Pethidine is one-tenth as potent as morphine and the dose is 1·5–2·0 mg/kg. Though sometimes taken by mouth in 25 or 50 mg tablets, it has no merit by this route and only about half reaches the systemic circulation unchanged (Moore and Nation, 1976).

Phenoperidine (Operidine) and Fentanyl (Sublimaze)

Both these agents produce profound analgesia and respiratory depression, and occasionally muscular rigidity. The action of phenoperidine is very long while that of fentanyl is considerably briefer. Thus while fentanyl may be used as a supplement to anaesthesia, phenoperidine has a place during controlled ventilation after major surgery. Both are used in conjunction with butyrophenones for neuroleptanalgesia. The dose of phenoperidine is 1–2 mg and that of fentanyl 0·1–0·2 mg. Brief though the action of fentanyl is, it will depress respiration in the post-operative period if used excessively during anaesthesia.

Methadone (Physeptone, Amidone)

Methadone is similar to morphine in potency and in many of its actions but in general the onset and cessation of its effects are more gradual, and the total duration is much longer. It is effective orally and sedation and constipation are less conspicuous. It is a powerful cough suppressant and may be taken in a linctus for severe intractable cough. It is useful orally in the treatment of severe chronic pain and is also used extensively in the treatment of heroin dependence. It can prevent withdrawal symptoms in an addict, while its own withdrawal symptoms are relatively gradual and mild. Although weaning from methadone which has successfully replaced heroin may not always be possible, the methadone addict can generally carry on a more normal life.

Dextromoramide (Palfium)

Dextromoramide is similar to morphine in most actions, but of briefer duration, less sedative and constipating and is as effective orally as parenterally. The adult dose is about 5 mg.

Dextropropoxyphene (Propoxyphene USP)

Propoxyphene is a mild analgesic, similar to codeine; the d-isomer possesses the analgesic activity. Dextropropoxyphene is present in Distalgesic tablets in a dose of 32·5 mg per tablet, in combination with 325 mg of paracetamol. The effect of 65 mg of dextropropoxyphene alone is better than that of placebo (Wang, 1974), and there is no doubt that as Distalgesic it has become extremely popular in Great Britain in recent years. A proportion of its effectiveness may stem from the marked placebo effect of the coffin-shaped tablets. Overdose of

Distalgesic can produce dangerous respiratory depression (Hunt, 1973), and once this is surmounted there is of course a risk of hepatic damage from the paracetamol it contains.

TOLERANCE AND DEPENDENCE

Tolerance to all the effects of morphine-like drugs, with the possible exception of constipation, is readily acquired with continuous but not with intermittent use. Tolerance to the emetic effects occurs very quickly, while that to respiratory depression occurs more slowly but is present to an extent anyway in the presence of severe pain. Tolerance to the analgesic and euphoriant effects usually heralds the onset of dependence. Although on occasion almost any drug may induce psychological dependence, a narcotic agonist will, after days or weeks of continuous administration, produce both psychological and physical dependence. On withdrawal, severe withdrawal symptoms result; these can be suppressed by the administration of another narcotic agonist. A partial agonist such as pentazocine cannot prevent withdrawal symptoms. If an addict is given a narcotic *antagonist*, withdrawal symptoms are precipitated. These typically consist of running eyes, nose and mouth, sweating, gooseflesh, anxiety, restlessness, dilated pupils, nausea, vomiting, abdominal and muscle cramps. When methadone is substituted for heroin in the treatment of addiction, and then withdrawn, symptoms are mild and rarely worse than an influenza-like illness.

NARCOTIC ANTAGONISTS

Nalorphine (N-allylnormorphine:Lethidrone) and Levallorphan (N-allylnorlevorphanol:Lorfan)

In these two compounds an allyl ($-CH_2CH = CH_2$) group replaces the $-CH_3$ group in the nitrogen atom of the parent compound. Such a change confers antagonist properties on the molecule; both these substances however are partial agonists, possessing some agonist properties when given alone or with therapeutic doses of pure agonists, but possessing antagonist activity when given with large doses of agonists. They possess more *antagonist* activity than does pentazocine. Each can antagonise the effects of any narcotic agonist (but not the effects of a partial agonist such as pentazocine). The explanation for such behaviour is that a partial agonist possesses higher affinity for opiate receptors than does a pure agonist, but lower efficacy. Thus its effects summate with those of a small dose of agonist, but after a large dose of agonist a partial agonist displaces many molecules of agonist from receptors thus substituting for a profound narcotic effect its own low-ceiling effect.

When given alone both nalorphine and levallorphan produce analgesia and mild respiratory depression, meiosis and some vomiting. These effects are not enhanced by increasing the dose. They are not useful as analgesics, however, as both usually produce dysphoria. When given with normal pain-relieving doses of a narcotic, the effects are variable, but adverse effects may be enhanced while analgesia is antagonised, thus necessitating bigger doses of the agonist. When given after toxic doses of a narcotic, respiratory depression is reduced to a non-life-threatening level and meiosis reversed. If given to an addict, marked dysphoria and severe withdrawal symptoms are precipitated.

The only clinical use of these two agents is therefore in the treatment of narcotic poisoning.

Levallorphan is more potent and longer-acting than nalorphine whose antagonism of morphine-induced respiratory depression lasts from 1 to 4 hours. The dose of nalorphine is 5–40 mg and that of levallorphan 1–2 mg. The latter, only, is effective orally.

Neonates are very susceptible to the respiratory depressant effects of narcotic analgesics given to mothers in labour. When neonatal respiratory depression can be attributed to this, nalorphine can be given in a dose of 0·2 mg into the umbilical vein after birth. It may however render the baby dysphoric for some hours. There can be no excuse, however, for giving the antagonist to the mother before delivery. This is simply asking her to make the appropriate dilution of the drug herself, before passing it across the placenta. She herself is not suffering from respiratory depression, and she needs all the analgesia she can get.

Nalorphine and levallorphan are contra-indicated in the treatment of respiratory depression due to drugs other than narcotic agonists, as their own depressant effect may summate with that of other drugs. They are also in-effective in pentazocine overdose.

Narcotic-antagonist combinations.—There are no indications for the use of narcotic analgesic-antagonist combinations, such as Pethilorfan (pethidine and levallorphan) in clinical practice. There is no reduction in side-effects or neonatal depression and slight antagonism of the analgesia may necessitate increasing doses (Telford and Keats, 1961).

Naloxone (Narcan)

Naloxone is the N-allyl derivative of oxymorphone and is a potent and highly effective narcotic antagonist that appears to be free from agonist activity. When given alone it produces neither analgesia nor respiratory depression and neither euphoria nor dysphoria.

Naloxone, unlike partial agonists, can reverse respiratory depression due to pentazocine overdose and has also been found useful in dextropropoxyphene (in Distalgesic) poisoning (Tarala and Forrest, 1973).

It would thus appear to be the agent of choice in obstetrics, anaesthesia and drug overdose because it rapidly reverses the effects of a narcotic and has no effect if depression is due to something else. Its one disadvantage is its somewhat brief duration of action, which may be as short as 20 minutes (Evans et al., 1974).

In obstetrics it is highly effective given to the neonate in whom it produces no dysphoria and even reverses such effects of pethidine as depression of the suckling reflex. As with nalorphine and levallorphan it should be given to baby rather than mother for the same reasons as are given above.

Naloxone may be given intramuscularly in a dose of 5–6 μg/kg or intra-venously in a dose of $1\frac{1}{2}$–3 μg/kg which may need to be repeated at intervals until the effects of the narcotic have worn off.

ADJUNCTS TO ANALGESIC DRUGS

Many drugs have been used from time to time in combination with analgesics, in an attempt to potentiate the analgesia and alleviate the side-effects. Antihistamines such as cyclizine, phenothiazines such as promazine and promethazine (Chapter 23) and anti-cholinergics such as hyoscine have all been used. All may combat nausea and vomiting, but enhance the respiratory depressant, sedative and hypotensive effects and constipation. Moreover promethazine has a mild anti-analgesic action (Keats *et al.*, 1961), and narcotic-induced emesis is not readily reversed by antihistamines, such as cyclizine or promethazine.

REFERENCES

ADRIAN, E. D. (1931). The messages in sensory nerve fibres and their interpretation. *Proc. roy. Soc. B.*, **109**, 1.

ARMSTRONG, D., DRY, R. M. L., KEELE, C. A., and MARKHAM, J. W. (1953). Observations on chemical excitants of cutaneous pain in man. *J. Physiol. (Lond.)*, **120**, 326.

ARMSTRONG, D., JEPSON, J. B., KEELE, C. A., and STEWART, J. W. (1957). Pain-producing substance in human inflammatory exudates and plasma. *J. Physiol. (Lond.)*, **135**, 350.

AYLWARD, M. (1973). Toxicity of benorylate (letter). *Brit. med. J.*, **2**, 118.

BEECHER, H. K. (1956). Relationship of significance of wound to pain experienced. *J. Amer. med. Ass.*, **161**, 1609.

BEECHER, H. K. (1957). The measurement of pain. *Pharmacol. Rev.*, **9**, 59.

BEECHER, H. K. (1959). *Measurement of subjective responses: quantitative effects of drugs.* New York: Oxford University Press.

BONNYCASTLE, D. D. (1962). *The Assessment of Pain in Man and Animals* (Proc. Internat. Symp. held under auspices of UFAW, Middlesex Hosp. Med. School, 1961), p. 231. Ed. by C. A. Keele and R. Smith. Edinburgh: E. & S. Livingstone.

BRAIN, R. (1962). *The Assessment of Pain in Man and Animals* (Proc. Internat. Symp. held under auspices of UFAW, Middlesex Hosp. Med. School, 1961), p. 9. Ed. by C. A. Keele and R. Smith. Edinburgh: E. & S. Livingstone.

BRUNK, S. F., and DELLE, M. (1974). Morphine metabolism in man. *Clin. Pharmacol. Ther.*, **16**, 51.

CHARPENTIER, J. (1968). In: *Pain* (Proc. Internat. Symp. organised by the Lab. of Psychophysiol., Faculty of Sciences, Paris, 1967), p. 171. Ed. by A. Soulairac, A. Cahn and J. Charpentier. New York: Academic Press.

COHEN, H., and JONES, H. W. (1943). The reference of cardiac pain to a phantom left arm. *Brit. Heart J.*, **5**, 67.

DEVINE, R., and MERSKEY, H. (1965). The description of pain in psychiatric and general medical patients. *J. psychosom. Res.*, **9**, 311.

DOUGLAS, A. P., HAMLYN, A. N., and JAMES, O. (1976). Controlled trial of cysteamine in treatment of acute paracetamol (acetaminophen) poisoning. *Lancet*, **1**, 111.

DUNDEE, J. W., CLARKE, R. S. J., and LOAN, W. B. (1965). A comparison of the sedative and toxic effects of morphine and pethidine. *Lancet*, **2**, 1262.

EVANS, J. M., HOGG, M. I. J., LUNN, J. N., and ROSEN, M. (1974). Degree and duration of reversal by naloxone of effects of morphine in conscious subjects. *Brit. med. J.*, **2**, 589.

FERREIRA, S. H. (1972). Prostaglandins, aspirin-like drugs and analgesia. *Nature (New Biol.)*, **240**, 200.

FORD, F. R., and WILKINS, L. (1938). Congenital universal insensitiveness to pain. *Bull. Johns Hopk. Hosp.*, **62**, 448.

FRASER, H. F., and HARRIS, L. S. (1967). Narcotic and narcotic antagonist analgesics. *Ann. Rev. Pharmacol.*, **7**, 277.

GASSER, H. S. (1943). Pain producing impulses in peripheral nerves. *Ass. Res. nerv. Dis. Proc.*, **23**, 44.

GELLHORN, E. (1953). *Physiological Foundations of Neurology and Psychiatry*. Minneapolis: Univ. Minnesota Press.

GONG, S. N. C., and ROGERS, K. J. (1973). Role of brain monoamines in the fatal hyperthermia induced by pethidine or imipramine in rabbits pretreated with a monoamine oxidase inhibitor. *Brit. J. Pharmacol.* **48**, 12.

GRUBER, C. M. (1962). The design of experiments evaluating analgesics. *Anesthesiology*, **23**, 711.

HAGBARTH, K. E., and KERR, D. I. B. (1954). Central influences of spinal afferent conduction. *J. Neurophysiol.*, **17**, 295.

HARDY, J. D., GOODELL, H., and WOLFF, H. G. (1951). Influence of skin temperature upon pain threshold as evoked by thermal radiation. *Science*, **114**, 149.

HARMAN, J. B. (1948). The localisation of deep pain. *Brit. med. J.*, **1**, 188.

HARMAN, J. B. (1951). Angina in the analgesic limb. *Brit. med. J.*, **2**, 521.

HEAD, H. (1920). *Studies in Neurology*. London: Oxford University Press.

HOLMES, T. H., and WOLFF, H. G. (1950). Life situations, emotions and backaches. *Ass. Res. nerv. Dis. Proc.*, **29**, 750.

HUNT, V. (1973). Treatment of dextropropoxyphene poisoning. *Brit. med. J.*, **1**, 554.

HUSKISSON, E. C., and WOJTULEWSKI, J. A. (1974). Measurement of side effects of drugs. *Brit. med. J.*, **2**, 698.

IGGO, A. (1972). In: *Pain*. Ed. Janzen, R., Keidel, W. D., Herz, A., and Streichele, C. London: Churchill-Livingstone.

JOYCE, C. R. B., ZUTSHI, D. W., HRUBES, V., and MASON, R. M. (1975). Comparison of fixed interval and visual analogue scales for rating chronic pain. *Europ. J. clin. Pharmacol.* **8**, 415.

KEATS, A. S., and TELFORD, J. (1964). Studies of analgesic drugs. VIII. A narcotic antagonist analgesic without psychotomimetic effects. *J. Pharmacol. exp. Ther.*, **143**, 157.

KEATS, A. S., TELFORD, J., and KUROSO, Y. (1961). "Potentiation" of meperidine by promethazine. *Anesthesiology*, **22**, 34.

KERR, F. W. L., and MILLER, R. H. (1966). The pathology of trigeminal neuralgia. *Arch. Neurol. (Chic.)*, **15**, 308.

KUNKLE, E. C., and CHAPMAN, W. P. (1943). Insensitivity to pain in man. *Ass. Res. nerv. Dis. Proc.*, **23**, 100.

LANDAU, W. M., and BISHOP, G. H. (1953). Pain from dermal, periosteal and fascial endings and from inflammation; electrophysiological study employing differential nerve blocks. *A.M.A. Arch. Neurol. Psychiat.*, **69**, 490.

LASAGNA, L. (1964). Clinical evaluation of morphine and its substitutes as analgesics. *Pharmacol. Rev.*, **16**, 47.

LASAGNA, L. (1970). Challenges in drug evaluation in man. *Ann. Rev. Pharmacol.*, **10**, 413.

LERICHE, R. (1949). *La Chirurgie de la Douleur*. Paris: Masson et Cie.

LOAN, W. B., and DUNDEE, J. W. (1967). The value of the study of postoperative pain in the assessment of analgesics. *Brit. J. Anaesth.*, **39**, 743.

MAJOR, V., ROSEN, M., and MUSHIN, W. W. (1966). Methoxyflurane as an obstetric analgesic: a comparison with trichloroethylene. *Brit. med. J.*, **2**, 1554.

MATTHEW, H., and LAWSON, A. A. H. (1970). *Treatment of Common Acute Poisonings*. Edinburgh: E. & S. Livingstone.

MELZACK, R., and WALL, P. D. (1965). Pain mechanisms: a new theory. *Science*, **150**, 971.

MELZACK, R., and WALL, P. D. (1968). Gate control theory of pain. In: *Pain* (Proc. Internat. Symp. organised by the Lab. of Psychophysiol., Faculty of Sciences, Paris, 1967), p. 11. Ed. by A. Soulairac, A. Cahn and J. Charpentier. New York: Academic Press.

MENDELL, J. L., and WALL, P. D. (1964). Presynaptic hyperpolarization: a role for fine afferent fibres. *J. Physiol. (Lond.)*, **172**, 274.

MERSKEY, H. (1968). Psychological aspects of pain. *Postgrad. med. J.*, **44,** 297.

MERSKEY, H., and SPEAR, F. G. (1967). The concept of pain. *J. psychosom. Res.,* **11**, 59.

MOORE, G., and NATION, R. (1976). Pharmacokinetics of meperidine in man. *Clin. Pharmacol. Ther.*, **19,** 246.

MULLER, J. (1840). *Handbuch der Physiologie des Menschen*, **2**, 249.

PARKHOUSE, J., and HOLMES, C. M. (1963). Assessing post-operative pain relief. *Proc. roy. Soc. Med.*, **56**, 579.

PAINTER, N. S., TRUELOVE, S. C., ARDRON, G. M., and TUCKEY, M. (1965). Effect of morphine, prostigmine, pethidine and probanthine on the human colon in diverticulosis. *Gut*, **6,** 57.

PRESCOTT, L. F., NEWTON, R. W., SWAINSON, C. P., WRIGHT, N., FORREST, A. R. W., and MATTHEW, H. (1974). Successful treatment of severe paracetamol overdosage with cysteamine. *Lancet*, **1,** 588.

RUCH, T. C., and FULTON, J. F. (1960). *Medical Physiology and Biophysics*. Philadelphia: W. B. Saunders Co.

SCHIFF, M. (1848). *Lehrbuch der Physiologie, Muskel und Nervenphysiologie*. Schavenburg., Fahr., **1,** 228.

SCHMIDT, R. F. (1972). In: *Pain*, Ed. Janzen, R., Keidel, W. D., Herz, A., and Streichele, C. London: Churchill-Livingstone.

SHERRINGTON, C. (1906). *The Integrative Action of the Central Nervous System*. London: Constable & Co.

SMITH, G. M., EGBERT, L. D., MARKOWITZ, R. A., MOSTELLER, F., and BEECHER, H. K. (1966). An experimental pain method sensitive to morphine in man: the submaximal effort tourniquet technique. *J. Pharmacol. exp. Ther.*, **154,** 324.

SOULAIRAC, A. (1968). In: *Pain* (Proc. Internat. Symp. organised by the Lab. of Psychophysiol., Faculty of Sciences, Paris, 1967), p. 5. Ed. by A. Soulairac, A. Cahn and J. Charpentier. New York: Academic Press.

SNYDER, S. H. (1975). Opiate receptor in normal and drug altered brain function. *Nature (Lond.)*, **257**, 185.

TARALA, R., and FORREST, J. A. H. (1973). Treatment of dextropropoxyphene poisoning. (Letter). *Brit. med. J.*, **2**, 550.

TELFORD, J., and KEATS, A. S. (1961). Narcotic-narcotic antagonist mixtures. *Anesthesiology*, **22**, 465.

VANE, J. R. (1971). Inhibitions of prostaglandin synthesis as a mechanism of action for aspirin-like drugs. *Nature (New Biol.)*, **231,** 232.

WALL, P. D. (1962). The origin of a spinal-cord slow potential. *J. Physiol. (Lond.)*, **164,** 508.

WALL, P. D. (1967). The laminar organisation of dorsal horn and effects of descending impulses. *J. Physiol. (Lond.)*, **188,** 403.

WANG, R. I. H. (1974). A controlled clinical comparison of the analgesic efficacy of ethoheptazine, propoxyphene and placebo. *Europ. J. clin. Pharmacol.*, **7,** 183.

WOLFF, H. G., and WOLF, S. (1958). *Pain*. Springfield, Illinois: Charles C. Thomas.

Chapter 33

THE TREATMENT OF PAIN

THE present chapter is concerned with the practical management of pain by the anaesthetist and may be considered under the headings of pre- and post-operative pain, and the symptomatic relief of chronic intractable pain. The last may be due to incurable malignant disease or to some condition such as post-herpetic neuralgia which does not immediately threaten the patient's life. Finally a brief comment is made on neuroleptanalgesia.

PRE-OPERATIVE PAIN

A patient suffering from some painful condition and awaiting surgery should receive the appropriate treatment, whether this necessitates morphine, some less potent analgesic, or merely sedation, rest and reassurance. In the immediate pre-operative period premedication affords the necessary pain relief and sedation, especially if morphine is used. Pain in the acute surgical emergency presents a more difficult problem. Analgesics should be withheld until a diagnosis has been reached and the course of action determined. Pain then having served its warning purpose, it is justifiable to relieve it with an opiate, given intravenously if necessary. Caution must be adopted in the elderly, toxic or shocked patient as a full therapeutic dose of morphine may cause collapse.

Patients in pain from acute trauma need and derive great benefit from morphine. A poor peripheral circulation from vasoconstriction may severely limit the absorption of drugs given by subcutaneous injection. The optimal dose of morphine can be given much more safely and rapidly by incremental intravenous injections until the desired effect is achieved. A period of 10 minutes should elapse between each injection so that the full effect of each dose can be assessed. Patients in severe pain often need much larger doses of narcotics than usual and the pain seems to antagonise the depressant effects of these drugs.

POST-OPERATIVE PAIN

The incidence of post-operative pain varies with the individual patient, but is largely governed by the site and nature of the operation. Upper abdominal and intrathoracic operations cause most pain and distress and are associated with an increased incidence of pulmonary complications. Post-operative hypoxaemia, which is also directly related to pain (Spence and Alexander, 1971) can persist up to five days and is more pronounced after upper abdominal surgery (Alexander et al., 1973). In a study on the incidence of post-operative pain after general surgical procedures, Parkhouse and his co-workers (1961) found that during the first 48 hours post-operatively, the greatest number of analgesic injections was required by patients after gastric surgery. Much less pain occurs after operations on the head and neck, the extremities, and on the superficial tissues.

Pain may arise from the skin, tendons, bones, muscles or viscera, but from the functional viewpoint may be divided into the dull, aching pain which persists at rest and the severe, sharp pain produced by movement or coughing. The former pain is readily relieved by morphine but the sharp, severe pain which is caused by the contraction of recently incised or injured muscle is much more difficult to relieve. Fear and anxiety may aggravate post-operative suffering by causing rigid muscle contractions in an attempt to splint the operative site. This leads to a self-perpetuating cycle of increased pain, fear, and muscle spasm.

Analgesics

The powerful effect of the placebo response must always be borne in mind when prescribing drugs for the easement of post-operative pain. Morphine sulphate in a dose of 10 mg has long been established as the standard drug for this purpose, despite its unpleasant side-effects, especially nausea and vomiting. Papaveretum is preferred by many clinicians because of a belief in its superiority as regards the incidence of side-effects. A dose of 20 mg is equivalent to 13·3 mg of morphine sulphate. In the immediate post-operative period, while the patient is still under the close supervision of the anaesthetist in the recovery room, it is often advantageous to give small incremental doses of these drugs intravenously until the desired degree of analgesia has been achieved. Anaesthetic techniques which include the use of intravenous analgesic drugs will postpone the need for post-operative analgesics and will reduce the total quantity required. The technique of neuroleptanaesthesia is often followed by a long period of post-operative analgesia and sedation. For patients who are intolerant of morphine, pethidine, is probably the most widely used alternative drug, and indeed is used as the routine post-operative analgesic by many anaesthetists. The dose of pethidine is 100 mg and as its duration of action is shorter than that of morphine it may have to be given more frequently. Promethazine in a dose of 25–50 mg is frequently combined with pethidine both pre- and post-operatively. It affords increased sedation and reduces the incidence of nausea and vomiting (Burtles and Peckett, 1957). Promethazine is one of the drugs which have been described as having an antanalgesic effect—see below (Moore and Dundee, 1961). However, the increased sedation provided by the promethazine does appear to reduce the need for post-operative analgesics.

Chlorpromazine has also been given to potentiate the effects of analgesics both pre- and post-operatively but its undesirable side-effects have led to its virtual abandonment. The dose of chlorpromazine is usually 25 mg three times a day. (For a description of individual analgesics see Chapter 32).

Increasing the dosage of analgesics enhances the severity of the side-effects but does not always produce more pain relief. The danger of addiction from the use of potent narcotic drugs in the relief of post-operative pain is small and is no reason for withholding their use. Nevertheless, non-addicting drugs should be substituted as soon as possible. If a series of painful operations is planned, the risk of dependence is increased, and for long-term pain therapy it may be useful to employ a non-addictive drug such as pentazocine which does not cause physical dependence.

The careful use of these pain-relieving drugs in the post-operative period will enable the patient to cough more effectively and to move more freely around the bed. Physiotherapy and breathing exercises should be timed to take place when the analgesia is at its maximum. Such a regime provides a safeguard against respiratory complications and thrombosis. The need of each patient for these drugs must be based on an assessment of his physical and mental state and the nature of the operation. Post-operative sedation must not be routine for all surgical patients as there is a considerable variation in prescribed therapeutic requirements.

Morphine and allied drugs, although relieving post-operative pain while the patient is lying quietly in bed, are unfortunately not as effective when the patient is coughing vigorously (Simpson and Parkhouse, 1961). The use of larger or more frequent doses of these drugs in an attempt to improve the analgesia can lead to a highly dangerous situation. Respiratory and circulatory depression together with immobility, increased drowsiness and lack of co-operation may contribute materially to post-operative morbidity and may even cost the patient his life. In these circumstances such drugs, instead of preventing, may contribute to the development of respiratory and thrombotic complications. Morphine antagonists have been used to prevent these dangers and have been discussed in the previous chapter.

Not all patients require potent analgesics to relieve their pain after major surgical operations. Milder analgesics such as dihydrocodeine, pentazocine, aspirin, paracetamol and Distalgesic are extremely useful and may be given freely during the first few days. Even patients who require morphine initially after operation can usually revert to simple remedies after the first 48 hours. Aspirin, if it is tolerated, is also very useful in relieving the stiffness and discomfort in back and limbs due to the unaccustomed and awkward positions which patients are forced to assume.

Children do not require the same scale of post-operative analgesia as an adult, perhaps because they have less fear of pain. Aspirin is often sufficient for children post-operatively. For severe pain, children may be given morphine (0·1–0·2 mg/kg), pethidine (1–2 mg/kg) or papaveretum (0·2–0·3 mg/kg).

Antanalgesia

Antanalgesia is the term applied to the action which certain drugs appear to have of lowering the pain threshold. This effect was first described by Clutton-Brock (1960) and is manifest even if an analgesic has been administered previously. Further observations were made by Dundee (1960) who found that small doses of thiopentone produced a transient fall in the pain threshold of patients premedicated with 100 mg of pethidine. Antanalgesia is in fact experimental confirmation of the clinical observations that sedatives and hypnotics, like phenothiazines and barbiturates, do not relieve pain unless administered in a dose which is large enough to produce unconsciousness. Smaller doses tend to produce an exaggerated response to pain and are clearly ineffective in relieving post-operative pain.

The post-operative restlessness which occurs so frequently in children who have been premedicated with barbiturates is almost certainly due to persistence of this antanalgesic effect. It is seen typically after painful operations like tonsillectomy and emphasises the advantages of an opiate as premedication or as part of the anaesthetic technique. Moreover, thiopentone which has been used for induction of anaesthesia, may exert an antanalgesic effect in the post-operative period. Low blood levels of thiopentone may persist for long periods and contribute to post-operative pain and restlessness. This effect may necessitate the use of larger doses of analgesics than would otherwise be required.

Local Anaesthetic Techniques

(a) **Intercostal block.**—Post-operative somatic pain in the chest or abdomen can be controlled effectively by blocking the intercostal nerves innervating the area of the incision and including one nerve above and below the appropriate dermatomes. It is most effective for superficial pain, but it does not block pain fibres from the viscera or peritoneum, thus deep pain may persist. The need for repeated multiple injections is the main disadvantage and it carries the risk of pneumothorax but, unlike extradural block, the fall in arterial blood pressure is minimal, as the block is distal to the sympathetic outflow. Bonica (1953) provided analgesia by repeating the injections daily for two to four days. The effect lasted for six to ten hours and the patients were able to breathe deeply and cough more effectively. Bridenbaugh et al. (1973) found the technique compared favourably to the opiates in the management of upper abdominal and thoracic cases.

(b) **Paravertebral block.**—Post-operative analgesia can be produced in any region of the body, except the head, by means of paravertebral block. Unlike intercostal block, it has the advantage of blocking all pain fibres (including those from the viscera) except for those in the vagus. It carries the risk of more severe complications including intrathecal injection, pneumothorax and hypotension.

(c) **Epidural block.**—A number of reports have stressed the superiority of epidural anaesthesia over other techniques for relieving post-operative pain (Bonica, 1953; Simpson et al., 1961; Bromage, 1967). Intermittent injections are given through an indwelling catheter. The complete pain relief which results from this block permits more effective coughing, better ventilation and increased mobility. After upper abdominal surgery the vital capacity is reduced to 25–30 per cent of the normal figure and to about 50 per cent after lower abdominal operations. This reduction in vital capacity is probably due to reflex muscle spasm because it is not augmented when the pain is relieved with morphine (Simpson et al., 1961). After epidural blockade there is a significant increase in vital capacity, which returns on average to 85 per cent of the pre-operative level. Spence et al. (1970) also found a marked improvement in respiratory function with epidural blockade following upper abdominal surgery.

For the adequate relief of pain in upper abdominal surgery the block should extend as high as the 4th–5th thoracic segments. To minimise the risk of postural hypotension from sympathetic blockade, the thoracic approach to the epidural space is recommended (Wallace and Norris, 1975), so that the tip of the catheter lies at the level of the thoracic roots to be blocked. This enables small volumes (4–6 ml) of local anaesthetic to be used, plain bupivacaine having replaced lignocaine as the agent of choice. Bromage (1972) suggested that the incidence of unblocked segments can be reduced by using carbonated local anaesthetics. The epidural technique affords excellent analgesia but requires special skill and training, strict asepsis and careful observation of the patient. It is unsuitable for routine use but is of great value in selected patients with respiratory disease.

Inhalational Techniques

The inhalation of known concentrations of volatile anaesthetic agents or nitrous oxide may be used to relieve post-operative pain and also for procedures such as changing dressings (Simpson and Parkhouse, 1961). Nitrous oxide-oxygen mixtures are of value when narcotic analgesics are contra-indicated or when the analgesia they afford is inadequate, and in patients who are already receiving oxygen therapy (Parbrook, 1967a). Because of the risk of leucopenia, nitrous oxide can only be administered for 24 hours.

Entonox, the premixed 50 per cent mixture of nitrous oxide and oxygen, is freely available in hospitals in the United Kingdom but if inhaled undiluted for prolonged periods it leads to somnolence, and if used in the immediate post-operative period it results in a continuation of the state of anaesthesia with immobility and lack of co-operation.

If Entonox is substituted for oxygen therapy in upper abdominal cases, it is possible to achieve some analgesia without cerebral depression because of the air-dilution that occurs if it is administered by an MC or Edinburgh type oxygen mask. These will provide 10–25 per cent nitrous oxide in 25–35 per cent oxygen depending on gas flow (Parbrook 1967b, 1972). The technique of deep breaths may help to cover movement, wound-dressing or post-operative physiotherapy.

Trichloroethylene 0·5 per cent and methoxyflurane 0·35 per cent vapour from self-administered draw-over vaporisers, can be used to provide analgesia equivalent to that obtained with narcotic analgesics for painful procedures such as physiotherapy in the post-operative period (Hovell et al., 1967; Yakaitis et al., 1972). Although devoid of significant respiratory depression, their pro-longed use may result in some clouding of consciousness. The volatile anaes-thetics have a limited application in the management of post-operative pain but nitrous oxide, which is cheap, convenient and rapidly eliminated, deserves much more extensive use (Wallace and Norris, 1975).

Discussion

There is usually a progressive reduction in the intensity of post-operative pain and after 48 hours narcotics are no longer required. Pain is the dominant factor in the production of post-operative chest complications and the effective relief of pain after surgery is not merely aimed at making the patient more comfortable, but is of vital importance in reducing the incidence and morbidity of such sequelae.

Morphine, papaveretum and pethidine have all been widely used in the relief of post-operative pain. They have the possible disadvantage of causing nausea and vomiting as a side-effect. Other analgesics such as phenazocine, methadone, levorphanol (see Chapter 32, p. 1054) have a lower incidence of side-effects, are longer lasting and orally effective but have not gained wide accep-tance in clinical practice.

THE MANAGEMENT OF CHRONIC OR INTRACTABLE PAIN

Severe intractable pain often presents a most difficult therapeutic problem. Many of the methods which are available for the symptomatic relief of pain are outside the sphere of the anaesthetist and are mentioned here only for the sake of completeness. These measures would include physiotherapy, psychotherapy, hormone therapy for hormone-dependent tumours, chemotherapy (including regional perfusion techniques), deep X-ray therapy, surgery including palliative removal of tumours, amputation of painful useless limbs, adrenalectomy and hypophysectomy for bone secondaries from carcinoma of the breast, cordotomy, leucotomy and rhizotomy.

The following methods will be discussed:

1. Local infiltration.
2. Injection of somatic nerves.
3. Injection of autonomic nerves and ganglia.
4. Intrathecal injection.
5. Hypertonic saline injection.
6. Barbotage of cerebrospinal fluid.
7. Epidural injection.
8. Percutaneous electrical cordotomy.
9. Systemic analgesic drugs.

1. Local Infiltration

One of the simplest ways of managing intractable pain is to inject 0·5 per cent lignocaine or 0·25 per cent bupivacaine, into the painful tissues. In addition to relieving pain locally, this technique may also cause the disappearance of referred pain, muscle spasm and vasomotor disturbances at some distance from the site of injection. Furthermore this secondary relief frequently lasts for a considerable time after the block has worn off. It has been postulated that in certain musculoskeletal disorders "trigger areas" act as a source of constant irritation and set up a vicious circle of impulses which produce the referred pain and other disturbances mentioned above. Local infiltration interrupts this vicious circle and may afford permanent relief of symptoms. This technique is widely used for a variety of disorders such as sprains and strains, painful undisplaced fractures, low back pain, bursitis, tendinitis, arthritis, muscle disorders including myalgia, contusions, torticollis, muscle contractions and "fibrositis". Nowadays injections of hydrocortisone are frequently given for these disorders, either by itself or in combination with a local anaesthetic. Painful scars following surgery and reflex dystrophies may also be treated successfully by local infiltration. It is often necessary to repeat the infiltration several times at intervals of three days to a week. The period of relief usually increases progressively after each injection.

2. Injection of Somatic Nerves

The injection of a local anaesthetic into a peripheral nerve, or its immediate vicinity, will cause complete analgesia in the area supplied by the nerve for a period of about one hour. In addition to its use in providing analgesia for surgery, it also has an important application for diagnostic purposes and for treating intractable pain. Like local infiltration, pain relief in the distribution of the nerve may persist long after the local anaesthetic has ceased to act and cutaneous sensation has returned. Post-herpetic neuralgia may be relieved by carrying out a paravertebral block on the appropriate spinal somatic nerve. Repeated nerve blocks may achieve long-lasting relief in this condition, particularly in patients with a short history of neuralgia. The mechanism by which prolonged relief is afforded in this way is not understood, but it has been suggested that nerve blocks may break up the vicious circle of pain by interrupting the reflexes which initiate or maintain the painful state. The accuracy of nerve blocking can be improved by using an insulated needle and electrical stimulation with a peripheral nerve stimulator. The specially insulated needle is covered with Teflon except at its tip and its correct placement adjacent to the nerve is indicated by muscle twitching when the stimulating current is switched on (Chapman, 1972). The increased accuracy achieved by this technique is especially useful when it is proposed to destroy the nerve with a neurolytic solution.

It is not proposed to describe all the therapeutic nerve blocks that may be practised. The following list merely sets out examples of conditions in which nerve blocks may be usefully employed. For a full description of the different blocks the reader is referred to Bonica's *Management of Pain* (1953) and Moore's *Regional Block* (1965). The use of nerve blocks in the management of chronic pain is well discussed in Mehta's *Intractable Pain* (1973).

(1) **Trigeminal nerve.**—Gasserian ganglion block with a local anaesthetic only relieves trigeminal neuralgia for a few hours, but it is an aid to the differential diagnosis of this condition and also allows patients to experience the anaesthesia of the face which would follow permanent relief with alcohol injection or surgery. In recent years phenol has been used as an alternative to alcohol. Very small quantities are injected at a time, the aim being to abolish sensation to pin prick yet retain light touch. If pain is limited to the distribution of one of the branches of the trigeminal nerve, then the individual branch can be blocked by the appropriate technique. The supra-orbital and supra-trochlear branches of the 1st division, the maxillary nerve in the pterygo-palatine fossa or its infra-orbital branch and the mandibular division after its emergence from the foramen ovale, can all be blocked by local anaesthetics or neurolytic solutions. Such procedures are particularly useful in patients with pain due to malignant disease or post-herpetic neuralgia. The pain of a fractured jaw can be relieved with a superior alveolar or mandibular block.

(2) **Glossopharyngeal nerve.**—It is sometimes necessary to block this nerve in patients with severe pain due to extensive malignant disease of the oropharynx. The nerve is injected at the base of the skull in the region of the jugular foramen but blockade may involve adjacent nerves such as the vagus, accessory and hypoglossal to which it is closely related.

(3) **Laryngeal nerves.**—Bilateral block of the internal laryngeal nerves will relieve the pain caused by laryngeal tuberculosis or malignancy.

(4) **Cervical nerves.**—The upper cervical nerves can be injected by a lateral approach as they lie in the sulci of the transverse processes. This block is useful with pain due to trauma, malignancy, neuralgia and osteoarthritis.

(5) **Thoracic nerves.**—Thoracotomies and renal operations are occasionally followed by pain and tenderness which are distributed segmentally and usually appear shortly after the wound has well healed. The aetiology of this postoperative neuralgia is uncertain but may well be due to the involvement of segmental nerves in scar tissue. Intercostal or paravertebral block, repeated at intervals, may prove helpful in such cases. Local anaesthetics may suffice for this procedure but often it is necessary to use 6 per cent aqueous phenol.

(6) **Fractured bones.**—A paravertebral block may help control the pain of fractured ribs, vertebrae or sternum. The acute pain and disability of the early stages are relieved and mobility encouraged.

(7) **Post-herpetic neuralgia.**—Repeated nerve blocks with a local anaesthetic are disappointing in the relief of this condition unless they can be carried out at an early stage of the disease. Often it is necessary to resort to a permanent block with alcohol or phenol and even then the success achieved is very limited. The pain and hyperaesthesia associated with this condition can sometimes be relieved by injecting the affected skin area with a mixture of a local anaesthetic and prednisolone.

(8) **Fibrositis and backache.**—In treating fibrositis and backache, Belam and Dobney (1957) describe the use of paravertebral block of the nerves which correspond with the area of greatest tenderness. These authors emphasise the importance of precise neurological diagnosis and of distinguishing between dermatomes and sclerotomes. Epidural blockade may also be found useful.

(9) **Lumbar nerves.**—Paravertebral block of the lumbar nerves is often performed for conditions such as post-herpetic neuralgia, disc protrusion and malignancy. The ilio-hypogastric and ilio-inguinal nerves often give rise to intractable pain from entrapment in the abdominal wall or in scars following hernia operations. Similarly the lateral cutaneous nerve of the thigh can cause pain due to entrapment in fascia in the thigh. Repeated blocks with bupivacaine will often relieve the pain in such cases.

Adductor spasm due to spasticity can be relieved by blocking the obturator nerve with 6 per cent aqueous phenol using a nerve stimulator to localise the nerve.

(10) **Abdominal wall pain due to nerve entrapment.**—A recently described cause of abdominal pain is entrapment of the intercostal nerves in the posterior wall of the rectus sheath (Mehta and Ranger, 1971; Applegate, 1972). The pain is sharp and burning in character and is associated with a localised area of tenderness along the outer border of the rectus sheath especially on coughing and straining or when the patient raises his head and shoulders off the pillow. Temporary relief can be achieved by infiltrating the tender area with a local anaesthetic and prolonged improvement often follows the injection of 6 per cent aqueous phenol.

Neurolytic agents—alcohol and phenol.—By injecting agents which destroy nerve fibres, it is possible to obtain prolonged and even permanent pain relief. This technique is used in patients with severe intractable pain due to malignant disease or conditions like post-herpetic neuralgia which have failed to respond to simpler measures.

Alcohol has been widely used as a neurolytic agent. Bonica (1953) concluded that with concentrations below 50 per cent only sensory fibres are involved. After an alcohol block the maximum analgesic effect is not apparent for several days. Regeneration of the fibres occurs in time unless the nerve cells are destroyed as well. If superficial nerves are injected, sloughing of the overlying skin may occur. Alcoholic neuritis is a serious complication of this technique and is due to failure to place the alcohol in exactly the right place. This leads to incomplete destruction of the somatic nerve and causes an intense burning pain which may be worse than the original. Absolute alcohol is frequently injected into the Gasserian ganglion for trigeminal neuralgia. A test injection of a small quantity of a local anaesthetic solution must produce perfect analgesia before the alcohol is given.

In recent years aqueous solutions of phenol (6 per cent) have been used as an alternative to alcohol. It seems to have little effect on tissues adjacent to the nerve and is more effective in blocking sympathetic fibres than somatic fibres. Phenol appears to diffuse less readily than alcohol. It used to be thought that these neurolytic agents destroyed the smaller fibres preferentially before the larger ones but it now seems that alcohol and phenol produce a patchy destruction of all sizes of fibres wherever contact with them occurs. The effect achieved is a quantitative reduction in the barrage of impulses emanating from the painful area rather than any specific qualitative change in the input.

3. Injection of Autonomic Nerves or Ganglia

There are many painful conditions in which the nerve impulses are carried by sympathetic pathways and in consequence sympathetic nerve blocks are among the most frequent that the anaesthetist is called upon to perform.

Vascular disorders.—An injury adjacent to a large vessel causes intense vasospasm which, if unrelieved, may progress to gangrene. Lesser degrees of vasospasm, whether due to trauma or vascular disease, are a frequent cause of pain. Disorders such as embolism, thrombophlebitis, Raynaud's disease, dissecting aneurysms and thromboangiitis obliterans all cause pain by vasospasm which may be relieved by the appropriate sympathetic block. The stellate ganglion may be blocked for disorders of the upper limb and is one of the easiest and most satisfactory blocks to perform. It has been advocated to relieve the vascular spasm caused by the intra-arterial injection of thiopentone and also spasm after angiography. For circulatory disturbances of the lower limb a lumbar sympathetic block is indicated. When it is desired to interrupt both the somatic and the sympathetic pathways a paravertebral block of the spinal nerves can be carried out.

Reflex sympathetic dystrophies (causalgic states).—This term is applied to a group of conditions all exhibiting a similar symptomatology. This consists of pain, hyperaesthesia, vasomotor disturbances and trophic changes. These conditions may be conveniently classified as follows:

1. *Major reflex dystrophies*
   - (a) Causalgia—following peripheral nerve lesions.
   - (b) Phantom limb pain.
   - (c) Central pain—e.g. thalamic syndrome.
2. *Minor reflex dystrophies*

This group includes many conditions such as the shoulder–hand syndrome (Steinbocker), post-traumatic dystrophy, Sudeck's atrophy, post-traumatic oedema and the post-frostbite syndrome.

It is believed that in all these conditions a reflex disorder involving the sympathetic nervous system is initiated by local damage. Conditions like Sudeck's atrophy and post-traumatic dystrophy follow injuries such as Pott's or Colles' fractures or contusion of a joint. The patient complains of a diffuse burning pain, often associated with cyanosis and sweating of the skin and decalcification of the bones. These syndromes may take eighteen months to two years to resolve but a lumbar sympathetic or stellate ganglion block usually affords complete but temporary relief of the pain and vasomotor disturbances.

Repeated blocks at weekly intervals on four to six occasions often result in a complete resolution of these distressing disabilities.

Causalgia is a distinct syndrome which develops after a peripheral nerve injury. It consists of a burning pain of varying severity which is exacerbated by minor stimuli, dryness, heat, or emotional disturbances, and often relieved by sympathectomy. Doupe and his co-workers (1944) put forward a theory that causalgia is due to fibre interaction or artificial synapses developing at the site of nerve injury. This results in efferent sympathetic impulses being short-circuited at the site of trauma into sensory afferent fibres, whence they return to the spinal cord and are eventually interpreted in the thalamus as pain. At the same time impulses from the artificial synapse can also travel peripherally, causing the release of bradykinin which induces a burning pain distally (Bergan and Conn, 1968). In any particular patient one or other of these processes may predominate but both are abolished by sympathectomy.

Cardiac pain.—Cardiac pain impulses travel via sympathetic fibres through the middle and inferior cervical cardiac nerves and the thoracic cardiac nerves, to reach the upper four or five thoracic sympathetic ganglia and the corresponding posterior spinal nerve roots. Nowadays most cases of angina can be satisfactorily controlled with beta-blocking drugs but in special circumstances the sympathetic pathways may be interrupted and pain relieved by stellate ganglion block or paravertebral block of the upper four or five thoracic spinal nerves. A left-sided stellate ganglion block is usually sufficient to achieve relief, otherwise the right side must be blocked as well.

Severe incapacitating angina occasionally requires surgical interruption of the pain pathways either by posterior rhizotomy or thoracic ganglionectomy, but good results are claimed for coronary artery by-pass grafting.

Cerebrovascular disease.—Bilateral stellate block produced no alteration in either cerebral blood flow or cerebral vascular resistance in a series of normotensive and hypertensive patients (Scheinburg, 1950). Nevertheless, vasospasm may be an important contributory factor in certain cerebrovascular accidents, typically thrombosis, embolus and haemorrhage, and good results have been claimed from stellate ganglion block following such episodes. Walsh (1956) found that 50 per cent of patients with cerebral thrombosis and hemiplegia could be improved with such treatment, although it may need to be repeated several times. Undoubtedly some patients do improve dramatically after stellate block, with a speed which suggests relief of spasm or increase in collateral blood flow. Assessment of this therapy is made difficult by the spontaneous, rapid and almost complete recovery which can occur after apparently serious cerebral vascular lesions even in the absence of any treatment (Brain, 1956). In a controlled trial on the treatment of cerebral embolus, Carter (1957) concluded that there was no significant difference between the control group of patients and those treated by repeated stellate block. Considerable doubt exists as to the precise value of stellate block in the treatment of these disorders. It should be avoided in patients with acute cerebral haemorrhage because of the risk of increasing the bleeding.

Cancer pain.—Sympathetic pathways are implicated in many cases of cancer pain and sympathetic nerve blocks are often effective in relieving a large component of the pain associated with inoperable or recurrent malignant disease.

Advanced carcinoma of the breast is often complicated by an uncomfortable oedematous arm and a severe burning pain in the shoulder and brachial plexus. To achieve complete pain relief by injection techniques, it is often necessary to interrupt the somatic pathways with a subarachnoid alcohol or phenol block and the sympathetic pathways with a stellate ganglion block. The use of subarachnoid and epidural techniques to block sympathetic pathways will be discussed in a later section.

TECHNIQUES

Stellate ganglion block is described in Chapter 35. When producing a prolonged block with alcohol the technique is modified to avoid the widespread diffusion of a large volume of solution. The procedure described in Chapter 35 is carried out and a marker is placed on the needle to indicate the depth of the fascial plane where the ganglion is located. The needle is then reinserted so that at the marked depth its tip is 1 cm below the original position. If a small test dose of lignocaine (1·5 ml) produces a Horner's syndrome, it can be assumed that the tip of the needle is adjacent to the ganglion and 1·5 ml of alcohol or phenol can then be slowly injected.

Lumbar sympathetic block.—This procedure will block the sympathetic pathways to the pelvic organs and lower limbs. It has a valuable diagnostic and therapeutic application, especially in vascular disorders of the lower limb, because of its effect in relieving vascular spasm and dilating blood vessels. Mandl's classical technique is described in Chapter 35.

Therapeutic sympathetic blocks using local anaesthetics may have to be repeated several times and, in the case of an arterial embolus in the lower limb, it may necessitate a block every day.

Phenol lumbar sympathetic block.—The injection of aqueous phenol solution into the lumbar sympathetic chain produces an effect equivalent to surgical sympathectomy and is an invaluable technique when surgery is contra-indicated. The limb becomes warm as a result of dilatation of the smaller vessels and sweating is abolished. The technique has proved of considerable value in ischaemic rest pain, established gangrene, especially prior to amputation, intermittent claudication and in conditions such as hyperhidrosis and pain due to Paget's disease (osteitis deformans) (Reid et al., 1970).

To facilitate a more accurate approach to the sympathetic chain, which lies on the antero-lateral aspect of the lumbar vertebral bodies, Reid and his co-workers advocate that the needles are introduced more laterally than in the conventional technique for lumbar sympathetic block using local anaesthetics. Needles inserted too near the midline are unable to negotiate the curve of the vertebral bodies to reach the sympathetic chain and success of the block depends on the volume of local anaesthetic (10 ml) injected. Such large volumes of neurolytic solutions are contra-indicated due to the risk of untoward damage caused by extensive spread.

The success of this modified technique is further enhanced by the use of the X-ray image intensifier. The patient is positioned with the side for injection uppermost and skin weals are raised 10 to 12 cm from the midline, opposite the bases of the 3rd and 4th lumbar spinous processes. Each needle is directed medially to the side of the vertebral body and then withdrawn and re-directed

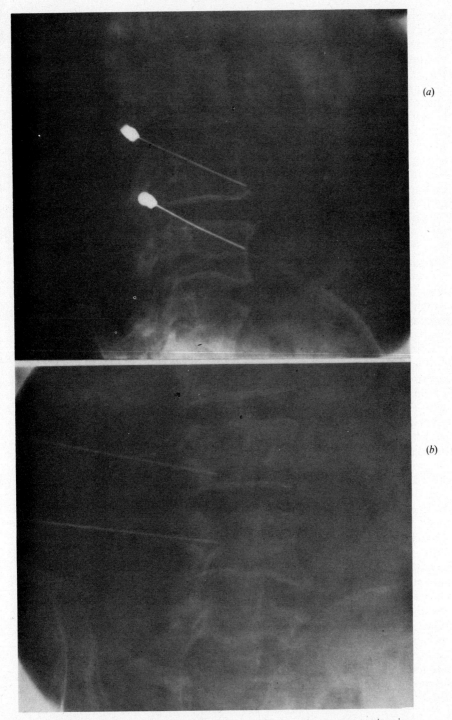

(a)

(b)

33/FIG. 1.—Phenol lumbar sympathetic block. (a) Lateral view; (b) antero-posterior view.

more laterally under image intensifier control, until in the lateral view (Fig. 1*a*) the tip of the needle is almost level with the anterior aspect of the vertebral body. The needle traverses the psoas muscle and a feeling of resistance is felt as the tip pierces the psoas fascia, at which point it is very close to the sympathetic chain. On screening (Fig. 1*a* and *b*) in the antero-posterior plane the needle should overlap the vertebral bodies by about a quarter of their total width. A drop of phenol solution is placed in the hub of the needle before complete withdrawal of the stylet. If the drop is sucked in, the pleural cavity may have been punctured. After waiting 20 seconds to exclude puncture of a blood vessel, the subarachnoid space, renal pelvis or ureter, the syringe containing the phenol solution is connected to the needle and with alternate aspiration and injection, a total of 3 ml of 6 per cent aqueous phenol is injected at each site in increments of 0·5 ml. Preliminary injection of local anaesthetic is not used, unless a local block is performed the previous day, as it merely dilutes the effect of the phenol solution.

Serious complications, such as paraplegia due to subarachnoid injection, are avoided by a meticulous technique and the use of the image intensifier. The only common complication is a temporary neuritis in the groin or thigh due to spread of the solution on to lumbar nerves.

Because the stellate ganglion and the lumbar sympathetic chain are readily accessible for surgery, most patients requiring permanent interruption of the sympathetic pathways at these sites are submitted to open operation. With the development of a safe and effective technique for chemical ablation of the lumbar sympathetic chain, however, many patients, especially those considered a poor risk for surgery, are being submitted to this alternative technique.

Coeliac plexus block.—The autonomic fibres innervating the upper abdominal viscera can be interrupted with a coeliac plexus block. Bridenbaugh and his co-workers (1964) described the use of bilateral coeliac plexus block with 40 to 50 ml of 50 per cent alcohol in 41 patients with intractable pain from advanced carcinoma of the stomach, pancreas, gall bladder or liver. All these patients, with one exception, were rendered free from pain for periods varying from six weeks to one year. The block is carried out with the patient in the prone position with a pillow under the abdomen. Marks are made at the inferior edge of the 12th thoracic spine and at the lower border of each 12th rib at a distance of 7 cm from the lumbar spine (Fig. 2). Lines are drawn between these three marks to form a triangle. The coeliac plexus lies at the level of the upper part of the body of the 1st lumbar vertebra, which coincides with the tip of the 12th thoracic spine. A 12 cm needle is inserted through the mark at the lower border of the 12th rib at an angle of 45 degrees to the skin, and advanced medially and upwards in the direction indicated by the side of the triangle marked on the patient's back. The depth at which the needle makes contact with the body of the 1st lumbar vertebra is noted. After withdrawing the needle, it is reinserted at a slightly steeper angle until it just slips off the body of the vertebra. After advancing the needle a further ½ inch (1·3 cm), its tip should lie adjacent to the coeliac plexus (Fig. 3). The distance to the plexus from the skin is between 7·6 and 10·2 cm. After a negative aspiration test, 25 ml of local anaesthetic is injected. These authors used 0·1 per cent tetracaine (Pontocaine) hydrochloride solution with 1 in 250,000 adrenaline, but 0·5 per cent lignocaine with 1 in 250,000 adrenaline or 0·25 per cent bupivacaine may be used as an alternative.

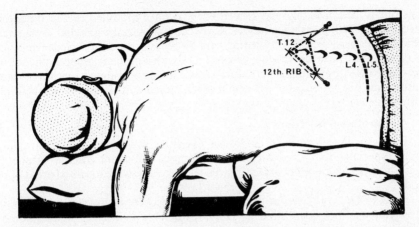

33/Fɪɢ. 2.—Coeliac plexus block. The position of the patient and skin markings for needle entries.

There should be no resistance to the injection of this solution. The other side is similarly blocked and this should produce pain relief for up to eight hours. If the block is successful it is repeated the following day using 25 ml of 50 per cent alcohol on each side. Initially 1 ml of alcohol is injected to exclude somatic nerve paraesthesia. If the patient complains of a feeling of pressure resembling "a kick in the solar plexus" and of being unable to get his breath, the needle is correctly sited.

A burning sensation lasting about one minute follows the injection of the alcohol. To prevent alcohol affecting the 1st lumbar nerve during withdrawal of the needle, the latter should be cleared by injecting 0·5 ml of air. The maximum effect from this block is not apparent for several days. Postural hypotension due to widespread interruption of vasomotor fibres may be a problem for a few days, especially in arteriosclerotic subjects. This may be prevented by wrapping the legs in elastic stockings and applying an abdominal binder before the patient

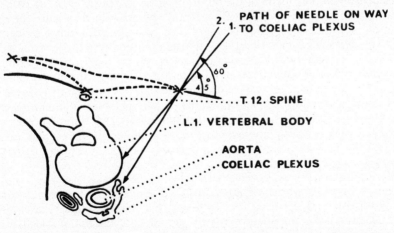

33/Fɪɢ. 3.—Coeliac plexus block. Oblique section to show the path of the needle.

gets out of bed. Gorbity and Leavens (1971) have modified this technique by introducing Teflon catheters under X-ray control onto the ganglia, using a trial of local analgesia before proceeding with 50 per cent alcohol. The development of paraplegia following a coeliac plexus block with 6 per cent aqueous phenol has been described by Galizia and Lahiri (1974). It was postulated that this complication was due to vascular ischaemia of the spinal cord from involvement of a lumbar artery.

4. Intrathecal Injections

The intrathecal route provides an excellent way of relieving intractable pain, especially that associated with incurable malignant disease. It enables neurolytic agents to be accurately placed so as to denervate localised areas of the body.

(a) *Alcohol.* —The use of intrathecal alcohol in the management of intractable pain was first introduced by Dogliotti in 1931 and it has since become a widely used and valuable technique. Alcohol is a tissue poison which may cause necrosis if injected into subcutaneous tissues. When injected into the intrathecal space, it acts as a neurolytic agent, destroying nerve fibres wherever it comes into contact with them until it is diluted by the cerebrospinal fluid. Absolute alcohol has a lower specific gravity (0·806) than cerebrospinal fluid (1·007), so that when it is slowly injected intrathecally it acts as a hypobaric solution and forms a layer on top of the cerebrospinal fluid. By careful positioning of the patient it is possible to limit the spread of the alcohol so that it only bathes those dorsal roots whose ganglia it is desired to block. Subarachnoid alcohol block may cause serious complications, so it is obligatory to pay the most careful attention to details of technique and selection of patients.

Selection and assessment of patients.—Because of the risk of complications, this technique is usually reserved for the management of intractable pain in patients with incurable malignant disease. It may at times be justifiable in non-malignant conditions, such as severe long-standing sciatica in a patient considered unfit for laminectomy. A careful history is taken from the patient, particular note being made of the duration, site and character of the pain. It is important to enquire if the patient has any disturbance of bladder or rectal function, as it would probably be aggravated by a block for pelvic or leg pain.

At the clinical examination detailed attention is paid to the nervous system and a note is made of any existing motor or sensory loss, muscle wasting, or alterations in the tendon reflexes. It is important to distinguish between difficulty in walking due to the aggravation of pain and that due to motor weakness.

The distribution of the pain should be plotted on a body dermatome chart. This serves as a guide to the nerve roots that need blocking but it is not accurate for pain arising in sclerotome structures such as bones, ligaments and muscles. Sympathetic pathways may also be implicated in carcinoma pain, particularly when viscera are involved.

The nature of the proposed treatment must be frankly discussed with the patient. A hopefully optimistic attitude should be adopted rather than a guarantee of success, and the need for a series rather than a single block must be stressed, otherwise the patient may be discouraged if the initial injection does not afford dramatic pain relief. The patient must be warned of possible complications such as numbness, weakness in the legs, and urinary retention. The low incidence of these complications must be pointed out, because if too black a picture is painted the patient may refuse treatment. In the more hopeless case, and especially if the patient is already partially incontinent, less emphasis should be placed on the risk of complications, although they should be fully discussed with a close relative and the reason for the treatment explained.

Most patients require more than one injection for complete relief, especially when the pain originates from a wide area. The response to the initial injection enables the anaesthetist to determine whether his assessment of the involved segments and site of block was correct.

Technique.—It is preferable to carry out the block on an operating table as it enables the patient to be positioned more accurately, but it can be carried out in the patient's bed with appropriately placed pillows. Morphine may be necessary beforehand to enable the patient to lie in the required position, but it is an advantage if the patient has some pain and is able to describe sensory changes during the block.

The patient lies in the lateral position with the painful side uppermost. The body is angulated by breaking the table so as to produce a scoliosis with the maximum curve corresponding to the site of the block. Both the head and legs should be lower than the point of injection. The patient is rolled forward 45 degrees into the semi-prone position so that the sensory posterior roots lie uppermost. Subarachnoid tap is made under strict aseptic conditions, the site of puncture depending on the roots involved. Bonica (1953) argued that it is better to deposit the alcohol at the point of emergence of the affected roots from the spinal cord. The spatial separation of the anterior and posterior roots is at a maximum at this point and, moreover, the expanded origin of the rootlets from the cord is thought to render them more susceptible to the action of the alcohol (Fig. 4). Blocking the roots at their exits through the intervertebral foramina carries an added risk of involving the anterior roots.

In carrying out the block an allowance must be made for the origin of the spinal nerves from the cord being above the level of the corresponding vertebra. It can be calculated as follows:

Cervical region: Spinal cord segments are one vertebra above the corresponding vertebra.
Upper thoracic region: Spinal cord segments are two vertebrae above the corresponding vertebra.
Lower thoracic region: Spinal cord segments are three vertebrae above the corresponding vertebra.
                         L 1 segment is opposite T 10 spine.

Using this technique it is unnecessary to do blocks below the T 12–L 1 interspace. The exact segment being blocked becomes apparent during the injection and any necessary adjustment in the level can then be made. Great care must be exercised when inserting the needle in the cervical or thoracic regions, owing to the risk of entering the spinal cord. As the epidural space is approached the stilette is withdrawn and, while slowly advancing the needle, either the hanging drop or the loss of resistance test is used to demonstrate entry into this space.

The needle is then very slowly advanced for a further 2 to 3 mm until its tip just enters the subarachnoid space.

The low pressure in the subarachnoid space may prevent the free flow of cerebrospinal fluid from the hub of the needle during a cervical tap. It is advisable therefore, to exert continuous suction with a syringe at this level so that the flow of fluid is immediately detected. It is important to position the patient with a slight head-down tilt to avoid spread of the alcohol to the medulla.

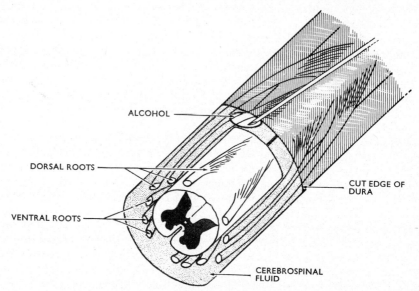

33/Fig. 4.—Intrathecal alcohol block. Diagram of lower thoracic cord region showing method of blocking dorsal roots as they emerge from the spinal cord (see text).

Absolute alcohol from a glass ampoule, the outside of which has been sterilised by autoclaving, is used and up to 0·5 ml is injected as an initial dose. The injection is made very slowly at a rate of about 0·1 ml per minute in order to localise the effect of the alcohol. The use of a 1 ml tuberculin syringe facilitates this procedure. Burning paraesthesiae are experienced by the patient and ideally these should be located in the centre of the painful area. By testing sensory and motor functions the extent of the block can be assessed. In the absence of motor impairment, further small increments of alcohol may be injected, but as a general routine not more than 1 ml should be injected at any one segment. If the paraesthesiae do not coincide with the painful area it may be possible, by tilting the table slightly in the appropriate direction, to float the hypobaric solution on to the involved nerve roots. If the disparity is more than one dermatome, it is preferable to change the position of the needle.

When pain arises from a wide area two or more needles should be inserted at different levels and small volumes of alcohol injected through each needle, rather than trying to produce an extensive block through one. In such cases, and especially when the pain arises from both sides, it may be preferable to carry out these blocks at intervals of a few days. After the injection the patient should lie in the same position for about half an hour to avoid spread of the alcohol and to enable it to be "fixed" to the correct nerve roots.

This technique is unsuitable for out-patients owing to the risks which attend any intrathecal technique.

Clinical effects and results.—An initial injection of 0·5 ml of alcohol affords some pain relief but in the majority of patients with severe pain the block has to be repeated, usually with a larger dose and perhaps in a different position. The maximum relief may be delayed as long as five days after the injection and a decision about a further block should be postponed until then. The larger the volume of alcohol injected, the greater the risk of side-effects. The precise dose in any individual patient can only be decided by a careful consideration of all the relevant factors, such as the severity and extent of the pain, and the willingness to accept the risk of side-effects. If the bladder sphincter is already paralysed, it may be permissible to use larger doses than usual. Incontinence is much more difficult to manage as a long-term problem in a woman than in a man, and hence it is possible to take more risks in a man.

Following the injection, a neurological examination will reveal a loss or diminution in sensation, especially to pin pricks and light touch. Tendon reflexes on the affected side are often absent and there may be a slight degree of motor weakness. These signs tend to disappear within a short time but areas of analgesia may persist for long periods. Some patients find this particularly distressing and complain vehemently.

The duration of pain relief ranges from six weeks to many months and even a year. The average duration is about three months, and if the pain does recur a further block can be carried out. Not all suitable patients are relieved by an intrathecal alcohol block.

Complications.—Some side-effects, such as headache and meningismus, are common to both spinal anaesthesia and subarachnoid alcohol block. The following complications are related to the neurolytic action of alcohol.

Motor paralysis.—This is due to involvement of the anterior roots and is more liable to occur when large volumes of alcohol are injected into the lumbar and lower cervical region. It may also result from bad positioning of the patient.

Bladder paralysis.—The injection of large volumes of alcohol into the lumbar region predisposes to this complication, which is due to involvement of the efferent parasympathetic fibres in the anterior sacral roots. These travel mainly in the second sacral nerve. Interrupting the sensory autonomic fibres, with consequent loss of bladder sensation, may lead to retention with overflow. Disturbance of bladder function occurs in about 5–10 per cent of cases but the incidence can be reduced by careful attention to technique. Spontaneous improvement usually occurs within a period of weeks or months.

Rectal incontinence.—The aetiology of this complication is the same as bladder paralysis but the incidence is less.

Cutaneous analgesia.—Areas of analgesia may persist for weeks and even months. It is particularly liable to occur when the block has been performed for a non-malignant condition in an otherwise healthy person.

Adhesive pachymeningitis.—Alcohol causes histological changes far beyond the point of injection, indicating that it diffuses widely in the subarachnoid space.

Transverse myelitis and cauda equina syndrome.—The risk of injecting alcohol into the cord can be avoided by ensuring that there is a free flow of cerebrospinal fluid before making the injection.

(b) **Phenol.**—Alcohol has the disadvantage of diffusing extensively in the sub-arachnoid space. This rapid diffusion, together with the difficulties of accurately controlling the flow of a hypobaric solution, have led to the search for alternative agents. Maher (1955 and 1957) described a technique for using intrathecal phenol in glycerine to alleviate the pain of incurable cancer. Aqueous phenol is a caustic substance, but when dissolved in glycerine it only diffuses slowly from solution to affect the nerve roots over which it is flowing (Nathan and Scott, 1958). Being a hyperbaric solution (Sp. G. glycerine 1·25: Sp. G. cerebrospinal fluid 1·007) it falls downwards in the subarachnoid space and is easier to control than alcohol. As Maher pointed out "it is easier to lay a carpet than to paper a ceiling". Maher concluded that 5 per cent phenol in glycerine is the optimal concentration to use as it will abolish pain without affecting other forms of sensation or disturbing motor function. These unwanted effects may result from the use of stronger solutions, while weaker solutions do not afford long-lasting relief. For patients unrelieved with phenol alone a phenol-silver nitrate solution can be used (silver nitrate 0·6 mg per ml of 4 per cent phenol in glycerine) (Maher, 1960). This is a more potent agent than phenol by itself but it may cause a meningeal reaction. With improvement in techniques, the need for this solution has decreased. Myodil (iophendylate) may also be used as a vehicle for phenol but it tends to protect the nerve roots and the phenol has to be used in a higher concentration (7 to 10 per cent) in order to achieve results comparable with 5 per cent phenol in glycerine.

These new techniques are being used extensively and in many centres phenol has replaced alcohol as the agent of choice in the relief of intractable pain.

Effect of phenol on the nervous system.—The belief that intrathecal phenol has a selective action on the small unmyelinated fibres of the posterior roots is no longer tenable, as a result of a study by Smith (1964). She carried out post-mortem studies on the nervous systems of patients who had received intrathecal injections of phenol and also on a control series of spinal cords from patients with malignant disease who had not been given this treatment. The effect of phenol in Myodil on healthy nervous tissue was investigated in cats by means of electrophysiological and histological studies carried out on nerve roots which had been exposed by laminectomy (Nathan et al., 1965). These investigators concluded that initially intrathecal phenol affects a large number of fibres of many roots, acting as a local anaesthetic. This effect comes on in 50 seconds and lasts about 20 minutes. Some fibres recover completely but others subsequently degenerate, depending on the concentration and duration of application of the phenol. It was concluded that phenol in glycerine or Myodil did not affect the spinal cord or posterior root ganglia but acted on the nerve roots, causing indiscriminate degeneration of all fibres, irrespective of their size, wherever it came into contact with them. Although the anterior roots were affected to some extent, the site of action of the solution was predominantly on the posterior roots between the ganglia and the spinal cord. A striking feature in the injected patients was a marked degeneration of nerve fibres in the posterior columns of the spinal cord, secondary to the action of the phenol on the posterior roots.

There was no suggestion of any marked meningeal reaction or direct damage to the cord. From these studies it was concluded that the effect of phenol in relieving chronic pain is not achieved by selectively destroying a particular type of nerve fibre (i.e. C fibres) because painful stimuli such as pricking and burning are still appreciated. The explanation is a quantitative rather than a qualitative one, depending on the destruction of a sufficient number of nerve fibres from the affected part of the body. This reduction in the sensory input and the lessening of the opportunity for summation between the opposing large and small fibre systems fits in with the Gate Control Theory of pain of Melzack and Wall (see Chapter 32).

Technique.—The selection of patients and the mapping out of the pain distribution on dermatome charts to determine the nerve roots that require blocking has already been discussed in the section on alcohol subarachnoid block. The needle should be inserted as near as possible to the roots it is desired to block with the phenol. A single injection of 1 ml of phenol in glycerine will usually block three nerve roots. The majority of patients require more than one injection and additional blocks are carried out at intervals of five days until all pain has been eradicated. With extensive bilateral pain it may be necessary to repeat the injections on three or four occasions.

Although Maher advocates carrying out this treatment at the bedside, the use of an operating table makes it easier to position the patient accurately and to control the flow of the solution after injection. With the patient lying on the painful side, subarachnoid puncture is performed with a 21-gauge needle, care being taken to ensure there is a free flow of cerebrospinal fluid. The needle is then withdrawn to the edge of the subarachnoid space so that the injected phenol does not affect the more centrally placed roots in the cauda equina, with a consequent risk to bladder or bowel control. Rotating the patient posteriorly to an angle of about 30° with the vertical helps to localise the effect of the phenol to the posterior roots. With the bevel of the needle directed downwards, an initial dose of 0·3 ml of 5 per cent phenol in glycerine is slowly injected. If the needle is correctly sited, the relief of pain is immediate, and is accompanied by a sensation of warmth and paraesthesiae in the distribution of the affected roots. If these sensory symptoms do not coincide precisely with the painful area, the table may be tilted so that the solution flows on to the appropriate nerve roots. Incremental doses each of 0·3 ml are given at intervals of 5 minutes until the desired effect has been achieved. The "end-point" for stopping the injections is determined by testing sensation immediately before each injection. The object is to diminish or abolish sensation to pin-pricks compared with the other side while leaving light touch unaffected.

The patient is kept lying still in the position of the injection for an hour afterwards in order to fix the phenol to the required roots. To minimise the risk of post-lumbar puncture headache, the patient is nursed lying flat in bed for 24 hours.

Details of technique and a guide as to the volume of solution required in each region of the vertebral column are set out below. Most patients suitable for an intrathecal phenol block have pain in the lower part of the body and, in consequence, most injections are carried out in the lumbar or lower thoracic regions.

Sacral region.—A common cause of intractable pain in the perineum and bottom of the coccyx is a recurrence of carcinoma, following an abdomino-perineal excision of the rectum. Subarachnoid puncture at the L5–S1 space is easier to perform with the patient sitting up. He is then made to lie on the most painful side with a 30° head-up tilt. Including the test dose of 0·3 ml, a total of 0·5 to 0·7 ml of 5 per cent phenol in glycerine is allowed to flow quickly down over the upper sacral roots, which supply the bladder, to form a pool at the bottom of the subarachnoid space. By slowly raising the patient to the vertical it is possible to block the lowermost sacral and coccygeal nerves on both sides. As the phenol does not diffuse through all the sacral roots with this technique, the risk of bladder involvement is much reduced. To block S 2–4 roots usually requires 0·7 ml and the injection is made with the patient lying with a slight head-up tilt (approximately 20°). If bladder control is normal prior to treatment no disturbance should occur after blocking the sacral roots unilaterally.

Lumbar region.—After a successful lumbar tap, the needle is withdrawn to the edge of the theca so that the injected phenol does not cross the nerve roots which are descending centrally in the cauda equina and emerging at a lower level. The average volume of solution required for this region is 1 ml and it is given in increments of 0·3 ml as described above. At times as little as 0·5 ml of solution is enough to produce the desired effect. If necessary, the table is tilted slightly to localise the effect of the phenol to the appropriate nerve roots. The occurrence of sensory symptoms in the upper leg after the initial injection indicates that the needle has been inserted too far towards the unaffected side, allowing the phenol to trickle over all the roots of the cauda equina. Unless the injection is abandoned the patient may have difficulty in controlling his bladder.

Dorsal region.—Great care must be exercised in carrying out a subarachnoid tap in this region because of the risk of inadvertantly transfixing the spinal cord. A short-bevelled needle is inserted initially into the epidural space, which may be recognised by the loss of resistance or hanging drop techniques. The needle is then advanced a millimetre at a time until cerebrospinal fluid just begins to flow. If the initial dose of 0·3 ml of 5 per cent phenol in glycerine causes no symptoms in the legs it is safe to give further increments until the pain has been relieved. The volume of solution required in this region is usually 1·5–3·0 ml.

Cervical region.—Because of the danger of phenol flowing into the cranium the patient must be positioned with a head-up tilt of 30° to 40°. The technique adopted is the same as in the thoracic region but as the spinal canal is narrow the needle must be inserted exactly in the midline. The results of intrathecal phenol are not so good in the cervical as in other regions, because the solution tends to flow away very quickly and also the cervical nerve roots are much shorter and hence the length available for absorption is less. Maher considers that subdural injections give better results in this area. The technique is to carry out a subarachnoid tap and then withdraw the needle until the cerebrospinal fluid is still just flowing. Reinserting the stilette helps to widen the subdural space prior to injecting 0·5 ml of 7·5 per cent phenol in Myodil. A honeycomb appearance on the X-ray, caused by the Myodil travelling down round the nerve roots, confirms the correct siting of the injection (Maher, 1957). A further injection of 0·5 ml of 7·5 per cent phenol in glycerine is then carried out in order to reach the upper cervical roots.

Preparation of solutions.—Phenol in Myodil must be prepared immediately before use. The outside of the Myodil ampoule cannot be sterilised by heat. The contents are drawn up and injected into a sterile ampoule containing phenol crystals.

Factors influencing results of treatment.—Most of the pain caused by cancer is of a constant, unremitting nature. It is carried by the small C fibres and can be eradicated by intrathecal phenol injections. A second type of pain, termed incident pain by Maher, is due to a sudden event such as a fracture or the collapse of a vertebra. This pain is not amenable to treatment by phenol, but as it is evoked by movement it can be relieved by complete rest.

Phenol has both a temporary and a permanent blocking effect (Nathan and Sears, 1960). When injected intrathecally it acts as a local anaesthetic, relieving all pain within a period of 50 seconds. Recovery takes place gradually after about 20 minutes but a varying number of pain fibres remain permanently damaged, so accounting for the relief of the constant pain in malignancy. Because of this dual effect phenol, unlike alcohol, destroys nerve fibres without causing pain.

Severe pain dominates a patient's whole existence, and if it cannot be relieved by analgesics it may materially shorten his life. Treatment of pain must not be an ordeal for these patients, as the majority have already endured operations and radiotherapy and many do not want anything further done. Good results can only be achieved if patients are referred early for treatment, preferably within two or three months of the pain becoming established. If it is long-standing and has been present for two or three years, the results are bound to be disappointing. Growth of tumour around the nerve roots may have a sheltering effect by preventing the phenol gaining access to them. Successful relief of pain in one part of the body frequently reveals pain in adjacent or more distant regions, which hitherto had been overshadowed by the patient's principal pain.

Long-lasting or even permanent relief can be anticipated if the patient is still pain-free three days after the phenol injection. Failure to obtain relief may be due to too few injections being given to cover adequately all the nerve roots innervating the painful area, or to the needle being inserted at the wrong place.

The return of pain after a period of relief may be due to the spread of tumour to another area or to the occurrence of incident pain.

Results.—The results of treatment depend largely upon the selection of patients and the other factors discussed above. Maher (1960) reported complete relief in 61 (75 per cent) out of 81 cases when intrathecal phenol was used below the level of T 3. Other workers have not achieved such a high success rate. Gordon and Goel (1963) used this technique on 37 patients and reported complete relief in 51 per cent and moderate to good relief in a further 30 per cent of patients. Nathan (1967) reported that 77 per cent of patients obtained relief after cordotomy compared with 54 per cent after phenol injections, but that after phenol motor function in the legs was less affected and the incidence of sphincter trouble was only 12 per cent.

Complications.—The possible complications of this technique are the same as those described in the section on subarachnoid alcohol block. The risk of interfering with the control of bladder or bowel function must always be borne in mind, but by using a meticulous technique the incidence can be kept down to an acceptable level. Temporary difficulty with micturition may occur necessitating the use of an indwelling catheter for a few days or a week.

Intrathecal phenol in the relief of spasticity.—Intrathecal phenol, using either glycerine or Myodil as a solvent, has a most useful application in the relief of spasticity and the pain associated with flexor spasms (Kelly and Gautier Smith, 1959; Nathan, 1959). 7·5 per cent–10 per cent phenol in Myodil is a suitable solution to use for these patients.

Intrathecal chlorocresol.—Maher (1963) suggested using a 1 in 50 solution of chlorocresol in glycerine as an alternative to phenol. Chlorocresol appears to have a delayed effect compared with phenol in glycerine and there are no immediate sensory changes or paraesthesiae. Fewer nerve roots are affected, so that a second injection may be required after three weeks. The higher proportion of success obtained with chlorocresol may be due to the diffusion affecting a greater length of nerve root.

For rectal, coccygeal and sacrosciatic pain the suggested dose of the solution is 0·5 ml; for the upper lumbar segments 0·75 ml; and for the thoracic segments 1·0 ml. This technique appears to be a more effective way of relieving the pain associated with carcinoma of the lung, especially that from a Pancoast tumour.

5. Hypertonic Saline Injection

Hitchcock (1967) described a technique for the relief of intractable pain based on the concept of the differential susceptibility of nervous tissue to hypothermia with the unmyelinated C fibres especially sensitive to the effects of cooling.

Further work has led to the belief that the results from this technique were due to the hypertonicity of the solution injected, which in practice was the supernatant liquid obtained from thawing frozen isotonic saline solution (Hitchcock, 1969). As a result of this conclusion, the technique was changed to the subarachnoid injection of hypertonic saline at room temperature (Hitchcock and Prandini, 1973).

After performing a lumbar puncture at L 3–4 or L 4–5 interspace and withdrawing a few millilitres of CSF, 20 ml of hypertonic saline are injected with the patient lying on the painful side. The concentration of saline used is between 10 and 15 per cent, depending on the build and condition of the patient, but in general 12·5 per cent is employed. The patient is rapidly tilted head up for lower body pain and head down for pain in the upper part of the body to encourage the flow of the hypertonic saline on to the appropriate nerve roots. The patient is kept in the same position for half an hour after the injection, and because of the unpleasant symptoms associated with this technique, especially paraesthesia and hyperventilation, it is customary to perform it under general anaesthesia. Compared with other methods, the duration of pain relief is short but at three months 50 per cent of cancer patients were still experiencing relief on the basis of their not requiring analgesics at all or only mild ones. At 6 months, 44 per cent of patients with benign conditions and 15 per cent of the malignant disease group were still experiencing relief. Sphincter disturbances occurred in 8 per cent and muscle weakness in 3 per cent of cases. The technique is contra-indicated in severe arterial disease and in the presence of intrathecal adhesions which may prevent dilution and diffusion of the injected solution. The technique is especially useful if there is a life expectancy of less than 3 months and widespread pain due to metastases.

6. Barbotage of Cerebrospinal Fluid

A similar technique to the use of saline in the management of severe chronic pain is barbotage, the alternate withdrawal and reinjection of the patient's own CSF (Lloyd et al., 1972). The procedure is carried out under premedication and intravenous diazepam, the spinal puncture being performed at the L3–4 space with the patient sitting up. A Tuohy epidural needle is employed to avoid blockage by nerve roots and 20 ml of CSF is withdrawn and replaced 15–20 times (Mehta, 1973). When inadequate pain relief is obtained with this technique, the aspirated CSF is cooled to $-5°$ C in a coil of drip tubing immersed in an alcohol bath.

Fifty per cent of patients were improved for periods varying from a few days to six months by this technique. The best results were obtained in the lumbosacral region and, not surprisingly in view of the large-bore needle used, headache occurred in 80 per cent of the patients but no adverse effects of other kinds were reported. The suggested mechanism of action is that pressure changes in the CSF cause peripheral demyelination in the spinal cord and so affect the spinothalamic fibres traversing this region. The place of this technique in the management of intractable pain has not yet been established but it deserves further trial.

7. Epidural Injection

The success achieved with intrathecal phenol solution has led to the use of this solution for epidural block. It has been particularly recommended by Maher for non-malignant forms of pain. Finer (1958) used 10 per cent phenol in glycerine epidurally for patients with incurable cancer. He injected 3 ml of the solution through a Tuohy needle at the L 4–5 space and simultaneously collapsed the dural sac by intrathecal puncture at L 1–2 space. By performing an epidural block with phenol at the T 12–L 1 space it is possible to interrupt sympathetic fibres and hence relieve cancer pain, particularly when it is due to involvement of viscera or blood vessels. Patients with perineal pain due to a carcinoma of the rectum are not always adequately relieved by a somatic block with intrathecal phenol. By performing an epidural block with phenol in glycerine at T 12–L 1 space, such cases can often be rendered pain-free. Doughty (1964) suggested a dose of 5 ml of 5 per cent phenol in glycerine. If necessary the injection can be repeated after a few days using 7·5 ml of $7\frac{1}{2}$ per cent or even 10 per cent phenol in glycerine. This block is especially effective in relieving the spasms of burning pain and tenesmus associated with advanced carcinoma of the rectum.

An epidural block may be preferred to an intrathecal one in the cervical or upper thoracic regions for patients with incurable malignant disease, but compared with subarachnoid injections, the technique is less precise in localising the solution to the affected nerve root. Moreover, because of the large doses of neurolytic agent used in the epidural approach, accidental dural puncture, if unrecognised, may lead to extensive neurological damage.

Intractable sciatica.—The injection of local anaesthetic into the epidural space has been used successfully in the last decade in the treatment of sciatica, and the results of a large series have been described by Swerdlow and Sayle Creer (1970). In the lumbar approach for this condition, 10 ml of 1 per cent lignocaine in 0·25 per cent bupivacaine are injected. Many clinicians prefer the caudal approach to the epidural space using up to 50 ml of 0·5 per cent ligno-caine, often with the addition of 80 mg of methylprednisone. The injection is repeated at weekly or fortnightly intervals.

8. Percutaneous Electrical Cordotomy

Anterolateral cordotomy is the most satisfactory technique for the long-term relief of intractable pain but it involves a major operation, with a variable mortality and morbidity, in patients who may be a poor operative risk.

The development of the technique of percutaneous electrical cordotomy (Mullan *et al.*, 1965; Rosomoff *et al.*, 1965; Lin *et al.*, 1966; Lipton, 1968) was an important advance in this field, as it affords satisfactory pain relief in patients who may be too ill to submit to open surgical cordotomy. Most patients undergoing this procedure can leave hospital within a few days and may well submit to this type of cordotomy when major surgery would be rejected.

The technique used by Lipton (1968) is to insert a spinal needle laterally, under X-ray control, between the first and second cervical vertebrae into the

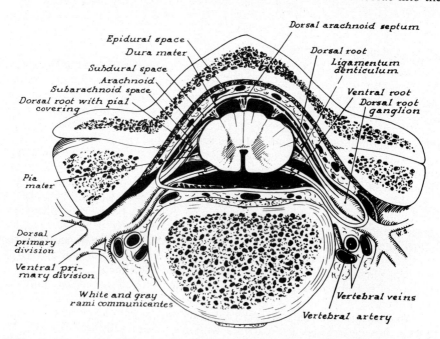

33/Fig. 5.—Cross-section of spinal cord in the spinal canal showing its meningeal coverings and the manner of exit of the spinal nerves (after Rauber).

subarachnoid space. The aim of the technique is to place the point of the needle in front of the dentate ligament (ligamentum denticulum) (see Fig. 5) which is identified by injecting a mixture of CSF and iophendylate injection BP. This emulsion sinks down on to the ligament, which is recognised as a line on the lateral X-ray. An electrode is introduced through the needle and inserted into the anterolateral column of the cord, the depth of penetration being assessed from an antero-posterior film.

If the tip of the electrode is situated too far posteriorly and is lying in the motor tract, stimulation of the cord by passing a current through the electrode causes movement of the limbs or body of the same side (ipsilateral). Movement of the neck of the same side indicates that the electrode tip is placed too far anteriorly and is in the anterior horn cells. With correct positioning there is no movement but there may be paraesthesiae on the opposite (contralateral) side. The anterolateral tract is then coagulated by a radio frequency current to produce analgesia in the contralateral side. With accurate placement of the electrode this analgesia can be localised to one quadrant of the body (body and arm or body and leg).

In fifty-two patients Lipton achieved effective pain relief in 67 per cent and partial relief in 13 per cent.

Percutaneous electrical cordotomy is relatively free from side-effects, although retention of urine may occur, especially after bilateral cordotomy. Headache is an almost invariable occurrence, while hyperalgesia and transient weakness may develop occasionally.

Respiratory embarrassment is a hazard of high cervical cordotomy and Mullan and Hosobuchi (1968) reported nine fatalities in 400 cases due to this complication. It occurs because fibres descending from the medullary centre to the respiratory muscles lie very close to the lateral spinothalamic tract and are damaged by the cordotomy. These patients are able to maintain adequate ventilation while they are awake but during sleep respiration becomes ineffective and may require assistance. Six of Mullan and Hosobuchi's patients died during their sleep.

This hazard exists when bilateral cordotomies are undertaken in the anterior quadrants of the cord and when unilateral lesions are produced in patients with impaired pulmonary function. Caution must be exercised in such cases as well as care and skill in localising the cordotomy to that part of the anterolateral column which is not essential for respiration.

In order to avoid this complication Lin et al. (1966) described an anterior approach to the lower cervical cord for percutaneous cordotomy. The spinal needle is inserted below the origin of the phrenic nerve between the carotid sheath and the oesophagus and trachea. Under X-ray control the needle traverses an intervertebral disc and enters the anterolateral quadrant of the cord. Analgesia is produced by inserting an electrode and applying radio frequency current. Using this technique these authors claim it is possible to produce segmental analgesia in the thoracic and lumbar regions, sparing the sacral segments and so having a lower incidence of bladder complications. The upper cervical approach, however, probably gives better pain relief.

9. Analgesic Drugs and their Adjuvants

The narcotic analgesics offer the only hope of pain relief in many advanced cases of malignant disease. The choice and dosage of analgesic depends on a number of factors:

1. Severity and fluctuation of the pain (this can be assessed by keeping a pain chart).
2. Likely duration of pain or the expectation of life.
3. Effect of drugs already administered.
4. Occurrence of undesirable side-effects.
5. Development of tolerance and addiction.
6. Domestic circumstances of the patient.

The effective use of these drugs requires a careful appraisal of each patient, with special reference to the history and any conditions which aggravate or relieve the pain. The aim of treatment is not merely to relieve pain but to make the patient more contented. There may be other distressing symptoms to alleviate as well, such as cough, dyspnoea, nausea and vomiting, paralysis and mental distress.

Analgesics should be administered orally for as long as possible and when there is a dull, steady background pain they should be given on a fixed time schedule. The aim should be to keep the patient free of pain, rather than treating it when it has occurred. Thus each dose is given while the previous one is still exerting its effect. The optimal dose of the drug should be prescribed (Denton and Beecher, 1949) and as tolerance develops the frequency of administration should be increased, rather than the dose. Large doses of analgesics cause a higher incidence of side-effects without affording much additional analgesia (Lasagna and Beecher, 1954). Side-effects, especially the emetic ones, are the limiting factor in narcotic analgesic therapy. There is considerable individual susceptibility but they are more common in ambulant patients. Side-effects, such as the sickness caused by pethidine, often persist longer than the analgesia.

Initially mild analgesics such as aspirin or, if it causes gastric irritation, paracetamol, may be sufficient. Once these fail, agents of intermediate efficacy such as dihydrocodeine, Distalgesic or pentazocine may be tried, but each may cause constipation and afford little better pain relief than aspirin. In advanced malignant disease there is no reason to withhold addictive narcotic drugs if other agents cannot provide analgesia. Particularly useful in this field are those that are well absorbed when taken by mouth and that produce little sedation and constipation. Suitable agents, therefore, include phenazocine and methadone (which have the added advantage of a duration of action longer than morphine) and heroin whose marked euphoriant property and relative freedom from nausea and constipation render it invaluable in this field.

Tolerance to narcotics is inevitable and may require increasing doses—which should on no account be withheld—within the first few weeks of use. Thereafter the dose requirement normally remains steady until death is near, when occasionally parenteral administration is needed.

Alcohol can be very useful in the management of intractable pain because it has both analgesic and sedative properties. The patient's own habits should be consulted in selecting the most suitable preparation, dosage and frequency of administration.

Cocaine is a very useful adjunct to narcotics in terminal illness, because it contributes its own euphoria while counteracting their sedative effect. Finally chlorpromazine may be added when nausea and vomiting are troublesome, and also for its tranquillising effect. Heroin and cocaine, with or without chlorpromazine, are frequently given in the form of an elixir (diamorphine and cocaine elixir BPC) in terminal disease, with excellent results.

Antidepressants

(a) **Tricyclics.**—Anxiety and depression are understandable and common accompaniments of intractable pain and Merskey and Hester (1972) recommended the administration of the antidepressant amitriptyline, together with the phenothiazine-pericyazine (Neulactil), for the management of intractable pain; this combination of drugs minimises the drowsiness and dry mouth caused by the phenothiazine and the antidepressant. Good relief occurs in conditions such as causalgia, post-herpetic neuralgia and phantom limb pain. The effectiveness of mild analgesics is enhanced but care must be taken to withdraw this treatment gradually or the symptoms may be exacerbated.

(b) **Monoamine oxidase inhibitors.**—These are the most effective antidepressant drugs available and also have analgesic properties, and can be used with striking success in certain selected patients with intractable pain from conditions such as post-herpetic neuralgia and intercostal neuralgia, when depression is the most prominent clinical feature. These patients have a meticulous obsessional type of personality and their lives become dominated by, and revolve around, their continuous pain. The most effective and popular of the monoamine oxidase inhibitors is phenelzine (Nardil) but it takes a month for the maximal elevation of mood and amelioration of symptoms to be obtained. The antidepressant effect is achieved by the accumulation of noradrenaline and other amines in the brain. Care must be taken to avoid tyramine-containing foods (cheese, yeast, extract, etc.) as this substance will no longer be inactivated in the gut by monoamine oxidase. Patients receiving monoamine oxidase inhibitors may also be sensitive to the analgesics—particularly pethidine (see p. 799).

PAIN CLINICS

In recent years anaesthetists have taken an increasing interest in the management of patients with chronic pain. This has led to the setting up of pain clinics where patients can be seen and assessed with a view to treatment. As it is impossible for one person to encompass all the techniques and procedures which can be applied to this problem, such a clinic should ideally be under the direction of a radiotherapist, a neurosurgeon, and an anaesthetist, with perhaps a neurologist and a psychiatrist in attendance as well. Most clinics do not conform to this pattern but are run by an anaesthetist who provides symptomatic treatment of pain with nerve blocks and analgesic drugs. Although the majority of patients referred for treatment are suffering from malignant disease, other conditions seen not infrequently include post-herpetic neuralgia and post-operative neuralgia.

A small group of patients, who are referred from time to time, appear to suffer from seemingly intractable pain and yet have no clear-cut aetiological cause. Before dismissing such patients as suffering from psychogenic pain, the possibility of a reflex sympathetic pain should be considered, particularly if it has developed after trauma or surgery.

The complete relief of pain, following the performance of a sympathetic block without an accompanying somatic block, enables the correct diagnosis to be made. A series of sympathetic blocks may lead to a complete cure or it may be necessary to refer the patient for surgical sympathectomy.

The anaesthetist, because of his skill and familiarity with local analgesic techniques, is ideally placed to help these patients. With increasing experience he can achieve worthwhile success in the relief of chronic pain by means of nerve blocks. Simple nerve blocks may be carried out on out-patients but the intrathecal or epidural injection of neurolytic agents should be confined to in-patients. The anaesthetist is at a disadvantage in having no hospital beds of his own, but an arrangement can usually be reached for the clinician referring the patient to provide a bed. Disappointments are not infrequent and relief is often partial or of short duration, but perseverance is rewarded with a worthwhile alleviation of suffering in this group of patients.

The second and equally important function of a pain clinic is to arrange the administration of analgesic drugs to patients who are unsuitable for a block, or who have failed to obtain adequate relief. The anaesthetist should be able to determine the most suitable analgesic regime for the particular patient, including any adjuvant drugs which may be indicated. The value of pain clinics for conducting controlled trials on new or established drugs is obvious, and anaesthetists have made many important contributions in this field. The extension of the anaesthetist's interests beyond the confines of the operating theatre is a significant and vital trend of current anaesthetic practice. The running of a pain clinic provides abundant clinical interest and a means of affording worthwhile relief to some patients whose suffering might otherwise remain unabated.

NEUROLEPTICS AND NEUROLEPTANALGESIA

Neuroleptic drugs such as the butyrophenone derivatives haloperidol and droperidol induce a state of apathy and mental detachment in which the patient is mildly sedated and uncaring about his surroundings. A technique introduced on the Continent for use in clinical anaesthesia termed "neuroleptanalgesia", is based on the combination of one of these neuroleptic drugs and an analgesic (Nilsson, 1963). The drugs used in this procedure have been developed by Janssen in Belgium. It is in reality a development of the technique of artificial hibernation based on the lytic cocktail, and differs from it in the greater emphasis placed upon analgesia and on the stability of the circulatory system.

The narcotic analgesics phenoperidine (Operidine) and fentanyl (phentanyl) (Sublimaze) used in this technique are very powerful, the latter being 100 times more potent than morphine, milligram for milligram. Complete general analgesia sufficient for surgical procedures can be achieved with these drugs, without disturbing the circulation or causing marked hypnosis. The analgesia is accompanied by an intense respiratory depression, which in the case of fentanyl is of short duration and disappears before the analgesia. Respiratory depression can be effectively reversed by giving nalorphine in doses of 2 to 10 mg or naloxone

0·2–0·4 mg, but then analgesia may also be counteracted. Doxapram may be preferable in this situation because it does not interfere with the analgesia.

In using the technique of neuroleptanalgesia, droperidol 2·5–5 mg is given intramuscularly 15–45 minutes pre-operatively as a premedication together with fentanyl 0·05–0·1 mg or phenoperidine 1 mg. This produces a calm patient, free from anxiety or pain, and it should enable procedures such as cardiac catheterisation, air encephalography or burns dressings to be performed without causing distress. Additional doses of the drugs can be given intravenously during the procedure if required. Neuroleptanalgesia has also been reported as affording excellent sedation during the surgical treatment of Parkinsonism, while retaining the patient's full co-operation for three hours or longer (Brown, 1964).

Thomas (1966) reported that neuroleptanalgesia combined with local analgesia provided very satisfactory conditions for intra-ocular surgery. After premedication with 25 or 50 mg of promethazine he gave a mixture of droperidol 3 mg and phenoperidine 1 mg intravenously. Smaller doses of phenoperidine were given to the frail or elderly. During the operation the patients remained placid and there was an absence of coughing, vomiting and fidgeting.

Holderness et al. (1963) and Aubry et al. (1966) described the use of these mixtures in combination with nitrous oxide and oxygen for general anaesthesia in a series of 400 patients and 1,000 patients respectively. They used droperidol combined with fentanyl, usually in a 50:1 mixture. This mixture is available as a proprietary preparation called Thalamonal, or Innovan, which contains droperidol 2·5 mg and fentanyl 0·05 mg in 1 ml. Conventional drugs can be used for premedication and anaesthesia is induced by the intravenous injection of 10–20 mg of droperidol together with fentanyl followed by the inhalation of nitrous oxide and oxygen to produce unconsciousness. For all but the gravest-risk patients a more rapid loss of consciousness is achieved by injecting a small sleep-dose of thiopentone (not more than 100 mg). Endotracheal intubation, if indicated, is performed after paralysis with suxamethonium or d-tubocurarine. For operations not requiring muscular relaxation spontaneous respiration is maintained but the initial dose of fentanyl should not exceed 0·2 mg or respiration will be unduly depressed. With assisted or controlled respiration, larger initial doses of fentanyl (0·4–0·6 mg) may be employed and when muscular relaxation is required d-tubocurarine is injected. Additional doses of fentanyl of 0·05 mg are administered if the patient shows signs of lessening analgesia such as movements or a rise in respiratory rate or blood pressure. Stability of the circulatory system is notable both during and after operation. The alpha-adrenergic blocking effect of droperidol may help prevent the development of shock and animal experiments have shown that it protects against adrenaline-induced arrhythmias. Respiratory depression similar to that seen after other potent narcotics may result from the use of fentanyl but is of shorter duration than with other drugs. The rapid intravenous injection of fentanyl may cause muscular rigidity during anaesthesia and lead to ventilatory insufficiency, but it responds rapidly to small doses of relaxants.

On discontinuing the nitrous oxide at the end of operation, patients rapidly respond to commands, and yet if left to themselves they sleep peacefully oblivious of uncomfortable catheters and suction tubes. The incidence of vomiting is low as droperidol has a potent anti-emetic effect, while in most instances analgesia continues into the post-operative period for several hours. The post-operative state following this technique makes it an ideal choice in patients who are undergoing major oral surgery, such as mandibular osteotomy, in which the jaws are wired together at the end of operation and contrasts with the restlessness which often follows more conventional methods of anaesthesia.

A rare complication of the butyrophenones such as droperidol is the occurrence of extrapyramidal type of movements 24 to 48 hours after administration. They occur most frequently in children or young adults and can be controlled by atropine or anti-Parkinson drugs such as orphenadrine (20–40 mg IM). Because minor central effects can last for up to 48 hours after the administration of droperidol, patients should be warned not to drive or operate machinery on the day following anaesthesia. As mental depression may be aggravated by droperidol, it should be avoided in depressed patients and care should be taken in patients with hepatic disease.

The value of neuroleptanalgesia in supplementing light general anaesthesia has now been established. The smooth post-operative course, protection against adrenaline-induced arrhythmias, the profound analgesia and minimal hypotension are all desirable features. There are objections, however, to the intravenous injection of mixtures of powerful drugs when there is inadequate human pharmacological data on the individual constituents (Dobkin *et al.*, 1963). Unlike an inhalational agent, there is no way of retrieving them once they have been administered. Nevertheless it has proved a useful technique, especially in geriatric surgery, in patients with haemodynamic disturbances, and those who might require ventilatory assistance in the post-operative period without recourse to tracheostomy. This technique now has an established place in the anaesthetist's armamentarium.

REFERENCES

ALEXANDER, J. I., SPENCE, A. A., PARIKH, R. K., and STUART, B. (1973). The role of airway closure in postoperative hypoxaemia: *Brit. J. Anaesth.*, **45**, 34.

APPLEGATE, W. V. (1972). Abdominal cutaneous nerve entrapment syndrome. *Surgery*, **71**, 118.

AUBRY, U., CARIGNAN, G., CHARETTE, D., KEERI-SZANTO, M., and LAVALLEE, J-P. (1966). Neuroleptanalgesia with fentanyl-droperidol: an appreciation based on more than 1,000 anaesthetics for major surgery. *Canad. Anaesth. Soc. J.*, **13**, 263.

BELAM, O. H., and DOBNEY, G. H. (1957). Persistent pain. Treatment by nerve block. *Anaesthesia*, **12**, 345.

BERGAN, J. J., and CONN, J. (1968). Sympathectomy for pain relief. *Med. Clin. N. Amer.*, **52**, 147.

BONICA, J. J. (1953). *The Management of Pain*. Philadelphia: Lea & Febiger.

BRAIN, R. (1956). Symposium on the treatment of cerebrovascular disease. *Proc. roy. Soc. Med.*, **49**, 164.

BRIDENBAUGH, L. D., MOORE, D. C., and CAMPBELL, D. D. (1964). Management of upper abdominal cancer. *J. Amer. med. Ass.*, **190**, 877.

BRIDENBAUGH, P. O., DUPEN, S. L., MOORE, D. C., BRIDENBAUGH, L. D., and THOMPSON, G. E. (1973). Postoperative intercostal nerve block analgesia versus narcotic analgesia. *Anesth. Analg. Curr. Res.*, **52**, 81.

BROMAGE, P. R. (1967). Extradural analgesia for pain relief. *Brit. J. Anaesth.*, **39**, 721.

BROMAGE, P. R. (1972). Unblocked segments in epidural analgesia for relief of pain in labour. *Brit. J. Anaesth.*, **44**, 676.

BROWN, A. S. (1964). Neuroleptanalgesia for the surgical treatment of Parkinsonism. *Anaesthesia*, **19**, 70.

BURTLES, R., and PECKETT, B. W. (1957). Postoperative vomiting. Some factors affecting its incidence. *Brit. J. Anaesth.*, **29**, 114.

CARTER, A. B. (1957). The immediate treatment of cerebral embolism. *Quart. J. Med.*, **26**, 335.

CHAPMAN, G. M. (1972). Regional nerve block with the aid of a nerve stimulator. *Anaesthesia*, **27**, 185.

CLUTTON-BROCK, J. (1960). Some pain threshold studies with particular reference to thiopentone. *Anaesthesia*, **15**, 71.

DENTON, J. E., and BEECHER, H. K. (1949). New analgesia: A clinical appraisal of the narcotic power of methadone and its isomers. *J. Amer. med. Ass.*, **141**, 1146.

DOBKIN, A. B., LEE, P. K. Y., BYLES, P. H., and ISRAEL, J. S. (1963). Neuroleptanalgesics: A comparison of the cardiovascular, respiratory and metabolic effects of Innovan and thiopentone plus methotrimeprazine. *Brit. J. Anaesth.*, **35**, 694.

DOGLIOTTI, A. M. (1931). Traitement des syndromes douloureux de la périphérie par l'alcoolisation sub-arachnoïdienne des racines postérieures à leur émergence de la moelle épinière. *Presse méd.*, **39**, 1249.

DOUGHTY, A. G. (1964). Personal communication.

DOUPE, J., CULLEN, G. H., and CHANCE, G. Q. (1944). Post-traumatic pain and the causalgic syndrome. *J. Neurol. Neurosurg. Psychiat.*, **7**, 33.

DUNDEE, J. W. (1960). Alterations in response to somatic pain associated with anaesthesia. II. The effect of thiopentone and pentobarbitone. *Brit. J. Anaesth.*, **32**, 407.

FINER, B. (1958). Epidural injection of carbolic acid in incurable cancer. *Lancet*, **2**, 1179.

GALIZIA, E. J., and LAHIRI, S. K. (1974). Paraplegia following coeliac plexus block with phenol. *Brit. J. Anaesth.*, **46**, 539.

GORBITZ, C., and LEAVENS, M. E. (1971). Alcohol block of the coeliac plexus for control of upper abdominal pain caused by cancer and pancreatitis. *J. Neurosurg.*, **34**, 575.

GORDON, R. A., and GOEL, S. B. (1963). Intrathecal phenol block in treatment of intractable pain of malignant disease. *Canad. Anaesth. Soc. J.*, **10**, 357.

HITCHCOCK, E. (1967). Hypothermic subarachnoid irrigation for intractable pain. *Lancet*, **1**, 1133.

HITCHCOCK, E. (1969). Hypothermic subarachnoid irrigation. *Lancet*, **1**, 1330.

HITCHCOCK, E., and PRANDINI, M. N. (1973). Hypertonic saline in management of intractable pain. *Lancet*, **1**, 310.

HOLDERNESS, M. C., CHASE, P. E., and DRIPPS, R. D. (1963). A narcotic analgesic and a butyrophenone with nitrous oxide for general anaesthesia. *Anesthesiology*, **24**, 336.

HOVELL, B. C., MASSON, A. H. B., and WILSON, J. (1967). Trichloroethylene for postoperative analgesia. *Anaesthesia*, **22**, 284.

KELLY, R. E., and GAUTIER SMITH, P. C. (1959). Intrathecal phenol in the treatment of reflex spasms and spasticity. *Lancet*, **2**, 1102.

LASAGNA, L., and BEECHER, H. K. (1954). Optimal dose of morphine. *J. Amer. med. Ass.*, **156**, 230.

LIN, P. M., GILDENBERG, P. L., and POLAKOFF, P. P. (1966). An anterior approach to percutaneous lower cervical cordotomy. *J. Neurosurg.*, **25**, 553.

LIPTON, S. (1968). Percutaneous electrical cordotomy in relief of intractable pain. *Brit. med. J.*, **2**, 210.

LLOYD, J. W., HUGHES, J. T., and DAVIES JONES, G. A. B. (1972). Relief of severe intractable pain by barbotage of cerebro-spinal fluid. *Lancet*, **1**, 354.

MAHER, R. M. (1955). Relief of pain in incurable cancer. *Lancet*, **1**, 18.

MAHER, R. M. (1957). Neurone selection in relief of pain. Further experiences with intra-thecal injections. *Lancet*, **1**, 16.

MAHER, R. M. (1960). Further experiences with intrathecal and subdural phenol. Observa-tions on two forms of pain. *Lancet*, **1**, 895.

MAHER, R. M. (1963). Intrathecal chlorocresol (parachlormetacresol) in the treatment of pain in cancer. *Lancet*, **1**, 965.

MEHTA, M. (1973). In: *Intractable Pain*. London: W. B. Saunders Co.

MEHTA, M., and RANGER, I. (1971). Persistent abdominal pain. Treatment by nerve block. *Anaesthesia*, **26**, 330.

MERSKEY, H., and HESTER, R. A. (1972). The treatment of chronic pain with psychotropic drugs. *Postgrad. med. J.*, **48**, 594.

MOORE, D. C. (1965). *Regional Block. A handbook for use in the clinical practice of medicine and surgery*, 4th edit. Springfield, Ill.: Charles C. Thomas.

MOORE, J., and DUNDEE, J. W. (1961). Promethazine. Its influence on the course of thio-pentone and methohexital anaesthesia. *Anaesthesia*, **16**, 61.

MULLAN, S., HEKMATPANAH, J., DOBBEN, G., and BECKMAN, F. (1965). Percutaneous, intramedullary cordotomy utilizing the unipolar anodal electrolytic lesion. *J. Neuro-surg.*, **22**, 548.

MULLAN, S., and HOSOBUCHI, Y. (1968). Respiratory hazards of high cervical percutaneous cordotomy. *J. Neurosurg.*, **28**, 291.

NATHAN, P. W. (1952). Newer synthetic analgesic drugs. *Brit. med. J.*, **2**, 903.

NATHAN, P. W. (1959). Intrathecal phenol to relieve spasticity in paraplegia. *Lancet*, **2**, 1099.

NATHAN, P. W. (1967). Some aspects of the cancer problem. *Brit. med. J.*, **1**, 168.

NATHAN, P. W., and SCOTT, T. G. (1958). Intrathecal phenol for intractable pain. *Lancet*, **1**, 76.

NATHAN, P. W., and SEARS, T. A. (1960). Effects of phenol on nervous conduction. *J. Physiol. (Lond.)*, **150**, 565.

NATHAN, P. W., SEARS, T. A., and SMITH, M. C. (1965). Effects of phenol solutions on the nerve roots of the cat: an electrophysiological and histological study. *J. neurol. Sci.*, **2**, 7.

NILSSON, E. (1963). Editorial: Origin and rationale of neurolept-analgesia. *Anesthesiology*, **24**, 267.

PARBROOK, G. D. (1967a). Techniques of inhalational analgesia in the postoperative period. *Brit. J. Anaesth.*, **39**, 730.

PARBROOK, G. D. (1967b). Comparison of trichloroethylene and nitrous oxide as anal-gesics. *Brit. J. Anaesth.*, **39**, 86.

PARBROOK, G. D. (1972). Entonox for postoperative analgesia. *Proc. roy. Soc. Med.*, **65**, 8.

PARKHOUSE, J., LAMBRECHTS, W., and SIMPSON, B. R. J. (1961). The incidence of post-operative pain. *Brit. J. Anaesth.*, **33**, 345.

REID, W., KENNEDY WATT, J., and GRAY, T. G. (1970). Phenol injection of the sympathetic chain. *Brit. J. Surg.*, **57**, 45.

ROSOMOFF, H. L., CARROLL, F., BROWN, J., and SHEPTAK, P. (1965). Percutaneous radio-frequency cervical cordotomy: technique. *J. Neurosurg.*, **23**, 639.

SCHEINBURG, P. (1950). Cerebral blood flow in vascular disease of brain, with observations on effects of stellate ganglion block. *Amer. J. Med.*, **8**, 139.

SHERLOCK, S. (1962). Jaundice. *Brit. med. J.*, **1,**, 1359.

SIMPSON, B. R. J., and PARKHOUSE, J. (1961). The problem of postoperative pain. *Brit. J. Anaesth.*, **33**, 336.

SIMPSON, B. R., PARKHOUSE, J., MARSHALL, R., and LAMBRECHTS, W. (1961). Extradural analgesia and the prevention of postoperative respiratory complications. *Brit. J. Anaesth.*, **33**, 628.

SMITH, M. C. (1964). Histological findings following intrathecal injections of phenol solutions for relief of pain. *Brit. J. Anaesth.*, **36**, 387.

SPENCE, A. A., and ALEXANDER, J. I. (1971). Mechanisms of postoperative hypoxaemia. *Proc. roy. Soc. Med.*, **65**, 12.

SPENCE, A. A., SMITH, G., HARRIS, R. (1970). The influence of postoperative analgesia and operative procedure on postoperative lung function: a comparison of morphine with extradural block. *Anaesthesia*, **25**, 126.

SWERDLOW, M., and SAYLE CREER, W. (1970). A study of extradural medication in the relief of the lumbosciatic syndrome. *Anaesthesia*, **25**, 341.

THOMAS, K. B. (1966). Neuroleptanalgesia for cataract surgery. *Acta anaesth. scand.*, Suppl., **24**, 229.

WALLACE, P. G. M., and NORRIS, W. (1975). The management of postoperative pain. *Brit. J. Anaesth.*, **47**, 113.

WALSH, R. C. (1956). Symposium on the treatment of cerebrovascular disease. *Proc. roy. Soc. Med.*, **49**, 161.

YAKAITIS, R. W., COOKE, J. E., and REDDING, J. S. (1972). Self-administered methoxyflurane on postoperative pain: effectiveness and patient acceptance *Anesth. Analg. Curr. Res.*, **51**, 208.

Chapter 34

THE PHARMACOLOGY OF LOCAL ANAESTHETIC DRUGS

A local anaesthetic drug reversibly blocks nerve conduction beyond the point of application, when applied locally in the appropriate concentration. Many drugs have local anaesthetic properties, notably quinidine-like anti-dysrhythmic drugs, antihistamines and tricyclic antidepressants, but this chapter refers only to those drugs used primarily for local anaesthesia.

History

For many centuries the inhabitants of the highlands of Peru and Bolivia chewed the leaves of the indigenous shrub *Erythroxylum coca* for the sake of their effects of diminishing fatigue and appetite. These effects are due primarily to the principal alkaloid, cocaine. Numbing of the oral mucosa was, of course, merely regarded as a side-effect; it was not until the second half of the nineteenth century that the possible nature of the active substances contained in the plant roused the interest of scientific investigators in Europe. Cocaine was first isolated in 1860 by Neimann, who noted its local anaesthetic effect. It was over a generation, however, before this discovery was exploited. In the 1880's Sigmund Freud studied the physiological effects of cocaine and used it to treat morphine addiction, thereby producing the first cocaine addict in Europe. While Freud was away visiting his fiancée in 1884, a colleague, Karl Köller introduced cocaine as a local anaesthetic for the eye at an ophthalmological congress, with immediate success. Freud was of course destined to become famous in other ways and so could afford to be magnanimous towards his colleague. Thereafter the field of local anaesthesia expanded quickly to include infiltration, nerve block and, later, spinal anaesthesia. Very soon the high systemic toxicity and addictive properties of cocaine stimulated the search for less toxic synthetic substitutes. A number of synthetic local anaesthetics emerged during this period, of which procaine, introduced by Einhorn in 1905, was the most important. It proved to be less toxic than cocaine, but somewhat unreliable and with a short duration of action. Numerous related compounds with few advantages over procaine emerged in the years that followed, but the major advance of the period was probably the production of cinchocaine in Germany in the late 1920's. The next milestone was the introduction of lignocaine in the 1940's: the forerunner of a new generation of chemically related and greatly improved local anaesthetics.

Chemistry

The local anaesthetics in current use have the following basic formula:

Aromatic lipophilic — Intermediate chain — hydrophilic group
group   (ester: —COO— or 2_{ary} or 3_{ary} amine.
amide—NH.CO—)

Individual formulae are:

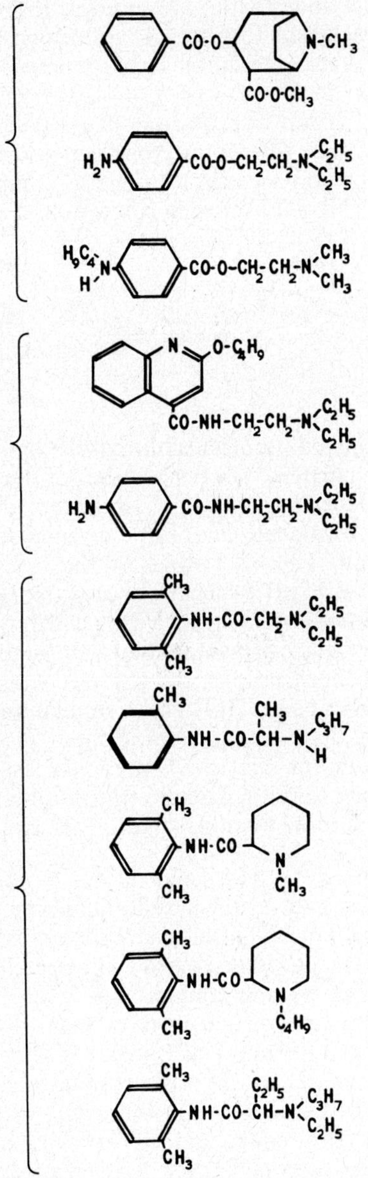

esters of
aromatic acids
with
amino-alcohols

amides of aromatic
acids with
aliphatic diamines
(*aminoalkyl amides*)

amides of amino
acids with
aromatic amines
(*aminoacyl amides*)

cocaine

procaine

amethocaine

cinchocaine

procainamide

lignocaine

prilocaine

mepivacaine

bupivacaine

etidocaine

34/Fig. 1.—The structural formulae of local anaesthetic drugs. Procainamide is included here, although used only as an anti-dysrhythmic, because it is mentioned in this chapter.

All modern local anaesthetics are amides. Esters are unstable in solution and cannot be autoclaved. Lignocaine, prilocaine, mepivacaine, bupivacaine and etidocaine all share a common basic structure that is sometimes termed aminoacyl amide.

The hydrophilic group in prilocaine is a secondary amine; the rest listed above are tertiary amines. The amine group confers on the molecule the property of a weak base (or proton acceptor) which can combine with an acid to form a water-soluble salt. This salt ionises in solution and is usually stable.

The non-ionised form of the molecule (the base) is lipid-soluble and consequently can penetrate tissue barriers. The proportions of the two forms of the molecule present in solution depend upon the pK_a of the molecule (see Chapter 21) and on the pH of the environment, and can be calculated from the Henderson-Hasselbalch equation. The pK_a values of the modern local anaesthetics are around 8 (see Table 3). At pH 7·4 a basic drug with pK_a of 7·86 such as lignocaine is 25 per cent non-ionised, whereas for a drug with a pK_a of the order of 9 such as procaine only 2·5 per cent is present in this form. At physiological pH, therefore, and at equal total concentrations, the concentration of lignocaine base is ten times that of procaine base. This factor contributes to the greatly enhanced penetrative power of lignocaine over procaine.

A local anaesthetic for injection is presented as a salt—usually the hydrochloride. The resulting solution is acidic, as the salt is derived from a strong acid and a weak base. In a more alkaline solution the drug is less soluble.

Nerve Conduction

A nerve fibre consists of a central semi-fluid core, the axoplasm, enclosed in a tube, the cell membrane. The cell membrane is believed to be built up of a bimolecular lipid palisade, interspersed with protein molecules and bounded inside and out by a monomolecular protein layer. Each fibre of a peripheral nerve is enclosed in a tube of neurilemma, from which it is separated by the myelin sheath, except at the nodes of Ranvier. The myelin sheath, an insulating layer, is absent—or nearly so—in non-medullated nerves. Nerve fibres so encased are collected in bundles within the *endoneurium*. The *perineurium* surrounds a collection of bundles, and the *epineurium* encloses a whole nerve. There is therefore a substantial barrier between a local anaesthetic injected into the extracellular compartment and its site of action at the nerve cell membrane.

During nerve conduction, changes occur in the cell membrane. In the *resting state* there is a potential difference across the cell membrane, inside negative, due to a higher concentration of sodium ions outside than in. The cell membrane is relatively impermeable to sodium ions whose gradient is maintained by the sodium pump.

Depolarisation phase.—When a nerve is stimulated, partial depolarisation of the membrane is accompanied by a release of calcium ions and leads to a large transient increase in permeability to sodium ions which therefore enter the fibre, resulting in massive depolarisation. Thus, the threshold required to produce the action potential is exceeded, with consequent propagation of the nerve impulse.

During the *neutralisation phase*, potassium ions pass out of the fibre to restore electrical neutrality.

In the *restoration phase* sodium ions return to the outside and potassium ions re-enter the fibre.

In myelinated nerves these changes take place only at the nodes of Ranvier, giving rise to saltatory conduction of the nerve impulse.

The Action of Local Anaesthetics on the Cell Membrane

The primary action of a local anaesthetic is on the cell membrane of the axon, on which it produces electrical stabilisation. The large transient increase in permeability to sodium ions, necessary for propagation of the impulse, is prevented, thus the resting potential is maintained and depolarisation in response to stimulation is inhibited. Initially the threshold for electrical excitation is raised, the rate of rise of the action potential reduced, and conduction slowed; eventually propagation of the impulse fails (Ritchie and Greengard, 1966).

Classical local anaesthetics probably have a dual action on the cell membrane to produce these effects (Takman, 1975).

(1) They have an action on the axoplasmic opening of the sodium channels;

(2) They produce a non-specific physicochemical effect within the lipid layer of the cell membrane.

Action on the interior or axoplasmic openings of sodium channels.—This is probably an action on specific receptors and is shared by quaternary analogues of lignocaine (Ritchie, 1975). Quaternary derivatives of lignocaine, being fully ionised, cannot penetrate the cell membrane, and produce nerve blockade only if applied to its inner surface. Similarly, amine local anaesthetics act principally in the cationic form (see below—Active Form of the Local Anaesthetic Molecule) and on the axoplasmic surface of the membrane (Narahashi *et al.*, 1970). This suggests that local anaesthetics impair sodium permeability by an action blocking the internal openings of sodium channels. This action accounts for about 90 per cent of the nerve conduction blocking effect of lignocaine.

Physicochemical mechanism (Seeman, 1972).—This is a non-specific action in contrast to a more specific drug-receptor interaction, and is analogous to the electrical stabilisation produced by a number of non-polar, purely lipid-soluble substances such as non-ionised barbiturates, general anaesthetics and benzocaine.

The production of nerve conduction blockade is associated with about a 3·5 per cent expansion of membrane volume; the actual volume of the anaesthetic occupying the membrane, however, is only about 0·3 per cent or less. The equivalent figures for general anaesthesia are a volume expansion of the membrane of 0·6 per cent compared with the volume of the anaesthetic of about 0·02 per cent. Since the volume occupied by the anaesthetic only accounts for about 10 per cent of this membrane expansion, a number of mechanisms have been suggested to account for the further 90 per cent. The most likely explanation is that there is an unfolding of membrane protein, together with a disordering of the lipid component of the cell membrane (Seeman, 1977), with consequent obstruction of the sodium channels. Displacement of membrane-bound calcium ions may also be involved; calcium is known to condense lipid layers and local anaesthetics to displace it. This mechanism may account for the major part of the effect of benzocaine and procaine, whose active form appears to be the uncharged base, but only the lesser part of the effect of lignocaine (Ritchie, 1975). Nevertheless, pressure has been shown to partially reverse nerve block by lignocaine, though not by procaine (Kendig and Cohen, 1977).

The Active Form of the Local Anaesthetic Molecule

In order to act, a local anaesthetic must first penetrate the surrounding tissues and the nerve sheath. Only the uncharged form, therefore, can gain access to the cell membrane.

According to the evidence of Ritchie *et al.* (1965), however, the cation is responsible for most of the nerve blocking effect. This they demonstrated in the following way. They suspended intact and desheathed nerves in bath fluids of different pH values and added different concentrations of lignocaine. By measuring the action potential produced by stimulation of the nerve they were able to find the minimum concentration of lignocaine necessary to produce conduction block in different pH conditions. They showed that while a high pH favoured block by lignocaine of an intact nerve, in a desheathed preparation the optimum pH for the action of lignocaine was neutral. Thus, where little or no penetration was required the lowest effective concentration was one which contained a predominance of the cationic form of the drug.

Carbonated local anaesthetics.—Research on carbonated local anaesthetics (Catchlove, 1972) provides further evidence that the cation is the active form of the local anaesthetic molecule and that it acts on the interior of the cell membrane. A number of factors may contribute to the enhanced effect of lignocaine carbonate over lignocaine hydrochloride:
  (i) the pH of the solution is higher than that of the hydrochloride, thereby increasing the concentration of uncharged base available for penetration.
 (ii) CO_2 is released and diffuses to the interior of the cell more rapidly than the local anaesthetic. Within the axon it lowers the pH thereby increasing the ionisation of the local anaesthetic. This has a two-fold effect:
     (a) the concentration of base is reduced, so increasing its gradient for diffusion into the cell, a phenomenon known as diffusion trapping:
     (b) the release of cation enhances the nerve blocking activity (*vide supra*).
(iii) CO_2 itself has some nerve blocking effect on desheathed preparations.

Clinically, carbonated lignocaine and prilocaine have both been shown to be superior to the hydrochlorides for epidural block in speed of onset, reduction in the incidence of missed segments and increased incidence of motor block (Bromage *et al.*, 1967).

Tachyphylaxis is also less evident with lignocaine carbonate than hydrochloride. Successive injections of the hydrochloride may lower the local pH, thus lignocaine becomes more ionised and less can penetrate to the site of action (Tucker and Mather, 1975). The carbonate, however, is a less acid salt. The advantages of carbonated *bupivacaine* are less clear (Atkinson and Nicholas, 1976). Tachyphylaxis is not evident with bupivacaine, in part perhaps because bupivacaine is a stronger base than lignocaine, thus the hydrochloride salt is less acid than lignocaine hydrochloride.

Potency and Duration of Action

Among local anaesthetics high potency and long duration of action tend to be directly related while the action of an individual drug can, to a certain extent, be prolonged by increasing the concentration and the dose.

In any one homologous series, for example in the mepivacaine-bupivacaine series, increasing the length of the side chain on the amine nitrogen increases potency, but beyond C_4 tissue irritancy becomes too high and aqueous solubility too low for usefulness (af Ekenstam, 1966).

High potency is associated with high lipid solubility because this property facilitates solution in and passage across the cell membrane. A high pK_a tends to reduce the concentration of base present at the site of injection, to increase the water solubility of the molecule and hence accelerate its removal from the site of action, as will the production of vasodilatation by the drug itself. Conversely vasoconstriction will enhance and prolong the effect.

Rapid biotransformation cannot shorten the action of amide local anaesthetics, which are only metabolised in the liver, while even the effect of pseudocholinesterase on procaine is negligible in the tissues.

The relationship between potency and toxicity is discussed below under Systemic Toxicity.

Some physicochemical properties mentioned above are listed for individual local anaesthetics in Table 3 (p. 1113).

Sensitivity of Different Fibre Types

All types of nerve fibres are affected by local anaesthetics, but within any one fibre type (see Table 1) there is a tendency for small, slower-conducting fibres to be more readily blocked than large, fast-conducting fibres (Franz and Perry, 1974).

34/TABLE 1

Fibre Type		Function		Fibre Diameter	Conduction Speed
		Sensory	Motor	µm	m/sec
A	α	proprioception	somatic	12–20	70–120
	β	touch, pressure		5–12	30–70
	γ		muscle spindle	3–6	15–30
	δ	pain, temperature		2–5	12–30
B			preganglionic	<3	3–15
C		pain, reflex	post-ganglionic	0·3–1·3	0·5–2·3

Between fibre types, however, these rules do not hold good. Heavner and de Jong (1974) showed that myelinated preganglionic B fibres which have a faster conduction time are about three times more sensitive to lignocaine than the slower non-myelinated postganglionic C fibres. In fact there is both experimental and clinical evidence that preganglionic fibres are the most sensitive of all: vasodilatation, with consequent hypotension if sufficiently widespread, is a

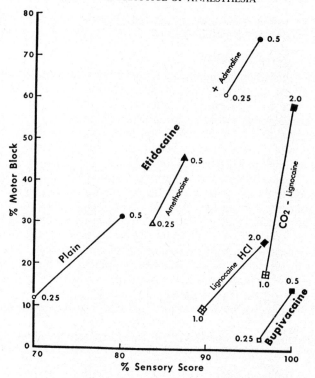

34/Fig. 2.—Comparison of average scores for motor and sensory blockade during epidural analgesia in obstetric patients (Bromage, 1975).

well-recognised early sequel to epidural, spinal or paravertebral block, which can all affect white rami communicantes of the sympathetic chain. The smaller A fibres, subserving pain and temperature sensation, are also more sensitive than C pain fibres, although more rapidly conducting (Strichartz, 1976; Nathan and Sears, 1961). Pathological pain (conducted by C fibres) such as that produced by impending uterine rupture or placental separation, may occasionally break through an epidural block which is relieving the physiological pain of labour: the "epidural sieve" (Crawford, 1976). The greater sensitivity of A δ than C fibres to local anaesthetic block could perhaps go some way to explain this phenomenon. Steinmann (1967) showed in the frog that sensory A fibres were more sensitive to blockade by a variety of specific and non-specific agents than were motor A fibres of the same conduction velocity. Franz and Perry (1974) suggest that because sensory fibres conduct at a higher frequency than motor fibres they are more susceptible to conduction block. Similarly, after epidural administration in man all local anaesthetics produce a higher incidence of sensory than of motor block, though the relationship between the two effects varies from one drug to another (see Fig. 2).

In summary the order of sensitivity to blockade appears to be (starting from the most sensitive): preganglionic, pain and temperature, touch, proprioception and motor fibres.

PHARMACOLOGICAL EFFECTS

The effects produced by local anaesthetics may be:

(a) *local:*   nerve blockade or a direct effect on smooth muscle (see below: vascular smooth muscle);

(b) *regional:* loss of pain and temperature sensation, touch, motor power, and vasomotor tone, in the region supplied by the nerves blocked;

(c) *systemic:* effects occurring as a result of systemic absorption, or intravenous administration. The production of nerve blockade requires a concentration about one thousand times higher than any that occurs systemically. Thus the so-called analgesic properties of a procaine infusion are due to central sedation and not to any peripheral nerve blocking action. The chief systemic effects of local anaesthetics are on the heart and the central nervous system, and are probably produced by the same action as is nerve blockade, that is by membrane stabilisation.

Cardiovascular System

The heart.—Local anaesthetics have a stabilising effect on the cell membrane of cardiac tissue. They tend to depress automaticity in abnormal or damaged fibres and thereby suppress cardiac dysrhythmias. Some, such as procaine and procainamide have quinidine-like effects; they prolong the action potential duration thus increasing the effective refractory period of cardiac cells, slowing conduction and so desynchronising ventricular contraction with a consequent depressant effect on myocardial contractility. Lignocaine in clinical doses appears not to possess a classical quinidine-like action. Its use as an anti-dysrhythmic is discussed on page 1117.

Vascular smooth muscle.—The effects local anaesthetics may have on vascular smooth muscle cause some confusion (Blair, 1975) since they may be local, regional or systemic. The *local* effects vary. While procaine is undoubtedly vasodilator and cocaine vasoconstrictor (due to its sympathetic potentiating effect), vasomotor effects among modern local anaesthetics vary depending upon the nature of the drug and upon its concentration (Reynolds *et al.*, 1976). Vasoconstriction is more frequent at lower concentrations and vasodilatation at higher (Åberg, 1972; Aps and Reynolds, 1976). Åberg (1972) suggested that vasoconstriction and vasodilatation were associated with stimulation and inhibition respectively of tissue-bound Ca^{++} release. Among the drugs in general use mepivacaine appears most likely to produce vasoconstriction at clinical concentrations, then prilocaine, lignocaine, and bupivacaine in that order. Of these drugs all but lignocaine exist as two stereoisomers, and the ability to produce vasoconstriction appears to be vested in one of the isomers (Luduena, 1969), concentration having the same effect as with the racemates (Aps and Reynolds, 1978). The *regional* effect is simply vasodilatation in the area supplied by blocked sympathetic nerves. *Systemic* effects may be produced in a variety of ways, reflexly and because of central nervous system involvement, but not as a result of any direct action on blood vessels outlined above, because the ambient concentration would be too low. Effects on the circulation of subconvulsive doses of modern local anaesthetics are variable but minimal (Jorfeldt *et al.*, 1968; Jewitt *et al.*, 1968), while large doses may produce circulatory collapse as a result of medullary depression and of convulsions causing respiratory impairment (Fink, 1973) and not because of any direct effect on the circulation.

Central nervous system.—The concept of local anaesthetics as central nervous system stimulants should be eschewed. It dates from the last century when cocaine was the only local anaesthetic. Cocaine has undoubted stimulant effects which are unrelated to its local anaesthetic action. With the synthetic agents, mild toxicity produces sedation, inebriation and sometimes disorientation. Less commonly, anxiety and apparent stimulation occur, in which case inhibitory neurones have proved more susceptible than excitatory ones to depression, a situation not unfamiliar with alcohol. With more marked toxicity there may be restlessness, pins and needles or tremors and twitching, which if severe proceed to convulsions and unconsciousness. Coma may be accompanied by apnoea and cardiovascular collapse, both of which can occur because of convulsions or medullary depression (Steinhaus, 1957). Convulsions and unconsciousness may occur unheralded in severe intoxication of rapid onset. While barbiturates may afford protection against cocaine convulsions (Fink, 1973) they may actually be harmful with other local anaesthetics. Treatment of intoxication is covered under Systemic Toxicity (p. 1106).

Both lignocaine and procaine have been used by intravenous infusion primarily to produce central sedation. The sedative effect of lignocaine absorbed after epidural administration, for example, is well recognised.

Autonomic nervous system.—Cocaine, by inhibiting catecholamine uptake, has an undoubted sympathetic potentiating effect. Some potentiating effect, albeit very weak and short-lived, has been observed with procaine and lignocaine (D'Amato and Truant, 1955) although neither mepivacaine nor lignocaine blocks noradrenaline uptake (Åberg et al., 1973). *Ganglia:* local anaesthetics are not ganglion blockers in clinical doses and any apparent block produced locally at extremely high concentrations is probably due to a stabilising action on the nerve terminals.

Neuromuscular junction.—Local anaesthetics can certainly block motor nerves if present in sufficient concentration, and the pre-synaptic blocking effect that has been observed under experimental conditions with high concentrations of procaine again simply reflects a membrane stabilising action.

Hypersensitivity.—This implies an abnormal antigen-antibody response, and not an exaggerated normal response, correctly termed *supersensitivity*. The term has also been misused to describe adverse reactions due to accidental intravenous injection and frank overdose, while the lay public frequently claim "sensitivity" to the local anaesthetic when they have suffered a classical faint or a typical adrenaline reaction. It appears that dentists encounter true hypersensitivity to modern local anaesthetics, though rarely, more frequently than do anaesthetists, probably because of the much larger number of patients given dental local anaesthesia. Hypersensitivity to a local anaesthetic is more frequent in atopic individuals and may be manifested as local oedema initially, as generalised urticaria, or as angioneurotic oedema with or without lymphadenopathy. Dermatitis may be encountered as a delayed reaction to skin applications and as contact dermatitis in dentists. Anaphylaxis appears less common than atopic reactions.

Hypersensitivity to procaine and other ester derivatives of benzoic acid is not uncommon. There is likely to be cross sensitivity within the ester group of drugs and with *p*-aminobenzoic acid (Gaul, 1955), widely used as a sunscreen, and *p*-hydroxybenzoic acid and its derivatives (paraben, methylparaben) which are preservatives and may be incorporated into amide local anaesthetic preparations (Aldrete, 1969). All these benzoic acid esters are relatively highly antigenic whereas the amide local anaesthetics are not, though true hypersensitivity to lignocaine has been reported (Waldman and Binkley, 1967; Eyre and Nally, 1971; Walker, 1971).

DISTRIBUTION AND FATE

Absorption.—A dose of local anaesthetic must eventually be absorbed virtually entirely into the systemic circulation. The rate of absorption depends on several factors. The pK_a and lipid solubility of the agent together determine the proportion remaining in the aqueous phase available for rapid removal by the blood, and the proportion taken up by the tissues and therefore only slowly released into the systemic circulation (see also sections on Chemistry and Mode of Action). The vascularity of the tissues influences removal and can be altered by the local anaesthetic itself and by adrenaline (see below). Absorption of some local anaesthetics from mucosal surfaces such as the trachea or an inflamed urethra, can give rise to plasma concentrations akin to those produced by direct intravenous injection (Adriani and Campbell, 1956). Absorption from the gastro-intestinal tract does occur, and for procainamide which is mainly excreted unchanged, oral antidysrhythmic therapy can be successful (Koch-Weser and Klein, 1971), but for lignocaine, of which 70 per cent may be metabolised in a single passage through the liver, this route is ineffective.

Distribution.—In the plasma, local anaesthetics are bound to plasma proteins (principally the globulin fraction) to an extent partly related to their potency and lipid solubility (see Table 3). A small proportion related to *free* concentration enters red cells. They are rapidly removed from the blood by the tissues. In general, distribution is so rapid that most of the drug has disappeared from the circulation before mixing in the blood is complete. Full equilibration with the tissues, however, may take many hours. Local anaesthetics readily cross lipid membranes such as cell membranes, the blood-brain barrier and the placenta (Chapter 44) and become more concentrated in tissues than in the blood. The volume distribution of lignocaine, for example, is about $2\frac{1}{2}$ l/kg but varies widely between individuals (Aps *et al.*, 1976).

Metabolism.—Metabolism of local anaesthetics produces in general more water-soluble compounds, which are therefore less concentrated in tissues and more rapidly excreted than the parent drugs. Amide local anaesthetics are metabolised in the liver, while most esters may also be hydrolysed in the plasma. In the liver, several pathways are involved. *N-dealkylation* of the tertiary amine has been shown to take place in a number of local anaesthetics (Reynolds, 1971*a*) producing a more water-soluble secondary amine, and in the case of lignocaine for example, rendering it more susceptible to amide hydrolysis (Hollunger, 1960), as is the more rapidly metabolised secondary amine prilocaine (Geddes, 1965). *Hydroxylation* of the aromatic nucleus is believed to occur in the case of lignocaine, mepivacaine and bupivacaine (Boyes, 1975), to produce a compound which can be conjugated and so become solely water-soluble. Owing to its wide use as an antidysrhythmic, the breakdown of lignocaine has been most extensively studied. As much as 70 per cent may be broken down during a single passage through the liver, this high first-pass clearance yielding mainly the N-dealkylated product monoethylglycine xylidine, itself a moderately toxic and effective antidysrhythmic. The high clearance rate of lignocaine is markedly reduced in the presence of a low cardiac output (Aps *et al.*, 1976) and hence by halothane (Difazio, 1975). Amino*alkyl* amides (cinchocaine and procainamide) are metabolised much more slowly than amino*acyl* amides (lignocaine etc.—see Chemistry) and a much larger proportion is consequently excreted unchanged (de Jong, 1975).

In the plasma, procaine is rapidly hydrolysed by pseudocholinesterase, but at a rate which is saturable (de Jong, 1975) and therefore subject to competition with suxamethonium. Amethocaine is hydrolysed at about a fifth the rate of procaine, while plasma cholinesterase appears unable to break down cocaine (de Jong, 1975).

Excretion.—With the exception of cinchocaine and procainamide, only a small fraction of the dose of a local anaesthetic is excreted unchanged in the urine. The water-soluble metabolites are readily excreted, but a lipid-soluble local anaesthetic base, once filtered in the glomerulus, can be re-absorbed in the renal tubule. In an acid urine it becomes highly ionised, tubular reabsorption is inhibited and renal clearance is high. However, with the high tissue uptake of the unchanged drug, renal excretion does not play a major role, even when the urine is acid.

SYSTEMIC TOXICITY

Drug factors.—The toxicity of many drugs such as barbiturates which act systemically, is dose-related and merely an extension of the therapeutic action. Such need not be the case with drugs which act locally and whose toxic effects depend upon systemic absorption. Not surprisingly, the potency of a local anaesthetic is directly related to its acute intravenous toxicity (Luduena *et al.*, 1958), that is when absorption is bypassed and the effect is so rapid that distribution and elimination cannot mitigate it. When a drug is used to produce local anaesthesia, the occurrence of systemic effects depends not upon the acute toxicity (since the dosage will be related to this) but upon the speed of absorption and elimination (see Distribution and Fate, p. 1105). As the rate of metabolism of a local anaesthetic cannot affect its duration of action or potency, but can affect its *chronic* toxicity especially during repeated administration, a drug with a favourable ratio between duration of action and speed of elimination has an advantage.

Other factors.—There is evidence that the occurrence of toxicity is not necessarily related to the concentration of solution injected (Scott *et al.*, 1972) as has been suggested, but rather to the total dose (Braid and Scott, 1966). The speed of epidural injection similarly appears not to affect systemic absorption, although if the drug is injected intravascularly, rapid injection is more likely to produce transient systemic effects. Clearly the site of injection and its vascularity will affect the speed of absorption as will the addition of a vaso-constrictor. The age and height of the patient may variably affect the occurrence of toxicity, and their importance in epidural blockade is dealt with in Chapter 36. Although overdose is rightly feared in the very young and the very old, they are probably no more sensitive to a given plasma level than are other patients. Those with disorders of acid-base balance, however, may be; Englesson and Matousek (1975) showed that local anaesthetic convulsions occur more readily in cats in the presence of a raised P_{CO_2} and reduced pH.

Why, then, does systemic toxicity occur in practice? True, the incidence has been reduced since the advent of bupivacaine and etidocaine. Nevertheless, before demanding the ideal local anaesthetic of long duration of action, slow absorption and rapid elimination, it must be pointed out that most cases of toxicity occur as a result of inadvertent intravascular administration, while rapid absorption from an inflamed urethra was a common cause of death from local anaesthesia before this hazard was realised (Deacock and Simpson, 1964). Moreover, some disasters have been due to gross overdosage (Sunshine and Fike, 1964). Widespread field blocks and excessive surface application of local anaesthetics, sources of trouble in the past, are no longer in vogue, so a single dose of a local anaesthetic should never cause toxicity. The principal danger of true intoxication from a correctly administered local anaesthetic probably lies in its continuous or repeated administration. For this purpose the long duration of bupivacaine and the rapid elimination of etidocaine offer clear advantages.

An attempt has been made to suggest maximum safe doses of the various local anaesthetics in Table 3 (p. 1113).

Manifestations.—Systemic intoxication from synthetic local anaesthetics affects the central nervous system. Severe intoxication is usually preceded by sedation and a feeling of inebriation, unless onset is very rapid because of massive intravenous injection. For an account of central nervous system effects, see under Pharmacological Effects (p. 1103). Even near-convulsant doses are not toxic to the cardiovascular system except through medullary depression.

Treatment.—If signs of minor central nervous system toxicity occur, administration of the local anaesthetic should be discontinued. In the case of an intravenous infusion, simply stopping it may be sufficient treatment. In more severe cases and after local administration (when absorption cannot be stopped) oxygen should be given. In many cases correcting the cerebral hypoxia by this means may be all that is necessary. With full convulsions, intravenous suxamethonium and artificial ventilation with oxygen via an endotracheal tube should be given. If convulsions return with recovery from suxamethonium, Moore and Bridenbaugh (1960) suggest that one more dose of suxamethonium should be given, followed if necessary by tubocurarine. Barbiturates alone should have no place in the treatment of a condition with so large a component of depression, nor do they appear to offer *protection* against convulsions due to any local anaesthetic except cocaine (Fink, 1973). It can be argued, however, that in addition to neuromuscular blockade, some protection of the brain from prolonged electrical discharges may be required, in which case diazepam may be the drug of choice. It has been shown to be effective in both prophylaxis and treatment of lignocaine convulsions (Ausinsch *et al.*, 1976), but pretreatment should offer no licence to use excessive doses.

VASOCONSTRICTORS

Adrenaline

Use.—Adrenaline, by virtue of its α-stimulant action, is used with a local

anaesthetic to prolong its action and delay absorption into the systemic circulation, thereby it is hoped, reducing the incidence of systemic toxicity. When
the very short-acting procaine was one of the few safe local anaesthetics the
use of adrenaline for anything but the shortest procedures was justified. It
increases the duration of action of lignocaine quite considerably, and when
prolonged blockade is required it may reduce the number of repeat doses
needed and delay the onset of chronic toxicity and tachyphylaxis. Its effects on
the long-acting drug bupivacaine, and on prilocaine, are less marked, although
it does prolong the action of etidocaine (see under individual local anaesthetics).
By delaying and reducing peak absorption it may diminish the toxicity of big
doses, even if local anaesthesia is not prolonged. It is more valuable in highly
vascular areas such as the intercostal space and pelvic floor than in the less
vascular epidural space, while in dentistry some form of vasoconstrictor is
essential with most agents. In other fields, however, its dangers may outweigh
its usefulness (*vide infra*), while in vascular areas it greatly increases the danger
from accidental intravenous injection.

For general purposes, adrenaline should not be used with local anaesthetic
solutions in a concentration higher than 5 µg/ml (1:200,000), while in some
cases an even lower concentration may be sufficient. In dentistry, however,
adrenaline 12·5 µg/ml (1:80,000) is still frequently used, though in this situation
of course the total dose is small.

Systemic effects.—Although adrenaline may reduce the systemic absorption
of a local anaesthetic, toxicity usually occurs because of accidental intravenous
injection. In this situation, adrenaline could be more dangerous than the local
anaesthetic itself. Adrenaline has been found to increase the toxicity of local
anaesthetics injected intravenously into mice (Henn and Brattsand, 1966). In
clinical practice, were the entire dose of local anaesthetic containing say 100–
150 µg of adrenaline to be inadvertently given intravenously, one might expect
marked tachycardia, palpitations, anxiety and sweating of brief duration. Such
a dose, however, absorbed slowly after a correctly placed block, would be
expected to have minimal systemic effects in the normal patient, with possibly
some redistribution of blood to areas rich in β-receptors, such as skeletal
muscle. Indeed Corall *et al.* (1975) found the addition of 5 µg/ml of adrenaline
to bupivacaine for obstetric epidurals to have no significant cardiovascular
effects, though it may reduce uterine blood flow (Wallis *et al.*, 1976). In patients
taking certain antihypertensive drugs (because of denervation supersensitivity)
and especially tricyclic antidepressants (Boakes *et al.*, 1973), and in those with
thyrotoxicosis, the systemic effects of adrenaline may be dangerously potentiated. In these situations adrenaline is contra-indicated.

Local effects.—The local α-vasoconstrictor effects of adrenaline may be
dangerous in certain situations. It increases the likelihood of anterior spinal
artery syndrome, a rare complication of epidural analgesia. If used for digital
block it may produce gangrene. If given into a restricted area such as the dermis
it may produce tissue anoxia because it also increases local oxygen consumption
(Klingenström and Westermark, 1964).

Noradrenaline

Noradrenaline is a less potent α-receptor stimulant than adrenaline, thus if used for local anaesthesia a higher concentration is required. It has been used in dentistry in concentrations of 20 or 40 µg/ml (1:50,000 or 1:25,000) and has given rise to dangerous hypertension (Boakes *et al.*, 1972). Tricyclic anti-depressants may cause a 4- to 8-fold potentiation of its pressor effects (Boakes *et al.*, 1973). It is contra-indicated in all those patients in whom adrenaline is contra-indicated, and in hypertension. There are thus no indications for its use in this field.

Felypressin

Felypressin (Octapressin) is a synthetic polypeptide related to vasopressin. It is a vasoconstrictor that may be used as a substitute for adrenaline in local anaesthesia. It is used with prilocaine in dentistry in which it is more effective in prolonging the action of prilocaine than is adrenaline (Goldman and Evers, 1969). Its systemic toxicity is less than that of adrenaline (Åkerman, 1969) and used in dentistry it produces no cardiovascular changes, where adrenaline 12·5 µg/ml is likely to produce tachycardia (Aellig *et al.*, 1970).

DESIRABLE PROPERTIES

There can be no such thing as the ideal local anaesthetic drug because different circumstances require different properties. However, certain characteristics are usually desirable. The first is good penetration. This tends to promote rapid onset of action, to eliminate patchy anaesthesia and to make topical application effective if this is required. A local anaesthetic should not produce local irritation, and systemic side-effects should be minimal. A safe therapeutic ratio is always necessary and not hard to achieve if the local anaesthetic is to be used in a single dose for most techniques in current use. In the past, paravertebral and intercostal block for tuberculosis surgery, for example, sometimes necessitated dangerously large doses. In the techniques commonly used at present, such as epidural blockade, it is relatively easy to keep within safe limits of dosage.

For the production of prolonged local anaesthesia many more properties are required. A long duration of action becomes an advantage for both convenience and safety, and it should be unnecessary to add adrenaline to achieve this. Tachyphylaxis should not occur and slow absorption but rapid elimination of the drug will tend to improve its therapeutic ratio (see discussion on Systemic Toxicity). Reversibility of action is stipulated by definition.

A local anaesthetic solution should be able to withstand repeated autoclaving and minor pH changes and should be stable in light and air.

ASSESSMENT

Most local anaesthetics are fairly satisfactory drugs and improvements gained in the manufacture of new drugs are likely only to be marginal. Therefore careful assessment of a new drug is mandatory if it is to be adopted in preference to a well-tried agent.

Local anaesthetics lend themselves to fairly accurate assessment as it is easier to measure their effects objectively than it is those of systemic analgesics. However, multifarious methods of testing have led to numerous conflicting reports of their relative efficacy and toxicity.

Before the first clinical trials of a new drug take place, extensive preliminary investigations in both animals and man will have established a number of facts. It behoves the clinician about to embark on a clinical study to acquaint himself with the relevant literature.

Laboratory Investigations in Animals and Man

Animal studies can be used to compare the acute and cumulative toxicity of drugs by various routes of administration (subcutaneous, intramuscular, intravenous, etc.) and to make a rough assessment of latency, potency and duration of action. The inhibition of the corneal reflex in the rabbit is used to measure surface anaesthetic activity. Inhibition of reaction to pinprick after intracutaneous injection in the guinea-pig can test infiltration analgesia. Conduction anaesthesia may be tested by sciatic nerve block in guinea-pig or frog, or by mouse tail root infiltration measuring inhibition of the pain reflex. In man a series of intradermal injections of different concentrations of the new drug, together with a standard drug and a blank (physiological saline) can be given in the forearm. A quantitative assessment of analgesia to pinprick can be made by counting the number of standard pinpricks that are felt as sharp out of a total of, say, five per intradermal weal, at regular intervals. This can give a crude estimate of latency, potency, duration of action and vasoactivity (Morgan and Russell, 1975; Reynolds *et al.*, 1976).

Given a source of willing or needy volunteers, other experimental tests may be carried out in man, such as bilateral ulnar nerve (Löfström, 1975) or brachial plexus block (Wencker *et al.*, 1975), one arm being used as control. Latency, potency, duration and penetration (patchy anaesthesia) of sensory and motor blockade may be tested.

Clinical Trials (Bonica, 1957; Covino and Bush, 1975)

In the light of the information so obtained, clinical studies may now be planned and these should attempt to establish potency, latency, penetration, duration and toxicity in clinical practice. It is generally considered advisable to use a new drug initially in a short series of cases without the use of a control or double blind technique: a "clinical impression" trial. In this way approximate potency may be confirmed and any major inadequacy detected. Having established feasibility, carefully planned and controlled double blind trials must be carried out (see Table 2) testing the agent against a standard drug such as lignocaine but not, of course, against a placebo. At this stage the help of an experienced organiser of clinical trials is valuable. The problem is simplified if a single type of local block is studied and the technique and rate of administration are standardised. When possible there should be a single operator and a single observer, to avoid minor variations in techniques of administration and assessment. A range of concentrations of the drug under scrutiny should be used and the volume of solution injected kept constant. If a vasoconstrictor is used, its concentration should be constant in all the test solutions. If its concentration varies, then the nature and concentration of the local anaesthetic it accompanies should be constant. Where possible, a subject should act as his own control—for example, when a bilateral block is required. During continuous epidural anaesthesia, different solutions may be compared sequentially. Otherwise, patients should be selected randomly for the different treatments,

34/TABLE 2

PLANNING A CLINICAL TRIAL

1. Search the literature.
2. Employ a double-blind technique using:
    reference drug (e.g. lignocaine)
    two or more concentrations of new drug
    patient as his own control where possible.
3. Standardise conditions:
    subjects
    route of administration
    technique of administration.
4. Standardise assessment of:
    artificial pain
    natural pain
    operating conditions
    side-effects
    and investigate potency, latency, spread and duration of action of the drug.
5. Evaluate results statistically where appropriate.

the series should be as large and as homogenous as possible, and parity of age, sex, etc., in the several groups should be checked at the end of the series.

There remains the actual assessment of the analgesia produced. Experimentally produced pain (for example, a pinprick) is preferable to natural pain, in so far as it can be standardised while natural pain waxes and wanes even in individual cases. Local anaesthesia lends itself better to testing with artificial pain than does systemic analgesia. Onset, duration and the area involved in the block, including any patchy analgesia, are recorded in each case. Ekblom and Widman (1966) produced a useful method of presenting these parameters graphically. The mean surface area involved in the block (e.g. the number of segments involved in the case of spinal or epidural analgesia) in each group is plotted graphically against the mean duration of action (Fig. 3). This supplies a visual means of instant comparison of two or more agents, showing the spread and completeness of analgesia and the onset and duration of action of each drug.

If natural pain is taken as a criterion for assessment of local anaesthetic effect—for example, in continuous analgesia for post-operative pain or labour —different local anaesthetics cannot easily be compared sequentially in a single subject because of the variability of the painful stimulus.

In practice, of course, the relief of labour or post-operative pain and the adequacy of operating conditions do provide useful supplementary evidence in a clinical trial. In addition to loss of pain, loss of sensation, weakness, loss of proprioception and the incidence of hypotension, systemic toxicity and other side-effects should be noted. As many data as possible should be recorded in each subject of a clinical trial, and measurements made at the same and sufficiently frequent time intervals.

With regard to toxicity, assessment in man presents a problem. The therapeutic ratio (that is, the ratio of mean toxic dose: mean effective dose) of a single local anaesthetic drug varies not only with species (owing to great differences in elimination rate) but also with route of administration, because of variation in the rate of absorption from different sites. Thus theoretically it should be determined in man for each different blocking technique. However, it is to be hoped and expected that, after the correct administration of a single dose of a local anaesthetic by any accepted route, the incidence of systemic toxicity will be nil. It is nevertheless essential to judge the margin of safety that may be expected from a drug in any given situation, as for instance with a large dose, an accidental intravenous injection, repeated injection after failed block, or for prolonged analgesia. Such assessment should not be made by trial and error as often happened in the past. It may be judged by measuring plasma concentrations of the local anaesthetic which occur in clinical practice in different situations and comparing these with the plasma concentration which gives rise to signs of systemic toxicity during experimental intravenous infusion in volunteers (Reynolds, 1971).

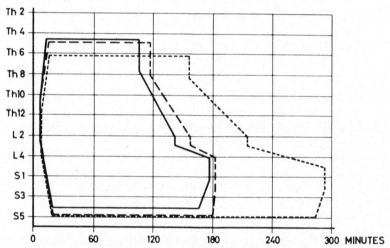

34/Fig. 3.—The extent and duration of epidural blockade using prilocaine (————), mepivacaine (– – –) and bupivacaine (- - - -).
(Ordinate—dermatomes. Abscissa—duration)
(After Ekblom and Widman, 1966)

Complete testing of a local anaesthetic may take a long time if this regime is followed. For many years local anaesthesia was regarded as a safe alternative to general anaesthesia for surgery in the sick, and only reports of increasing numbers of deaths gave the lie to this idea. Now, with better techniques, safer drugs and a better understanding of their behaviour, local anaesthesia should be very much safer than it was in the past.

INDIVIDUAL LOCAL ANAESTHETIC DRUGS

The number of drugs that have been marketed as local anaesthetics is legion, and only products in current use by anaesthetists, or those of historical importance, are included here. They are presented in chronological order. Numerical data are often misleading, because they may have been calculated from experiments under varying conditions by different workers. However, in Table 3, an

34/TABLE 3

PHYSICOCHEMICAL AND TOXICOLOGICAL DATA

	pKa	Protein binding at clinical Concentrations	Partition Coefficients		Anaesthetic Concentration Relative to Lignocaine†	Maximum* Safe Dose	LD_{50} mg/kg mice and rats	
			Heptane/ buffer	Oleyl Alcohol/ buffer			IV	SC
COCAINE	8·4				2·0	?2 mg/kg	17·5	
PROCAINE	9·0	35%		0·6	3·0	10 mg/kg	55	370–630
CINCHOCAINE	8·5			530	0·1	0·4 mg/kg	2·5–4·7	
AMETHOCAINE	8·4			80	0·25	1·0 mg/kg	4·3–8·0	32–62
LIGNOCAINE	7·86	60–75%	2·9	25–30	1·0	7 mg/kg	15–38	300–400
MEPIVACAINE	7·7	75%	0·8	10–17	1·0	7 mg/kg	27–40	260–270
PRILOCAINE	7·9	55%	0·4	11	1·0	8 mg/kg	18–62	600–900
BUPIVACAINE	8·1	90–97%	28	212–890	0·25	2 mg/kg	7·8	83
ETIDOCAINE	7·7	94–97%	142	>1000	0·4	4 mg/kg	5·8–7·2	89–102

From: Luduena *et al.* (1958), Truant and Takman (1959), Henn (1960), Sawinski and Rapp (1963), af Ekenstam (1966), Henn and Brattsand (1966), Tucker (1975), Messrs. Astra Pharmaceuticals, *Merck Index*, Reynolds (personal observation) IV = intravenous; SC = subcutaneous.

† These figures are only approximate. Relative potencies vary with site and especially with nerve fibre type.
* There is no single maximum safe dose for an individual local anaesthetic. The figures suggested here relate to plain solutions given by single shot into a non-vascular area such as the epidural space. These doses may often have been exceeded with impunity when adrenaline is added, while smaller doses of plain solutions may be toxic in vascular areas. If the doses were injected rapidly intravenously, severe toxicity might be expected.

attempt has been made to supply such as enable some quantitative comparison of different local anaesthetics. The pharmacological actions of the various drugs are covered mainly in earlier sections (p. 1103). The ensuing text deals principally with usage.

COCAINE

This drug is now little used owing to its toxic and addictive properties. In addition to its nerve-blocking action it enhances the effect of sympathetic stimulation and of catecholamines.

Sympathetic activity is normally terminated because transmitter substance is removed from the region of the receptor by its re-uptake into sympathetic nerve endings. Cocaine inhibits this re-uptake process and therefore allows accumulation of transmitter at the receptor site. The marked difference between the effects of cocaine and of other local anaesthetics is largely a reflection of this property. Cocaine is not a markedly potent or long-acting local anaesthetic and its therapeutic ratio in clinical use is substantially lower than that of the more modern drugs. It is active as a surface anaesthetic and the vasoconstriction it produces may delay its systemic absorption and, furthermore, has made it popular for ear, nose and throat work.

Although first used for eye surgery, the dangers of precipitating glaucoma and of causing corneal damage make it unsuitable in this field.

Central nervous system effects.—Cocaine, unlike modern local anaesthetics, has a stimulant effect like that of amphetamine, even in low doses. It produces excitement, euphoria and garrulousness and is prone to abuse. Medullary stimulation may cause hypertension, increased respiratory rate and vomiting. Body temperature may rise. In severe intoxication, coma, convulsions and medullary depression usually precede death.

Cardiovascular system.—Because of vasoconstriction and a sympathomimetic effect on the heart, the arterial pressure is initially raised by cocaine. Ventricular fibrillation may cause sudden death without premonitory signs of severe intoxication.

Use.—As a local anaesthetic, cocaine should be used only for surface application, if at all. A 10 per cent solution is used for endotracheal spraying and other surface application to the nose and throat, while some ENT surgeons use 20 per cent cocaine paste in the nose. Fortunately it appears to be fairly slowly absorbed in this form, though an element of risk in its use is undeniable.

For systemic use, it makes the perfect partner for heroin in Brompton mixture. It offsets the sedative effect of heroin, while the euphoriant properties summate most satisfactorily.

PROCAINE AND PROCAINAMIDE

Procaine is a local anaesthetic of short duration and poor penetrative powers. These properties stem from its vasodilator activity and relatively high pK_a, which renders it highly ionised at physiological pH. It is therefore rapidly absorbed into the circulation when injected, and is inactive as a surface anaesthetic. It is of lower potency than lignocaine, and carries a lower incidence of successful nerve blockade. Its duration is about half that of lignocaine, but can be greatly prolonged by the addition of adrenaline.

Procaine, once in the circulation, is hydrolysed by pseudocholinesterase in the plasma and liver to *p*-aminobenzoic acid and diethylaminoethanol. It is therefore effectively of low toxicity. Several drug interactions, however, are possible:

1. Procaine may prolong the effect of suxamethonium by competing with it for the same enzyme.

2. One product of hydrolysis, *p*-aminobenzoic acid, is a potent inhibitor of the bacteriostatic effects of sulphonamides, as well as being allergenic.

3. Diethylaminoethanol potentiates the effect of digitalis and therefore might precipitate intoxication in patients on digitalis-type drugs.

4. Anti-cholinesterase drugs may increase the toxicity of procaine.

It has been stated that procaine should not be given to patients with myasthenia gravis. A reason for this is that such patients are likely to be taking anti-cholinesterase drugs, rather than because of any enhancement by procaine of neuromuscular blockade. Neither procaine nor any other local anaesthetic should be regarded as a ganglionic or neuromuscular blocker in therapeutic doses.

Cardiovascular system.—Procaine was early found to be an effective anti-dysrhythmic drug, but procainamide soon replaced it as it is less likely to produce central nervous system toxicity and because it is not broken down by pseudocholinesterase it has a more prolonged cardiac effect. Both drugs have an anti-dysrhythmic effect like that of quinidine (see under Pharmacological effects, p. 1103). Because conduction is readily depressed, a wide QRS complex may herald ventricular extrasystoles and fibrillation. Asynchronous contraction of the ventricle may be associated with a fall in cardiac output. Oral procainamide is used in the treatment of supraventricular dysrhythmias, and occasionally for ventricular dysrhythmias (Koch-Weser and Klein, 1971). There is great individual variation in dosage requirement dependent partly upon absorption from the gastro-intestinal tract, and partly upon renal function, because procainamide is excreted at least 50 per cent unchanged. Monitoring the plasma concentration is therefore indicated to avoid the risk of overdose and consequent myocardial depression.

Use.—There are now no indications for the use of procaine as a local anaesthetic. It appears, however, to have a specific therapeutic effect in malignant hyperpyrexia (Moulds and Denborough, 1972). In the treatment of dysrhythmias, procainamide tablets must be taken three-hourly in whatever dosage is required to maintain therapeutic plasma levels, starting at say 250 mg.

CINCHOCAINE (DIBUCAINE (USP), NUPERCAINE)

Cinchocaine is the most potent local anaesthetic that has been used medically. Although more potent than bupivacaine, its duration of action is not as great, as it produces vasodilatation and has a higher pK_a. The importance of cinchocaine lies in the pride of place it has held over many years for spinal analgesia. For some time three solutions of cinchocaine were made for this purpose: light (1:1,500 or 0·06 per cent), isotonic (1:200 or 0·5 per cent) and heavy (1:200 or 0·5 per cent in 6 per cent glucose). The light spinal technique, involving a subarachnoid injection of a large volume of dilute solution, was associated with chronic adhesive arachnoiditis and other serious neurological sequelae, and should not be used. Now only the heavy technique is employed. For some years heavy cinchocaine was supplied for this purpose in response to a demand so limited that there could be no commercial advantage in its production. It is now no longer available and its place has been taken principally by prilocaine 5 per cent (Citanest heavy).

Other uses of cinchocaine.—Under its USP name, dibucaine, this drug is used in the detection of atypical pseudocholinesterase (see Chapter 26).

AMETHOCAINE (TETRACAINE (USP), DECICAINE, PONTOCAINE)

Amethocaine is a potent, long-acting local anaesthetic, and is a very effective surface anaesthetic. It is used in a 0·5 per cent concentration in the eye, and a 1 to 2 per cent solution for application to mucous membranes. Amethocaine hydrochloride for injection is usually presented as a dry powder and has been added to lignocaine solution to prolong the action of the latter in nerve blocks and epidural anaesthesia. It has also been used alone, in a 0·25 per cent or occasionally a 0·5 per cent concentration, 15–20 ml, for epidural anaesthesia, with or without adrenaline, when its duration of action is similar to that of bupivacaine. It appears that 0·5 per cent is no more effective or long-acting than 0·25 per cent (Bromage, 1969). Amethocaine has also been used for spinal anaesthesia.

Both cinchocaine and amethocaine are described as very toxic local anaesthetics, yet they have been ascribed toxicity and potency values such that their therapeutic ratios would be higher than that of procaine (Gray and Geddes, 1954). The reason for this is probably that intravenous toxicity is taken to represent clinical toxicity, which it does not (see Systemic toxicity, p. 1106). Such a calculation would indicate that they were exceptionally safe local anaesthetics; a moment's reflection suggests that this is not the case, although admittedly many cases of toxicity have occurred through their being given in unnecessarily large doses. There can now be few indications for the use of amethocaine.

LIGNOCAINE (LIDOCAINE (USP), XYLOCAINE)

Lignocaine was synthesised in 1943 in Sweden, by Löfgren of AB Astra, and it was introduced into clinical practice in 1948. It has numerous advantages over many of its predecessors, and has been popular ever since.

Lignocaine is a local anaesthetic of moderate potency and duration, but of good penetrative powers and rapid onset of action. It is effective by all routes of administration and its advent was partly responsible for the increased popularity of epidural anaesthesia, because its excellent penetration renders blockade by this method highly successful.

It sometimes causes local vasodilatation. Adrenaline prolongs the action of lignocaine and also reduces its rate of systemic absorption. Thus the duration of action epidurally is about $\frac{3}{4}$–1 hour, prolonged up to $2\frac{1}{2}$ hours with adrenaline. With repeated injection, tachyphylaxis often occurs: indeed it may occasionally be practically impossible to produce analgesia after some hours. Adrenaline can reduce but not abolish this feature.

The carbonate of lignocaine has remarkable penetrative powers, a rapid onset of action, a high incidence of motor block (Bromage and Gertel, 1970) and a reduced incidence of missed segments (Bromage, 1972) when used for epidural anaesthesia (see also p. 1100).

Lignocaine is very effective as a surface anaesthetic. Absorption from mucosal surfaces, however, is rapid and may give rise to high blood levels unless the dose is carefully controlled. For this reason, laryngo-pharyngeal and laryngeal spraying may be preferred to tracheal spraying, since they are as effective and lower plasma lignocaine levels result (Curran et al., 1975).

Absorption from the inflamed urethra can take place at a rate equivalent to intravenous injection.

Cardiovascular system (see general section, p. 1103).—Lignocaine is a useful drug in the treatment of cardiac dysrhythmias. It stabilises the membrane of damaged and excitable cells, tending to suppress ectopic foci. In therapeutic doses it causes no consistent rate change, and does not depress conduction in Purkinje tissue (Bigger and Heissenbuttel, 1969). Widening of the QRS complex is not seen and there is usually no apparent myocardial depression. Even an improvement in cardiac output and blood pressure has been observed when it is used in the treatment of cardiac dysrhythmias (Harrison et al., 1963). It is less useful than quinidine or procainamide in the treatment of supraventricular dysrhythmias, in which the myocardial depressant action of the two latter drugs is often of little importance. The great value of lignocaine, however, is in the acute treatment of ventricular dysrhythmias, after myocardial infarction or cardiac surgery. Its lack of depressant effect in the myocardium is valuable in these circumstances. Toxicity affects the central nervous system producing sedation initially which, with an intravenous infusion, should give ample warning of more serious sequelae. Toxic effects are more likely in the presence of hepatic under-perfusion (Prestcott et al., 1976), such as may accompany a reduced cardiac output.

Dosage.—Concentrations of lignocaine hydrochloride of 0·25–0·5 per cent are used for infiltration. If extensive block is required 0·25 per cent with adrenaline should be used. Up to 40 ml of 0·5 per cent lignocaine without adrenaline is usually used for intravenous regional analgesia. 1 per cent lignocaine suffices for most nerve blocks. A concentration of 2 per cent, with adrenaline 12·5 µg/ml (1:80,000) is popular in dentistry. Concentrations of 1·2–2 per cent are used for epidural analgesia, sometimes with the addition of adrenaline 5 µg/ml (1:200,000). For surface application lignocaine may be used in solution as a liquid (4 per cent) for spraying or application on wool pledgets, or in a lubricating gel for the urethra (2 per cent) or on instruments, endotracheal tubes and oropharyngeal airways (4 per cent).

In the treatment of cardiac dysrhythmias, 1 mg/kg is usually given as a bolus dose intravenously, followed by an infusion of 1–2 mg/minute. Such a regime gives rise to a short-lived high blood concentration initially, followed by one which may be too low to be effective for 4–6 hours. Therefore infusion should be rapid at first (e.g. 4 mg/minute for 20 minutes) then gradually slowed down to 1 mg/min as the tissues begin to take up lignocaine less rapidly. Such an infusion continued at a steady rate for days is liable to give rise to systemic toxicity. A low infusion rate, and caution throughout, should be used in the presence of a low cardiac output and after cardiac surgery (Aps et al., 1976).

The safe dose limit for lignocaine has been much disputed. After the publication by Deacock and Simpson (1964) of a series of fatalities from lignocaine, the upper safe dose ascribed to it was 200 mg plain and 500 mg with adrenaline. However, this decision failed to take into account differences in weight of patients and different absorption rates from various sites of injection. The maximum safe dose in man is probably about 7 mg/kg—possibly less than this for plain solutions in vascular areas—while more than this has often been given with impunity with adrenaline into less vascular areas. Toxic symptoms may occur at plasma levels of 3 (Jewitt et al., 1968) to 5 (Foldes et al., 1960) μg/ml (12·8–21·4 μmol/l) yet such levels are not uncommonly produced after a single shot epidural block (Braid and Scott, 1965 and 1966).

During continuous epidural blockade to maintain analgesia in labour, toxic plasma concentrations are almost inevitable beyond eight hours (Reynolds and Taylor, 1970) by which time 1–2 g will have been given.

Mepivacaine (Carbocaine, Scandicaine)

Mepivacaine was synthesised by Bo af Ekenstam of AB Bofors in Sweden (af Ekenstam et al., 1956), as one of a large homologous series. Mepicavaine is similar to lignocaine in local anaesthetic potency and speed of onset; it has good penetrative powers and a slightly longer duration of action. It produces vasoconstriction more readily than lignocaine (de Rochemont and Hensel, 1960) and prilocaine (Reynolds et al., 1976), but its duration of action is increased by adrenaline. It has been used for all types of blockade, in doses and concentrations akin to those of lignocaine, and like lignocaine has caused death when used in excessive dosage (Sunshine and Fike, 1964). Moreover, it is markedly cumulative when given epidurally (Moore et al., 1968). The toxic plasma level may be slightly higher than that of lignocaine (Jorfeldt et al., 1968) but it is readily produced by repeated doses. Therefore for long-continued use it is certainly less safe than bupivacaine. It has nevertheless been used extensively in obstetrics in the United States, with reports of fetal intoxication during caudal epidurals, accidental fetal injections and paracervical blocks. Whether any of these troubles can be directly laid at the door of mepivacaine remains debatable, but during caudal and lumbar epidural block there is no doubt that mepivacaine gives rise to relatively higher fetal blood concentrations than do other local anaesthetics that have been measured (Morishima et al., 1966; Moore et al., 1968; Reynolds, 1971b).

Mepivacaine has undoubted value in dentistry. Unlike lignocaine, it has an acceptable success rate when used without adrenaline and a duration of dental anaesthesia of about 20 minutes (Mumford and Gray, 1957; Mumford and Geddes, 1961) which is prolonged to 30–40 minutes by the addition of adrenaline.

Prilocaine (Citanest, Propitocaine, L67)

Prilocaine emerged in 1960, shortly after mepivacaine, from the same stable as lignocaine—AB Astra—having been synthesised some years previously by Löfgren.

Its potency and speed of onset as a local anaesthetic are similar to, or very slightly less than, those of lignocaine and its penetrative powers good. It can be used for all types of blockade, in concentrations similar to those of lignocaine. It is a moderate vasoconstrictor; its vasoactivity is intermediate between that of mepivacaine and lignocaine (Reynolds *et al.*, 1976). When used for epidural blockade it may produce a higher incidence of motor block than does lignocaine and a slightly longer duration of action. After the addition of adrenaline its duration is only slightly prolonged, and is equal to that of lignocaine with adrenaline (Bromage, 1965). For spinal anaesthesia it may be used as a 5 per cent solution with 5 per cent glucose (Citanest heavy), and its duration of action is about 1–1½ hours, less than that of cinchocaine and only slightly longer than that of lignocaine (Fisher and Bryce-Smith, 1971).

It is used in dentistry in a 3 per cent solution. Its somewhat brief action can be more effectively prolonged by felypressin than by adrenaline (Goldman and Evers, 1969). It may be recommended in this field with felypressin (as Citanest with Octapressin) when a long duration of dental block is required in patients taking tricyclic antidepressants in whom adrenaline is contra-indicated.

The administration of prilocaine gives rise to much lower plasma concentrations than does an equal dose of lignocaine (Scott *et al.*, 1972). This is in part accounted for by more rapid metabolism and possibly also by greater tissue uptake (Eriksson, 1966) because it is less protein-bound. It is therefore only about two-thirds as toxic as lignocaine after a single dose, and considerably less cumulative.

Although it may be relatively unlikely to cause central nervous system toxicity, one product of its rapid metabolism *o*-toluidine, induces methaemoglobinaemia. This is a dose-related phenomenon; when 600 mg of prilocaine have been given, the methaemoglobin level, normally about 1 per cent, may rise to 5 per cent or more. Levels greater than 10 per cent have been observed in mothers and their babies after delivery, when prilocaine has been used for epidural analgesia (Arens and Carrera, 1970). The maximum methaemoglobin concentration is normally seen four to six hours after prilocaine administration and declines to normal in about 24 hours. Methaemoglobinaemia can be treated successfully in this situation with methylene blue, 1 mg/kg. Nevertheless, its occurrence may contra-indicate prilocaine in many situations, though a slight, transient rise in methaemoglobin level is harmless to most people.

BUPIVACAINE (MARCAIN, MARCAINE, LAC 43)

Bupivacaine is one of the homologous series synthesised by Bo af Ekenstam to which mepivacaine belongs. First reports of its use were made in 1963 (Telivuo, 1963). Bupivacaine is three to four times as potent as lignocaine, and considerably longer lasting. Its speed of onset may be marginally slower than that of lignocaine and mepivacaine. It has been used for all manner of nerve blocks, lumbar and caudal epidurals, paracervical block, and intravenous regional anaesthesia (Ware, 1975). It has become very popular for providing long-lasting analgesia, especially by continuous epidural blockade, when tachyphylaxis is much less likely than with lignocaine and it appears that safe and effective analgesia can be provided almost indefinitely (Duthie *et al.*, 1968). For the relief of pain in labour its duration of action is from two to four hours, while it has produced post-operative analgesia for more than twelve hours (Telivuo, 1963). It produces a low incidence of motor blockade (see Fig. 2, p. 1102).

Bupivacaine is less likely than lignocaine to produce vasoconstriction (Aps and Reynolds, 1976) unless sufficiently dilute. Nevertheless adrenaline prolongs its action only marginally (Waters *et al.*, 1970) if at all (Telivuo, *et al.*, 1971) and is unnecessary even to provide prolonged continuous epidural blockade in obstetrics. Bupivacaine crosses the placenta but little, owing to the marked disparity between maternal and fetal protein binding (Thomas *et al.*, 1976; see also Chapter 44). For an account of its unique value in obstetrics see page 1327.

Dosage.—Concentrations of 0·125–0·5 per cent of bupivacaine may be used for epidural blockade. A concentration of 0·25 per cent has been found by some workers to fail to give complete blockade occasionally, while 0·5 per cent bupivacaine invariably achieves successful analgesia. Others have found 0·25 per cent satisfactory and the lack of motor blockade advantageous (Duthie *et al.*, 1968). Adrenaline 2·5–5·0 µg/ml (1 : 400,000–1 : 200,000) is sometimes added, though it is of little value (Reynolds and Taylor, 1971) and introduces an added risk. For intravenous regional anaesthesia, a concentration of 0·2 per cent bupivacaine and a maximum dose of 1·5 mg/kg, have been found satisfactory (Ware, 1975).

Clinically occurring blood levels of bupivacaine are usually well below those likely to produce toxic symptoms (Jordfelt *et al.*, 1968) and it is a less cumulative drug than lignocaine or mepivacaine. For a single-shot epidural, the maximum safe dose is about 2 mg/kg. To provide prolonged analgesia, if 25–30 mg 2-hourly suffices, this dose rate can probably be given almost indefinitely. Geerinckx *et al.* (1974) found bupivacaine not to accumulate in obstetric patients when 0·125 per cent was used. Reynolds, Hargrove and Wyman (1973) showed that if 50 mg doses were repeated every 2–3 hours, a maximum dose without adrenaline of 320 mg and with adrenaline of about 500 mg, could probably be given with safety.

A few isolated cases of prolonged blockade have been noted following epidural bupivacaine (Guerden *et al.*, 1977), but these have always recovered and it is doubtful if the incidence is any higher than with other agents, in view of the extensive use of bupivacaine in obstetrics.

ETIDOCAINE (DURANEST)

Etidocaine is Astra's most recent addition to the field of local anaesthetic drugs. It has been used for ulnar nerve block (Radtke *et al.*, 1975), axillary plexus block (Hollmen and Mononen, 1975) and intercostal nerve block (Bridenbaugh *et al.*, 1973), but principally for epidural block (Niesel and Munch, 1975; Gitschmann and Nolte, 1975), for induction of labour (Phillips, 1975), delivery (Moore *et al.*, 1975), pain relief in labour (Poppers *et al.*, 1975; Wilson, 1975), surgery (Moore *et al.*, 1974) and post-operative pain relief (Abdel-Salam and Scott, 1975).

It is generally used in concentrations double those of bupivacaine, because it is less potent than bupivacaine in producing sensory block and also less reliable (Moore *et al.*, 1974), though more potent for motor block (see Fig. 2). Its onset of action is sometimes quicker than that of bupivacaine. Although longer acting than lignocaine, its duration of action is less than that of bupivacaine unless adrenaline is added, when duration of sensory blockade is only slightly briefer than that of bupivacaine, although some degree of motor block may occasionally outlast it.

Etidocaine is of value when prolonged epidural blockade is required for surgery, in which the high degree of motor blockade is an advantage. For this purpose 20 ml of 1 per cent etidocaine with adrenaline 5 µg/ml (1:200,000) may be given, and should last 2–5 hours. A 1·5 per cent solution with adrenaline has been found to have a briefer action (Bridenbaugh et al., 1973). For obstetric pain relief it is less suitable than bupivacaine (although it crosses the placenta but little) because no concentration can produce reliable sensory block without an unacceptably high incidence of motor block.

Etidocaine is more rapidly eliminated than bupivacaine (Scott et al., 1973), and less toxic after equal single doses. Thus for a single dose the therapeutic ratios of the two drugs are similar (Munson et al., 1975). For continuous use, as etidocaine has to be given at double the dose of bupivacaine, and at a greater frequency unless adrenaline is added, it may have as great a cumulative tendency (Poppers, 1975). Accumulation, however, is not likely to be dangerous with either drug.

REFERENCES

ABDEL-SALAM, A., and SCOTT, B. (1975). Bupivacaine and etidocaine in epidural block for post-operative relief of pain. Acta anaesth. scand., Suppl. 60, 80.

ÅBERG, G. (1972). Myogenic action of local anaesthetics on smooth muscle; role of Ca^{++} and cyclic AMP. Acta pharmacol. (Kbh.), 31, Suppl. 1, 46.

ÅBERG, G., MORCK, E., and WALDECK, B. (1973). Studies on the effects of some local anaesthetics on the uptake of ^{3}H-1-noradrenaline into vascular and cardiac tissues in vitro. Acta pharmacol. (Kbh.), 33, 476.

ADRIANI, J., and CAMPBELL, D. (1956). Fatalities following topical application of local anesthetics to mucous membranes. J. Amer. med. Ass., 162, 1527.

AELLIG, W. H., LAURENCE, D. R., O'NEIL, R., and VERRILL, P. J. (1970). Cardiac effects of adrenaline and felypressin as vasoconstrictors in local anaesthesia for oral surgery under diazepam sedation. Brit. J. Anaesth., 42, 174.

AKERMAN, B. (1969). Effects of felypressin (Octapressin) on the acute toxicity of local anaesthetics. Acta pharmacol. (Kbh.), 27, 318.

ALDRETE, J. A. (1969). Allergy to local anesthetics. J. Amer. med. Ass., 207, 356.

APS, C., BELL, J. A., JENKINS, B. S., POOLE-WILSON, P. A., and REYNOLDS, F. (1976). Logical approach to lignocaine therapy. Brit. med. J., 1, 13.

APS, C., and REYNOLDS, F. (1976). The effect of concentration on the vasoactivity of bupivacaine and lignocaine. Brit. J. Anaesth., 48, 1171.

APS, C., and REYNOLDS, F. (1978). An intradermal study of the local anaesthetic and vascular effects of the isomers of bupivacaine. Brit. J. clin. Pharmacol., 5 (in press).

ARENS, J. F., and CARRERA, A. E. (1970). Methemoglobin levels following peridural anesthesia with prilocaine for vaginal deliveries. Anesth. Analg. Curr. Res., 49, 219.

ATKINSON, R. E., and NICHOLAS, A. D. G. (1976). A comparison of bupivacaine hydrochloride and bupivacaine carbonate during labour. Communication to the Obstetric Anaesthetists Association.

AUSINSCH, B., MALAGODI, M. H., and MUNSON, E. S. (1976). Diazepam in the prophylaxis of lignocaine seizures. Brit. J. Anaesth., 48, 309.

BIGGER, J. T., and HEISSENBUTTEL, R. H. (1969). The use of procaine amide and lidocaine in the treatment of cardiac arrhythmias, Progr. cardiovasc. Dis., 11, 515.

BLAIR, M. R. (1975). Cardiovascular pharmacology of local anaesthetics. *Brit. J. Anaesth.*, **47**, S 247.

BOAKES, A. J., LAURENCE, D. R., LOVEL, K. W., O'NEIL, R., and VERRILL, P. J. (1972). Adverse reactions to local anaesthetic/vasoconstrictor preparations. A study of the cardiovascular responses to Xylestesin and Hostacain with noradrenaline. *Brit. dent. J.*, **133**, 137.

BOAKES, A. J., LAURENCE, D. R., TEOH, P. C., BARAR, F. S. K., BENEDIKTER, L. T., and PRICHARD, B. N. C. (1973). Interactions between sympathomimetic amines and antidepressant agents in man. *Brit. med. J.*, **1**, 311.

BONICA, J. J. (1957). Clinical investigation of local anesthetics. *Anesthesiology*, **18**, 110.

BOYES, R. N. (1975). A review of the metabolism of amide local anaesthetic agents. *Brit. J. Anaesth.*, **47**, 225.

BRAID, D. P., and SCOTT, D. B. (1965). The systemic absorption of local analgesic drugs. *Brit. J. Anaesth.*, **37**, 394.

BRAID, D. P., and SCOTT, D. B. (1966). Dosage of lignocaine in epidural block in relation to toxicity. *Brit. J. Anaesth.*, **38**, 596.

BRIDENBAUGH, P. O., TUCKER, G. T., MOORE, D. C., BRIDENBAUGH, L. D., and THOMPSON, G. (1973). Etidocaine: clinical evaluation for intercostal nerve block and lumbar epidural block. *Anesth. Analg. Curr. Res.,* **52**, 407.

BROMAGE, P. R. (1965). A comparison of the hydrochloride salts of lignocaine and prilocaine for epidural analgesia. *Brit. J. Anaesth.*, **37**, 753.

BROMAGE, P. R. (1969). A comparison of bupivacaine and tetracaine in epidural analgesia for surgery. *Canad. Anaesth. Soc. J.*, **16**, 37.

BROMAGE, P. R. (1972). Unblocked segments in epidural analgesia for relief of pain in labour. *Brit. J. Anaesth.*, **44**, 676.

BROMAGE, P. R. (1975). Mechanism of action of extradural analgesia. *Brit. J. Anaesth.*, **47**, S 199.

BROMAGE, P. R., BURFOOT, M. F., CROWELL, D. E., and TRUANT, A. P. (1967). Quality of epidural blockade III: carbonated local anaesthetic solutions. *Brit. J. Anaesth.*, **39**, 197.

BROMAGE, P. R., and GERTEL, M. (1970). An evaluation of two new local anaesthetics for major conduction blockade. *Canad. Anaesth. Soc. J.*, **17**, 557.

CATCHLOVE, R. F. H. (1972). The influence of CO_2 and pH on local anesthetic action. *J. Pharmacol. exp. Ther.*, **181**, 298.

CORALL, I. M., BROADFIELD, J. B., KNIGHTS, K. M., NICHOLSON, J. R., and STRUNIN, L. (1975). Cardiovascular effects of extradural analgesia in labour: comparison of bupivacaine with lignocaine. *Brit. J. Anaesth.*, **47**, 1297.

COVINO, B. G., and BUSH, D. F. (1975). Clinical evaluation of local anaesthetic agents. *Brit. J. Anaesth.*, **47**, 289.

CRAWFORD, J. S. (1976). The epidural sieve and MBC (minimum blocking concentrations) an hypothesis. *Anaesthesia*, **31**, 1277.

CUERDEN, C., BULEY, R., and DOWNING, J. W. (1977). Delayed recovery after epidural block in labour. A report of four cases. *Anaesthesia*, **32**, 773.

CURRAN, J., HAMILTON, C., and TAYLOR, T. (1975). Topical analgesia before tracheal intubation. *Anaesthesia*, **30**, 765.

D'AMATO, H. E., and TRUANT, A. P. (1955). Potentiation of epinephrine and norepinephrine blood pressure responses by local anesthetic agents. *Arch. int. Pharmacodyn.*, **101**, 113.

DEACOCK, A. R., and SIMPSON, W. T. (1964). Fatal reactions to lignocaine. *Anaesthesia*, **19**, 217.

DIFAZIO, C. A. (1975). Biotransformation of lidocaine. In: *Biotransformation of Local Anesthetics, Adjuvants, and Adjunct Agents*, p. 21. Ed. by dal Santo, G. Boston: Little Brown & Co. *Internat. Anesthesiol. Clinics*, **13**, no. 4.

DUTHIE, A. M., WYMAN, J. B., and LEWIS, G. A. (1968). Bupivicaine in labour. Its use in lumbar extradural analgesia. *Anaesthesia,* **23,** 20.

EKBLOM, L., and WIDMAN, B. (1966). A comparison of the properties of LAC 43, prilocaine and mepivacaine in extradural anaesthesia. *Acta anaesth. scand.,* Suppl. **21,** 33.

EKENSTAM, B. af (1966). The effect of the structural variation on the local analgesic properties of the most commonly used groups of substances. *Acta anaesth. scand.,* Suppl., **25,** 10.

EKENSTAM, B. af, EGNÉR, B., ULFENDAHL, H. R., DHUNÉR, K. G., and ALJELUND, O. (1956). Trials with carbocaine: a new local anaesthetic drug. *Brit. J. Anaesth.,* **28,** 503.

ENGLESSON, S., and MATOUSEK, M. (1975). Central nervous system effects of local anaesthetic agents. *Brit. J. Anaesth.,* **47,** 241.

ERIKSSON, E. (1966). Prilocaine: an experimental study in man of a new local anaesthetic with special regards to efficiency, toxicity and excretion. *Acta chir. scand.,* Suppl. **358.**

EYRE, J., and NALLY, F. F. (1971). Nasal test of hypersensitivity—including a positive reaction to lignocaine. *Lancet,* **2,** 264.

FINK, B. R. (1973). Acute and chronic toxicity of local anesthetics. *Canad. Anaesth. Soc. J.,* **20,** 5.

FISHER, A., and BRYCE-SMITH, R. (1971). Spinal analgesic agents: a comparison of cinchocaine, lignocaine and prilocaine. *Anaesthesia,* **26,** 324.

FOLDES, F. F., MOLLOY, R., MCNALL, P. G., and KOUKAL, L. R. (1960). Comparison of toxicity in intravenously given local anesthetic agents in man. *J. Amer. med. Ass.,* **172,** 1493.

FRANZ, D. N., and PERRY, R. S. (1974). Mechanisms for differential block among single myelinated and non-myelinated axons by procaine. *J. Physiol. (Lond.),* **236,** 193.

GAUL, L. E. (1955). Cross sensitization for para-aminobenzoate in sunburn preventives. *Anesthesiology,* **16,** 606.

GEDDES, I. C. (1965). Studies of the metabolism of Citanest C^{14}. *Acta anaesth. scand.,* Suppl. **16,** 37.

GEERINCKX, K., VANDERICK, G. G., VAN STEENBERGE, A. L., BOUCHE, R., and DE MUYLDER, E. (1974). Bupivacaine 0·125 per cent in epidural block analgesia during childbirth: maternal and foetal plasma concentrations. *Brit. J. Anaesth.,* **46,** 937.

GITSCHMANN, J., and NOLTE, H. (1975). Comparative study with etidocaine and bupivacaine in epidural block. *Acta anaesth. scand.,* Suppl. **60,** 55.

GRAY, T. C., and GEDDES, I. C. (1954). A review of local anaesthetics. *J. Pharm. Pharmacol.,* **6,** 89.

GOLDMAN, V., and EVERS, H. (1969). Prilocaine-felipressin: a new combination for dental analgesia. *Dent. Practit. dent. Rec.,* **19,** 225.

HARRISON, D. C., SPROUSE, J. H., and MORROW, A. G. (1963). Antiarrhythmic properties of lidocaine and procaine amide: clinical and physiologic studies of their cardiovascular effects in man. *Circulation,* **28,** 486.

HEAVNER, J. E., and DE JONG, R. H. (1974). Lidocaine blocking concentrations for B- and C-nerve fibers. *Anesthesiology,* **40,** 228.

HENN, F. (1960). Determination of toxicological and pharmacological properties of Carbocaine, lidocaine and procaine by means of simultaneous experiments. *Acta anaesth. scand.,* **4,** 125.

HENN, F., and BRATTSAND, R. (1966). Some pharmacological and toxicological properties of a new long-acting local analgesic, LAC-43 (Marcaine), in comparison with mepivacaine and tetracaine. *Acta anaesth. scand.,* Suppl. **21,** 9.

HOLLMEN, A., and MONONEN, P. (1975). Axillary plexus block with etidocaine. *Acta anaesth. scand.,* Suppl. **60,** 25.

HOLLUNGER, G. (1960). On the metabolism of Lidocaine II. The biotransformation of Lidocaine. *Acta pharmacol. (Kbh.),* **17,** 365.

JEWITT, D. E., KISHON, Y., and THOMAS, M. (1968). Lignocaine in the management of arrhythmias after acute myocardial infarction. *Lancet*, **1**, 266.

JONG, R. H. DE (1975). Biotransformation of local anesthetics: general concepts. *Internat. Anesthesiol. Clinics*, **13**, no. 4, 1.

JORFELDT, L., LÖFSTRÖM, B., PERNOW, B., PERSSON, B., WAHREN, J., and WIDMAN, B. (1968). The effect of local anaesthetics on the central circulation and respiration in man and dog. *Acta anaesth. scand.*, **12**, 153.

KENDIG, J. J., and COHEN, E. N. (1977). Pressure antagonism to nerve conduction block by anesthetic agents. *Anesthesiology*, **47**, 6.

KLINGENSTRÖM, P., and WESTERMARK, L. (1964). Local tissue oxygen tension after adrenaline, noradrenaline and Octapressin in local anaesthesia. *Acta anaesth. scand.*, **8**, 261.

KOCH-WESER, J., and KLEIN, S. W. (1971). Procainamide dosage schedules, plasma concentrations, and clinical effects. *J. Amer. med. Ass.*, **215**, 1454.

LÖFSTRÖM, J. B. (1975). Ulnar nerve blockade for the evaluation of local anaesthetic agents. *Brit. J. Anaesth.*, **47**, 297.

LUDUENA, F. P. (1969). Duration of local anesthesia. *Ann. Rev. Pharmacol.*, **9**, 503.

LUDUENA, F. P., HOPPE, J. O., and BORLAND, J. K. (1958). A statistical evaluation of the relationships among local anesthetic activity, irritancy and systemic toxicity. *J. Pharmacol. exp. Ther.*, **123**, 269.

MOORE, D. C., and BRIDENBAUGH, L. D. (1960). Oxygen: the antidote for systemic toxic reactions from local anesthetic drugs. *J. Amer. med. Ass.*, **174**, 842.

MOORE, D. C., BRIDENBAUGH, L. D., BAGDI, P. A., and BRIDENBAUGH, P. O. (1968). Accumulation of mepivacaine hydrochloride during caudal block. *Anesthesiology*, **29**, 585.

MOORE, D. C., BRIDENBAUGH, P. O., BRIDENBAUGH, L. D., THOMPSON, G. E., BALFOUR, R. I., and LYSONS, D. F. (1974). A double-blind study of bupivacaine and etidocaine for epidural (peridural) block. *Anesth. Analg. Curr. Res.*, **53**, 690.

MOORE, D. C., BRIDENBAUGH, P. O., BRIDENBAUGH, L. D., THOMPSON, G. E., BALFOUR, R. I., and LYSONS, D. F. (1975). Bupivacaine compared with etidocaine for vaginal delivery. *Anesth. Analg. Curr. Res.*, **54**, 250.

MORGAN, M., and RUSSELL, W. J. (1975). An investigation in man into the relative potency of lignocaine, bupivacaine and etidocaine. *Brit. J. Anaesth.*, **47**, 586.

MORISHIMA, H. O., DANIEL, S. S., FINSTER, M., POPPERS, P. J., and JAMES, L. S. (1966). Transmission of mepivacaine across the human placenta. *Anesthesiology*, **27**, 147.

MOULDS, R. F. W., and DENBOROUGH, M. A. (1972). Procaine in malignant hyperpyrexia. *Brit. med. J.*, **4**, 526.

MUMFORD, J. M., and GEDDES, I. C. (1961). Trial of Carbocaine in conservative dentistry. *Brit. dent. J.*, **110**, 92.

MUMFORD, J. M., and GRAY, T. C. (1957). Dental trial of Carbocaine—a new local anaesthetic. *Brit. J. Anaesth.*, **29**, 210.

MUNSON, E. S., TUCKER, W. K., AUSINSCH, B., and MALAGODI, M. H. (1975). Etidocaine, bupivacaine and lidocaine seizure thresholds in monkeys. *Anesthesiology*, **42**, 471.

NARAHASHI, T., FRAZIER, D. T., and YAMADA, M. (1970). The site of action and active form of local anesthetics I. Theory and pH experiments with tertiary compounds. *J. Pharmacol. exp. Ther.*, **171**, 32.

NATHAN, P. W., and SEARS, T. A. (1961). Some factors concerned in differential nerve block by local anaesthetics. *J. Physiol. (Lond.)*, **157**, 565.

NIESEL, H. C., and MUNCH, I. (1975). Experience with etidocaine and bupivacaine in epidural analgesia. *Acta anaesth. scand.*, Suppl. **60**, 60.

PHILLIPS, G. (1975). A double blind trial of bupivacaine (Marcain) and etidocaine (Duranest) in extradural block for surgical induction of labour. *Brit. J. Anaesth.*, **47**, 1307.

POPPERS, P. J. (1975). Evaluation of local anaesthetic agents for regional anaesthesia in obstetrics. *Brit. J. Anaesth.*, **47**, 322.

POPPERS, P., COVINO, B., and BOYES, N. (1975). Epidural block with etidocaine for labour and delivery. *Acta anaesth. scand.*, Suppl. **60**, 89.

PRESTCOTT, L. F., ADJEPON-YAMOAH, K. K., and TALBOT, R. G. (1976). Impaired lignocaine metabolism in patients with myocardial infarction and cardiac failure. *Brit. med. J.*, **1**, 939.

RADTKE, H., NOLTE, H., FRUHSTORFER, H., and ZENZ, M. (1975). A comparative study between etidocaine and bupivacaine in ulnar nerve block. *Acta anaesth. scand.*, Suppl. **60**, 17.

REYNOLDS, F. (1971*a*). Metabolism and excretion of bupivacaine in man—a comparison with mepivacaine. *Brit. J. Anaesth.*, **43**, 33.

REYNOLDS, F. (1971*b*). A comparison of the potential toxicity of bupivacaine, lignocaine, and mepivacaine during epidural blockade for surgery. *Brit. J. Anaesth.*, **43**, 567.

REYNOLDS, F., BRYSON, T. H. L., and NICHOLAS, A. D. G. (1976). Intradermal study of a new local anaesthetic agent: aptocaine. *Brit. J. Anaesth.*, **48**, 347.

REYNOLDS, F., HARGROVE, R. L., and WYMAN, J. B. (1973). Maternal and foetal plasma concentrations of bupivacaine after epidural block. *Brit. J. Anaesth.*, **45**, 1049.

REYNOLDS, F., and TAYLOR, G. (1970). Maternal and neonatal blood concentrations of bupivacaine: a comparison with lignocaine during continuous extradural analgesia. *Anaesthesia*, **25**, 14.

REYNOLDS, F., and TAYLOR, G. (1971). Plasma concentrations of bupivacaine during continuous epidural analgesia in labour: the effect of adrenaline. *Brit. J. Anaesth.*, **43**, 436.

RITCHIE, J. M. (1975). Mechanism of action of local anaesthetic agents and biotoxins. *Brit. J. Anaesth.*, **47**, 191.

RITCHIE, J. M., and GREENGARD, P. (1966). On the mode of action of local anaesthetics. *Ann. Rev. Pharmacol.*, **6**, 405.

RITCHIE, J. M., RITCHIE, B., and GREENGARD, P. (1965). The effect of the nerve sheath on the action of local anesthetics. *J. Pharmacol. exp. Ther.*, **150**, 160.

ROCHEMONT, W. DU M. DE, and HENSEL, H. (1960). Messung der Hautdurchblutung am Meschen bei Einwirkung verschiedener Lokalanaesthetica. *Naunyn-Schmiedeberg's Arch. exp. Path. Pharmak.*, **239**, 464.

SAWINSKI, V. J., and RAPP, G. W. (1963). Interaction of human serum proteins with local anesthetic agents, *J. dent. Res.*, **42**, 1429.

SCOTT, D. B., JEBSON, P. J. R., and BOYES, R. N. (1973). Pharmacokinetic study of the local anaesthetics bupivacaine (Marcain) and etidocaine (Duranest) in man. *Brit. J. Anaesth.*, **45**, 1010.

SCOTT, D. B., JEBSON, P. J. R., BRAID, D. P., ÖRTENGREN, B., and FRISCH, P. (1972). Factors affecting plasma levels of lignocaine and prilocaine. *Brit. J. Anaesth.*, **44**, 1040.

SEEMAN, P. (1972). The membrane actions of anesthetics and tranquillizers. *Pharmacol. Rev.*, **24**, 583.

SEEMAN, P. (1977). Anesthetics and pressure reversal of anesthesia. Expansion and re-compression of membrane proteins, lipids and water. *Anesthesiology*, **47**, 1.

STEINHAUS, J. E. (1957). Local anesthetic toxicity: a pharmacological re-evaluation. *Anesthesiology*, **18**, 275.

STEINMANN, J.-M. (1967). Anesthésie différentielle de fibres A alpha motrice et sensorielles de la grenouille. *J. Physiol. (Paris)*, **59**, 175.

STRICHARTZ, G. (1976). Review article: Molecular mechanisms of nerve block by local anesthetics. *Anesthesiology*, **45**, 421.

SUNSHINE, I., and FIKE, W. W. (1964). Value of thin layer chromatography in two fatal cases of intoxication due to lidocaine and mepivacaine. *New Engl. J. Med.*, **271**, 487.

TAKMAN, B. (1975). The chemistry of local anaesthetic agents: classification of blocking agents. *Brit. J. Anaesth.*, **47**, 183.

TELIVUO, L. (1963). A new long-acting local anaesthetic solution for pain relief after thoracotomy. *Ann. Chir. Gynaec. Fenn.*, **52**, 513.

TELIVUO, L., SVINHUFVUD, U., and NUUTTILA, K. (1971). An infrared thermography study on duration of intercostal nerve blocks using bupivacaine with and without adrenaline. *Acta anaesth. scand.*, **15**, 131.

THOMAS, J., LONG, G., MOORE, G. and MORGAN, D. (1976). Plasma protein binding and placental transfer of bupivacaine. *Clin. Pharmacol. Ther.*, **19**, 426.

TRUANT, A. P., and TAKMAN, B. (1959). Differential physical-chemical and neuropharmacologic properties of local anesthetic agents. *Anesth. Analg. Curr. Res.*, **38**, 478.

TUCKER, G. T. (1975). Plasma binding and disposition of local anesthetics. *Internat. Anesthesiol. Clinics*, **13**, no. 4, 33.

TUCKER, G. T., and MATHER, L. E. (1975). Pharmacokinetics of local anaesthetic agents. *Brit. J. Anaesth.*, **47**, 213.

WALDMAN, H. B., and BINKLEY, G. (1967). Lignocaine hypersensitivity: report of a case. *J. Amer. dent. Ass.*, **74**, 747.

WALKER, R. T. (1971). Hypersensitivity reaction to local anaesthetic. *Brit. dent. J.*, **130**, 2.

WALLIS, K. L., SHNIDER, S. M., HICKS, J. S., and SPIVEY, H. T. (1976). Epidural anesthesia in the normotensive pregnant ewe. *Anesthesiology*, **44**, 481.

WARE, R. J. (1975). Intravenous regional analgesia using bupivacaine. *Anaesthesia*, **30**, 817.

WATERS, H. R., ROSEN, N., and PERKINS, D. H. (1970). Extradural blockade with bupivacaine. *Anaesthesia*, **25**, 184.

WENCKER, K. H., NOLTE, H., and FRUHSTORFER, H. (1975). Brachial plexus blockade for evaluation of local anaesthetic agents. *Brit. J. Anaesth.*, **47**, 301.

WILSON, J. (1975). A double-blind comparison of single doses of etidocaine 1% and bupivacaine 0·5 per cent during continuous lumbar epidural block in obstetrics. *Acta anaesth. scand.*, Suppl. **60**, 97.

Chapter 35

LOCAL ANAESTHETIC TECHNIQUES

THIS chapter is not meant to be comprehensive. The object has been to present some of the ways in which local anaesthesia can be usefully and simply produced. Local anaesthesia is not commonly practised in the United Kingdom but there are occasions, typically for unprepared out-patients and certain very poor-risk patients, when it may be preferable to general anaesthesia. It is also useful for diagnostic and therapeutic reasons.

Spinal and epidural analgesia are described in Chapter 36 and 42. Some local anaesthetic techniques not described here are discussed in other parts of the book.

STELLATE GANGLION BLOCK

The cervical sympathetic chain normally consists of three ganglia, called the superior, middle, and inferior, according to their position in the neck, which are connected and through which the sympathetic supply to the upper limb, the neck, and the head is transmitted. A branch also runs to the cardiac plexus of nerves. The inferior cervical ganglion is frequently joined with that from the first thoracic nerve and is then known as the stellate ganglion. Sometimes the second thoracic ganglion is also included and occasionally either the fifth or sixth cervical ganglion, or both, are also incorporated, in which case the middle cervical ganglion is correspondingly smaller or absent.

The stellate ganglion is situated on the anterior surface of the neck of the first rib behind the subclavian artery and origin of the vertebral artery, and just superior to the dome of the pleura.

Technique

The anterior approach to the ganglion is satisfactory in practice. The patient lies supine with the head fully extended at the atlanto-occipital joint. The point of insertion of the needle is determined by measuring two fingers' breadth lateral to the jugular notch of the sternum and then a similar distance above the clavicle. The skin weal, which is raised in this position, should lie on the medial border of the sternomastoid muscle and over the transverse process of the seventh cervical vertebra. As a further check, the prominent tubercle (Chassaignac's) of the sixth cervical vertebra can be palpated behind the lateral border of the sternomastoid muscle. The cricoid cartilage also lies at the level of the sixth cervical vertebra so the skin weal should lie on a plane about 1·3 cm below these landmarks. The sternomastoid muscle and the carotid sheath are retracted laterally by two fingers of the left hand which press backward and laterally while a fine 5–8 cm needle is inserted at right angles to the skin until it comes in contact with the bone of the seventh cervical transverse process. If the needle is now withdrawn about 0·5 cm, its point will lie in the tissue plane anterior to the fascia which covers the pre-vertebral muscle and in which the sympathetic fibres run (Macintosh and Ostlere, 1955). After aspiration for blood and cerebrospinal fluid, 10 ml of 1 per cent lignocaine or 0·5 per cent bupivacaine should be injected and this will diffuse up and down the fascial plane blocking the sympathetic ganglia from C2 to T4. The patient should not cough, talk or move while the injection is being carried out.

The signs of a successful block have been recapitulated by Macintosh and Mushin (1954). They are enophthalmos, ptosis, myosis (the original triad of Horner's syndrome), unilateral blockage of the nose due to congestion of the nasal mucosa, absence of sweating and flushing of the skin due to vasodilatation in the head and neck vessels and those in the arm, all of which occur on the side of the block.

Indications

Stellate ganglion block may be of diagnostic and prognostic value in the treatment of Raynaud's disease of the upper limb. It is also useful in assessing a phantom limb, and as an emergency measure in the treatment of accidental intra-arterial injection of thiopentone, arterial injuries, crushing injuries and embolism of the upper extremity. It is of value in the so-called post-traumatic syndrome and Sudeck's atrophy, when pain, swelling and vasomotor disturbances are present. A recent indication for stellate ganglion block is to produce vasodilatation in the vessels of the arm and so make the surgery easier when an arteriovenous fistula is being created to enable haemodialysis to be undertaken in patients with renal failure. It is worth a trial in the treatment of severe angina at rest, and if successful may be repeated with a neurolytic agent such as phenol. Successful block does not produce dilatation of cerebral vessels, and its value for patients with cerebral thrombosis or embolism has not been proven.

Brachial Plexus Block

The brachial plexus arises from cervical roots 5, 6, 7 and 8 and the greater part of thoracic 1. It may also receive some supply from cervical 4. Brachial plexus block is useful for fractures, dislocations, and skin and muscle injuries of the forearm and hand, and—provided it is complete—will suffice for the reduction of a dislocated shoulder. It also provides anaesthesia of the skin over the outer side of the upper arm, but not of the superior part of the inner side which is supplied by thoracic 2. Should anaesthesia of the latter be required, the block must be combined with an intradermal and subcutaneous infiltration of local anaesthetic solution in the form of a ring around the top of the upper arm.

Supraclavicular Technique

The simplest technique for injection of the plexus is to approach it by the supraclavicular route as described by Macintosh and Mushin (1954). Lignocaine 1 per cent should be used and adrenaline may be added (on the basis of 0·5 ml of adrenaline 1:1,000 to each 100 ml of local anaesthetic solution) if anaesthesia lasting more than 45 to 60 minutes is required. For prolonged operations 0·5 per cent bupivacaine gives good results. The patient lies in the dorsal position with a pillow under his shoulders and his head turned away from the side to be injected. The affected arm must be by his side and the shoulder lowered so that the subclavian artery can be easily palpated above the clavicle. A skin weal is raised about a third of an inch above the midpoint of the clavicle just lateral to the area where the subclavian artery can be felt, and avoiding the external

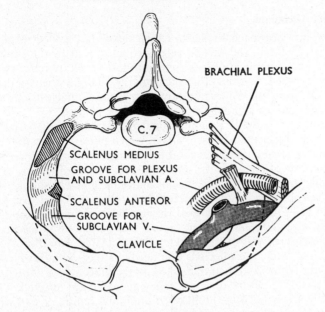

BRACHIAL PLEXUS

C.7

SCALENUS MEDIUS
GROOVE FOR PLEXUS
AND SUBCLAVIAN A.

SCALENUS ANTEROR
GROOVE FOR
SUBCLAVIAN V.

CLAVICLE

35/Fig. 1.—The first rib.

jugular vein. A 5 cm (2 inch) 22-gauge needle is then introduced through the skin weal in a backward, inward and downward direction toward the upper surface of the first rib over which the plexus runs (Fig. 1). While inserting the needle with one hand, it is helpful to push the subclavian artery medially with the first two fingers of the other, thus avoiding the risk of arterial puncture. Paraesthesia in the hand or forearm will most likely be felt by the patient as the point of the needle enters the plexus; at this stage 30 ml of local anaesthetic should be injected. If no paraesthesia is elicited, then the point of the needle must be advanced until it touches the upper surface of the first rib and local anaesthetic solution injected as it is withdrawn towards the skin. Repeated injections made in this manner, and with the needle point gradually moved along the upper surface of the first rib towards the subclavian artery, will block the plexus.

Puncture of the subclavian artery is not harmful provided local anaesthetic solution is not injected, but pressure should be temporarily applied to the vessel after removal of the needle to prevent the formation of a haematoma. The pleural cavity may also be entered if the direction of insertion of the needle is wrong.

Ball (1962) has described a modified supraclavicular approach to minimise the risk of accidental puncture of the pleura. In this technique the needle is inserted and advanced *vertically downwards* and *inwards*. This is a two-dimensional approach compared with the three-dimensional backward, inward and downward one previously described. Should the rib be missed the needle's position is anterior to the rib and outside the thoracic cage. If contact with the rib is not achieved at the first placing of the needle, it is withdrawn and reintroduced slightly more posteriorly but still vertically downwards.

Axillary Technique

The axillary approach to the brachial plexus has gained in popularity in recent years. Using it, the success rate is equal to that by the supraclavicular route, and the complications of pneumothorax and phrenic paralysis are completely avoided. It is therefore particularly valuable when a bilateral block of the plexus is needed. It does not, however, produce analgesia of the shoulder. If this is required, the supraclavicular route must be used.

The arm is abducted at a right angle from the body and the axillary artery palpated. The highest part in the axilla at which pulsation can be felt is the site for injection of local anaesthetic solution through a short, fine needle of 24 SW gauge. Such a needle lessens the risk of damage to the divisions of the plexus in the axillary sheath, and makes a haematoma unlikely should the axillary artery or vein be accidentally punctured. A finger is placed over the axillary artery, and after raising a skin weal the needle is advanced to one side of the artery until a definite and sudden "give" is experienced as the needle passes through the fascial wall of the axillary sheath. After aspiration, 15–20 ml of 1 per cent lignocaine are injected. The needle is then withdrawn as far as the subcutaneous tissues and then reinserted on the other side of the axillary artery where a further 15–20 ml of 1 per cent lignocaine are injected. The axillary sheath is effectively filled by 40 ml of solution and failure or partial block can follow the use of too small a volume of solution. In order to prevent the distal spread of the local anaesthetic solution and force it upwards into the axilla, it is advisable to apply a tourniquet to the upper arm immediately below the axilla. This should remain in place for about ten minutes.

INTRAVENOUS REGIONAL ANAESTHESIA

Holmes (1963) has described a useful method of producing analgesia of either an arm or leg by a modification of Bier's (1908) original intravenous analgesia technique.

Technique

A Gordh needle or plastic intravenous cannula is placed in a suitable vein toward the extremity of the limb. The limb is then elevated and an Esmarch bandage applied from the fingers or toes inwards to reach a sphygmomanometer cuff on the upper arm or leg. This is now blown up to a level above the patient's systolic blood pressure, the Esmarch bandage is removed, and a solution of 0·5 per cent lignocaine is injected intravenously through the Gordh needle. Bupivacaine (1·5 mg/kg of 0·5 per cent) diluted to 0·2 per cent with normal saline has proved satisfactory (Ware, 1975). About 40 ml of solution are required for an adult arm and up to 80 ml for an adult leg. The onset of anaesthesia is rapid and accompanied by paraesthesia and a feeling of warmth in the limb. Muscular paralysis occurs. The technique can usually be carried out successfully without an Esmarch bandage provided the limb is elevated long enough to allow some drainage of blood. The sphygmomanometer must be kept above the level of the systolic blood pressure until the operation is completed. Holmes suggests that if this is uncomfortable for the patient, a second cuff should be used below it on the analgesic part of the limb, and the original cuff removed. The use of a double-ballooned sphygmomanometer cuff has been advocated as a refinement of this technique (Hoyle, 1964).

The manner in which local anaesthesia and muscle paralysis are produced by this technique is unknown, but sensation and muscle power return within a matter of minutes after release of the sphygmomanometer cuff.

At the end of the operation, at least 15 minutes should have elapsed since giving the injection of local anaesthetic before deflating the cuff, because of the increased risk of toxic reactions after short periods of circulatory occlusion. Some workers believe that the risk of toxic reactions to the local anaesthetic released into the circulation at the end of the procedure can be reduced by intermittent release, that is deflating the tourniquet for only a few seconds at a time on several occasions. The pharmacokinetic aspects of intravenous regional anaesthesia have been described in a recent study (Tucker and Boas, 1971). This showed that after cuff release the peak plasma levels of lignocaine were 20 to 80 per cent lower than when the same dose of lignocaine was given by direct intravenous injection. The peak levels achieved were inversely proportional to the total time the tourniquet was applied and tended to be lower when the same dose was given by 0·5 per cent rather than 1·0 per cent solution. The release of the lignocaine into the circulation was noted to be biphasic, with an initial fast release of about 30 per cent of the dose, the remainder appearing by a gradual wash-out. 50 per cent of the dose of lignocaine can remain in the arm 30 minutes after release of the cuff, so it is possible to re-establish anaesthesia within 10–30 minutes of the initial deflation of the tourniquet by reinflating and injecting half of the original dose of the drug.

DIGITAL NERVE BLOCK

The digital nerves to a finger or toe can be blocked by infiltration of local anaesthetic solutions on either side of the base of the proximal phalanx. Lignocaine, 0·5 per cent, should be used, but without the addition of adrenaline in case marked vasoconstriction of the digital vessels should lead to gangrene.

COELIAC PLEXUS BLOCK

The object of this block is to deposit local anaesthetic solution in the vicinity of the coeliac ganglia and plexus of nerves, as they lie in the retroperitoneal tissues anterior to the body of the first lumbar vertebra.

The technique is described in Chapter 33, page 1074. A successful block is always followed by some fall in systemic blood pressure, due to dilatation of the splanchnic vessels. This can be controlled by the intravenous infusion of Ringer Lactate solution or a vasopressor if this is considered necessary.

Coeliac plexus block is required when upper abdominal surgery is performed under local anaesthesia alone. It is nowadays principally of value to relieve the severe pain of acute pancreatitis and of carcinoma of the pancreas or stomach. For the latter two indications a block with alcohol or phenol is necessary.

BLOCKS FOR ABDOMINAL OPERATIONS

Paravertebral and intercostal blocks for abdominal surgery are now rarely used. This is directly due to improvements in general anaesthesia, and, where a strong indication for local anaesthesia exists, to the many advantages of epidural block. To prepare a patient for an upper abdominal operation under intercostal combined with splanchnic block requires fifteen separate injections which in a psychologically unsuitable subject is difficult and not devoid of the risks of accidental pneumothorax and toxic reaction. However, as recently as 1962, Moore and Bridenbaugh listed seven reasons why this technique, or intercostal block with light general anaesthesia, might be considered the anaesthetic of choice for upper abdominal surgery.

For purposes of discussion, these seven reasons are quoted below:

1. Relaxation is equivalent to spinal or epidural anaesthesia or general anaesthesia plus relaxants.
2. Hypotension does not result unless the coeliac plexus is blocked, and even so, the hypotension is easily corrected.
3. The extent of anaesthesia is more predictable than that due to spinal or epidural block.
4. The duration of anaesthesia using amethocaine with adrenaline is longer than single-dose epidural or spinal block. Anaesthesia for 5–7 hours can be achieved.
5. The technique is ideal for a patient in a poor physical state, as it produces the minimum of psychological disturbance.
6. There are no neurological sequelae.
7. There are unlikely to be medico-legal objections on the part of the patient.

If each of these reasons is taken in turn and compared with modern general anaesthetic techniques using muscle relaxants, it is difficult to find any distinct or great advantage in their favour. When light general anaesthesia is used in addition to the intercostal nerve blocks, the morbidity of the local technique compared to that of the muscle relaxant is likely to be greater. Moore backed his opinions with a successful series of 4,333 patients and a low incidence of pneumothorax of only 0·092 per cent. This implies that the blocks were done by experts, but similar considerations would apply to the morbidity of relaxants given by experts.

Intercostal and other nerve blocks may in special circumstances still have a useful part to play. In some parts of the world few specialist anaesthetists are available and reliance must be placed on regional anaesthetic techniques performed by the surgeon himself. Farman and his colleagues (1962) describe a technique suitable for a single-handed surgeon. After inducing anaesthesia and intubating the patient, the general anaesthetic management of the patient is handed over to a relatively unskilled person by the surgeon, who then performs the intercostal nerve blocks.

A local nerve block technique may be useful in a very aged or poor-risk patient with a strangulated hernia to avoid hazards of regurgitation and vomiting under general anaesthesia.

Technique of Intercostal Block

Upper abdominal operations require bilateral intercostal block of the 6th–12th segments and lower abdominal operations the 7th to the 12th segments. Angle intercostal block is undertaken, four fingers' breadth from the midline of the back. At this point the rib is free from the cover of the erector spinae muscles and is easily palpable. The patient is placed in the lateral position with the scapula of the side to be blocked drawn as far as possible away from the midline. For patients in very poor condition for whom the minimum of movement is desirable, intercostal block can be performed with the patient supine. The arms are drawn up to expose the axillae and the injections performed just posterior to the mid axillary line to include the lateral cutaneous branches of the intercostal nerve. The lower border of the rib is palpated and a skin weal raised. The skin overlying the rib is drawn upwards and a 5 cm needle is passed down to the lower border of the rib. Having made contact with bone, the needle is angulated so that the tip is pointing in a slight upward direction and then the needle is slowly moved down on the rib until it slips under its lower edge. The needle must not be allowed to advance to a depth greater than 3 mm from the lower border of the rib, where its position is fixed. After aspiration, 5 ml of 1 per cent lignocaine with adrenaline are injected while the needle is advanced and withdrawn 1–2 mm, to ensure that some of the injected solution is deposited in the correct plane between the internal intercostal muscles and the intercostales intimi (Fig. 2). The most important complication of intercostal nerve block is a pneumothorax caused by the needle advancing too far and puncturing the lung. A tension pneumothorax may ensue and as these blocks are often performed in poor-risk patients the whole value may be lost by this complication. Lignocaine 1 per cent with adrenaline produces satisfactory anaesthesia for up to two hours. For operations of longer duration bupivacaine should be used. If multiple intercostal blocks are being undertaken for abdominal surgery, it may be necessary to reduce the concentration of local anaesthetic used in order to avoid exceeding the permitted maximum dose.

Local Block for Herniorraphy

This can be very useful for a strangulated hernia in an aged or otherwise poor-risk patient.

A single epidural injection will do just as well in many cases, but in some circumstances it may be particularly desirable to avoid a fall in blood pressure or the risk of dural puncture in, for example, a severe bronchitic where repeated coughing may lead to severe post-spinal headache.

An iliac crest block of the twelfth thoracic, the ilio-inguinal and ilio-hypogastric nerves (Fig. 3), as they lie between the transverse abdominis and internal oblique muscles, is performed as follows. A skin weal is raised two fingers' breadth from the iliac crest along a line joining the anterior superior spine to the xiphisternum. A needle is then passed through this to strike the inner surface of the ilium just below the crest. Ten ml of 1 per cent lignocaine solution are deposited as the needle is slowly withdrawn. The injection is then repeated with the needle reinserted at a slightly steeper angle. The contents of the inguinal canal are catered for by a separate injection into the neck of the peritoneal sac one finger's breadth above the mid-inguinal point. The needle is inserted perpendicularly until it pierces the aponeurosis of the external oblique, and the needle then advanced a further 2–3 cm through the extra-peritoneal fat in this region. Ten ml of solution are deposited at this depth and a further 10 ml as the needle is withdrawn over 2 cm (Macintosh and Bryce-Smith, 1953). This ensures block of the neck of the peritoneal sac and the genital branch of the

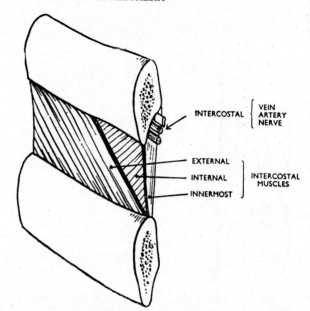

35/Fig. 2.—The intercostal space.

genito-femoral nerve. The block is then completed by a subcutaneous infiltration of the line of the surgical incision.

Discussion

It is difficult to define precisely the place of regional analgesia for abdominal surgery. Some points have already been touched on in the general description of the blocks. Undoubtedly, in the whole field of regional analgesia, its use for

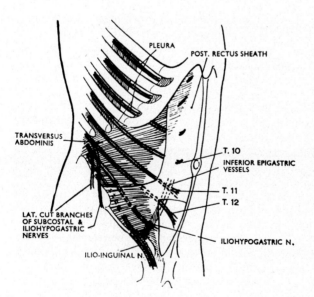

35/Fig. 3.—The lower intercostal, subcostal and first lumbar nerves.

abdominal surgery has suffered the greatest decline. Several factors contribute to this. The techniques are exacting for anaesthetist and patient, and are time-consuming. A considerable element of anxiety always exists for the whole surgical team when the patient is conscious. Anyone familiar with a patient nauseated and hiccupping from traction on upper abdominal viscera appreciates what the difficulties are. When a "light general anaesthetic" is given as well, conditions are certainly much improved, but if a light general anaesthetic can be given, why not a relaxant and controlled respiration? A specific contra-indication to a relaxant may be present, for example an anatomical abnormality which prevents intubation, or, in some types of patient, the risk of an abnormal response to the relaxant.

Some patients with abdominal disease, such as poor-risk prostatectomies, can be managed by a combination of regional and spinal anaesthesia—rectus sheath block and saddle block spinal. This is a valuable method, since the blocks are technically easy to do and such a technique avoids the fall of blood pressure that is a concomitant of either spinal or epidural anaesthesia sufficient to cover the whole operation field itself.

Much depends on individual circumstances. In abstract discussion it is often easy to decide the ideal anaesthetic management of a patient, but surgical preferences play a part, as does the skill of the anaesthetist in regional anaes-thesia. Present-day general anaesthesia has the supreme advantage of speed, and is a hundred per cent effective. Oxygenation, so important in the ill patient, and carbon dioxide elimination can often be best assured by controlled respiration using a high oxygen percentage in the gas mixture. All these factors must be assessed by the individual anaesthetist in the circumstances in which he finds himself.

LUMBAR SYMPATHETIC BLOCK

The lumbar sympathetic ganglia can be blocked where they lie against the vertebral bodies. The conventional approach was described by Mandl in 1926. The patient lies on his side and skin weals are raised 3 fingers' breadth or 5 cm lateral to the upper border of the 2nd, 3rd and 4th lumbar spinous processes. A needle is inserted at right angles to the skin through each weal and at a depth of 4–5 cm it strikes the transverse process. After slight withdrawal it is directed inwards and upwards for another 3–4 cm until it slides off the antero-lateral aspect of the vertebral body. Aspiration is carried out to ensure that no blood or cerebrospinal fluid enters the syringe and 10 ml of local anaesthetic solution, such as 1 per cent lignocaine, is then injected. By keeping the needle just above the transverse process in this manner the lumbar nerves will be missed but the solution will track up and down retroperitoneally.

The objection to this method is the uncertainty of placing the point of the needle at the right depth to miss the great vessels and the psoas muscle. Bryce-Smith (1951) overcame this difficulty by aiming the needle inwards from the start at an angle of 60–70° to the skin surface so as to strike the body of the vertebra on its lateral aspect. One injection only is made, namely from the middle weal in the original technique. The local anaesthetic tracks forwards beneath the tendinous arch bridging the sides of the vertebrae. Successful block is evidenced by a subjective sensation of warmth in the lower extremity with flushing and absence of sweating.

Chemical lumbar sympathectomy with alcohol or phenol is often of value in patients with chronic vascular disorders of the lower limb who are unfit for operation on general grounds. The technique is described in Chapter 33, page 1072. Temporary blocks with a local anaesthetic solution are not helpful in assessing the place for surgical sympathectomy, since the maximum benefits of operation are often not apparent for a long time—months in some patients. Temporary lumbar sympathetic block is useful when deciding whether sympathectomy will benefit phantom limb pain.

REFERENCES

BALL, H. C. J. (1962). Brachial plexus block. A modified supraclavicular approach. *Anaesthesia*, **17**, 269.

BIER, A. (1908). Ueber einen neuen Weg Localanasthesie an der Gliedmasse zu erzeugen. *Verh. dtsch. Ges. Chir.*, **37**, 204 (Part II).

BRYCE-SMITH, R. (1951). Injection of the lumbar sympathetic chain. *Anaesthesia*, **6**, 150.

FARMAN, J. V., GOOL, R. Y., and SCOTT, D. B. (1962). Intercostal block in abdominal surgery. A method for the singlehanded surgeon. *Lancet*, **1**, 879.

HOLMES, C. McK. (1963). Intravenous regional analgesia. A useful method of producing analgesia of the limbs. *Lancet*, **1**, 245.

HOYLE, J. R. (1964). Tourniquet for intravenous regional analgesia. *Anaesthesia*, **19**, 294.

MACINTOSH, R. R., and BRYCE-SMITH, R. (1953). *Local Analgesia: Abdominal Surgery.* Edinburgh: E. & S. Livingstone.

MACINTOSH, R. R., and MUSHIN, W. W. (1954). *Local Analgesia: Brachial Plexus*, 3rd edit. Edinburgh: E. & S. Livingstone.

MACINTOSH, R. R., and OSTLERE, M. (1955). *Local Analgesia: Head and Neck.* Edinburgh: E. & S. Livingstone.

MANDL, F. (1926). *Die Paravertebrate Injektion, Anatomie und Tecknik, Begründung, und Anwendung.* Wien: J. Springer.

MOORE, D. C., and BRIDENBAUGH, L. D. (1962). Intercostal nerve block in 4,333 patients: indications, technique and complications. *Anesth. Analg. Curr. Res.*, **41**, 1.

TUCKER, G. T., and BOAS, R. A. (1971). Pharmacokinetic aspects of intravenous regional anaesthesia. *Anesthesiology*, **34**, 538.

WARE, R. J. (1975). Intravenous regional anaesthesia using bupivacaine. *Anaesthesia*, **30**, 817.

Chapter 36

SPINAL AND EPIDURAL BLOCK

Section One

ANATOMY AND PHYSIOLOGY

THE ANATOMY OF THE SPINAL COLUMN, SPINAL CANAL, SPINAL CORD AND COVERINGS

THE vertebral column is made up of 33 vertebrae: 7 cervical, 12 thoracic, 5 lumbar, 5 sacral, and 4 coccygeal. A typical vertebra is composed of the following parts. (Fig. 1):

1. *The Body*, which is weight-bearing and separated from adjoining vertebral bodies by the intervertebral disc.
2. *The Vertebral Arch*, composed of pedicles and laminae which surround and protect the spinal cord and its coverings.
3. *The Transverse and Spinous Processes*, which give attachment to ligaments and to muscles acting on the vertebral column.
4. *The Superior and Inferior Articular Processes*.

Each pedicle is grooved, especially on the lower surface. These grooves are termed the superior and inferior vertebral notches and together make up the intervertebral foramen for the passage of the spinal nerve. The transverse process arises at the junction of the pedicle and the lamina.

The vertebral arch, its processes and connecting ligaments are the anatomical parts of greatest interest to the anaesthetist, for it is in this region that the needle is passed to introduce the local anaesthetic solution into the subarachnoid or epidural space.

The posterior surface of the vertebral bodies together with the vertebral arches, intervertebral discs and the connecting ligaments collectively form the

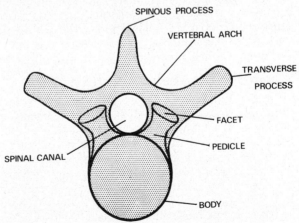

36/FIG. 1.—Diagram of a typical vertebra showing its components.

vertebral canal containing the spinal cord and its investing membranes. Deficiences occur in the lateral and posterior walls of the vertebral canal, the former being the intervertebral foramen while posteriorly is situated the interlaminar foramen. This foramen is bounded below by the upper edge of the laminae of the lower vertebra and, at the sides, by the inner aspect of the inferior articular process of the vertebra above. In extension the interlaminar foramen is small and triangular shaped but it elongates in flexion and provides access for passage of the spinal needle in performing lumbar puncture.

Although the lumbar region is the commonest site for the introduction of local anaesthetic solutions to the spinal or epidural space, the cervical and thoracic regions may in certain circumstances be used.

The spines of the thoracic vertebrae are of anaesthetic interest because they necessitate oblique placing of an epidural needle in the mid-thoracic region (Fig. 2). The spincs of T5–8 are almost vertical and in consequence their tips lie at the level of the body of the vertebra below. The spines of T1 and 2 and of T11 and 12 are almost horizontal, while those of T3 and 4, and of T9 and 10 are somewhat oblique.

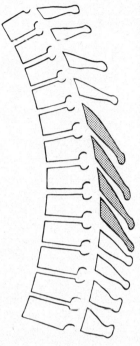

36/FIG. 2.—The inclination of the thoracic vertebral spines.

The lumbar vertebrae.—These are five in number, with large and massive kidney-shaped bodies because of their weight-bearing function, and are distinguished from cervical vertebrae by having no foramen in the transverse process and from thoracic by having no articular facets for ribs on the vertebral bodies (Fig. 3). The bodies are slightly taller anteriorly than posteriorly and the intervertebral discs are similarly shaped, producing the lumbar curve. The pedicles are directed backwards and laterally as in the cervical region. The superior intervertebral notch is small and the inferior large. The laminae are thick and sloping, as in the thoracic region, and the spinal canal is triangular. The spine is a thick oblong plate which projects backwards nearly horizontally.

Important Ligaments of the Vertebral Column

It is essential for the anaesthetist practising spinal and epidural anaesthesia to have an accurate knowledge of those ligaments in the spine through which the spinal or epidural needle passes. The different sensations of resistance that these ligaments impart to the advancing needle can with practice be appreciated by the operator and are an invaluable aid to successful technique.

The vertebrae are held together by a series of overlapping ligaments which not only bind together the vertebral column but assist in protecting the spinal cord (Fig. 4).

The anterior longitudinal ligament.—This ligament is more of anatomical

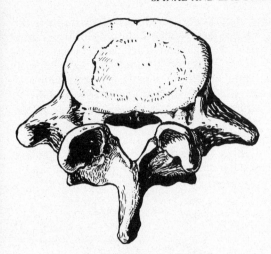

SUPERIOR VIEW

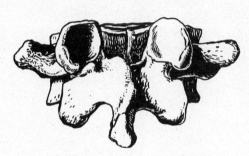

POSTERIOR VIEW

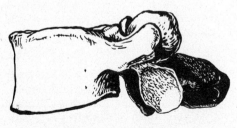

LATERAL VIEW

36/Fig. 3.—A lumbar vertebra.

than anaesthetic interest. It begins at the axis (C2) as a continuation of the atlanto-axial ligament and extends down the entire front of the bodies of the vertebrae to the sacrum, closely attached to the margins of the vertebral bodies. It is thickest in the thoracic and lumbar regions.

The posterior longitudinal ligament.—This ligament begins on the posterior surface of the vertebral body of the axis and extends down through the entire length of the vertebral column, fanning out at the vertebral margins to reinforce the intervertebral discs. The ligament is thinnest in the cervical and lumbar regions. It is possible for this ligament to be pierced by a too-far-advancing lumbar-puncture needle, and for damage to the intervertebral disc to result.

The ligamentum flavum.— This ligament is of considerable importance to the anaesthetist and must be described in detail. It is composed entirely of yellow elastic fibres, which account for its name. It is placed on either side of the spinous process and extends laterally to blend with the capsule of the joints between the superior and inferior articular processes. It runs from the anterior and inferior aspects of the lamina above to the posterior and superior aspect of the lamina below. In the midline is a cleft between it and the ligamentum flavum of the opposite side for the passage of veins. A spinal needle accurately placed in the midline would only pass through a few thin fibres of the ligamenta flava and impart very little change of resistance to the anaesthetist. In practice, however, the needle is probably always a little off centre and passes through the full thickness of the ligament. The ligamenta flava comprise over half of the posterior wall of the vertebral canal, the bony laminae accounting for the remainder. The ligament is thinnest in the cervical region and thickest in the lumbar region, where powerful stresses and strains have to be countered. Functionally, these ligaments are muscle sparers, assisting in the recovery of the erect posture after bending, and in maintaining the erect posture.

Interspinous ligaments.—These ligaments connect adjoining spinous processes from their tips to their roots. They fuse with the supraspinous ligament posteriorly and with the ligamentum flavum anteriorly. In the lumbar region they are wide and dense.

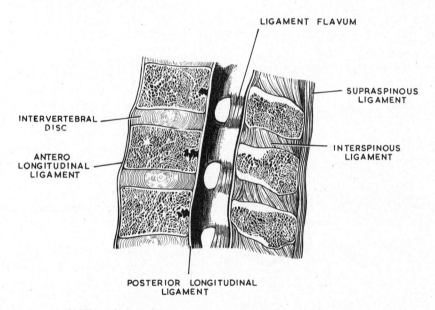

36/Fig. 4.—Important ligaments of the vertebral column.

Supraspinous ligament.—This ligament is a continuation of the ligamentum nuchae and joins together the tips of the spinous processes from the seventh cervical vertebra to the sacrum. It increases in thickness from above downwards and is thickest and widest in the lumbar region.

The Intervertebral Discs

These discs are responsible for a quarter of the length of the spinal column, and, functionally, are shock absorbers placed between the vertebral bodies. They are thicker in the cervical and lumbar regions, where they allow of great mobility, than in the thoracic parts of the column. Each disc consists of a peripheral fibrous portion—the annulus fibrosus—and a gelatinous central portion —the nucleus pulposus—which accommodates itself to changes in shape during movement between the vertebrae. If a lumbar-puncture needle is accidentally pushed too far through the subarachnoid space and into the annulus, the nucleus pulposus may prolapse and cause sciatica.

The Spinal Cord and its Coverings

The spinal cord, a direct continuation of the medulla oblongata, begins at the upper border of the atlas and ends at the lower border of the 1st lumbar vertebra. It is 42–45 cm in length. It is not uncommon for the cord to extend to the second lumbar vertebra, particularly in African races. Exceptionally the cord can reach the 3rd lumbar vertebra. In order to avoid possible damage to the cord, lumbar puncture should, if possible, be made in the L4–5 interspace. In the new-born child the cord ends at the 3rd lumbar vertebra, and in fetal life the cord extends the entire length of the vertebral canal and the spinal nerves run in a horizontal direction. As the vertebral column elongates with growth, the spinal cord does not keep pace and the nerve roots assume an increasingly oblique and downward direction towards their foramina of exit. Consequently, below the 1st lumbar vertebra the canal is occupied by a leash of lumbar, sacral and coccygeal nerve roots, termed the cauda equina. The difference between the cord level of a given spinal root and the vertebral level has important practical

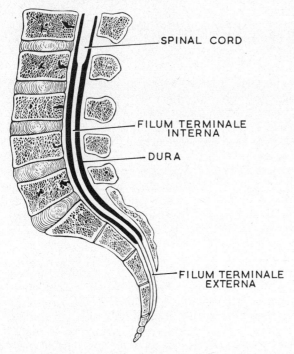

SPINAL CORD

FILUM TERMINALE INTERNA

DURA

FILUM TERMINALE EXTERNA

36/Fig. 5.—The termination of the vertebral canal.

consequences when it is desired to block accurately spinal nerve roots with small volumes of neurolytic agents. Failure to appreciate this point and the choice of the vertebral level rather than the cord level for injection will result in destruction of nerve roots below the desired levels.

From the lower end of the spinal cord extends a thread-like structure known as the filum terminale interna which ends with the dura and the arachnoid mater at the level of the second sacral vertebra (Fig. 5). It pierces the dura and arachnoid and is continued below this level as the filum terminale externa, eventually blending with the periosteum on the back of the coccyx. The 31 spinal nerves emerge from the spinal cord in pairs, 8 cervical, 12 thoracic, 5 lumbar, 5 sacral, and one pair of coccygeal nerves. The spinal nerves are composed of the anterior and posterior roots which unite in the intervertebral foramina to form the spinal nerve trunks. The cord has two enlargements, cervical and lumbar, corresponding to the nerve supply of the upper and lower limbs. The cervical enlargement extends from C3 to T2 and the lumbar enlargement from T9–12.

The spinal cord is enveloped by three membranes, dura, arachnoid, and pia mater, which are direct continuations of those surrounding the brain.

Blood Supply of the Spinal Cord

The viability of the spinal cord depends on its receiving an adequate blood supply and impairment of this, by either thrombosis, clamping of the aorta, or prolonged vasoconstriction, may lead to ischaemia of the cord. Such a mechanism may explain the occasional neurological disaster following spinal or epidural analgesia.

There are two posterior spinal arteries on each side which arise from the posterior inferior cerebellar arteries at the base of the brain. They supply the posterior columns of the spinal cord.

There is a single anterior spinal artery lying in front of the anterior median fissure in the pia mater. It arises at the level of the foramen magnum by the union of a small branch from each vertebral artery. It passes down the whole length of the spinal cord, receiving communications from the intercostal and lumbar arteries. Those at the level of T1 and L2 are larger than the others (the arteries of Adamkiewicz) in order to supply the cervical and lumbar enlargements. The anterior spinal artery supplies the anterior and lateral columns of the cord. Thrombosis of this vessel causes the anterior spinal artery syndrome in which there is paraplegia without loss of posterior column sensation (joint position, touch and vibration sense). The anterior and posterior spinal arteries do not anastomose with each other so that there are three distinct vascular areas within the cord, two posterior and one anterior (Djindjian, 1970).

The spinal veins comprise anterior and posterior plexuses which drain through the intervertebral foramina into the vertebral, azygos and lumbar veins.

The spinal dura mater.—In the cranial cavity the dura is arranged in two layers, "periosteal" and "investing", which are firmly adherent except where they split to enclose venous sinuses. The outer periosteal layer is the periosteum of the inner surface of the skull bones which, in the spine, acts as the periosteum lining the spinal canal. The inner or investing layer is continued from the cranium into the spinal canal. Between the two layers in the spinal canal is the extra- or epi-dural space which anatomically would be better termed the *inter-dural* space.

The inner layer of dura is firmly adherent to the margins of the foramen magnum where it blends with the outer or periosteal layer. Hence solutions deposited correctly in the spinal epidural space cannot enter the cranial cavity or produce nerve block higher than the 1st cervical nerves. The inner layer is loosely attached to the posterior longitudinal ligament by fibrous strands anchoring it in place. The epidural space is narrower anteriorly and wider posteriorly where the inner layer of dura is unattached; its greatest width (6 mm) occurs in the mid-thoracic region.

The anterior and posterior nerve roots issuing from the spinal cord pierce the investing layer of dura and carry tubular prolongations (dural cuffs) which blend with the perineurium of the mixed spinal nerve (Fig. 6).

The investing layer of dura ends as a tube at the 2nd sacral vertebra, and so also does the arachnoid, so that cerebrospinal fluid is not found below this level. The dura ends by giving an investment to the filum terminale externa which blends eventually with the periosteum on the back of the coccyx.

The arachnoid mater.—The spinal arachnoid is a continuation of the cerebral arachnoid. An incomplete and inconstant septum divides the spinal subarachnoid space along the midline of the dorsal surface of the cord. The arachnoid is the middle of the three investing membranes covering the brain and spinal cord and is closely applied to the dura mater. The subdural space between the dura and the arachnoid is a capillary interface containing a little serous fluid, but has no connection with the subarachnoid space.

The pia mater.—In the vertebral canal the pia is closely applied to the spinal cord and extends into the anterior median fissure. The blood vessels going to the brain and spinal cord lie in the subarachnoid space before piercing the pia. They carry with them into the brain and spinal cord a double sleeve of meninges; the inner wall of the sleeve is derived from the pia, and the outer from the arachnoid.

The Epidural Space

The formation of the epidural space by the splitting of the two layers of the

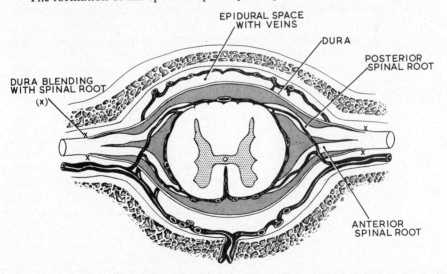

36/Fig. 6.—Dural cuffs and the venous plexus of the epidural space.

spinal dura mater has been described. It remains to define the space and its contents anatomically and in greater detail. The space is limited superiorly by the fusion of the two layers of dura at the foramen magnum, and inferiorly by the sacrococcygeal ligament closing the sacral hiatus. The 31 pairs of spinal nerves with their dural prolongations traverse the space on the way to their exit at the intervertebral foramina. The intervertebral foramina are the passageways between the epidural and paravertebral spaces, and solutions of local anaesthetic injected into them are free to travel from one to the other, except in old age when the foramina may become blocked by fibrous tissue. It is difficult to predict the extent of spread of local anaesthetic solutions injected into the epidural space because of the variability in the patency of the 58 intervertebral foramina, but the height of the block achieved by a given volume of solution will be appreciably higher in the elderly than in the young (Bromage, 1969).

The venous plexuses of the vertebral canal lie in the epidural space (see Fig. 6). These veins receive tributaries from the adjacent bony structures and the spinal cord. They form a network running vertically within the epidural space and can be subdivided into a pair of anterior venous plexuses which lie on either side of the posterior longitudinal ligament, into which the basivertebral veins empty and a single posterior venous plexus which connects with the posterior external veins. These veins, although divided into anatomical groups, all interconnect with one another and form a series of venous rings at the level of each vertebra. They connect with the intervertebral veins which pass out through the intervertebral foramina and so communicate with the vertebral, ascending cervical, deep cervical, intercostal, iliolumbar and lateral sacral veins. These veins have no valves and afford a connection between the pelvic veins below with the intracranial veins above, so explaining the frequency of cerebral and vertebral metastases from primary lesions in the pelvis. Similarly, air or local anaesthetic solutions injected into the epidural veins may track up to the brain.

The epidural veins become distended during coughing and straining and also when the inferior vena cava is obstructed by large abdominal tumours or in late pregnancy. Fatty tissue lies between the arteries, veins and nerves in the epidural space. The greatest depth of fat within the epidural space is situated posteriorly and antero-laterally; it is continuous with the fat in the intervertebral foramina around the spinal nerves.

The Paravertebral Space

The paravertebral spaces in the thoracic region lie between the heads of the ribs and because they are in direct contact with the pleura they are subject to the same fluctuations as occur in intrathoracic pressure (Fig. 7a). The fat in the epidural space surrounds the intercostal nerves as they pass through the intervertebral foramina and so is in direct continuity with the fat in the paravertebral space. The negative intrathoracic pressure is thus conducted via the paravertebral spaces to the thoracic epidural space and to a diminishing extent to the cervical and lumbar regions.

THE PHYSIOLOGY OF SPINAL AND EPIDURAL BLOCK

Following the introduction of a local anaesthetic solution into the subarachnoid space, pre-ganglionic sympathetic fibres are blocked first. After these

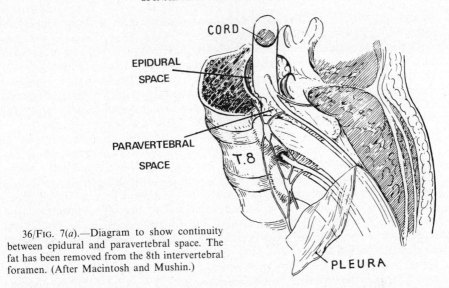

CORD

EPIDURAL
SPACE

PARAVERTEBRAL
SPACE

T.8

PLEURA

36/Fig. 7(a).—Diagram to show continuity between epidural and paravertebral space. The fat has been removed from the 8th intervertebral foramen. (After Macintosh and Mushin.)

the sensory fibres (in order of increasing diameter) transmitting the sensations of temperature, pain, touch, and finally pressure, cease to function. The largest fibres are motor and proprioceptive, and these too will be ultimately blocked if the concentration of anaesthetic drug is high enough. This sequence of events can be observed in the conscious patient during spinal anaesthesia. When sensory blockade is complete, skeletal muscle movement may still be possible,

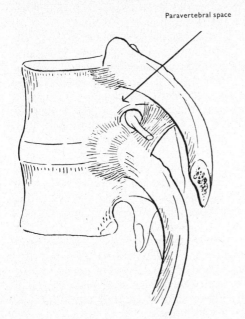

Paravertebral space

36/Fig. 7(b).—Diagram to illustrate the boundaries of the paravertebral space (see text).

though this in turn will disappear if the concentration of drug is high enough to affect the larger fibres of the motor roots.

The site of action of local anaesthetics in the subarachnoid space is assumed to be on the fibres of the dorsal and ventral roots. At what particular point on the dorsal root is not certain: it could be on the cells of the dorsal root ganglia, their axons, or both. Frumin and his co-workers (1953a) have produced evidence that the site of action of minimally effective concentrations of procaine, which block sensory but not motor impulses, is the dorsal root ganglion.

While the precise site of action of local anaesthetic drugs introduced into the subarachnoid space is of scientific interest, the site of action of drugs introduced into the epidural space is of practical importance. The one common factor to all the neurological sequelae of spinal analgesia is the introduction of a drug into the subarachnoid space, and it is commonly argued that the use of drugs epidurally will avoid these neurological sequelae. But if epidurally placed anaesthetic solutions do diffuse across the dura into the cerebrospinal fluid—and there is now considerable evidence that they do—the use of epidural blocks might be expected to be followed by neurological sequelae similar to those of spinal analgesia. The exact site of action of a local anaesthetic placed in the epidural space is, however, still not certain. For a long time only two possible sites of action were considered. First, the drug diffuses across the dura into the subarachnoid space and effects a true "spinal" analgesia, acting on either nerve roots or dorsal root ganglia. Secondly, the drug diffuses from the epidural space through the intervertebral foramina and produces nerve block in the paravertebral space. Evidence for the first hypothesis is conflicting, but a great deal of laboratory work, both in man and animals, has demonstrated that local anaesthetics cross the dura and enter the subarachnoid space. In many cases the concentration of procaine was greater than the level necessary to block the myelinated fibres in the spinal nerve roots (Frumin et al., 1953b).

Bromage (1975) has produced a working hypothesis reconciling all the clinical and experimental evidence available for the mode of action of epidural anaesthesia (Table 1). The longitudinal spread of solutions injected into the epidural space is dependent on the volume injected. The patent intervertebral foramina, present in young subjects, permit the local anaesthetic solution to pass out freely into the paravertebral spaces along the spinal nerves, producing multiple paravertebral blocks of the nerve trunks. Diffusion of the solution through the epineurium and perineurium and so into the subperineural spaces results in some centripetal diffusion back towards the neuraxis and hence to the subpial space. This paravertebral block is probably unimportant in elderly subjects and with small volumes of solution. There is an increased permeability to local anaesthetics in the dural cuffs surrounding the spinal roots and they constitute the principal pathway for diffusion and blockade after epidural injection.

Sensitive radioassay techniques using ^{14}C-labelled lignocaine or mepivacaine showed that the concentration of local anaesthetics was nearly as high in intradural roots as in the extradural portion after epidural injection (Bromage et al., 1963; Bromage and Burfoot, 1964). Radioactivity could also be demonstrated around the periphery of the cord and extended up as high as the medulla. High extradural pressure on injection, which tends to occur in elderly subjects, favours diffusion through the pia arachnoid root villi in the region of the dural cuffs.

36/TABLE 1

THE FATE OF AN EPIDURAL INJECTION

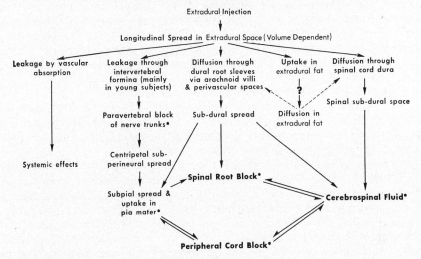

* = Sites where experimental measurement has demonstrated local anaesthetic concentrations in excess of the minimal effective concentration (Cm.).

From this area, further spread of the solution can follow into the subdural space and hence to the subpial and subarachnoid spaces with accompanying blockade of the spinal roots and peripheral tracts of the spinal cord. After an epidural injection, the intradural spinal nerve roots are the initial and probably the main site of blockade, followed by the incoming tracts of the spinal cord in the dorsal horn. Penetration of the cord depends on the physico-chemical properties of the local anaesthetic itself, etidocaine, for example, being much more effective in this respect than lignocaine.

The concept of neuraxial spread is a most important one, because if it is correct and if the view is taken that some neurological sequelae of spinal anaesthesia are due to the anaesthetic itself, then it follows that epidural anaesthesia cannot be regarded as potentially free from the same risks.

Bromage's views are summarised in Table 1.

The amount of drug available to diffuse along the neuraxis will depend on the state of the neural coverings and the physical laws of diffusion. These factors have an important bearing on the height of epidural anaesthesia and will be discussed later.

Fate of Local Anaesthetics in the Subarachnoid and Epidural Spaces

Following the injection of a local anaesthetic into the subarachnoid space, the concentration falls rapidly in the cerebrospinal fluid at the point of injection. The rate of fall is quickest during the first five minutes after injection and is then more gradual. The initial steep fall is due to diffusion of the drug away from the point of injection which in turn depends on such factors as the speed of injection, the specific gravity of the solution, the posture of the patient and the rate of absorption into nerve roots. These factors will shortly be discussed. It is during this period that spinal analgesia is said to become "fixed".

Local anaesthetics are not destroyed in the cerebrospinal fluid, and so the more gradual decrease in concentration reflects the removal of the drug by vascular absorption. Detoxication takes place after systemic absorption. Detectable amounts of local anaesthetic drug remain in the cerebrospinal fluid during the effective duration of the analgesia and even up to the point when the block is waning.

There are three possible mechanisms of absorption.

1. *Absorption through the spinal arachnoid villi.*—Elwan, in 1923, demonstrated cell clusters in the regions where the arachnoid is reflected proximally on to the segmental nerves as they leave the subarachnoid space. Some absorption probably occurs through these cells.

2. *Absorption through capillaries.*—Figure 6 shows the numerous vascular channels that lie within the subdural and epidural spaces. Cerebrospinal fluid is probably absorbed by this capillary network. Such a mechanism would therefore play an important part in the removal of drugs from the subarachnoid space.

3. *Absorption through the cranial arachnoid villi into the venous sinuses.*— Absorption undoubtedly takes place in effective amounts before the solution reaches the cranium. Koster and his co-workers (1936 and 1938) showed in man, by means of serial taps above the lumbar puncture injection, a rapidly decreasing concentration of drug in the subarachnoid space.

Studies with radioactive dibromoprocaine in animals indicate that the greater portion of local anaesthetic leaves the subarachnoid space by the venous drainage, and a much smaller proportion by the lymphatics (Howarth, 1949).

As might be expected, the use of a vasoconstrictor in conjunction with the local anaesthetic results in considerable prolongation of the duration of analgesia. Moore and Bridenbaugh (1966) showed in a large series of subarachnoid blocks that adrenaline increases the duration of analgesia by 50 per cent. Phenylephrine also has a similar effect in prolonging analgesia (Meagher *et al.*, 1966). The use of intrathecal adrenaline carries the theoretical risk of causing neural ischaemia and for this reason is avoided by many anaesthetists.

Absorption of epidural solutions is largely by way of the epidural vessels and is delayed if vasoconstrictors are added. The ultimate clearance of an epidural solution is complex, for it is now appreciated that apart from spreading longitudinally in the epidural space, it also traverses meningeal and perineural barriers to reach the cerebrospinal fluid. Thus it will be cleared to some extent by mechanisms that apply to drugs directly introduced into the cerebrospinal fluid.

Pathological states may also influence clearance of drugs both in the epidural space and the cerebrospinal fluid. Decreased blood flow to the vessels surrounding the subarachnoid space could explain the longer duration of analgesia in arteriosclerotic patients. Hypotension will also prolong both spinal and epidural analgesia.

Factors Controlling the Height of Spinal Anaesthesia

The upward passage of a local anaesthetic solution in the subarachnoid space depends upon a number of factors. The following are the most important which control the subsequent level of analgesia:

1. **Specific gravity of the solution.**—Of the many factors which influence the spread of solutions in the cerebrospinal fluid, gravity is the most important. Spinal solutions are classed as hyperbaric, isobaric, and hypobaric according to whether their specific gravity is higher, the same, or lower than that of cerebrospinal fluid. The movement of hyperbaric and hypobaric solutions in the CSF depends in turn upon the position of the patient during injection, and any change in position after the injection is completed.

2. **Volume of solution.**—The greater the volume of solution injected into an area of fixed volume, such as the subarachnoid space, the more extensive is the subsequent spread. The effect of volume is independent of concentration and specific gravity. The extent to which this variable is used in clinical practice will be discussed under the description of spinal anaesthetic techniques.

3. **Total dose of drug injected.**—In general, the larger the dose of drug injected the longer the duration of blockade and the greater the height to which it rises.

4. **Speed and force of injection.**—The faster the rate of injection, the higher the level of analgesia obtained. Turbulent currents are set up by rapid injection and these cause spread of the solution. Macintosh and Lee (1973) have described experiments with saline-filled "glass spines" and shown that rapid injection with the production of eddies is facilitated by the use of small syringes and large-bore needles. With the fine needles now recommended to diminish the incidence and severity of post-lumbar puncture headache it is difficult to inject sufficiently rapidly to set up big enough eddies to spread the drug widely in the cerebrospinal fluid.

5. **Barbotage.**—The term is derived from the French *barboter*—to puddle, to mix. The word "barbotage" was coined by Le Filliotre and the technique was popularised in spinal anaesthesia by Labat. The basis of the technique is to leave the injecting syringe attached to the spinal needle and make repeated aspirations and injections, thus mixing and dispersing the original dose of local anaesthetic. The spread of a given dose of a local anaesthetic is closely related to the amount of barbotage used, a much higher level of blockade resulting from its use.

6. **Site of injection.**—It is of course possible to use any spinal interspace for the introduction of a local anaesthetic, but in order to avoid possible damage to the spinal cord it is safer to restrict lumbar puncture to the interspaces at L3–4 or L4–5, other variables being then responsible for the ultimate height of the block.

7. **Position of patient during and after injection.**—The movement of a hyperbaric solution in the CSF depends in turn upon the position of the patient during injection and any change after the injection is completed. If the patient remains sitting during and after the injection, the effect of a hyperbaric solution will be localised to the sacral nerve roots. Allowing the patient to remain on his side will facilitate a more pronounced block on the dependent side. For abdominal surgery, the patient is turned on his back after injection which leads to puddling in the thoracic and sacral regions and, as described in Section II, the upward spread is determined by the degree of head-down tilt.

Factors Controlling the Height of Epidural Analgesia

Some of the principles which control the spread of local anaesthetic in the subarachnoid space also apply to spread in the epidural space.

1. **Site of injection.**—Any interspace of the spine may be used for epidural injection. If it is desired to keep the dose down to the minimum, injection should be made at the level of the spinal segment corresponding to the middle of the area to be blocked. Thus puncture at levels between C7 and T3 has been used for upper thoracic operations, and between T4 and T10 for upper abdominal operations. In general the lumbar region is the easiest route technically and from it the desired level can usually be reached by using an appropriate volume of solution.

2. **Volume of solution.**—This is a very important factor in the spread of epidural solutions. The larger the volume used the greater the area blocked. The height to which a given volume may rise depends also on the patency of the intervertebral foramina which, as previously explained, are the normal escape route for epidural solutions. In the elderly these foramina tend to become blocked by fibrous tissue and a given volume of solution produces a much greater area of analgesia than in a young person with widely patent intervertebral foramina.

3. **Position of the patient after injection.**—Position is important since epidural solutions flow under the influence of gravity and will diffuse cephalad in the Trendelenburg position and caudally in a patient sitting up.

4. **Speed of injection.**—Rapid injection spreads the solution upwards and downwards in the epidural space. A given volume injected rapidly will produce a more extensive block than the same volume injected slowly, though the duration will be shorter, since the volume of solution is widely dispersed and more rapidly removed by venous absorption (Bromage, 1954).

5. **Pregnancy and intra-abdominal tumours.**—In the presence of inferior vena caval compression from a gravid uterus or an intra-abdominal tumour, the venous return from the lower part of the body is diverted to the vertebral and epidural venous plexuses. The resultant distension of the epidural veins causes a reduction in the capacity available in the epidural space so that a given volume of local anaesthetic will spread more extensively than in a normal subject.

6. **Concentration of the solution.**—A more concentrated solution of local anaesthetic will produce blockade over a wider area than an equal volume of a lower concentration of the same drug.

7. **Other factors.**—As has been previously outlined, two mechanisms are involved in the ultimate spread of an epidural injection; these are, longitudinal spread in the epidural space governed by factors 1 to 5, and neuraxial spread. Again it is to Bromage that we owe an understanding of this very important mechanism.

Neuraxial spread itself will depend on the state of the neural coverings and the physical laws of diffusion across these coverings. The important facts here in relation to the epidural space are the nature of the drug (see Chapter 34), the area of contact between neural coverings and the drug, the concentration of the local anaesthetic, and the duration of contact.

The area of contact will depend on the volume of solution injected and the patency of the intervertebral foramina. The duration of contact will depend on the rate of removal of the drug from the epidural space, which in turn will depend again on the patency of the intervertebral foramina and the physical state of the epidural vessels. Diffusion gradients appear to be very important even in relation to volume, and small volumes of concentrated solutions— 4 to 5 per cent lignocaine—can produce widespread blockade. With these small volumes of concentrated solution, longitudinal spread in the epidural space is presumably confined to a few segments, but neuraxial spread is extensive owing to the high concentration gradient.

Bromage (1962) has also drawn attention to the exaggerated spread of epidural anaesthesia in arteriosclerotic patients. Fifty-six patients who were severely arteriosclerotic reacted to 2 per cent lignocaine as if they had received a solution of 3 per cent, 4 per cent, or 5 per cent. It is probable that the degenerative changes in connective tissue associated with arteriosclerotic disease produce increased permeability of neural coverings. Furthermore, sclerosis of the vasa nervorum hastens the normal degeneration of myelin sheaths that occurs with increasing age, thus bringing the solution more readily into contact with the axons of the posterior nerve roots.

This concept of a neuraxial spread that is exaggerated in arteriosclerotic patients provides a rational explanation of some previously unexplained cases of total spinal blockade. A number of patients have been reported in whom identification of the epidural space seemed certain, and from which neither cerebrospinal fluid nor blood could be aspirated, and yet total spinal anaesthesia resulted from the injection of a comparatively small volume of anaesthetic solution. In some reported instances total spinal anaesthesia was delayed for 30 to 40 minutes, or even longer (Morrow, 1959). Severe arteriosclerotic disease is the only common feature of all such cases.

Thus the spread in the epidural space of an anaesthetic solution is the result of a number of complex interrelated factors, with age and pathological processes probably playing an important part. Bromage has aptly stated that our ideas on this subject need to be more sophisticated than hitherto. These factors will be considered further in the discussion of dosage for epidural block.

Circulatory Effects of Spinal and Epidural Block

The pre-ganglionic sympathetic fibres arise from the spinal cord between T1 and L2 and run in the corresponding anterior roots across the subarachnoid and epidural spaces. It is a good working rule to regard the fall in blood pressure that accompanies spinal or epidural analgesia as correlated with the height of the block and therefore with the number of sympathetic fibres blocked. The resultant sympathetic blockade leads to dilatation of both resistance and capacitance vessels with consequent decreased peripheral vascular resistance and hypotension. The peripheral venous pooling causes a reduction of venous return to the heart with a subsequent fall in stroke volume and in the amount of work performed by the left ventricle. Pugh and Wyndham (1950) measured the cardiac output of hypertensive and control subjects under high spinal anaesthesia and found the main factor in the fall of blood pressure was a fall in cardiac output without significant change in the peripheral resistance. Their conclusion was that the fall in cardiac output might be due to relaxation of venous tone, and the role of the sympathetic nervous system in the control of blood pressure depended on the control of the veins, at least as much as in the control of the arterioles. The degree of hypotension induced by vasomotor blockade to the same segmental level with both epidural and subarachnoid anaesthesia was studied by Defalque (1962). He found that the fall in arterial pressure had a linear relation to the height of the block.

Segmental blockade of the sympathetic nerves up to the level of T5 can be compensated in normovolaemic man by vasoconstriction in the upper part of the body (Shimosato and Etsten, 1969; Bonica *et al.*, 1971). This compensation occurs with little change in cardiac output and with little more than a 5–16 per cent fall in mean arterial pressure (Stanton Hicks, 1975). Thus it is possible for a large part of the arteriolar bed to be dilated under the influence of the sympathetic blockade while the total peripheral resistance changes little due to compensatory vasoconstriction elsewhere.

If blockade extends above the level of T5 and more of the sympathetic outflow is blocked, it becomes progressively more difficult to compensate for these haemodynamic changes and the blood pressure falls. The sympathetic block invariably extends higher than the level of the accompanying sensory block as the small sympathetic fibres are susceptible to the action of a lower concentration of local anaesthetics. Greene (1969) in a review of the cardiovascular effects of spinal anaesthesia regards the fall in blood pressure as the result of pre-ganglionic sympathetic blockade. Minor degrees of arterial hypotension are principally due to changes in peripheral resistance but if the pressure continues to fall below a certain critical level, there is probably an associated reduction of venous return and hence in cardiac output.

This critical level is about 90 mm Hg (12·0 kPa) systolic in a normal patient. The position of the patient during spinal anaesthesia has an important effect on the cardiac output. A patient with a pre-anaesthetic systolic blood pressure of 120 mm Hg (16·0 kPa) who is given high spinal anaesthesia and tipped into the head-down position to maintain the cardiac output will often only have a fall in systolic blood pressure to 100 or 90 mm Hg (13·3 kPa or 12·0 kPa). If the same patient is placed horizontal or in the foot-down position, the cardiac output falls due to gravitational pooling of blood, and severe hypotension develops.

The baroreceptors in the carotid sinus and aortic arch normally respond to a fall in blood pressure by producing a compensatory tachycardia (Marey's law) through vagal afferent and efferent pathways. Most patients under spinal or epidural anaesthesia, however, exhibit bradycardia and hypotension (Greene, 1969) and it would appear that the Bainbridge reflex predominates. This reflex is mediated by receptors in the great veins and right atrium which adjust the heart rate according to the venous filling pressure. An increase in venous return is believed to stimulate the volume receptors and this activity is then signalled to the brain via vagal *afferents*. The cardiac sympathetic nerves (arising from T1–4 segments) carry the *efferents* so that the heart rate increases in response to a rise in venous return. Conversely, in spinal or epidural anaesthesia there is venous pooling in the periphery, a reduction in stimulation of the volume receptors, and therefore diminished activity of the cardiac sympathetic nerves. The result is vagal preponderance and a *slowing* of the heart rate. Block of the cardiac sympathetic nerves by either high spinal or epidural block may also be an additional factor causing bradycardia. It is important to remember that sympathetic blockade may extend two to three dermatomes higher than analgesia.

Many authorities in the past have claimed that the fall in blood pressure from an epidural block is less than from a spinal of comparable height (Odom, 1936; Gutierrez, 1939; Dogliotti, 1939; Dawkins, 1945). In more recent work, however (Bromage, 1954; Bonica et al., 1957; Defalque, 1962), it has been found that the incidence and extent of the fall in blood pressure is similar in both forms of anaesthesia but the speed of onset is slower in epidural analgesia. Bromage (1954) has pointed out that in a few patients the blood pressure is maintained at normal levels after a moderately high epidural block, but that as soon as light general anaesthesia is induced the mean arterial pressure falls to a level determined by the segmental extent of the block, and rises again immediately the patient awakes. Toxic doses of local anaesthetics absorbed into the circulation may depress the vasomotor centre.

In conclusion, it is fair to say that a variety of factors contribute to the fall in blood pressure produced by spinal and epidural block. These are all due to paralysis of the pre-ganglionic sympathetic nerves with arteriolar dilatation and compensatory vasoconstriction elsewhere, a fall in venous return due to vaso-dilatation causing a fall in cardiac output, block of the pre-ganglionic nerve fibres to the adrenal medulla, and psychological influences. To these basic physiological changes must be added the effects of the operation, the position and age of the patient, the pre-operative blood volume and the circulatory effects of hypoxia, hypercarbia, general anaesthesia and tranquillisers such as diazepam. The individual importance of each factor will vary considerably under clinical conditions. The responsibility of assessing these various factors, and their relationship to one another, rests with the anaesthetist in his management of the patient.

Respiratory Effects of Spinal and Epidural Block

Spinal block can depress respiration centrally and peripherally. As the drug diffuses upwards in the cerebrospinal fluid, the intercostal nerves become progressively blocked and the diaphragm steadily takes over respiration. If the local anaesthetic reaches the phrenic roots, respiration ceases altogether. This combination of circumstances is only likely to arise when gross errors of dosage and technique have occurred, for, as has already been outlined, the removal of the local anaesthetic by normal absorption mechanisms and adsorption on to nervous tissue is so rapid that high concentrations of it are unlikely to reach the phrenic roots (C3, 4 and 5). Moreover the large motor fibres are not readily blocked by low concentrations of local anaesthetic drugs. In a correctly managed spinal anaesthetic it is even less likely that an effective concentration of local anaesthetic could reach the fourth ventricle, though it could occur with gross overdosage and the use of excessive barbotage. Should respiratory and cardio-vascular collapse occur despite a correct technique, it is nearly always due to an inadequate circulation in the brain stem as the result of severe hypotension. With an accidental total spinal from an epidural injection, it is possible that the concentration of local anaesthetic may rise sufficiently high to depress the medullary centres directly.

Spinal and epidural blocks are characterised by quiet unobtrusive respiratory movements and yet measurements of tidal and minute volumes show minimal changes in ventilatory function (Moir, 1963). Likewise, measurements of blood gas tensions show only negligible changes from normal values (Moir and Mone, 1964; De Jong, 1965; Ward *et al.*, 1965). Quiet respiration is undertaken by the diaphragm and the 5th–9th intercostal muscles. Paralysis of the intercostal nerves during spinal or epidural block causes complete relaxation of the abdominal wall which will aid the descent of the diaphragm and the abdominal contents. Because expiration is passive, this is unaffected, although there is inability to cough effectively and increase intrapulmonary pressure (Egbert *et al.*, 1961).

Despite the fall in pulmonary arterial pressure and pulmonary blood volume during high spinal block due to the reduced venous return to the heart, there is little change in pulmonary gas exchange (De Jong, 1965) even although there is some increase in alveolar dead space. Other factors such as respiratory depressant drugs, steep head-down tilt and the use of retractors and packs may interfere adversely with pulmonary gas exchange.

Respiratory failure is the great risk of high spinal anaesthesia when this is required for thoracic and upper abdominal operations. During the critical first few minutes of spinal anaesthesia when the solution is being "fixed" the anaesthetist should be constantly on the watch for signs of it. These signs are the progressive failure of intercostal respiration, with increasing diaphragmatic activity, reduction of the voice to a whisper, dilatation of the alae nasae, the use of the unparalysed accessory muscles of respiration, and a tracheal tug. The anaesthetist must be prepared to clear the airway, intubate, ventilate the lungs with 100 per cent oxygen, and restore the blood pressure by a combination of the head-down position, the intravenous infusion of fluids, atropine and the possible use of vasopressor drugs. The restoration of blood pressure is the primary physiological consideration since most cases of apnoea during spinal block are due to hypotension rather than spread of the drug to the brain stem. Should the apnoea be due to phrenic paralysis the same treatment is needed. Speed is vital in treatment as cardiac arrest rapidly follows respiratory arrest in cases of ischaemic medullary paralysis.

The term "fixed" implies that the concentration of local anaesthetic has fallen below the minimum concentration necessary to depress the functional activity of the spinal nerve roots, phrenic roots, and the medullary centres. This dilution is produced by the normal absorptive mechanisms and the uptake of local anaesthetic by nervous tissue. Once the drug is fixed the patient can be postured to meet the needs of the particular surgical procedure and surgeon, as alterations in position no longer cause changes in the level of anaesthesia. Fixing normally takes about 5 to 6 minutes.

The mechanism of respiratory failure with epidural block is somewhat different. It used to be thought that provided the blockade solution is correctly placed in the epidural space, the highest level to which analgesia can extend is the first cervical nerve, due to the fusion of the two layers of the dura at the foramen magnum. Spread to the fourth ventricle was therefore regarded as impossible unless there was massive intrathecal injection. This view must now be modified in the light of Bromage's concept of "neuraxial" spread within the central nervous system (see p. 1146). However, in most cases the dangers of intercostal and—more important—phrenic paralysis are slight with epidural block provided the correct strength of solution is employed and excessive volumes are not injected, e.g. 1·5 per cent lignocaine gives good sensory block but leaves the motor side of respiration relatively unimpaired. The use of excessive volumes of 2 per cent lignocaine might well result in intercostal and phrenic paralysis.

Apart from the effects of spinal and epidural anaesthesia on the respiratory muscles, the effects of autonomic block on the bronchial tree are important. Bromage (1954) has pointed out that it might be expected with the sympathetic blockade present during epidural block that there would be a tendency to bronchial constriction. Daly and Schweitzer (1951) have shown that vascular hypotension is accompanied by bronchodilatation brought about through baroreceptors in the carotid sinus. The hypotension of epidural block may thus be the underlying cause of the bronchial dilatation. The reduced pulmonary blood volume due to the reduced venous filling of the heart may also contribute to this effect by increasing the space available for air in the lungs (Macintosh and Lee, 1973).

These same results might also be extended to follow a fall in blood pressure from spinal blockade.

Effects of Spinal and Epidural Blockade on the Gastro-intestinal Tract and Related Structures

Sympathetic blockade, whether produced by spinal or epidural anaesthesia, results in a contracted bowel with relaxed sphincters. There is an increase in peristalsis and also in the pressure within the lumen of the bowel (Eckenhoff and Cannard, 1960). The contracted bowel is one of the main factors responsible for the popularity with surgeons of spinal and epidural anaesthesia for abdominal operations, although it may cause some difficulty in performing end-to-end anastomosis of bowel. It must be clearly understood that the vagus is not blocked in spinal anaesthesia so that, in a conscious patient, handling of the viscera may stimulate nausea and retching. A separate vagal block is advisable during operations such as gastrectomy under spinal or epidural anaesthesia alone to prevent these complications.

The spleen enlarges two or three times in high spinal anaesthesia due to blockade of the splanchnic nerves.

Bromage (1952) has observed swelling and a change in colour of the liver under high epidural block when the blood pressure falls to about 60 mm Hg (8·0 kPa). He attributes this to local tissue hypoxia consequent upon the hypotension.

THE CEREBROSPINAL FLUID

Physical Characteristics and their Relation to Spinal Anaesthesia

Cerebrospinal fluid (CSF) is a clear, colourless liquid with a slight opalescence due to the presence of globulin, and has a pH of 7·4. The average volume in the adult is about 135 ml of which 35 ml is within the ventricles, 25 ml in the cerebral subarachnoid space and 75 ml in the spinal subarachnoid space (O'Connell, 1970).

An important factor determining the spread of drugs in the subarachnoid space is the specific gravity of the drug compared with that of the CSF. The specific gravity of CSF at body temperature referred to water at 4° C is 1·003 (Macintosh and Lee, 1973).

The Sp.G of "heavy" cinchocaine (Nupercaine) 1 in 200 in 6 per cent glucose is 1·024 at 37° C (body temperature) and that of the heavy solution prilocaine 5 per cent ("Citanest" Heavy) is 1·022. The difference in Sp.G between these figures and that of CSF is in the second decimal place, so that these solutions are certainly hyperbaric.

Cerebrospinal fluid pressure in health varies between 70–180 mm H_2O (0·7–1·8 kPa) in the lateral position to 375–550 mm H_2O (3·7–5·4 kPa) in the vertical position. While there is a positive pressure in the dural envelope, there is a negative pressure in the epidural space. The injection of solutions into the epidural space converts its negative pressure to a positive pressure, which is transmitted to the CSF. A conscious patient will often notice a sensation of dizziness during the performance of epidural block, which can be attributed to a transient rise in CSF pressure.

The normal protein content of CSF is 20 mg per cent (mg/dl) with equal albumin and globulin fractions, and glucose 45–80 mg per cent (2·5–4·4 mmol/l). After spinal block there is a rise in both the albumin and globulin content: the albumin level rises until about the 18th day, when it is nearly double the normal level.

Section Two

TECHNIQUE AND COMPLICATIONS

GENERAL CONSIDERATIONS

THE anaesthetist should always visit patients for whom spinal or epidural anaesthesia is planned, in order that he may examine the spine for any points of difficulty, and, if general anaesthesia is not also to be used, explain to the patient some important details. A few words about flexion of the spine and lying still during the procedure (particularly important for epidural anaesthesia) are of great assistance in securing the patient's co-operation at the time of injection. The psychological background to local anaesthesia cannot be over-emphasised. In units where operations are performed under local anaesthesia, preparation begins in both the out-patient department and the ward, so that by the time the patient arrives in the theatre most of his fears have been dealt with. For patients who are to remain awake during operation it may be advisable to give a heavy premedication, especially if they are likely to be unco-operative or nervous. The value of the pre-operative visit is that all these things can be assessed beforehand.

The choice of drugs for premedication before spinal and epidural anaesthesia varies widely from one anaesthetist to another. Papaveretum (10–20 mg) has been widely used, but the dosage must of course be reduced for elderly and poor-risk patients. There is nowadays a very good case to be made for a neuroleptic drug such as droperidol in combination with an analgesic. For elderly and poor-risk patients 5 mg of droperidol with 0·1 mg of fentanyl one hour before anaesthesia produces tranquillity without hypotension. Young, fit patients require doses of the order of 10 mg and 0·2 mg respectively, and these can be safely supplemented by a further intravenous injection of 5–10 mg of droperidol with 0·05–0·1 mg of fentanyl according to the patient's response to the initial dose given as premedication. Neuroleptic drugs, producing as they do analgesia for needle pricks and a loss of awareness for surroundings, produce particularly satisfactory conditions for a patient who is to have an operation under block anaesthesia. Intravenous diazepam in a dose of 10–20 mg is also a useful agent for inducing additional sedation after an opiate premedication.

So few operations in this country are performed under local anaesthesia with the patient awake, that there is a tendency for theatre teams to neglect the elementary points of care of the conscious patient. There should be complete silence in the operating theatre, essential conversations being carried on in whispers. The anaesthetist must be in attendance to answer any questions from the patient and to give encouragement. A surgeon experienced in operating under local anaesthesia—be it epidural, spinal, or intercostal—handles tissues gently and never clatters instruments or specimens.

Sterilisation

All spinal and epidural sets of equipment should be packed in such a manner that steam and air are able to penetrate the packaging material when they are autoclaved. Metal drums are often used for this purpose but the distortion and damage they can suffer after prolonged use may lead to contamination occurring after sterilisation. The common practice now in many central sterile supply departments is to use special cardboard trays and to wrap the equipment in paper packages. Care must be taken to prevent these packs becoming wet after sterilisation or organisms may penetrate to the interior.

It is important to stress the danger of inadequate washing of syringes and needles after previous use and before sterilisation, particularly if they have been in contact with any chemical solution. Needles, ampoules, syringes, files, sterile towels, swabs, swab-holding forceps and gallipots for skin-cleansing solution should be included in the packs. Each anaesthetist will have his own individual ideas on equipment, and everything which might be needed should be included in the pack. It is not uncommon for a sterile technique to break down because some vital piece of equipment is missing and has to be sterilised separately before the anaesthetic can proceed. Infection is the one completely preventable complication of spinal and epidural block, so that the anaesthetist practising these techniques should personally take pains to avoid it. Only in this way can a breakdown of sterile technique, such as occurs when an ampoule is opened with an unsterile file, or a local anaesthetic solution for the skin weal drawn up from a rubber capped bottle, be prevented. Disposable spinal and epidural packs, which have been sterilised by gamma radiation, are now available commercially and although more expensive than locally produced packs, they have proved to be very satisfactory.

The anaesthetist should scrub up as for a surgical operation, and wear cap, mask, sterile gown and gloves. The contents of the pack should be laid out on a sterile trolley by an experienced assistant using sterile forceps. The skin should be cleaned with sterile swab-holding forceps, using two lots of 2 per cent iodine in spirit; the use of a coloured antiseptic helps to avoid contamination of the fingers on unsterile skin. The site of the puncture should be surrounded by sterile towels as it is very easy, while palpating bony prominences and concentrating on the introduction of the needle, to dirty the hands against unsterile areas. These techniques are contra-indicated if there is evidence of infection of the skin of the back.

The Blood Pressure

It is sometimes said that patients under spinal anaesthesia should not be disturbed by frequent blood pressure recordings, but this kindness seems unwise. The control of the blood pressure under a high spinal or epidural block is vital, and an adequately premedicated and sedated patient does not find repeated recordings disturbing. The anaesthetist performing spinal or epidural blockade must be prepared to deal with hypotension; but there is a considerable difference of opinion as to the extent to which the blood pressure is allowed to fall before corrective measures are undertaken. The use of vasopressors to maintain blood pressure within normal limits will nullify the advantages which accrue from the dry operative field and the reduced blood loss, and may also reduce tissue perfusion to vital organs.

In a patient lying supine during spinal or epidural anaesthesia the tissues usually remain well perfused despite the low blood pressure and the coronary circulation is adequate for the reduced work level of the heart. A systolic pressure of 60 mm Hg (8·0 kPa) or less is dangerously low and immediate measures should be taken to raise it. For previously normotensive subjects a range of systolic pressure of 60–80 mm Hg (8·0–10·7 kPa) is satisfactory but it needs to be monitored carefully so as to detect at once any further drop. Hypertensive patients should be maintained at higher levels of systolic pressure. In conscious patients restlessness, due to the accompanying cerebral hypoxia, is often associated with hypotension, and may be mistaken for incomplete analgesia. Should the anaesthetist fail to recognise the true cause of the restlessness, he may be tempted to quieten the patient with a small intravenous dose of thiopentone; such treatment may easily be fatal in the circumstances. When the systolic pressure falls below 80 mm Hg (10·7 kPa) in conscious patients, a vasovagal attack may be triggered leading to profound hypotension, with accompanying bradycardia, nausea and vomiting (Scott, 1975). In anaesthetised patients the hypotension is usually well tolerated, provided the block does not reach the upper thoracic segments and so cause bradycardia (Stephen, et al., 1969).

An intravenous infusion should be set up in all patients having spinal or epidural anaesthesia and in the event of a dramatic fall of blood pressure, an infusion of Hartmann's solution or dextran can be given. It also provides access to the circulation for vasopressors should they be considered necessary. Blood loss is tolerated badly during spinal anaesthesia, as the normal physiological responses to haemorrhage are absent and the loss should be made good with blood or other fluid. It is important to maintain the blood pressure in elderly patients, who may have associated cerebrovascular and coronary atheroma, if cerebral or myocardial damage from hypotension is to be avoided (Morris and Candy, 1957).

It is important for the anaesthetist to remember that while managing the level of blood pressure during spinal or epidural block, he is also directly controlling the cerebral circulation and he must be aware of the possible morbidity which may follow from a fall in cerebral blood flow due to hypotension. Severe arterial hypotension under spinal anaesthesia is certain to be associated with dangerous decreases in cerebral blood flow (Greene, 1969), and Wyke (1960), in a review of the changes in the cerebral circulation during anaesthesia, warns of the dangers of arterial hypotension. Cerebral vasodilatation, even when maximal, will be unable to maintain an adequate blood flow to the brain when the blood pressure has dropped beyond a critical level. As a clinical rule of thumb, it is wise to assume that in the supine position levels of mean arterial blood pressure below 55 mm Hg (7·3 kPa) are associated with dangerous decreases in cerebral blood flow in normal patients, and should be avoided. In patients with arteriosclerotic changes involving cerebral vessels the blood pressure must be maintained considerably above this level in order to ensure an adequate cerebral blood flow (Shanbrom and Levy, 1957).

Should severe arterial hypotension develop during spinal or epidural blockade, the oxygen concentration of the inspired mixture should be increased and either the legs raised or the patient tilted into a head-down position. The tilt increases the venous return from the lower limbs and trunk thus raising the cardiac output and hence the arterial pressure. There is no evidence that the Trendelenburg position improves the cerebral vascular perfusion (Taylor and Weil, 1967). The supine hypotensive syndrome caused by compression of the inferior vena cava by a pregnant uterus at term, can be relieved by tilting the patient on to one side.

When hypotension is associated with bradycardia, it can be effectively treated in most cases by giving small doses of atropine (0·2 mg) intravenously until the pulse is raised to a more normal rate. After these initial measures, the most rational and effective treatment of severe hypotension is the rapid infusion of fluids intravenously, using either compound sodium lactate solution (Hartmann's) or dextran. The rapid infusion of 500–1000 ml will fill the enlarged vascular bed produced by the spinal or epidural block and so raise the blood pressure to an acceptable level.

The role of vasopressors in the management of hypotension is controversial. If despite a fall in blood pressure the patient remains pink, well perfused, has a good capillary circulation, constricted pupils and a palpable peripheral pulse such as the superficial temporal, then he is unlikely to be in immediate danger. The use of vasopressors will raise the pressure but the benefit that results is difficult to evaluate as the vasoconstriction may reduce tissue perfusion and so accentuate the tissue hypoxia and metabolic acidosis (Macintosh and Lee, 1973). Vasopressors stimulate alpha and beta adrenergic receptors to a varying degree, increasing arteriolar tone and the force of cardiac contraction respectively. The anaesthetist should restrict himself to two or three of these drugs so as to be thoroughly familiar with their pharmacological actions. Suitable drugs include ephedrine, metaraminol (Aramine) mephentermine (Mephine) all of which have both α and β actions while pure α-stimulants such as phenylephrine and methoxamine may be dangerous because they commonly cause reflex cardiac depression and tissue underperfusion. Vasopressors should only be used if the patient's condition continues to deteriorate and the blood pressure remains persistently at very low levels, despite the other measures previously described. Particular care must be taken to guard against a sudden fall in blood pressure when the position of a patient is altered especially from the lithotomy position. It is also an important part of spinal and epidural techniques that the blood pressure should be recorded in the recovery room and ward, and should be maintained at adequate levels while the block is wearing off.

Respiration

The anaesthetist must constantly be on the alert for the effects of high epidural and spinal block on the respiration. The effects of hypoxia on the respiratory and cardiac centres of the brain stem consequent upon severe falls of blood pressure have already been discussed. The use of the head-down position must again be stressed. The commonest cause of hypoxic paralysis of the brain stem is use of a foot-down tilt in the presence of arterial hypotension. This is the commonest cause of death under spinal or epidural anaesthesia and is completely preventable with correct management. The anaesthetist must think of the blood pressure and respiration together. Hypoxia from a failing respiration will aggravate hypoxic effects on the brain and heart from severe arterial hypotension. Low blocks present no problem, as the intercostal muscles and the sympathetic chain are not affected. With a high spinal block the intercostal muscles are paralysed and only the diaphragm and possibly a few of the upper intercostals remain for ventilation. The Trendelenburg position, abdominal packs and retractors, or the presence of an abdominal mass, ovarian cyst or pregnancy may add to the respiratory difficulties. Macintosh and Lee (1973) have emphasised strongly how important it is to give oxygen to these patients. One of the advantages of an epidural block is that satisfactory analgesia and complete relaxation can be obtained without impairing respiration. For example, 1·5 per cent lignocaine will give profound analgesia, excellent relaxation, and leave the respiration relatively unaffected. It must not be supposed, however, that supplementary oxygenation is never necessary during epidural anaesthesia, since some degree of motor loss may occur even with this strength of solution, though on the whole it is slight. As with spinal block, the effect of posture, abdominal packs and retractors on the respiration must also be taken into account.

Sickness

Nausea may be experienced by the patient under epidural or spinal block, and is due either to a fall in blood pressure or to traction on a hollow viscus during an abdominal operation. The nausea is vagal in origin, and is particularly likely to occur during the operation of gastrectomy, especially when the left and right gastric arteries are tied. The most satisfactory way to prevent it and those conditions with which it is associated, is for the surgeon to do a para-oesophageal vagal block with a local anaesthetic on opening the abdomen. This symptom sometimes responds to the intravenous injection of atropine 0·2–0·6 mg and the inhalation of oxygen, but if it persists it may be necessary to administer a light general anaesthetic.

Hiccup

Hiccup may occur during upper abdominal surgery under spinal or epidural anaesthesia. Like sickness it may well have its origin in the stimulation of vagal nerve endings, due to traction on the mesentery or handling the viscera, so that local infiltration of these nerves should be carried out. Occasionally deep general anaesthesia is necessary to restore tranquillity to the operative field.

Supplementary Anaesthesia

Whether the patient remains awake during the operation depends on the wishes and condition of the patient and the practice and preference of the anaesthetist and surgeon. In the United Kingdom most patients prefer to be asleep during surgery but in certain areas of the world fear of loss of consciousness adds to the attraction of spinal and epidural anaesthesia.

Intravenous thiopentone or methohexitone are very useful in small doses for maintaining light sleep during epidural or spinal anaesthesia. With a lignocaine epidural block the patient tends to become drowsy and only very small quantities of thiopentone or methohexitone are required. When a patient has been tranquillised with droperidol only the minutest quantities should be used, doses about 25 mg of thiopentone and 10 mg of methohexitone being sufficient to maintain a light sleep with an active eyelash reflex. The use of supplemental general anaesthesia during spinal or epidural blocks will ensure that the patient suffers no discomfort during the operation. Because 100 per cent success cannot be guaranteed with these techniques, general anaesthesia enables any deficiency, due to inadequate spread throughout the operative field to be readily overcome. The risk of toxic reactions to local anaesthetic agents are markedly reduced while vasovagal attacks are prevented (Scott, 1975). General anaesthesia can be induced before or after performing the block, depending on whether or not assistance is available. A technique of thiopentone, nitrous oxide and oxygen, with the patient breathing through a mask is satisfactory, but to ensure smooth anaesthesia it is usually advisable to supplement this with diazepam (10 mg) or a low concentration of halothane (0·5 per cent). For long procedures, especially when the patient is in a steep head-down position, as in an abdomino-perineal excision of the rectum, endotracheal intubation is to be commended for the added safety it provides and the ease with which respiration can be assisted manually.

Management of the Total Spinal

Accidental massive subarachnoid injection occurring during epidural block should not be regarded as a catastrophe, but as a reversible complication. Within three minutes of the injection the patient will develop severe hypotension, apnoea and dilated pupils. The basis of treatment is two-fold—efficient ventilation and oxygenation via an endotracheal tube and the maintenance of blood pressure by vasopressors and the intravenous infusion of fluid. The incidence of this distressing occurrence can be reduced to negligible proportions by careful technique, but the means of resuscitation must always be at hand when epidural blocks are being done. The following figures are quoted for the incidence of a total spinal following an epidural injection in the lumbar area:

Moore . . .	. 0 in 1,700 cases	0·00 per cent
Bonica . . .	. 1 in 2,290 cases	0·04 per cent
Selva de Assis .	. 2 in 1,000 cases	0·20 per cent
Bromage . .	. 1 in 1,000 cases	0·10 per cent

The duration of respiratory paralysis depends on the local anaesthetic used but is unlikely to be more than 1–2 hours. In most cases the operation should not be abandoned because an accidental total spinal has been given.

SPINAL ANAESTHESIA

Lumbar Puncture

Macintosh and Lee (1973) have described and illustrated in great detail the anatomical points concerned in successful lumbar puncture. The chief points to be remembered are:

1. In median puncture the needle passes through the skin, subcutaneous tissue, supraspinous ligament and interspinous ligament, between the ligamentum flava, and then through the epidural space and finally the dura, to enter the subarachnoid space. A successful lumbar puncture will be followed by a free flow of CSF, usually at the rate of 1 drop a second. Median puncture is the easiest to use, but if the needle goes off centre it will pass through the dura having pierced the ligamentum flavum, since in the lateral parts of the epidural space these and the dura lie adjacent. In elderly osteoarthritic subjects the supraspinous and interspinous ligaments may be fused and heavily calcified, making the introduction of a fine spinal needle extremely difficult. For such patients the lateral approach may be advisable.

2. In lateral puncture the needle passes through the skin, subcutaneous fat, lumbar aponeurosis and lumbar muscles, and then with correct angulation through the ligamentum flavum.

3. The interlaminar foramen is a bony ring formed between two vertebrae, the upper border bounded by the laminae and root of the spine of the vertebra above, the lower border by the laminae and root of the spine of the vertebra below and the sides by the articulation between the superior and inferior facets. The foramen is closed by the ligamentum flavum. An incorrectly angulated spinal needle may impinge on any part of this bony ring. Flexion of the spine increases the diameter of the ring, so that the advancing needle is then less likely to be arrested by the bony margin. The lumbar spines have a slight downward inclination and the needle must be advanced inclined slightly upwards.

The distance from the skin to the epidural space is reasonably constant in the average individual, and any variation is largely dependent on the thickness of the subcutaneous fat. It is usually 3·5–5 cm, thus the subarachnoid space lies at a deeper level.

In lumbar puncture the differing resistance of the ligaments can often be appreciated—the resistance increasing as the needle enters the ligamentum flavum—and a "give" occurring as the needle enters the epidural space. Sometimes an audible click can be heard as the needle passes through the dura. With the fine spinal needles at present in use, these sensations have become more difficult to appreciate. In epidural work, however, it is almost essential to use a thicker needle (18 SWG) so that the feel of the ligaments can be appreciated. Needles for both spinal and epidural block are illustrated in Figs. 8 (*a*) and (*b*).

In some cases there are good reasons for using a Sise spinal needle introducer. For instance, in midline puncture when the supraspinous and interspinous ligaments are very tough, the introducer is advanced for about 1 inch down to the ligamentum flavum and then a fine spinal needle (passed through the introducer) has only to pierce the ligamentum flavum and dura.

A Sise introducer probably offers an additional safeguard against infection, since it and the stilette pierce the epidermis so that no part of the spinal needle comes into contact with the skin. An introducer is also of value in an elderly patient whose lumbar vertebrae are fixed in extension, so that the interlaminar foramen is small, necessitating repeated attempts to get the angle just right. It eliminates the need to touch the skin and removes the temptation to touch the shaft of the needle (Macintosh and Lee, 1973). The size of the needle has an important bearing on the incidence of postspinal headache (see p. 1179). An introducer makes it possible to use a very fine spinal needle.

Types of Technique

Hyperbaric technique.—A very useful technique for anorectal operations for haemorrhoids, fissures and the like, and for a bladder-neck operation such as transurethral prostatectomy, is to inject 1 ml of a heavy solution (*vide infra*) at the L4–5 interspace, with the patient sitting up. For operations about the anus where only the 4th and 5th sacral roots require to be blocked, 0·6 ml of solution is sufficient. The patient should be kept sitting up for five minutes after the injection while the heavy solution sinks rapidly to the bottom of the dural sac,

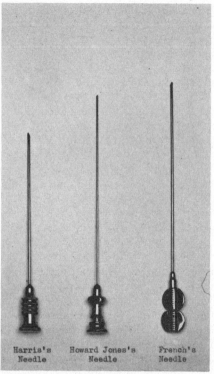

36/FIG. 8(*a*)—Spinal needles.

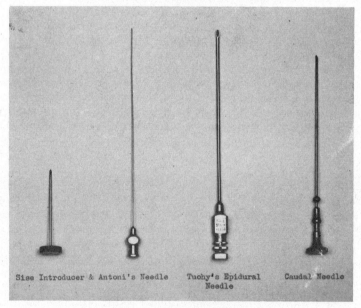

36/FIG. 8(*b*)—Epidural needles.

blocking the necessary sacral nerves. There is little or no fall in blood pressure so that a vasopressor is very seldom required.

For lower abdominal operations such as appendicectomy, prostatectomy and Caesarean section, 1·4–1·8 ml of solution is injected at the L2–3 interspace with the patient on his side and in a slight but definite head-down tilt. Immediately after the injection the patient is turned on his back. The heavy solution then spreads under the influence of gravity to the 7th or 8th thoracic segment. Mushin (1943) has pointed out that while in the average patient in the lateral position the vertebral column is more or less horizontal, in some women it may incline downwards towards the head because of the width of the pelvis relative to the shoulders, and in some men towards the coccyx because of the width of the shoulder relative to the pelvis. Thus the solution may spread in the wrong direction until the patient is rolled supine and tipped into the correct position. It is therefore best when using a heavy solution for an upper abdominal operation in a man, to tip the table until it is obvious that the vertebral column inclines towards the head. With the spine exactly horizontal the solution may not run high enough when injected at L3–4, the apex of the lumbar curve, and tends to spread down towards the coccyx when the patient is rolled on to his back.

For upper abdominal operations where analgesia to the 4th or 5th thoracic segment is required, 2 ml of solution are injected at the L2–3 interspace with the patient head-down. The spine should be in about 5 degrees of Trendelenburg position. As before, the solution spreads by gravity, and any excess of unfixed drug pools in the hollow of the thoracic curve, opposite the 4th and 5th nerve roots.

In planning the height to which analgesia is required for a particular operation it is useful to remember the following segmental levels:

Nipple line	T4–5
Xiphisternum	T7
Umbilicus	T10
Groin	L1
Perineum	S1–4

For upper abdominal operations anaesthesia must not only be sufficient to reach the xiphisternum at T7, but also to include the splanchnic nerves (greater splanchnic nerve—T4, 5, 6, 7, 8), since an incomplete block of these makes surgical handling of the omentum and mesentery uncomfortable for a conscious patient. Moreover, as already mentioned, it is advisable to combine the spinal block with para-oesophageal block of the vagus.

A point frequently not appreciated about such lower abdominal operations as abdomino-perineal resection of the rectum is that while the incision may not extend to the costal margin, nevertheless anaesthesia up to this region is needed, since the surgeon requires to push the lower abdominal contents into the upper abdomen and may want to palpate the liver.

Hyperbaric solutions.—The introduction of new drugs has contributed to the current practice of spinal analgesia.

Cinchocaine (Nupercaine, dibucaine USP) 0·5 per cent dissolved in 6 per cent glucose (sp. gravity at 37° C 1·024) is still very popular in Britain.

Amethocaine hydrochloride (Pontocaine, Pantocaine, tetracaine USP) is used either as a 1 per cent solution or in ampoules containing 20 mg of crystals to which are added 5–10 per cent dextrose to produce a hyperbaric solution. The maximal intrathecal dose is 20 mg. This local anaesthetic is widely used in the United States.

Mepivacaine (Carbocaine) has been successfully used as a 4 per cent solution in 10 per cent glucose (Siker *et al.*, 1966).

Lignocaine (Lidocaine USP) 5 per cent with glucose 7·5 per cent has a specific gravity of 1035 at 37° C.

Prilocaine (Citanest) 5 per cent with glucose 5 per cent has a specific gravity of 1022 at 37° C.

In a study of three different drugs for spinal analgesia, Fisher and Bryce-Smith (1971) reported that prilocaine was very satisfactory for this purpose and they considered it superior to lignocaine and as good as Nupercaine.

Hypobaric techniques.—Techniques using solutions of local anaesthetic drugs with a lower specific gravity than that of CSF are no longer recommended.

Continuous spinal analgesia.—Any place that continuous spinal anaesthesia may have had in anaesthetic practice has been lost. A technique with such potential morbidity from the introduction of catheters into the subarachnoid space should not be used, particularly when safer alternatives are readily available.

EPIDURAL ANAESTHESIA

There is a tendency to think of epidural anaesthesia as a recent development. This can probably be accounted for by the decline in the popularity of spinals since the late forties and a search for methods with the advantages of the spinal, but without its dangerous sequelae. In point of fact the approach to the epidural space is of some antiquity and as long ago as 1901 the French investigators Sicard and Cathelin described epidural injections through the sacral hiatus. By 1920 the technique had become popular and Zweifel was able to analyse the incidence of fatalities encountered in 4,200 caudal epidural blocks recorded in the literature. Although the interspinous approach to the epidural space had also been demonstrated at the beginning of the century, Poges (1921) was the first to describe the practical application of lumbar epidural anaesthesia. Later Dogliotti (1931–33) in Italy popularised the technique, followed by other clinical exponents, Hess (1934), Odom (1936) and Harger *et al.* (1941) in the USA, and Gutierrez (1939) in South America.

The next important development was the adaptation of Tuohy's (1945) catheter technique—developed for continuous spinal anaesthesia—to epidural anaesthesia by Curbello (1949).

Methods of Identifying the Epidural Space

The technique of the sacral approach to the epidural space will be discussed later and only the lumbar approach dealt with here. Methods can be regarded as falling into two groups, those dependent on the loss of resistance as the needle pierces the ligamentum flavum and enters the epidural space, and others relying upon a negative pressure in the epidural space.

The loss-of-resistance sign.—This is the most widely used technique and is based on the fact that there is considerable resistance to injection through the epidural needle as it is advanced through the interspinous ligament and ligamentum flavum. As the point emerges from the ligamentum flavum and enters the epidural space, the resistance disappears almost completely. The simplest way of appreciating these changes in resistance is to exert continuous pressure on the plunger of a syringe filled with fluid or air. The advantage of fluid, which should be saline rather than local anaesthetic solution, is that being incompressible, the changes in resistance are transmitted more directly to the anaesthetist's fingers than is the case with an air-filled syringe. In either case, the plunger of the syringe should move very freely within its barrel.

In order to reduce the risk of dural puncture, a Tuohy needle which has a curved rather blunt point is recommended. Although designed for the passage of a catheter in continuous epidural anaesthesia, this needle is equally suitable for single-shot techniques. Some workers prefer a conventional thin-wall 18-gauge needle which ideally should be marked so that the depth of the point can be calculated. The patient is placed in the lateral position with the spine and neck flexed to open up the interlaminar space and so make it easier to enter the epidural space. In obese patients or for thoracic epidurals, it may be easier to perform the block with the patient in the sitting position. In conscious patients a skin weal of local anaesthetic solution is raised in the selected interspace which should be upper lumbar for a high block and a lower one for a low block. The infiltration is extended into the interspinous ligament. A Sise introducer is used to pierce the skin and supraspinous ligament and so facilitate the passage of the blunter epidural needle. The Tuohy needle is inserted into the interspace in the midline in a slightly cephalad direction with its bevel directed laterally. To achieve maximum control of the needle its hub is grasped by the thumb and index finger, while the other fingers and back of the hand rest against the patient's back. A syringe filled with saline or air is attached to the hub of the needle and as the needle is slowly advanced, continuous pressure is applied to the plunger with the other hand. The interspinous ligament offers only moderate resistance to the injection through the needle: resistance increases sharply as the ligamentum flavum is reached and in a large man this may be as much as 7·0 mm thick. The needle should not be allowed to deviate to one side and enter the lumbar muscles, as a false loss of resistance will be obtained and the solution deposited outside the epidural space. The advance of the needle is stopped immediately the loss of resistance is detected. The main points in favour of this technique are its essential simplicity, and that it concentrates the attention of the anaesthetist on the feel of the ligaments the whole time, while visual and mechanical aids have a tendency to distract the anaesthetist from the essential feel of the ligaments. Its disadvantage is that it cannot be used for the lateral approach to the epidural space, as the lumbar muscles will not satisfactorily block the point of the needle.

Mechanical aids to the loss-of-resistance sign.—In general these are not to be recommended. When they work at a demonstration they are dramatic and convincing, but the sense of touch is really the key to successful epidural blockade. Macintosh's (1953) needle with the spring-loaded stilette is better than Brunner and Ilké's (1949) spring-loaded syringe. The latter is far too heavy in practice, while both it and Macintosh's stilette—as with all mechanical devices—are only reliable if kept in perfect working order. Both these devices of necessity need very large-bore needles, which, if pushed on through the dura cause a large dural hole, so that a post-lumbar puncture headache is likely. For general hospital use a simple needle and syringe is the best.

Macintosh's (1950) balloon technique must be mentioned here. A tiny balloon is attached to the epidural needle, and, when the point of the needle is lying in the interspinous ligament, inflated by injecting air through its thick self-sealing neck. Deflation occurs as soon as the epidural space is entered.

The negative-pressure sign.—A negative pressure is present in 80 per cent of epidural spaces (Dawkins and Steel, 1971) and three explanations have been put forward to account for it.

First, that it is an artefact simply created by indentation of the dura by the point of the advancing needle. Janzen (1926) from a careful investigation came to the conclusion that the negative pressure depended on the type of needle used. Blunt needles, which tended to push the dura away for some distance, before piercing it, gave a greater negative pressure than sharp needles and a needle with a side opening and closed end gave a greater negative pressure than an open-ended one. He observed that the negative pressure could be increased or decreased by advancing or withdrawing the needle.

The second explanation is that the negative pressure is created by flexion of the spine (Odom, 1936). Dawkins (1954) describing his technique of epidural injection with Odom's indicator, stated that should localisation of the space take longer than three minutes, the spine should be extended for one minute and then reflexed in order to restore the negative pressure. The third explanation of the negative pressure is that it is created by transmission of the negative intra-pleural pressure via the paravertebral spaces to the epidural space (Macintosh and Mushin, 1947). Because the epidural space is filled with fat, connective tissue and venous plexuses, the negative pressure is poorly transmitted caudal to the thoracic region. Macintosh (1950) further showed that with his balloon indicator attached to a needle in the epidural space, a cough by the patient would reinflate the balloon. Dawkins (1963) pointed out that no experimental proof of the theory has been produced. In his own experience of a series of 1,176 cases using Odom's indicator, a negative pressure was present in 72·8 per cent in the lumbar region, but only 51·8 per cent in the thoracic region.

The hanging-drop sign.—This is a very simple technique first described by Gutierrez (1933). The epidural needle is placed in the interspinous ligament, and a drop of fluid deposited on the hub; as the needle enters the epidural space the drop is sucked in.

Odom's indicator.—Odom (1936) described a similar device to that of Gutierrez, the drop of fluid being contained in a small glass capillary tube attached to the needle. As the epidural space is entered there is a movement inwards of the fluid: in some cases it disappears entirely.

Both these methods are positive in about 85 per cent of cases. In the remaining 15 per cent, provided the anaesthetist concentrates on the feel of the ligaments as well as on watching the movements of the drop of liquid, the loss of resistance on entering the epidural space can be noted and a spinal tap prevented despite no movement of the indicator. When both signs—the sense of "give" on piercing the ligamentum flavum and the sucking in of the indicator fluid—occur together, the anaesthetist can be completely certain the epidural space has been correctly identified. The negative-pressure sign has the advantage that it can be used with a lateral approach to the epidural space, since it does not depend on the continuity of ligaments to block the needle point as is the case with the loss-of-resistance sign.

Brooks (1957) devised an Odom's indicator with an air-filled bulb at the end which was modified subsequently by Dawkins (1969). The indicator is partially filled with coloured sterile water so that the capillary tube shows one or more menisci. The bulb is momentarily heated with a spirit lamp creating a slight positive pressure as the air expands. This is released when the epidural space is entered as is shown by the movement of the meniscus. Dawkins (1969) reported that this modified indicator was superior to any other device in identifying the epidural space with a dural puncture rate of 0·4 per cent.

Summary.—It matters little that there are so many methods for locating the epidural space, each with its advantages and disadvantages. That there are so many simply underlines the fact that no one method is completely satisfactory and that much depends on the anaesthetist's personal preference. Lightness of control is most important, particularly in the thoracic region where ligaments are less well defined. If special indications exist to warrant puncture in the thoracic region, the modified Brooks indicator is the most satisfactory device for identifying the epidural space (Dawkins, 1971).

The Epidural Injection

While the consequences of epidural infection are possibly less disastrous than those of subarachnoid infection, they are nevertheless serious enough to warrant a scrupulous aseptic technique.

Those for whom an epidural block is indicated will often be unsuitable for general anaesthesia, and it is therefore better for the anaesthetist to develop his technique with conscious patients. Sudden and unexpected movements during the injection are, however, not only irritating but dangerous, and though a co-operative patient can avoid these, an unco-operative one may not. For the latter a general anaesthetic is desirable if it is practicable, but it is well to remember that a patient will often respond actively to a pin prick under light anaesthesia. The Tuohy needle should be advanced through the ligaments with the opening facing laterally, but before injecting the solution it is rotated through 90° either upwards or downwards depending upon the area to be blocked.

Only when the epidural space has been identified with certainty should any injection of anaesthetic solution be made. Confirmation that the needle is in this space can be made in several ways. If the loss-of-resistance sign is being used, then at the moment when the syringe is detached, a little fluid may drip back from the hub of the needle. A few drops should be allowed to fall on the bare skin of the anaesthetist's forearm, when injected saline solution at room temperature will feel cold while cerebrospinal fluid will be warm. In some cases this drip back is considerable, and it is therefore important that the first few drops are tested, as the anaesthetic solution rapidly becomes warm after injection. Other confirmatory tests, that can be applied before injection, are aspiration (nothing should return if the needle point lies in the epidural space) and injection of a little air followed once more by aspiration. A helpful sign of a satisfactory position for the needle is the commonly noticed increase in the rate and depth of respiration during epidural injection, which can be attributed to the stimulating effect of the cold anaesthetic solution on the intercostal nerve roots. Finally, when injecting into the epidural space—having been satisfied that the dura is not punctured—the solution runs very freely with no sense of resistance. The sensation is quite characteristic and readily appreciated after a little practice with this technique. If there is the slightest doubt about the position of the needle, the epidural space should be identified again at a different level, as only in this way can an accidental total spinal be avoided.

A percentage of spinal taps is inevitable in any series of epidural blocks. It is particularly liable to occur in old people with tough ligaments where a good deal of pressure on the advancing needle is required. The "give" of the ligamentum flavum is then very sudden and difficult to arrest. Once spinal tap occurs all attempts to locate the epidural space at that level should stop and another convenient space be used. There is only a remote possibility that the solution spreading in the epidural space will pass through such a dural puncture hole against the CSF pressure. Once a dural tap occurs, however, one of the main advantages of an epidural is lost, because the patient is liable to a post-operative headache—especially with the size of hole made by an epidural needle.

It is difficult to lay down precise rules for avoiding a total spinal. Never inject when in doubt is the best rule, and doubt can only be converted to certainty by practice. A few anaesthetists regard epidural blocks as a formidable undertaking, but the technique is easily learned by anyone with the interest and patience to do so. Injection into the epidural space should be slow, 10 ml at a time, and the patient carefully observed. Any untoward signs can be detected before a massive intrathecal dose is given should the needle have pierced the dura. This is one of the advantages of doing an epidural block on a conscious patient.

Posture.—Positioning of the patient during injection varies with the operative requirements. For saddle blocks the sitting position can be used if the anaesthetist prefers, or the lateral position with the table tilted into the reverse Trendelenburg position. The spread of solution in the epidural space is not so certain as with subarachnoid injection and even in saddle epidural blocks, with the patient sitting up, a fall in blood pressure can occur. For lower abdominal cases the lateral position is used with the spine tilted slightly head down as for hyperbaric spinal solutions. For upper abdominal operations, after the injection has been completed, the patient must be turned on his back and the table tilted into about 15 degrees Trendelenburg position.

Drugs.—Lignocaine has been used extensively for epidural anaesthesia with very satisfactory results. It has a very rapid onset of action, produces complete analgesia and has a reasonable duration of action (about $1-1\frac{1}{2}$ hours). A concentration of 1·5 per cent causes effective sensory and autonomic blockade but it is unlikely to produce motor paralysis. More recently, bupivacaine (0·5 per cent) has tended to supplant lignocaine as the drug of choice in epidural anaesthesia. There are three reasons. Firstly, its duration of action is longer ($2-2\frac{1}{2}$ hours); secondly it has better affinity for the tissues so that less will be absorbed into the circulation, thus reducing the risk of a toxic reaction; thirdly, when used with a continuous technique there is much less chance of a tachyphylaxis.

For full details of the local anaesthetic drugs the reader is referred to Chapter

32. However, the anaesthetist is primarily concerned with producing a spread of anaesthesia of high quality sufficient to cover the operative area without achieving a toxic blood level or severe respiratory or circulatory complications. The following scheme is offered as a rough guide to dosage for the anaesthetist who only occasionally practises epidural anaesthesia. It must be remembered that many factors such as the amount of fat in the epidural space, the presence of osteo-arthritis, and the volume, concentration and total mass of drug injected will influence the response.

36/TABLE 2

GUIDE TO DRUG DOSAGE (LIGNOCAINE OR BUPIVACAINE) FOR EPIDURAL ANAESTHESIA

Site of Operation	Dose		Position
	1·5 per cent Lignocaine	0·5 per cent Bupivacaine	
Upper abdominal	30 ml	30 ml	15–20° Head↓
Lower abdominal	20 ml	20 ml	10° Head↓
Herniae and varicose veins	20 ml	20 ml	Horizontal
Perineal and bladder-neck operations	15 ml	15 ml	Sitting-up

N.B. All injections are made between L1–2.

In some cases, half the required dose of lignocaine is combined with half the dose of bupivacaine in an attempt to obtain the benefit of rapid onset of anaesthesia (lignocaine) with the longer duration of action of bupivacaine.

Continuous Epidural Anaesthesia

Continuous epidural anaesthesia dates from the adoption of Tuohy's (1945) catheter technique—developed for continuous spinal anaesthesia—to epidural anaesthesia by Curbello (1949). The need for a continuous technique using catheters has been reduced in recent years with the advent of the long-acting local anaesthetics, bupivacaine and etidocaine. It is only when the operation is expected to last more than two or three hours or it is proposed to continue epidural analgesia into the post-operative period that it is necessary to use a catheter technique.

Two types of needle can be used—a straight, wide-bore needle or a Huber point Tuohy needle. The latter, which has a slightly curved pointed end with the orifice laterally set, is the most suitable as the catheter can be directed either up or down the epidural space from the point of insertion of the needle. With a straight needle the catheter passes straight across the epidural space and it is difficult to get it to slide to either side of the dura without damage to the latter. The incidence of spinal taps is less with the Tuohy than with a straight needle, while the likelihood of it puncturing the dura from inadvertent movement during injection is eliminated. Continuous epidural blockade has made great strides since the introduction of polyvinyl or nylon catheters which are of uniform thickness and supplied ready sterilised by gamma radiation, and calibrated at 5, 10 and 15 cm from the tip (Lee, 1962). The technique of introducing the catheter is described in Chapter 43.

The use of the catheter technique would seem to be ideal, but unfortunately there are snags. The passage of a catheter for any distance in the epidural space containing, as it does, delicate venous plexuses and nerve roots, may result in an epidural haematoma and the possible injection of analgesic solution into open veins. Post-mortem examination of patients dying from other causes who have had a catheter passed for epidural anaesthesia, has shown some degree of venous damage (Bromage, 1954). Catheters may run for short distances in the epidural space and then double back on themselves or pass out through an intervertebral foramen. There has even been one report of a catheter tying itself in a knot in the epidural space (Nash and Openshaw, 1968). The knot was thought to be caused by the catheter forming a loop in the epidural space, then doubling back on itself and through the loop. The tendency of an epidural catheter to curl up at the site of introduction limits an important theoretical advantage of the catheter technique. It is tempting to assume that a catheter can be threaded to a predetermined level cephalad or caudad to the centre of the segments to be blocked, thus eliminating blockade of unnecessary segments and reducing dosage when the lumbar route is used. Bridenbaugh et al. (1968) have shown convincingly that it is well-nigh impossible to thread a catheter up the lumbar epidural space as it almost always curls up at the site of introduction. In their hands only about 12 per cent of catheters could be threaded up to the desired levels. By way of contrast they demonstrated that 70 per cent of catheters introduced into the subarachnoid space could be threaded to the anticipated levels. Sterility must be maintained during continuous lumbar epidural blockade and this is usually achieved by introducing a bacterial filter (e.g. a millipore) between the catheter and the syringe. Continuous epidural blockade is generally maintained by intermittent injection, but a continuous infusion can be employed.

THERAPEUTIC APPLICATION OF SPINAL AND EPIDURAL ANALGESIA

The therapeutic use of a single subarachnoid injection is now almost confined to the management of pain from inoperable carcinoma. Phenol in glycerine or Myodil is the agent most commonly employed (see Chapter 34).

Many conditions which can be treated by subarachnoid block require repeated injections over a long period. The greater safety of the epidural catheter over the subarachnoid catheter with its risk of meningitis and trauma has been responsible for the greater application of continuous epidural techniques to therapeutic problems.

Therapeutic Application of Epidural Blocks

The concentration of drugs required for sympathetic block are:

Procaine	0·5–1·00 per cent
Lignocaine	0·5–0·75 per cent
Bupivacaine	0·25 per cent

Relief of pain in child-birth.—This is discussed in Chapter 42.

Relief of post-operative pain.—By using a continuous epidural technique, complete analgesia can be given for the first 48 hours after operation. The patient is able to cough, expectorate and carry out breathing exercises unhampered by wound pain. Simpson and his colleagues (1961) published a detailed description of the technique based on their experience with sixty patients subjected to abdominal operations. They found that the injection of local anaesthetic solution through an epidural catheter inserted through a lumbar intervertebral space led to widespread block and marked hypotension. The use of a mid-thoracic intervertebral space made small volumes of solution effective and rendered hypotensive complications insignificant. Vital capacity measurements during the first twenty-four hours after the operation showed an average return to 85 per cent of the pre-operative level. Bromage (1967) reported on the use of this technique to provide early ambulation after major abdominal procedures. The patient can be walked around the recovery room within an hour of leaving the operating theatre. For success the technique must provide a narrow band of analgesia sufficient to cover the wound area, and leave the lower limbs unaffected.

A continuous epidural technique is useful for patients after thoracotomy, and for the post-operative management of patients with bronchitis and emphysema. But the technique is exacting and unsuitable for routine use except where the facilities of a post-operative recovery ward or intensive care unit are available.

Crush injury of the chest.—Continuous epidural analgesia is increasingly used in the treatment of chest injuries. The complete relief from pain that it affords reduces paradoxical respiration and allows the patient to clear the lower airways by coughing freely. As a result many patients can be spared a tracheostomy. This value of epidural analgesia is, however, limited to the "mild" case of chest injury or Group I in the classification of Lloyd *et al.* (1965). In this group there are perhaps two or three fractured ribs but the patient is unable to breathe easily or cough because of the pain. Group I patients who also have concomitant chest diseases, such as chronic bronchitis or emphysema, are particularly suitable for epidural analgesia. Patients with moderate or severe chest injuries (Groups II and III of Lloyd *et al.*) usually require tracheostomy and intermittent positive-pressure ventilation and because of the number of fractured ribs they are unsuitable for epidural analgesia. The extensive block needed would very likely be followed by marked hypotension, particularly in a patient who has suffered blood loss. Epidural analgesia is worth considering after resuscitation when the bony injury is limited to the lower part of the thoracic cage and to help wean the patient off the ventilator after a period of intermittent positive-pressure ventilation.

Intractable pain.—Dogliotti and Ciocatto (1953) reported that when a mixed nerve is repeatedly subjected to concentrated solutions of a local anaesthetic the pain fibres are selectively destroyed. Using 2 per cent lignocaine injected every 3 hours for 72–96 hours, they obtained pain relief lasting over two years in 50 per cent of patients. Other workers have been unable to repeat these results (Bonica *et al.*, 1957). Any long-term relief of pain achieved by this method is perhaps due to reorganisation of sensory input at a higher level (Melzack and

Wall, 1965). Cases of intractable root pain are better managed by intrathecal injections of neurolytic agents (see Chapter 33).

Sciatic nerve pain.—The use of epidural analgesia for the relief of sciatic pain was reported many years ago (Evans, 1936; Kelman, 1944). Cyriax (1957) advocates it as the conservative treatment of choice for those patients who have a low lumbar disc lesion causing nerve-root pressure with neurological signs in the affected leg. Coomes (1961), from a comparison of the results of treatment by epidural injection with those from rest in bed, has reinforced this view.

Peripheral vascular disease.—A single epidural injection is a convenient way of assessing the likely effects of a subsequent sympathectomy and saves the discomfort of blocking the sympathetic ganglia by several paravertebral injections. The block of sympathetic fibres produced by a sacral epidural injection of local anaesthetic may be used in the relief of vasospastic states. The prompt treatment by this technique may save a limb endangered by arterial embolism or traumatic injuries, as it will open up the collateral vessels that are in spasm. A white leg of pregnancy may also respond. Here the deep vein thrombosis is thought to produce a reflex spasm of the small veins and arterioles, resulting in hypoxia and transudation of fluid from the capillaries into the tissue, where it increases the oedema further by pressing on the lymphatics. An early sympathetic block may free the vicious circle, but it usually has to be repeated or maintained over several days for successful treatment.

Visceral pain.—The severe pain of acute pancreatitis, and the agonising pain of dissecting aneurysm of the aorta, can be successfully relieved by continuous epidural analgesia.

Eclampsia.—The value of epidural block for eclampsia is described in Chapter 43.

CAUDAL EPIDURAL ANAESTHESIA

Anatomy of the Sacrum, Sacral Canal and Hiatus

The sacrum represents the fusion of 5 sacral vertebrae. Variations of this fusion are common and have an important bearing on the failure rate of caudal epidural anaesthesia. Indeed the comparative anatomical constancy of the lumbar compared with the sacral region is a strong argument in favour of using the former approach to the epidural space whenever possible.

The sacrum is triangular in shape; the apex, below, articulates with the coccyx, while the base, above, has median and lateral portions. The median part represents the body of the 1st sacral vertebra and articulates with the corresponding surface of the body of the 5th lumbar vertebra. The lateral portions, known as the alae, represent fused costal and transverse elements.

The anterior surface is concave and ridged at the sites of fusion between the five sacral vertebrae. Lateral to the ridges are the large anterior sacral foramina through which the anterior primary rami of the first four sacral nerves pass. Local anaesthetic solutions injected into the sacral epidural space can pass freely through these foramina, and this is a factor in the unpredictable height to which caudal anaesthesia may extend.

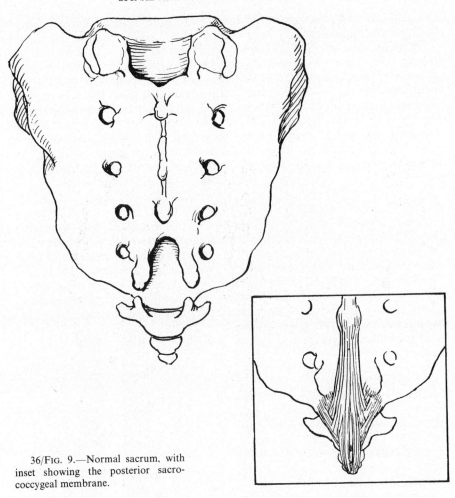

36/Fig. 9.—Normal sacrum, with inset showing the posterior sacrococcygeal membrane.

The posterior surface has greater interest for the anaesthetist (Fig. 9). It is convex, and in the midline runs a bony ridge, the median sacral crest, with three or four rudimentary spinous processes. The sacral hiatus is a deficiency of the posterior wall formed by the failure of fusion of the laminae of the 5th sacral vertebra and is triangular in shape, with its apex at the spine of the 4th sacral vertebra. The lateral margins of the space each bear a prominence—the sacral cornu—which represent the inferior articular processes of the 5th sacral vertebra. The base of the hiatus is the superior surface of the coccyx. The posterior sacrococcygeal membrane, which in elderly subjects may be ossified, is attached to the bony margin and fills in the hiatus. In some cases the apex of the hiatus is the 3rd sacral spine, due to the absence of the 3rd and 4th laminae, and occasionally the whole of the bony posterior wall is deficient. When the laminae of the 5th sacral vertebra are present, the hiatus may be very small in size—with a diameter as narrow as 2 mm—making the introduction of a caudal needle almost impossible.

There are four pairs of posterior sacral foramina corresponding with the anterior ones. The sacral canal (Fig. 10) is triangular, containing the cauda equina, the filum terminale, and the dural sac which terminates opposite the lower border of the 2nd sacral vertebra. Below this the canal contains only the lower sacral nerve roots, the coccygeal nerve and filum terminale, together with their dural coverings. Fibrous bands may be present in the sacral epidural space dividing it into loculi which prevent the spread of solutions, and these may account for occasional incomplete anaesthesia. As in the spinal epidural space, fatty tissue, varying with the obesity of the subject, and venous plexuses are also present.

Needles

A malleable steel needle (Fig. 8b) is best, as this will adapt itself to the curve of the sacrum and will not break. Such needles are likely to come apart where the hub joins the shaft, and for this reason there is placed near the hub a small round enlargement which ensures that a portion of shaft must always stick out of the skin. The length of the shaft, between point and enlargement, should be between 2 or 3 inches (5 and 7·5 cm). As with spinal epidural anaesthesia, however, the wider-bore needles give a better feel of the structures they pass through, while a short bevel at the point minimises the risk of puncturing the dura.

Technique

The block can be done with the patient either in the prone or left lateral position. For obstetric patients the latter position is the more convenient. A scrupulous aseptic technique, as described for spinal anaesthesia, must be observed.

The sacral hiatus is identified by feeling for the sacral cornu with the tip of the index finger; a skin weal of local anaesthetic solution is then raised over it using a fine needle. In obese patients it is difficult to feel, and in others it may be smaller than normal. When in difficulty Galley (1949) recommended identifying the tip of the coccyx and placing the tip of the index finger over this with the rest of the finger in the intergluteal fold. The hiatus should then coincide in position with the proximal interphalangeal joint. The caudal needle is passed through the

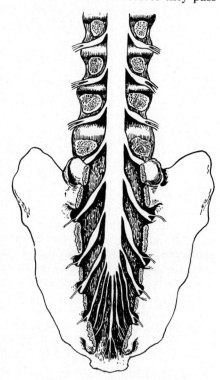

36/Fig. 10.—The sacral canal.

skin weal to pierce the sacrococcygeal membrane at right angles to the skin surface. The hub of the needle is then depressed until it is almost in the inter-gluteal fold parallel to the skin over the sacrum. The needle is then pushed cephalad into the sacral canal, taking care that the point does not ascend any higher than a line joining the posterior superior iliac spines at which level the subarachnoid space begins.

Aspiration tests for blood and CSF are made. A drop or so of blood is no contra-indication to proceeding with the injection, but if CSF is aspirated the block must be abandoned or converted to spinal anaesthesia. Free bleeding from the needle hub means that an epidural vein has been pierced and the needle should be withdrawn for 0·5 cm. A test dose is then injected—say 5–8 ml of solution—and if the patient can move his toes at the end of 5 minutes the needle can be assumed to be safely in the epidural space and the main dose is injected.

In spite of careful technique the needle may pass into sites other than the epidural space: it may miss the sacrococcygeal membrane and pass dorsal to the sacrum. If this is suspected it can be tested for by injecting a few ml of air and palpating the skin over the tip of the needle for crepitus. The main danger is if the needle slips past the base of the coccyx into the rectum, or even to pierce the fetal skull. Marked resistance to injection, with complaint of backache, suggests the needle point has run beneath the periosteal layer of the sacral canal, and this can be corrected by slightly withdrawing the needle. When the needle is correctly placed in the epidural space the solution should run freely without any sensation of resistance as with lumbar epidural injection. Any feeling of resist-ance suggests the needle is not correctly placed.

Drugs.—Lignocaine is recommended, as for lumbar epidural work, but bupivacaine is an excellent alternative when a long period of anaesthesia is required.

Dosage.—The level of anaesthesia depends on the volume of solution in-jected, the speed of injection, and the position of the patient. The average capa-city of the sacral canal is 34 ml in males and 32 ml in females.

About 20–30 ml of solution are required for blocks up to L4–5 for opera-tions on the anus, perineum or vagina. About 40 ml of solution plus a slight Trendelenburg position will give a block up to the umbilicus. Larger doses than this, which would be necessary for upper abdominal operations are not recom-mended, due to the definite risk of toxic reactions. For upper abdominal surgery the lumbar epidural route should be used.

Indications for Caudal Epidural Blockade

Surgical operations.—The main value of this route is for the production of anaesthesia of the sacral nerves for such procedures as cystoscopy, operations on and near the anus, and gynaecological operations on the vulva and vagina. In obese patients for whom a local block is likely to provide better operating conditions in these regions of the body than a general anaesthetic, the sacral approach to the epidural space may be technically difficult. For such cases it is easier and more satisfactory to perform a lumbar epidural block with the patient sitting up to allow the local anaesthetic solution to diffuse down into the sacral canal.

Obstetrical analgesia.—The motor and sensory innervation of the whole birth canal lends itself to the use of epidural analgesia for the relief of pain in labour (see Chapter 43). The whole sensory supply to the uterine body, cervix, vagina, perineum and vulva arises from the level of T11 and below, while the motor innervation of the uterine body arises from T10 and above. This arrangement enables pain relief to be provided without affecting the motor supply of the uterine body by an epidural block up to the level of T11.

The use of continuous caudal epidural analgesia has never been very popular in this country. One disadvantage is the large volume of local anaesthetic required to produce a block up to the level of T11 for relief of pain in the first stage of labour. Modern practice now veers towards using the lumbar route for continuous epidural analgesia in labour (see Chapter 42).

The Complications of Spinal and Epidural Blockade

Traumatic Results of Subarachnoid and Epidural Puncture

Backache.—This is caused by damage to the supraspinous and interspinous ligaments and the ligamentum flavum through which the spinal or epidural needle passes, and is also occasionally due to damage of an intervertebral disc. With the fine spinal needles in use today backache is very uncommon, but it is the commonest post-analgesia complication of epidural anaesthesia. Foldes and his associates (1956) have reported an incidence of 3 per cent in 422 cases, using the Tuohy needle and catheter technique. The condition is due to trauma inflicted by the wide-bore needles essential for epidural work.

It seems remarkable that damage to an intervertebral disc can occur, but it undoubtedly can and Dripps and Vandam (1951) reported gelatinous material dripping from a needle which entered the nucleus pulposus in a 14-year-old girl during lumbar puncture. Prolapse of the disc may follow damage to the annulus fibrosus (Everett, 1941). It is possible that the flexion of the spine needed during lumbar puncture increases the pressure in the discs and causes them to bulge into the spinal canal.

Damage to epidural arteries, veins and nerves.—Injury to the epidural plexus of vessels is a common cause of "bloody tap". Bleeding can be severe enough to result in the formation of an epidural haematoma, and if blood reaches the subarachnoid space signs of meningeal irritation will follow. Damage to the epidural vessels is more likely to occur with an epidural catheter technique than with a simple lumbar puncture. Anticoagulant therapy should be considered a contra-indication to epidural block owing to the risk of epidural haematoma and the possible occurrence of paraplegia. More than one hundred cases of epidural haematoma associated with epidural block have been reported (Cousins, 1972). An epidural haematoma can act as a nidus for infection if a bacteraemia occurs. Damage to the nerve roots in the epidural space during attempted lumbar puncture can occur if the needle is deviated in a lateral direction, and will be associated with pain in the appropriate distribution.

Damage to the spinal cord and nerve roots in the subarachnoid space.— Although in 94 per cent of cases the cord terminates in the region of the 1st lumbar vertebra, in some cases it may end as low as the 3rd and can be damaged by a lumbar puncture needle inserted above the L3–4 interspace. This applies particularly in infants and young children where the cord terminates relatively lower in the spinal canal than in the adult. Dripps and Vandam (1951) reported contact with sensory roots of the cauda equina in 13 per cent of cases in a series of lumbar punctures performed by them.

Headache

(a) **Leakage.**—There is considerable evidence that most post-spinal headaches are due to a low CSF pressure consequent upon seepage of CSF through the dural puncture hole. Headache can also result from aseptic meningeal irritation or it may herald the onset of infective meningitis. Typical post-spinal headache comes on within an hour or two of the anaesthesia. It is not, however, generally appreciated that its onset may be delayed for 7–10 days, and may last for weeks or even months, although these protracted headaches are difficult to explain on a simple leakage theory.

Headache from the continued leakage of cerebrospinal fluid through a hole in the dura has certain well-defined characteristics. The patient recognises that the headache is different from any other previously experienced and is made worse by sitting up and relieved by lying down or abdominal compression. Pain may spread across the whole frontal area or be localised behind the eyeballs or in the nuchal region. In the latter case it is often accompanied by a stiff neck and is difficult to distinguish from meningeal irritation. Nausea and vomiting not uncommonly accompany the headache and the patient may find difficulty in focusing his eyes on an object. Tinnitus and deafness may occur— these are explicable on the basis of a low CSF pressure resulting in a fall in intralabyrinthine pressure.

Strong supporting evidence comes from the fact that a dural puncture hole can persist for as long as 14 days after injection (Franksson and Gordh, 1946). Macintosh also reports that he has seen—at laminectomy—CSF escape through a dural puncture hole made 36 hours previously (Macintosh and Lee, 1973). With a cerebrospinal fluid pressure of about 150 mm of water and a subatmospheric pressure in the epidural space, fluid will continue to leak after lumbar puncture until the dural hole becomes sealed. Franksson and Gordh (1946) in experiments on human beings showed that a leakage of 0·17 ml/min of CSF into the epidural space is possible, which in 24 hours could amount to a loss of 240 ml. In post-spinal headaches the pressure is invariably below 50 mm of water. Anything which is likely to increase the leak through the dura may increase the incidence of headache. Thus, the high incidence of post-spinal headache in obstetric patients can be accounted for by the straining during normal labour and the early ambulation in the puerperium. Similarly, patients with a cough often develop a severe post-spinal headache. Reduction in the size of the dural hole by the use of fine spinal needles significantly reduces the incidence of spinal headache. Dripps and Vandam (1951) showed from their series that with a 16-gauge needle the incidence of headache was 24 per cent while with a 24-gauge needle it fell to 6 per cent. The latter is the smallest size needle which can in practice be used without the aid of an introducer.

If it is accepted that the underlying cause of spinal headache is low CSF pressure, the question arises what structures are responsible for the pain. Wolff (1948) and his co-workers showed that the venous sinuses, basal parts of the dura, and basal dural cerebral arteries are sensitive to pain. Painful stimuli arising from the superior surface of the tentorium cerebelli and above are transmitted via the 5th nerve and referred to the anterior half of the head. Pain from below the tentorium is transmitted by the 9th and 10th cranial nerves and upper three cervical nerves and referred to the posterior half of the head. Traction on all these structures would arise when the normal cushioning effect of CSF is lost; this is the probable reason for the severe headache that occurs after an air-encephalogram, in which a large volume of CSF is removed and replaced by air.

The high incidence—nearly double that of general surgical patients—of spinal headache in obstetric patients calls for further comment. A number of factors contribute. General surgical patients are often confined to bed for a few days after operation. Howe and Chen (1951) in a series of 400 spinals found that the incidence of headache in patients ambulant on the first post-operative day was 42·7 per cent, and in patients not allowed up until the fourth day 4·3 per cent. Analgesics required for post-operative pain of general surgical operations during the first 36–48 hours may mask a mild spinal headache. Fluid balance is carefully attended to in general surgical patients and therefore CSF pressure is not likely to be further lowered from dehydration. This factor is difficult to evaluate since patients in labour are enthusiastically given fluids to drink, but may retain large volumes of fluid in the stomach. Finally, the straining of vaginal deliveries may raise CSF pressure and increase the loss of fluid through the dural puncture hole. As a Tuohy needle is commonly used this hole is likely to be large.

Although the basic cause of low-pressure headache is seepage of CSF through the dural puncture hole, it is not surprising when so many additional factors play a part that the reputed incidence varies on average between 3 and 30 per cent. It must be remembered, too, that there is a definite incidence of headache after general anaesthesia.

(b) **Aseptic meningeal reaction.**—The second cause of post-spinal anaesthetic headache is the development of an aseptic inflammatory meningeal reaction caused by the injected solution or perhaps blood or antiseptic from the skin. The cause of the headache is thought to be due to engorgement and distension of the blood vessels.

(c) **Infective meningitis.**—The third cause of headache is that due to an infective meningitis from the introduction of organisms into the CSF. Fortunately this complication is rare and should not occur with the use of a strict aseptic technique.

These last two causes are sometimes referred to as "high-pressure headaches" but although the CSF pressure is usually raised in these conditions, it is doubtful whether the pressure itself is responsible for the symptoms.

Treatment.—The treatment of low-pressure headache begins with the prophylactic use of a fine spinal needle and the horizontal position for the first 24 hours post-operatively. Simple measures, such as the maintenance of this posture with the foot of the bed raised, the avoidance of coughing and straining and the use of mild analgesics like aspirin and paracetamol, are often sufficient for the established headache. The patient should be encouraged to drink plenty of fluids. The antidiuretic vasopressin in a dose of 20 units intramuscularly at twelve-hourly intervals has been recommended in the prevention of lumbar puncture headaches (Aziz et al., 1968). The rationale of this treatment is to retain fluid within the extracellular spaces including the cerebrospinal fluid pathways. Deoxycorticosterone acetate in a dose of 5 mg three times a day in the form of sublingual tablets has also been recommended for this condition (Wolfson *et al.*, 1970). Occasionally the headache may be so severe as to warrant more vigorous treatment, which should be directed towards decreasing the dural leak and raising the CSF pressure to compensate for the continual loss of fluid until the puncture hole in the dura heals. Intrathecal or epidural injections of saline will both produce relief of headache (Rice and Dobbs, 1950). Intrathecal injections may, however, only make a further dural leak, so that the headache is ultimately worse, while both it and the epidural injection are unfortunately only likely to be temporarily successful. For an intractable headache epidural saline with a continuous catheter technique would seem the better method.

Intravenous hypotonic solutions have been recommended with the object of increasing the production of CSF. Kreuger (1953) suggests 2·5 per cent dextrose in 0·45 per cent saline, to each 500 ml of which has been added 100 mg of nicotinic acid to dilate the vessels of the choroid plexus.

Epidural Blood Patch

Gromley (1960) reported that the epidural injection of 2–3 ml of autologous blood at the site of dural puncture formed a gelatinous tampon which sealed the dural opening and relieved, post-lumbar puncture headache. Ostheimer *et al.* (1974) in a series of 185 patients, used an average of 10 ml of autologous blood as an epidural blood patch four days after the onset of headache and reported that 98 per cent of cases were completely and permanently relieved of symptoms. There were no severe or permanent complications but transient side-effects included backache, neckache and paraesthesia in the legs. This would appear to be a safe and effective treatment for refractory post-lumbar puncture headache.

Meningitis

This is the dreaded complication of lumbar puncture, but is completely preventable if a rigid aseptic technique is used. All the equipment used for spinal or epidural anaesthesia should be autoclaved or sterilised by gamma radiation.

Paralysis of the 6th Cranial Nerve (Abducens)

This is an unusual complication of spinal anaesthesia and causes double vision from impaired action of the external rectus muscle of the eye. With the exception of the 1st (olfactory), and 10th (vagus) nerves, paralysis of every cranial nerve has been reported following spinal anaesthesia, but the 6th nerve is affected most commonly.

The recorded facts indicate that low CSF pressure is the likely cause of 6th nerve palsy (Bryce-Smith and Macintosh, 1951). In the majority of cases diplopia is preceded by severe headache and often dizziness and photophobia. The time of onset of palsy varies from anything between 3 to 21 days.

Dripps and Vandam (1951) claim to have correlated the incidence of the condition with the size of lumbar puncture needle used. In a total series of 6,147 patients they used a 16-gauge spinal needle in 637, and found an incidence of headache of 22 per cent and diplopia in 5 patients. In the remaining patients a fine needle was used and no further cases of 6th nerve palsy occurred. Low pressure is assumed to result in descent of the medulla and pons and to cause stretching of the nerve—since it is anchored between its position in the cavernous sinus and origin from the pons—as it passes over the apex of the petrous temporal bone. All patients suffering post-spinal headaches should take plenty of fluid as a prophylaxis against the development of this paresis.

The treatment of the lesion is to cover the affected eye to eliminate diplopia and prevent nausea. Spontaneous recovery can be expected in 50 per cent of cases in about a month, but muscle exercises and fusion training may help. Any surgical correction should be postponed for two years as spontaneous recovery has been known to be delayed for as long as this.

Other Permanent Neurological Sequelae to Spinal Anaesthesia

That permanent neurological damage may occur as a direct consequence of spinal anaesthesia has been shown beyond doubt, but whether this is due, as is the opinion of neurologists such as Walshe and Critchley, to the anaesthetic agent or to some error in technique is still debated.

The cauda equina syndrome.—Lesions of the cauda equina characterised by retention of urine, incontinence of faeces, loss of sensation in the perineal region and loss of sexual function are not uncommon. Most of these cases recover spontaneously but some residual lesions may persist for many years. Courville (1955) describes a case operated on in error for spinal tumour, which ultimately came to autopsy, in which the arachnoid at operation was very congested and adherent to the roots of the cauda equina. At autopsy only a mild arachnoiditis was found, but the nerve roots showed advanced degenerative changes. Courville concluded from a review of the literature and his own personal experience, that the cauda equina syndrome constitutes the most common permanent neurological sequel to spinal analgesia.

More serious neurological lesions have been reported including radiculitis, transverse myelitis, adhesive arachnoiditis, meningo-encephalitis and bulbar involvement (Kennedy et al., 1950). The light spinal (Hypobaric) technique was abandoned because it was believed to be associated with neurological complications.

It is difficult to determine the aetiology of these neurological disorders. It may be due to the action of the local anaesthetic drug on the meninges and spinal cord. Eminent neurologists, such as Walshe and Critchley strongly support this view pointing out that the only common factor to permanent neurological damage is the introduction of a spinal anaesthetic drug into the subarachnoid space. The review of Courville (1955) of the pathological changes on the meninges and spinal cord after spinal anaesthesia lends strong support to this opinion. It is possible that some cases of chronic adhesive arachnoiditis may be due to some unidentified virus infection which could occur in the absence of a drug being introduced into the subarachnoid space.

Another theory suggests that contaminants may be introduced into the subarachnoid space at the time of the spinal injection. In the now famous Roe and Wooley case (*Times*, 1953), the court accepted the view that paraplegia resulted from phenol that had reached the local anaesthetic solution through minute cracks in the ampoules during their sterilisation by immersion in a solution of this disinfectant.

Pre-existing neurological disease may be exacerbated after spinal anaesthesia (Fleiss, 1949). Although this probably is not of great significance, it is inadvisable to use this technique in a patient suffering from multiple sclerosis because of the tendency of this disease to undergo spontaneous exacerbations and remissions.

The development of hypotension and ischaemia in patients with occlusive arterial disease may lead to neurological sequelae. There is some experimental evidence for this in that dogs subjected to severe hypotension and the intravenous infusion of large volumes of non-colloid fluids deficient in electrolytes, such as 5 per cent dextrose, showed an increased incidence of neurological signs (Funquist, 1967). The anterior spinal artery syndrome (Wells, 1966), a rare neurological disorder, is a recognised complication of extradural anaesthesia (Macintosh and Lee, 1973). Paraplegia develops as a result of ischaemia of the cord but without involvement of the posterior columns so that joint, touch and vibration sense are retained. A period of hypotension will predispose to thrombosis of the anterior spinal artery, which travels a great length with few communicating branches. Adrenaline added to the local anaesthetic solution may also be a factor by causing vasoconstriction and for this reason many workers avoid intrathecal adrenaline.

Local damage to the spinal cord and nerve roots due to trauma from the lumbar puncture needle may also be a factor in these neurological disorders. Electromyographic studies enable lower motor neurone lesions due to spinal anaesthesia to be differentiated from myopathies and other pre-existing neurological disorders (Marinacci and Courville, 1958).

Comment.—The neurological sequelae of spinal anaesthesia remains a controversial subject and for this reason there has been a swing against this very effective technique in recent years. Large series of spinals without major complications, however, have been reported to show what can be achieved with meticulous technique and strict asepsis (Dripps and Vandam, 1954; Moore and Bridenbaugh, 1966). Gordh (1969) reported that 50,000 spinals had been performed in the Karolinska Hospital without any serious neurological complications.

Incidence of Complications of Epidural Anaesthesia

Dawkins (1969), in a survey of the world literature, has summarised the complications and their incidence that may follow epidural anaesthesia as follows: *Lumbar and thoracic epidural analgesia*

	Number of recorded analgesias	*Number of times complication occurred*
Dural puncture	43,152	1,090 (2·5 per cent)
Accidental spinal	48,287	102 (0·2 per cent)
Blood vessel puncture	6,578	189 (2·8 per cent)
Toxic reaction	66,366	144 (0·2 per cent)
Massive epidural	16,644	28 (0·1 per cent)
Severe hypotension	42,900	797 (1·8 per cent)
Backache	9,107	185 (2·0 per cent)
Transient paralysis	32,718	48 (0·1 per cent)
Permanent paralysis	32,718	7 (0·02 per cent)

Sacral epidural analgesia

	Number of recorded analgesias	Number of times complication occurred
Dural puncture	13,639	171 (1·2 per cent)
Accidental spinal	6,334	9 (0·1 per cent)
Blood vessel puncture	639	4 (0·6 per cent)
Failure to find sacral hiatus	2,803	87 (3·1 per cent)
Toxic reaction	3,332	6 (0·2 per cent)
Sepsis	3,767	8 (0·2 per cent)
Breakage of needle	850	12 (1·4 per cent)
Breakage of catheter	5,379	6 (0·1 per cent)
Severe hypotension	3,189	201 (6·3 per cent)
Transient paralysis	22,968	5 (0·02 per cent)
Permanent paralysis	22,968	1 (0·005 per cent)

Permanent Neurological Sequelae to Epidural Anaesthesia

Such complications following epidural anaesthesia are certainly rare. As with subarachnoid anaesthesia, large series of cases have been published without serious neurological sequelae. Cyriax (1961), who used epidural injections in over 20,000 cases, stated he has had no permanent complications. In two patients an aseptic meningitis was produced but both recovered within a week and the complications were attributed to contamination of the syringes used for injection by acriflavine that had found its way into the steriliser (see p. 1157). Paraplegia has, however, been recorded following an epidural (Davies *et al.*, 1958), the signs being those normally associated with thrombosis or spasm of the anterior spinal artery and often referred to as the anterior spinal artery syndrome. This may be associated with hypotension and with the use of adrenaline (see Chapter 34). Other factors that could account for neurological sequelae following epidural anaesthesia are inadvertent puncture of the dura and subsequent subarachnoid injection of some of the local anaesthetic solution, diffusion of local anaesthetic solution through the dura and even into the central nervous system itself, pressure on the spinal cord by a large haematoma in the epidural space and the spasm of the anterior spinal artery from the effects of adrenaline, when this vasoconstrictor is added to the local anaesthetic solution.

SPINAL AND EPIDURAL ANAESTHESIA VERSUS GENERAL ANAESTHESIA

The conflicting views on the subject of permanent paralysis have been presented and in the last analysis only the individual anaesthetist with the anaesthetic problem before him can decide whether he will use a spinal or not. If he adopts the view of neurologists such as Kennedy, Critchley and Walshe, then only very rarely will he give a spinal. If he takes the view of Macintosh that a patient has no more tendency to develop paralysis after spinal anaesthesia than he has to die after thiopentone, then he may use a spinal frequently. The notoriety given to these complications is undoubtedly one of the principal reasons for the decline in popularity of spinal anaesthesia in Great Britain. But equally important are the muscle relaxants, hypotensive and newer anaesthetic agents, and the general availability of trained anaesthetists who are able to satisfy the needs of most patients and surgeons by general methods and with few troubles. The swing away from spinal anaesthesia has, however, produced a situation in which anaesthetists undergoing their training are unable to learn the basic technique—yet there are undoubtedly individual patients who are better anaesthetised by spinal (or epidural) anaesthesia than by general methods. The operating conditions and physiological changes in the patient are almost identical in the two methods but technically epidural block is slightly more difficult. Patients with severe chest disease and marked impairment of respiratory reserve are especially suitable for these techniques. Lee (1967) considered that spinal anaesthesia was indicated in certain cases including amputation of the lower limb in old and diabetic patients, genito-urinary surgery, operations in the vicinity of the anus and in operative obstetrics. In general, local anaesthetic drugs exert their effect more quickly in the subarachnoid space than in the epidural space—and this is an advantage for long operating lists since it minimises delay between cases. Drugs such as lignocaine and prilocaine in some measure overcome this difficulty. With lignocaine, only 10 minutes is required for the development of a satisfactory epidural block.

REFERENCES

Aziz, H., Pearce, J., and Miller, E. (1968). Vasopressin in the prevention of lumbar puncture headaches. *Brit. med. J.*, **4**, 677.

Bonica, J. J., Akamatsu, T. J., Berges, P. U., Morikawa, K., and Kennedy, W. F. (1971). Circulatory effects of peridural block. II: effects of epinephrine. *Anesthesiology*, **34**, 514.

Bonica, J. J., Backup, P. H., Anderson, C. E., Hadfield, D., Crepps, W. F., and Monk, B. F. (1957). Peridural block: analysis of 3,637 cases and a review. *Anesthesiology*, **18**, 723.

Bridenbaugh, L. D., Moore, D. C., Bagdi, P., and Bridenbaugh, P. O. (1968). The position of plastic tubing in continuous-block techniques. An X-ray study of 552 patients. *Anesthesiology*, **29**, 1047.

Bromage, P. R. (1952). Effect of induced vascular hypotension on the liver: alterations in appearance and consistence. *Lancet*, **2**, 10.

Bromage, P. R. (1954). *Spinal Epidural Analgesia*. Edinburgh: E. & S. Livingstone.

Bromage, P. R. (1962). Exaggerated spread of epidural analgesia in arteriosclerotic patients. Dosage in relation to biological and chronological ageing. *Brit. med. J.*, **2**, 1634.

Bromage, P. R. (1967). Extradural analgesia for pain relief. *Brit. J. Anaesth.*, **39**, 721.

Bromage, P. R. (1969). Ageing and epidural dose requirements. *Brit. J. Anaesth.*, **41**, 1016.

Bromage, P. R. (1975). Mechanism of action of extradural analgesia. *Brit. J. Anaesth.*, **47**, 199.

Bromage, P. R., and Burfoot, M. F. (1964). Further studies in the distribution and site of action of extradural local anaesthetic drugs using 14C-labelled lidocaine in dogs. *Third World Congr. of Anaesth.*, **1**, 371.

Bromage, P. R., Joyal, A. C., and Binney, J. C. (1963). Local anaesthetic drugs: penetration from the spinal extradural space into the neuraxis. *Science*, **140**, 392.

Brooks, W. (1957). An epidural indicator. *Anaesthesia*, **12**, 227.

Brunner, C., and Ilké, A. (1949). Beitragzen peridural anästhesia. *Schweiz. med. Wschr.*, **79**, 799.

BRYCE-SMITH, R., and MACINTOSH, R. R. (1951). Sixth nerve palsy after lumbar puncture and spinal analgesia. *Brit. med. J.*, **1**, 275.

CATHELIN, F. (1901). Une nouvelle voie d'injection rachidienne. Méthode des injections épidurales par le procédé du canal sacré. Applications à l'homme. *C.R. Soc. Biol. (Paris)*, **53**, 452.

COOMES, E. N. (1961). A comparison between epidural anaesthesia and bed rest in sciatica. *Brit. med. J.*, **1**, 20.

COURVILLE, C. B. (1955). Untoward effects of spinal anaesthesia on the spinal cord and its investments. *Curr. Res. Anesth.*, **34**, 313.

COUSINS, M. J. (1972). Hematoma following epidural block. *Anesthesiology*, **37**, 263.

CURBELLO, M. M. (1949). Continuous peridural segmental anesthesia by means of a urethral catheter. *Curr. Res. Anesth.*, **28**, 12.

CYRIAX, J. H. (1957). *Textbook of Orthopaedic Medicine*, 3rd edit. London: Cassell & Co.

CYRIAX, J. H. (1961). Lumbar disc lesions. *Acta orthop. belg.*, **27**, 442.

DALY, M. DE B., and SCHWEITZER, A. (1951). Reflex broncho-motor responses to stimulation of receptors in the region of the carotid sinus and arch of the aorta in the dog and the cat. *J. Physiol. (Lond.)*, **113**, 442.

DAVIES, A., SOLOMON, B., and LEVENE, A. (1958). Paraplegia following epidural anaesthesia. *Brit. med. J.*, **2**, 654.

DAWKINS, C. J. M. (1945). Discussions on extradural block. *Proc. roy. Soc. Med.*, **38**, 302.

DAWKINS, C. J. M. (1954). The present position of spinal and extradural analgesia. *Proc. roy. Soc. Med.*, **47**, 311.

DAWKINS, C. J. M. (1963). The identification of the epidural space. A critical analysis of the various methods employed. *Anaesthesia*, **18**, 66.

DAWKINS, C. J. M. (1969). An analysis of the complications of extradural and caudal block. *Anaesthesia*, **24**, 554.

DAWKINS, C. J. M., and STEEL, G. C. (1971). Thoracic extradural (epidural) block for upper abdominal surgery. *Anaesthesia*, **26**, 41.

DEFALQUE, R. J. (1962). Compared effects of spinal and extradural anesthesia upon the blood pressure. *Anesthesiology*, **23**, 627.

DE JONG, R. H. (1965). Arterial carbon dioxide and oxygen tensions during spinal block. *J. Amer. med. Ass.*, **191**, 698.

DJINDJIAN, R. (1970). Selective spinal cord arteriography in cord compression by tumour. *Proc. roy. Soc. Med.*, **63**, 181.

DOGLIOTTI, A. M. (1931). Eine neue Methode der regionares Anästhesia: "Die peridurale segmentäre Anästhesia". *Zbl. Chir.*, **58**, 3141.

DOGLIOTTI, A. M. (1932). Un nuovo metodo di anestesia tronculare: la rachianestesia peridurale segmentaria. *Arch. ital. Chir.*, **38**, 797.

DOGLIOTTI, A. M. (1933). A new method of block anesthesia; segmental peridural spinal anesthesia. *Amer. J. Surg.*, **20**, 107.

DOGLIOTTI, A. M. (1939). *Anesthesia: narcosis, local, regional, spinal.* Chicago: S. B. Debour.

DOGLIOTTI, A. M., and CIOCATTO, E. (1953). Our method of selective antalgic block for the therapy of intractable pains. (Presented at the Annual Meeting of the Amer. Soc. of Anesthesiologists in Seattle, Washington. Oct. 7th, 1953).

DRIPPS, R. D., and VANDAM, L. D. (1951). Hazards of lumbar puncture. *J. Amer. med. Ass.*, **147**, 1118.

DRIPPS, R. D., and VANDAM, L. D. (1954). Long-term follow-up of patients who received 10,098 spinal anesthetics; failure to discover major neurological sequelae. *J. Amer. med. Ass.*, **156**, 1486.

ECKENHOFF, J. E., and CANNARD, T. H. (1960). Influence of anesthetic agents and adjuvants upon intestinal tone. *Anesthesiology*, **21**, 96.

EGBERT, L. D., TAMERSOY, K., and DEAS, T. C. (1961). Pulmonary function during spinal anesthesia: the mechanism of cough depression. *Anesthesiology*, **22**, 882.

ELWAN, R. (1923). Spinal arachnoid granulations with especial reference to the cerebro-spinal fluid. *Bull. Johns Hopk. Hosp.*, **34**, 99.

EVANS, W. (1936). Intrasacral epidural injection in the treatment of sciatica. *Lancet*, **2**, 1225.

EVERETT, A. D. (1941). Lumbar puncture injuries. *Proc. roy. Soc. Med.*, **35**, 208.

FISHER, A., and BRYCE-SMITH, R. (1971). Spinal analgesic agents. A comparison of cincho-caine, lignocaine and prilocaine. *Anaesthesia*, **26**, 324.

FLEISS, A. N. (1949). Multiple sclerosis appearing after spinal anaesthesia. *N.Y. St. J. Med.*, **49**, 1076.

FOLDES, F. F., COLAVINCENZO, J. W., and BIRCH, J. H. (1956). Epidural anesthesia: a reappraisal. *Curr. Res. Anesth.*, **35**, 33 and 89.

FRANKSSON, C., and GORDH, T. (1946). Headache after spinal anesthesia and a technique for lessening its frequency. *Acta chir. scand.*, **94**, 443.

FRUMIN, M. J., SCHWARTZ, H., BURNS, J. J., BRODIE, B. B., and PAPPER, E. M. (1953a). Sites of sensory blockade during segmental spinal and segmental peridural anesthesia in man. *Anesthesiology*, **14**, 576.

FRUMIN, M. J., SCHWARTZ, H., BURNS, J. J., BRODIE, B. B., and PAPPER, E. M. (1953b). The appearance of procaine in the spinal fluid during peridural block in man. *J. Pharmacol. exp. Ther.*, **109**, 102.

FUNQUIST, B. (1967). Influence of arterial hypotension and intravenously administered non-colloid solutions on the incidence of spinal cord lesions in experimental spinal analgesia. *Acta anaesth. scand.*, **11**, 237.

GALLEY, A. H. (1949). Continuous caudal analgesia in obstetrics. *Anaesthesia*, **4**, 154.

GORDH, T. (1969). In: *Illustrated Handbook on Local Anaesthesia*. Ed. Eriksson, E. Copen-hagen: Munksgaard.

GREENE, N. M. (1969). *Physiology of Spinal Anaesthesia*, 2nd edit. Baltimore: Williams and Wilkins.

GROMLEY, J. B. (1960). Treatment of postspinal headache. *Anesthesiology*, **21**, 565.

GUTIERREZ, A. (1933). Valor de la aspiracion liquida in el espacio peridural en la anestesia peridural. *Rev. Cirug. (B. Aires)*, **12**, 225.

GUTIERREZ, A. (1939). *Anestesia extradural*. Buenos Aires.

HARGER, J. R., CHRISTOFFERSON, E. A., and STOKES, A. J. (1941). Peridural anesthesia: a consideration of 1,000 cases. *Amer. J. Surg.*, **42**, 25.

HESS, E. (1934). Epidural anesthesia in urology. *J. Urol. (Baltimore)*, **31**, 621.

HOWARTH, F. (1949). Studies with radio-active spinal anaesthetic. *Brit. J. Pharmacol.*, **4**, 333.

HOWE, Y. L., and CHEN, C. E. (1951). Headache following spinal anesthesia. *Chin. med. J.*, **69**, 251.

JANZEN, E. (1926). Der negative Vorschlog bei lumbal Punktion. *Dtsch. Z. Nervenheilk.*, **94**, 280.

KELMAN, H. (1944). Epidural injection therapy for sciatic pain. *Amer. J. Surg.*, **64**, 183.

KENNEDY, F., EFFROM, A. S., and PERRY, G. (1950). The gross spinal paralysis caused by spinal anaesthesia. *Surg. Gynec. Obstet.*, **91**, 385.

KOSTER, H., SHAPIRO, A., and LEIKENSOHN, A. (1936). Procaine concentrations at the site of injection in subarachnoid anesthesia. *Amer. J. Surg.*, **33**, 245.

KOSTER, H., SHAPIRO, A., and LEIKENSOHN, A. (1938). Concentration of procaine in the cerebro-spinal fluid of the human being after subarachnoid injection. *Arch. Surg. (Chic.)*, **37**, 603.

KREUGER, J. E., (1953). Etiology and treatment of postspinal headaches. *Curr. Res. Anesth.*, **32**, 190.

LEE, J. A. (1962). A new catheter for continuous extradural analgesia. *Anaesthesia*, **18**, 66.

LEE, J. A. (1967). Twenty years ago. *Anaesthesia*, **22**, 342.

LLOYD, J. W., CRAMPTON SMITH, A., and O'CONNOR, B. T. (1965). Classification of chest injuries as an aid to treatment. *Brit. med. J.*, **1**, 1518.

MACINTOSH, R. R. (1950). Extradural space indicator. *Anaesthesia*, **5**, 98.

MACINTOSH, R. R. (1953). Extradural space indicator. *Brit. med. J.*, **1**, 398.

MACINTOSH, R., and LEE, J. A. (1973). *Lumbar Puncture and Spinal Analgesia*, 3rd edit. Edinburgh: Churchill Livingstone.

MACINTOSH, R. R., and MUSHIN, W. W. (1947). Observations on the epidural space. *Anaesthesia*, **2**, 100.

MARINACCI, A. A., and COURVILLE, C. G. (1958). Electromyogram in evaluation of neurological complications in spinal anesthesia. *J. Amer. med. Ass.*, **168**, 1337.

MEAGHER, R. P., MOORE, D. C., and de VRIES, J. C. (1966). Phenylephrine: the most effective potentiator of tetracaine spinal anesthesia. *Anesth. Analg. Curr. Res.*, **45**, 134.

MELZACK, R., and WALL, P. D. (1965). Pain mechanisms: a new theory. *Science*, **150**, 971.

MOIR, D. D. (1963). Ventilatory function during epidural analgesia. *Brit. J. Anaesth.*, **35**, 3.

MOIR, D. D., and MONE, J. G. (1964). Acid-base balance during epidural analgesia. *Brit. J. Anaesth.*, **36**, 480.

MOORE, D. C., and BRIDENBAUGH, L. D. (1966). Spinal (subarachnoid) block. A review of 11,574 cases. *J. Amer. med. Ass.*, **195**, 907.

MORRIS, D. D. B., and CANDY, J. (1957). Anaesthesia for prostatectomy. *Brit. J. Anaesth.*, **29**, 376.

MORROW, W. F. K. (1959). Unexplained spread of epidural anaesthesia. *Brit. J. Anaesth.*, **31**, 359.

MUSHIN, W. W. (1943). Gravity control in spinal anaesthesia. *Postgrad. med. J.*, **19**, 175.

NASH, T. G., and OPENSHAW, D. J. (1968). Unusual complication of epidural anaesthesia (C). *Brit. med. J.*, **2**, 700.

O'CONNELL, J. E. (1970). Cerebrospinal fluid mechanics. *Proc. roy. Soc. Med.*, **63**, 507.

ODOM, C. B. (1936). Epidural anesthesia. *Amer. J. Surg.*, **34**, 547.

OSTHEIMER, G. W., PALAHNIUK, R. J., and SHNIDER, S. M. (1974). Epidural blood patch for post-lumbar puncture headache. *Anesthesiology*, **41**, 307.

POGES, F. (1921). Anaesthesia metamerica. *Rev. Sanid. milit. argent.*, **11**, 351.

PUGH, L. G. C., and WYNDHAM, C. L. (1950). The circulatory effects of high spinal anaesthesia in hypertensive and control subjects. *Clin. Sci.*, **9**, 189.

RICE, G. G., and DOBBS, C. H. (1950). The use of peridural and subarachnoid injections of saline solutions in the treatment of severe post-spinal headache. *Anesthesiology*, **11**, 17.

SCOTT, D. B. (1975). Management of extradural block during surgery. *Brit. J. Anaesth.*, **47**, 271.

SHANBROM, E., and LEVY, L. (1957). The role of systemic blood pressure in cerebral circulation in carotid and basilar artery thrombosis: clinical observations and therapeutic implications of vasopressor agents. *Amer. J. Med.*, **23**, 197.

SHIMOSATO, S., and ETSTEN, B. E. (1969). The role of the venous system in cardiocirculatory dynamics during spinal and epidural anaesthesia in man. *Anesthesiology*, **30**, 619.

SICARD, A. (1901). Les injections médicamenteuses extradural par voie sacrococcygienne. *C.R. Soc. Biol. (Paris)*, **53**, 396.

SIKER, E. S., WOLFSON, B., STEWART, W. D., PAVILOCK, P., and PAPPAS, M. T. (1966). Mepivacaine for spinal anesthesia: effects of changes in concentration and baricity. *Anesth. Analg. Curr. Res.*, **45**, 191.

SIMPSON, B. R., PARKHOUSE, J., MARSHALL, R., and LAMBRECHTS, W. (1961). Extradural analgesia and the prevention of postoperative respiratory complications. *Brit. J. Anaesth.*, **33**, 628.

STANTON-HICKS, M. D. A. (1975). Cardiovascular effects of extradural anaesthesia. *Brit. J. Anaesth.*, **47**, 253.

STEPHEN, G. W., LEES, M. M., and SCOTT, D. B. (1969). Cardiovascular effects of epidural block combined with general anaesthesia. *Brit. J. Anaesth.*, **41**, 933.

TAYLOR, J., and WEIL, M. H. (1967). Cerebral circulation in the head-down position. *Surg. Gynec. Obstet.*, **124**, 1005.

Times (1953). Law Report. November 13th.

TUOHY, E. B. (1945). Continuous spinal anesthesia: a new method utilising a urethral catheter. *Surg. Clin. N. Amer.*, **25**, 834.

WARD, R. J., BONICA, J. J., FREUND, F. G., AKAMASTU, T., DANZIGER, F., and ENGLESSON, S. (1965). Epidural and subarachnoid anesthesia: cardiovascular and respiratory effects. *J. Amer. med. Ass.*, **191**, 275.

WELLS, C. E. C. (1966). Clinical aspects of spinovascular disease. *Proc. roy. Soc. Med.*, **59**, 790.

WOLFE, H. G. (1948). *Headache and Other Head Pain.* New York: Oxford Univ. Press.

WOLFSON, B., SIKER, E. S., and GRAY, G. H. (1970). Post-pneumoencephalography headache. *Anaesthesia*, **25**, 328.

WYKE, B. D. (1960). *Principles of General Neurophysiology, relating to Anaesthesia and Surgery*, pp. 98–9. London: Butterworth & Co.

ZWEIFEL, E. (1920). Die Todesfälle bei Sakrolanästhesie. *Zbl Gynäk.*, **44**, 140.

Section Four

THE METABOLIC, DIGESTIVE AND EXCRETORY SYSTEMS

Chapter 37

ANAESTHESIA AND THE GASTRO-INTESTINAL TRACT

SOME ASPECTS OF THE ANATOMY AND PHYSIOLOGY OF THE OESOPHAGUS
AND STOMACH

Valves and Sphincters

THE oesophagus which is about 25 cm long in the adult, extends from the cricopharyngeal sphincter at the level of the sixth cervical vertebra to the gastro-oesophageal junction which is called the cardia. It is surrounded by an outer layer of longitudinal muscle with an inner circular layer. Around the upper third of the oesophagus the latter muscle is striated while the lower part consists of smooth muscle. There is a sphincter at the pharyngo-oesophageal junction and another at the oesophago-gastric junction. Each sphincter extends over a length of approximately 3–4 cm and is capable of resisting a pressure of 15–20 cm water. The upper sphincter is formed by the cricopharyngeus muscle while the lower one is formed by thickening of the longitudinal and circular muscle coats of the oesophagus. There is no anatomical sphincter in man (Hightower, 1974).

The nerve supply to the oesophagus is both extrinsic and intrinsic. The former is derived from parasympathetic fibres from the vagi with sympathetic fibres from the superior and inferior cervical, and fourth and fifth thoracic, sympathetic ganglia. The intrinsic nerve supply includes the plexus of Auerbach and Meissner.

In the normal person a short segment of the lower oesophageal sphincter lies above the diaphragm, the remainder lying within the abdominal cavity. It used to be thought that the part of the sphincter below the diaphragm played an important part in preventing regurgitation as the increased intra-abdominal pressure would increase the tone in that part of the sphincter lying below the diaphragm. However, Cohen and Harris (1971) showed that displacement of the oesophago-gastric sphincter into the thoracic cavity in patients with a hiatus hernia did not necessarily result in reflux. The latter only occurred if the normal muscular tone of the sphincter was significantly reduced.

Sphincteric pressure is controlled not only by the intrinsic nerve plexus of the oesophagus but is also influenced by gastrin, gastric acidity and cigarette smoking (Dennish and Castell, 1971).

Abnormalities.—While the primary factor in preventing reflux of gastric content into the oesophagus is the pressure in the lower sphincter, the oblique angle at which the oesophagus enters the stomach may play a supportive role in those patients with a lowered sphincter pressure. Thus a number of factors may play a part in increasing the likelihood of regurgitation including a hiatus hernia, a distended stomach (Robson and Welt, 1959), the presence of an oesophageal tube, or with a physiological abnormality produced during the induction of anaesthesia. Airway obstruction and attempted inflation of the lungs by positive-pressure ventilation following paralysis (before intubation of the trachea) can precipitate reflux from the stomach or oesophagus because the distension of the oesophagus that can occur may be greater than the lower sphincteric pressure (Ruben *et al.*, 1961). Coughing and straining may also precipitate reflux, if the mechanism to prevent it be weak or abnormal (Marchand, 1957).

Dinnick (1961) has drawn the attention of the part that inspiratory obstruction during the induction of anaesthesia may play in causing regurgitation from the stomach of a patient with a previously unsuspected hiatus hernia, a condition which is common in pregnant women. It is tempting to speculate on the part that progesterone may play at the gastro-oesophageal junction during pregnancy. A high level of this hormone is present in the body during late pregnancy, and the relaxing effect that this produces on smooth muscle might conceivably affect the efficiency of the sphincter mechanism.

Posture.—Although changes in position from supine to foot-down or to head-down produce alterations in intragastric pressure, they do not in a normal, unanaesthetised person, affect the proper functioning of the gastro-oesophageal junction. The effects of the position of a patient during the induction of anaesthesia and paralysis must be considered in relation to the action of the drugs administered at the time and to the possible responses of that patient. All that can be said with any degree of objectivity is as follows: a steep foot-down tilt prevents the passive flow of fluid towards the oropharynx once paralysis is complete, but it renders tracheal aspiration probable should gastric or oesophageal contents reach the oropharynx by any other means, either before or during the onset of paralysis. A foot-down tilt lowers intragastric pressure, and enhances any adverse effects that the drugs used may have on the patient's circulation. A steep head-down tilt raises intragastric pressure and encourages the passive flow of fluid towards the oropharynx, but makes tracheal aspiration improbable in the presence of total paralysis. The supine, horizontal position combines in some measure the disadvantages of the two positions described, while the lateral position (left or right) used with a head-down tilt assists fluid to drain away from the area of the glottis.

Sickness

The syndrome of nausea, retching and vomiting is known as sickness, and each part of it can be distinguished as a separate entity (Knapp and Beecher, 1956). Nausea is the subjective sensation of the desire to vomit but without any attempt at expulsive movements. It is frequently accompanied by such objective signs as the secretion of saliva, sweating and an increase in pulse rate, and variations in the rate, depth and regularity of respiration. Retching and vomiting, both active expulsive mechanisms, are differentiated by the results of the process, the latter always producing some gastric contents, the former nothing. The mechanism consists of a series of movements designed to squeeze the relaxed stomach between the descending diaphragm and contracting abdominal muscles. The gastro-oesophageal junction and the cricopharyngeal sphincter are open and the oropharynx is enlarged, the palate raised and the larynx held forward with the glottis closed. The act of vomiting is controlled by the vomiting centre situated near the respiratory centre in the medulla.

Discussion.—A knowledge of these mechanisms is important to the anaesthetist, particularly when dealing with patients who are likely to have fluid or food in either the oesophagus or stomach when anaesthesia is essential. The cricopharyngeal sphincter is affected both by anaesthetic drugs and muscle relaxants, becoming progressively incompetent as anaesthesia deepens or muscle paresis increases. A fully relaxed sphincter aids the surgeon during oesophagoscopy. Any degree of relaxation, should the position favour it or the intrathoracic pressure be high, may allow fluid retained in the oesophagus to flow or be forced into the pharynx. Pulmonary inflation with high pressures or coughing may cause oesophageal reflux of this type under anaesthesia. The gastro-oesophageal junction is not affected by anaesthetics, muscle relaxants, local infiltration with analgesic solutions, or autonomic blocking agents (O'Mullane, 1954). The use of suxamethonium is associated with a rise in intragastric pressure in some patients (La Cour, 1969). Since there is no evidence to suggest that suxamethonium has a direct effect on the smooth muscle of the stomach, this rise in intragastric pressure is presumably secondary to a rise in intra-abdominal pressure caused by the fasciculations of skeletal muscles during depolarisation. Quite remarkable pressures can be applied directly to the stomach when it is full of air or fluid without evidence of reflux into the oesophagus in normal patients. During anaesthesia, provided the active processes of retching or vomiting are entirely suppressed and the gastro-oesophageal valve is not made incompetent, stomach contents will not enter the oesophagus in normal patients, even when postural changes, which would normally aid their movement, are taking place. Should a patient, however, be able to bring into action any part of the active mechanism of vomiting, then aspiration of stomach or oesophageal contents into the respiratory tract is always a potential danger due to the depressant effect of the anaesthetic or relaxant drugs upon laryngeal activity.

The syndrome of sickness may be initiated centrally by the effects of drugs or of hypoxia, or by stimulation of afferents throughout the body. Typically, these impulses arise from the stomach or other parts of the gastro-intestinal tract, and, during light anaesthesia, they may be started by surgical manipulation or by the anaesthetist inserting an airway or trying to introduce an irritant vapour too quickly. Afferent impulses can arise from almost any part of the body, and an important source is in the vestibular apparatus of the labyrinth.

Gastric Emptying Time

The time that the stomach takes to empty after a meal is very variable, even in a normal person. It is influenced principally by the following factors (Best and Taylor, 1955): the consistency of the gastric contents, their quantity and osmotic pressure, and the motility of the stomach itself.

The more fluid the meal, the quicker it leaves the stomach, so that a slow emptying time is usually associated with food such as meat which contains proteins and can only slowly be rendered fluid or semi-fluid. Large quantities need a long time, and if the meal follows soon after a previous one, a full duodenum may delay stomach emptying.

Hypertonic solutions are delayed in the stomach until they are rendered more nearly isotonic. A marked prolongation of emptying time has been demonstrated by Hunt and his colleagues (1951) who added sucrose in varying concentrations up to 25 per cent to a standard test meal.

The motility of the stomach is affected by numerous factors, such as disease, fear, many drugs and foods containing fats. King (1957) demonstrated the influence of some of these factors by comparing a group of fasting but healthy young adults with a series of patients (diabetic and non-diabetic), none of whom had any clinical or radiological evidence of delay in stomach emptying. A volume of 200 ml of fluid containing 50 g of glucose and a little phenol red was given to the young adults. Gastric aspiration was then performed at intervals of 15 minutes up to 2 hours. On average the meal was diluted to about twice the volume, but after two hours an average of 46 ml of fluid containing 0·3 g of glucose remained. Similar solutions, but containing no phenol red, were given to twenty patients two hours before operation and gastric aspiration performed just before anaesthesia was due to be induced. These patients were prepared in the normal manner and premedicated. In ten of them volumes ranging from 100 to 265 ml (average 146 ml) and containing 2–10·2 g of glucose were removed from the stomach, thus demonstrating the influence of such factors as anxiety and premedication upon gastric function.

An easily digested meal will have left the stomach of a normal person in from one and a half to three hours, whereas a more solid one may take as long as four hours. Water, on the other hand, will pass into the duodenum almost as quickly as it is drunk. The introduction of metoclopramide has added a new dimension to gastric emptying. This agent has been shown to increase the rate at which the stomach empties and also to increase intestinal motility (Eisner, 1971). Despite some enthusiastic reports on the use of metoclopramide (Armstrong, 1973; Fry, 1974) to reduce the period of fluid deprivation before operation, there are (as yet) *no* clear-cut indications that this practice is entirely safe—particularly when applied to the emergency situation.

It is probable that the stomach is never truly "empty", since normal secretions are continuously produced, although only in very small quantities—up to approximately 50 ml in one hour—unless stimulated by food, by the presence of a gastric tube, or by emotion. Gastric secretions contain, amongst other things, about 0·5 per cent free hydrochloric acid.

Discussion.—The interplay of fear, disease and drugs on gastric emptying must at all times be present in the mind of an anaesthetist. Normality in this respect is so variable that the potential risk of even a small quantity of gastric secretion entering the respiratory tract must always be borne in mind when a patient's normal protective reflexes are depressed or abolished.

Although the risk of pulmonary aspiration is widely appreciated to be a potential complication of anaesthesia, it is less widely known as a hazard of feeding or vomiting in severely ill patients. Yet Gardner (1958), who has investigated the problem in both the living and the dead, considers that aspiration of food or vomit is often the *coup de grâce* in an ill patient who might otherwise recover. When such a complication arises it is usually labelled an agonal phenomenon, and very often the subsequent discovery of vomit in the lungs at a postmortem is ignored. There is, in fact, no doubt that the gastric contents can reach the lungs after death, so that the trachea must be blocked at death if autopsy evidence of ante-mortem aspiration is to be considered conclusive. Gardner not only demonstrated such facts, but also studied a series of adult patients of both sexes who were either debilitated for a variety of reasons or who had undergone a recent major operation. He was able to show that about 9 to 10 per cent of the patients studied aspirated food while feeding and about 1 to 2 per cent aspirated vomit. Some of the patients died as a result of aspiration, but most did not, although a few developed a pulmonary complication. Gardner found it difficult to diagnose aspiration clinically—his investigation was carried out radiographically and with the aid of barium sulphate, which was placed in the patient's stomach or added to the food or fluid—but he thought that the aspiration of fluid was facilitated by the use of standard hospital feeding cups. These have a spout, which enables fluid to be poured into the trachea, and a hood that prevents the patient from seeing the level of the contents. An ordinary cup or glass is safer, and—for patients in the recumbent posture—the addition of a straw is helpful.

Preparation for Anaesthesia

Patients for elective operations should be prepared for anaesthesia—local or general—by pre-operative starvation for five hours. The last meal taken prior to this period should be light, preferably containing very little protein, and small in quantity. When the patient is to be anaesthetised as an out-patient, these instructions must be carefully explained, and it may be advisable to emphasise them by enlarging upon the unpleasantness, and perhaps even upon the danger, of sickness if they are not observed. Children need special care since they are unlikely to co-operate. When they are out-patients it is safest to give the parent or responsible person written instructions so that no doubt can exist, and to stress that starvation includes both food and fluid. Out-patient operations are best performed in the early morning.

Unless the patient is known to have been prepared in the manner described, it must be assumed that the stomach is not empty and all non-urgent operations must be postponed until it is. An exception may be made for relatively minor operations which can be easily performed with local analgesia. If an operation is delayed, the physical condition and mental state of the patient must be taken into account when estimating how long to wait for normal emptying to be completed.

A surprisingly large number of factors can be responsible for the presence of material in the oesophagus or stomach of a patient presented for anaesthesia. The anaesthetist must be aware of these possibilities, which are listed in Table 1 (Morton and Wylie, 1951).

The Hazards of Vomiting or Regurgitation

The active process of vomiting has already been described. Regurgitation can be considered as a passive process (Morton and Wylie, 1951), so that when the patient is horizontal or in the head-down position fluid will come out of the oesophagus and the stomach—if the gastro-oesophageal junction has been rendered incompetent by the presence of a tube—as a gravitational effect. Vomiting or regurgitation are dangerous when the patient is unconscious or the protective glottic reflexes are depressed. Edwards and his colleagues (1956), in an investigation of anaesthetic deaths, record 110 deaths as due to this hazard.

These represent about 18·6 per cent of a total of 589 patients in whom anaesthesia was thought to be responsible for death.

Mechanism of Death

This may be due to respiratory obstruction caused by an overwhelming quantity of vomit. In an ill patient, unless pre-induction oxygenation has been carried out, sudden vomiting—even though no material enters the respiratory tract—may cause a sufficient duration of anoxia to kill the patient. Commonly, quantities of fluid vomit are aspirated into the trachea and major bronchi. Relatively small quantities of vomit may induce laryngeal spasm in lightly anaesthetised patients, and this may cause sufficient hypoxia to harm the patient. This situation is often accentuated on the one hand by attempted removal of the

37/Table 1

Conditions in which the Stomach may not be Empty

Material in the oesophagus	Oesophageal obstruction or pouch. Pyothorax with oesophageal fistula.
Material introduced into the stomach from above	Food and drink given, i.e. lack of pre-operative "preparation". Fluids given for medical reasons, e.g. to diabetics, or stomach washouts not completely removed. Swallowed blood. Bleeding from nose, mouth or pharynx, due to accident or operation.
Material introduced into the stomach from below	Intestinal obstruction. Ileus.
Material from the stomach itself	Normal or hypersecretion. Bleeding from ulcer, neoplasm, or site of operation.
Prolonged emptying time of the stomach	A. Pyloric obstruction (including congenital pyloric obstruction). B. Dilatation of the stomach. C. Reflex I. Emotional states. Pain. Parturition. Shock. Accidents—e.g. cuts, fractures, burns. II. Peritoneal irritation, e.g. perforated ulcer, twisted ovarian tumour. D. Abdominal distension, e.g. large tumours, pregnancy at term. Gross ascites. E. Severe illness. Toxaemia. Near-moribund patients. F. Drugs. Morphia, papaveretum, pethidine, scopolamine, atropine. Most anaesthetic agents.

Several causes are often present together, e.g. a patient brought to the theatre for resuture of a "burst abdomen" may be in poor general condition and may have taken food or fluids just before the incident. There will be shock, emotional disturbance, and peritoneal irritation, and morphine may have been given.

vomit with sucker, laryngoscope or perhaps bronchoscope, and on the other, by the addition of intravenous anaesthesia or a muscle relaxant in an endeavour to enable this treatment to be carried out more easily. Death may be delayed and follow the late results of aspiration into the lungs. Bronchopneumonia, collapse of lung tissue and abscess formation are well-known; the condition of acute exudative pulmonary oedema described by Mendelson (1946) may also occur (see Chapter 43).

Vomiting or regurgitation may occur during the induction of anaesthesia, while the operation is in progress, or during the immediate recovery period while the patient emerges from anaesthesia.

Preparation for Emergency Operations

It is possible to differentiate surgical emergencies into those which are true and will brook no delay in their treatment, or at the very most a short period for essential preparation, and those which are relative in their acuteness and can safely be delayed while the essential points of normal preparation are carried out. The final decision upon the time for operation can only be taken by the surgeon, but part of the responsibility for adequate preparation must fall upon the anaesthetist. The importance of this division of emergency cases lies in the increased safety that goes with adequate preparation before anaesthesia and operation—and furthermore in the greater comfort for the patient. In the true emergency, when there is any doubt about the oesophagus or stomach being empty, steps must be taken to drain them.

In most patients—92 out of the 110 patients investigated by Edwards and his colleagues (1956)—the material is likely to be liquid, so that a small-bore stomach tube is helpful. A 6-gauge (4 mm) tube or a Ryle's tube (4 mm) which has not become flabby from repeated boiling, will cause little discomfort to the patient and enable a lot of information to be gleaned about the stomach contents. Moreover, the surgeon may well require such a tube for the post-operative period. A double lumen tube (the Salem Sump, Fig. 1) is largely replacing the old single lumen tube in popularity. It is plastic and disposable and allows fluid to be instilled down the narrow bore whilst suction drainage can be applied to the larger lumen. Ideally these tubes are passed through the nose whilst the patient is still conscious and can aid the process with their swallowing reflex. However, these tubes can be passed satisfactorily in the anaesthetised patient particularly if the plastic tube is stiffened by keeping in a refrigerator prior to use.

Patients with early acute appendicitis and women in labour are often treated as exceptions to the general rule for gastric lavage—the former because nausea, vomiting and then a period of anorexia are typical of the disease, so that the patient is usually presented for anaesthesia with an empty stomach. If the inflammation has progressed to peritonitis, however, there may be some ileus, when full precautions must be taken. Obstetrical patients are considered in greater detail in Chapter 43.

Even after apparently successful preparation, an anaesthetic technique must be chosen so as to lessen any risk of aspiration into the respiratory tract should any material remain in the oesophagus or stomach.

Whenever it is proposed to induce anaesthesia with the risk of vomiting or regurgitation present, the essential apparatus must be checked beforehand. This

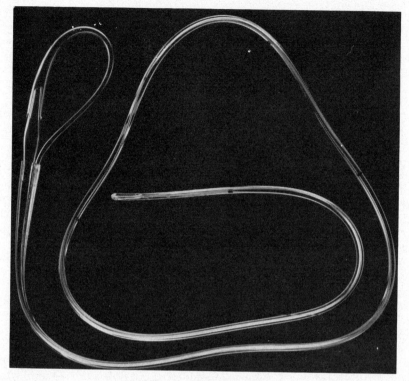

37/Fig. 1.—Salem sump tube.

must include an efficient suction apparatus. The patient should be induced on the operating table or a trolley which can be rapidly tilted head-down.

General Anaesthesia

Safety during general anaesthesia for these cases can only be assured by a cuffed endotracheal tube. The most critical period is that between the loss of the patient's protective pharyngeal reflexes and the inflation of the cuff of the endotracheal tube in the trachea. It is this interval that must be kept to an absolute minimum. Pre-oxygenation with 100 per cent oxygen with a well-fitting face mask for 3 minutes is mandatory and an open vein must be available. In a patient with a stable cardiovascular system induction may be carried out with an intravenous agent followed by suxamethonium. Cricoid pressure should be applied immediately prior to induction of anaesthesia by a competent assistant who has been told exactly what is required. All too often pressure is applied too late and released before the endotracheal cuff has been inflated.

In the very sick even a small dose of an intravenous inducing agent may be considered unsafe and an inhalational technique may be advisable. The use of cyclopropane and oxygen can be invaluable under these circumstances. In some centres this situation is considered a suitable justification for an awake intubation, whilst in others, ketamine has been recommended for the induction of anaesthesia. Once anaesthesia has been achieved suxamethonium may be given intravenously and intubation carried out. In all cases the dose of suxamethonium that is given must always be adequate to produce complete paralysis, because attempts to intubate a partially paralysed patient will greatly increase not only the risk of regurgitation but also of active vomiting. If cricoid pressure is being carried out, the latter may result in oesophageal rupture (Sellick, 1961).

The position of the patient at the time of induction will depend on the technique that has been chosen. Cricoid pressure which compresses the oesophagus between the back of the cricoid cartilage and the anterior surface of the body of the sixth cervical vertebra is best applied with the patient supine and horizontal. If competent assistance is not available, induction and intubation are best carried out with the patient head down in the left lateral position. Induction may be achieved with either of the two methods already described. The advantages of this position are firstly, should any regurgitation occur tracheal soiling will not result. It is well known that position *per se* does not affect the intersphincteric pressure of the cardio-oesophageal junction. Secondly, the tongue will fall to the side of the mouth allowing easy insertion of the laryngoscope blade with a clear view of the cords. Thirdly, in the pregnant patient compression of the inferior vena cava is prevented.

Discussion

The most important aspect of the management of a patient with a potentially full stomach is the awareness of the dangers. These include the realisation that despite the passage of a tube into the stomach, irrespective of the bore, both liquid and solid material may still be present within the stomach, and that the presence of a tube in the oesophagus at the time of induction is more likely to result in regurgitation from incompetence of the lower oesophageal junction and failure of cricoid pressure to be fully effective.

The consequences of inhalation of gastric contents are essentially those of chemical pneumonitis and pneumonia. In the former it is the pH of the gastric contents that is of critical importance for if this value is above 2·5, a severe reaction within the lungs is unlikely (Bannister and Sattilaro, 1962). In consequence oral antacids are often given prior to induction, to lower the gastric acidity particularly in the obstetric patient (Taylor and Pryse-Davies, 1966; Peskett, 1973). Their use will be discussed more fully in Chapter 43.

Treatment of Vomiting or Regurgitation Occurring during Anaesthesia

If stomach or oesophageal contents enter the pharynx when the trachea is unprotected, urgent treatment is necessary. The patient must be quickly tilted into the head-down position, if not already in it, the obstructing material aspirated to clear the airway, and oxygen given. Priority for oxygen or suction will depend upon the particular state of affairs—obviously it will be a waste of time giving oxygen if the airway is completely blocked. Nevertheless, when the patient is breathing, and there is some sort of airway, it may be wiser to oxygenate first, with intermittent or continuous suction beneath the mask when possible, rather than risk death from anoxia. An oral airway will be a help if the jaw is relaxed. Attempts to intubate the patient before oxygenation, can be helpful only when the obstruction cannot be relieved by other methods or when the trouble arises in a paralysed patient. Attempted intubation in the presence of laryngeal spasm aggravates the situation; deliberate paralysis at this stage runs the risk of death before intubation and oxygenation can be completed, but may be the only step left.

Tracheal toilet down a bronchoscope may be necessary but should only be considered after the emergency treatment has been carried out, and the patient restored to a state in which the procedure can be justified. As an immediate measure it is very dangerous; an endotracheal tube is quite adequate for suction. As soon as the patient improves, bronchoscopy should be considered if it seems likely that material has been aspirated. Obvious food or fluid should be removed by suction and, if the fluid portion is considerable, 20 to 30 ml of a weak solution of bicarbonate or saline should be squirted into the bronchi and, if possible, sucked back again, repeating the procedure two or three times in an endeavour to neutralise or dilute any hydrochloric acid that may remain. (Further treatment is discussed in Chapter 43.) Critics of this technique will point out that additional fluid may wash inhaled substances further down the bronchial tree and also increase the risk of infection.

When possible the proposed operation should be postponed if the patient has suffered a long period of hypoxia or has aspirated material into the lungs.

Local Anaesthesia

Many emergency operations can be performed under local anaesthesia, and those on the extremities often lend themselves well to nerve block procedures. Operations upon, or within, the abdomen can be performed under more extensive blocks, such as epidural anaesthesia, and the risk of the dangers associated with a full stomach can usually be circumvented, but other dangers and considerations must be assessed. Other factors besides the risk of aspiration alone— a bad chest, for example—may suggest a local technique, but provided precautions are taken general anaesthesia matches up to local anaesthesia in safety and is most often preferred by the patient and the surgeon.

Intubation of the trachea with a cuffed endotracheal tube may be undertaken with local anaesthesia and, once effected, general anaesthesia can be induced with safety. But this, like other local anaesthetic techniques in the presence of a full stomach, does not guarantee that vomiting or regurgitation will not occur, so that the risk of tracheal aspiration persists until intubation is accomplished.

Post-operative Care

The risk of aspiration returns at the termination of the operation when the endotracheal tube is removed. For this reason the tube must be left in place until the patient has been turned on the side and placed head down. This position should be maintained until the patient is fully conscious and the pharyngeal reflexes are active. All patients must be carefully observed during the period of recovery preferably in an area specifically designated for this purpose with highly trained staff who will recognise any deleterious change in the patients condition.

Some Anaesthetic Considerations for Intraperitoneal Operations

It is not proposed to consider every operative procedure that can be performed on the gastro-intestinal tract or abdominal viscera, nor the differing types of general or local anaesthesia that have been employed for them from time to time.

Muscle Relaxation

In no other part of the body is muscle relaxation more important for the surgeon. Inadequate relaxation not only hampers the surgeon's work but, in the long run, harms the patient. An important fundamental principle of anaesthesia is the provision of adequate reflex suppression in advance of surgical stimulation. Depression of sensory or motor reflexes before their threshold is lowered, besides enabling suitable conditions to be maintained with smaller quantities of drugs than would otherwise be the case, tends to prevent the end-results of those repetitive and harmful surgical manipulations, such as forceful pulling and retracting, which are made necessary by poor operating conditions.

The muscle relaxants have a special part to play in this area of the body. When the simple spinal reflex is broken completely by motor paralysis, severe depression and chemical disturbance from potent anaesthetic drugs in order to facilitate surgical access becomes unnecessary. This is particularly important for major and prolonged operations, and the control of respiration that of necessity follows, leads to a quiet and helpful operation site. Inflammable agents can be avoided and the surgeon enabled to use the diathermy with safety. Although similar principles apply for restricted or short procedures, such as appendicectomy, less importance need be attached to the value of the muscle relaxants.

The Operative Incision

Some incisions are more helpful to the anaesthetist than others. Generally, the surgical incision chosen is that which offers the most convenient approach to the site of the disease, but in doubtful cases a less direct approach may be necessary. Paramedian and midline incisions sometimes result in quite extensive retraction to enable the surgeon to reach laterally placed organs, and this despite complete relaxation. Oblique incisions, such as that of Kocher for operations on the biliary system, avoid this. They are more comfortable for the patient in the post-operative period than longitudinal incisions, but because the muscles are cut across they are liable to be followed by a higher incidence of incisional hernia. The difficulties of access that may be associated with a small incision must not be confused with inadequate anaesthetic conditions.

Shock

A number of procedures—most of which cannot be avoided even when well-accepted standards of anaesthesia are practised—may lead to some degree of peripheral circulatory depression, irrespective of obvious haemorrhage. Manipulating and freeing from the posterior abdominal wall a large carcinoma of the caecum or an extensive length of bowel affected with ulcerative colitis, common bile duct surgery, and operations in the region of the coeliac plexus, are typical examples. Although some patients sweat a little or show variations in pulse rate, blood pressure and capillary refill time, the majority usually have little discernible reaction to an operation, yet, *in all*, fundamental, but normally reversible, changes occur. Many of these changes can be objectively recorded. Alterations in peripheral blood flow, in the distribution and elimination of electrolytes and the output of endocrine glands have all been measured at one time or another. The results are of little immediate value to the clinical anaesthetist who must strive from more simple and constantly observable data to maintain or improve the state of his patient.

All potent anaesthetic agents tend to increase circulatory depression *pari passu* with the depth of anaesthesia obtained. Light anaesthesia ensures that the normal compensatory mechanisms remain essentially intact, yet it must be adequate to suppress noxious stimuli, or an attempt made to prevent these by using special techniques such as local blocks, or drugs with more or less specific properties.

Anaesthesia

The choice of technique will depend on the state of the patient, the length and type of the operation and the surgical requirements. In general, elective surgery for abdominal procedures may be carried out with induction using thiopentone, intubation with either suxamethonium or a non-depolarising muscle relaxant followed by maintenance with nitrous oxide-oxygen analgesic sequence and intermittent positive-pressure ventilation. The choice of muscle relaxant for intubation will depend on the problems that are anticipated with the passage of the endotracheal tube. The aphorism that a patient should never be paralysed unless he can be ventilated must not be forgotten (Greene, 1976). However, the introduction of pancuronium which has a comparatively rapid onset of action has resulted in its frequent use for intubation when required for elective surgery of long duration. It obviates not only the misery of post-operative muscle pains associated with suxamethonium but may also be of use in conditions associated with abnormal serum potassium levels. However, in emergency situations (where there is a vital necessity to insert a cuffed endotracheal tube rapidly) suxamethonium still remains the agent of choice. Factors such as those discussed in the previous section, which suggest a deterioration in the patient's condition, demand special attention but there is no unanimity as to their treatment, other than to ensure that replacement of blood loss is adequate. In this respect, all estimates must allow for internal loss from the circulation—transfusion still remains the best method of combating incipient circulatory failure (see Chapter 18). With regard to cholecystectomy, two points are worth bearing in mind. Firstly, the assistant retracting the liver may, as he becomes more tired, allow the retractor to rest on and thus obstruct the inferior vena cava with a consequent sharp fall in cardiac output and systemic pressure, and secondly traction on the vagal fibres in the hepatic region may cause a marked bradycardia. This will respond to atropine. The choice and necessity for supplementation of the nitrous oxide-oxygen anaesthetic will depend on the premedication and response of the patient. Incremental doses of narcotic agents, for example pethidine, are frequently used. Fluid replacement should be given as required.

Intestinal obstruction.—An ageing population with a high incidence of chronic pulmonary and circulatory disease, and the associated disorders of fluid and electrolyte balances that result from the obstruction, account for some of the problems of anaesthesia. Vomiting, regurgitation and distended bowels present practical difficulties. It is probably no coincidence that this type of patient has been largely associated with prolonged periods of apnoea following the use of non-depolarising relaxants, intermittent positive-pressure respiration and antidotes. The use of suxamethonium (Morton, 1957), rather than a non-depolarising agent, enables complete relaxation of the abdominal musculature to be produced without the special risk of prolonged apnoea, or side-effects upon the circulation. However, if the procedure is a particularly lengthy one the problems of a Phase II block in association with large doses of suxamethonium must always be remembered. Seriously ill patients often require only very small doses of a non-depolarising relaxant to produce excellent abdominal-muscle relaxation. The correct dose for each situation can only be ascertained by careful titration using a peripheral nerve stimulator before the commencement of surgery. Provided an overdose is not administered and other factors such as anuria, metabolic acidosis, etc. are not present, then the neuromuscular block is readily reversible.

Obesity

The problems associated with the anaesthetic management of the overweight patient essentially involve all physiological systems. During the past years surgical treatment has been added to the list of methods of attempting to correct obesity, and thus the anaesthetist has been faced with the many difficulties associated with its management.

Obese patients are more prone to a number of diseases including gall-stones, hiatus hernia, osteoarthritis, varicose veins, fractures, prolapse, diabetes with associated arterial disease and renal calculi (Bliss, 1973). They also have a mortality rate some 2–3 times that of a normal patient even for comparatively minor surgery, for example appendicitis.

The surgical procedures that may be undertaken include apronectomy and intestinal bypass. The latter may involve a number of different techniques, the most common of which is currently the production of a blind loop of small intestine which results when the proximal 14 inches of jejunum are anastomosed to the last 4 inches of the terminal ilium. This is the 14/4 operation described by Payne and DeWind (1969).

In considering the anaesthetic management of the obese surgical patient, the respiratory and circulatory systems are of particular importance. Many of the patients cannot lie down because of the decreased inspiratory capacity that ensues. It is known that the functional residual capacity is decreased and the closing volume increased in the obese (Fisher et al., 1975) and with the addition of anaesthesia in the supine position, the alveolar arterial oxygen tension gradient will be increased even further. While pre-operative physiotherapy and breathing exercises are of benefit, the great danger is of hypostatic pneumonia post-operatively. The lung compliance is decreased by the cuirass of fat surrounding the chest. The Pickwickian syndrome associated with hypoventilation and a raised carbon dioxide tension is less common than originally believed (Farebrother and McHardy, 1974).

Obesity is associated with an increase in cardiac output, hypertension and cardiomegaly with a strong correlation with sudden death (Kannel et al., 1967).

The explanation of this increase in cardiac output (essentially stroke volume as the heart rate remains constant) is probably not due so much to the cuirass effect of the fat on the chest wall but to the overall increased body mass of fat. In fact, it has been estimated that 13·5 kg of fat contain five miles of blood vessels (Smart, 1956).

The anaesthetic management of the obese patient requiring surgery will necessitate a full clinical, biochemical and radiological assessment. Blood gas analysis and pre-operative lung function studies are particularly important. Evidence of existing cardiac disease must be sought.

Induction may be hindered by the absence of suitable veins although a small indwelling needle can usually be inserted on the ventral aspect of the wrist. Pre-oxygenation should be carried out prior to induction because inflation of the lungs may be difficult and a coincidental hiatus hernia is common. Thiopentone followed by intubation using suxamethonium may be used. As intubation is often technically difficult, a laryngoscope with a long blade and a stilette for introduction of the tube should always be available.

Maintenance of anaesthesia essentially requires a technique that will allow rapid return of consciousness at the end of the operation while permitting full relaxation of the abdominal muscles during the procedure. Pancuronium with small incremental doses of narcotic analgesic (e.g. pethidine) has been found to be satisfactory. The inspired oxygen concentration should not be less than 30 per cent.

Post-operatively the important considerations include oxygen therapy with blood gas determinations to ensure adequate ventilation. The patient should be sat up as soon as possible and chest physiotherapy commenced. Wound infections are more common and the incidence of deep venous thrombosis is twice that found in the normal patient. Post-operative pain must be adequately treated. Vaughan and Wise (1975) have shown that the post-operative arterial oxygen tension is lower in those patients in whom surgery is carried out through a vertical incision rather than a transverse one; the former resulting in prolonged shallow respiration as a consequence of pain with resultant patchy pulmonary atelectasis.

Post-operative Sickness

Post-operative sickness is generally no more than a temporary, but unpleasant, malady for the patient. Occasionally in severe cases it can be incapacitating, leading to serious disturbance of fluid and electrolyte balance, and to a considerable strain on some operation wounds.

Incidence

This is so dependent upon the differing circumstances of individual series that quoted figures must be considered in relation to the type of premedication, anaesthesia, and operation, as well as to many other factors, if they are to have any practical meaning. Thus Knapp and Beecher (1956), using a standard anaesthetic sequence of nitrous oxide, oxygen and ether for many different operations, had an incidence of sickness of all kinds as high as 82 per cent, whereas Dent and his associates (1955) showed an incidence of only 27·2 per cent with a series of 2,000 patients undergoing all types of surgery with many anaesthetic sequences, and, in a comparable investigation, Burtles and Peckett (1957) had a total incidence of 32 per cent.

The last two series, being based on unselected material and methods, may be usefully compared with an overall incidence of 40·6 per cent quoted by Waters in 1936, and give a fair indication of the general decline of the complication.

The severity of post-operative sickness has also decreased, and in the series of Burtles and Peckett, severe vomiting—defined as vomiting on more than four occasions—occurred in only 2·8 per cent of cases.

Aetiology

A multitude of factors may play a part in the production of post-operative sickness, but the anaesthetic agents themselves are of greatest importance. Thus the effects of ether and chloroform are well known, and no inhalational agent—not even nitrous oxide—can be exonerated. Gold (1969) showed that in a series of some 1,200 gynaecological patients those induced with thiopentone and maintained with halothane or cyclopropane had a significantly lower incidence of post-operative vomiting than those induced and maintained with cyclopropane or halothane. Some patients are very easily upset, and a history of vomiting after a previous anaesthetic should always be an indication for special care and perhaps the use of precautionary measures of treatment. Females are notoriously more susceptible to this complication than males. Sensitivity to the emetic effects of opiates and related analogues is a very real problem for some patients, while others are undoubtedly psychologically attuned to the attitude that all anaesthetics make them sick. The technique of anaesthesia is also of some importance, since hypoxia and carbon dioxide retention predispose to sickness, as does inflation of the stomach with air!

The site and type of operation have always been considered to play some part in the aetiology of post-operative sickness, but Knapp and Beecher (1956) found no evidence that intraperitoneal operations are more likely to produce this complication than non-abdominal cases. There is, however, no doubt that operations on or in the region of the semi-circular canals can produce sickness, particularly following movement, for a period of days afterwards.

Sickness is sometimes induced by the early or too liberal use of sweetened fluid in the immediate post-operative period.

Treatment

Carefully selected and administered anaesthesia, including both pre- and post-operative medication, will limit both the incidence and severity of sickness. Specific anti-emetics can be used routinely to prevent sickness or more selectively to treat the severer cases, but since none of the powerful anti-emetics is without side-effects, their routine use can only be justified if these other actions are thought to be reasonable and acceptable in the circumstances.

Drugs of the phenothiazine and associated groups are the most effective anti-emetics. A specific effect on the vomiting centre in the medulla is claimed for them, while their general sedative action also plays a part. Prevention of sickness is most usefully attempted by combining the chosen drug with the premedication, and then administering further doses at 3- to 4-hourly intervals in the post-operative period. Alternatively, they can be used as the main component of premedication instead of an opiate or one of its analogues, and only combined with atropine or scopolamine. Yet another way is to give a dose intramuscularly just before the patient leaves the operating theatre, and then to repeat the dose at intervals during the next 24 hours. All these methods will tend to prolong the period of unconsciousness or semi-consciousness which follows general anaesthesia, while the selective effect on the respiratory tract reflexes and autonomic ganglia may increase the hazards of the immediate post-operative period. It is therefore probably safer, and not much less effective, to use them when indicated in the post-operative period and only after the initial recovery of consciousness—though even then the induced hypotension is not without its dangers. Occasional patients who are known to have a severe sickness after anaesthesia might be counted as the exceptions and treated more thoroughly.

The effectiveness of these anti-emetics can be gauged from the published results of large investigations. Burtles and Peckett (1957) were able to reduce their incidence of post-operative sickness by approximately 50 per cent, using either chlorpromazine or promethazine in the premedication, while Knapp and Beecher (1956) converted an overall incidence of 82 per cent to 59 per cent, using a single intramuscular injection of chlorpromazine at the end of the operation.

Many drugs are useful anti-emetics, but the choice of a particular preparation depends upon a knowledge of its relative effectiveness in different circumstances and of its side-effects (Riding, 1963). These drugs are described in Chapter 23, but those most favoured are promethazine in a dose range of from 25–50 mg and perphenazine in 5 mg doses. Metoclopramide (10 mg) has been shown to produce significantly less nausea, retching and vomiting in a comparative trial with perphenazine (5 mg) (Breivik and Lind, 1970). Other compounds have their advocates for the prevention and treatment of post-operative sickness. Dimenhydrinate (Dramamine) and promethazine-8-chlorotheophyllinate (Avomine) are best used for cases of motion sickness typified in the post-operative period after operations on on near the labyrinth. The dose is from 25 to 50 mg. They are not of great use for other types of sickness. N-benzhydryl-N-methyl piperazine dihydrochloride (Marzine) is said to have fewer side-effects than other antihistamines, but to have an equally effective control of sickness, and should be used in single doses of up to 50 mg intramuscularly.

The relative mildness of much post-operative sickness suggests that some of the old-fashioned remedies may still have their place in treatment. Moreover, even the special drugs fail to control sickness in some patients, so that less specific and homely, but none the less practical, procedures may be helpful. Sips of cold water to which a little bicarbonate or iodide has been added are often beneficial.

A small-bore tube (Ryle's or similar type of 4 mm diameter) for gastric suction is often a useful ancillary in the treatment of severe cases, and can also be helpful if used prophylactically in cases known to be liable to this complication. Occasionally, especially in episodes following operations upon children, intravenous replacement of fluid, food and electrolytes may be an essential part of treatment.

No case of persistent or severe post-operative vomiting should be treated by routine therapy until a surgical cause has been excluded.

REFERENCES

ARMSTRONG, R. F. (1973). Metoclopramide and gastric emptying. *Brit. J. Anaesth.*, **45**, 123.

BANNISTER, W. K., and SATTILARO, A. J. (1962). Vomiting and aspiration during anesthesia. *Anesthesiology*, **23**, 251.

BEST, C. H., and TAYLOR, N. B. (1955). *The Physiological Basis of Medical Practice*, 6th edit. Baltimore: Williams & Wilkins.

BLISS, B. P. (1973). The surgical management of obesity. *Brit. J. hosp. Med.*, **10**, 19.

BREIVIK, H., and LIND, B. (1971). Anti-emetic and propulsive peristaltic properties of metoclopramide. *Brit. J. Anaesth.*, **43**, 400.

BURTLES, R., and PECKETT, B. W. (1957). Postoperative vomiting. Some factors affecting its incidence. *Brit. J. Anaesth.*, **29**, 114.

COHEN, S., and HARRIS, L. D. (1971). Does hiatus hernia affect competence of the gastro-oesophageal sphincter? *New Engl. J. Med.*, **284**, 1053.

DENNISH, G. W., and CASTELL, D. O. (1971). Inhibitory effect of smoking on the lower oesophageal sphincter. *New Engl. J. Med.*, **284**, 1136.

DENT, S. J., RAMACHANDRA, V., and STEPHEN, C. R. (1955). Post-operative vomiting: incidence, analysis and therapeutic measures in 3,000 patients. *Anesthesiology*, **16**, 564.

DINNICK, O. P. (1961). Hiatus hernia: an anaesthetic hazard. *Lancet*, **1**, 470.

EDWARDS, G., MORTON, H. J. V., PASK, E. A., and WYLIE, W. D. (1956). Deaths associated with anaesthesia. A report on 1,000 cases. *Anaesthesia*, **11**, 194.

EISNER, M. (1971). Effect of metoclopramide in gastrointestinal motility in man: a manometric study. *Amer. J. dig. Dis.*, **16**, 409.

FAREBROTHER, M. J. B., and MCHARDY, G. J. R. (1974). Respiratory complications of obesity. *Brit. med. J.*, **3**, 469.

FISHER, A., WATERHOUSE, T. D., and ADAMS, A. P. (1975). Obesity: its relation to anaesthesia. *Anaesthesia*, **30**, 633.

FRY, E. N. S. (1974). Metoclopramide and drinking before general anaesthesia. *Anaesthesia*, **29**, 754.

GARDNER, A. M. N. (1958). Aspiration of food and vomit. *Quart. J. Med.*, **27**, 227.

GOLD, M. I. (1969). Post-anaesthetic vomiting in the recovery room. *Brit. J. Anaesth.*, **41**, 143.

GREENE, N. M. (1976). Familiarity as a basis for the practice of anesthesiology. *Anesthesiology*, **44**, 101.

HIGHTOWER, N. C. (1974). Applied anatomy and physiology of the stomach. In: *Gastroenterology*, Vol. 1. Ed. Bockus, H. L. Philadelphia: Saunders.

HUNT, J. N., MACDONALD, I., and SPURRELL, W. R. (1951). The gastric response to pectin meals of high osmotic pressure. *J. Physiol. (Lond.).*, **115**, 185.

KANNEL, W. B., LEBAUER, E. J., DAWBER, T. R., and MCNAMARA, P. M. (1967). Relation of body weight to development of coronary heart disease: the Framingham Study. *Circulation*, **35**, 734.

KING, R. C. (1957). The control of diabetes mellitus in surgical patients. *Anaesthesia*, **12**, 30.

KNAPP, M. R., and BEECHER, H. K. (1956). Postanesthetic nausea, vomiting and retching. Evaluation of the antiemetic drugs dimenhydrinate (Dramamine), chlorpromazine, and pentobarbital sodium. *J. Amer. med. Ass.*, **160**, 376.

LA COUR, D. (1969). Rise in intragastric pressure caused by suxamethonium fasciculations. *Acta anesth. scand.*, **13**, 255.

MARCHAND, P. (1957). A study of the forces productive of gastro-oesophageal regurgitation and herniation through the diaphragmatic hiatus. *Thorax*, **12**, 189.

MENDELSON, C. L. (1946). Aspiration of stomach contents into lungs during obstetric anesthesia. *Amer. J. Obstet. Gynec.*, **52**, 191.

MORTON, H. J. V. (1957). Intestinal obstruction and anaesthesia. *Brit. med. J.*, **2**, 224.

MORTON, H. J. V., and WYLIE, W. D. (1951). Anaesthetic deaths due to regurgitation or vomiting. *Anaesthesia*, **6,** 190.

O'MULLANE, E. J. (1954). Vomiting and regurgitation during anaesthesia. *Lancet*, **1,** 1209.

PAYNE, J. H., and DEWIND, L. T. (1969). Surgical treatment of obesity. *Amer. J. Surg.*, **118,** 141.

PESKETT, W. G. H. (1973). Antacids before obstetric anaesthesia. *Anaesthesia*, **28,** 509.

RIDING, J. E. (1963). The prevention of postoperative vomiting. *Brit. J. Anaesth.*, **35,** 180.

ROBSON, J. G., and WELT, P. (1959). Regurgitation in anaesthesia; report on some exploratory work with animals. *Canad. Anaesth. Soc. J.*, **6,** 4.

RUBEN, H., KNUDSEN, E. J., and CARUGATI, G. (1961). Gastric inflation in relation to airway pressure. *Acta anaesth. scand.*, **5,** 107.

SELLICK, B. A. (1961). Cricoid pressure to control regurgitation of stomach contents during induction of anaesthesia. *Lancet*, **2,** 204.

SMART, G. A. (1956). In: *Price's Textbook of the Practice of Medicine*, 9th edit., p. 450. Ed. D. Hunter. London: Oxford Med. Publishers.

TAYLOR, G., and PRYSE-DAVIES, J. (1966). The prophylactic use of antacids in the prevention of the acid-pulmonary-aspiration syndrome. *Lancet*, **1,** 288.

VAUGHAN, R. W., and WISE, L. (1975). Choice of abdominal operative incision in the obese patient: a study using blood gas measurements. *Ann. Surg.*, **181,** 829.

WATERS, R. M. (1936). Present status of cyclopropane. *Brit. med. J.*, **2,** 1013.

Chapter 38

ANAESTHESIA AND THE LIVER

ANATOMY

THE liver, which is the largest glandular organ of the body, lies below the right costal margin under the diaphragm. In the adult the liver constitutes approximately one-fortieth of the body weight ranging between 1000–1500 g, and is divided imperfectly into two lobes—a large right and a small left one. Neither of these two lobes is derived exclusively from the right and left hepatic buds of the embryo nor do they receive their blood supply solely from one or other of the two hepatic arteries. On the inferior and posterior surface between the right and left lobes are two smaller lobes—the caudate and the quadrate. The falciform ligament consists of two layers of peritoneum which are closely united until they reach the upper surface of the liver, where they part company to cover the peritoneal surface of the right and left lobe. This ligament joins the liver to the diaphragm and the anterior abdominal wall. In its free edge stretching from the umbilicus to the lower border of the liver is the ligamentum teres containing small para-umbilical veins. At its upper end the two layers of the falciform ligament separate widely to expose a small triangular area—the bare area of the liver. The right fold of the ligament joins the upper layer of the coronary ligament and the left fold sweeps away to become continuous with the anterior layer of the left triangular ligament.

The porta hepatis is found on the inferior surface of the liver lying between the quadrate lobe in front and a process of the caudate lobe behind. This structure is important because it consists of a deep fissure containing most of the essential structures of the liver. Viewed from below these structures, from right to left, are the common hepatic duct, which gives off a branch—the cystic duct—leading to the neck of the gall bladder, the bile duct, the portal vein and finally the hepatic artery with a plexus of hepatic nerves.

The minute structure of the liver comprises a whole mass of neatly arranged lobules. Each lobule consists of numerous cells arranged in columns which radiate from around a central vein. Irregular blood vessels or sinusoids can be found between the columns of cells. The blood supply to these lobules comes from the hepatic artery and the portal vein. Both these vessels, soon after entering the porta hepatitis, divide into right and left branches. Each branch then undergoes dichotomy many thousands of times to supply all the lobules. The hepatic artery, which arises from the coeliac axis, brings fresh oxygenated blood for the liver cells almost directly from the aorta, whereas the portal vein carries all ingested material in the venous blood from the gastro-intestinal tract and spleen. These two vascular supplies are carried throughout the liver on the periphery of the lobules. Small branches are given off from both vessels which encircle the lobule as the interlobular plexus and from these plexuses small capillary-like vessels (sometimes described as sinusoids) run between the column of cells of the lobule and finally drain into the vein in the centre of the lobule—the central vein. All the central veins join up to form the hepatic veins which finally drain into the inferior vena cava.

The nerve supply of the liver—the hepatic plexus—consists of non-medullated fibres from the sympathetic ganglia of T_7 and T_{10} which synapse in the coeliac axis, and fibres from both vagi and the right phrenic nerve. The nerves ramify around the vessels and bile ducts and finally terminate in the liver cells.

PHYSIOLOGY

The blood flow to the liver is about 1,500 ml per minute. Of this total, about 80 per cent (1,200 ml) reaches the liver through the portal vein and the remaining 20 per cent (300 ml) passes along the hepatic artery. However, the blood in the hepatic artery is about 95 per cent saturated with oxygen whereas that in the portal vein is around 85 per cent.

It has been estimated that the liver normally requires about 60 ml of oxygen per minute, of which about 17 ml are supplied by the hepatic artery and the remainder by the portal vein. The total amount of oxygen available to the liver cells can be reduced by a number of conditions:

1. Anaesthesia. Due to (a) reduced hepatic blood flow;
   (b) reduced arterial oxygen saturation through pulmonary shunting.
2. Lowered cardiac output, as in shock, haemorrhage or hypotension.
3. Inhalation of a low inspired concentration of oxygen.
4. Hypermetabolic states, e.g. pyrexia.
5. Hepatotoxic substances.
6. Obstruction of the portal vein or hepatic artery.
7. Portal hypertension, with extensive extrahepatic collateral circulation or internal portal hepatic venous shunts.

It is clear, therefore, that as the cells surrounding the central lobular vein are the last to receive nourishment, they are the first to suffer from any deprivation. With toxic substances one might expect the cells surrounding the hepatic artery to receive the worst damage, but it is liver toxins which cause the hepatic cells to swell, and it is their swelling which further interferes with the blood supply of the central cells and causes them to suffer the worst damage.

Functions of the Liver

General metabolism.—Ingested carbohydrates are broken down in the intestine and the resulting monosaccharides are absorbed and stored in the liver in the form of glycogen (glycogenesis). The breakdown of glycogen (glycogenolysis) is through the Embden-Meyerhof pathway to pyruvic acid and then via the citric acid cycle to carbon dioxide and water. Any excess glucose not converted to glycogen may be converted to fatty acids.

Fats pass from the depots throughout the body to the liver and are broken down, almost as fast as they arrive, into glycerol and fatty acids under the influence of the enzyme liver lipase.

The end-products of protein digestion are amino acids which play such an important part in cellular structure. The "amino acid pool" is composed not only of the fresh supplies from the gut, but also from the continual breakdown and rebuilding of the tissues. The amino acids number about twenty and each protein molecule is a composite group of most of them. Amongst the more important of these amino acids are glycine, cystine, methionine, tyrosine and leucine. About one half of the body protein synthesis and resynthesis takes place in the liver and it is here that the surplus amino acids undergo oxidative deamination. In this process the amine group (NH_2) is released as ammonia (NH_3): the latter substance is either excreted as urea or is used again for building other amino acids. The remainder of the molecule (the non-nitrogenous part) is broken down to produce energy for the general metabolism.

The amino acid methionine is of special interest because it is concerned in the synthesis of choline; it generously donates three methyl groups to ethanolamine to form choline, and this may then become acetylated in the presence of the enzyme choline acetylase to form the essential substance of neuromuscular transmission—acetylcholine. Another of methionine's important functions is to supply a methyl group to noradrenaline to synthesise adrenaline.

Storage.—Fats, protein and glycogen and likewise certain vitamins—such as vitamin B which plays such an important part in pernicious anaemia—are all stored in the liver.

Production and destruction.—Amongst its tasks the liver synthesises plasma proteins, prothrombin, fibrinogen and heparin. In early life it plays an important part in red blood cell formation and later becomes one of the principal places where the breakdown products of old red blood corpuscles are dealt with.

Formation of the bile secretion.—This is carried out in the liver.

Detoxication of drugs.—The liver is able to remove many foreign substances by oxidation. For example pethidine is removed in this manner and, therefore, liver function is important in any assessment of drug activity. Barbiturates in common with many other drugs metabolised in the liver have the ability to stimulate the microenzyme systems within the hepatic cells. The effect of this "Enzyme Induction" results in an increase in the amount of enzyme present in the cells, with the result that repeated doses of the same drug are metabolised with increasing speed and in consequence have a decreasing effect. The enzymes stimulated by a particular drug are not specific to that drug and may thus increase the rate of metabolism of other drugs given at the same time. For example the alcoholic patient will tolerate barbiturates very well. However, once the liver begins to fail such a patient becomes extremely sensitive to barbiturates particularly the short-acting group, because there is insufficient functioning hepatic tissue to metabolise them.

LIVER FUNCTION TESTS

In attempting to assess the functional state of the liver a number of points must be remembered. Because the liver carries out such diverse functions, a great variety of biochemical tests have been used to assess the overall state of the organ and many of these may be normal in the presence of liver disease while factors other than liver disease may cause abnormal results.

Serum Bilirubin Estimations

Bilirubin is formed mainly from the breakdown of the haem part of the haemoglobin molecule. This occurs in the reticulo-endothelial cells of the liver and spleen. The unconjugated bilirubin (which is carried in the plasma bound to albumin) is taken up by the liver cells which convert it from a fat-soluble to a water-soluble form by conjugating it with glucuronic acid.

The Van den Bergh reaction determines the conjugated level of bilirubin [normal value 0·2 mg/100 ml (3·4 μmol/l) or less] and by the addition of methyl alcohol also the total concentration of the serum bilirubin, that is the sum of the conjugated and unconjugated bilirubin [normal value 0·8 mg/100 ml (13·7 μmol/l) or less].

Bromsulphthalein Test

This dye, consisting of phenol and tetrabromphthalein disodium sulphonate, is taken up by the liver cells and excreted unchanged in the bile. The test is based upon a study of the concentration remaining in the blood after the intravenous injection of this dye and is expressed as a percentage of the control value. The patient is given 5 mg/kg body weight of 5 per cent bromsulphthalein intravenously, and if normal, should have 0 to 3 per cent of it left in the blood after forty-five minutes. In patients with hypoalbuminaemia a normal result may be found even in the presence of liver disease. This is in consequence of an inverse relationship that exists between the rate of removal from the plasma of bromsulphthalein and plasma albumin concentration (Grauz and Schmid, 1971).

Serum Enzyme Tests

The multiplicity of tests for liver function is evidence of the complexity of processes carried out by this organ and the inadequacy in consequence of a single test to give an overall picture of the state of the liver. Enzymes are present in most of the cells of the major organs throughout the body and the serum of the blood contains a steady level of each, because there is a constant small breakdown of cells. However, if an organ such as the heart or liver suddenly undergoes an ischaemic episode, then cellular breakdown will increase precipitously and this will be reflected in a dramatic elevation of the serum level of the corresponding enzymes. Similarly, if obstruction to the biliary tract occurs, the enzymes normally excreted by this route will spill into the blood stream with a marked increase in serum levels. For this reason these enzyme tests play an important role in distinguishing jaundice due to hepatic cellular damage and that following early obstruction of the common bile duct.

The enzymes in question include transaminases, dehydrogenases and phosphatases.

(A) **The transaminases.**—Transamination is a chemical reaction in which an amino group of an amino acid replaces the keto group of another acid to form a new amino acid, with the enzyme for this process being a transaminase. There are two principal hepatic transaminases:

1. *Aspartate aminotransferase* (*glutamic oxaloacetic transaminase*).—This is present in large quantities in the liver, heart, kidney and skeletal muscle. High serum values for this enzyme are found in both hepatocellular necrosis and myocardial infarction. Normal serum value 5 to 17 International units/dl.*

---

* There is a wide variation in the normal range quoted by different laboratories. This is because each uses its own technique, and there are no generally agreed standards for temperature, pH or buffering solutions. Though there are International units, there is no International technique.

2. *Alanine aminotransferase* (*glutamic pyruvic transaminase*).—This is also present in many organs but there is relatively less in the liver cells as compared with the heart and skeletal muscle. Normal serum value 4 to 13 International units/dl (Sherlock, 1975).

In severe liver disease such as acute hepatitis, the level of these enzymes in the serum may rise to 800 International units/dl or more, whilst in the presence of simple obstructive jaundice the level is usually in the region of 50 to 100 International units/dl.

(B) **The dehydrogenases.**—These enzymes catalyse an oxidation-reduction reaction in the presence of a co-enzyme which serves as a hydrogen donor or acceptor.

The principal enzymes of this group include lactic dehydrogenase (LDH) and isocitric dehydrogenase (ICD). The former is a relatively insensitive index of hepatocellular injury although the serum level may be greatly raised in association with hepatic neoplasms. In the latter case raised levels are found in hepatic damage but normal values occur in the presence of myocardial infarction (Sherlock, 1975). Other diagnostic procedures for assessing liver function include needle biopsy and hepatic scanning using a gamma-emitting isotope.

Normal values for LDH are up to 500 International units/dl. This figure is considerably raised in infective or toxic hepatitis but is usually within normal limits in early obstructive jaundice.

(C) **The phosphatases.**—The serum alkaline phosphatase is also useful in helping to diagnose the cause of jaundice, as a low figure in King Armstrong units (0–15 units/dl) suggests either a normal response or the presence of inflammation of the liver cells. A high figure (35 or more units/dl), on the other hand, signifies an obstruction to the flow of bile. Other phosphatases that may be affected by liver disease include serum glucose 6-phosphatase and serum 5-nucleotidase.

Pseudo (Plasma) Cholinesterase Test

Pseudocholinesterases are responsible for the breakdown of acetylcholine and also suxamethonium. These esterases are believed to be formed mainly in the liver, and in the presence of damage to this organ or starvation low values may be expected. Nevertheless, a low pseudocholinesterase level may be present in otherwise healthy subjects and this is one of the first points that comes to mind if a prolonged apnoea follows suxamethonium. It must be assumed, therefore, that there are other causes of a low pseudocholinesterase reading besides liver damage; and it is known that merely altering the protein intake in the diet is rapidly reflected in the level of the esterase in the blood (see Chapter 27).

Pseudocholinesterase (*Michael's Method*).—40 to 100 units/dl. (For details of the paper test see Chapter 27.)

JAUNDICE AND ITS DIFFERENTIAL DIAGNOSIS

The cause of the yellow tinge in the skin, which is so characteristic of jaundice, is an increase in the concentration of bilirubin in the blood. This may occur for a variety of reasons:

(*a*) **Haemolytic jaundice** is due to an excessive destruction of red blood cells with the consequent accumulation of large quantities of unconjugated bilirubin, which is formed so fast that the liver cells are simply unable to remove it quickly enough, so that the concentration in the blood rises. This type of jaundice most commonly occurs after the transfusion of incompatible blood or the injection of haemolytic drugs and sera. It also occurs in association with a number of hereditary defects of the red cell membrane (e.g. hereditary spherocytosis) or its haemoglobin content (sickle-cell anaemia).

(b) **Hepatic jaundice.**—This results from failure of the liver cell to conjugate the bilirubin and excrete it into the biliary system. This may be the direct result of toxic damage to the cell (e.g. drugs). The cells surrounding the central part of the lobule are the most susceptible to damage because they are supplied with the lowest saturation of oxygen and are thus the first to suffer. Damage to these central cells often introduces an element of "obstruction" into this type of jaundice. Alternatively, there are a number of comparatively rare conditions, often familial, in which there is an abnormality of bilirubin conjugation (e.g. Gilbert's syndrome).

(c) **Obstructive jaundice** signifies some form of blockage in the biliary system preventing the outflow of bile. A rare type of this condition occurs in the newborn where the congenital abnormality is some failure in the cannulation of the bile duct system. More commonly it is seen in adults as an acquired condition following obstruction of the common bile duct by a stone or by carcinoma of the head of the pancreas.

Bilirubin being the essential cause of jaundice, a description of its formation and fate is important in any attempt to differentiate between the various types of jaundice described above.

Normally the red blood cells are broken down by the reticuloendothelial system. The globin portion of the molecule is split off and returns to the metabolic protein pool. The haem is then broken down to iron and porphyrin. The iron is carried to the bone marrow where it is used again for further haemoglobin synthesis. The porphyrin is broken down to bilirubin which is carried in the blood bound to albumin which is insoluble in water and cannot pass into the urine. A rise in red cell destruction, therefore, will lead to a corresponding rise in the protein-bound bilirubin. On reaching the liver the latter is conjugated with glucuronic acid to form the water-soluble bilirubin glucuronide which passes from the liver cell down the bile duct to the intestines where it is acted upon by bacteria and forms urobilinogen. Some of this is then reabsorbed and passes into the blood stream, but about half passes on down to join the faeces and in contact with air it becomes oxidised to form urobilin. Of that part of urobilinogen that is reabsorbed some returns to the liver to complete the cycle, whilst the rest passes to the kidney and is excreted in the urine. Ultimately it is likewise oxidised in the presence of air to form urobilin.

In haemolytic jaundice the total quantity of protein-bound bilirubin is greatly increased. The liver cells just cannot manage to deal with the huge quantities that are reaching them and a rise in concentration is inevitable. The urine does not contain any bilirubin because the bilirubin in the blood is insoluble in water. The concentration of urinary urobilinogen is increased. In obstructive jaundice the water-soluble bilirubin cannot be excreted down the bile duct into the intestine and it overflows from the liver cell back into the blood stream. The concentration of the serum water-soluble bilirubin rises and it appears in the urine. As no urobilinogen is able to be formed in the intestine the stools are pale and the urine contains no urobilinogen. In hepatic jaundice which has resulted from toxic damage to the liver the biochemical picture is more confused giving usually an initial obstructive type picture with a haemolytic element superimposed a little later. Assessment of liver function tests will show evidence of hepatic cell damage.

Liver Blood Flow

The splanchnic vascular system supplies all the blood passing to the intestines from which it finally drains into the portal system and is carried to the liver. The liver blood flow, however, receives another contribution in the hepatic artery so that variations in the splanchnic flow and in that of the hepatic artery are reflected in the final amount of blood which passes through the liver.

Measurement of Liver Blood Flow

This is a complex procedure based on the extraction of bromsulphthalein by the liver cells (Bradley *et al.*, 1945). This technique has been adapted for use in anaesthetised patients by Shackman and his associates (1953). The conscious patient is first screened and a radio-opaque catheter is passed under vision up an arm vein via the superior vena cava into the inferior vena cava and from there into a branch of the right hepatic vein. This provides samples of portal blood *after* it has passed through the liver. Bromsulphthalein is injected intravenously, first as an initial primary dose and then as a continuous infusion of a 3 per cent solution in saline at an average of about 1·4 ml/minute. Once stabilisation has been reached the concentration in a peripheral artery is taken to equal that in the blood reaching the liver cells. A comparison between this concentration and that in the hepatic vein will reveal a relative drop due to the extraction by the liver cells. Since the arteriovenous difference can also be determined for similar samples, the actual amount of blood flowing through the liver can be calculated. Caesar and his colleagues (1961) have described a technique using indocyanine green in order to measure the splanchnic blood flow. Other substances which have also been used include galactose and ethanol.

Flow in the Conscious State

Measurements made on conscious subjects suggest that the average liver blood flow is about 1·25 to 1·5 litres per minute. As the normal cardiac output for a patient at rest is about 5 litres/minute this means that about 25 per cent of this output passes to the liver. Under certain conditions, however, the liver has to sacrifice some of this flow in order to protect the homeostatic mechanism, maintain the systolic pressure, and ensure a blood supply to the most "vital" centres. Haemorrhage, congestive heart failure and severe exercise are amongst these causes.

Flow in the Anaesthetised Patient

The induction and maintenance of general anaesthesia is sufficient to produce a drop of up to 50 per cent in the amount of blood flowing through the liver (Thorshauge, 1970). As the average flow in the conscious patient is about 1500 ml/min it follows that the onset of anaesthesia reduces this flow to around half (750 ml/min). Deeper planes of anaesthesia produce an even greater fall. Price and his colleagues (1965) used indocyanine green to measure the splanchnic blood flow during anaesthesia in a group of volunteers who were not undergoing surgery. When cyclopropane was the anaesthetic used, the liver blood flow was significantly reduced by splanchnic vasoconstriction. If, at this point, a small dose of hexamethonium (i.e. one insufficient to lower the blood pressure yet capable of some ganglion blockade) was also given, then both the hepatic and the splanchnic flow could be returned to normal. On the basis of these findings the authors concluded that the reduced liver blood flow of cyclopropane anaesthesia is probably secondary to increased sympathetic activity in the splanchnic vascular bed.

In contrast, halothane anaesthesia produces a fall in liver blood flow *without* altering the splanchnic vascular tone. In this case the fall in hepatic blood flow parallels the decrease in cardiac output (Ahlgren *et al.*, 1967). The latter has been shown to vary with arterial carbon dioxide tension (Prys-Roberts *et al.*, 1968) and Juhl and Einer-Jensen (1974) have shown that as a consequence of this response hypercapnia may lessen the fall in hepatic blood flow and hypocapnia increase it.

In other words, a rise in arterial P_{CO_2} leads to an increase in cardiac output, which in view of the unaltered splanchnic tone, will lead to an increase in liver blood flow. Conversely, a fall in arterial P_{CO_2} leads to a reduction in cardiac output and a diminution of hepatic blood flow.

Methoxyflurane anaesthesia causes an even more marked reduction in splanchnic blood flow than either halothane or cyclopropane (Price and Pauca, 1969). This seems to result from an increase in splanchnic resistance and decreased mean arterial pressure. Epstein *et al.* (1961) found that general anaesthesia using thiopentone, nitrous oxide, oxygen and succinylcholine, with intermittent positive-pressure ventilation and maintenance of normal arterial carbon dioxide tension, altered splanchnic blood flow very little. Recently, Cowan *et al.* (1975) have measured hepatic blood flow under conditions of routine general anaesthesia and they state: "Studies in man using hepatic vein catheters have shown that blood flow through the liver falls significantly after induction with various anaesthetic agents, but returns to pre-anaesthetic levels during the subsequent abdominal surgery. This fall, which is greater with trichloroethylene than with halothane, may be large enough in some patients to contribute to post-operative liver dysfunction". Their results suggest that though *induction* of anaesthesia can cause a sharp fall in hepatic blood-flow, the *trauma* of surgery could be responsible for a rapid return to normal levels in the lightly anaesthetised patient.

Any reduction in hepatic blood flow must be considered in the light of the tremendous increase in flow that takes place in the skin and muscle vessels at the same time. As there is no compensatory increase in the cardiac output in most forms of anaesthesia, it follows that the liver—ably helped by the kidney—is the source for this extra amount of blood passing to the periphery. In fact, active vasoconstriction may take place. There is no evidence to suggest that this reorganisation of the blood flow is in any way beneficial to the patient, and certainly it is extremely troublesome for the surgeon.

Flow during Autonomic Blockade

The effects of autonomic blockade depend in part on the technique by which it is produced. Kennedy *et al.* (1971) have shown in conscious volunteers that epidural anaesthesia (to the level of T_5) using lignocaine solutions containing adrenaline, results in an initial fall in splanchnic vascular resistance while the hepatic blood flow decreased by about 25 per cent 30 minutes after T_5 anaesthesia had been achieved and then slowly returned to normal. When plain lignocaine was used, the splanchnic vascular resistance rose significantly with a rapid fall in hepatic blood flow also of about 25 per cent which gradually returned to normal. The difference in effect between the two solutions used may depend on a splanchnic vasodilator action of adrenaline (Bearn *et al.*, 1951).

In high spinal anaesthesia hepatic blood flow decreased by an amount similar to that with epidural anaesthesia. However, the splanchnic vascular resistance did not alter significantly, the decrease in flow being associated with a fall in mean arterial pressure (Kennedy *et al.*, 1970). It would thus appear that the high serum levels of lignocaine that are found in epidural anaesthesia when adrenaline is not used may have specific action on splanchnic vasculature.

Ganglionic blockade does not cause any change in splanchnic vascular resistance but a fall in flow proportional to the fall in mean arterial pressure (Cooperman, 1972) .

Flow during Hypotension associated with Vasoconstriction

This follows oligaemia from severe blood loss. The splanchnic bed attempts to compensate for this alteration in the haemodynamics by vasoconstriction which, in turn, results in a drop in the portal flow. When the systemic pressure falls the flow through the hepatic artery also drops. Thus the combination of vasoconstriction in the splanchnic bed with hypotension—as occurs after severe haemorrhage—may lead to a serious depletion of liver blood flow.

Flow during Hypothermia

Hypothermia causes both a fall in blood pressure and a reduction in liver blood flow, but it has the great advantage that in this case the metabolism (oxygen requirements) of the hepatic cells are reduced *pari passu* with the fall in temperature and blood pressure. There is little evidence to suggest that the liver cells suffer any damage from hypothermia alone, but if a period of cardiac arrest is also included then severe congestion of the liver cells may result from temporary occlusion of the inferior vena cava.

Flow and Vasoconstrictor Drugs

The administration of such drugs may reduce the liver blood flow. While the local action of adrenaline on the liver is one of vasoconstriction, the effects of a raised systemic blood pressure and splanchnic vasodilatation predominate, and the result is that hepatic blood flow increases. Noradrenaline, on the other hand, is such a powerful vasoconstrictor that the liver flow usually shows a slight fall despite the rise in systemic pressure. Cases of damage to the liver cells following the infusion of noradrenaline have been reported. Other vasopressors, like methylamphetamine, which stimulate cardiac output increase the hepatic flow.

ANAESTHESIA AND THE HEPATIC CELLS

Most anaesthetic drugs can be classed as protoplasmic poisons of lesser or greater degree, so that it is not surprising that they figure prominently in any study of liver function. As has already been mentioned, the liver cells surrounding the central lobular vein are working with a low oxygen saturation; it is hardly surprising, therefore, that they are the first to suffer damage if the saturation falls even lower. This, if coupled with the action of any anaesthetic drug used, may be sufficient to produce signs of liver damage. In essence the two causes—hypoxia and drugs—are inseparable and complementary.

Hypoxia may be the result not only of a fall in the oxygen content of the hepatic blood but also of a fall in the absolute amount of blood arriving at the liver in a given time. While the oxygen consumption of the liver may decrease during general and regional anaesthesia the splanchnic blood flow is reduced to a greater degree (Cooperman *et al.*, 1968). Price *et al.* (1966) examined the effects of cyclopropane and halothane anaesthesia to see if this disproportionate reduction in oxygen requirement and splanchnic blood flow caused any evidence of hepatic cell anoxia but found none. However, as Cooperman (1972) pointed out, the problem remains of applying this data, obtained in general from fit, healthy young volunteers, to the ill and aged patient undergoing surgery.

One added factor that is often not considered is the effect on splanchnic circulation of surgical trauma and stimulation which occurs during intra-abdominal surgery. Torrance (1957) showed that hepatic blood flow could fall markedly as a result of even the most minor surgical manoeuvre such as manipulation of the peritoneum, and it is not difficult to see how hypoxia of the centrilobular cells of the liver could arise. It seems surprising that hepatic dysfunction does not occur more commonly after intra-abdominal surgery.

Sherlock (1975) has divided therapeutic agents that may effect the liver into two broad groups, the predictable and the unpredictable.

In the *predictable* group are included drugs that interfere with bilirubin metabolism and those with a direct hepatotoxic effect. The hepatic effects of drugs in this group can be reproduced in animals. Novobiocin is an example of a substance that interferes with the conjugation of bilirubin and this may be of particular relevance in the neonate, while carbon tetrachloride produces a direct dose-dependent action on the liver. Large doses of intravenous tetracycline are also directly hepatotoxic.

In the *unpredictable* group only a small number of those receiving the drug concerned will be affected. The incidence is unrelated to the dose though it is more common after multiple exposures suggesting a sensitivity reaction. Furthermore, the liver lesion cannot be reproduced in animals. This hypersensitivity type of reaction is either hepatitic, being indistinguishable from viral hepatitis (for example, isoniazid), or cholestatic with obstruction to the excretion of bilirubin as may be seen with the phenothiazine group of drugs. Recently, much interest has centred on the effects of inhalational agents, particularly halothane, on the liver. An association has been described between its use and the occurrence of hepatitis (Sherlock, 1971). While the U.S. National Halothane Study (1966) and the British Committee on the Safety of Medicines (Inman and Mushin, 1974; Medical Research Council, 1974) have suggested a low incidence of severe liver disease following surgery, the former found the mortality when halothane was used to be less than that found with all other agents. The possible mechanisms of "halothane hepatitis" have been debated at length but no clear explanation has been given (Simpson *et al.*, 1973).

It has also been suggested that hepatic damage is more likely to occur in patients who are exposed to halothane on multiple occasions (Hughes and Powell, 1970; Davis and Holdsworth, 1973) but this has been disputed (Dykes *et al.*, 1972; McPeek and Gilbert, 1974; Simpson *et al.*, 1975*a*). Since at present there are no clinical or histological findings that are pathognomonic of "halothane hepatitis", the problem remains unanswered. However, Simpson *et al.* (1975*b*) have stated that in their view "if other equally suitable techniques are available for anaesthetising the patient with a history of unexplained jaundice following a previous halothane anaesthetic, halothane should not be used".

It may seem strange that 20 years after its introduction and having been used for over 100 million anaesthetics, controversy still exists. However, as Kalow *et al.* (1976) have pointed out "evidence directly relating halothane exposure to liver damage in a cause and effect relationship continues to be unconvincing because of the high selectivity of the cases reported and the impossibility of excluding other causes of the hepatocellular damage".

Hepatic reactions have also been reported after methoxyflurane anaesthesia (Katz, 1970).

Comment

It seems unlikely that the current enigma will be solved rapidly as the evidence is so conflicting. In the meantime, any patient exhibiting a mild pyrexia and leucopenia after operation must be regarded with particular suspicion; in most circumstances, if a further anaesthetic is required in the four weeks following surgery, then it is advisable to use a different volatile anaesthetic agent (assuming one is necessary). On the other hand, if there are specific indications for the use of a particular agent then the risk of hepatitis is so small that its use on a repeat occasion can be considered justifiable.

The muscle relaxants and liver damage.—The exact relationship between *d*-tubocurarine and the metabolism of the liver is still obscure. Dundee and Gray (1953) drew attention to the observation that patients with liver dysfunction required more *d*-tubocurarine to produce complete muscular paralysis than was normally required in similar healthy subjects. They have suggested that the reason for this relationship may be associated with the pseudocholinesterase level. It is first assumed that if this is low, the cholinesterase at the motor end-plates is likewise affected; in this event it is reasonable to suppose that the concentration of acetylcholine ions is higher than normal because it is not being destroyed so rapidly. Thus, more *d*-tubocurarine than usual will be required to bring about paralysis. A more likely explanation is that many patients with liver disease have raised serum globulin levels, and because *d*-tubocurarine is bound to gamma globulin (Aladjemoff *et al.*, 1958) the dose of this drug that will be required depends on the plasma protein concentration. Pancuronium, which is less affected by an abnormality of liver function, is also bound by serum proteins particularly the gamma globulin fraction (Thompson,

1976). Nevertheless, Farman *et al.* (1974) have suggested it is the muscle relaxant of choice in patients with liver dysfunction.

The relationship between suxamethonium and pseudocholinesterase is now firmly established. Since the pseudocholinesterase level is a test of liver function it follows that it will be low in cases of hepatic failure. In this event the action of suxamethonium may be prolonged.

ACUTE LIVER FAILURE IN RELATION TO ANAESTHESIA AND SURGERY

In clinical anaesthesia liver damage may result from a number of different causes, the most important of which is probably a period of severe hypotension occurring during or immediately after major surgery. The extent of the hepatic changes will depend on the degree and duration of the hypotension.

The onset of post-operative jaundice may be due to a number of other causes which may be subdivided into those producing increased serum levels of unconjugated bilirubin, impaired hepatocellular function and extrahepatic obstruction (LaMont and Isselbacher, 1973).

The increase in serum bilirubin may be the result of blood transfusion. One unit of 14-day-old stored blood may contain 250 mg of bilirubin which is the normal daily production. Jaundice after massive transfusions of blood, for example after cardiac surgery, is generally of the order of 10 per cent. The reabsorption of massive haematomata may also result in post-operative jaundice.

Hepatocellular damage may result from drugs that have been administered either pre- or intra-operatively, from sepsis or from pre-existing liver disease, for example, anicteric hepatitis. Extrahepatic biliary obstruction may arise from bile duct injury during surgery or post-operative cholecystitis.

One of the important associations with hepatocellular failure is renal failure which occurs even in the presence of previously normal renal function from an alteration in renal cortical perfusion (Kew *et al.*, 1971) in conjunction with a reduction in effective renal blood flow (Lieberman, 1970). The exact aetiology of this phenomenon is not known.

The symptoms and signs of hepatic failure are rather vague and indefinite at first but gradually become more obvious. At the start the patient complains of lassitude, malaise, anorexia and headache. Vomiting and pyrexia are often prominent. At about the third day vomiting is persistent and at the end of a week jaundice may be present. This heralds the final stages when the mental state becomes confused, with periods of delirium, and finally drifts into coma and death.

Treatment

The management of hepatic failure (Sherlock, 1975) is essentially supportive with treatment of the biochemical abnormalities that occur. Great care must be taken to see that nothing is given that might increase the degree of failure or coma that may be present. If sedation is essential a small dose of barbitone, which is not metabolised by the liver, may be used. Essentially protein intake is stopped and intestinal absorption of protein minimised by oral neomycin in order to prevent or decrease the encephalopathy. Hypoglycaemia is treated with i.v. 50 per cent glucose if the blood sugar falls below 100 mg/100 ml (5·6 mmol/l).

Electrolytic disorders, particularly hyponatraemia, must be corrected and renal failure may necessitate dialysis. Bleeding tendencies and anaemia may require vitamin K, fresh frozen plasma and fresh blood. In general, the complications of corticosteroid therapy outweigh the benefits. Finally, temporary hepatic support either by exchange transfusion, cross-circulation or extracorporeal liver perfusion may be necessary.

HEPATIC DISEASE AND ANAESTHESIA

The reserves of the liver are so great that unless the patient is rapidly approaching hepatic failure, there are few agents that cannot be used in small dosage. Two factors, must, however, always be kept in mind. First the extent to which any particular agent depends upon liver function for its breakdown and removal from the body, and secondly the effect of the agent, and indeed of the anaesthetic and surgical procedure as a whole, on liver function.

In practice, minor surgical procedures in the presence of hepatic disease are best performed under local anaesthesia. It must be borne in mind that amide local anaesthetic drugs are metabolised in the liver. Thus with single-dose spinal and epidural anaesthesia the low doses used cannot lead to a toxic concentration. However, if these drugs are infused (or given continuously) then the presence of severe hepatic dysfunction (with delayed metabolism) can rapidly lead to a toxic concentration accumulating in the plasma. Similarly, the barbiturates, the opiates, and the phenothiazines must only be used in small quantities (if at all) as they primarily rely on the hepatic cells for their metabolism or conjugation.

If general anaesthesia is mandatory then a light level in association with full muscular paralysis is the method of choice, as the volatile agent and relaxant can be excreted unchanged. In selecting a particular anaesthetic agent or technique in the patient with hepatic disease, it should be remembered that the cardiac output, the hepatic blood flow and the oxygen saturation are probably more important factors than the effect of a particular agent on liver function. For extensive operations in association with severe liver disease particular problems arise from the dangers of hypoxaemia and myocardial depression. The patients concerned tend to have a hyperdynamic circulation with a high cardiac output and depressed total peripheral resistance (Kaplan et al., 1971). A high inspired oxygen concentration is essential throughout the procedure if desaturation is to be avoided. Both systemic and pulmonary shunting of blood occur which contributes to the hypoxaemia. The pulmonary shunting in liver disease is particularly important being associated with a marked increase in ventilation/perfusion imbalance (Ruff, 1971).

The risk of concomitant renal failure in patients with cirrhosis even without obvious precipitating cause is greater than normal and this appears to be the result of renal vasomotor instability (Epstein et al., 1970). Prophylactic use of intravenous mannitol to maintain an adequate urinary output throughout the surgical procedure is advisable.

Hepatitis

The outbreak of hepatitis particularly in dialysis and transplant units has become a recognised hazard in recent years. The aetiology is in almost all cases one of two viral agents known as Virus A and Virus B. Hepatitis A and B which results from infection with the respective virus produce two distinguishable clinical diseases, the differences between which are summarised in Table 1. The pathology of the two diseases is essentially the same with acute inflammation of the entire liver. In hepatitis B, antibodies are produced against an antigen that was initially found in an Australian aborigine (Blumberg *et al.*, 1965). This antigen was initially called *Australia antigen* but has now been redesignated as

38/TABLE 1
VIRAL HEPATITIS IN MAN

	Hepatitis A	Hepatitis B
Synonym	Infectious hepatitis	Serum hepatitis
HB antigen in serum	Negative	Positive
Transmission	Faecal-oral	Parenteral transfer or close
	By food or water	physical contact
		Blood and blood products
Incubation period	3–5 weeks	More variable, generally longer
	(mean 28 days)	
Presumed infective particle	27 nm, enterovirus-like	44 nm, double-shelled virion
	RNA (probably)	(Dane particle) DNA
Found mainly in	Faeces	Blood
Small laboratory animal	None	None
Cell culture technique	None	None

Waterson, A. P. (1976).

38/TABLE 2
PATIENTS UNDER SUSPICION AS HEPATITIS B CARRIERS

(1) All patients with liver diseases, however acute or chronic.
(2) Patients undergoing haemodialysis, or who have had a renal transplant.
(3) All patients with leukaemia, reticuloses, polyarteritis nodosa or polymyositis.
(4) Patients being treated with radiotherapy or immunosuppressive drugs.
(5) Immigrants or visitors from countries with a high background of carriers.
(6) Persons who have been transfused in, or recently returned from, countries with a high background incidence (namely tropical and sub-tropical areas and Greenland).
(7) Patients who have received blood or a blood product in the last 6 months, or who have been transfused with blood or blood products from paid blood donors.
(8) Inmates of prisons or institutions for the mentally defective.
(9) Drug addicts, prostitutes, and homosexuals.
(10) The tattooed.
N.B. This list should not be regarded as exhaustive.

Waterson, A. P. (1976).

Hepatitis B antigen (HBAg.). It is found in 83 per cent of sera tested within 12 days of the onset of symptoms of type B hepatitis and has usually been cleared by 3–4 weeks (Sherlock, 1975).

It is hepatitis B rather than A that is of importance to the anaesthetist

(Waterson, 1976). It may be transmitted in the blood or secretions of a patient who may either have acute hepatitis clinically or be a symptom-free carrier. It is the latter group that are the great danger. It is not possible at the present time to test blood from every patient for the presence of hepatitis B antigen. There are, however, "certain categories of patient who should be regarded with suspicion, treated with respect, and tested without fail" (Waterson, 1976), and these are shown in Table 2.

In patients who are hepatitis B antigen-positive or in whom time does not allow screening tests to be carried out, full precautions must be taken from the time the patient leaves the ward. All staff entering theatre should be gowned, gloved and masked, preferably in disposable material that can be incinerated after the operation. The anaesthetist must take particular care to see that contamination does not arise from blood spilt at the time when intravenous infusions are set up or from syringes and needles that have been used. The practical details of the management of hepatitis B antigen-positive patients who require surgery has recently been fully reviewed by Waterson (1976).

There is no specific treatment for hepatitis B infections but for those who have been contaminated to an extent which is highly likely to result in the disease, a preparation of concentrated specific hepatitis B antigen antiserum (500 mg i.m.) should be given.

LIVER TRANSPLANTATION

The indications for this operation have been summarised by Williams (1970) as a primary hepatoma (without extrahepatic metastases), advanced cirrhosis without severe bleeding tendency in patients under the age of 60, and inoperable biliary atresia in children over the age of 1 year.

The selection and preparation of a patient for liver transplantation is an extremely important and difficult task. Sherlock (1972) has described the problems in detail, which in summary include general investigations with emphasis on assessment of liver function; methods of determining the hepatic vasculature and anatomy of the biliary system; tissue compatibility tests and control of hepatocellular failure.

The difficulties associated with anaesthesia have been discussed by Samuel (1972) and Farman et al. (1974). The latter report their experiences in a series of 27 orthoptic liver allografts. In summary they emphasise the effect of hepatic dysfunction on drug metabolism and conclude that a conventional technique using nitrous oxide, oxygen and pancuronium is best. Two particular problems arise, firstly, the rapid loss of blood that may occur in the initial stages of the operation, and secondly the fall of cardiac output that results from clamping of the inferior vena cava. Both may be corrected by blood transfusion. The donor liver releases cold acid perfusate which is rich in potassium. The effects of the latter on the myocardium can be reversed by intravenous calcium chloride while sodium bicarbonate will reverse the acidosis. In the post-operative period it is essential that good oxygenation is maintained and repeated examinations made for biochemical abnormalities.

REFERENCES

AHLGREN, I., ARONSEN, K.-F., ERICSSON, B., and FAJGELJ, A. (1967). Hepatic blood flow during different depths of halothane anaesthesia in the dog. *Acta anaesth. scand.*, **11**, 91.

ALADJEMOFF, L., DIKSTEIN, S., and SHAFRIR, E. (1958). The binding of *d*-tubocurarine chloride to plasma proteins. *J. Pharmacol. exp. Ther.*, **123**, 43.

BEARN, A. G., BILLING, B., and SHERLOCK, S. (1951). The effect of adrenaline and noradrenaline on hepatic blood flow and splanchnic carbohydrate metabolism in man. *J. Physiol. (Lond.)*, **115**, 430.

BLUMBERG, B. S., ALTER, H. J., and VISNICH, S. (1965). A "new" antigen in leukemia sera. *J. Amer. med. Ass.*, **191**, 541.

BRADLEY, S. E., INGLEFINGER, F. J., BRADLEY, G. P., and CURRY, J. J. (1945). The estimation of hepatic blood flow in man. *J. clin. Invest.*, **24**, 890.

CAESAR, J., SHALDON, S., CHIANDUSSI, L., GUEVARA, L., and SHERLOCK, S. (1961). The use of indocyanine green in the measurement of hepatic blood flow and as a test of hepatic function. *Clin. Sci.*, **21**, 43.

COOPERMAN, L. H. (1972). Effects of anaesthetics on the splanchnic circulation. *Brit. J. Anaesth.*, **44**, 967.

COOPERMAN, L. H., WARDEN, J. C., and PRICE, H. L. (1968). Splanchnic circulation during nitrous oxide anesthesia and hypocarbia in normal man. *Anesthesiology*, **29**, 254.

COWAN, R. E., JACKSON, B. T., and THOMPSON, R. P. H. (1975). The effects of various anaesthetics and abdominal surgery on liver blood flow in man. *Gut*, **16**, 839.

DAVIS, P., and HOLDSWORTH, G. (1973). Jaundice after multiple halothane anaesthetics administered during the treatment of carcinoma of the uterus. *Gut*, **14**, 566.

DYKES, M. H. M., GILBERT, J. P., and McPEEK, B. (1972). Halothane in the United States. An appraisal on the literature on "halothane hepatitis" and the American reaction to it. *Brit. J. Anaesth.*, **44**, 925.

DUNDEE, J. W., and GRAY, T. C. (1953). Resistance to *d*-tubocurarine chloride in the presence of liver damage. *Lancet*, **2**, 16.

EPSTEIN, M., BERK, D. P., HOLLENBERG, N. K., ADAMS, D. F., CHALMERS, T. C., ABRAMS, H. L., and MERRILL, J. P. (1970). Renal failure in the patient with cirrhosis. The role of active vasoconstriction. *Amer. J. Med.*, **49**, 175.

EPSTEIN, R. M., WHEELER, H. O., FRUMIN, M. J., HABIF, D. V., PAPPER, E. M., and BRADLEY, S. E. (1961). The effect of hypercapnia on estimated hepatic blood flow, circulating splanchnic blood volume, and hepatic sulfobromophthalein clearance during general anesthesia in man. *J. clin. Invest.*, **40**, 592.

FARMAN, J. V., LINES, J. G., WILLIAMS, R., EVANS, D. B., SAMUEL, J. R., MASON, S. A., ASHBY, B. S., and CALNE, R. Y. (1974). Liver transplantation in man. *Anaesthesia*, **29**, 17.

GRAUZ, H., and SCHMID, R. (1971). Reciprocal relation between plasma albumin level and hepatic sulfobromophthalein removal. *New Engl. J. Med.*, **284**, 1403.

HUGHES, M., and POWELL, L. W. (1970). Recurrent hepatitis in patients receiving multiple halothane anesthetics for radium treatment of carcinoma of the cervix uteri. *Gastroenterology*, **58**, 790.

INMAN, W. H., and MUSHIN, W. W. (1974). Jaundice after repeated exposure to halothane; an analysis of Reports to the Committee on Safety of Medicines. *Brit. med. J.*, **1**, 5.

JUHL, B., and EINER-JENSEN, N. (1974). Hepatic blood flow and cardiac output during halothane anesthesia: an animal study. *Acta anaesth. scand.*, **18**, 114.

KALOW, B., ROGOMAN, E., and SIMS, F. H. (1976). A comparison of the effects of halothane and other anaesthetic agents on hepato-cellular function in patients submitted to elective operations. *Canad. Anaesth. Soc. J.*, **23**, 71.

KAPLAN, J. A., BITNER, R. L., and DRIPPS, R. D. (1971). Hypoxia, hyperdynamic circulation, and the hazards of general anesthesia in patients with hepatic cirrhosis. *Anesthesiology*, **35**, 427.

KATZ, S. (1970). Hepatic coma associated with methoxyflurane anesthesia. *Amer. J. dig. Dis.*, **15**, 733.

KENNEDY, W. F., EVERETT, G. B., COBB, L. A., and ALLEN, G. D. (1970). Simultaneous systemic and hepatic hemodynamic measurements during high spinal anesthesia in normal man. *Anesth. Analg. Curr. Res.*, **49**, 1016.

KENNEDY, W. F., EVERETT, G. B., COBB, L. A., and ALLEN, G. D. (1971). Simultaneous systemic and hepatic hemodynamic measurements during high peridural anesthesia in normal man. *Anesth. Analg. Curr. Res.*, **50**, 1069.

KEW, M. C., BRUNT, P. W., VARMA, R. R., HOURIGAN, K. J., WILLIAMS, R., and SHERLOCK, S. (1971). Renal and intrarenal blood-flow in cirrhosis of the liver. *Lancet*, **2**, 504.

LAMONT, J. T., and ISSELBACHER, K. D. (1973). Postoperative jaundice. *New Engl. J. Med.*, **288**, 305.

LIEBERMAN, F. L. (1970). Functional renal failure in cirrhosis. *Gastroenterology*, **58**, 108.

MCPEEK, B., and GILBERT, J. P. (1974). Onset of post-operative jaundice related to anaesthetic history. *Brit. med. J.*, **3**, 615.

MEDICAL RESEARCH COUNCIL (1974). *Brit. med. J.*, **3**, 268.

NATIONAL HALOTHANE STUDY (Summary). (1966). *J. Amer. med. Ass.*, **197**, 775.

PRICE, H. L., DEUTSCH, S., COOPERMAN, L., CLEMENT, A. J., and EPSTEIN, R. M. (1965). Splanchnic circulation during cyclopropane anesthesia in normal man. *Anesthesiology*, **26**, 312.

PRICE, H. L., DEUTSCH, S., DAVIDSON, I. A., CLEMENT, A. J., BEHAR, M. G., and EPSTEIN, R. M. (1966). Can general anesthetics produce splanchnic visceral hypoxia by reducing regional blood flow? *Anesthesiology*, **27**, 24.

PRICE, H. L., and PAUCA, A. L. (1969). Effects of anesthesia on the peripheral circulation. *Clin. Anesth.*, **3**, 674.

PRYS-ROBERTS, C., KELMAN, G. R., GREENBAUM, R., KAIN, M. L., and BAY, J. (1968). Hemodynamics and alveolar-arterial Po_2 differences at varying $Paco_2$ in anesthetized man. *J. appl. Physiol.*, **25**, 80.

RUFF, F. (1971). Regional lung function in patients with hepatic cirrhosis. *J. clin. Invest.*, **50**, 2403.

SAMUEL, J. R. (1972). Anaesthesia for liver transplantation. In: *Anaesthesia in Organ Transplantation*. Basel: Karger.

SHACKMAN, R., GRABER, I. G., and MELROSE, D. G. (1953). Liver blood flow and general anaesthesia. *Clin. Sci.*, **12**, 307.

SHERLOCK, S. (1971). Halothane hepatitis. *Gut*, **12**, 324.

SHERLOCK, S. (1972). Selection and preparation of the patient for liver transplantation. In: *Anaesthesia in Organ Transplantation*, p. 32. Basel: Karger.

SHERLOCK, S. (1975). *Diseases of the Liver and Biliary System*, 5th edit. Oxford: Blackwell Scientific Publications.

SIMPSON, B. R., STRUNIN, L., and WALTON, B. (1973). Halothane hepatitis—fact or fallacy? *Proc. roy. Soc. Med.*, **66**, 56.

SIMPSON, B. R., STRUNIN, L., and WALTON, B. (1975b). Halothane and jaundice. *Brit. J. hosp. Med.*, **13**, 433.

SIMPSON, B. R., WALTON, B., and STRUNIN, L. (1975a). The halothane dilemma—three years on. *Proc. roy. Soc. Med.*, **68**, 769.

THOMPSON, T. M. (1976). Pancuronium binding of serum proteins. *Anaesthesia*, **31**, 219.

THORSHAUGE, C. (1970). Hepatic blood flow during anaesthesia. *Acta anaesth. scand.*, Suppl. **37**, 205.

TORRANCE, H. B. (1957). Liver blood flow during operations on the upper abdomen. *J. roy. Coll. Surg. Edinb.*, **2**, 216.

WATERSON, A. P. (1976). Hepatitis B as a hazard in anaesthetic practice. *Brit. J. Anaesth.*, **48**, 21.

WILLIAMS, R. (1970). Transplantation of the liver in man. *Brit. med. J.*, **1**, 585.

Chapter 39

ANAESTHESIA AND THE KIDNEY

ANATOMY

THE two kidneys lie retroperitoneally in the abdomen on either side of the vertebral column. Each weighs between 120 and 170 g normally and measures $12 \times 7 \times 3$ cm. In the cadaver the upper and the lower poles are at the level of the twelfth thoracic and third lumbar vertebrae respectively. The right kidney may lie slightly lower than the left due to the mass of the liver. During normal inspiration each kidney moves up and down over a distance of one vertebral body.

The anterior surface of each kidney bears important relationships to many intra-abdominal structures, the upper pole is closely attached to the adrenal gland, and the renal vessels and ureter join the hilum at its medial border. The kidney itself is covered in a fibrous capsule which may easily be removed, exposing a layer of smooth muscle fibres beneath. A cross-section of the kidney reveals the outer cortical and the inner medullary substance.

Vascular System

The main renal arteries pass directly from the abdominal aorta to the kidneys. After giving off small branches to the capsule and pelvis, each main artery then enters the hilum and divides into five segmental arteries which in turn divide into interlobar arteries as they run through the renal medulla towards the cortex. Each of the segmental arteries is an end artery which means that it does not anastomose with its neighbouring artery and if one should become occluded the segment of the kidney which it supplies will become infarcted. On reaching the point of junction between medulla and cortex at the base of the pyramids each interlobar artery divides into two, and in a T-shaped fashion each branch runs at right angles to the parent stem between cortex and medulla. These vessels give off important branches, the interlobular arteries. These run through the cortex giving off a large number of branches which pass directly to the glomeruli (the afferent glomerular arterioles) and finally terminate as perforating arteries which supply the surface of the kidney. Although the renal veins follow the same course as the arteries the larger veins anastomose freely through the arcuate veins.

Urinary System

Each individual renal tubule and its glomerulus is called a nephron and each adult kidney has approximately $1\frac{1}{2}$ million of these structures. The glomerulus consists of a mass of capillary vessels surrounded by the blind end of an expanded renal tubule called Bowman's capsule. This apparatus is concerned with the filtering of substances from the blood stream. Bowman's capsule leads to the proximal convoluted tubule, down the descending limb of the loop of Henle and bends sharply back as the ascending limb to become the distal convoluted tubule which finally drains into the collecting tubule. The function of this tubular system is both selective reabsorption and excretion so that the material that finally reaches the ureters is urine.

At the point where the distal tubule begins, it lies close to the arterioles which enter and leave its own glomerulus and is modified histologically being known as the macula densa. The area formed by these cells, the arterioles and the few cells lying between these structures is called the juxtaglomerular apparatus from which renin is secreted.

Nerve Supply

The kidney has a sympathetic supply which is derived from the 12th thoracic to the 2nd lumbar segments of the spinal cord. The adrenergic fibres enter the renal substance along the renal arteries and are predominantly vasoconstrictor in action being distributed to the afferent and efferent glomerular arteries. Nerve fibres have also been shown to terminate close to the cells of the juxtaglomerular apparatus. Cholinergic fibres have also been found in the kidney but their exact function is not known.

PHYSIOLOGY

Under normal resting conditions about 20–25 per cent of the total cardiac output passes through the renal circulation each minute. In other words, the two kidneys between them receive a blood flow of 1,100–1,200 ml/minute. Approximately half of this total consists of plasma and the rest is made up of cells. Although the distribution of blood flow to the glomeruli in different parts of the cortex may alter there do not appear to be any arteriovenous shunts present. However, not all the blood which enters the interlobular arteries in the cortex passes to the glomeruli since these arteries may emerge on the surface of the kidney and anastomose with the capsular vessels. In the glomerular capillaries the arterial pressure which is probably some 10–20 mm Hg (1·3–2·6 kPa) below the systemic pressure, tends to drive the fluid across the glomerular membrane being opposed by the osmotic pull of the proteins in the blood and the hydrostatic pressure in Bowman's capsule. Thus of the original total of about 1000 ml of blood that enters the kidneys every minute about 1/10th or 100 ml is filtered off and passed down the tubules. At this point the selective reabsorption mechanism plays a major role and almost all the fluid content passes back into the circulation again. Of each 100 ml of fluid entering the tubules, 99 ml is reabsorbed. Put in another way, this means that 1 ml of urine is formed from every 1,000 ml of blood that goes to the kidneys.

Glomerular Filtration

The glomerular membrane is permeable to both fluid and electrolytes, but not to protein or cells. In fact a small amount of protein does pass through even in the normal kidney but is reabsorbed in the proximal tubules. The driving force across this membrane is called the effective filtration pressure (EFP) and is calculated as the glomerular capillary pressure minus the sum of the osmotic pressure of the plasma proteins and the hydrostatic pressure in Bowman's capsule. In man this value has been estimated to be about 20 mm Hg (2·7 kPa) (Lambert et al., 1971). The fraction that passes across the glomerular membrane is normally about one-sixth of the renal plasma flow or one-tenth of the renal blood flow.

Thus:

If the renal blood flow is	1,200 ml/minute,
and the renal plasma flow is	750 ml/minute,
the total reaching the tubules is one-sixth of 750 ml/minute,	
i.e.	125 ml/minute.

There are a number of factors which influence the EFP which include the systemic blood pressure, alterations in the osmotic pressure of the plasma proteins and increase in the pressure within Bowman's capsule resulting from obstruction in the tubules lower down the nephron. While the kidney is able to maintain the glomerular capillary pressure at a constant level over a wide range of systemic pressures it is very vulnerable if the latter falls markedly. Clinically, it is known that in cases of severe hypotension during or immediately after surgery renal excretion ceases altogether, and this may be associated with signs of renal damage in the post-operative period.

In renal disease there is a close relationship between the severity of the damage and the number of functioning glomeruli, so that any further damage by anaesthetic agents or the like becomes of prime importance. The glomerular membrane itself is particularly susceptible to damage by hypoxia, ischaemia and drugs. Normally molecules with a weight of 69,000 or more cannot pass through the membrane while those of lower weight pass through with increasing ease as their size diminishes. For example, albumin, with a molecular weight of 69,000 is essentially impermeable to the membrane while, if present, free haemoglobin with a molecular weight of 68,000 passes through in appreciable quantities. Ischaemia of the glomerulus destroys this semi-permeability, hence the value of albumin in the urine as a guide to renal damage.

Tests of glomerular filtration.—In normal circumstances the glomeruli filter the plasma contents without showing any favours. Substances with large molecules pass across more slowly than those with small ones. The glomerular filtration rate is described as the amount of fluid passing from the capillaries in the glomerular tuft into the lumen every minute.

Precise measurements of GFR are not usually carried out because of the technical difficulties of the methods available, but reasonably accurate values may be obtained by determination of the "clearance" of a substance from the plasma. If a substance is completely filtered into Bowman's capsule from the glomerular capillaries and is neither absorbed nor excreted during its passage through the renal tubules then the volume of plasma which initially held the amount of substance excreted will be equal to the GFR.

The calculation is made from the following equation:

$$\frac{\text{Concentration of substance in urine} \times \text{volume of urine}}{\text{Concentration of substance in plasma}} = \text{clearance in ml/min}$$

1. *Inulin clearance.*—The most accurate method of assessing glomerular filtration rate is by the use of inulin, as this substance is filtered unchanged by the glomeruli but is not reabsorbed by the tubules. Despite this, such measurements are usually reserved for estimations requiring great accuracy, as the continuous infusion of inulin and the repeated blood sampling make this method unsuitable for routine clinical testing.

2. *Creatinine clearance.*—As creatinine is a normal constituent of the blood which is filtered rapidly by the glomeruli yet is not reabsorbed in the tubules, it has become a popular means of assessing glomerular function. Unfortunately a very small quantity is secreted by the tubules, but this can be taken into account in the final assessment. Fortunately the blood level of creatinine remains remarkably constant, so that a long period of study can be contemplated yet it is only necessary to measure the blood level once during this period. The concentration of creatinine is determined spectroscopically, based on the intensity of the orange colour produced in the sample by picric acid.

Details of test.—The patient first empties his bladder thoroughly and this specimen is discarded. A 24-hour save of all the urine passed is then commenced. Creatinine in the blood and in the urine is known, together with the total volume of urine passed during the period, hence the total quantity of glomerular filtrate can be calculated.

Although the creatinine clearance test is not quite as accurate as that with inulin (see below), its simplicity makes it much more convenient in routine clinical practice, and even with advanced renal disease the differences between inulin and creatinine clearances are not of clinical importance.

The normal value in an adult patient of the creatinine clearance (i.e. glomerular filtration rate) is approximately 120 ml/minute.

There is a wide variation of about $\pm$ 15 ml/minute, and as the age of the patient increases so the glomerular filtration rate declines steadily until by the time the age of 90 or over is reached, the rate has fallen by approximately 50 per cent to 60 ml/minute.

3. *Urea clearance.*—Like creatinine, urea is a normal constituent of the blood and therefore it is easy to measure the clearance simply by determining its blood and urine concentrations and measuring the total volume of urine passed. Since some of the urea that enters the tubules is reabsorbed into the circulation an allowance must be made for this and if the glomerular filtration rate is 120 ml/minute, then the urea clearance is 60 per cent of 120, or 75 ml/minute. Furthermore, the urea clearance is very dependant on the rate of urine flow and when the flow drops below 2 ml/minute the inaccuracies are considerable. Then a figure can only be calculated with the use of a complex formula and is sometimes referred to as the *standard urea clearance*, but in clinical practice it is rarely used. Under normal conditions of the test, the fluid intake of the patient is so adjusted that the total quantity of urine passed exceeds 2 ml/minute. The result may then be termed a *maximal* urea clearance. Although once popular this test is now very seldom used having been replaced by creatinine clearance or radio-isotope studies.

4. ^{51}Cr-*EDTA.*—Recently a number of substances have been introduced which have radio-active markers. Initially these included labelled forms of inulin but these tended to be expensive and relatively unstable. The most widely used alternative is ^{51}Cr-EDTA (ethylene diaminetetracetate) which is readily available and can be stored satisfactorily (Lingardh, 1972). This is filtered and passes through the renal tubule in exactly the same way as inulin. The usual calculation may be applied either by using a constant intravenous infusion or a single-shot technique in which the fall of plasma concentration of the gamma-emitting isotope, during a 2-hour period, is determined.

5. *Blood urea and creatinine levels.*—As both urea and creatinine clearance values are useful methods of assessing glomerular filtration rates, so the level of these substances in the blood gives some indication of renal function.

The normal blood values are:

Urea   15·0–40·0 mg per cent (2·5–6·7 mmol/l)
Creatinine   0·7–1·5 mg per cent (62–132 μmol/l)

A rise in blood urea is a relatively late sign of renal damage. Unfortunately, as both urea and creatinine are produced in the body their concentrations in the blood can be altered by other factors. For example the effect of high- and low-protein diets can be seen in Fig. 1. As GFR decreases the blood urea rises

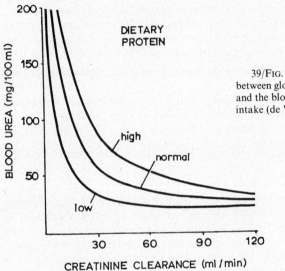

39/FIG. 1.—Schema of the relationship between glomerular rate (creatinine clearance) and the blood urea at varying levels of protein intake (de Wardener, 1973).

quite slowly and even a fall of 50 per cent in GFR will only result in a blood urea of 30 mg/100 ml (5 mmol/l) if a low-protein diet is being eaten, and this value is within the normal range for the population. Serum creatinine concentrations are less affected by dietary protein being in general proportional to the muscle mass so that a slightly raised serum level in a patient with a very small muscle mass may mask a severely decreased GFR.

6. *Proteinuria.*—The presence of significant quantities of protein in the urine denotes the presence of glomerular or tubular damage. Normally about 10–20 mg per cent of protein passes across the glomerular membrane, but almost the entire quantity is reabsorbed by the tubules. The method of detection of protein in the urine depends either on simple precipitation by boiling or by flocculation with 25 per cent salicyl sulphonic acid.

SALICYL SULPHONIC ACID TEST

Trace of precipitate—approximately equivalent to a concentration of 0·2 g protein/litre.

Heavy precipitate—approximately equivalent to a concentration of 5·0 g protein/litre.

The significance of a positive result to this test is influenced by the dilution of the urine. Thus a positive response in a very concentrated urine is of less importance than the same result in a dilute one. Macroscopic blood or pus will be responsible for some precipitate and care should be taken to avoid this error.

The exact type of proteins excreted is sometimes of significance in diagnosis of the underlying renal disease. Thus electrophoretic separation can be used to distinguish between albumin and globulin. In acute nephritis both protein types are excreted in the same proportions as in the plasma, whereas in myelomatosis a protein of low molecular weight (22,000) may appear with albuminuria (de Wardener, 1973).

7. *Blood cells and casts.*—Small amounts of blood cells (red and white) and hyaline casts may be found in the urine of normal subjects. Nevertheless, if a 4-hour save of urine is taken and the phosphates in it precipitated by glacial acetic acid, then when the resultant fluid has been centrifuged, the number of cells recognised microscopically in a counting chamber can be determined:

Normal urine contains 50,000 cells, with a range of 0–200,000 white cells per hour.

Abnormal urine contains over 200,000 white cells per hour (de Wardener, 1973), and the rate of excretion of red cells is approximately the same.

The only casts that are of any clinical importance are the blood and granular types and both these denote renal damage.

Tubular Reabsorption

The contents of the glomerular filtrate are identical with that of the plasma lying across the glomerular membrane inside the tuft of capillaries. But although this liquid starts out on its journey through the tubular system resembling plasma, by the time it reaches the end it bears no relation to it at all. On its way down, enormous quantities of water and certain electrolytes are reabsorbed. This process is selective, so that the kidney tubules play an important part in controlling the electrolyte balance of the body. For example, for every 100 litres of water that enters the tubules less than 1 litre reaches the urine. Reabsorption may be either an active process requiring energy or a passive process which depends on diffusion along a concentration gradient. A single substance may be reabsorbed by both processes in different parts of the nephron. Substances which are actively absorbed include calcium, amino acids and uric acid. There are specific mechanisms controlling the reabsorption of salts and water. In the latter case the water content of the body is controlled through the antidiuretic hormone of the posterior pituitary, and it is well known that nearly all anaesthetic drugs stimulate the release of this substance. Adrenal corticoid excretion controls sodium and chloride levels and again this would appear to be slightly stimulated by anaesthetic drugs.

Tubular Secretion

The secretion of substances into the tubular lumen may also be either active or passive. In man active secretion appears to be limited to a number of steroid metabolites while potassium and urea are examples of passive secretion.

Tests of tubular function.—As the role of the tubules is largely one of selective reabsorption, most of the tests are based on the concentration of solids in the urine. Similarly, as the primary function of the tubules is to withdraw most of the water from its lumen, the ability to pass a concentrated or dilute urine under different conditions can be used as a gauge of tubular activity.

(i) *Urine concentration test.*—The specific gravity of the urine can be measured with a hydrometer. Normally, the range lies between 1003–1030 depending on the fluid intake. In diabetes, when large quantities of glucose are reaching the urine, the specific gravity is high, whereas tubular damage leads to a very dilute urine.

The ability of the kidney to concentrate urine may be studied in two ways: (*a*) complete abstinence from fluids for a 24-hour period has been used. This method is extremely unpleasant for the patient. A normal kidney should produce one specimen during this period with a specific gravity of 1,020 or more. (*b*) An intramuscular injection of pitressin tannate (5 mg) in oil is found to be a much more satisfactory alternative because it does not interfere with the patient's normal fluid intake. The action of the pitressin is to inhibit diuresis, so again a 24-hour urine save is instituted. The patient is allowed to eat and drink in a normal manner. One sample during this period should have a specific gravity of 1,020 or more if normal tubular function is present.

(ii) *Urine dilution test.*—For this test the patient consumes a known quantity of water (1 litre) and the ability of the kidney to excrete most of this intake is then studied. First the bladder is emptied and the contents discarded in the usual manner. Samples are then taken hourly for the next four hours. Normally at least 750 ml out of the 1 litre drunk by the patient should be recovered in the urine and the specific gravity will be less than 1,004 in at least one specimen. Smoking and extreme emotion, however, may limit the diuresis.

Other methods that are used to study tubular function are more complex and involve the measurement of sodium, potassium, calcium, phosphate, and ammonium excretion.

MEASUREMENT OF RENAL BLOOD FLOW (RBF)

The renal blood flow is the total quantity of blood passing to both kidneys each minute. In order to measure this amount of blood it is necessary to find a substance which is completely removed from the plasma during a single passage through the glomerular tuft yet is neither reabsorbed nor excreted by the tubules. Then the plasma flow can be measured, and from this the blood flow to the kidney can be calculated. Diodrast and para-amino-hippuric acid (PAH) nearly fulfil these criteria, but PAH is technically easier to use. In fact only 90 per cent of it passes across the membrane and the remaining 10 per cent recirculates. Nevertheless allowances can be made for this fraction in the final calculation. The exact proportion of PAH that is removed by a normal kidney has been confirmed in patients by simultaneous sampling of the concentration in the renal artery and vein during a steady infusion. Theoretically, if this substance was completely removed the concentration in the renal vein would be nil. In practice is was found that a small percentage (10 per cent) eluded filtration. Thus, measurements using PAH give an estimation of the "effective" renal plasma flow (ERPF) and this is converted to the true renal plasma flow by multiplying the results obtained by 1·1. ·

Measurement of renal plasma flow is made by first giving the patient a priming dose of PAH followed by an infusion of it given at a rate which just compensates for its loss in the urine. In these circumstances the concentration of PAH in the peripheral venous plasma is essentially the same as that in the arterial plasma of the glomerular capillaries, so that venous samples may be used in the estimation.

Thus:

PAH clearance $\times 1\cdot 1 =$ Renal plasma flow in ml/minute.

The plasma flow can be converted to blood flow if the value for the haematocrit is known:

$$\text{RBF} = 1,100\text{--}1,200 \text{ ml/minute.}$$

In renal disease the extraction of PAH may well be lower than the normal value of 90 per cent and unless the renal vein is catheterised at the same time an accurate value for RBF cannot be calculated. More commonly ^{125}I-Hippuran and ^{131}I-Hippuran are now used instead of PAH. A single shot of the substance is given and the rate at which it disappears from the plasma measured. It is usual to estimate ERPF and GFR simultaneously using ^{131}I-Hippuran and ^{51}Cr-EDTA.

RENAL BLOOD FLOW IN THE CONSCIOUS PATIENT

In normal circumstances the flow through the renal vessels does not vary widely. This constancy is maintained largely by alteration in the calibre of the renal arterioles. The kidney has its own "regulating" mechanism which ensures that it receives as adequate a supply of blood as possible despite variations in the systemic pressure. The range of mean systemic pressures over which auto-regulation acts has been shown to be 70–200 mm Hg (9·3–26·7 kPa) in the dog (Hatch, 1969). There are many factors which can reduce the renal blood flow in a conscious patient and prominent amongst them are haemorrhage, fainting, asphyxia and cardiac failure.

The mechanism by which these various conditions reduce the renal blood flow is not the same in each case.

(a) *In hypovolaemia*, as is evidenced by haemorrhage, the mechanism is complex. In man there is a profound fall in renal blood flow and glomerular filtration. This fall is out of all proportion to the drop in blood pressure and is caused by severe renal vasoconstriction. One of the principal features of this condition is that even if the patient is thoroughly transfused and the blood volume and pressure returned to normal levels, the vasoconstriction does not wear off for several hours (Lauson *et al.*, 1944).

The cause of this vasoconstriction has been thoroughly investigated and is now believed to be one of two factors—one nervous, the other humoral. Following severe haemorrhage with renal ischaemia, transfusion will slowly reverse the vasoconstriction if it is given within the first four hours. During this period the vasoconstriction is believed to be nervous in origin.

After four hours of renal ischaemia produced by hypotension the vasoconstriction may take many days to pass off even after suitable transfusion therapy; alternatively it may be irreversible. This persistent vasoconstriction is thought to be humoral in origin. Various substances have been suggested, and the most likely is renin (Wright, 1965).

(*b*) *In the faint reaction*, there is essentially a slowing of the heart rate with marked peripheral vasodilatation. The cardiac output falls and the renal blood flow is reduced.

(*c*) *A high concentration of carbon dioxide or a low oxygen tension* in the blood reaching the kidneys causes the renal vessels to constrict. The latter response is induced reflexly through the sympathetic nervous system from stimulation of the carotid chemoreceptors and is markedly increased if the hypoxia is associated with a fall in systemic blood pressure which will also stimulate the carotid baroreceptors (Pelletier and Shepherd, 1975).

(*d*) *In denervation*, as in autonomic block due to spinal analgesia or to the use of ganglion-blocking drugs, the renal vessels are dilated and the renal flow closely follows any changes in the systemic blood pressure. If the pressure remains unchanged the renal flow will do likewise: if it falls, so will the flow through the kidney. The decrease in GFR is parallel to the fall in mean arterial pressure. The ERPF falls slightly less than the GFR suggesting that the decrease in renal vascular resistance is greater in the post-glomerular capillary bed (Kennedy *et al.*, 1970).

RENAL BLOOD FLOW IN THE ANAESTHETISED PATIENT

Effect of Anaesthesia

It would appear that all general anaesthetic agents commonly employed cause a decrease in renal blood flow to a greater or lesser extent. The degree of depression of the flow will depend upon the depth of anaesthesia. Thus, under very light anaesthesia the flow will be about 800 ml/minute (*cf* conscious = 1,200 ml/minute), but under deep anaesthesia it falls to 200 ml/minute or even less. So fine and rapid is this change in flow in relation to alterations in the depth of anaesthesia with both ether and cyclopropane, that the renal blood flow could easily be used as an accurate sign of anaesthetic depth. During a long operation with a constant level of anaesthesia the flow remains unaltered, and as soon as the anaesthetic is withdrawn the blood flow starts to return to normal. Thus in lightly anaesthetised patients the fall will be moderate, while in those in whom the alpha-blocking agents (for example, droperidol) are used in conjunction with a balanced anaesthetic technique no significant alteration in renal blood flow may occur (Gorman and Craythorne, 1966).

The mechanism of this reduction in flow has been studied in animals (Miles and de Wardener, 1952) using ether and cyclopropane. Dogs were anaesthetised by a continuous intravenous infusion of pentobarbitone sodium, which produces little change in the renal circulation. The kidney was then perfused with a constant volume pump. The inhalation of ether and cyclopropane resulted in a pronounced and sustained rise in the perfusion pressure. Since this effect no longer occurred after denervation of the kidney it was concluded that the fall in blood flow was due to neurogenic vasoconstriction. Halothane, like most other general anaesthetic agents, brings about a fall in renal blood flow in premedicated patients (Mazze *et al.*, 1963). However, at comparable depths of anaesthesia the reduction with cyclopropane and ether is greater than that with halothane. This could be explained on the basis that halothane produces less catecholamine excretion (leading to renal vasoconstriction) than either ether or cyclopropane.

Methoxyflurane produces a decrease in renal blood flow (RBF) by two different mechanisms. Firstly it modifies autoregulation so that RBF is directly dependent on the systemic pressure and secondly it depresses RBF by a separate mechanism which is pressure independent (Leighton *et al.*, 1973).

Effect of Surgery

Habif and his co-workers (1951) have shown that most operative procedures do not produce any change in the renal circulation. de Wardener (1955) has confirmed these findings, but referred to one case where severe traction upon the large bowel had produced temporary vasoconstriction. Since there is considerable difficulty in obtaining adequate data on patients undergoing major surgery, it would at present seem advisable to conclude that major surgical stimulation—particularly under very light anaesthesia—may lead to depression of renal blood flow.

Effect of Ganglion-blocking Drugs

Since the introduction of the hypotensive technique many authors have strongly condemned this method of reducing bleeding during surgery, on the grounds that it leads to increased damage to the kidney. It is difficult to gather from a simple comparative study of patients under anaesthesia with and without hypotension whether any renal damage occurs. Hampton and Little (1953) stated that the incidence of renal complications following the use of hypotensive drugs during anaesthesia was no greater than in a comparable control series. Evans and Enderby (1952) in a similar study based upon fluid excretion, proteinuria and the appearance of casts and red cells in the urine found, in a small series of 50 patients, that although the incidence of damage was slightly greater in the hypotensive group it was statistically insignificant. Miles and his colleagues (1952) produced valuable evidence by measuring the renal blood flow and glomerular filtration rate of patients undergoing hypotension without surgery. They used pentamethonium bromide and found in a series of 10 patients that although the systemic pressure fell by an average of 34 per cent, the average fall in the renal blood flow was only 5 per cent. In one of their cases the mean blood pressure fell below 40 mm Hg (5·3 kPa) yet the renal blood flow—though depressed—was still greater than they had found under deep anaesthesia in the absence of ganglion-blocking drugs.

From these observations it is concluded that renal vasodilatation must occur in the presence of hypotensive anaesthesia due to ganglion-blocking drugs. The experimental evidence available suggests that as the systemic pressure falls, so the renal vessels dilate to keep an almost steady flow of blood. On this basis it can be said that the normal kidney does not suffer damage from relatively short periods of hypotensive anaesthesia. It must be emphasised, however, that no data are available for very long periods of hypotension or the pathological kidney.

Moyer and McConn (1956), in a group of anaesthetised patients receiving pentamethonium, hexamethonium, and trimetaphan, were unable to confirm these results obtained by Miles and his colleagues. In their patients the fall in blood pressure was followed by a reduction in the renal blood flow and the glomerular filtration rate in both normal and hypertensive patients. Associated with the fall in glomerular filtration rate was a marked reduction in the excretion of water and sodium. This was so great that they emphasised the dangers of overloading such a patient with fluids. Wakim (1955), using a flow meter inserted into the renal vein of dogs, also found a fall in their renal blood flow during hypotension with hexamethonium.

This evidence completely contradicts that of Miles and his colleagues (1952), but on close scrutiny of the figures the actual reduction in blood flow is not very great. Most significant of all, little or no mention is made by Moyer and McConn of steps taken to prevent any fluctuation in depth of anaesthesia or to prevent a rise in the carbon dioxide tension of the blood. Since the smallest change in anaesthetic depth or carbon dioxide tension is sufficient to produce marked changes in the renal blood flow, variations in either of these measurements may account for the fundamental differences in these results.

Effect of Haemorrhage

On purely theoretical grounds it might be reasoned that the renal vessels would constrict in the presence of increasing blood loss. de Wardener and his associates (1953) have shown that this is not the case. In the anaesthetised subject the renal vessels dilate as the systemic pressure falls, so that they maintain an even flow of blood to the renal tissue despite the obvious paucity of flow in other parts of the body.

In their study these investigators measured the cardiac output, right auricular pressure, forearm blood flow, systemic pressure, heart rate, glomerular filtration and renal blood flow in a series of patients under light anaesthesia. The anaesthetic agents used were ether and cyclopropane. Haemorrhage was produced by venesection in amounts varying from 800–1,500 ml at a rate of 70–200 ml/minute. In the whole group the average fall in the estimated blood volume was 23 per cent. The only frequent change that they observed was a small reduction in renal flow during the actual venesection, but this rapidly returned to the previous level after the bleeding was completed. In twelve out of their fourteen patients venesection produced no *significant* change in the renal blood flow. In the two remaining patients the blood pressure fell to such a low level (below 40 mm Hg; 5·3 kPa) that the flow of urine ceased. When it started again the data available suggested, however, that the renal blood flow had continued during the period of anuria and that this flow had been reduced far less than would have been expected. The severe hypotension and bradycardia that occurred in these two patients was corrected immediately by rapid transfusion.

There are two important facts that emerge from this work on haemorrhage in the anaesthetised patient. First, the normal kidney does not apparently suffer acute ischaemia from severe hypotension under anaesthesia, and any reduction in flow that may occur can quickly be restored by transfusion therapy. Secondly, it is possible for the normal anaesthetised patient to lose up to 25–30 per cent of his total circulating blood volume without showing any significant changes in blood pressure or heart rate. This finding is of particular importance in any discussion upon the aetiology of post-operative renal failure.

In man, complete renal ischaemia lasting longer than 30 minutes is usually followed by tubular damage and such an event is most likely to occur during the removal of an aortic aneurysm. This damage can be largely prevented by hypothermia; periods of up to two hours of total occlusion with only minor signs of renal damage at a body temperature of 28° C have been reported (Churchill-Davidson, 1955).

Auto-regulating mechanism.—In the conscious subject even a relatively small haemorrhage is followed by a vasovagal attack where the blood pressure falls largely due to widespread dilatation of the muscle vessels. At the same time the renal vessels dilate (de Wardener and McSwiney, 1951). Under anaesthesia, even after a relatively massive haemorrhage, the renal vessels still dilate, but now the muscle vessels are found to be constricted. It was originally thought that the renal dilatation that occurred on fainting might be part of a widespread neurogenic vasodilating mechanism. The finding that under anaesthesia the muscle vessels constrict whilst the renal vessels dilate supports, however, the concept that the kidney has its own auto-regulating mechanism which tends to maintain an even level of renal blood flow despite alterations in the cardiac output and systemic pressure. The presence of such an intrinsic mechanism has been confirmed in animals (de Wardener and Miles, 1952). Phillips and his associates (1945), working with dogs, also commented upon the relative stability of the renal circulation after haemorrhage, and they stated "the kidneys appear now to be favoured at the expense of the other peripheral circulation". Severe renal vasoconstriction occurred, however, after 4 to 6 hours of oligaemia.

Therefore, on the basis of all this evidence, it seems improbable that a transient reduction in blood volume, as may occur during surgery, can be responsible for the ischaemic renal damage that occasionally follows operations. Nevertheless, it is important to stress that all these measurements were made upon people with good kidney function and these deductions certainly do not hold when severe renal disease is already present.

Effect of Vasopressor Drugs

When hypotension develops during anaesthesia a vasopressor drug is often used to restore the systemic pressure to a normal level. Two assumptions are usually made when considering the injection of these drugs. First, that the low blood pressure is necessarily associated with a reduced flow to the vital organs, and secondly, that raising the blood pressure by pressor drugs will automatically improve the flow. When considering the kidney both these assumptions may be unwarranted.

In the conscious patient, raising the blood pressure either with adrenaline (Smith, 1943) or noradrenaline (Barnett *et al.*, 1950) is associated with a pronounced renal vasoconstriction and fall in renal blood flow.

In the anaesthetised patient, the action of adrenaline, noradrenaline and methylamphetamine upon the renal blood flow have been studied (Churchill-Davidson *et al.*, 1951). These pressor drugs were given to both a group of patients with a normal blood pressure and a group with induced hypotension produced by pentamethonium bromide. The effect of the drugs upon the renal vessels was essentially the same, whether a low blood pressure was present or not. Adrenaline and noradrenaline both produced a rise in blood pressure accompanied by a consistent fall in the renal blood flow. On the other hand, methylamphetamine led to a rise in blood pressure and an overall increase in renal blood flow. No information is available about the action of these drugs upon the renal circulation in cases of hypotension due to haemorrhage. Moyer and

McConn (1956) studied the effects of vasopressor drugs on a group of hypertensive patients. Their results showed an increase in renal flow when the blood pressure was raised by noradrenaline after an injection of pentamethonium.

Dopamine possesses a selective renal vasodilatory action and also has positive inotropic cardiac activity. It, therefore, might be considered the most suitable agent for use in the presence of poor renal perfusion (see page 669). If, however, the latter was mainly due to reduced cardiac output then isoprenaline (with its stronger inotropic action) might be preferable.

RENAL FAILURE IN RELATION TO ANAESTHESIA AND SURGERY

Following major surgery it is commonplace to find traces of albumin, red cells and casts in the urine during the first three post-operative days. In fact, Evans and Enderby (1952) found that 78 per cent of a small series of normal patients developed proteinuria on the day after operation and in 34 per cent this persisted for more than three days. Cases of severe renal damage are fortunately rare, but when they occur they are often attended by a fatal result. The clinical picture of post-operative renal damage may be classed as either mild or severe.

In the mild condition the patient passes a plentiful supply of water in the first few days after operation. If it were accurately measured a polyuria would be noticed. Around the 7th–10th day the patient becomes mentally difficult or drowsy, and it is this change in the patient's mental attitude that often draws attention to the underlying condition. A blood urea taken at this stage reveals a level of 250 mg (41·7 mmol/l) or more. In all probability these patients had underlying renal damage before operation and a careful history usually reveals that they had polyuria at the same time. This can most easily be ascertained by a history of rising in the night to pass water with the absence of any prostatic enlargement on examination.

The severe type is the commoner condition and usually oliguria or anuria are noticed on the first post-operative day. Anuria is exceptional. The blood urea shows a steadily rising value and the rate of this rise is often taken as an indication of the severity of the condition. Vomiting and diarrhoea are early signs, together with restlessness, a wandering mind, and severe headache. Insomnia may be a marked feature and in the later stages muscle twitches and cramps may occur.

Causative Factor

Many factors have been blamed in the past, but at the present time the general opinion favours a prolonged period of hypotension leading to renal ischaemia as the principal cause. Anaesthesia, surgery, and even haemorrhage hardly affect the normal kidney, but then it is rare for the patient with normal kidney function to suffer failure post-operatively. During major surgery, particularly on the heart, a period of severe hypotension may occur. The resulting hypoxia of the renal cells is believed to lead to damage which is only revealed during the post-operative period. In the immediate post-operative period, when consciousness has been regained, a low blood volume state—as occurs after blood loss—is the most likely cause of intense renal vasoconstriction. Experimental data have shown that it is possible for a patient under light anaesthesia to lose 25 per cent of his blood volume without obvious circulatory signs. When consciousness has been regained, however, a hypovolaemia of this extent may be sufficient to cause intense renal vasoconstriction while producing only a slight fall in blood pressure.

Under normal circumstances the renal blood flow in the conscious patient remains remarkably constant despite considerable fluctuations in the perfusion pressure. This intimate control is believed to be exerted through neural and hormonal influences as part of the homeostatic mechanism controlling the extracellular fluid volume. In severe haemorrhage there is an immediate increase in intrarenal vascular resistance, presumably due to vasoconstriction (Parsons *et al.*, 1963). In turn, this leads to a decrease in renal blood flow, a fall in the amount of sodium and water excreted and possibly a reduction in glomerular filtration rate. These changes, which are at first reversible but eventually lead to tubular damage, are more severe in those patients with pre-existing renal disease.

The induction of general anaesthesia causes a fall in the renal blood flow which is roughly proportional to the depth of anaesthesia. The exact mechanism of renal ischaemia in the surgical patient is still unknown but it is probably similar to that in the conscious state. The most widely held view is that cellular damage takes place either during or immediately after a period of hypotension. On the re-establishment of a normal blood flow these cells either recover completely or their permeability is damaged so that they swell with oedema and partially or totally occlude the lumen of the tubule. This theory is the basis for the use of mannitol in the prophylactic treatment of suspected cases of renal damage. As mannitol is excreted virtually unchanged it is presumed that a hypertonic solution not only tends to keep the lumen of the tubules patent but may also withdraw some of the water from the tubule cells, thus diminishing the effects of the oedema (Flores *et al.*, 1972).

Evidence to support the hypotensive theory of post-operative renal failure is mostly clinical. Certainly oliguria and anuria are very rare complications in patients undergoing routine minor surgery with general anaesthesia. Yet in major surgery—particularly in association with the extracorporeal circulation with a poor total perfusion—the signs of renal damage are frequently observed.

Diagnosis

The first indication of renal damage in the post-operative period is oliguria. This is a term used to denote a total urinary output in twenty-four hours of less than 500 ml. Nevertheless, oliguria in the post-operative period is not always due to renal failure for it is commonly brought about by dehydration. This form of renal failure is often referred to as "pre-renal" and if not treated will progress to true renal failure. If a patient's fluid intake by mouth is curtailed or abandoned for many hours before operation, yet the "insensible" loss of sweating, humidification and alimentary secretions continues, it is not surprising that dehydration rapidly occurs. The "insensible" loss is usually estimated at about 1 litre per 24 hours. To this must be added any haemorrhage at the time of operation together with the extrusion of fluid into the lumen of bowel during surgical manipulations. If adequate precautions are not taken to maintain the circulating fluid volume by infusion then dehydration will result. This will lead to haemoconcentration with a raised haematocrit and haemoglobin level.

In attempting to differentiate between oliguria due to dehydration and that due to intrinsic renal failure, the determination of two ratios are of greatest value, namely the urine/plasma ratio of urea and osmolality.

In the dehydrated group a high urine/plasma osmolality ratio greater than 1·8–2·0 and a urine/plasma urea ratio greater than 20 are usually found while in those patients with established renal failure values of these ratios are less than 1·15 and less than 10 respectively (Luke et al., 1970). The distinction is not however cast-iron and between the two groups fall those with intermediate values who may well respond to the institution of a forced diuresis with either mannitol or diuretics. Contrast radiography may also be invaluable as it may show the presence of treatable extrarenal obstruction.

In a clinical situation it is often difficult to differentiate between oliguria due to a low circulating blood-volume and oliguria due to renal damage. The administration of 25 g of mannitol (i.e. 250 ml of 10 per cent solution) should rapidly produce a diuresis in the low blood-volume state whereas it will have little effect in the presence of renal damage. Such a low dose should not significantly overload the circulation.

Treatment

In patients with pre-renal failure any deficit in blood volume should be rapidly corrected. Alpha-adrenergic blocking drugs have been used to overcome the intense renal vasoconstriction and thus restore renal output (Fromm and Wilson, 1969). Metabolic acidosis, if present, should be corrected by administration of bicarbonate because it increases renal vasoconstriction (Zimmerman, 1969).

If this treatment fails to restore urine output and the urine/plasma osmolality and urea ratios are greater than 10 and 1·15 respectively, a diuretic and/or mannitol should be given. The amount of mannitol should not exceed 25 g (i.e. 250 ml of 10 per cent solution) given in a single dose (Luke and Kennedy, 1967). If greater than this dose is given, it can cause over-expansion of the blood volume with pulmonary oedema, red cell damage and hyponatremia (Morgan et al., 1968). In the presence of incipient circulatory overload diuretics may be particularly valuable. Ethacrynic acid may produce deafness but 200–400 mg frusemide can be used satisfactorily.

A patient with severe, acute post-operative renal failure rarely survives for more than ten days unless effective treatment is employed quickly. In the less severe type of case which responds fairly rapidly to therapy the oliguria gives way to polyuria.

The basic principle, therefore, of any treatment of this condition is twofold. First, since the cells of the collecting tubules are damaged, the fluid intake of the patient must be kept as nearly as possible equal to the fluid output. This latter figure must take into account any insensible loss from sweating, vomiting and diarrhoea, besides any small amount of urine that is passed. Secondly, the diet must be so arranged that protein metabolism is kept as low as possible, because the waste products of nitrogen metabolism soon mount to toxic levels. In normal subjects it is known that a carbohydrate intake of 100 g depresses protein metabolism and it is assumed that the same process takes place under the conditions of acute renal failure.

The present-day management of patients with early post-operative renal failure is based on a strict surveillance of body weight and the biochemical changes in both blood and urine.

Preliminary measures.—1. The *weight* of the patient is accurately determined, as this will give an indication of gain or loss of fluids in the future treatment.

2. *Biochemical data* are also obtained as a baseline for the effectiveness of the therapy. The measurements made are:

(*a*) Blood. Values for urea, calcium, potassium, sodium, chloride and bicarbonate are obtained. The haematocrit is also measured.

(*b*) Urine. Values for urea, sodium and potassium are estimated.

3. *An indwelling catheter* is inserted into the bladder so that a close watch can be kept on the exact amount of urine that is excreted.

4. *Restriction of fluids.*—The vital importance of the water obtained from metabolism within the body must be remembered. This sum amounts to approximately 600 ml daily. The total fluid required for a perfect balance of fluid therapy is composed of the sum of fluid lost by "sensible" and "insensible" loss. The "sensible" loss is the fluid which leaves the body either as urine or vomit. The "insensible" is the amount of fluid used up in sweating, humidification of the air in the lungs, and secretions into the bowel lumen which are lost in the faeces, and is usually taken as 1 litre per day. Thus a patient's fluid requirements will be 400 ml of sugar solution which together with the 600 ml produced within the body will provide for the 1,000 ml lost from "insensible" sources. To this total intake must also be added exactly the amount lost through urinary excretion and vomit.

The basis for restricted fluid therapy in acute renal failure can be expressed as:

$$
\begin{array}{ll}
\text{Insensible} & 400 \text{ ml of sugar solution} \\
\text{loss (1,000 ml)} & + \ 450 \text{ ml from tissue metabolism} \\
+ \quad = & + \ 150 \text{ ml from carbohydrate metabolism} \\
\text{sensible loss} & + \text{ sensible loss (urine or vomit)}
\end{array}
\left. \begin{array}{l} \\ \\ \end{array} \right\} = \begin{array}{l} 600 \text{ ml from} \\ \text{body} \\ \text{metabolism} \end{array}
$$

In this way fluid intake and output can be finely balanced. However, a small steady weight loss of 200–500 g daily will occur when a balance has been achieved, presumably due to a loss of body proteins.

Further measures.—1. *Carbohydrate* in the form of laevulose is most commonly used because not only is the sugar more easily metabolised than the others but it is also believed to be the least nauseating when given by mouth in high concentration. Normally 100 g of laevulose are added to 400 ml of water, and this can be taken orally. If vomiting occurs as a complication, then a sterile solution of fructose can be infused into a large vein. As high concentrations of sugar solutions produce a severe reaction with thrombosis in small veins, it is advisable to insert a polythene catheter into the lumen of the vena cava (inferior or superior) before starting the infusion. Nevertheless the oral route is preferable because of the risk of infected emboli from the use of intravenous catheters.

2. *Anabolic steroids* (i.e. testosterone) are given to reduce the breakdown of protein within the body.

3. *Antibiotics* and *anticoagulants* must only be used with caution as many tend to accumulate in the circulation if renal function is poor. For example, streptomycin is contra-indicated in such circumstances as even small doses may lead to VIIIth cranial nerve damage. Similarly, the sulphonamides should not be used as they tend to form crystals in the renal tubules, thus increasing the renal damage. Crystalline and the various oral penicillins have been found to be satisfactory.

Most of the long-acting anticoagulants (e.g. dicoumarin) tend to accumulate in the presence of renal failure but heparin can be used with safety because it is detoxicated in the liver.

4. *Ion-exchange resins* can be used to control the serum potassium level which tends to rise steadily in the presence of acute renal failure. These resins are in powder form and can be given either orally or rectally. They act by accepting potassium and releasing sodium in exchange. Using Resonium 15 g four times a day, it is often possible to keep the serum potassium level between 3·5 and 4·0 mEq/litre (mmol/l). Alternatively in an emergency the administration of glucose (40 g) and insulin (20 units) tends to lower the serum potassium level by holding the electrolyte within the cell and also actively promoting its uptake by the cell.

Once this regime has been fully established it is then only necessary to observe closely the effects of this therapy. The future progress will reveal the extent and severity of the renal damage. If it is clear that restriction of fluids alone is not preventing a gradual deterioration in the patient's state then the question of dialysis must be considered.

Indications for dialysis are:

(a) Worsening of the clinical state of the patient—particularly the appearance of pre-uraemic features together with mental retardation.

(b) Blood urea nitrogen (BUN) over 150–170 mg per cent (25–28 mmol/l) or a blood urea over 300 mg per cent (50 mmol/l/).

(c) A rise in the serum potassium level over 7·0 mEq/litre (mmol/l).

(d) A fall in the plasma bicarbonate to 12 mEq/litre (mmol/l) or below.

Dialysis.—There are two principal methods of trying to remove the waste products of metabolism from the circulation in the presence of poor renal function.

(a) *Peritoneal dialysis* necessitates the introduction of a large volume of fluid of known composition into the peritoneal cavity. Those electrolytes and nitrogenous substances which are in excess in the circulation can then diffuse out into the fluid and so finally be removed. This technique requires an intra-peritoneal catheter with numerous fine holes in the terminal 4 cm. The tubing is inserted under local analgesia about one-third of the way along a line drawn from the umbilicus to the pubic symphysis; 2·5 litres of either an isotonic (if the patient is not overloaded already with water) or hypertonic (if waterlogged) solution are run in and left *in situ* for about 40 minutes, after which it is all drained out again. Antibiotics and heparin are added to the solution to prevent infection and the formation of fibrin clots. The whole technique is simple and effective in mild or moderate cases. It can be repeated frequently without much trouble. The only disadvantage is that it removes the plasma proteins and also exposes the patient to the risk of infection.

(*b*) *Haemodialysis* is based on the principle of passing the blood through semi-permeable Cellophane tubing in its passage from an artery to a vein. The tubing or membrane is surrounded by a solution of known concentration so that during the passage of the blood the electrolytes and other waste products can diffuse out. Such an apparatus is often described as an "artificial kidney". The development of these machines has now progressed to a stage where it is perfectly feasible to keep a patient alive indefinitely without renal function provided his blood is dialysed at least twice weekly.

Histological Findings in a Fatal Case of Post-operative Renal Failure

The glomerular membrane is less sensitive to hypoxia and ischaemia than is the tubular system, so that it is not surprising that the latter structures suffer most in cases of acute post-operative renal failure. The distal convoluted tubules show dilatation with flattening of the epithelium, and pigmented casts may be found in the lumen of these tubules and also that of the loop of Henle and the collecting tubule (Brun and Munck, 1957). Necrosis of the tubules is not a common finding in this condition, but the cells of the tubules show cellular infiltration and oedema. The anuria or oliguria is clearly not due to any damage to the glomerular apparatus but rather to alteration in the function of the tubules. Biopsy specimens have failed to confirm that swelling of the tubules occurs and blocks the flow of urine. The most acceptable explanation is that the tubules lose their semi-permeability and almost all the water passing down the lumen is reabsorbed.

KIDNEY TRANSPLANTATION

For many years it has been established that in man tissues can easily be transferred from one region of the body to another, yet great difficulty is experienced if an attempt is made to transfer this same tissue to another person. This failure to accept the tissues of other human beings is due to the immune response. A significant advance in our knowledge of the mechanism of this response has been made by the contributions of Medawar (1958) and Burnet (1959), both of whom were jointly awarded the Nobel Prize for Medicine in 1962. These authors demonstrated that the immune reaction is a protective mechanism possessed by every animal and is most easily illustrated as the inflammatory response to an invading organism or the allergic reaction to a foreign protein. Without this protection, man would have succumbed to the microbe many centuries ago.

The treatment of chronic renal failure by means of renal transplantation has now become a well-established practice, with well over 8300 transplants being recorded by the International Transplant Registry (Hulme, 1975). Analysis of the results has shown that the number of grafts functioning at the end of the first and third year for cadaveric kidneys was 53 per cent and 40 per cent while for kidneys taken from living related donors the number was 73 per cent and 58 per cent respectively (Gurland *et al.*, 1973).

The Immune Response

This is generated mainly by lymphoid tissue. It is most easily studied by observing the reaction to a homologous skin graft, though the same principle applies to transplanted organs such as the kidney. At first the new graft thrives, so that during the initial five days or so it becomes vascularised and pink with a really healthy appearance. On about the 5th to 7th day, the homograft takes on a discoloured appearance, and soon the evidence of necrosis begins to appear, until by the 12th day it is obviously dead. Pathological examination of the grafted region will reveal a lymphocytic reaction with also, but to a lesser degree, a proliferation of plasma cells. If a second attempt is now made to repeat the grafting process then the time taken for the rejection phenomenon to reveal itself is even faster.

It is clear, therefore, that the immune response is a fundamental law permitting the body to recognise self from non-self and involves two factors, cellular and humoral. The cellular factor is believed to be more important than the humoral one. The whole process is intimately linked with the lymphoid tissue throughout the body, and this system is known to be closely concerned with the production of antibodies. Burnet (1962) has suggested that the probable role of the thymus gland is to organise the immune response and this takes place around the time of birth. Once achieved, the thymus no longer has a function to fulfil so that it atrophies and shrinks. In mice, if the thymus gland is removed soon after birth this immune response does not develop. Thus it is established that if a successful homologous tissue transplantation is to be achieved in man, it is vital to try and match the donor and recipient tissues as nearly as possible and also to suppress the immune response.

Tissue Typing

The antigens (which are on the surface of grafted cells and are responsible for the immune response in patients receiving grafts) are called histocompatibility antigens. It is the immune response of the recipient against these antigens that results in the rejection of the tissue that has been grafted. In man the most important histocompatibility antigens are called the HL-A antigens and these are found in all nucleated cells of the body including leucocytes. Each person can carry up to 6 different HL-A antigens.

There are two general methods that are used to determine the compatibility between the donor and the recipient of grafted tissue. The first involves the determination *in vitro* of the histocompatibility antigens in both donor and recipient and only if there are some antigens common to both are the tissues for grafting considered acceptable. In the second method donor and recipient tissues are mixed *in vivo* and observed for signs of incompatibility.

Suppression of the Immune Response

Although there are numerous methods, the principal difficulty is to achieve a delicate balance between a lethal dose on the one hand and yet an adequate one on the other.

Genetic compatibility.—A number of successful kidney transplant operations have been reported between identical twins. Because of the genetic compatibility between these two beings, the immune response is not present. However, some of these patients have developed glomerulo nephritis (the initial disease of the host) in the grafted kidney, but this complication is less likely to occur if the diseased kidney is removed first. The genetic relationship between children and parents and between siblings enhances the chance of successful transplantation in these groups.

Current methods of treatment.—1. *Corticosteroids.* These are usually given in the form of prednisone or prednisolone. Three general schemes are in current use. In the first, high doses are given from the time of transplantation and then gradually reduced until either signs of rejection occur or a maintenance level of 10–15 mg daily is reached (Straffan *et al.*, 1966). Secondly minimal steroid therapy is given until signs of rejection are seen when the dosage is rapidly increased (Mowbray *et al.*, 1965). Thirdly, over and above a maintenance dose of steroids a large bolus of methyl prednisolone (10–30 mg/kg) is given as a single dose or on several occasions. This must be injected slowly as there have been reports of cardiac irregularities and even arrest.

2. *Azathioprine.* This is an antimetabolite which interferes with nucleic acid synthesis in the cell. It only becomes active after conversion in the liver to 6-mercaptopurine. Azathioprine and its metabolites are excreted by the kidney and the dosage is dependent on renal function which is assessed by creatinine clearance. With normal renal function the dosage currently in use (3 mg/kg) does not depress bone-marrow function but the white cell and platelet counts must be checked regularly. Treatment with azathioprine is usually continued indefinitely.

3. *Antilymphocytic globulin.* This is an antiserum produced in a foreign species against the recipient's lympocytes. It inhibits cellular delayed-type sensitivity and will prevent or delay graft rejection. It is usually given at the time of transplantation.

4. *Cyclophosphamide.* This is an alkylating agent which may be used in place of azathioprine.

5. *Radiotherapy.* Local radiation of the graft with 150 rads on 3 occasions over a 4-day period has been used (Hume *et al.*, 1963) and this has replaced whole-body irradiation.

6. *Anticoagulants.* During the rejection period of a graft, it has been shown histologically that platelets and fibrin are deposited in the small renal vessels. Treatment of the recipient with heparin, oral anticoagulants and the platelet de-aggregating agent dipyridamole, has shown that these lesions can be prevented (Kincaid-Smith, 1969).

The Rejection Phenomenon

The success or failure of a graft to "take" is determined by histocompatibility factors which are inherited. For this reason it follows that the nearer the donor tissue is to that of the recipient the more likely is the grafting to be successful. Ideally, therefore, the most suitable donor tissue is that taken from an identical twin. Next comes a close family relationship such as the mother for her son. Finally, a donor with as many HL-A antigens as possible similar to those of the patient should be selected.

The rejection response is a very complicated process and the signs can first be observed at any time from a few days to even months after the grafting. Sometimes the process can be halted and even reversed by local irradiation or increasing the dose of drugs if the diagnosis is established sufficiently early.

Diagnosis of the rejection response.—The initial finding is deterioration of renal function with decreasing urine output, reduced urinary concentration of urea and sodium, and increased protein excretion. The creatinine clearance falls and the serum creatine and urea rise. The graft may swell and become tender and hypertension and pyrexia may occur. Urine examination may show an increased number of lymphocytes, and blood examination a leucocytosis, eosinophilia and a thrombocytopenia. Although a number of enzyme estimations may show evidence of an immunological reaction, clinical examination and simple laboratory tests are usually adequate to confirm that rejection is occurring (Merrill, 1971).

Treatment

The most common method of treatment of the rejection episode is with large doses of methylprednisolone given intravenously (Woods *et al.*, 1973). 1–2 g of methylprednisolone are given twelve-hourly for 36 hours. In this dosage which is lymphocytic, the long-term side-effects of steroid therapy are not seen. Alternatively either the oral steroid therapy or, less often, the dose of azathioprine may be increased.

RENAL DISEASE AND ANAESTHESIA

Anaesthesia for patients with renal disease may be broadly divided into four categories:

1. Insertion of arteriovenous shunt or construction of an arteriovenous fistula.
2. Nephrectomy related to transplantation.
3. Kidney transplantation.
4. Surgery unrelated to the coincidental renal disease.

The choice of anaesthetic agents is dependent on the degree of remaining renal function because it is necessary to limit the drugs to those in which the degree of reduction of renal excretion will not lead to prolonged action. If the drugs are metabolised to inactive substances before excretion no difficulties will arise from their use. The metabolism of the inhalational agents, with exception of methoxyflurane, do not affect renal function. The latter has been shown to produce an impairment of renal concentrating power directly related to the total dose given and to the resulting serum levels of ionic fluoride which are formed from the metabolism of the methoxyflurane (Cousins and Mazze, 1973). It has also been suggested that enflurane which is also a fluorinated methylethyl ether may also cause renal damage (Loehning and Mazze, 1974), although these findings have not been confirmed by other workers.

The non-inhalational anaesthetic agents are essentially dependent on the kidney for their excretion either unchanged or as active or inactive end-products, and each drug must be considered on its own merits. In some instances the presence of renal failure may result in alternative metabolic pathways being used, for example an increased amount being excreted in the bile as is found with tubocurarine (Cohen et al., 1967).

General Considerations

In patients with advanced renal failure the major problems are those of uraemia, anaemia, hypertension, infection and electrolyte disorders, especially hyperkalaemia. In those awaiting transplantation, uraemia can be satisfactorily treated by dialysis and most patients will have been attending a dialysis unit twice weekly, or more frequently in the acute stage. Dialysis will ensure normal fluid balance as well as correcting electrolyte disturbances and eliminating urea. Haemodialysis is performed through an arteriovenous shunt placed on the forearm or lower leg. The Scribner teflon shunt has been widely used for this purpose but recently the Cimino-Brescia shunt has become increasingly popular. This involves the establishment of a direct arteriovenous fistula between the radial artery and an adjacent vein by open operation. The marked dilatation of the veins in the forearm that results from this shunt enables frequent and easy access to be established with the circulation, using needles of sufficient calibre to carry the blood flow required for haemodialysis. Once a satisfactory shunt has been established, dialysis can be performed whenever required.

Almost all patients presenting for transplantation are severely anaemic, as the anaemia associated with uraemia is very resistant to treatment. The infusion of large volumes of blood carries a risk of precipitating pulmonary oedema and moreover could stimulate the production of antibodies in patients who are awaiting a transplanted kidney. Blood is only added sparingly during dialysis, as the stimulus to the patient's own erythrocyte production would be thereby reduced and moreover each transfusion carries the risk of introducing serum hepatitis, and infection is liable to spread rapidly in dialysis units.

Most patients will have a haemoglobin level in the region of 7 g/dl when they present for operation, a figure which would be regarded as totally unacceptable for other operative procedures. Nevertheless patients undergoing renal transplantation seem to survive surgery and anaesthesia remarkably well despite this severe degree of anaemia. Because of the frequency of infections during chronic renal failure many patients having renal transplants will be receiving antibiotic therapy. The potentiation of the action of non-depolarising muscle relaxants following the intraperitoneal administration of polymyxin, streptomycin and neomycin is well known. This phenomenon may also become manifest in patients with a low urinary output who are receiving these antibiotics by injection, because their requirements for these drugs are considerably reduced (Samuel and Powell, 1970).

Arteriovenous Shunts and Fistulae

While anaemia and some degree of uraemia will usually be present, the use of peritoneal dialysis and cation exchange resins should have resulted in the patient having normal electrolytes. The initial procedure that is usually carried out is the insertion of a teflon/silastic shunt. At the same time or at a subsequent operation, a subcutaneous arteriovenous fistula is formed. It is necessary to insert the shunt first, because the fistula may take some weeks before it may be used satisfactorily.

Renal Transplantation

With the exception of transplantation from a living (related) donor, this procedure is usually undertaken as an emergency. The donor kidney is removed from the cadaver as soon as possible after death has been certified. The warm ischaemic time—that is the time between the cessation of renal perfusion until the kidney has either been surface cooled or perfused with a cold solution at 4° C (for example Hartmann's solution), should ideally be less than thirty minutes. Although subsequent storage for up to 16 hours has been reported without severe tubular necrosis (Hulme, 1975), this should be kept to an absolute minimum. Tissue cross-matching between donor and intended recipient is carried out and, if satisfactory, blood is taken for full blood count, urea and electrolyte estimation and cross-matching.

Bilateral Nephrectomy

This has been carried out after renal transplantation when the grafted kidney is functioning well. The problems are essentially the same as those for transplantation although the problem of renal excretion of drugs will be of less importance in the presence of an adequate renal output. The patient will still be receiving both steroids and immunosuppressive drugs and the dosage of these should be increased over the period of surgery.

Anaesthetic management.—Initial pre-operative examination of the patient is vital with particular emphasis to see if any signs of fluid overload are present. A full explanation of what may be expected post-operatively is essential, for the patient may understandably be extremely apprehensive.

Either regional or general anaesthesia techniques may be suitable. In many instances regional anaesthesia may not appear acceptable to the patient, but a full explanation of what such a technique would involve, with adequate sedation (for example, oral diazepam), will usually result in the patient's agreement. For surgery involving the arms brachial plexus block has been used. The problem of post-operative clotting of the arteriovenous fistula has resulted in the use of infiltration with local anaesthetic of the operative site and sympathetic blockade which in the arm is achieved by stellate ganglion block. The latter may be carried out with 10 ml of 0·5 per cent bupivacaine because its length of action will ensure continued dilatation of the forearm vessels well into the post-operative period.

When multiple procedures are being performed, or in very apprehensive patients, general anaesthesia will be required. Induction with thiopentone or methohexitone followed by maintenance with nitrous oxide, oxygen and minimal amounts of halothane has proved satisfactory. However, the latter may cause marked hypotension and trichloroethylene should be used in such cases. As blood levels of thiopentone are altered by redistribution and tissue uptake (Saidman and Eger, 1966) its length of action is unaffected by the degree of renal failure.

If it is necessary to intubate the patient the dangers associated with the use of suxamethonium in patients with renal failure must be considered. It has been shown that injection of suxamethonium causes a small but statistically significant rise in serum potassium (Striker and Morrow, 1968), and it has been suggested that this may be the cause of cardiac arrest in uraemic patients (Roth,

1969). The maximum increase in two separate studies was 0·5 mEq/l (Koide and Waud, 1972) and 0·7 mEq/l (Millar *et al.*, 1972) and no difference was found between normal patients and those in renal failure. In Millar's series none of his patients with renal failure was uraemic although the highest serum potassium was 6·6 mEq/l (mmol/1). He concluded that suxamethonium is not contra-indicated in patients with renal failure in the absence of uraemia. Samuel and Powell (1970) used suxamethonium for intubation in 97 patients for renal transplantation without a problem. Measurements of serum potassium and blood urea ranged between 3·0–7·2 mEq/l (mmol/l) and 15–256 mg/100 ml (2·5–42·5 mmol/l) respectively in this series.

Although the antigenic profile of the recipients awaiting transplant will already be on record it will take approximately two hours to determine for which recipient the donor kidney is suitable. In consequence it is likely that the acceptable recipient will have eaten recently and thus have a full stomach. Although attempts to empty the stomach by gastric aspiration have been advocated, the results are usually incomplete and the procedure both time-consuming and distressing to the patient. Because the time factor is critical in emergency transplantation, premedication with oral antacids alone (magnesium trisilicate 30 ml) has been recommended (Samuel and Powell, 1970).

Immediately prior to *induction* oxygen should be given for at least 3 minutes. An open vein should be secured with a small-gauge indwelling needle in the dorsum of the hand. Great care must be taken of any fistula or shunt that is present, so the limb should be wrapped in cotton-wool, kept immobile and in extension. The blood-pressure cuff should be placed on another limb to minimise any chance of clotting in the shunt. ECG electrodes should be positioned on the chest.

The patient may be induced with a small dose of thiopentone or methohexitone mixed with a normal premedicant dose of atropine and followed by suxamethonium and rapid intubation. Cricoid pressure should be applied to prevent regurgitation of gastric contents. The potential hazards of using suxamethonium have already been discussed; in patients who have been adequately starved intubation may be carried out using either tubocurarine or pancuronium. However, not only does the onset of laryngeal paralysis take longer to supervene but the large dose required for intubation increases the risk of administering an overdose. It is advisable, therefore, to titrate each patient with a peripheral nerve-stimulator (Chapter 25). In view of the high risk of infection in patients receiving corticosteroids and immunosuppressive drugs all equipment used for intubation and ventilation should have been sterilised. Maintenance of anaesthesia with nitrous oxide/oxygen/tubocurarine and minimal doses of halothane has been reported by Samuel and Powell (1970) in 100 patients. In six of these a small dose of either morphine or pethidine was added. They noted that halothane when used as the main anaesthetic agent could cause unpredictable hypotension in patients with potentially abnormal plasma volumes after dialysis. It would seem that halothane and tubocurarine can decrease renal blood flow (Deutsch *et al.*, 1969). As about 90 per cent of doses of morphine, pethidine and fentanyl are inactivated before excretion, these drugs may be used as the main agent for maintaining anaesthesia, with halothane being confined to the treatment of any acute hypertensive episodes that may occur.

While gallamine is contra-indicated because it is excreted by the kidney in an active form, both tubocurarine and pancuronium have been used satisfactorily as neuromuscular blocking agents. The total dose should be kept to the minimum requirements because prolonged action has been reported with both agents. Incremental doses of suxamethonium have also been used satisfactorily for providing muscular relaxation during transplantation. A supplementary dose of atropine should be given to protect the heart against the effect of reflex bradycardia. Once anaesthesia has been established a nasogastric tube is passed and an intravenous infusion commenced. At this stage both corticosteroids and immunosuppressive drugs are usually given, the exact dosage depending on the renal unit concerned. Intravenous heparin is given prior to anastomosis of the renal vessels. The kidney is usually placed retroperitoneally in the pelvic cavity with anastomosis of the renal artery and vein to the iliac vessels. The heparin may be reversed at the end of the operation with protamine sulphate. The latter should be given by slow intravenous injection because marked hypotension may occur. On completion of the anastomosis either diuretics or mannitol may be given and antibiotic therapy may be started. At the end of the operation non-depolarising muscle relaxants are reversed in the usual way with atropine and neostigmine. The ECG should be carefully observed during this period because dysrhythmias may occur which may lead to cardiac arrest particularly in patients with hyperkalaemia. Post-operatively patients are transferred to a specialised unit and nursed in as near a sterile condition as possible.

REFERENCES

BARNETT, A. J., BLACKET, R. B., DEPOORTER, A. E., SANDERSON, P. H., and WILSON, G. M. (1950). The action of noradrenaline in man and its relation to phaeochromocytoma and hypertension. *Clin. Sci.*, **9**, 151.

BRUN, C., and MUNCK, O. (1957). Lesions of the kidney in acute renal failure following shock. *Lancet*, **1**, 603.

BURNET, F. M. (1959). *The Clonal Selection Theory of Acquired Immunity*. (Abraham Flexner Lectures). Nashville: Vanderbilt University Press.

BURNET, F. M. (1962). Role of the thymus and related organs in immunity. *Brit. med. J.*, **2**, 807.

CHURCHILL-DAVIDSON, H. C. (1955). Hypothermia. *Brit. J. Anaesth.*, **27**, 313.

CHURCHILL-DAVIDSON, H. C., WYLIE, W. D., MILES, B. E., and DE WARDENER, H. E. (1951). The effects of adrenaline, noradrenaline and methedrine on the renal circulation during anaesthesia. *Lancet*, **2**, 803.

COHEN, E. N., WINSLOW BREWER, H., and SMITH, D. (1967). The metabolism and elimination of *d*-tubocurarine H³. *Anesthesiology*, **28**, 309.

COUSINS, M. J., and MAZZE, R. I. (1973). Methoxyflurane nephrotoxity: a study of dose-respone in man. *J. Amer. med. Ass.*, **225**, 1611.

DEUTSCH, S., BASTRON, R. D., PIERCE, E. C., and VANDAM, L. D. (1969). The effects of anaesthesia with thiopentone, nitrous oxide, narcotics and neuromuscular blocking drugs on renal function in normal man. *Brit. J. Anaesth.*, **41**, 807.

DE WARDENER, H. E. (1955). Renal circulation during anaesthesia and surgery. *Anaesthesia*, **10**, 18.

DE WARDENER, H. E. (1973). *The Kidney. An outline of normal and abnormal structure and function*, 4th edit. London: Churchill Livingstone.

DE WARDENER, H. E., and MCSWINEY, R. R. (1951). Renal haemodynamics in vasovagal fainting due to haemorrhage. *Clin. Sci.*, **10**, 209.

DE WARDENER, H. E., and MILES, B. E. (1952). The effect of haemorrhage on the circulatory autoregulation of the dog's kidney perfused *in situ*. *Clin. Sci.*, **11**, 267.

DE WARDENER, H. E., MILES, B. E., LEE, G. DE J., CHURCHILL-DAVIDSON, H. C., WYLIE, W. D., and SHARPEY-SCHAFER, E. P. (1953). Circulatory effects of haemorrhage during prolonged light anaesthesia in man. *Clin. Sci.*, **12**, 175.

EVANS, B., and ENDERBY, G. E. H. (1952). Controlled hypotension and its effect on renal function. *Lancet*, **1**, 1045.

FLORES, J., DI BONA, G. F., BECK, C. H., and LEAF, A. (1972). The role of cell swelling in ischemic damage and the protective effect of hypertonic solute. *J. clin. Invest.*, **51**, 118.

FROMM, S., and WILSON, R. F. (1969). Phenoxybenzamine in human shock. *Surg. Gynec. Obstet.*, **129**, 789.

GORMAN, H. M., and CRAYTHORNE, N. W. B. (1966). The effects of a new neuroleptanalgesic agent (Innovar) on renal function in man. *Acta anaesth. scand.*, Suppl. **24**, 111.

GURLAND, H. J., BRUNNER, F. P., DEHN, H., HARLEN, H., PARSONS, F. M., and SCHARER, K. (1973). Combined report on regular dialysis and transplantation in Europe. *Proc. Europ. dial. & transpl. Ass.*, **10**, 42.

HABIF, D. V., PAPPER, E. M., FITZPATRICK, H. F., LOWRANCE, P., SMYTHE, C. McC., and BRADLEY, S. E. (1951). The renal and hepatic blood flow, glomerular filtration rate and urinary output of electrolytes during cyclopropane, ether and thiopental anesthesia, operation and the immediate postoperative period. *Surgery*, **30**, 241.

HAMPTON, L. J., and LITTLE, D. M. (1953). Complications associated with the use of "controlled hypotension" in anesthesia. *Arch. Surg.*, **67**, 549.

HULME, B. (1975). Medical aspects of renal transplantation. In: *Recent Advances in Renal Disease*, ed. Jones, N. F. London: Churchill Livingstone.

HUME, D. M., MAGEE, J. M., KAUFMAN, H. M., RITTENBURY, M. S., and PROUT, G. R. (1963). Renal homotransplantation in man in modified recipients. *Ann. Surg.*, **158**, 608.

KENNEDY, W. F., SAWYER, T. K., GERBERSHAGEN, H. U., EVERETT, G. B., CUTLER, R. E., ALLEN, G. D., and BONICA, J. J. (1970). Simultaneous systemic cardiovascular and renal hemodynamic measurements during high spinal anaesthesia in normal man. *Acta anaesth. scand.*, **14**, Suppl. 37, 163.

KINCAID-SMITH, P. (1969). Modification of vascular lesions of rejection in cadaveric renal allografts by dipyridamole and anticoagulants. *Lancet*, **2**, 920.

KOIDE, M., and WAUD, B. E. (1972). Serum potassium concentrations after succinylcholine in patients with renal failure. *Anesthesiology*, **36**, 142.

LAMBERT, P. P., GASSEE, J. P., VERNIORY, A., and FICHEROULLE, P. (1971). Measurement of the glomerular filtration pressure from sieving data from macromolecules. *Pflügers Arch. ges. Physiol.*, **329**, 34.

LAUSON, H. D., BRADLEY, S. E., and COURNAND, A. (1944). Renal circulation in shock. *J. clin. Invest.*, **23**, 381.

LEIGHTON, K. M., KOTH, B., and WENKSTEIN, B. M. (1973). Autoregulation of renal blood flow: alteration by methoxyflurane. *Canad. Anaesth. Soc. J.*, **20**, 173.

LINGARDH, G. (1972). Renal clearance investigations with 51 Cr-EDTA and 125 I-Hippuran. *Scand. J. Urol. Nephrol.*, **6**, 63.

LOEHNING, R. W., and MAZZE, R. I. (1974). Possible nephrotoxicity from enflurane in a patient with severe renal disease. *Anesthesiology*, **40**, 203.

LUKE, R. G., BRIGGS, J. D., ALLISON, M. E. M., and KENNEDY, A. C. (1970). Factors determining response to mannitol in acute renal failure. *Amer. J. med. Sci.*, **259**, 168.

LUKE, R. G., and KENNEDY, A. C. (1967). Prevention and early management of acute renal failure. *Postgrad. med. J.*, **43**, 380.

Mazze, R. I., Schwartz, R. D., Slocum, H. C., and Kevin, G. B. (1963). Renal function during anesthesia and surgery. 1. The effects of halothane anesthesia. *Anesthesiology*, **4**, 279.

Medawar, P. B. (1958). *The Immunology of Transplantation*, p. 144. (Harvey Lectures No. 52). New York: Academic Press Inc.

Merrill, J. P. (1971). Diagnosis and management of rejection in allografted kidneys. *Transplant. Proc.*, **3**, 287.

Miles, B. E., and de Wardener, H. E. (1952). Renal vasoconstriction produced by ether and cyclopropane anaesthesia. *J. Physiol. (Lond.)*, **118**, 141.

Miles, B. E., de Wardener, H. E., Churchill-Davidson, H. C., and Wylie, W. D. (1952). The effect on the renal circulation of pentamethonium bromide during anaesthesia. *Clin. Sci.*, **11**, 73.

Miller, R. D., Way, W. L., Hamilton, W. K., and Layzer, R. B. (1972). Succinylcholine-induced hyperkalaemia in patients with renal failure. *Anesthesiology*, **36**, 138.

Morgan, A. G., Bennett, J. M., and Polark, A. (1968). Mannitol retention during diuretic treatment of barbiturate and salicylate overdosage. *Quart. J. Med.*, **37**, 589.

Mowbray, J. F., Cohen, S. L., Doak, P. B., Kenyon, J. R., Owen, K., Percival, A., Porter, K. A., and Peart, W. S. (1965). Human cadaveric renal transplantation: report of twenty cases. *Brit. med. J.*, **2**, 1387.

Moyer, J. H., and McConn, R. (1956). Renal hemodynamics in hypertensive patients following administration of pendiomide. *Anesthesiology*, **17**, 9.

Parsons, F. M., Blagg, C. R., and Williams, R. E. (1963). Chemistry, therapy and hemodialysis of acute renal failure. *Biochem. Clin.*, No. **2**, p. 457.

Pelletier, C. L., and Shepherd, J. T. (1975). Effect of hypoxia on vascular responses to the carotid baroflex. *Amer. J. Physiol.*, **228**, 331.

Phillips, R. A., Dole, V. P., Hamilton, P. B., Emerson, K., Jr., Archibald, R. M., and van Slyke, D. D. (1945). Shock and renal function. *Amer. J. Physiol.*, **145**, 314.

Roth, F., and Wuthrich, H. (1969). The clinical importance of hyperkalaemia following suxamethonium administration. *Brit. J. Anaesth.*, **41**, 311.

Saidman, L. J., and Eger, E. L. (1966). The effect of thiopental metabolism on the duration of anaesthesia. *Anesthesiology*, **27**, 118.

Samuel, J. R., and Powell, D. (1970). Renal transplantation. *Anaesthesia*, **25**, 165.

Smith, H. W. (1943). *Lectures on the Kidney*. (Porter Lectures, Series IX, and the William Henry Walch Lectures.) Lawrence, Kan.: Univ. of Kansas Press.

Straffan, R. A., Hewitt, C. B., Kiser, W. S., Stewart, B. H., Nakamoto, S., and Kolff, W. J. (1966). Clinical experience with the use of 79 kidneys from cadavers for transplantation. *Surg. Gynec. Obstet.*, **123**, 483.

Striker, T. W., and Morrow, A. G. (1968). Effect of succinylcholine on the level of serum potassium in man. *Anesthesiology*, **29**, 214.

Wakim, K. G. (1955). Certain cardiovasculorenal effects of hexamethonium. *Amer. Heart. J.*, **50**, 435.

Woods, J. E., Anderson, C. F., De Weerd, J. H., Johnson, J. H., Donadio, W. J., Leary, F. J., and Frohnert, P. P. (1973). High dosage intravenously administered methylprednisolone in renal transplantation: a preliminary report. *J. Amer. med. Ass.*, **223**, 896.

Wright, S. (1965). *Applied Physiology*, 10th edit. London: Oxford Univ. Press.

Zimmerman, W. E. (1969). Metabolic disorders, renal and hepatic blood flow in shock and the effect of infusion fluids on parameters of acid-base balance. *Bibl. haemat. (Basel)*, **33**, 408.

Section Five

THE ENDOCRINE SYSTEM

Chapter 40

ANAESTHESIA AND THE ENDOCRINE GLANDS

THE STRESS RESPONSE

THE concept that the body possesses a defence mechanism with which to combat aggression is not new. Claude Bernard placed emphasis upon the maintenance of a *status quo* or the *milieu intérieur* of the bodily functions. Almost any kind of initial stimulus—infection, trauma (surgical or accidental), burns or even anaesthesia alone—can be considered as an aggression upon the body tissues, and thus constitutes a form of stress. The body's response to this wide range of stimuli is remarkably constant and, although the functional changes set in motion are complex, they may be summarised as occurring in the following sequence:

1. Immediate circulatory adjustment.
2. The metabolic response.
   (*a*) The catabolic phase.
   (*b*) The anabolic phase.

The immediate circulatory changes are considered more fully elsewhere. Briefly, they may be seen as a generalised increase of adrenergic activity, resulting in tachycardia and vasoconstriction most marked in the splanchnic and cutaneous vascular beds. The apparent aim of these changes is to maintain adequate perfusion of vital centres.

The ensuing catabolic phase of the metabolic response is characterised by breakdown of the body proteins and negative nitrogen balance. Potassium is also lost, presumably being released from the cells as protein is metabolised. Oliguria with sodium retention—disputably obligatory—occurs and the blood picture shows a polymorphonuclear leucocytosis with lymphopenia and eosinopenia. The duration of this phase is variable, depending chiefly on the severity of the initial injury, but is usually about 48 hours. In the subsequent anabolic phase, there is nitrogen retention and restoration of the body proteins.

Mechanism of the Stress Response

The initial vascular response appears to be neurogenic, mediated by the sympathetic system, whose post-ganglionic nerve endings release noradrenaline as a chemical transmitter. The adrenal medulla may be regarded as a modified sympathetic ganglion, and it is believed that it participates in this increased sympathetic activity by releasing catecholamines, both noradrenaline and adrenaline, into the circulation. The mechanisms underlying the catabolic and anabolic phase are not fully understood, but it is generally considered that, in the former at any rate, the release of hormones from the adrenal cortex plays an important part. That this is in fact so, has been shown by the increased plasma concentrations of adrenocortical hormones during the catabolic phase of the metabolic response to injury. Further evidence that the secretion of hormones is involved is shown by the finding that the adrenals enlarge after injury and also that both adrenalectomy and hypophysectomy in animals abolishes the negative nitrogen balance.

It was believed that adrenaline, released immediately after trauma, stimulated the hypothalamus which in turn triggered the release of ACTH from the anterior pituitary. However, it is now known that circulating adrenaline and noradrenaline do not increase ACTH secretion in man (Ganong, 1975).

Anaesthesia and Stress

An assessment of the effect of stress may be made by determination of the plasma level of adrenocortical hormones. There is a marked increase in plasma cortisol levels on the day of operation and this can be prevented by a number of premedication drugs, for example diazepam and barbiturates. Pethidine did not inhibit adrenocortical stimulation when given 1 hour, pre-operatively in a dose of 2 mg/kg (Oyama et al., 1969).

In considering the individual effects of plasma cortisol level of general anaesthetic agents, Oyama (1973) has shown that ether, halothane and cyclopropane increase plasma cortisol levels, whilst methoxyflurane has an insignificant effect and enflurane causes a decrease. However, the addition of a surgical stimulus increased plasma cortisol levels above normal with all these agents. Of the induction agents, thiopentone produced a decrease in cortisol levels, propanidid and Althesin produced no significant change. Both ketamine and gamma-hydroxybutyric acid increase plasma cortisol levels while neuroleptanaesthesia with droperidol and fentanyl supplemented with oxygen and nitrous oxide did not alter levels during anaesthesia alone, but failed to prevent the rise associated with surgical stimulus. While it had been thought in the past that both spinal and epidural anaesthesia would completely prevent the effects of surgical stress it appears that although the response (determined by cortisol levels) is much less than that seen during general anaesthesia, there is a small but significant rise in plasma cortisol levels (Oyama and Matsuki, 1970 and 1971). The muscle relaxants have not been shown to have any effect on adrenocortical response.

Hypothermia depresses the hypothalamic pituitary system. Below 28°C the response to surgical stimulus is progressively reduced (Van Brunt and Ganong, 1963). Above 30°C it appears that the type of anaesthetic agent used affects the cortisol response (Sarajas et al., 1958).

In conclusion, it would seem that although premedication may abolish the increase in adrenocortical hormone output resulting from fear and anxiety, no form of general anaesthetic can fully prevent the stressful effects of surgery, although spinal and epidural anaesthesia may lessen them considerably. However, it must be remembered that while the anaesthetist is endeavouring to limit the response of the patient to the stress of surgery, as some patients cannot respond in a normal manner (for example those with physical disease), there may be a necessity for steroid therapy if they are to survive.

The Pituitary Gland

The pituitary gland lies in the sella turcica, a small cavity in the body of the sphenoid bone and is connected to the hypothalamus by a neural stalk. The posterior pituitary is derived embryologically from the hypothalamus with which it has direct neural connections while the anterior pituitary is derived from oropharyngeal tissue and has no such connections.

The two hormones released from the posterior pituitary (antidiuretic hormone and vasopressin) are secreted by nuclei in the hypothalamus. The hormones of the anterior pituitary are produced within this part of the gland and their output controlled by individual "releasing factors" derived from the hypothalamus.

Anterior pituitary hormones include:

Adrenocorticotrophic hormone   (ACTH)
Growth hormone   (GH)
Thyroid-stimulating hormone   (TSH)
Gonadotrophic hormones*
Melanocyte-stimulating hormone   (MSH)

With the exception of GH and MSH all these hormones act on specific target glands.

Failure of the pituitary may occur due to pituitary tumours, postpartum infarction (Sheehan's syndrome), hypophysectomy or pituitary irradiation, following the implantation of radioactive material.

Pituitary ablation may be carried out in the treatment of primary tumours (for example Cushing's syndrome and acromegaly), in the treatment of metastatic cancer of the breast or prostate, or in the management of severe diabetic retinopathy. The surgical technique that is often used is the implantation of Yttrium-90.

In man some 80 per cent of the pituitary must be destroyed before clear evidence of pituitary insufficiency is seen. The clinical findings in hypopituitarism reflect the loss of function of the individual endocrine glands which are normally stimulated by the pituitary. The severity of the disease will depend on the speed of onset and progression of the lesion.

The majority of patients with pituitary insufficiency who require surgery will have been stabilised with adequate doses of adrenocortical and thyroid hormones. In these patients supplementary doses of corticosteroids should be given. The number of days post-operatively during which this increased dosage should be continued will depend on the severity of the operation. It is not normally necessary to increase the dose of thyroid hormone.

The management of patients undergoing elective hypophysectomy, for example by the implantation of Yttrium-90, will depend on the functional activity of their adrenal glands at the time of surgery. This must be assessed preoperatively not only by determinations of the normal cortisol output but also by the ability of the adrenal cortex to respond to stress which may be determined by the insulin tolerance test (Whitwam *et al.*, 1973). Post-operative replacement therapy will depend on the extent of the surgery and the pre-operative findings, but in those patients with decreased adrenal reserve or those in whom the entire pituitary is to be removed, initial supplementary doses of corticosteroids will be required (see p. 1266) and life-long therapy continued with prednisone

---

* These comprise (1) Follicular-stimulating hormone
                         (2) Luteinising hormone, and
                         (3) Prolactin.

or a similar preparation. The onset of diabetes insipidus may require treatment with pitressin tanate in oil and assessment for the necessity of the thyroxine will be required during follow-up.

In patients with diabetes in whom hypophysectomy is carried out, an increase in their insulin requirement (covered by intravenous glucose) will be needed during the time when large doses of corticosteroids are being given. However, on reduction of the steroids the requirement of insulin will usually fall to less than that needed pre-operatively (Whitwam et al., 1973).

Acromegalic patients requiring anaesthesia may present problems of airway management and intubation (Kitahata, 1971) and pre-operative tracheostomy may be necessary.

In untreated hypopituitarism it is essential prior to surgery to attempt to correct the lack of adrenocortical and thyroid hormones. Patients with severe hypothroidism are very poor operative risks. Any hypoglycaemia or hypothermia should be corrected before surgery. Patients with panhypopituitarism are liable to sudden attacks of coma. The cause is endocrine failure, but the precipitating factors are often comparatively minor, thus emphasising the borderline level at which consciousness is maintained in such people. Analgesics and anaesthetics, even in small doses, can precipitate coma. The diagnosis of hypopituitarism need not be difficult, if it is remembered that (at such a severe state of the disease) pubic and axillary hair will probably have long since disappeared, and the sexual organs atrophied.

THE THYROID GLAND

The normal thyroid comprises of two lobes joined by an isthmus which lies at the level of the second and third tracheal ring. It consists of multiple spherical follicles which contain colloid and are surrounded by a single layer of cells. In the gland iodine is linked to tyrosine molecules which are attached to thyroglobulin (a glycoprotein), to form initially mono- and then di-iodotyrosine. The latter are coupled to form tri-iodothyronine (T_3) and thyroxine (T_4) which are released into the circulation as active hormones by the thyroid-stimulating hormone from the anterior pituitary.

Hyperthyroidism results from excess secretion of T_4 and/or T_3 either from a simple "toxic nodule" or more often from a diffuse hyperplasia of the thyroid. Thyrotoxicosis is the clinical result of hyperthyroidism. Nowadays, a very large proportion of patients suffering from this disease are cured by planned medical treatment with radioactive iodine or one of the antithyroid drugs, but some, on account of a relapse, intolerance to the specific drugs, secondary thyrotoxicosis in an adenoma, progressive exophthalmos, general enlargement of the gland with medical therapy, and perhaps obstructive symptoms, or more simply for personal reasons, need the surgeon's aid.

None should be operated upon until the thyrotoxicosis has been controlled to the fullest extent. This is usually done with one of the antithyroid drugs. The commonly used antithyroid drugs include the thioamides which block the incorporation of iodine into the precursors of thyroid hormone, and those drugs that interfere with concentration of iodide ion by the thyroid gland and include potassium perchlorate. In view of the greater incidence of aplastic anaemia with the latter the thioamides are used almost exclusively in the drug treatment of thyrotoxicosis. This group includes propylthiouracil, methyl-thiouracil and carbimazole. These drugs are given in an increased dosage for about 8 weeks by which time the patient should be euthyroid and a maintenance level is continued for life. Side-effects include allergic reactions which may vary from rashes to leucopenia or even aplastic anaemia and blood counts are essential during the first two months of treatment. When the thyrotoxicosis is mild, simple iodine alone for a week or two immediately before operation may suffice. Iodine can be given as Lugol's solution which is an aqueous solution of 5 per cent w/v of iodine and 10 per cent w/v of potassium iodine; 0·5 ml is usually given 8-hourly. Antithyroid compounds tend to enlarge the thyroid gland and make it more vascular—disadvantages for the surgeon—but a ten-day course of iodine before operation after the antithyroid drug may be useful in offsetting this increased vascularity. If preparation of the patient by such means is carefully carried out, the risk of a thyroid crisis following the operation is extremely slight. Thyroid crisis or storm which may be considered as the most severe form of uncontrolled thyrotoxicosis, is most likely to be seen nowadays if a patient with previously undiagnosed and therefore uncontrolled thyro-toxicosis has to have an emergency operation for some unrelated condition. In such circumstances the thyrotoxicosis may be recognised pre-operatively and treatment should consist of alpha- and beta-blocking agents, corticosteroids and iodine (Stehling, 1974).

Because these patients tend to be excitable, special consideration must be given to the pre-operative sedation, which may with benefit be started days, rather than hours, before the expected time. Usually a small dose of pheno-barbitone (30 to 60 mg) for a day or two is sufficient, but the choice of drug and its dose depends upon the patient, who already may have tried several during medical treatment. Phenothiazine drugs have a special application and may be particularly useful for immediate premedication.

Anaesthesia

Although the operation can be very satisfactorily performed under local analgesia provided the surgeon is gentle, general anaesthesia is preferable for all concerned. The choice of anaesthetic depends very much on personal preference. Deep anaesthesia is unnecessary except in patients whose hyperthyroidism has not been fully controlled pre-operatively, when it will prevent a marked increase in catecholamine production which may not be suppressed if the pre-operative adrenergic blockade is inadequate. Badly administered anaesthesia, particu-larly with inadequate oxygenation, may be more hazardous than usual. Thio-pentone, nitrous oxide-oxygen with supplementation either by inhalational agents such as enflurane or halothane, or a judicious use of an intravenous analgesic with spontaneous respiration is satisfactory. Alternatively, many anaesthetists prefer to control respiration throughout with a muscle relaxant and avoid the use of a potent inhalational agent. Pre-operative oxygenation of the patient is advisable and, after induction, the trachea and glottis should be carefully sprayed with 4·0 per cent lignocaine before an oral armoured endo-tracheal tube is passed. Infiltration in the area of the proposed incision with a solution of 1:200,000 adrenaline, or 1:400,000 noradrenaline, in saline mark-edly reduces the vascularity of the skin flaps, but must be carried out before the introduction of a volatile agent to the anaesthetic mixture. Pharmacological evidence would suggest that the risk of exogenous adrenaline is less with enflurane than halothane anaesthesia (see Chapter 6). Induced hypotension is not recommended, since—merely to prevent bleeding—the advantages do not seem to outweigh the potential hazards for this type of operation; bleeding from the gland and its immediate surroundings depends very much on the adequacy of the surgical technique and, in competent hands, is surprisingly small. A little foot-down tilt will assist the venous drainage.

Three further points should be noted. It is not necessary to over-extend the patient's head upon a sandbag or hard pillow to give the surgeon good access; hyperextension puts the strap muscles on the stretch and produces occipital headache post-operatively. It may be helpful to the surgeon to watch the vocal cords during extubation and make certain that the recurrent laryngeal nerves are not damaged. A patient at rest even with bilateral palsies may yet have an adequate airway, but returning consciousness with pain stimuli can lead to obstruction. Abductor palsy is even more dangerous. A little care at this stage may save an acute emergency later. Finally, the patient's eyes must be carefully protected during the operation.

Post-operative Care

This is normally routine, but the immediate progress of the patient must be observed in case a thyroid crisis or respiratory obstruction develop. The patient should be kept at a moderately cool temperature and be adequately sedated. A rapidly rising pulse rate, pyrexia, sweating, hypertension followed by hypotension with cardiac failure and excessive restlessness are the predominant signs of a crisis. The latter usually develops within the first post-operative day. Treatment with antithyroid drugs, iodine, steroids and adrenergic blocking agents must be started at once (Stehling, 1974). The concentration of inspired oxygen should be increased and hypothermia may be of special value in these cases.

Respiratory obstruction is uncommon, but may be caused in several ways. Damage to the recurrent laryngeal nerves has already been mentioned, but laryngeal oedema, tracheal collapse and reactionary haemorrhage can lead to respiratory obstruction, each of which will require urgent treatment.

THE ADRENAL GLANDS

These paired organs lie on the superior pole of each kidney and comprise of an outer cortex and a central medulla. Each weighs approximately 6 g.

The adrenal cortex is composed of three zones, each of which produces a distinctly separate form of hormone. The outer layer, the zona glomerulosa, secretes mineralocorticoids, the middle layer, the zona fasciculata secretes glucocorticoids, and the inner layer, the zona reticularis, secretes sex hormones.

Functions of the Adrenal Corticoid Hormones

All these hormones are derivatives of cholesterol and may be divided into three groups:

1. *Glucocorticoids.*—Hydrocortisone is the principal glucocorticoid produced by the adrenal cortex. It has an effect on carbohydrate metabolism

opposed to that of insulin. In excess, it stimulates gluconeogenesis and produces a negative nitrogen balance associated with muscle-wasting, osteoporosis and atrophy of the skin. It also has an anti-inflammatory effect, associated with lymphopenia and eosinopenia. Both hydrocortisone and other glucocorticoids also possess weak mineralocorticoid properties.

2. *Mineralocorticoids.*—The principal naturally-occurring hormone is aldosterone. It promotes the retention of sodium and excretion of potassium by the kidneys, its secretion being stimulated by a fall in extracellular fluid volume.

3. *Sex hormones.*—Adrenal androgens have weak virilising activity compared with testosterone, which is secreted by the testes. They are also believed to have anabolic effects. Progesterone and oestrogens are possibly secreted in small amounts by the adrenal cortex in women.

TREATMENT WITH HORMONES

Aldosterone and hydrocortisone are the principal natural steroids produced by the adrenal cortex, but for therapeutic purposes a number of substances are available, most of which have been produced synthetically and with chemical changes in their structure designed to increase their clinical value. The steroids that are commonly used therapeutically are classified in Table 1.

Corticotrophin (ACTH) may be given to stimulate adrenal cortical activity

40/TABLE 1

SOME HORMONES IN COMMON USE, AND THEIR DOSAGE

Corticotrophin (ACTH)	Administered by subcutaneous or intramuscular injection, but as this hormone is very short-acting when continuous therapy is indicated, the total dose must be divided and given at four-hourly intervals. Dose from 20 to 200 mg a day.
Hydrocortisone Sodium Succinate	Prepared immediately before use for intramuscular or intravenous injection. Dose 50 to 100 mg or larger as required.
Cortisone Acetate	Can be administered orally in tablet form or intramuscularly as a suspension. Dose 25 to 400 mg a day.
Prednisone and Prednisolone	Derivatives respectively of cortisone and hydrocortisone, but five times more potent in respect of glucocorticoid activity and with similar potency for mineralocorticoid activity. Administered orally in a dose of from 10 to 100 mg daily.
Dexamethasone and Betamethasone	Approximately thirty-five times more potent than cortisone but with virtually no mineralocorticoid activity. Administered orally in a dose of from 0·5 to 10 mg daily. Dexamethasone in doses of 50–100 mg has been recommended for the treatment of malignant hyperpyrexia (see Chapter 28).
Fludrocortisone Acetate	This is a fluorinated hydrocortisone with enhanced mineralocorticoid activity, and is used in place of deoxycortone. Administered orally in a dose range of from 0·1–0·2 mg daily.

either when this has been suppressed by previous steroid administration or more simply as a means of treatment in some inflammatory and allergic disorders. It is, however, not commonly used for these purposes, but rather as a test of adrenal cortical activity.

The principal indications for therapy with cortisone and similar corticosteroids are physiological replacement of the secretions of the adrenal cortex, suppression of some inflammatory and allergic disorders, and depression of adrenal cortical function. Prednisone and prednisolone are most commonly used for these purposes, but for emergency use hydrocortisone sodium succinate should be injected intravenously. When a specific control of water and electrolyte balance is required deoxycortone or fludrocortisone acetate are often preferred. The requisite dose depends on the therapeutic indication, the degree of urgency and the size of the patient. Although a relatively large initial dosage may be justified in certain circumstances, graded doses may be necessary to find the patient's essential requirements, and it is important to bear in mind that there are disadvantages in prescribing corticosteroids, particularly too much for too long a time.

The normal physiological output of the adrenal is put at about the equivalent of 20–25 mg of cortisone a day, so that routine therapy in the absence of any adrenal function need rarely exceed this dose or its equivalent in terms of other steroids, and can be administered by mouth. Cortisone can, if necessary, be supplemented by 0·1 mg of fludrocortisone a day. When replacement therapy is planned for either the removal of a pituitary or both adrenal glands it is usual to provide a larger initial dosage to cover the possible immediate and post-operative stress of the surgical and anaesthetic procedures. While a number of different regimens have been advocated, the results of Plumpton and his colleagues (1969) suggest that adequate replacement therapy will be achieved by the following scheme:

Pre-operatively: Hydrocortisone hemisuccinate 100 mg i.m. with pre-medication.

Intra-operatively: Repeat above if operation over 6-hours duration.

Post-operatively: Hydrocortisone hemisuccinate 100 mg i.m. 6-hourly for 1–3 days depending on severity of operation. Restart oral corticosteroid therapy with dose given pre-operatively when possible.

There does not appear to be any good evidence for the necessity slowly to decrease steroid levels post-operatively to pre-operative levels. If the patient is undergoing stress, for example requiring nasogastric aspiration, hydrocortisone hemisuccinate 100 mg should be continued 6-hourly intramuscularly. As soon as the stressful stimulus is removed, pre-operative steroid requirements will be adequate.

Effects of Corticosteroid Therapy

Apart from the useful results of treatment with corticosteroids, side-effects may occur, especially when large doses are used. Several are of particular importance and of interest to the anaesthetist. The patient frequently has a marked sense of well-being and is inclined to euphoria, which may mask the true physical state of affairs. There is evidence that corticosteroids produce a tendency to thrombosis and delayed wound healing, and that they diminish the normal response to infection. Thus they should not normally be given to patients suffering from tuberculosis. These effects are, however, very slight in clinical or surgical practice, but when an operation is contemplated they must be weighed against the benefits of the steroid, though they do not contra-indicate their essential use. The effect of corticosteroids on the electrolytes is weak, but they quite commonly produce glycosuria and they may lead to water and salt retention. This is especially likely to occur when they are used for replacement therapy during and after an operation on a patient already receiving treatment with the same or similar-acting steroids. In such circumstances the dose must be adjusted accordingly, and if a large dose is considered necessary to cover the operative period, it must be reduced as soon as possible post-operatively. Long-continued therapy causes some osteoporosis and weakening of the bones.

Cortisone and barbiturate poisoning.—Dhunér and Nordquist (1957) have drawn attention to the danger of administering cortisone to patients recovering from an overdose of a barbiturate, since this may result in the reinduction of unconsciousness. The danger also exists with promethazine poisoning. A similar phenomenon has been known to occur following the injection of hypertonic glucose into animals awakening from barbiturate narcosis (Lamson *et al.*, 1949). The explanation of this action of cortisone and glucose is not known. It may, however, have clinical importance not only when patients are treated for over-dosage of barbiturates or promethazine, but also in routine anaesthesia.

Hormone suppression of adrenal cortical activity.—The therapeutic use of adrenal cortical hormones in doses that are equivalent to or more than the patient's normal physiological requirements, will lead to suppression of this part of the gland's function. Ingle and Kendall (1937) showed that this effect is due to decreased secretion of the ACTH and similar hormones produced by the anterior pituitary. This is a form of pituitary inhibition and it eventually leads to adrenal cortical atrophy. This effect may outlast the original treatment for a considerable period of time—perhaps for as long as a year or more (Salassa *et al*, 1953; Slaney and Brooke, 1957)—and does not necessarily only follow heavy or prolonged treatment with cortisone or similar compounds. A week of treatment may be long enough. The clinical significance of such a reduction in the function of the adrenal cortex is variable, but it is always potentially important. Such a patient's response to a period of stress—say, even to a minor anaesthetic and operation—may be inadequate, and acute adrenal insufficiency will then occur. This is characterised by sudden and severe hypotension, progressing to other signs of shock, coma and anuria, and may lead to death. It usually takes place in the immediate post-operative period, but there seems no reason why it should not occur during the operation and anaesthetic.

Nowadays, very many patients—particularly those suffering from one or other of the collagen diseases, such as rheumatoid arthritis—receive a course of corticosteroid therapy, and despite the fact that many of them are in all proba-bility subjected to many differing forms of stress after treatment ceases, very few indeed go into acute adrenal failure. It is, however, important to remember the possibility when faced with sudden circulatory failure during or following an operation, particularly if the response to treatment with intravenous fluids and drugs is unexpectedly poor, or when the operative procedure seems unlikely to have been the major cause of the collapse.

Pre-operatively it is rational and wise to consider carefully any history of treatment with corticosteroid during the previous twelve months, the more so if the proposed operation is likely to be extensive. Certain facts may support the possibility of adrenal cortical inactivity in a patient. Fatigue, weakness and irritability are the typical symptoms which become more suspect with the history of corticosteroid treatment previously. Objectively estimation of adrenal hypo-function can be carried out by measuring the increase in cortisol output achieved by the intravenous injection of a synthetic form of ACTH called Synacthen. Blood can be collected 30 minutes later and the alteration in plasma cortisol level determined. In general, however, this test is not used as a routine pre-operatively because the risk of acute adrenal insufficiency, in those patients who have had corticosteroid therapy and cannot be assessed or treated pre-operatively on clinical grounds, is very small. Moreover, the only really adequate test is the response of the patient to the anaesthetic and operation. If in doubt the patient should always be covered by a course of corticosteroid therapy for the period of operation and a day or two afterwards. Many authorities advocate this routinely for all patients who have had treatment with it within one year of the proposed operation, especially when this is of any magnitude. But an alternative approach is to bear in mind the risk, deliberately omit a routine cover and keep hydrocortisone available at the patient's bedside, so that it can be given intravenously if needed (Nelson, 1963) or to give an injection of hydrocortisone hemisuccinate (100 mg) with the premedication and further doses only if required. Bearing in mind that very few patients who have been previously submitted to steroid therapy are, in practice, at risk, this method has at least the merit of objectivity and avoids any potential complications from the routine use of corticosteroids. When corticosteroid treatment is already being given to a patient—either for surgical reasons or because of some incidental disease—and an operation is contemplated, the dose should be increased to cover the period of stress in case the physiological response is inadequate. Plumpton *et al.* (1969) advised that intramuscular hydrocortisone hemisuccinate 100 mg 6-hourly, be given from the time of premedication and continued for up to 3 days after major surgery and 24 hours after minor operations, while a single dose is adequate for very short procedures. A very serious collapse may follow from discontinuing corticosteroid therapy during this critical period.

The treatment of acute adrenal insufficiency should be by intravenous hydrocortisone since the patient has usually collapsed, and is often semiconscious. For less urgent occasions, and provided the patient can tolerate it without sickness, a corticosteroid can be given by mouth, since it will be very rapidly absorbed from the stomach. Both glucose and sodium usually need replacement in this condition, and should be combined and given intravenously as a 5 per cent dextrose, 0·9 per cent saline drip.

CONDITIONS AFFECTING THE ADRENAL GLANDS

Adrenal Cortex

Addison's disease.—This disease is usually caused by simple atrophy or by tuberculosis affecting both the cortex and medulla of the adrenals. The symptoms and signs, however, result from the absence of cortical secretions and principally consist of pigmentation, weakness, hypotension, and electrolyte changes due to the patient's inability to retain sodium. Many such patients are maintained by means of a high-salt diet, cortisone (or a more potent equivalent) and, if necessary, fludrocortisone, but this may be inadequate for cases of more than average severity, or in the presence of exceptional stresses. A patient with Addison's disease, who is to be submitted to anaesthesia and an operation, should always be prepared with cortisone and fludrocortisone. Cortisone itself does little to maintain a normal electrolyte balance, so that it cannot be regarded as a substitute for fludrocortisone. There are no special points concerning anaesthesia, other than the intolerance of these patients to more than minimal doses of potent agents. Thiopentone is especially likely to precipitate an acute hypotensive episode, while its metabolism is slower than normal.

An Addisonian crisis may occur after operation. Typically, acute and marked hypotension is associated with nausea, vomiting, vague pains, hypoglycaemia, coma, and unless rapidly treated, death. Treatment of a crisis should consist of the intravenous injection of 100 mg of hydrocortisone and the infusion of isotonic sodium chloride solution to replace the extracellular fluid volume deficit which may be very severe. Additional mineralocorticoids are not usually required. Hypoglycaemia may occur and should be treated with intravenous injections of 50 per cent glucose. The hydrocortisone will have to be repeated possibly at three- to four-hourly intervals. Intravenous fluids will be required until they can be taken by mouth. In the early stages of the crisis, vasoconstrictors may be necessary to assist in maintaining a reasonable blood-pressure level.

Adrenal Medulla

The adrenal medulla consists largely of chromaffin cells which are the equivalent of post-ganglionic nerve fibres. Indeed, the medulla can be considered as a post-ganglionic nerve since it receives only pre-ganglionic fibres from the sympathetic nervous system and it is activated by the release of acetylcholine at the synapse. The chromaffin cells can be divided into two types, those which store adrenaline and those which store noradrenaline. In humans the normal adrenal medulla contains about 80 per cent adrenaline and 20 per cent noradrenaline. The synthesis of these hormones is shown in Fig. 1 and the metabolism in Fig. 2.

Phaeochromocytoma.—This is a tumour of chromaffin tissue which usually arises in the adrenal medulla, but may also be found in any part of the body where there is sympathetic nervous tissue, with the exception of catecholamine-producing cells within the central nervous system. Thus, it may be found on the sympathetic chain in the abdomen or chest, and in the bladder wall. The tumours are most frequently benign in the sense that less than 10 per cent behave in a malignant manner by producing secondaries elsewhere in the body. They are, however, not necessarily single, since in up to 20 per cent of cases more than one tumour is found. Most phaeochromocytomata are physiologically active, though this may be intermittent in occurrence; and while all tumours arising in the adrenal medulla secrete both noradrenaline and adrenaline, fifty per cent of those arising outside the medulla secrete only noradrenaline.

Clinical symptoms and signs.—The classical picture is of paroxysmal hypertension, but this may take the form of a maintained high blood pressure with intermittent episodes when it rises even higher. In an attack, apart from having a very high blood pressure, the patient will complain of sweating, palpitations and headache. But the symptomatology may be unusual, and phaeochromocytomata have presented in bizarre ways with features suggesting primary renal disease, oligaemia with hypotension, toxaemia of pregnancy and even a cerebral tumour (Leather *et al.*, 1962). The presence of a phaeochromocytoma may only be suspected at operation for some incidental disease or during parturition when the blood pressure becomes markedly unstable (Ross, 1962). A phaeochromocytoma may present unexpectedly during aortography for the differential diagnosis of hypertension. It may also initially be mistaken for such other diseases as thyrotoxicosis and anxiety state, and it may cause glycosuria, but this is not of clinical significance (Robertson, 1965).

When undiscovered, the presence of a phaeochromocytoma eventually leads to a permanently sustained high blood pressure, which makes the disease difficult to differentiate from essential hypertension on clinical grounds. Structural changes in the heart and vessels occur sooner or later and death may follow from cardiac failure or cerebrovascular accident.

Diagnosis.—The history is frequently suggestive of the diagnosis, but the sight of a conscious patient during a bout of hypertension from the sudden liberation of catecholamines into the circulation may be diagnostic. The patient is anxious, pallid, sweating and complaining of headache and palpitations. Indeed, one clinical test for a tumour is to compress the area of the patient's loins in an attempt to induce such an attack. An alternative, but dangerous, method that is not commonly used nowadays is to inject intravenously a very small dose of histamine (0·025 to 0·05 mg). A safer test is to try the effect of a blocking drug such as phentolamine during a period of hypertension. The intravenous injection of 5 mg should produce a marked fall in blood pressure in a matter of two or three minutes, if the raised blood pressure is due to circulating catecholamines. Phentolamine has no effect on the level of blood pressure in patients with essential hypertension. However, the best method of establishing the diagnosis is by measurements of urinary levels of catecholamines and their metabolites. Accurate determinations of the concentration of adrenaline, noradrenaline, met- and nor-metadrenaline and vanillylmandelic acid (VMA) may be made and in almost all patients who have a phaeochromocytoma an increased level of all these substances will be found in a 24-hour urine specimen. The determination of plasma catecholamines is a difficult measurement and 24-hour urinary results are not always diagnostic. Normal values for urine are shown below:

1. Catecholamines—less than 0·1 mg
2. Met- and nor-metadrenaline—less than 1·3 mg
3. VMA—less than 6·8 mg

The diagnosis can also be established by radiological techniques, but these are most useful for localisation of the tumour. The range of procedures is large and includes straight X-rays of the thorax and abdomen, and intravenous pyelography which, though simple, may yet be helpful. Presacral injection of carbon dioxide or oxygen (the former is safer, but is absorbed so quickly that

TYROSINE

Tyrosine hydroxylase ← − − − α METHYL-P-TYROSINE

DIHYDROXYPHENYLALANINE (DOPA)

Aromatic-L-amino-acid decarboxylase ← − − − − α METHYLDOPA

DIHYDROXYPHENYLETHYLAMINE (DOPAMINE)

Dopamine β-hydroxylase

NORADRENALINE

Phenylethylamine N-methyl transferase

ADRENALINE

40/Fig. 1.—Diagram to illustrate the biosynthesis of catecholamines. The sites of action of α methyltyrosine and α methyldopa are shown with dotted arrows.

the series of X-rays necessary may not be possible) will outline the kidneys and the adjacent adrenals, and the presence of a tumour may be demonstrated either on account of its size or, in the case of a small tumour, because of an alteration in the normal shape of the adrenal (Edwards, 1962). Retrograde catheterisation

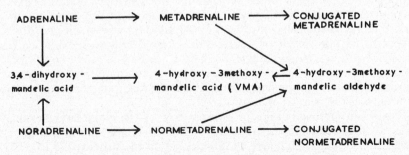

ADRENALINE ⟶ METADRENALINE ⟶ CONJUGATED METADRENALINE

3,4-dihydroxy-mandelic acid ⟶ 4-hydroxy-3methoxy-mandelic acid (VMA) ← 4-hydroxy-3methoxy-mandelic aldehyde

NORADRENALINE ⟶ NORMETADRENALINE ⟶ CONJUGATED NORMETADRENALINE

40/Fig. 2.— The metabolic pathways of adrenaline and noradrenaline.

of the aorta with the injection of a dye to delineate the tumour, which is vascular, is also of value (Edwards, 1962). Catheterisation of the inferior vena cava with sampling for plasma catecholamines at different levels is a safe manipulation and helpful in the localisation of a tumour.

Preparation for operation.—Surgical removal is the only method of treatment but before it is attempted certain investigations must be carried out to determine the general physical state of the patient, particularly in relation to the heart and circulation, and the patient must be prepared for operation.

Apart from routine examination of the heart, electrocardiographs must be taken and blood volume studies may well be of considerable value. When the phaeochromocytoma is of long standing the patient may have a marked reduction in blood volume due to continuous vasoconstriction (Brunjes *et al.*, 1960), but this is the exception rather than the rule (Sjoerosma *et al.*, 1966; Walters, 1969). If the blood volume is low, removal of the tumour may be followed by acute hypotension due to vasodilatation in the presence of chronic hypovolaemia. Leather and his colleagues (1962) have drawn attention to the high haemoglobin values that may be found during and for a day or two after a hypertensive crisis. They explain them on a similar basis to the reduction in blood volume, since catecholamines reduce plasma volume and raise the venous haematocrit (Kalreider *et al.*, 1942; Finnerty *et al.*, 1958).

Preparation for operation should include special consideration of the adminstration of α and β blockers. Of the α blockers phenoxybenzamine is the most popular, and its pre-operative administration to control symptoms and blood pressure levels is recommended by many. Johns and Brunjes (1962) consider that if it is administered for a sufficiently long period of time pre-operatively the blood volume of the patient may be restored to normal and acute hypotension following removal of the phaeochromocytoma avoided. Although Sjoerosma and his colleagues (1966) consider the blood volume to be normal in most patients with a phaeochromocytoma they recommend adrenergic blockade to stabilise the blood pressure and to prevent dysrhythmias. This can be done by the use of an α and a β blocker for two to three days pre-operatively. Harrison *et al.* (1968) suggest that α-blocking agents are indicated if the blood pressure is constantly in excess of 200/130, there are frequent paroxysms of uncontrolled hypertension or if the patient is receiving beta blockers. The latter are indicated if the pulse rate is in excess of 140 beats per min, there is a history of dysrhythmias or there are frequent premature ventricular contractions. Fanning *et al.* (1970) recommend that when an alpha blocker is indicated phenoxybenzamine, 30 mg/day, should be given in divided doses and when a beta blocker is indicated propranolol, 60 mg/day, also in divided doses. As hypotension may result on giving α blockers due to vasodilatation in the presence of a low blood volume, the beta blockers should not be started until 24 hours later, by which time the vascular volume can if necessary have been corrected. Where indicated alpha-blocking agents are usually commenced about four days before surgery (Csanky-Treels *et al.*, 1976).

Another approach to this problem is to block the synthesis rather than the effects of catecholamines. α-methyl-p-tyrosine blocks the first step in the formation of catecholamines by inhibiting tyrosine hydroxylase (see Fig. 1), the enzyme which catalyses the hydroxylation of tyrosine to 3,4-dihydroxyphenylalanine (DOPA). Its use in pre-operative preparation of patients with phaeochromocytomas has been discussed by Jones *et al.* (1968).

Anaesthesia and operation.—In essence the anaesthetic agents which should be chosen are those which stimulate the release of catecholamines least and do not sensitise the myocardium to catecholamines. For premedication droperidol and fentanyl have been used satisfactorily (Csanky-Treels *et al.*, 1976). Droperidol reduces the pressor response to adrenaline in man (Whitwam and Russell, 1971) and has also been shown to increase the threshold of adrenaline-induced dysrhythmias. Unlike morphine and pethidine, fentanyl does not cause histamine release (Dobkin *et al.*, 1965).

With regard to anaesthetic technique the essential prerequisite is a smooth induction and maintenance without straining, hypoxia or carbon dioxide retention. Suxamethonium should be avoided if possible because it may cause ventricular dysrhythmias (Stoner *et al.*, 1968) and pancuronium which does not cause histamine release, would appear to be the relaxant of choice for both intubation and maintenance (James, 1970). Because cyclopropane, trichloroethylene and halothane sensitise the myocardium to catecholamines they should be avoided as should ether which like trichloroethylene and cyclopropane stimulate the release of endogenous catecholamines. Enflurane, therefore, may prove to be useful in these circumstances (see Chapter 6). Anaesthesia may be induced with droperidol and fentanyl and maintained with nitrous oxide, oxygen, pancuroniun and fentanyl. The occurrence of paroxysms of hypertension during the operation can be treated with phentolamine 1–2 mg intravenously and severe ventricular dysrhythmias with propranolol 2–3 mg intravenously. If excessive hypertension occurs during the operation this may be controlled by intravenous phentolamine 1–2 mg. Cardiac dysrhythmias may present a problem, but unless they arise in the ventricles and are continuous, suggesting the likelihood of the onset of ventricular fibrillation, they are probably best left untreated, since they usually subside. Indeed, the pre-operative use of propranolol make the occurrence of more than a minimal disturbance of this nature unlikely. Treatment, when necessary, should be with an intravenous injection of 2–3 mg of propranolol but the drug must be used with great caution during anaesthesia.

Measurement of the arterial and central venous pressures should be performed throughout the operation and in the post-operative period until stability of the circulation is ensured. Similarly a continuous electrocardiograph should be monitored. Blood loss must be measured and replacement carried out. Hypotension is likely to occur soon after the tumour is removed, or in the immediate post-operative period, but it is not by any means invariable. Just occasionally persistent hypertension may suggest a second tumour in the patient. Almost always hypotension can be combated by the administration of a blood transfusion, and such treatment, usually in excess of the actual quantity of blood lost during the operation, is the best therapy for the low blood pressure. Noradrenaline is best avoided but may occasionally be required. It is as well to note that this agent may be ineffective if the patient's α receptors have been previously blocked. When a noradrenaline infusion is used, care must be taken to ensure that this does not cause or mask any persistent haemorrhage from the operation site, particularly in the post-operative period. The patient must be weaned as quickly as possible from the noradrenaline as the blood pressure stabilises itself. Patients who have had a phaeochromocytoma for a long time—particularly if structural changes have developed in their vessels—may well retain their hypertensive blood pressure level and never revert to normal.

Bilateral Adrenalectomy

Bilateral adrenalectomy is usually undertaken for the treatment of Cushing's syndrome or of patients with metastases from a breast carcinoma. For the former it can be expected to ensure remission of the disease whether the hyperadrenalism is due to a cortical tumour or to hyperplasia. Hypophysectomy is certainly the more logical treatment for hyperplasia and is becoming more popular. For the latter it is combined with bilateral oöphorectomy, either at the same or another operation, in an attempt to remove all the hormone-producing tissue on which these tumours to some extent depend. A successful operation is usually associated with marked symptomatic improvement, particularly when pain has been a severe factor, and in many patients there is evidence of tumour regression.

The anaesthetic problem is created by the general state of the patient, who is usually seriously ill, often emaciated, and generally with multiple secondaries. A pleural effusion, not infrequently bilateral, often complicates the situation and may hamper respiration sufficiently to warrant aspiration before operation. Even small effusions create mechanical difficulties during anaesthesia when the patient is postured. When anaesthesia can be safely induced in spite of their presence, it is kinder, however, to aspirate as soon as the patient is anaesthetised rather than in the ward. The patient's tolerance for anaesthetic drugs is likely to be reduced, and, when large doses of opiates or other analgesics have been administered, great care is needed to avoid an overdose. Unless the patient is moved into the necessary position for operation with caution, bones may be broken at the site of secondary deposits.

A course of cortisone on the lines previously suggested must be given. Although hypotension may occur in this type of patient, both during and after operation, it appears to be more an indication of the weak general condition than of loss of adrenal medullary secretions. Provided blood loss is adequately replaced and the anaesthetic sequence and dosage are chosen to avoid circulatory depression, vasoconstrictors such as noradrenaline are unnecessary.

Bilateral adrenalectomy alone has also been advocated and performed for the treatment of malignant hypertension, but with a singular lack of success in improving the symptoms or course of the disease, and for this condition the operation carries a high mortality in spite of supportive therapy for the circulation.

THE PANCREAS

The greater part of the pancreas consists of alveoli in which acinous cells secrete a digestive juice, but situated between the alveoli are occasional groups of cells known as the islets of Langerhans. The islets contain three distinguishable types of cell, alpha, beta, and delta. The alpha cells secrete *glucagon*, the beta cells *insulin* and the delta cells *gastrin*. These cells have an excellent blood supply and their venous drainage is into the portal vein.

Insulin is intimately concerned with carbohydrate metabolism. Its most important function is the promotion of glucose utilisation by the tissues, probably by stimulating the transfer of the carbohydrate across the cell wall by activating enzymes concerned in its metabolism. Insulin increases the process of glycogen formation in the liver (glycogenesis), its storage in both the liver and other body tissues—principally the muscles—and the rate of formation of fatty acids from glucose in the liver. It inhibits the breakdown of glycogen to glucose (glycogenolysis) in the liver, and also the formation of both glycogen and glucose from the end-products of protein metabolism (gluconeogenesis). Finally, the ultimate breakdown of glucose in the tissues, to provide energy for the body, is increased by insulin (Table 2).

Many other factors are concerned in the metabolism of carbohydrates. Hormones from the anterior pituitary and the adrenal cortex tend to antagonise the effect of insulin on peripheral glucose utilisation and to increase the break-down of glycogen to glucose and the formation of glucose from protein meta-bolism. They are, therefore, antagonistic to insulin. Thyroid and posterior pituitary hormone, and adrenaline from the adrenal medulla, have a similar effect—the mobilisation of sugar. Glucagon causes hyperglycaemia by pro-moting hepatic glycogenolysis, and catecholamines may block insulin secretion in response to rises in blood sugar. A rising blood sugar inhibits the liver's action in producing more glucose, while a falling blood sugar stimulates this. The blood sugar, in a normal person, represents the balance between these several factors. When insulin is absent, diabetes mellitus results; when it is present in excess, as may be the case in certain tumours of the pancreas, spon-taneous hypoglycaemia occurs.

40/TABLE 2

SUMMARY OF ACTIONS OF INSULIN ON LIVER, MUSCLE AND FATTY TISSUE

LIVER	MUSCLE
1. Increased protein and fat synthesis	1. Increased glucose uptake and glycogen synthesis
2. Decreased glucose output	2. Increased amino acid uptake and protein synthesis
3. Increased glycogen synthesis	3. Decreased protein breakdown
4. Decreased glycogen breakdown	4. Increased uptake of ketones

FAT

1. Increased glucose uptake
2. Increased fatty acid synthesis

Diabetes Mellitus

The primary result of the absence of insulin is a rise in blood sugar caused by the liver failing to make and store glycogen, and increasing the production of glucose from protein metabolism. Sugar eventually appears in the urine. The secondary result is a rise in the level of ketones in the blood, caused by an increase in the release of free fatty acids (FFA) from adipose tissue. Insulin plays a major part in the control of the release of FFA into the plasma which are then utilised by the liver. However in the absence of insulin the liver cannot cope with the excessive amount of FFA released and the result is an increase in the keto acids—acetoacetic and beta-hydroxybutyric acid—in the blood and then in the urine. A subsidiary result of the body's failure to break down carbo-hydrate is that ingested carbohydrate food merely adds to the already raised blood sugar.

The clinical syndromes associated with insulin lack are variable, but the classical immediate results of a high blood sugar (hyperglycaemia) are thirst, and marked polyuria, due to the high osmotic pressure exerted by the sugar in the urine preventing tubular reabsorption. The effect of a rising ketone level in the blood (ketosis) is to produce acidosis. This leads to hyperventilation (in its extreme the classical Küssmaul respiration), loss of sodium due to the combina-tion of these acids with body base and, as a result, more loss of fluid. Ultimately the patient becomes comatose, the blood pressure falls, and death follows. Peripheral neuritis and peripheral vascular disease are often associated with long-standing diabetes, and are probably the end results of associated metabolic deficiencies brought about by the absence of insulin.

The diagnosis of diabetes mellitus rests on the history, on examination of the urine and the blood sugar level.* The urine must be tested for sugar and for ketone bodies; while a glucose tolerance curve will give evidence of the glucose metabolism (see Fig. 3). A number of commercial tests are available for the rapid determination of blood and urine sugar and keto-acid concentrations. The normal renal threshold for glucose in blood is about 180 mg per 100 ml (10 mmol/l). Patients with a low renal threshold may leak glucose into the urine, even though their carbohydrate metabolism is normal. An alimentary lag in the absorption of glucose from the blood into the liver accounts for an abnormally high rise in the blood sugar with glycosuria in some people after a glucose meal, but the level falls to normal again as rapidly as it rises.

Diabetic patients broadly form two distinct types; those who are young, tend to be thin, are sensitive to insulin and easily made ketotic, and those who are elderly, perhaps well covered, insensitive to insulin and rarely ketotic. This is an important differentiation for purposes of treatment, since the first group need insulin and are easily controlled with it, enabling them to lead a normal life with few, if any, restrictions in diet. The second group are better controlled by some restriction of diet, since insulin is not always necessary and extremely large doses of it may have little effect upon them. Oral hypoglycaemic com-pounds may have a part to play in the treatment of patients in the second group.

These compounds are of two types—sulphonyl ureas and diguanides. They are valuable in the treatment of mild diabetic patients who do not have ketosis. Most patients in this group develop diabetes late in life and tend to be fat, and many of them can be controlled by dietetic measures alone. It is only as a supplement to dietetic control that oral hypoglycaemic agents should be used.

The *sulphonyl ureas* are tolbutamide (Rastinon) and chlorpropamide (Diabinese), the former having a short action and necessitating multiple (1–4)

---

* Dextrostix and the Blood Sugar

An approximate blood sugar level can be gauged simply and quickly by the use of Dextrostix. These consist of a buffered mixture of glucose oxidase, peroxidase and a chromogen system covered with a semi-permeable membrane on the end of plastic strip. A large drop of blood is spread over the reactive area on the strip, and washed off exactly one minute later by a jet of cold water. The presence of glucose is shown by the formation of a blue colour, and the quantity of glucose can be gauged by comparison with a colour chart.

daily doses, while the latter is usually effective for twenty-four hours. Both are thought to produce hypoglycaemia by causing the release of insulin from the beta cells of the pancreatic islets.

The *diguanides* are not often used, nor is their mode of action fully understood.

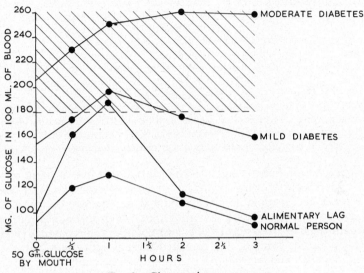

40/Fig. 3.—Glucose tolerance curves.

Excess of insulin in the sensitive patient may lead to symptoms of hypoglycaemia. These are sweating and tachycardia due to the release of adrenaline in an attempt to mobilise more glucose, and irritability of the central nervous system, due to lack of glucose. This takes the form of excitability, anxiousness, tremor, hunger, occasionally twitching, and rarely a fit. When treatment with intravenous glucose is not instituted quickly, marked mental changes occur followed by coma and death. Hypoglycaemic and hyperglycaemic coma are contrasted in Table 3 as the differential diagnosis is important to the anaesthetist, and may have to be dissociated from the effects of anaesthesia postoperatively.

Treatment.—It is not proposed to discuss the details of treatment, but only to stress the working principle that a young diabetic is best controlled with adequate doses of insulin—preferably a long-acting preparation such as protamine zinc insulin†—and allowed a free diet. Such treatment is amply justified by

† There are many types of insulin available, the three commonly used being soluble insulin (SI), protamine zinc insulin (PZI) and insulin zinc suspension (IZS). SI has a short action of up to twelve hours, while PZI is effective for twenty-four hours or longer. The duration of action of IZS varies from about twelve to thirty-six hours depending upon the particular suspension used.

A mild or moderately severe case of diabetes can usually be controlled with a single dose of PZI given in the morning, or by a morning and evening dose of SI. A severe case is unlikely to be completely controlled by PZI alone and may need SI as well in the morning to limit glycosuria during the day; both these insulins can, however, be combined in the same syringe and injected together. A suitable suspension of IZS may be as effective as a combined injection of PZI and SI.

40/Table 3

THE CLINICAL SIGNS OF HYPERGLYCAEMIA AND HYPOGLYCAEMIA

	Hyperglycaemia	*Hypoglycaemia*
General . .	Cold, dehydrated, smell of acetone, sunken eyeballs, pupils not specific, may be vomiting. Reflexes all sluggish.	Sweating, pallor, large pupils generalised twitching and reflexes hyperactive (unless terminal).
Respiration .	Deep, sighing hyperventilation.	Unaffected.
Circulation .	Low blood pressure, tachycardia.	Blood pressure normal in early stages, but tachycardia marked.

A blood sugar always establishes the diagnosis. Sugar may be present in the urine in hypoglycaemic coma if there has been a sudden swing due to insulin. Ketone bodies signify hyperglycaemia, but it should not be forgotten that causes other than diabetes can account for it, i.e. ether or chloroform anaesthesia and prolonged vomiting.

the large number of diabetic patients who lead normal lives without restriction of activity and without being any more upset by everyday illnesses than non-diabetic patients. Treating the diabetic patient as a normal patient is also the key to safe anaesthesia when it is needed. The fat, probably elderly patient is usually controlled by a restricted diet in terms of both calories and carbohydrate but if this does not succeed, and provided there is no ketosis, an oral hypoglycaemic agent should be tried. All diabetics must be maintained with ketone-free urine; a trace of sugar is satisfactory. A summary of the different types of insulin that are in common use and their approximate onset and duration of action are shown in Table 4.

40/Table 4

PREPARATIONS OF INSULIN

Name	*Strength of solution (units/ml)*	*Approx. onset action (hr)*	*Approx. duration action (hr)*
Insulin Injection BP (Sol. Insulin)	20,40,80	1	6
Insulin Zinc Suspension (Amorphorous) BP (Semilente)	40,80	1	14
Insulin Zinc Suspension (Crystalline) BP (Lente Insulin)	40,80	3	22
Protamine Zinc Insulin Injection BP	40,80	7	36

The blood sugar and anaesthesia.—Three sets of facts need consideration:

1. The effects of the anaesthetic drugs and technique.

2. The effects of operation.

3. The effects of pre- and post-operative complications.

1. *The effects of anaesthetic drugs and techniques.*—At one extreme are drugs such as ether which produce hyperglycaemia in some degree, and at the other, thiopentone, nitrous oxide (with sufficient oxygen), methoxyflurane and enflurane which do not affect blood glucose levels. Between them are halothane, trichloroethylene, cyclopropane and many other agents which tend to cause a slight, though varying, rise in blood sugar. A badly administered anaesthetic—particularly if associated with hypoxia—is very likely to produce hyperglycaemia.

The exact cause of this increase in blood sugar differs with each agent. It probably does not represent a direct effect on the liver of the agent concerned but an indirect action mediated by the alteration of insulin secretion and the output of adrenal cortical and medullary hormones. Direct action by growth hormone may also play a significant part (Oyama, 1973). Other factors which may also lead to sympathetic stimulation and the release of adrenaline such as fear, hypoxia and a difficult induction may also cause hyperglycaemia.

2. *The effects of operation.*—These may be more profound than those of the anaesthetic, but are surprisingly slight. Griffiths (1953) showed a statistically significant, but clinically unimportant, maintained rise in blood sugar during upper abdominal sections, when sympathetic stimulation might be expected to be the cause. In superficial operations the blood sugar was not affected. On the other hand, removal of the cause of a hyperglycaemic response, such as the baby from a pregnant diabetic woman, may result in a hypoglycaemic tendency—particularly if the insulin dosage is not modified post-operatively (Foster and Francis, 1955).

3. *The effects of pre- and post-operative complications.*—The severity of the surgical condition, and any associated disease, are most important here. Acute infective processes in particular lead to an increased blood sugar as the energy requirements of the patient rise. Post-operatively similar considerations hold, but vomiting may be an additional complication. Protracted vomiting (pre- or post-operative) can lead to ketosis in otherwise normal people, but even more moderate nausea and emesis may lead to hypoglycaemia in a diabetic patient by preventing an adequate carbohydrate intake.

The diabetic patient, operation and anaesthesia.—People with diabetes live normal lives. For them the risks associated with anaesthesia and operation are very little more than for a normal person, but certain essentials must be assumed for such a statement to be substantiated. The anaesthetic must be properly chosen and administered, adequate facilities for blood and urinary sugar estimations must be available, and the state of the diabetes at the time when the operation is proposed must be understood.

The management of diabetic patients requiring surgery will depend essentially on the nature of the operation, the severity of the diabetes and its degree of control. Many regimes have been advocated (King, 1957; Steinke, 1970; Malins and Sulway, 1972; Maw, 1975), and although the general principles are often similar, their papers confirm the difficulty of laying down specific guide lines which will always be applicable to any given patient. It is only by careful management of each patient individually that metabolic complications can be prevented.

Diabetic patients may be divided into those treated with either diet or oral hypoglycaemic agents and those treated with insulin. In the former group in whom elective minor surgery is necessary no difficulties should arise. Patients receiving oral hypoglycaemic agents should not take these on the day of operation, and if the agent is chlorpropamide this is usually stopped 24 hours before operation because it has a long half-life of approximately 36 hours and may thus cause hypoglycaemia during surgery. In all diabetics a routine estimation of the blood sugar level should be made both pre- and post-operatively. If a patient in this group is undergoing major surgery, particularly if this is an emergency procedure, it may be necessary to treat their diabetes with insulin and care must always be taken to see that hyperglycaemia and ketosis does not occur.

In the second group of diabetics are all those patients who are receiving insulin whether on a short-term basis—as mentioned above—until oral therapy can be recommenced, or for life. Their management will depend on the severity of the metabolic disturbance caused by the surgery, and not necessarily on the extent of the surgery. Thus an amputation of a limb under regional anaesthesia may result in only minimal metabolic disturbance.

Operation, whenever possible, should be arranged at the start of the morning, programme because the management of the therapy will be based on a specific time schedule and full laboratory facilities will be available throughout the remainder of the day for all estimations required. No patient should receive any oral glucose within 6 hours of operation. The hypertonicity of the solution will delay gastric emptying and give rise to the grave danger of aspiration (King, 1957).

All elective operations must be performed on patients whose diabetes is fully controlled. For minor procedures carried out early in the morning insulin may be withheld until the patient is in the recovery room when two-thirds of the normal daily dose is given and fluid taken orally. For major elective procedures two regimes of therapy will be considered. In the diabetic who does not normally require more than 60 IU of insulin a day and who is not prone to ketosis, one-third of the normal morning insulin dosage, of whatever type, may be given pre-operatively with intravenous 5 per cent dextrose being given during the operation; post-operatively the same dose of insulin is again given and if the blood sugar is above 250 mg per cent (15·5 mmol/l) or the urine showing 4+ test for sugar additional soluble insulin is given (Steinke, 1970).

If intravenous feeding is continued on the following day one-third of the insulin dose can be given in the morning and one-third in the afternoon. Measurements of blood sugar are continued and any adjustments necessary to the total insulin dosage are made. This regime allows the patient to be maintained on the same forms of insulin during the operative period as was being received prior to admission.

In diabetics who are unstable and require high daily insulin dosage or have a tendency to become ketotic, treatment should be with soluble insulin given t.d.s. 2–3 days before surgery to achieve full control pre-operatively. On the morning of surgery two-thirds of the normal morning insulin dose on which the patient has been stabilised is given and a 5 per cent dextrose drip set up and 500 ml given every 6 hours until oral fluids are again being taken. In order not to increase the rate of protein catabolism that will occur normally post-operatively at least 100 g of glucose should be given intravenously every 24 hours.

Post-operatively the patient can be given the remaining one-third of the morning dose provided the blood sugar is greater than 110 mg/100 ml (6·1 mmol/l). If oral fluids cannot be taken the following day soluble insulin may be given on a sliding-scale basis related to the urine or blood sugar estimations (Maw, 1975).

The uncontrolled diabetic should never undergo surgery until stabilisation has been achieved unless the surgical condition is life-threatening. The operative morbidity and mortality of patients who are ketotic is greatly in excess of normal. The major metabolic problems in this type of patient include severe hyper-glycaemia, hyperkalaemia, acidosis and ketosis (although this is not found in the hyperosmolar, hyperglycaemic, non-ketotic form of diabetic coma— McCurdy, 1970). Insulin may be given intramuscularly in small repeated doses (Alberti *et al.*, 1973; Page *et al.*, 1974) by continuous infusion (Sonksen *et al.*, 1972) or by large bolus doses intravenously (Soler *et al.*, 1974). Isotonic saline is given and after the first litre potassium supplements added, approximately 30–40 mmol/hour. An untreated patient with diabetic ketoacidosis may have a normal or only moderately raised serum potassium. However, insulin causes a shift of potassium from the extracellular to the intracellular fluid so that the serum level can fall dramatically. It is essential, therefore, to monitor serum K^+ levels during treatment to prevent a dangerous hypokalaemia. If there is a severe metabolic acidosis intravenous bicarbonate (1 per cent or 1·26 per cent) may be necessary (Soler *et al.*, 1975). Throughout the management of diabetic ketoacidosis repeated measurements of blood sugar, serum potassium and acid-base status are essential.

Anaesthetic Technique

When possible, regional techniques of anaesthesia (properly conducted) will result in the least metabolic disturbance. In those patients requiring general anaesthesia thiopentone, nitrous oxide/oxygen and muscle relaxants (when necessary supplemented with an inhalational agent or intravenous narcotic), will have little effect *per se* on the diabetes. The mild hyperglycaemia that may occur during general anaesthesia is of little significance when compared with the rapid and dangerous consequences of hypoglycaemia.

Pancreatic Tumours

A rare tumour of the pancreas, arising from the islets of Langerhans, may cause symptoms of hypoglycaemia due to the excessive secretion of insulin. These tumours may be benign or malignant, and the attacks they cause tend to be paroxysmal. They are frequently amenable to surgery. Hypoglycaemia may occur as a result of fasting during the pre-operative period (Fraser, 1963; Bourke, 1966) and if untreated can lead to circulatory collapse during the induction of anaesthesia and before the tumour is handled. This may be mini-mised by treatment with 100–200 mg of hydrocortisone per day pre-operatively with an increase in carbohydrate intake. The blood sugar level should therefore be gauged, at least approximately, just before induction of anaesthesia. An intravenous infusion of 5 per cent dextrose should be used throughout the operation, which may be associated with hypoglycaemia during the handling of the tumour. The only clinical evidence of this is likely to be an increasing tachycardia with perhaps sweating. Removal of the tumour may be associated with some post-operative suppression of insulin formation by the remaining normal pancreatic tissue, so that a temporary hyperglycaemia occasionally results.

REFERENCES

ALBERTI, K. G. M., HOCKADAY, T. D. R., and TURNER, R. C. (1973). Small doses of intramuscular insulin in the treatment of diabetic "coma". *Lancet*, **2**, 515.

BOURKE, A. M. (1966). Anaesthesia for the surgical treatment of hyperinsulinism. *Anaesthesia*, **21**, 239.

BRUNJES, S., JOHNS, V. J., Jr., and CRANE, M. G. (1960). Pheochromocytoma: post-operative shock and blood volume. *New Engl. J. Med.*, **262**, 393.

CSANKY-TREELS, J. C., LAWICK VAN PABST, W. P., BRANDS, J. W. J., and STAMENKOVIC, L. (1976). Effects of sodium nitroprusside during the excision of phaeochromocytoma. *Anaesthesia*, **31**, 60.

DHUNÉR, K. G., and NORDQUIST, P. (1957). Sleep reinduced by cortisone and glucose in patients intoxicated with barbiturates and related drugs. *Acta anaesth. scand.*, **1**, 55.

DOBKIN, A. B., BYLES, P. H., and CHO, M. H. (1965). Neuroleptanalgesics 3: Effect of innovar—nitrous oxide anaesthesia on blood levels of histamine, serotonin, epinephrine and norepinephrine, and on urine excretion. *Canad. Anaesth. Soc. J.*, **12**, 349.

EDWARDS, D. (1962). Radiological investigation of phaeochromocytoma. *Proc. roy. Soc. Med.*, **55**, 428.

FANNING, G. L., DYKES, M. H. M., and MAY, A. G. (1970). Anaesthetic management of phaeochromocytoma. A case report. *Canad. Anaesth. Soc. J.*, **17**, 261.

FINNERTY, F. A., BUCHHOLZ, J. H., and GUILLAUDEU, R. L. (1958). The blood volumes and plasma protein during levarterenol-induced hypertension. *J. clin. Invest.*, **37**, 425.

FOSTER, P. A., and FRANCIS, B. G. (1955). An operation for the diabetic? *Brit. J. Anaesth.*, **27**, 291.

FRASER, R. A. (1963). Hyperinsulinism under anaesthesia. *Anaesthesia*, **18**, 3.

GANONG, W. F. (1975). *Review of Medical Physiology*, 7th edit. Los Altos, Cal.: Lange.

GRIFFITHS, J. A. (1953). The effects of general anaesthesia and hexamethonium on the blood sugar in non-diabetic and diabetic surgical patients. *Quart. J. Med.*, **22**, 405.

HARRISON, T. S., BARTLETT, J. D., Jr., and SEATON, J. F. (1968). Current evaluation and management of pheochromocytoma. *Ann. Surg.*, **168**, 701.

INGLE, D. J., and KENDALL, E. C. (1937). Atrophy of adrenal cortex of rat produced by administration of large amounts of cortin. *Science*, **86**, 245.

JAMES, M. L. (1970). Endocrine disease and anaesthesia. *Anaesthesia*, **25**, 232.

JOHNS, V. J., Jr., and BRUNJES, S. (1962). Pheochromocytoma. *Amer. J. Cardiol.*, **9**, 120.

JONES, N. F., WALKER, G., RUTHVEN, C. R. J., and SANDLER, M. (1968). α-methyl-p-tyrosine in the management of phaeochromocytoma. *Lancet*, **2**, 1105.

KALREIDER, N. L., MENEELY, G. R., and ALLEN, J. R. (1942). The effect of epinephrine on the volume of the blood. *J. clin. Invest.*, **21**, 339.

KING, B. C. (1957). The control of diabetes mellitus in surgical patients. *Anaesthesia*, **12**, 30.

KITAHATA, L. M. (1971). Airway difficulties associated with anaesthesia in acromegaly. *Brit. J. Anaesth.*, **43**, 1187.

LAMSON, P. D., GREIG, M. E., and ROBBINS, B. H. (1949). Potentiating effect of glucose and its metabolic products on barbiturate anesthesia. *Science*, **110**, 690.

LEATHER, H. M., SHAW, D. B., CATES, J. E., and MILNES WALKER, R. (1962). Six cases of phaeochromocytoma with unusual clinical manifestations. *Brit. med. J.*, **1**, 1373.

McCURDY, D. K. (1970). Hyperosmolar, hyperglycaemic nonketotic diabetic coma. *Med. Clin. N. Amer.*, **54**, 683.

MALINS, J. M., and SULWAY, M. J. (1972). Management of diabetes in pregnancy, surgery and intercurrent illness. *Brit. J. hosp. Med.*, **7**, 201.

MAW, D. S. J. (1975). The emergency management of diabetes mellitus. *Anaesthesia*, **30**, 520.

NELSON, D. H. (1963). Present status of the problem of iatrogenic adrenal cortical insufficiency. *Anesthesiology*, **24**, 457.

OYAMA, T. (1973). *Anesthetic Management of Endocrine Disease*. Berlin: Springer-Verlag.

OYAMA, T., and MATSUKI, A. (1970). Plasma levels of cortisol in man during spinal anaesthesia and surgery. *Canad. Anaesth. Soc. J.*, **17**, 234.

OYAMA, T., and MATSUKI, A. (1971). Plasma cortisol levels during anaesthesia and surgery in man. *Anaesthesist*, **20**, 140.

OYAMA, T., TAKIGUCHI, M., TAKAZAWA, T., and KIMURA, K. (1969). Effect of meperidine on adrenocortical function in man. *Canad. Anaesth. Soc. J.*, **16**, 282.

PAGE, M. McB., ALBERTI, K. G. M. M., GREENWOOD, R., GUMAA, K. A., HOCKADAY, T. D. R., LOWRY, C., NABARRO, J. D. N., PYKE, D. A., SÖNKSEN, P. H., WATKINS, P. J., and WEST, T. E. T. (1974). Treatment of diabetic coma with continuous low-dose infusion of insulin. *Brit. med. J.*, **2**, 687.

PLUMPTON, F. S., BESSER, G. M. and COLE, P. V. (1969). Corticosteroid treatment and surgery. *Anaesthesia*, **24**, 12.

RIDDELL, V. (1970). Thyroidectomy: prevention of bilateral recurrent nerve palsy. *Brit. J. Surg.*, **57**, 1.

ROBERTSON, A. I. G. (1965). Pre- and postoperative care in patients with phaeochromocytomas. *Postgrad. med. J.*, **41**, 481.

ROSS, E. J. (1962). Phaeochromocytoma: medical aspects. *Proc. roy. Soc. Med.*, **55**, 427.

SALASSA, R. A., BENNETT, W. A., KEATING, F. R., and SPRAGUE, R. G. (1953). Postoperative adrenal cortical insufficiency occurrence in patients previously treated with cortisone. *J. Amer. med. Ass.*, **152**, 1509.

SARAJAS, H. S., NYHOLM, P., and SUOMALAINEN, P. L. (1958). Stress in hypothermia. *Nature (Lond.)*, **181**, 612.

SJOEROSMA, A., ENGELMANN, K., WALDMANN, T. A., COOPERMANN, L. H., and HAMMOND, W. G. (1966). Phaeochromocytoma: current concepts of diagnosis and treatment. *Ann. intern. Med.*, **65**, 1302.

SLANEY, G., and BROOKE, B. N. (1957). Postoperative collapse due to adrenal insufficiency following cortisone therapy. *Lancet*, **1**, 1104.

SOLER, N. G., BENNETT, M. A., FITZGERALD, M. G., and MALINS, J. M. (1974). Successful resuscitation in diabetic ketoacidosis: a strong case for the use of bicarbonate. *Postgrad. med. J.*, **50**, 465.

SOLER, N. G., FITZGERALD, M. G., WRIGHT, A. D., and MALINS, J. M. (1975). Comparative study of different insulin regimens in management of diabetic ketoacidosis. *Lancet*, **2**, 1221.

SÖNKSEN, P. H., SRIVASTAVA, M. C., TOMPKINS, C. V., and NABARRO, J. D. N. (1972). Growth hormone and cortisol responses to insulin infusion in patients with diabetes mellitus. *Lancet*, **2**, 155.

STEHLING, L. C. (1974). Anesthetic management of the patient with hyperthyroidism. *Anesthesiology*, **41**, 585.

STEINKE, J. (1970). Management of diabetes mellitus and surgery. *New Engl. J. Med.*, **282**, 1472.

STONER, T. R., and URBACH, K. F. (1968). Cardiac arrythmias associated with succinyl-choline in a patient with pheochromocytoma. *Anesthesiology*, **29**, 1228.

VAN BRUNT, E. E., and GANONG, W. F. (1963). The effects of preanesthetic medication, anesthesia and hypothermia in the endocrine response to injury. *Anesthesiology*, **24**, 500.

WALTERS, G. (1969). Secretory characteristics of phaeochromocytoma and related tumours: their diagnostic and clinical significance. *Ann. roy. Coll. Surg. Engl.*, **45**, 150.

WHITWAM, J. G., and RUSSELL, W. J. (1971). The acute cardiovascular changes and adrenergic blockade by droperidol in man. *Brit. J. Anaesth.*, **43**, 581.

WHITWAM, J. G., TUNBRIDGE, W. M. G., and FULLER, W. I. (1973). Management of patients for yttrium-90 implantation of the pituitary gland. *Brit. J. Anaesth.*, **45**, 1121.

Section Six

THE REPRODUCTIVE SYSTEM

Chapter 41

THE PHYSIOLOGY OF CHILDBIRTH

Innervation of the Genital Tract (Fig. 1)

The female pelvic viscera are under both nervous and hormonal control. The nervous control is derived primarily from the hypothalamus through the reticular formation where the descending pathways interact with ascending influences from the pelvis. Thus the higher centres are concerned with the control of the balance between the effects of the two peripheral autonomic divisions, the sympathetic and the parasympathetic systems. They should not be considered as antagonistic to each other as in many instances they are synergistic and work harmoniously under the control of the descending pathway to achieve their physiological function.

The sympathetic centres for the female pelvic viscera lie in the lower thoracic and upper lumbar segments of the spinal cord. From here pre-ganglionic fibres pass through the ganglia of the sympathetic trunk to the *aortico-renal plexus* where they finally synapse. A part of the aortico-renal plexus extends along the ovarian artery as the *ovarian plexus*. The *superior hypogastric plexus* or *pre-sacral nerve* is the continuation of the aortico-renal plexus passing down over the bifurcation of the aorta where it divides in front of the sacrum into two trunks, the *right* and *left hypogastric nerves*. Each hypogastric nerve is joined by the parasympathetic, *pelvic splanchnic nerves* (nervi erigentes) of the corresponding

INNERVATION OF THE GENITAL TRACT

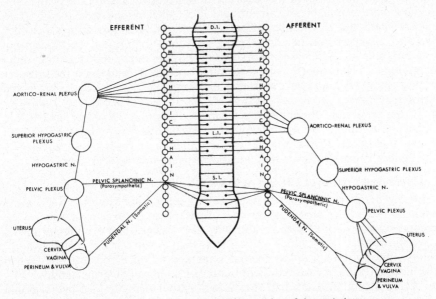

41/Fig. 1.—Diagram of the principal innervation of the genital tract.

side to form the right or left *pelvic* (inferior hypogastric; Frankenhauser's) *plexus*. The pelvic plexus thus contains a mixture of sympathetic and para-sympathetic elements. The *paracervical* or *utero-vaginal plexus* on each side is an extension of the pelvic plexus along the course of the uterine artery within the base of the broad ligament.

Nervous Control of Uterine Activity

In the cervix and lower part of the body of the uterus numerous adrenergic and cholinergic nerve fibres are associated with muscle bundles also forming an adventitial plexus around the blood vessels. The endometrial glands in this region are richly innervated by cholinergic fibres and only very sparsely with adrenergic fibres. The lamina propria of the vaginal cervix contains both adrener-gic and cholinergic fibres. In the remainder of the body and fundus of the uterus the myometrium is innervated with adrenergic nerve fibres and only occasional cholinesterase-positive fibres are seen in these regions (Coupland, 1969).

Jeffcoate (1969) states "There is difficulty in deciding to what extent auto-nomic nerves demonstrated in the pelvic organs carry impulses to and from the blood vessels and to what extent they are motor or sensory to other tissues . . . It is not known whether the uterus receives both parasympathetic (cholinergic) and sympathetic (adrenergic) nerves or whether it has only a sympathetic component". In a summary of the present state of knowledge on these matters Wendell-Smith (1970) states "The pharmacological events which follow the arrival of an impulse at post-ganglionic sympathetic nerve endings are complex and not completely understood. The uterus was one of the first organs for which it was demonstrated that sympathetic stimulation releases acetylcholine as well as adrenergic substances. There is increasing evidence that the release of acetyl-choline is the first event in the sequence that makes the membrane of the sym-pathetic fibre permeable to calcium ions. The calcium ions enter the fibre and release adrenergic transmitter substances from the bound form in which they are held. Furthermore the adrenergic transmitters are not pure substances but are mixtures of adrenaline, noradrenaline, dopamine and possibly other compounds. The proportions and amounts of these depend upon the intensity of nervous activity, and their synthesis, in the myometrium at least, is promoted by oestrogens".

From the welter of conflicting evidence concerning the motor innervation of the uterus, opinion seems to favour the view that the parasympathetic system contributes little to myometrial activity, and that the uterus is mainly affected by the inhibitory and stimulatory influences of the sympathetic system.

Hormonal Control of Uterine Activity

It is generally agreed that an intact nerve supply is not essential to the initia-tion and progress of labour. A number of paraplegic patients have reached the second stage of labour without difficulty and Vasicka and Kretchmer (1961) have shown that spinal block extending as high as the cervical region will not inhibit uterine activity unless there is a marked fall of blood pressure. When the blood pressure is restored there is a return to normal uterine activity.

There is good evidence that the onset of labour is determined by hormonal changes that take place in the fetus (Robinson and Thorburn, 1974). This would seem a logical arrangement as the timing of delivery should depend upon fetal maturity.

The fetal pituitary/adrenal axis is believed to be important because pituitary ablation in fetal lambs prolongs gestation indefinitely; in the human, anencephaly in the absence of hydramnios may be associated with prolonged gestation. Furthermore, a marked increase in the growth rate of fetal adrenals has been observed near term and in otherwise unexplained prematurity. A large increase in fetal cortisol concentration precedes spontaneous labour. Cortisol is believed to be principally concerned with fetal lung maturation, but may also increase the production of oestrogens by the feto-placental unit.

Oestrogens.—A dramatic increase in unbound oestrogens of fetal origin, in particular 17 β oestradiol, has been observed near term. 17 β oestradiol is synthesised in the feto-placental unit from precursor steroids of adrenal origin, under the control of fetal ACTH. High doses of synthetic glucocorticoids given to the mother during pregnancy may therefore suppress this fetal oestrogen production. 17 β oestradiol is believed to stimulate the synthesis and release of prostaglandins in the myometrium, and to increase uterine sensitivity to oxytocin.

Oxytocin has no physiological role in the initiation of labour, nor do endogenous levels appear to increase markedly until the second stage, when stretching the birth canal associated with expulsive efforts promotes reflex release of oxytocin from the maternal posterior pituitary (Bisset, 1976). Oxytocin may be involved in the release of prostaglandin $F_{2\alpha}$ and certainly acts synergistically with prostaglandins and oestrogen in stimulating uterine contractility. Exogenous oxytocin can accelerate normal labour although it cannot induce abortion without simultaneous prostaglandin administration. The important physiological role of oxytocin is in stimulating milk ejection (Bisset, 1976), while oxytocin of fetal origin may play a synergistic role in myometrial stimulation.

Progesterone is the key factor in inhibiting uterine activity in pregnancy. In the first few months it is produced by the corpus luteum but later its site of production shifts from the ovary to the placenta. A gradual fall in progesterone level precedes the onset of labour. Progesterone may act by blocking the release or the effect of prostaglandins on the myometrium. The presence of a high concentration of progesterone may prolong gestation, while an intermediate level may delay cervical dilatation.

Prostaglandins (PGs) are a large series of unsaturated hydroxy fatty acids widely distributed in minute amounts in the tissues. Their primary action seems to be in regulating adenylate-cyclase activity and producing smooth-muscle stimulation, but they have a wide variety of effects in the body, and appear to be involved in the inflammatory response. They comprise several families of related compounds designated alphabetically A to H, which differ from each other chemically and in biological activity. Those of the E and the F series particularly are uterine stimulants. As well as playing a role in conception, they may form an essential step in the final common path of all modes of uterine stimulation. In the uterus they are formed in the decidual cells following disruption of the lysosomes. Lysosomal disruption can be promoted by oestrogens, by lower segment stretching and by sweeping the membranes off the lower segment. Uterine contraction, causing further lysosomal disruption, therefore becomes auto-accelerating. Hibbard *et al.* (1974) showed that there was a progressive rise in PG concentration in amniotic fluid from the 36th week of gestation and a further rise during the first stage of labour. $PGF_{2\alpha}$ has been found to be present in large amounts in the uterine vein in normal labour, in concentrations varying directly with those of 17 β oestradiol (Robinson and Thorburn, 1974) which triggers its synthesis and release.

Prostaglandins have been used clinically in therapeutic termination of pregnancy and in the induction and maintenance of labour (Embrey, 1969; Karim *et al.*, 1969). They are administered orally or by intravenous infusion but the dosage may be limited by troublesome side-effects such as nausea, vomiting, diarrhoea or tissue irritation and erythema at the infusion site. When higher doses are required to empty the uterus in cases of intra-uterine death, anencephaly or hydatidiform mole, the infusion may be given extra-amniotically and the side-effects avoided (Embrey *et al.*, 1974).

Catecholamines do not play a major role in the initiation or maintenance of labour but they may modify the uterine response to oxytocic agents. In the non-pregnant uterus *noradrenaline* is thought to be active in closing the isthmic canal during the late menstrual cycle to reduce the chance of abortion or low implantation of a fertilised ovum. The primary effect of *adrenaline* on the uterus is to inhibit uterine contraction. However, if a β-blocking agent, propranolol, is given with adrenaline, uterine activity is enhanced. This suggests that only the β-activity is inhibitory while the less dominant α-activity is excitatory.

The myometrial inhibitory effect of β-receptor stimulation has been used clinically to suppress premature labour with orciprenaline, but the dosage is limited by maternal tachycardia (Baillie *et al.*, 1970). More recently, the more specific β_2 stimulants salbutamol (Liggins and Vaughan, 1973) and ritodrine (Zuspan, 1972) have been used to inhibit labour with less tendency to cause maternal tachycardia, which in any case may be controlled by practolol (McDevitt *et al.*, 1975), or one of the newer cardioselective β_1-receptor blockers.

ONSET OF LABOUR

These considerations suggest a possible explanation of the events leading to the onset of labour. During the first and second trimesters of pregnancy, uterine activity is normally inhibited by the stimulation of the β_2-adrenoreceptors. As a result of other hormonal changes associated with the rise of oestrogen activity in late pregnancy, the myometrial inhibition by progesterone is reduced and the threshold of the β_2-adrenoreceptors rises. The threshold of the α-adrenoreceptors falls, increasing the excitatory effect of adrenergic stimulation. The uterus is thus prepared for the production of the strong regular contractions in response to the release of oxytocin from the posterior pituitary or administered by the buccal or intravenous route. Following the initiation of uterine contractions there is an increased secretion of prostaglandin which assists in sustaining the progress in labour.

Sensory Pathways

Sensory stimuli from the uterine body are transmitted through the pelvic, superior hypogastric and aortico-renal plexuses to the 11th and 12th thoracic segments (Cleland, 1933), but there is reason to believe that the severe pain of the late first stage and of the second stage is also mediated through the two adjacent segments (Bonica, 1972*a*).

Sensory stimuli from the *cervix* pass through the pelvic plexus along the pelvic splanchnic nerves to sacral segments 2, 3 and 4 and to the sacral portion of the sympathetic chain. The sensory supply of the *vagina* is derived partly from parasympathetic and partly from somatic nerves. Stimuli from the upper vagina run through the pelvic plexuses and the pelvic splanchnic nerves to sacral roots 2, 3 and 4 through the pudendal nerve. Other sensory pathways are derived from the terminal branches of the ilio-inguinal and genito-femoral nerves supplying the labia majora. The perineal branch of the posterior cutaneous nerve of the thigh communicates with the pudendal nerve in giving terminal branches to the perineal body.

Practical Implications (Fig. 2)

Sensation of the processes of labour are transmitted through dual pathways to the central nervous system. Uterine contraction is perceived via the sympathetic afferent nerves entering at the lower thoracic segments while the sensations of rectal pressure and vaginal, perineal and vulval distension are transmitted via sacral roots 2, 3 and 4. The significance of the afferent pathway from the cervix to sacral segments 2, 3 and 4 via the pelvic plexus and pelvic splanchnic nerves is less easy to determine but it is thought to be the route by which severe backache is felt in labours with inco-ordinate uterine action, cervical dystocia or a persistent occipito-posterior position of the infant's head. An explanation of the low backache of very early labour is that during a uterine contraction the fundus of the uterus comes forward causing pressure on the posterior segment of the pelvic brim. This sensation would therefore be transmitted by somatic nerves to sacral roots 2, 3 and 4 (Crawford 1965).

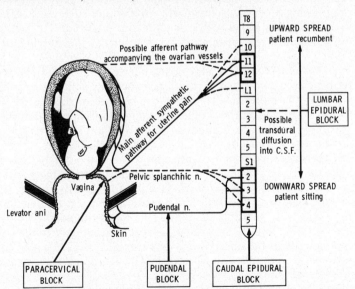

41/Fig. 2.—Schematic representation (simplified) of the effect of nerve blocks used in labour.

The degree of pain suffered in labour by individual women varies in intensity. For practical purposes it may be considered to be of *uterine* and *perineal* origin. Uterine pain is transmitted mainly by the lower thoracic roots and can be relieved by a blockade affecting these segments while perineal sensation, if it becomes painful, may be relieved by a block of sacral roots 2, 3 and 4. In the early part of labour, only uterine pain is felt but even when the head is pressing on the perineum and is distending the vulva the complaint may be only that associated with uterine pain. If the mother complains of perineal pain it will be relieved by a block affecting the sacral roots. Occasionally the severe backache associated with inco-ordinate action of the uterus or a posterior position of the occiput will only be relieved by a block affecting the sacral roots (Moir and Willocks, 1967).

Pudendal block, when used for forceps delivery, does not relieve the pain of labour but merely affords perineal analgesia and relaxation. Low subarachnoid (saddle) block would have a similar but more intense effect and in addition would relieve pain perceived via sacral roots 2, 3 and 4. It should not be forgotten that block of the pudendal nerve is insufficient by itself for episiotomy and forceps delivery. Perineal infiltration is needed to block the endings of the perineal branch of the posterior cutaneous nerve of the thigh. In addition infiltration of the labia majora may be required to block the labial branches of the ilio-inguinal and genito-femoral nerves.

Paracervical block interrupts the nerve pathways by which uterine and cervical pain are perceived but it leaves perineal, vaginal and vulval sensation unimpaired. Its variable success may be due to the alternative afferent pathway from the fundus via the nerves accompanying the tubo-ovarian vessels.

Caudal epidural block up to the 11th thoracic segment abolishes all sensation of labour by blocking both the sacral and the lower thoracic pain pathways—the sacral roots being blocked preferentially long before such block is needed by the mother. Reduction of pelvic floor muscle tone predisposes to malrotation of the baby's head and, in primigravidae, the virtual inevitability of assisted delivery.

Lumbar epidural block with large doses of local anaesthetic spreads up to the lower thoracic roots and down to the sacral roots thus obliterating all the sensations of labour. In smaller doses the effect can be made more selective (Doughty, 1969). If given with the mother in the horizontal position or with a slight head-down tilt the block can be limited to the lower thoracic roots thus blocking uterine pain without affecting perineal sensation or the tone of the perineal muscles. If perineal analgesia is required later in labour a further injection may be directed to the sacral roots by placing the mother in a sitting position. Some degree of sacral block may be obtained quite fortuitously with a small-dose epidural block given at the 2nd–3rd lumbar interspace without any formal attempt to direct the solution caudally. This raises the possibility of a direct transdural diffusion into the subarachnoid space affecting the cauda equina and is in accordance with the observations of Frumin *et al.* (1953) who found that procaine injected epidurally can be recovered in significant concentrations from the cerebrospinal fluid.

Implications of sympathetic blockade.—While it is necessary to block the sympathetic afferent impulses entering at the 11th and 12th thoracic segments to relieve the pain of uterine contraction, any extension of the block to a higher level will affect the motor nerve supply to the uterus. Although the role of the motor nerves in the regulation of uterine activity in labour is very doubtful, any diminution of the strength and frequency of contractions following epidural block may be compensated by buccal or intravenous oxytocin.

Blockade of the sympathetic efferent nerves will cause arteriolar relaxation and fall of blood pressure which may be responsible for some diminution of uterine activity (Vasicka and Kretchmer 1961). This effect can be minimised by using doses just sufficient to produce relief of labour pain. The extent of the rise of the block in the thoracic region may be checked by testing the level of analgesia to pinprick on the anterior abdominal wall although it should be remembered that sympathetic block is likely to be effective for 2 to 3 segments above the level of sensory block.

The effect of the limitation of venous return to the heart caused by the backward pressure of the gravid uterus on the inferior vena cava may be made manifest by even a small degree of sympathetic block. A normal level of blood pressure with a diminished cardiac output can only be maintained by an increased peripheral resistance due to compensatory sympathetic vasoconstriction. Even the small degree of sympathetic blockade accompanying caudal or lumbar epidural analgesia may be followed by a sudden fall of blood pressure which may be expected at any time up to 45 minutes from the initial injection or after any subsequent top-up The remedy is the immediate relief of caval compression by turning the mother on to her side or by manual lateral displacement of the uterus (see Chapter 43).

PAIN IN LABOUR

The uterus itself can be cut or compressed without discomfort but traction on the supporting ligaments is painful. During the latter part of pregnancy the uterus contracts rhythmically but without evoking any unpleasant sensation. Genuine labour begins when contraction of the muscles of the upper segment stretches the longitudinal fibres of the lower segment of the uterine body and cervix. Simultaneously the circular fibres of the cervix relax.

The pains are analogous to those produced by distension and stretching of other hollow viscera and are usually felt in the hypogastrium over the area supplied by the cutaneous branches of the 11th and 12th thoracic nerve roots with a contribution from L.1. In other labours—particularly those in which the occiput is posterior—pain is felt in the back over the sacrum and occasionally on the posterior aspect of the thighs. Late in the first stage of labour the sensation of pressure on the rectum and levatores ani muscles may become painful as may the distension of the vagina, perineum and vulva in the second stage.

At the start of labour the contractions are ill-defined, infrequent and of short duration. As labour progresses they become more frequent, occur at fairly regular intervals and persist for longer periods. Towards the end of the first stage they are likely to occur every three to four minutes and persist for about one and a half minutes. During the first stage there is normally little or no desire to bear down, but towards full dilatation of the cervix, a local pelvic reflex may come into play, making pain appear purposive. At this stage a voluntary bearing down effort can be of no value and may result in oedema of the rim of the cervix.

This is a most difficult pain for the mother to bear. With the onset of the second stage the contractions become more purposive and normally lead to active voluntary efforts to expel the infant. The bearing-down character of the contractions now raises the threshold of the mother to their stimuli, so that by comparison with those of the late first stage they seem less severe. This may account for the observation (Doughty, 1969) that many mothers given an epidural block for the relief of first stage labour pain will happily tolerate the purely somatic sensation of parturition even to tearing the perineum without complaint. As this stage progresses, the strength and frequency of the contractions are, in fact, not less intense, but more so. They last for up to one minute and occur at approximately two-minute intervals.

The intensity of pain bears little relationship to the strength of uterine contraction, nor to the consequent increased uterine pressure. Each uterine contraction slowly mounts to a maximum which is sustained for a few seconds and then rapidly falls away. Pain commences at a variable interval following the start of the contraction and the length of this interval depends on the mother's individual threshold to pain (Fig. 3).

In the diagram uterine contraction is represented by a curve ascending until maximum intensity is reached; it is held for a short time at maximum intensity and then diminishes until the contraction ceases at, say, one minute from its commencement. At a variable degree of intensity of contraction the pain threshold is crossed. In the diagram the "normal" pain threshold is represented by a line which is crossed by the curve 15 seconds after the start of the contraction. The pain threshold is crossed again as the contraction diminishes in intensity 45 seconds from its start. Thus with the "normal" threshold to pain the mother would experience 15 seconds of painless contraction, 30 seconds of painful con-

RELATIONSHIP OF PAIN TO UTERINE CONTRACTION

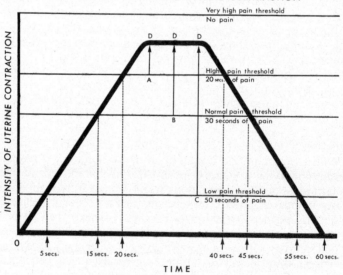

41/FIG. 3.—Relationship of pain to uterine contraction (see text).

traction followed by 15 seconds of painless contraction as its intensity diminishes below the threshold. The intensity of pain suffered may be represented by the vertical distance BD.

The threshold to pain varies widely in different women. A few may deny suffering any pain whatever in labour. These would be represented on the diagram as having a "very high pain threshold" which is never crossed by the contraction curve. A uterine contraction in a woman with a "high pain threshold" would be painless for the first 20 seconds, painful for the next 20 seconds and painless for the last 20 seconds. The intensity of pain felt is represented by the vertical distance AD.

Unhappily a fair number of mothers can be regarded as having a "low pain threshold". Here the interval between the start of the contraction and the crossing of the pain threshold is only 5 seconds, the painful section of the contraction lasts 50 seconds and the intensity of pain suffered can be represented by the vertical distance CD.

Practical Implications

In circumstances where midwives assume responsibility for the management of analgesia, the progress of labour rather than the pain itself conditions the choice and use of analgesic agents. As the first stage of labour may be long, varying from a few hours to 24 hours or more, relief of pain is commonly sought in the use of narcotic analgesic agents. These can be simply administered by injection in doses adequate to raise the mother's threshold to pain for several hours yet without undue effect on uterine contractions. The greatest intensity of labour pain occurs just before full dilatation of the cervix, when traditionally the residue of narcotic analgesia is supplemented by the more cumbersome inhalational methods. These can be controlled

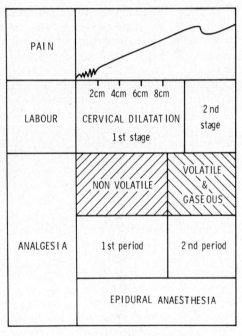

41/Fig. 4.—Diagram to illustrate use of drugs in labour.

to meet the particular and variable needs of the mother as the last and most painful part of labour progresses and, it is hoped, with minimal effect on the child's respiratory centre. For purposes of pain relief, therefore, labour can be artificially divided into two periods, according to whether non-inhalational agents or volatile and gaseous agents are used. These two periods overlap and do not bear any exact relationship to the stages of labour, although they are superimposed upon them (Fig. 4).

It is fortunate that there is a brief interval between the onset of uterine contraction and the perception of pain, as this enables the midwife to compensate in some measure for the lag between the inhalation of nitrous oxide and the onset of analgesia. However, failure to start the inhalations as soon as the contractions begin will result in less than adequate pain relief being obtained by the time that the contractions become painful. Nitrous oxide analgesia, from which the mother recovers completely between the contractions, has to be re-induced in association with each subsequent contraction. In a woman with a low threshold to pain the contractions become painful before the inhalations of nitrous oxide become effective. In these cases, nitrous oxide may be supplemented with or replaced by trichloroethylene or methoxyflurane, both of which have cumulative and therefore continuous analgesic effects. Alternatively, in most modern maternity departments, the mother would be afforded more effective relief by means of an epidural block which may be given at any time in labour irrespective of the degree of cervical dilatation.

Physiological Changes in Pregnancy

Normal pregnancy results in numerous changes in maternal physiology affecting all the major systems and it is not possible accurately to judge the functions of pregnant women by the criteria used for males and non-pregnant females. Lind (1975) lists some of the physiological changes that occur during pregnancy, together with the clinical diagnoses they might indicate and draws an admittedly exaggerated picture of "an overweight, starving, myxoedematous, thyrotoxic, infected, anaemic wreck—the healthy pregnant woman!"

Salt and water retention is a normal phenomenon of pregnancy. There is also an increase in blood volume which may eventually be 50 per cent above normal and this is accompanied by a significant but smaller increase of 18 per cent in total red cell mass. The net result is the apparent "physiological anaemia of pregnancy" which may be exacerbated by the demand for iron by the growing fetus. With the increase in blood volume is a marked rise in cardiac output which may eventually be 30 per cent above normal. The rise in output is progressive until the 6th month, after which it was thought to fall to near normal values by the time labour starts. This fall in late pregnancy is not seen if the measurement is made with the woman lying on her side, thus suggesting that inferior vena caval occlusion by the gravid uterus is mainly responsible for the apparent reduced cardiac output. The blood pressure is not significantly changed during normal pregnancy, but rises during labour and increases still further with each uterine contraction. As the uterus retracts after delivery, the pulmonary circulation becomes temporarily loaded with blood from the placenta. This sudden auto-transfusion may not be well tolerated by a woman with a restricted cardiac output (for example from mitral or aortic stenosis) in whom a sudden increase in venous return may lead to congestive cardiac failure. In these cases intravenous oxytocin is preferred to ergometrine because oxytocin is free from any vasoconstrictor effect. Although both drugs cause contraction of uterine muscle, oxytocin is less likely to increase venous return. In the presence of a restricted cardiac output a modest blood loss may be permitted (without replenishment) to reduce the circulating blood volume.

As the uterus increases in size the diaphragm rises, but this is compensated by transverse and antero-posterior enlargement in the thoracic cage. Tidal volume is increased to an even greater extent resulting in a fall of $Paco_2$ to about 30 mm Hg (4·0 kPa). The respiratory alkalosis is partially compensated by a fall in buffer base so that the pH of the blood remains at about 7·44 during pregnancy.

Despite the increase in vital capacity and a reduction in airway resistance due to bronchiolar relaxation, dyspnoea tends to occur in late pregnancy particularly on exercise. During labour the stimulus of pain leads to a great increase in the tidal volume and peak inspiratory flow rate (Crawford and Tunstall, 1968). Any apparatus designed for use in inhalational analgesia should be able to meet a demand of a peak inspiratory flow of 350 l/min and tidal volumes up to 3 litres without imposing a resistance to inspiration.

Among the serum enzyme changes in late pregnancy is a 30 per cent reduction in pseudocholinesterase activity (Shnider, 1965). The high frequency of the use of suxamethonium in obstetric anaesthesia and rarity of prolonged apnoea in pregnant patients suggest that this enzyme change has little clinical significance.

THE FETUS AND FETAL DISTRESS (see also Chapter 44)

With each uterine contraction the placental circulation is diminished, and the maternal placental blood flow may fall to a very low level, even though the maternal blood pressure itself rises. Thus the transfer of oxygen to the fetal circulation falls with, and rises again after, each uterine contraction. Abnormal states of the placenta—such as partial or complete separation from the uterine wall or infarction with loss of surface area—diminish the oxygen-saturation level in the fetal circulation. The normal progress of the second stage of labour leads to a progressive diminution in the placental circulation, thus submitting the fetus to an increasing degree of hypoxia and acidosis (Pearson and Davies, 1974). In ordinary circumstances this is compatible with the birth of a living child. Unduly prolonged labour or continuous uterine hypertonus may lead to such a degree of fetal hypoxia as to cause permanent cerebral damage. This hazard can be compounded by the uncontrolled use of oxytocin particularly if the fetus is otherwise at risk.

The fetal heart rate.—The normal fetal heart rate varies from 120 to 160 beats per minute. Bradycardia is the response of the fetal heart and circulation to oxygen lack which may cause a sharp fall in rate to about 60 beats per minute. To some degree the fetal heart may be expected to slow during uterine contractions but the failure to return rapidly to its normal rate between contractions may be a cause for concern. When hypoxia is particularly severe, irregularity may follow bradycardia.

Fetal tachycardia is sometimes noted as an early sign of distress but this had been thought unlikely to be due to hypoxia since, unlike bradycardia, it is not readily relieved by maternal oxygen inhalations. Nevertheless it should be taken as implying the need for a closer monitoring of the fetal heart rate as tachycardia has been shown to be associated with fetal acidosis and may be followed later by bradycardia (Coltart et al., 1969).

Cardiotocography.—The limitations of intermittent auscultation of the fetal heart are generally recognised and fetal welfare is now monitored by continuous recording of the fetal heart rate (FHR) and uterine contractions

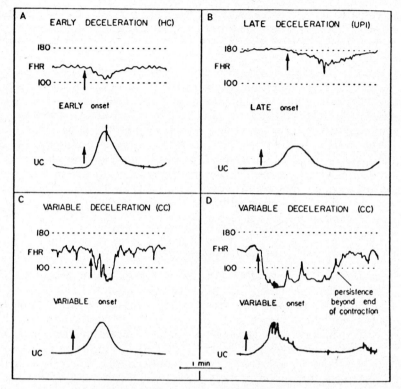

41/FIG. 5.—Fetal heart rate deceleration patterns (after Bonica, 1972b).

(Hon, 1969). The FHR patterns comprise *baseline changes* from normal which occur independently of uterine contractions and in *periodic changes* which are closely associated with them. The important baseline recordings are the *fetal heart rate* itself which is normally between 120 and 160 beats per minute and the *beat-to-beat variation* of the FHR which normally varies by 5 to 25 beats per minute. A loss of the beat-to-beat variation is considered to be of particularly serious significance.

The periodic changes are the three deceleration patterns observed in association with the uterine contractions (Fig. 5—Bonica, 1972b). *The early deceleration pattern*, otherwise known as "Type I dip", is a slowing of the FHR, the lowest point of which coincides with the peak of the uterine contraction, the normal FHR being restored when the uterus relaxes. This change is thought to be due to compression of the fetal head and is considered to be physiological and not of serious significance. However, a slow recovery of the FHR to normal level following uterine relaxation might be interpreted as an early warning of possible fetal distress.

The late deceleration pattern, otherwise known as "Type II dip", is a fall of the fetal heart rate occurring after the peak of the uterine contractions. This is held to be due to utero-placental insufficiency and is usually accepted as a reliable sign of fetal distress. It should be understood that the deceleration may occur within the normal baseline limits of the FHR, namely 120–160 beats per minute. It is the time-lag between the start of the contraction and the beginning of the dip in the FHR which gives the late deceleration pattern its serious significance.

The variable deceleration pattern is a slowing of the FHR persisting for unequal periods and irregularly co-ordinated with the uterine contractions. It is thought to be due to umbilical cord compression but, unless prolonged and severe, it is not considered to be of serious significance, as in the early stages it is not associated with biochemical changes in the fetus. However, it should be taken as a warning of the possible development of the late deceleration pattern.

The interpretation of baseline and periodic variations in the FHR has been a matter of considerable debate. For instance, Emmen *et al.* (1975) claimed to identify a "terminal" pattern of tracings obtained in labours ending in intra-uterine death. The baseline FHR was within the normal range but there was a decrease or disappearance of beat-to-beat variation together with late decelera-tion patterns in relation to the uterine contractions. It was, nevertheless, pointed out that a suppression of beat-to-beat variations may occur when diazepam is used as a sedative in labour and it has also been reported for a short period following the injection of lignocaine in epidural analgesia. In these cases supportive measures such as a change from the supine to the lateral posture together with an infusion to increase circulating blood volume were effective in restoring normal baseline variability (Boehm *et al.*, 1975).

On the other hand, late deceleration patterns were observed by Thomas (1975) in 8·4 per cent of labours but the fetal pH was less than 7·25 in only 41 per cent of cases and the one-minute Apgar score was less than 7 in only 47 per cent. Epidural anaesthesia and the supine position were associated with late deceleration in 71 per cent of cases, but in spite of this the fetal scalp pH and the 1-minute Apgar scores were identical in the epidural and non-epidural cases.

It is generally agreed that cardiotocography should be regarded only as a screening method of fetal monitoring; fetal blood sampling should be used as the final arbiter of the need for urgent delivery. Used alone, cardiotocography is likely to result in unnecessary operative deliveries.

Fetal blood sampling.—The measurement of the pH of fetal blood has provided the most accurate and reliable means of assessing the condition of the fetus during labour (Saling and Schneider, 1967). If the fetus is deprived of oxygen its glycogen metabolism proceeds anaerobically to the formation of lactic acid rather than through the normal aerobic metabolic cycle via pyruvic acid to carbon dioxide and water. The accumulation of lactic acid in the fetal blood lowers its pH and results in metabolic acidosis. Thus a fall of the fetal blood pH can be an index of fetal asphyxia.

The mean range of variability of the fetal blood pH during labour is from 7·35 to 7·26. This should remain constant until shortly before delivery; then a fall in pH occurs due not only to the natural interruption of placental flow during the uterine contraction but also to an accumulation of lactic acid in the mother which is transferred to the fetus. In general a fall in fetal pH to below 7·25 would be considered abnormal and a fall in pH to 7·20 suggests that early delivery would be desirable.

Some caution is needed in the interpretation of these figures. An abnormally low pH value can be caused by errors of technique in collecting the sample from the fetal scalp, such as contamination with liquor, inadequate mixing of the sample or a delay of more than a few minutes before taking the measurement. Ideally, the pH measuring apparatus should be sited within the labour ward area, not only to avoid the delay in obtaining the result but also for the convenience of repeated tests, as clinical action on the basis of only one measurement may not be justified. Serial estimations at short intervals showing a steady fall in pH might suggest the need for some positive action to deliver the baby.

Before taking action on the basis of a low fetal pH it should be remembered that any degree of metabolic acidosis in the mother will be reflected in the fetus. For instance if the mother herself is dehydrated and ketotic, a pH of below 7·25 in her infant may not be viewed as seriously as if her own acid-base status had been normal. In practice a maternal blood sample should be taken together with the fetal sample and any base deficit in the mother corrected with a bicarbonate infusion. Normally the maternal-fetal base deficit difference is 3 mEq/litre (mmol/l). A progressive increase of this difference in serial samples would indicate fetal asphyxia.

The benefits derived from fetal blood sampling are shown by the reduction in the number of Caesarean sections done for fetal distress at Queen Charlotte's Hospital from 86 cases in 1964/65 to 27 in 1966/67. It was unusual to perform the operation solely because of the clinical signs of fetal distress if the pH remained within normal limits (Beard and Morris, 1969).

REFERENCES

BAILLIE, P., MEEHAN, F. P., and TYACK, A. J. (1970). Treatment of premature labour with orciprenaline. *Brit. med. J.*, **4**, 154.

BEARD, R. W., and MORRIS, E. D. (1969). *Modern Trends in Obstetrics*, p. 298. London: Butterworths.

BISSET, G. W. (1976). Neurohypophyseal hormones. In: *Peptide Hormones*. Ed. J. A. Parsons. London: Macmillan Press.

BOEHM, F. H., WOODRUFF, L. F., and GROWDON, J. H. (1975). The effect of lumbar epidural anesthesia on fetal heart rate baseline variability. *Anesth. Analg. Curr. Res.*, **54**, 779.

BONICA, J. J. (1972a). *Obstetric Analgesia and Anaesthesia*, p. 50. Berlin: Springer Verlag.

BONICA, J. J. (1972b). *Principles and Practice of Analgesia and Anesthesia*, p. 1248. Philadelphia. F. A. Davis, Co.

CLELAND, J. G. P. (1933). Paravertebral anaesthesia in obstetrics. *Surg. Gynec. Obstet.*, **57**, 51.

COLTART, T. M., TRICKEY, N. R. A., and BEARD, R. W. (1969). Foetal blood sampling. Practical approach to management of foetal distress. *Brit. med. J.*, **1**, 342.

COUPLAND, R. E. (1969). The distribution of cholinergic and other nerve fibres in the human uterus. *Postgrad. med. J.*, **45**, 78.

CRAWFORD, J. S. (1965). *Obstetric Anaesthesia*, 2nd edit., p. 23. Oxford: Blackwell Scientific Publications.

CRAWFORD, J. S., and TUNSTALL, M. E. (1968). Notes on respiratory performance in labour. *Brit. J. Anaesth.*, **40**, 216.

DOUGHTY, A. (1969). Selective epidural analgesia and the forceps rate. *Brit. J. Anaesth.*, **42**, 1058.

EMBREY, M. P. (1969). The effect of prostaglandins on the human pregnant uterus. *J. Obstet. Gynaec. Brit. Cwlth.*, **76**, 783.

EMBREY, M. P., CALDER, A. A., and HILLIER, K. (1974). Extra-amniotic prostaglandins in the management of intra-uterine fetal death, anencephaly and hydatidiform mole. *J. Obstet. Gynaec. Brit. Cwlth.*, **81**, 47.

EMMEN, L., HUISJE, S., AARDOUDSE, J. G., VISSER, G. H. A., and OKKEN, A. (1975). Antepartum diagnosis of the "Terminal" fetal state by cardiotocography. *Brit. J. Obstet. Gynaec.*, **82**, 353.

FRUMIN, M. J., SCHWARTZ, H., BURNS, J. J., BRODIE, B. B., and PAPPER, E. M. (1953). The appearance of procaine in the spinal fluid during peridural block in man. *J. Pharmacol. exp. Ther.*, **109**, 102.

HIBBARD, B. M., SHARMA, S. C., FITZPATRICK, R. J., and HAMLETT, J. D. (1974). Prostaglandin $F_2\alpha$ concentrations in amniotic fluid in late pregnancy. *Brit. J. Obstet. Gynaec.*, **81**, 35.

HON, E. H. (1969). *An Introduction to Fetal Heart Rate Monitoring.* New Haven: Harty Press Inc.

JEFFCOATE, T. N. A. (1969). Pelvic pain. *Brit. med. J.*, **3**, 431.

KARIM, S. M. M., TRUSSELL, R. R., HILLIER, K., and PATEL, R. C. (1969). Induction of labour with prostaglandin $F_2\alpha$. *J. Obstet. Gynaec. Brit. Cwlth.*, **76**, 769.

LIGGINS, G., and VAUGHAN, G. S. (1973). Intravenous infusion of salbutamol in the management of premature labour. *J. Obstet. Gynaec. Brit. Cwlth.*, **80**, 29.

LIND, T. (1975). The assessment of normal pregnancy. *Brit. J. hosp. Med.*, **14**, 253.

MCDEVITT, D. G., WALLACE, R. J., ROBERTS, A., and WHITFIELD, C. R. (1975). The uterine and cardio-vascular effects of salbutamol and practolol during labour. *Brit. J. Obstet. Gynaec.*, **82**, 442.

MOIR, D. D., and WILLOCKS, J. (1967). Management of inco-ordinate uterine action under continuous epidural analgesia. *Brit. med. J.*, **3**, 396.

PEARSON, J. F., and DAVIES, P. (1974). The effect of continuous lumbar epidural analgesia upon fetal acid-base status during the second stage of labour. *J. Obstet. Gynaec. Brit. Cwlth.*, **81**, 975.

ROBINSON, J. S., and THORBURN, G. D. (1974). The initiation of labour. *Brit. J. hosp. Med.*, **21**, 15.

SALING, E. E., and SCHNEIDER, D. (1967). Biochemical supervision of the foetus during labour. *J. Obstet. Gynaec. Brit. Cwlth.*, **74**, 799.

SHNIDER, S. M. (1965). Serum cholinesterase activity during pregnancy labor and the puerperium. *Anesthesiology*, **26**, 335.

THOMAS, G. (1975). The aetiology, characteristics and diagnostic relevance of late deceleration patterns in routine obstetric practice. *Brit. J. Obstet. Gynaec.*, **82**, 126.

VASICKA, A., and KRETCHMER, H. E. (1961). Effect of conduction and inhalational anesthesia on uterine contractions. *Amer. J. Obstet. Gynec.*, **82**, 600.

WENDELL-SMITH, C. P. (1970). *Scientific Foundations of Obstetrics and Gynaecology*, p. 88. Ed. by E. E. Philipp, J. Barnes, and M. Newton. London: Heinemann Medical Books.

ZUSPAN, F. (1972). Premature labor: its management and therapy. *J. Reprod. Med.*, **9**, 93.

Chapter 42

THE RELIEF OF PAIN IN LABOUR

ALTHOUGH drugs play an important role in the relief of pain in labour it must not be supposed that they are necessarily of greater importance than proper preparation and training for childbirth. Normal labour can be an easy, trouble-free and deeply satisfying experience for many women provided that a rational and understanding approach is made to the matter by the mother and her medical attendants.

The normal process of childbirth must be explained simply and the discomfort involved should be mentioned and logically justified. The mother must be told that pain can be controlled, and it is always worth while describing the methods by which this relief will be given. Since some women do not need any form of analgesia, and others do not desire it, they should be assured that they are not obliged to accept it unless they wish to do so. Many women prefer to give birth to their child with their consciousness unclouded by drugs. The moment of birth is the longed-for climax of their months of pregnancy and they may regard as a disservice the imposition of heavy sedation or of a general anaesthetic merely for the crowning of the baby's head. Finally, the ability to relax during labour can be assisted by antenatal preparation with exercises designed to improve the voluntary control of the abdominal and pelvic muscles.

A more recent development is the establishment of classes for antenatal education independent of the hospital where parturition will ultimately take place. Most antenatal teachers appreciate that efforts to instil self-confidence in the mother antenatally must never be made at the expense of the confidence in those who are responsible for the well-being of the mother and baby during labour. Nevertheless, it must be recorded that the opportunity is sometimes taken to foster prejudice in the mother against certain aspects of the modern management of labour such as amniotomy, oxytocin stimulation, fetal monitoring and epidural analgesia. This creates confusion in the mind of the mother and militates against the principle of successful preparation which should create a bond of mutual confidence between the mother and her attendants.

Minimising the pain of labour depends to some extent upon the sympathy and assurance given by the attending doctor or midwife; it is certainly not beyond the capacity of anyone willing to spend the necessary time with the mother. Apart from drugs, she may be helped by such simple remedies as change of posture, changing a sodden sheet, rubbing of the lower part of the back together with kind words of encouragement. The tendency to welcome husbands or other close relatives to stay with the mother during labour may help to avoid the loneliness which, to many women, is the most distressing memory of childbirth. The presence of any "outsider" may make the professional attendants more alert to the needs of the parturient for more adequate analgesia.

It is when the ordinary remedies fail that the obstetric anaesthetist may play a major role in relieving pain and thus saving the mother's morale.

HYPNOSIS IN CHILDBIRTH

The advantages claimed for hypnosis during childbirth are that the mother can be kept pain-free but awake and co-operative; if desirable, sleep can be induced; there are no complications attributable to the method; and post-hypnotic suggestion can help to prevent after-pains and the expected post-partum depression. The best results are undoubtedly achieved in selected patients, and, perhaps one should add, by selected hypnotists. Unfortunately the method is too unreliable to be considered as a satisfactory routine alternative to chemical analgesia.

Obstetrical patients usually make good subjects for hypnosis, being open to suggestion and needing only a slight trance state to relieve their labour pains. There is moreover, a special value in the method since it enables the mother to remain awake and relaxed and consciously to participate in the birth of her child unaffected by depressant drugs.

To achieve a reasonable chance of success the mother must be trained by undergoing hypnosis on a number of occasions during pregnancy. She is then prepared for the onset of labour when hypnosis can be induced immediately. This training is time-consuming, although after at least one personal interview a number of selected mothers may be hypnotised in antenatal clinics (Michael, 1952). During the course of the actual labour, personal attention is essential if the best results are to be obtained. It may be possible to teach a patient auto-hypnosis so that she can be independent of the hypnotist (Davidson, 1962).

ACUPUNCTURE

Since the current wave of interest in acupuncture, attempts have been made to assess its value in analgesia for vaginal and abdominal delivery. The insertion of the intracutaneous needle alone has been effective in some patients but more consistent results have been obtained following the application of an electric current (Bonica, 1972). Abouleish and Depp (1975) used acupuncture in 12 parturients and obtained partial analgesia in early labour. When it became ineffective, a spinal or epidural block was given to produce complete analgesia. Acupuncture did not adversely affect the fetus or uterine contractions and there were no harmful after-effects. However, the analgesia was inconsistent, unpredictable and incomplete, the technique was time-consuming, it limited the patient's movement, added more wires and machinery and interfered with the electronic monitoring of the mother and fetus. One would not wish to condemn a technique which may suffer from being incompletely understood but its few advantages do not appear to be sufficiently attractive in the face of the frequent need to supplement its inadequacies by more reliable and well-tried methods.

GENERAL ANALGESIC DRUGS

The threshold to pain varies from patient to patient, so that each mother must be assessed individually. Some patients experience severe pain despite relative weak uterine contractions—indeed it seems likely that, in some, the acuteness of the pain inhibits the normal relaxation of the cervix and the contractions of the uterus. For this type of patient it was considered preferable to control the pain with narcotics to ensure sleep even at the expense of a temporary depression of uterine action. A far better modern alternative is to use epidural analgesia and to enhance the uterine contractions with an oxytocin infusion.

Normal multiparous women are usually more rapidly delivered than the primiparae and generally need less analgesia particularly in the second stage owing to the added relaxation of the previously stretched birth canal. This is not invariably so as many multiparae experience tumultuous, painful though rapid labours. The pattern of a previous childbirth may yield useful information as to what might be expected in the next.

The maturity of the child must be considered. Prematurity must be an indication for minimal doses of all central nervous system depressants. The small premature infant seldom causes difficulty at delivery, so that adequate analgesia can be produced without resort to high doses of any drug. In these cases it is better to avoid general analgesia and to use some form of conduction block rather than to increase the risk of neonatal asphyxia—a risk much greater than in full-term infants irrespective of analgesic drugs.

First Period—Sedative and Analgesic Drugs

The theoretical background of the control of pain in labour has been discussed in the previous chapter and as a guide to the selection of a general analgesic drug an artificial division of labour into two periods has been suggested. The pain of the first period, from the commencement of labour up to three-quarters dilatation of the cervix, may be controlled by non-inhalational agents, and that of the second period, from three-quarters dilatation to delivery, by inhalational agents (p. 1308).

In the early stages of labour and before the development of severe pain it has been customary to give mothers sub-hypnotic doses of chloral, barbiturates or other drugs as "sedation". The principal disadvantage of hypnotic drugs is their tendency to cause delirium if the pain becomes severe. It is now recognised that the *primary* need of a mother in labour is for *pain relief* either by an adequate dose of narcotic or by conduction block. Once the pain is adequately relieved the majority of mothers need no sedation and may go to sleep if they are so disposed. Occasionally some mothers show signs of anxiety or agitation and may require sedatives or tranquillisers in addition to analgesics but these are exceptions against the background of the over-riding need for effective analgesia.

Pethidine (Meperidine USP, Demerol)

Pethidine is the most generally used analgesic in the first period of labour. It is indicated when the discomfort of early labour merges into regular, frequent and painful contractions that are beginning to cause distress to the mother. The onset of genuine pain may be quite sudden and usually occurs at 3–4 cm dilatation of the cervix. The initial dose of 100 mg should be given by intramuscular injection; its effect will be apparent in 10–15 minutes and should last for two to three hours. When the pains are more severe or if the woman is unduly obese or anxious, the initial dose should be raised to 150 mg.

The subjective effect of pethidine varies widely in different women. To some it gives a pleasurable euphoria coupled with relief of pain, to some a positive dysphoria with nausea and vomiting, while others will deny any analgesic effect at all.

The dose should be repeated as the effect of the first dose is beginning to wane rather than after waiting for the distress to become fully re-established. If the labour has reached the second period when inhalational analgesia would be more appropriate, the administration of respiratory depressant drugs such as pethidine must be discontinued for fear of subsequent neonatal asphyxia.

The incidence of neonatal asphyxia severe enough to warrant active resuscitation is difficult to assess, and, in view of the almost universal acceptance of pethidine in labour for use by the unsupervised midwife, it has been assumed that the risk must be small enough to be outweighed by the benefits received. Nevertheless as long ago as 1954 the Medical Research Council's Committee on Analgesia in Midwifery showed that while infant survival was unaffected, the use of pethidine was followed by an increased need for active resuscitation. Roberts et al. (1957) found some diminution of the respiratory minute volume of most babies for several hours after birth when the mothers had received pethidine. Koch and Wandel (1968) showed carbon dioxide retention persisting for up to 5 hours in the infants of mothers who had received only one dose of 100 mg pethidine. Unexpectedly, infants whose mothers had received intramuscular pethidine less than one hour before birth were less likely to show respiratory depression than those whose mothers had been given pethidine 2 to 3 hours before birth (see also Chapter 44).

Evans et al. (1976) have drawn attention to the disadvantages of pethidine given intramuscularly. The onset of analgesia is slow, there is a short-lived peak level of effect, the individual tolerance of pain and response to analgesic drugs is variable and the mother's analgesic requirements during labour are quite unpredictable. They reported on the development of an apparatus for the intravenous self-administration of pethidine. Subject to an overall clinical control of the maximum dose, size of increment, maximum frequency of administration and infusion rate, the mother herself was free to control the timing of the increments according to her need. The opinion of mothers significantly favoured the use of the patient-controlled apparatus as it provided more effective analgesia than was obtained by a group of patients receiving pethidine intramuscularly; the mean total dose of 2·5 mg/kg was similar in the two groups as were the umbilical venous plasma pethidine concentrations.

Pethidine is believed to have an additional beneficial effect in labour quite apart from its analgesic action. Lindgren (1959) and Filler et al. (1967) have shown that when labour was well-established, pethidine reduced uterine hypertonus and frequency of the contractions but enhanced their amplitude. In cases of uterine dystocia the decreased frequency of contractions was associated with an increase in the rate of cervical dilatation. However, in modern practice, epidural analgesia would probably be preferred in these circumstances.

Pentazocine (Fortral)

Pentazocine is of particular interest because it is the first clinically useful analgesic which is pharmacologically related to the narcotic antagonists. Because it rarely causes drug dependence, it is free from narcotic legislation. Given intramuscularly, in a dose of 40 mg, pentazocine is equivalent to 100 mg pethidine (Moore et al., 1970), but analgesia cannot be enhanced by increasing the dose. Pentazocine has a more rapid onset of action of somewhat shorter duration and causes some respiratory depression which is not generally progressive with increasing dosage. It causes less sedation, nausea and vomiting. In common with all narcotic analgesics, pentazocine crosses the placenta. While the fetal/maternal ratio is not as high as that of pethidine (Moore *et al.*, 1970 and 1973), none of the comparative trials of the two drugs has shown important differences in the infants' Apgar scores (see also Chapter 44).

In contrast to pethidine, nalorphine and levallorphan do not reverse the effect of pentazocine but naloxone is an efficient and reliable antagonist for both analgesics.

The Central Midwives Board has approved the use of pentazocine by midwives in doses of 30–45 mg.

NARCOTIC ANTAGONISTS (see also Chapter 32)

The allyl derivatives of morphine or levorphanol, nalorphine and levallorphan, have been used to offset the respiratory depressant effects of pethidine and other narcotics. For many years a combination of pethidine 100 mg with levallorphan 1·25 mg in a 2 ml ampoule was commercially available as Pethilorfan. The mixture was recommended as providing maximal antagonistic effect to respiratory depression with minimal interference with the analgesic effect of pethidine. Following the work of Telford and Keats (1965), Campbell *et al.* (1965) and Rouge *et al.* (1969), it is now accepted that the combination of pethidine with a narcotic antagonist produces no less respiratory depression than pethidine given alone, but the incidence of unwanted side-effects is increased.

Nalorphine and levallorphan have both agonist and antagonist activity. Given alone they cause drowsiness, sweating, nausea and respiratory depression with some analgesia, but when given after an overdose of a narcotic analgesic, they antagonise both respiratory depression and analgesia. In the case of nalorphine the antagonism is of short duration and the subject may relapse into respiratory depression (Payne, 1954).

Naloxone (Narcan), the allyl derivative of oxymorphone, has narcotic antagonist properties but, unlike nalorphine or levallorphan, is devoid of agonist activity. Unlike nalorphine or levallorphan, it is capable of antagonising the agonist effects of pentazocine (Kallos and Smith, 1968) and even those of nalorphine and levallorphan (Blumberg *et al.*, 1966). Its duration of action, however, is rather brief.

When a mixture of pethidine 100 mg with naloxone 0·4 mg is given in labour, the analgesic effect of pethidine is antagonised without abolishing its side-effects (Girvan *et al.*, 1976). It seems therefore that the search for a satisfactory pethidine-antagonist mixture is likely to be unavailing.

The place of naloxone in obstetrics is to antagonise the effect of narcotics given to the mother should the labour proceed more rapidly than anticipated. A dose of 0·4 mg should be given intravenously and may be repeated at 3-minute intervals until the desired effect is obtained. If the infant is born with narcotic depression, a dose of 0·01 mg/kg should be injected into the umbilical vein and repeated if necessary. There have been no reports of overdosage with naloxone and large and repeated doses have been given without producing respiratory depression.

Narcotic-Tranquilliser Combinations

Despite modern efforts to achieve true analgesia in labour without affecting the mother's consciousness and ability to co-operate, interest still persists in the search for an "ideal state" of analgesia, somnolence and amnesia that has continued since the time when "twilight sleep" was in vogue. This involved the supplementation of the analgesic and soporific actions of an opiate with the cerebral sedative and amnesic effects of hyoscine. The disadvantages of hyoscine were the tendency to delirium in the mother when the analgesic effect of the opiate had worn off, and the discomfort of its antisialogogue effect. More recently the combination of pethidine with the phenothiazines, chlorpromazine, promazine or promethazine have been used in the belief that they potentiate the analgesic action of pethidine without increasing its respiratory depressant effect. They also tend to produce somnolence, mental detachment, anti-emesis and amnesia. Of the three phenothiazines mentioned, promazine (Sparine) has become the most popular because it is shorter-acting than chlorpromazine although it lasts 2 to 3 times as long as pethidine and because it has a mild analgesic effect in contrast to the anti-analgesic action found with promethazine by Dundee and Moore (1961).

Comparing pethidine and promazine with pethidine and a placebo, Matthews (1963) showed that the potentiating effect of promazine, as measured by the reduced amount of pethidine given, was evident only in labours lasting more than 12 hours. The retrospective maternal assessment of satisfaction showed no significant difference between the two groups. Even if a difference had been shown it could have been attributed to the amnesic effect of the promazine. Although no fall of blood pressure was recorded some tendency to tachycardia was observed.

A disadvantage of promazine and other phenothiazines is that, by virtue of their adrenolytic action, they tend to block the vascular response to loss of blood volume which may manifest itself in severe hypotension following quite a modest postpartum haemorrhage. Unexpectedly severe falls of blood pressure may occur with the subsequent induction of epidural analgesia or with halothane anaesthesia. A further disadvantage of promazine is that the mother may be so sleepy in the second stage of labour that she will be unable to summon up sufficient co-operation for the spontaneous delivery of her child. These drawbacks may be reduced by cautious dosage of no more than 25 mg and if the patient appears unduly sleepy when the next dose of pethidine is required, it should be given without promazine.

Diazepam (Valium) had a brief vogue as a supplement to pethidine analgesia. In a dose of 10–15 mg it has sedative and amnesic properties but is not anti-emetic; it is less likely to produce hypotension than the phenothiazines. It has been used in larger doses in the management of pre-eclampsia and in attempts to suppress premature labour. It also prevents the rise of central venous pressure and precipitation of pulmonary oedema following intravenous ergometrine in patients with mitral stenosis or arteriovenous shunts (Vaughan-Williams et al., 1974).

Some anxiety has been expressed concerning fetal welfare following placental transfer of diazepam (Cree et al., 1973). While a total dose of 30 mg to the mother had little effect on the infant's state, larger doses were associated with low Apgar scores at birth, apnoeic spells, muscular hypotonia, hypothermia, reluctance to feed and impaired metabolic response to cold and stress. Measurements of plasma levels of diazepam and its active metabolite, N-desmethyl diazepam showed that both were detectable in significant concentrations in some infants for up to eight days after birth. Hence great care should be taken in the use of this otherwise useful drug, particularly in the management of pre-eclampsia.

Other Narcotic Drugs

Despite the introduction of other narcotic analgesics such as alphaprodine, phenazocine and oxymorphone, none seems likely to displace pethidine and pentazocine as analgesics for the routine relief of pain in the early part of labour. Mention should be made, however, of the place of morphine and diamorphine (heroin) in the management of prolonged labour with severe pain. Either morphine 15 mg or diamorphine 10 mg reliably relieves pain and induces sleep and so enables an exhausted mother to rest and recover her morale. It should be remembered that when either of these drugs has been used the infant's respiratory centre could be affected if delivery occurs within five hours of their administration. In this event, naloxone given to the mother before delivery would guard against neonatal asphyxia.

It is doubtful whether morphine or diamorphine should ever be used in labour where facilities exist for epidural analgesia.

Second Period—Inhalational Agents

In 1934 Minnitt described a nitrous oxide/air apparatus which enabled parturients to administer analgesia to themselves. It was approved by the Central Midwives Board in 1936. Since then midwife-supervised self-administration has become the pattern of all the other "approved" inhalational methods of alleviating pain in the latter part of labour when narcotic analgesia should cease because of the risk of delivery of a depressed infant within the time of action of the drug.

Nitrous Oxide and Air

Nitrous oxide and air were given from a relatively simple type of intermittent flow apparatus of which the Minnitt, the Talley and the Jecta are examples and, even now, many thousands of these machines must still be in use all over the world. They are designed to deliver 50 per cent nitrous oxide in air and thus the mother's inspired gases contain no more than 10·4 per cent of oxygen.

For many years after its introduction, nitrous oxide/air was considered safe and satisfactory. It is surprising that there are so few published criticisms of the practice of allowing women in labour to respire an oxygen-deficient mixture particularly in view of the increasing preoccupation with the maintenance of adequate fetal oxygenation. Since the introduction of nitrous oxide/oxygen mixtures and with the current concern for fetal welfare, nitrous oxide/air machines must now be considered obsolete. The final seal was set on the fate of nitrous oxide/air analgesia by the withdrawal of approval by the Central Midwives Board in 1970.

Pre-mixed Nitrous Oxide and Oxygen

Barach and Rovenstine (1945) drew attention to the hazards of the practice of using hypoxic mixtures of nitrous oxide and oxygen in anaesthesia. In order to avoid hypoxia they proposed the use of 80 per cent nitrous oxide with 20 per cent oxygen pre-mixed in a single cylinder. The total cylinder pressure 700 psig (4826 kPa) was deliberately kept below the liquefaction pressure of nitrous oxide. This seriously limited the capacity of the cylinders because filling them to more than approximately one-third of their full pressure would result in liquefaction of the nitrous oxide as its saturation vapour pressure was exceeded.

Following a request by Tunstall (1961) the British Oxygen Company produced mixtures of 50 per cent and 60 per cent nitrous oxide with oxygen at total cylinder pressures of 2000 psig (13790 kPa) without liquefaction of the nitrous oxide.

Theoretically liquefaction of pure nitrous oxide should begin when its partial pressure exceeds the following values:

at 20° C	750 psig (5171 kPa)
10° C	600 psig (4137 kPa)
0° C	470 psig (3241 kPa)
−10° C	370 psig (2551 kPa)

According to Dalton's Law of Partial Pressures it should be possible, in a cylinder at or below these pressures to increase the cylinder pressure by adding oxygen without causing liquefaction of the nitrous oxide; the total cylinder pressure rises but the partial pressure of the contained nitrous oxide does not. Thus in a 50 per cent nitrous oxide/oxygen mixture at a total cylinder pressure of 1500 psig (10342 kPa), the nitrous oxide partial pressure is 750 psig (5171 kPa) and provided that the temperature stays at 20° C, the mixture should remain entirely gaseous.

In practice it has been found that the total pressure in a cylinder containing 60 per cent nitrous oxide can be raised to 3000 psig (20684 kPa) without liquefaction despite the fact that the theoretical nitrous oxide partial pressure would be 1800 psig (12411 kPa). It is clear that the cylinder contents do not behave as an "ideal" two-component system in compliance with Dalton's Law. This phenomenon, due to the solution of nitrous oxide in the gaseous oxygen to form a homogeneous gas mixture, is well demonstrated in the classical experiment by the British Oxygen Company scientists (Figs. 1a–d).

A transparent cylinder contains a measured quantity of nitrous oxide at a pressure of 660 psig (4551 kPa) at 15·6° C. The liquid level of the compressed nitrous oxide is visible (Fig. 1a). This cylinder is connected through a tap to a supply of oxygen kept at a constant pressure of 2000 psig (13790 kPa). The tap is opened allowing oxygen to bubble through the liquid nitrous oxide; the pressure in the transparent cylinder slowly rises (Fig. 1b). By the time that the pressure in the cylinder has reached 1300 psig (8963 kPa) the liquid level has disappeared and the two gases exist together in a single gas phase. The approximate proportion of nitrous oxide to oxygen is now 4:1 (i.e. cylinder content 80 per cent N_2O and 20 per cent O_2) (Fig. 1c). More oxygen is admitted to the

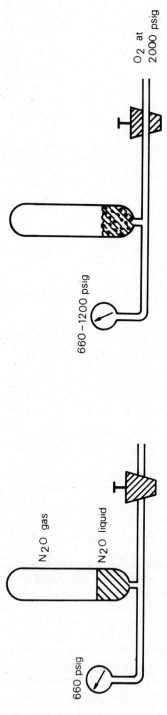

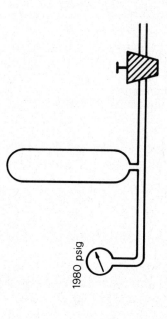

(a) The cylinder has been filled with the correct amount by weight of nitrous oxide.

(b) Oxygen is bubbled through liquid nitrous oxide—the cylinder pressure rises.

(c) The liquid nitrous oxide is now converted into gas. The cylinder pressure is 1300 psig and the composition of the mixture is 80 per cent/20 per cent $N_2O + O_2$.

(d) Oxygen continues to pass into the cylinder until the pressure has reached 1980 psig. The composition of the mixture is now 50 per cent/50 per cent $N_2O + O_2$.

42/Fig. 1.—The mixing of nitrous oxide and oxygen at 15·6° C.

cylinder until the pressure reaches 1980 psig (13652 kPa). The proportion of nitrous oxide to oxygen is now 50 per cent/50 per cent (Fig. 1d).

This phenomenon is not unique to nitrous oxide and oxygen. It has been observed with other gas mixtures including carbon dioxide and oxygen or nitrous oxide and nitrogen. It occurs most readily when the liquid phase is near its critical point, that is the temperature above which the gas can no longer be liquefied however great the pressure applied.

Such a nitrous oxide and oxygen mixture is stable as long as the cylinder contents remain above the separation temperature of the mixture. Below this point some nitrous oxide liquefies and separates from the oxygen. Separation in a full cylinder originally at a pressure of 1980 psig (13652 kPa) occurs at $-7°$ C with 50 per cent, and 1° C with 60 per cent and at 13° C with 70 per cent nitrous oxide. If the cylinder is used in the *vertical* position with the valve uppermost the early samples drawn off will be deficient in nitrous oxide and give inadequate analgesia, while the samples taken when the cylinder is near exhaustion will be oxygen-deficient and cause hypoxia, undue sleepiness and loss of co-operation.

Excessive cooling of the cylinder is liable to occur in exceptionally cold weather while in transit from the factory to the consumer premises. Although records show that prolonged severe winter weather is unusual in the United Kingdom (Gale *et al.*, 1964) this takes no account of conditions which may occur in many other countries. The cylinders may also remain exposed to cold after delivery to the consumer who must accept the responsibility for taking them immediately into relatively warm storage.

Another cause of cooling is the fall of cylinder temperature while the gas mixture is running owing to the heat absorption which occurs when a compressed gas is released. However, experiments have shown that even under conditions of high gas flow the temperature fall is never sufficient to change the composition of the emergent gas mixture (Crawford *et al.*, 1967). While cylinders containing nitrous oxide 50 per cent with oxygen would not contain separate gases until the temperature falls below $-7°$ C, cylinders nominally of this composition have been found to contain mixtures with an oxygen content varying between 48 per cent and 56 per cent from cylinder to cylinder. Any increase in the proportion of nitrous oxide could raise the separation temperature of the mixture and therefore the frequency of occasions when the weather conditions would predispose towards separation. The manufacturers now take special precautions to ensure that the gas mixtures are reliable within a tolerance of ± 2 per cent.

Mere re-warming of the cylinder is insufficient to guarantee *immediate* adequate re-mixing of separated gases; the cylinders must be agitated by inverting them three times (Cole, 1964). This is reasonably practicable with the portable 500 litre cylinders, very difficult with the heavy hospital size 2000 litre cylinders and virtually impossible with the 5000 litre cylinders intended for pipeline use. However storage of cylinders in the *horizontal* position at a temperature above 5° C for 24 hours will re-constitute mixtures which have been separated by cooling down to $-40°$ C. The more rapid distribution of the cylinder contents in the horizontal as compared with the vertical position is due to the larger area of interface between the liquid and the gaseous phase and the smaller distance between the surface of the liquid and the cylinder wall. This facilitates a more rapid evaporation and diffusion (Bracken *et al.*, 1968).

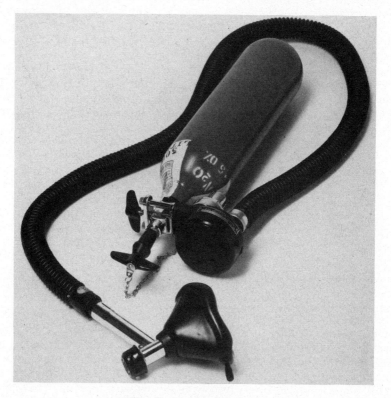

42/Fig. 2.—The "Entonox" apparatus.

Because of the difficulty of handling the 5000 litre cylinder intended for pipeline use and because they are outside the direct control of the user the manufacturers have, as an added safety precaution, fitted them with an internal tube extending from the valve to the further end of the cylinder cavity similar to that in a soda-water siphon. If storage and handling instructions have been ignored and some of the nitrous oxide is liquefied it will contain at least 20 per cent oxygen in solution and this sample would be drawn off first without serious danger to the patient. Without an internal tube an oxygen-rich sample would be drawn off first with the risk of leaving an oxygen-deficient mixture when the cylinder is approaching exhaustion (MacGregor *et al.*, 1972).

Apparatus.—The pre-mixed nitrous oxide and oxygen mixture is delivered by means of the "Entonox" apparatus (Fig. 2) which comprises a two-stage valve fitted to a cylinder head. A pressure gauge indicates the quantity of gas mixture in the cylinder and the gases pass on demand through a corrugated hose to a mask fitted with an expiratory valve.

The first stage consists of a simple reducing valve which decreases the full cylinder pressure of 1980 psig (13652 kPa) to 200 psig (1379 kPa) (Fig. 3). The slight negative pressure of inspiration opens the second stage tilting valve and the mixture is drawn into the corrugated hose. The slight positive pressure of expiration pushes down the sensing diaphragm and the tilting valve connected with it closes the flow of gases from the reducing valve.

The inspiratory resistance is extremely low; indeed if the corrugated hose

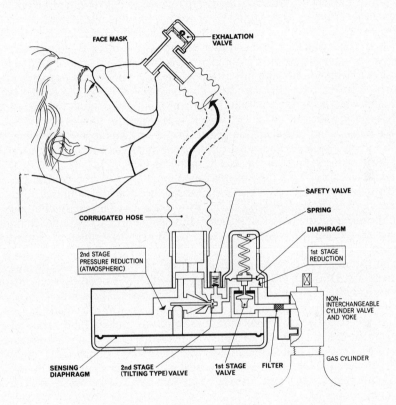

42/Fig. 3.—Mechanism of the "Entonox" apparatus.

is removed from the apparatus the gas mixture will continue to flow unless the outlet is momentarily occluded to make the tilting valve close. The design also ensures that no gas mixture can flow when the cylinder pressure falls below the first stage pressure of 200 psig (1379 kPa). Although this means that the final 10 per cent of the cylinder contents is inevitably wasted it does represent an added safety factor. If some separation of gases has occurred due to cooling below −7° C the wasted gases would be a portion containing higher than 50 per cent nitrous oxide.

The Entonox machine is very suitable for domiciliary practice, being compact and portable. It weighs 13½ lb (6·1 kg) with one full 500 litre cylinder. It is recommended that at least one spare cylinder should be carried for multiparous labours and two for primiparous (Crawford and Tunstall, 1968).

Not the least advantage of the pre-mixture of nitrous oxide and oxygen is that the mother, throughout the latter part of her labour, is breathing oxygen at a concentration near to that considered optimal for fetal welfare (Rorke et al., 1968; Phillips and MacDonald, 1971).

Nitrous oxide and oxygen from separate cylinders.—The advantages of a single concentration of nitrous oxide are less obvious in hospital practice where more bulky and less portable machines can be used to deliver nitrous oxide and oxygen either from separate cylinders or from a pipeline installation.

The "Lucy Baldwin" apparatus (Fig. 4) is a modification of the "Walton Five" dental gas machine (see Chapter 9) and is calibrated to deliver a range of mixtures from 80:20 nitrous oxide/oxygen to pure oxygen. The machine operates on demand only and has a stop at 70:30 nitrous oxide/oxygen so that mixtures stronger than this can only be obtained by using a special key. A safety device has been fitted so that the patient breathes room air only when the supply of either nitrous oxide or oxygen fails. Pressure gauges are provided for both oxygen and nitrous oxide and it should be remembered that while the pressure in an oxygen cylinder is proportional to its gas content, the pressure in a nitrous oxide cylinder is not (see Chapter 6).

The advantage of this type of machine is that the inspired concentrations of nitrous oxide and oxygen can be changed not only to suit the needs of different patients whose responses to nitrous oxide may be variable but also to match the needs of an individual patient whose pain may vary with the changing intensity of the uterine contractions and to the waning influence of narcotic analgesics previously received.

In an attempt to determine the optimum proportion of the two gases, McAneny and Doughty (1963) gave either 50, 60, 70, 75 or 80 per cent nitrous oxide with oxygen to five groups each of 100 mothers. The numbers of those receiving satisfactory analgesia rose as the proportion of nitrous oxide increased from 50 to 70 per cent. Higher concentrations of nitrous oxide showed no improvement in analgesia but an increased tendency to cause unconsciousness. However, a trial conducted by the Medical Research Council (1970) showed little difference in analgesic effect between 50 per cent and 70 per cent in normal labours but that 70 per cent nitrous oxide appeared to be more effective in abnormal labours.

Variable mixture nitrous oxide/oxygen machines are not "approved" by the Central Midwives Board unless they are locked so that they cannot deliver concentrations in excess of 50 per cent nitrous oxide. The Board has given limited approval for midwives in hospital practice to use varying mixtures provided that the responsibility is accepted by a doctor.

Administration of nitrous oxide/oxygen analgesia.—In common with all inhalational agents the characteristics of nitrous oxide/oxygen analgesia depend on certain physical properties. Being gaseous at room temperature but relatively insoluble in blood, a high alveolar concentration and arterial partial pressure can be attained very rapidly. On discontinuing the inhalation the gas is rapidly eliminated. This means that nitrous oxide/oxygen can only provide intermittent analgesia unless it is respired continuously. Normally the mother breathes it in association with each uterine contraction and she should be instructed to start the inhalation with the onset of the sensation of contraction and not to wait

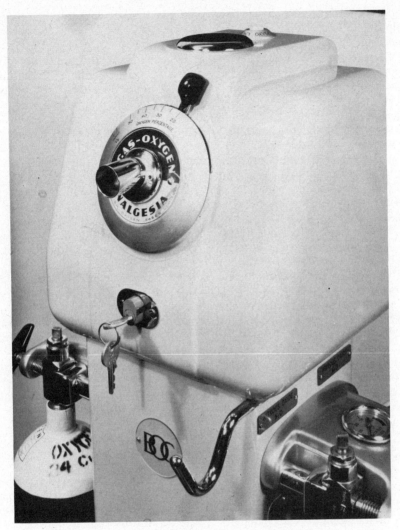

42/Fig. 4.—The head of the "Lucy Baldwin" apparatus.

until the contraction becomes painful. It is important that she should understand that there is a time lag of about 15 seconds between the inhalation and the onset of analgesia. If the mother has a low threshold to pain the contraction becomes distressing very soon after its commencement and she has no time to attain an analgesic blood level of nitrous oxide (41/Fig. 3). This type of patient is not satisfied by nitrous oxide and is probably better suited by trichloroethylene or methoxyflurane. On the other hand, nitrous oxide/oxygen inhalation may be started much earlier in labour than trichloroethylene or methoxyflurane as there is no fear of a cumulative effect depressing the baby at birth.

Other factors contributing to optimum results from nitrous oxide analgesia are firstly, an immediate air-tight fit of the mask on the face followed by rapid deep inhalations and secondly, a vigilant eye on the pressure gauge so that analgesia does not fail owing to cylinder exhaustion.

Latto *et al.* (1973) considered that more effective analgesia with nitrous oxide/oxygen might be achieved by variations in the technique of administration. If the uterus was contracting at regular intervals, each inhalation could be started well in advance of the onset of the contractions; thus a higher blood level of nitrous oxide would be attained. Alternatively, a raised blood level of nitrous oxide could be maintained by intermittent inhalations between contractions or by continuous inhalation of 20–25 per cent of nitrous oxide by a nasal catheter; this would not cause unconsciousness and the analgesia could then be boosted with 50:50 per cent nitrous oxide/oxygen by face-piece during the contractions. This method would risk the mother becoming unconscious unless the mask were removed immediately upon the conclusion of the contractions.

Thus the major disadvantage of nitrous oxide/oxygen analgesia is that its efficacy depends on meticulous and probably unattainable attention to the details of administration. Other disadvantages are its relative unsuitability for mothers with a low threshold to pain, the discomfort of the mouth and throat caused by the prolonged forced inhalation of dry gases and the exhaustion of the mother due to the muscular effort demanded by hyperventilation.

Hyperventilation is a common response to the pain of uterine contractions. Excessive hyperventilation may be due to compliance with antenatal training in "breathing exercises", to inadequate pain relief, or to the desire of the mother rapidly to attain an analgesic blood level of nitrous oxide. An excessive fall in carbon dioxide tension has been shown to be associated with fetal distress (Fadl and Utting, 1969), who advise discretion in encouraging hyperventilation with nitrous oxide/oxygen.

Trichloroethylene (Trilene)

Trichloroethylene in a concentration of 0·5 per cent in air was approved by the Central Midwives Board in 1955 for administration by the unsupervised midwife. Some ingenuity in the design of the "approved" machines was needed to ensure that the inspired vapour concentration does not exceed 0·5 per cent under all conditions of use despite changes in the ambient temperature, agitation of the apparatus and changes in the respiratory minute volume of the patient. The standards required of an approved inhaler drawn up by the Medical Research Council (1954) are as follows:

1. The concentration of trichloroethylene vapour delivered should be 0·5 per cent volume/volume in air with a permissible variation of ±20 per cent. If possible, there should be available also a weaker setting, delivering 0·35 per cent of trichloroethylene, to allow for the increased susceptibility of some patients after prolonged inhalation.
2. The concentration of trichloroethylene vapour should remain within these limits with variations of room temperature from 12·5° C to 35° C (55° F to 95° F); a respiratory rate of 12–30 per minute; a tidal volume of 250–1000 ml; and a minute volume of 7–10 litres.
3. Where the respiratory minute volume falls to 7 litres or less, the concentration of vapour should also fall.

4. The resistance to air drawn through the apparatus should be not more than 1·25 cm $H_2O \, L^{-1}$ sec (0·13 kPa L^{-1} sec) at a flow of 30 litres a minute.

5. The weight and bulk of the apparatus should be as small as possible. It should weigh not more than 15 lb (6·1 kg), should hold 60 ml of liquid trichloroethylene, and should be sufficiently robust to stand up to reasonable wear and tear.

6. The apparatus must comply with these specifications in all working positions and after shaking and inversion. It must not be possible for liquid trichloroethylene to leak out.

In order to comply with the regulations of the Central Midwives Board trichloroethylene inhalers must be checked annually by the British Standards Institution to ensure that they continue to function in accordance with specification. The date of testing is stamped on the machine and a certificate is issued to its owner.

The Automatic Emotril Inhaler (Fig. 5*a* and *b*).—This inhaler was designed by Epstein and Macintosh (1949). There are two separate entries for air, one directly into the vaporising chamber and the other through a bypass to dilute the mixture of trichloroethylene and air emerging from the vaporising chamber. Changes in temperature are compensated by a bellows type thermostat which varies the size of the air exit. The surface from which the trichloroethylene evaporates consists of a wick which dips into the liquid agent below the chamber which is kept at a fairly constant temperature by means of a water jacket. The amount of trichloroethylene remaining in the inhaler may be estimated by the level in a gauge. The vapour passes to the patient through a non-return valve through an exit port. By opening a second bypass and allowing more air to be drawn into the machine, a weaker concentration of vapour—0·35 per cent in air—may be obtained if desired.

The Tecota Mark 6 Inhaler (Fig. 6).—Air is drawn through an opening where it divides into two streams. One stream passes through the vaporising chamber where it collects trichloroethylene vapour from the wicks and passes to an aperture, the size of which is controlled by a valve which is actuated by a bi-metallic temperature-sensitive strip. The valve tends to open the aperture when the apparatus is cool and to close it when warm. Thus a greater or lesser proportion of vapour can leave the vaporising chamber according to the temperature. A constant bypass stream mixes with this and passes through a non-return valve to the patient. As with the Emotril inhaler the amount of trichloroethylene remaining in the inhaler can be estimated by the level in the gauge. A weaker mixture—0·35 per cent—may be obtained by increasing the flow of air through the bypass.

Administration of trichloroethylene analgesia.—Trichloroethylene has physical properties totally dissimilar to nitrous oxide. A liquid at room temperature, with a boiling point of 87° C, its vapour pressure is low but varies with changes in the ambient temperature. It is much more readily soluble in blood and has a high lipid solubility. Because of the low inspired concentration, uptake by the body is slow and because of its high blood solubility alveolar-blood equilibrium is unlikely to be reached in labour. This same property prevents a rapid recovery from its effects when inhalation ceases as the venous blood is not easily cleared of trichloroethylene during its passage through the lungs. With prolonged administration its accumulation in the body fats will further delay complete recovery.

When trichloroethylene is given in labour, the onset of analgesia is slow and

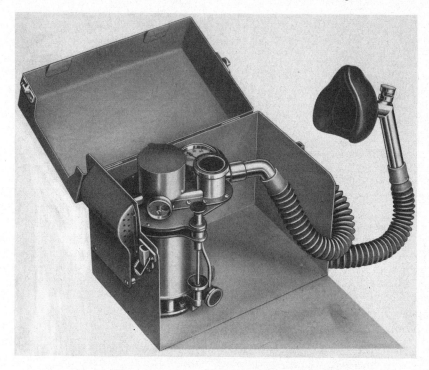

(*a*)

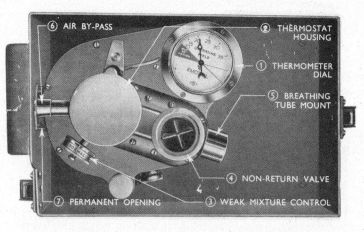

(*b*)

42/Fig. 5.—The automatic Emotril inhaler.

inhalation in association with several uterine contractions is required before a satisfactory level of pain relief is achieved. However, the patient does not recover from the effects of the drug between inhalations so that trichloro-

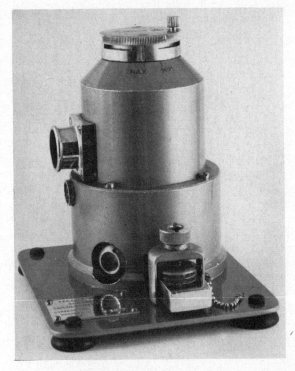

42/FIG. 6.—The Tecota Mark 6 Inhaler.

ethylene can be regarded as conferring continuous analgesia in contrast to the intermittent effect of nitrous oxide. It has therefore an advantage for mothers with a low threshold to pain for whom nitrous oxide is unsuitable.

Its cumulative effects are a disadvantage. The mother may become unduly sleepy with prolonged administration and while this effect may produce amnesia, the length of both first and second stages of labour tend to be prolonged. Because of the rapid placental transfer of trichloroethylene the infant is more likely to require resuscitation at birth, particularly after the use of pethidine earlier in the labour (Medical Research Council, 1954).

Phillips and MacDonald (1971) compared the effect of pethidine, trichloroethylene and 50 per cent nitrous oxide/oxygen on fetal and neonatal acid-base state and Po_2. They reported that the normal progressive fetal acidosis and hypoxia during the second stage was aggravated by trichloroethylene analgesia, particularly when pethidine had been used earlier in labour. By contrast, nitrous oxide/oxygen analgesia was associated with *less* acidosis and hypoxia following pethidine than when pethidine had been used alone. At birth the "Entonox" babies had higher Apgar scores than the "Trilene" babies and, within an hour of birth, had achieved a significantly higher Po_2 and pH and a greater reduction in base deficit.

A further caution that should be mentioned is that mothers given trichloro-ethylene who subsequently require operative delivery must not be given an anaesthetic through a soda-lime absorber. Dichloracetylene may be formed by the reaction of trichloroethylene with warm soda-lime and the re-inhalation from the absorber may result in cranial nerve palsies (see Chapter 6).

Methoxyflurane (Penthrane)

Methoxyflurane in a concentration of 0·35 per cent was approved by the Central Midwives Board for use by the unsupervised midwife in 1970. It is given by means of the "Cardiff" Inhaler (Fig. 7) which is an adaptation of the Tecota Mark 6 trichloroethylene inhaler (Fig. 6). The only differences between the two machines are that the thermostat has been redesigned to suit methoxyflurane's vaporising characteristics, the control for the administration of a weaker strength has been removed and a charging device has been incorporated so that the inhaler can be filled only from the manufacturer's methoxyflurane bottle. As with the trichloroethylene machine, the "Cardiff" Inhaler must be subjected to an annual test by the British Standards Institution to ensure that it continues to function in compliance with the specifications which, apart from the difference in concentration of vapour delivered, are essentially similar to those which apply to trichloroethylene inhalers.

Like trichloroethylene, methoxyflurane is a liquid of low volatility (B.P. 104·8° C) and is administered in a low inspired concentration. It has a high blood and lipid solubility and it might be expected to provide a similar type of analgesia with a relatively slow onset, slow recovery and a tendency to accumulation after prolonged administration.

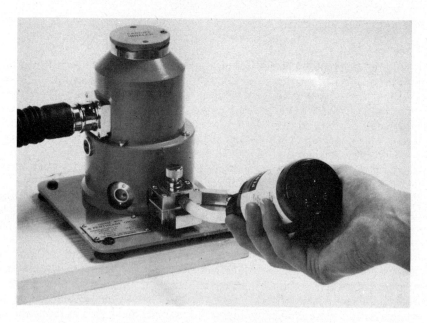

42/Fig. 7.—The "Cardiff" Inhaler.

Opinions concerning the efficacy of methoxyflurane and its place in obstetrical analgesia remain confused. Boisvert and Hudon (1962) state that the
intensity and rapidity of onset of analgesia is "remarkable", occurring within
two minutes of the start of inhalation. On the other hand, Torda (1963) in tibial
pressure studies, found a variable response with half his subjects showing an
anti-analgesic effect after 4 minutes, which only disappeared after a further 8
minutes' inhalation. Dundee and Love (1963) in similar experiments were unable to show any analgesic effect in sub-narcotic doses. In earlobe algesimetric
studies Siker et al. (1967) found significant increases in pain threshold in 12 out
of 14 volunteers inhaling variable concentrations of methoxyflurane up to 0·4
per cent. In two subjects however, there was little initial effect followed by minimal to marked falls in threshold at the point of onset of drowsiness. While the
blood levels remained raised for some time after discontinuing administration
4 subjects during the recovery period showed a threshold to pain lower than
before the start of the inhalations. These findings underline not only the expected
biological variability of response to drugs but also the wisdom of having
available a variety of analgesic agents rather than expecting a single one to suit
all patients.

Bodley et al. (1966), using methoxyflurane 0·5 per cent as an analgesic in
labour, reported that initially after six to ten breaths the mothers became
relaxed and drowsy, indifferent to their pain and detached from the processes
of labour. Later, analgesia could be induced after two or three breaths. The
possibility was raised that analgesia might not be produced in the absence of
drowsiness.

Siker et al. (1968) reported that, as expected from its high lipid solubility
(see Chapter 44), methoxyflurane crossed the placenta rapidly but there was a
low incidence of fetal depression.

A detailed investigation of methoxyflurane in comparison with other
inhalational analgesics is given in five publications from Cardiff:

(a) Major et al. (1966) compared methoxyflurane with trichloroethylene
given continuously in labour by an anaesthetist who was able to vary the
inspired concentrations according to the needs of the mother. They defined
satisfactory analgesia not only by the suppression of the responses to painful
uterine contractions, but also took account of the retention of consciousness
and absence of restlessness between contractions. In the opinion of the anaesthetist, methoxyflurane appeared to maintain the more satisfactory state of objective analgesia for the period of the administration. The answers given by the
mothers, when questioned directly, suggested that both drugs produced a
comparably high standard of pain relief.

It was found that the mean inspired concentration of trichloroethylene
necessary to give satisfactory analgesia fell from 0·4 per cent to 0·08 per cent
over 85 minutes of administration while that of methoxyflurane fell only from
0·32 per cent to 0·16 per cent. The steeper slope of the trichloroethylene curve
confirms the necessity for two fixed concentrations delivered by the inhalers,
while the flatter slope obtained with methoxyflurane suggests that, for intermittent administration, only one fixed concentration is necessary.

(b) Major et al. (1967) reported that a single fixed concentration of 0·35 per
cent methoxyflurane was superior to 0·25 per cent as a self-administered anal-

gesic, not only in the opinion of the observing anaesthetist but also in the opinion of the midwives and the mothers concerned. A higher concentration of 0·45 per cent produced an unacceptable degree of drowsiness.

(c) Jones *et al.* (1969a) compared varying concentrations of methoxyflurane with nitrous oxide/oxygen 50 per cent/50 per cent given continuously by an anaesthetist in an attempt to maintain the ideal analgesic state. Under these conditions the two agents were almost equally effective although nitrous oxide induced semi-consciousness too easily from which some patients awoke in confusion and distress complaining of unpleasant dreams. Nitrous oxide was also associated with a higher frequency of nausea and vomiting.

(d) Jones *et al.* (1969b) compared nitrous oxide/oxygen (50 per cent/50 per cent) with methoxyflurane 0·35 per cent in air self-administered by the mothers in midwife-conducted labours. From the observer's point of view methoxyflurane was the more satisfactory, mainly because it suppressed the mothers' reaction to the uterine contractions. The previous administration of pethidine appeared to improve the efficacy of methoxyflurane, but not that of nitrous oxide/oxygen. When midwives and mothers were questioned no difference could be found between the two agents except for an association of nitrous oxide with nausea and vomiting.

(e) Rosen *et al.* (1969) reported on the results of a field trial on 1257 patients receiving methoxyflurane 0·35 per cent, trichloroethylene 0·5 per cent and nitrous oxide/oxygen (50 per cent/50 per cent) in eight maternity units. According to the mothers' opinions there was little difference between the three; the midwives' opinion was that both methoxyflurane and trichloroethylene gave better pain relief than nitrous oxide, but that mothers receiving nitrous oxide and trichloroethylene were more co-operative than those inhaling methoxyflurane. An association of nitrous oxide with nausea and vomiting was not confirmed. Pethidine given in early labour was found to increase the incidence of neonatal asphyxia with all three agents.

In view of reports of kidney damage following methoxyflurane anaesthesia, Rosen *et al.* (1972) studied the renal function of 200 mothers, some of whom had methoxyflurane 0·35 per cent and others who had nitrous oxide/oxygen analgesia. No significant differences were found between the two groups and it was concluded that methoxyflurane is not nephrotoxic when used as a self-administered analgesic. It was pointed out that nephrotoxicity is dose-dependent and that blood concentrations during methoxyflurane *analgesia* are only one-sixth of those attained during methoxyflurane anaesthesia (see Chapter 6).

REGIONAL ANALGESIA IN OBSTETRICS

Narcotic and inhalational analgesics alone cannot ensure a painless childbirth nor can they make labour tolerable when the pain is exceptionally severe. It is on these occasions that the obstetric anaesthetist can help by giving some form of regional analgesia.

The need for a more effective method of pain relief was shown by a survey in Sheffield by Beazley *et al.* (1967) who made special efforts to ensure that the established sedative and analgesic drugs together with inhalational agents were given as soon as needed and with the closest possible attention to the details of their administration. Morphine, diamorphine and even paracervical block were freely used when the simpler methods failed. Despite this intensive effort only 23 per cent of women admitted having a pain-free labour and there remained 40 per cent whose childbirth was unacceptably painful. More recently, Holdcroft and Morgan (1974) reported that 75 per cent of mothers received little or no relief from intramuscular pethidine while pre-mixed nitrous oxide/oxygen (Entonox) gave satisfactory analgesia in only 50 per cent of parturients.

Apart from the limited effectiveness of narcotic analgesics there are other disadvantages which should be considered. For example, La Salvia and Steffen (1950) reported that all the narcotics used in labour delayed the gastric emptying time, thus adding to the danger of general anaesthesia which might be used for subsequent operative delivery. This observation was confirmed more recently by Nimmo et al. (1975) who showed that gastric emptying was normal in patients who had not received a narcotic analgesic but was markedly delayed in women given pethidine, diamorphine or pentazocine. This effect was not reversed by metoclopramide. It could be argued that the stress of labour itself could inhibit gastric emptying but the same effect was produced by narcotics given to healthy non-pregnant volunteers.

The hazards of narcotic respiratory depression of the fetus in combination with the inhalational analgesics are well-recognised (Rosen et al., 1969). Huch et al. (1974) recorded reduction in transcutaneous oxygen tension to between 40 and 50 mm Hg (5·3 and 6·7 kPa) after only 50 mg of pethidine given intravenously. This was due to hypoventilation between contractions following a period of hyperventilation during the contractions. If the mother was positively encouraged to breathe normally between contractions her Po_2 remained normal. It was conceded that normal fetuses may be reasonably tolerant of some degree of hypoxia but obviously pethidine must be contra-indicated where fetal welfare is already compromised. Chang et al. (1976) reported respiratory acidosis in the mother and metabolic acidosis in the fetus following narcotic analgesia with pethidine, morphine or diamorphine. Pearson and Davies (1974) observed similar changes with narcotic analgesia but noted less alteration in fetal and maternal acid-base status when the mother had been given epidural analgesia in the first stage of labour.

The quality of obstetric analgesia has been assessed by estimations of free fatty acid mobilisation (Maltau et al., 1975). Free fatty acid in the serum is increased following lipolysis of fatty tissues in response to catecholamine release associated with muscular effort, pain, fear and anxiety. Even when patients were under the influence of conventional sedatives and analgesics they showed a degree of lipolysis comparable to that resulting from severe trauma. A similar increase was not observed in those given epidural analgesia.

It is clear not only that there is a limit to the relief that can be obtained with techniques based mainly on central depression but there is also reason to believe that the more effective relief obtained from regional analgesia is in the better interests of maternal and fetal welfare quite apart from the more obvious compassionate considerations.

In view of the predominant current interest in continuous lumbar epidural analgesia this technique will be described in some detail. Caudal epidural analgesia and paracervical block will be considered more briefly.

LUMBAR EPIDURAL ANALGESIA

The anatomical basis of the practice of continuous lumbar epidural analgesia in labour has been discussed in Chapter 41 (41/Fig. 2), and numerous techniques for achieving it have been described. Duthie *et al.* (1968) aimed to block sensation from the 11th dorsal to the 4th sacral segments for the duration of labour. The dose given was 10–15 ml 0·5 per cent bupivacaine with adrenaline or 15–20 ml 0·25 per cent bupivacaine with adrenaline, the patient lying in the horizontal position. It was stated that the weaker solution was as reliable as the stronger but with less liability to cause muscle paresis. Moir and Willocks (1968) performed epidural puncture in the sitting position to achieve greater spinal flexion and gave 6 to 10 ml 2 per cent lignocaine as the initial dose.

Bromage (1961) aimed to block the lower thoracic segments with 7 ml of local anaesthetic with the mother in the horizontal position and then to give a larger dose in the sitting position to block the sacral roots when the labour had reached the second stage. The object was to avoid relaxation of the muscles of the pelvic floor in order to facilitate the rotation and full flexion of the fetal head and avoid the undue frequency of assisted delivery. It has been observed that many mothers experienced little or no perineal discomfort in the second stage of labour even though the aim had been only to block the lower thoracic segments (Doughty 1969*a*). No formal attempt was made to block the sacral roots unless the mother specifically complained of vaginal or perineal pain. The intention was to provide relief of pain without depriving her of the sensations of labour. Only when dictated by the mother's need was 10 ml of local anaesthetic solution given in the sitting position. This technique was named "selective epidural block" and it was reported that as few as 19 per cent of mothers delivering spontaneously demanded a formal attempt to block the sacral roots in the second stage. Some diminution of perineal sensation must have been produced quite fortuitously by a spread of the effect of the top-up doses given in the recumbent position.

Advantages claimed for selective epidural analgesia include:

1. Preservation of the tone of the muscles of the pelvic floor and hence the normal mechanism of labour thus achieving a reasonably low incidence of assisted delivery.
2. Retention by the mother of the sensation of the baby's head in the vagina, thus preserving her reflex expulsive efforts.
3. The smaller doses of local anaesthetic given imply a reduced frequency of toxic side-effects, hypotension and paresis of the legs and a lesser quantity of drug transferred across the placenta to the fetus.
4. In the rare event of an inadvertent subarachnoid injection, recovery from a small dose would be more rapid than from a larger one.

Technique of Lumbar Epidural Analgesia

The anaesthetist should first obtain the mother's consent to receive epidural analgesia and should give her a brief explanation of what he proposes to do, the effect intended and the co-operation that he requires. The degree of dilatation of the cervix, the character of the labour pain, the mother's blood pressure and pulse and the fetal heart rate should already have been recorded by the labour ward staff.

The anaesthetist must take full aseptic precautions as for a surgical operation. The smooth running of all syringes must be checked and the patency of the Portex epidural cannula must be established, as must the capability of the cannula to pass through the Tuohy needle.

Assuming the operator to be right-handed, the patient should lie horizontally on her left side with the knees drawn up towards the chest and the neck fully flexed. The back is swabbed with 1 per cent chlorhexidine in spirit. The sterile towels are applied. A weal is raised in the midline immediately caudal to the 2nd lumbar spine and some local anaesthetic injected up to 3 cm deep to the skin weal. A puncture through the skin and supraspinous ligament is made with a thick sharp needle to facilitate the passage of the blunter epidural needle. A Tuohy needle with centimetre markings is passed through the skin and supraspinous ligament and a 20-ml syringe charged with 10 ml normal saline is attached. The Tuohy needle is advanced in a slightly cephalad direction until the resistance of the ligamentum flavum is identified. The point of the needle with attached syringe is very cautiously advanced through the ligamentum flavum, a slight pressure being maintained on the plunger by the palm of the right hand.

In some patients considerable force may be required to advance the point of the needle through the ligament. To avoid inadvertent dural puncture, the left hand should control the passage of the needle point into the epidural space once the ligamentous resistance has been overcome.

As soon as the needle enters the epidural space the loss of resistance to injection will be appreciated. The 20-ml syringe is detached from the Tuohy needle, a smoothly running 2-ml syringe is attached and *gentle* aspiration made for cerebrospinal fluid. The 2-ml syringe is then filled with air and an attempt made to elicit a "pneumatic" bounce which would be apparent if the bevel of the needle were not completely in the epidural space. The 2-ml syringe is then set aside and the marked cannula is fed into the epidural space through the Tuohy needle until the 3-band (15 cm) mark reaches the hub. The length of the needle shaft visible from the skin to the hub is noted and the cannula is fed into the needle as the needle is extracted from the patient's back. The Tuohy needle is then slid up the cannula to its proximal end and the cannula is pulled out even further until the 2-band (10 cm) mark is at the same distance from the skin as was the hub of the Tuohy needle when the epidural space was penetrated. By this means exactly 2 cm length of cannula should lie in the epidural space (Fig. 8; Doughty, 1974). The site of the puncture is sprayed with Nobecutane, a dressing applied and the cannula strapped to the mother's back with waterproof adhesive tape. The cannula is led over the mother's shoulder and attached to a "Millex" filter unit which enables injections to be given without cumbersome sterile precautions.

The mother is then turned on to her back and a dose of 2 ml 0·5 per cent bupivacaine is injected through the cannula to test whether the cannula tip has punctured the dura and has inadvertently entered the subarachnoid space (Moir and Hesson, 1965). If, after two minutes there is no evidence of paresis of the legs, a further 5 ml of local anaesthetic is injected to complete the first dose. Relief of pain should follow within 10 minutes. The mother's blood pressure, pulse rate and the fetal heart rate should be recorded at 15 and 30 minutes following the onset of analgesia. A slight fall of blood pressure of 10–20 mm Hg (1·3–2·6 kPa) is to be expected as severe pain tends to cause some

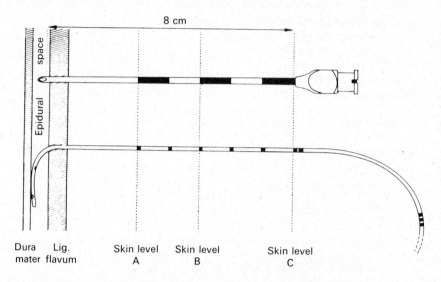

42/Fig. 8.—Needle and cannula graduated to facilitate precise placement of cannula tip in the epidural space.
Skin level A—Epidural space at 3 cm depth, 5 cm graduations withdrawn from skin.
Skin level B—Epidural space at 5 cm depth, 3 cm graduations withdrawn from skin.
Skin level C—Epidural space at 8 cm depth, 2-band (10 cm) mark fixed at skin level.

hypertension above the level measured before the mother's distress became apparent. Any fall should be maximal within 30 minutes but, as a precaution the patient should be turned on to her side to counteract the effects of vena caval occlusion. Those in attendance on the mother should be warned that any tendency to supine hypotension should be treated immediately by turning her on to her side with the onset of the premonitory symptoms of pallor, vertigo, nausea, faintness or ringing in the ears, without waiting for the actual measurable fall of blood pressure. On questioning, some mothers may admit that such symptoms have arisen in late pregnancy and that they have found lying on the side more comfortable than on the back. In these patients it is essential to avoid the supine position throughout labour. The doses of local anaesthetic should be given through the cannula, half with the mother lying on one side and half, five minutes later, with her lying on the other side.

Confirmation of Efficacy of Epidural Analgesia

It must be admitted that successful relief of pain cannot be guaranteed in every case. To some extent it depends on the experience of the operator (Romine et al., 1970); it depends too, on the determination of the operator to make subsequent adjustments to achieve success in the initially unsuccessful case; but above all, it depends on the competent and conscientious management of the analgesia once the initial pain relief has been obtained (Doughty, 1975).

It is reasonable to predict continuous and effective analgesia if, 15 minutes after the first injection, all pain has been relieved and if, after a further 15 minutes, bilateral cutaneous analgesia extends to the 11th thoracic dermatome and both feet are dry and warm with dilatation of the superficial veins.

THE CHOICE OF LOCAL ANAESTHETIC

Which Agent?

Bupivacaine has become established as the most suitable agent for obstetric epidural blockade for the following reasons:—

(a) *It has a long duration of action* and tachyphylaxis does not occur (Duthie *et al.*, 1968).

(b) *It is less cumulative* than lignocaine (Reynolds and Taylor, 1970; Reynolds, 1971) or mepivacaine (Moore *et al.*, 1968). All are eliminated at approximately the same rate from the plasma but the need for top-up doses occurs at more frequent intervals with lignocaine and mepivacaine than with bupivacaine. Thus toxic effects in the mother are extremely rare with bupivacaine in contrast with the other two agents.

(c) *It is less liable to cause motor blockade.* Etidocaine, which also has a moderately long duration of action and little cumulative tendency (Poppers, 1975) causes a high incidence of motor blockade, an undesirable feature in obstetrics (Bromage, 1975).

(d) *It crosses the placenta only to a limited extent* (see Chapter 44); umbilical cord levels at delivery after comparable therapeutic doses to the mother, are similar to those of etidocaine, about one-tenth those of lignocaine and one-twentieth those of mepivacaine. Its effect on the baby is therefore minimal.

What Concentration?

Bupivacaine has been used for obstetric analgesia in percentage concentrations from 0·5, 0·375, 0·25 down to 0·125 per cent. Generally speaking, weakening the concentration sacrifices the length and reliability of action of bupivacaine for the advantages of reduced side-effects and maternal and fetal blood levels. Choice of concentration is therefore a matter of personal preference. Because in most hospitals the maintenance of anaesthesia is heavily dependent on topping-up by midwives, the present writer opts for maximum reliability and length of action and recommends the use of bupivacaine 0·5 per cent.

Should Adrenaline be Added?

Adrenaline has a negligible effect in prolonging the action of bupivacaine (Reynolds and Taylor, 1971; Reynolds, 1972) though the effect may be enhanced with bigger doses, possibly because a high concentration of bupivacaine causes less vasoconstriction than a lower one (see Chapter 34). In any case, adrenaline is not required to prevent tachyphylaxis or cumulative toxicity. Reynolds *et al.* (1973) using 10-ml increments of 0·5 per cent bupivacaine without adrenaline calculated that a total dose of up to 320 mg may safely be given without approaching a toxic maternal blood level. This represents 64 ml of solution, sufficient to provide continuous analgesia for well over 20 hours particularly if the smaller incremental doses of 7 ml (35 mg) are used as prescribed in this chapter.

As the addition of adrenaline to bupivacaine is not essential it should be avoided because:

(a) it increases the systemic toxicity of an accidental intravenous injection;

(b) its systemic effects might be dangerous in severe pre-eclampsia;

(c) local vasoconstriction coupled with vascular hypotension may predispose to interference with the arterial supply to the spinal cord (Braham and Saia, 1958; Davies et al., 1958; Urquhart-Hay, 1969);

(d) owing to the presence of a preservative, the commercially available adrenaline solution is more acid (pH 3·8) than the plain solution (pH 6·0); thus injection into the tissues and epidural space can be more painful. The risk of neurological damage following inadvertent subarachnoid injection would be increased;

(e) it may reduce uterine blood flow (Wallis et al., 1976).

NOTES ON TECHNIQUE

1. Full sterile precautions are taken not only on general principles but also because there is always the remote possibility of dural puncture.

2. The importance of checking equipment cannot be overstressed. Sticky syringes detract from the delicacy of the loss of resistance test. Epidural cannulae have been known to be supplied kinked or without lumen. Tuohy needles may have been damaged by previous use and may not allow the cannula to pass. The bevel may be rough which could result in damage to the cannula.

3. The needle should not be advanced during a uterine contraction as the mother cannot be expected to co-operate at this time; the epidural veins are distended and dural pressure is raised; failure to observe this precaution may result in haemorrhage in the epidural space or in dural puncture.

4. The test of identification of the epidural space described is that using the loss of resistance to fluid injection. An alternative is to use an air-filled syringe. The supposed advantage of air is that there should be no confusion as to the nature of any fluid emerging from the hub of the Tuohy needle. However, confusion may be caused by the trickle back of a pool of local anaesthetic previously placed in the region of the interspinous ligament. This may give a false impression of inadvertent dural puncture and cause the unnecessary application of the treatment of this complication. The advantage of fluid in the syringe lies in its incompressibility so that the loss of resistance on penetrating the epidural space is more striking than with air. Other advantages of fluid are that any leaks between the syringe and the needle or between the barrel and the plunger will be evident, the fluid helps to lubricate a sticky syringe and it is believed that the jet of fluid produced in the epidural space on penetration may help to push the dura away from the point of the needle. Whatever technique is used, whether it be with air or fluid, there is no substitute for the tactile identification of the ligamentum flavum and the certain expectation of the imminence of loss of resistance to injection.

5. The epidural cannula should not be passed through the Tuohy needle during a uterine contraction owing to the risk of puncturing the temporarily tense dura or the congested epidural veins. It should always be filled with local analgesic solution before threading it through the needle as occasionally there is a small reflux of blood from the epidural space which, if not diluted, would clot and block its lumen. If, during the course of labour a blood reflux is noted it should be pushed back by an injection of 2 ml 3·8 per cent sodium citrate B.P. through the cannula. If the reflux of blood is persistent the possibility of intra-vascular penetration by the cannula tip should be considered; the epidural puncture and cannula insertion should be repeated in an adjoining lumbar interspace.

6. The epidural cannula should be fixed so that only 2 cm of its length lies within the epidural space (see Fig. 8). Thus the operator can be certain that anal-gesia will take effect from the level at which the cannula has been inserted. Usu-biaga et al. (1970) have shown that an excessive length of cannula passed into the epidural space may account for one-sided analgesia. Bromage (1954), Sanchez et al. (1967) and Bridenbaugh et al. (1968) have demonstrated by radiography that a flexible cannula passed into the epidural space cannot be relied upon to travel for any distance in accordance with the direction of the bevel of the Tuohy needle. The cannula may pass out of the epidural space through an intervertebral foramen, curl up at the site of insertion or be diverted by an obstruction and turn caudally. Only about one in four cannulae pursue a straight upward course within the epidural space.

7. The epidural injection must be made slowly and between contractions. An injection made rapidly or during a contraction may result in a widespread but patchy analgesia.

Difficulties

1. *Lack of co-operation by the mother.*—It has already been stated that epidural puncture should not be attempted during a uterine contraction. Occasionally the mother may be so distressed by pain and co-operation made impossible by sedatives and hypnotics that she cannot be relied upon to lie still even between contractions. In this event she may be given an effective intramuscular analgesic and the epidural puncture attempted when the drug becomes effective. The oxytocin infusion should be temporarily discontinued.

2. *Bony obstruction to the passage of the needle.*—There is no doubt that even the most practised operators sometimes find difficulty in penetrating the epidural space at the selected site. However, attention should be paid to the following details of technique:

   (a) The patient's back should be fully flexed, the knees well drawn up and the neck flexed so that the chin touches the chest.

   (b) The spine must not be in rotation: thus the line joining the shoulder tips should be parallel with that joining the hips.

   (c) The needle must be advanced in the midline at right angles to the patient's back possibly with a slight cephalad inclination. A very common error is to insert the needle parallel with the floor when the patient is lying in a slightly prone position.

3. *Identification of bony landmarks.*—Occasionally the mother is so obese

that the lumbar spines cannot be palpated with certainty, but they may be sought by percutaneous exploratory puncture with fine hypodermic needles, and the midline may be more easily identified with the patient in the sitting position. It should be remembered that in such patients it may be necessary to advance the Tuohy needle into the back as far as its hub before the epidural space is penetrated.

4. *Difficulty in passing the cannula through the needle.*—The shaft of the Tuohy needle is 8 cm long. If the cannula will not pass through the hub to the 10-cm mark the obstruction is at the tip of the needle and this should have been noted by the preliminary test of equipment before the epidural puncture. Needle and cannula should be withdrawn together and the puncture attempted with another needle tested against the cannula. Once the 10-cm mark has passed through the hub any obstruction to the passage of the cannula must be in the epidural space. Pressure on the cannula with a plain dissecting forceps rather than with finger and thumb, together with slight rotation of the Tuohy needle, usually succeeds, but if obstruction is absolute the needle with cannula must be withdrawn and the puncture performed in a neighbouring space. On no account should the cannula be withdrawn through the needle as there is a risk of a portion shearing off and remaining in the epidural space. Occasionally there is an absolute obstruction after a length of only 12 cm has passed through the hub. In these cases, if the cannula is very carefully fed into the hub as the needle is withdrawn, a sufficient minimal length of cannula will have been introduced into the epidural space.

5. *Prevention of top-ups by cannula obstruction.*—The importance of avoiding blockage of the cannula by blood clot has already been mentioned above. If this occurs the epidural puncture must be repeated in an adjoining lumbar interspace and a new cannula inserted. Kinking of the cannula may also cause obstruction to the top-ups. Inspection of cannulae that have become so blocked has shown that the kink is nearly always about 1 cm below skin level, that is, at the point where the cannula would pass through the supraspinous ligament. At the time of epidural puncture the patient's back is flexed and the points where the cannula passes through the skin and through the supraspinous ligament are opposite each other. When the mother straightens her back the skin moves upwards in relation to the ligament, thus causing the cannula to bend sharply. The kink may be straightened out by asking the mother to flex her back, the skin of the back may be pushed caudally or the cannula may be withdrawn very slightly. If none of these remedies succeeds there is no alternative to repeating the epidural puncture.

6. *Failure of block.*—Occasionally, despite apparently impeccable technique, the single epidural injection given in the horizontal position fails to relieve the pain of uterine contractions. If the pain relief is unilateral the mother should be turned to the unaffected side and a further injection of 3 ml of local anaesthetic solution given through the cannula.

If labour has been prolonged or the baby's head is in a posterior position or the cervix is near full dilatation a dose of 8–10 ml should be given through the cannula in the sitting position to direct the solution towards the sacral roots. Following the injection the mother should remain upright for 5 minutes. Occasionally a top-up in the sitting position fails to achieve adequate perineal analgesia; a single epidural injection of 15 ml 0·5 per cent bupivacaine at the lumbosacral interspace or through the caudal canal will provide complete analgesia for spontaneous or instrumental delivery although the obstetrician should be warned to wait 15 minutes for the full effect of the injection. Alternatively, the obstetrician may be willing to give a pudendal nerve block.

The pain relief may be patchy and small areas of the central hypogastrium may continue to be painful. In this case the passage of a catheter to empty the bladder may bring relief. The rare possibility of placental abruption (accidental haemorrhage) or rupture of the uterus may be considered; the pain of these and most other forms of pathological pain are unlikely to be masked by a small-dose epidural block.

If the block continues to be unsatisfactory it should be repeated through an adjacent lumbar interspace without further delay. Early recognition of the probable misplacement of the cannula tip would reduce the risk of accumulation and toxicity from repeated ineffective doses of local anaesthetic. The readiness to set up an epidural again should be regarded as essential to the running of an effective obstetric analgesia service (Doughty, 1975).

THE TIMING OF INDUCTION OF EPIDURAL ANALGESIA

In the past elective epidural analgesia was given when the mother was well established in labour and the cervix 5–6 cm dilated in primigravidae and 3–4 cm dilated in multigravidae. This rule was probably dictated by the desire to minimise the time that the anaesthetist was obliged to be in personal attendance on the patient. The practice of topping-up by midwives has enabled epidural analgesia to be given throughout the painful part of labour unless the patient wishes to bear some pain or to test the adequacy of more conventional methods of pain relief.

When a patient is in strong spontaneous labour the epidural should be given without delay. When the epidural is elective the cannula should be inserted well in advance of pain or as soon as the premonitory contractions begin.

Thus, five variations of technique may be practised:

1. The epidural cannula may be inserted before surgical induction. A dose of 10 ml bupivacaine plain 0·5 per cent is injected in the sitting position and rupture of membranes carried out 30 minutes later.
2. If the membranes are already ruptured and the contractions are not painful the epidural cannula is placed in position and a 2 ml test dose injected. The main pain-relieving dose may be given later when the contractions become painful.
3. When the patient is in painful first stage labour the cannula is inserted and the test and therapeutic doses are given consecutively.
4. If the labour has progressed to near full dilatation both uterine and perineal pain demand relief. A dose of 7 ml bupivacaine 0·5 per cent including a 2 ml test dose is given through the cannula in the recumbent position followed after 5 minutes by 8 ml in the sitting position.
5. If the labour has progressed to the second stage a single dose of 15 ml local anaesthetic solution should be given through the Tuohy needle to obtain rapid relief of all labour pain before delivery.

INDICATIONS FOR EPIDURAL ANALGESIA

The primary effect of epidural analgesia is to relieve pain and thereby to preserve the morale and to prevent exhaustion of the mother. As the method has now become fairly well established, the view is widely held that epidural analgesia may be given to any mother prepared to accept it provided there are no contra-indications to its use. The frequency with which it is used varies from hospital to hospital according to the availability, aptitude and enthusiasm of the anaesthetic service and the local predilections of the obstetricians.

Assuming the service to be readily available and that the local facilities will allow its application to more than 30 per cent of mothers, the conditions in which epidural analgesia may be particularly helpful are as follows:

1. Pre-eclampsia.
2. Slow, painful labour with obstetric abnormality, such as inco-ordinate uterine action and cervical dystocia.
3. Cardiac and respiratory disease.
4. Premature or high-risk fetus.
5. Trial of labour.
6. Operative delivery where the stomach is known to be full.
7. Failure of conventional analgesia and impending loss of morale in an otherwise normal labour.
8. Fear of a repetition of a particularly painful experience in a previous labour.
9. Wish expressed by the patient to have a painless labour, irrespective of past experience.

These indications are given in order of probable acceptance by obstetricians and midwives. Most would accept the first seven but some might hesitate to accede to a request from the patient for an epidural.

Comment

Continuous epidural analgesia may be used to control blood pressure in pre-eclampsia. An injection of 8–10 ml bupivacaine 0·5 per cent without adrenaline, given at the 2nd–3rd lumbar interspace should produce analgesia up to the 9th–10th thoracic dermatome. Further injections through the cannula may be given until the desired fall of blood pressure has been attained. Care should be taken to monitor the blood pressure closely as severe hypotension may occur necessitating the use of infusion fluids to expand the blood volume.

Despite initial success, attempts to control hypertension with epidural blockade over long periods are often disappointing as the blood pressure may continue to rise even though the sensory block has reached a level well above the costal margin. It has therefore no place in treatment before labour has begun. Given during labour it will not only temporarily help to lower the blood pressure by sympathetic blockade but will reduce afferent stimuli simply by relief of pain. The fetus, already at a disadvantage with prematurity and placental insufficiency, is given time to recover from any depressant drugs already given to the mother and will stand a better chance of survival at birth.

Among the situations that arise during labour, epidural analgesia should be given whenever there is severe pain inadequately relieved by the conventional methods. With inco-ordinate uterine action it has been shown to increase the rate of cervical dilatation in 70 per cent of cases, it will gain time for the treatment of associated electrolyte imbalance, dehydration and keto-acidosis, and obstetricians need not be pressed by maternal distress to deliver by Caesarean section (Moir and Willocks, 1967, 1968). Any severe intractable pain in labour should be treated by epidural analgesia as the memory of a harrowing experience may prejudice a woman against any further childbearing. There is a tendency to use the method more readily to reduce psychological stress in those with intra-uterine death, in the victims of rape and in the unmarried mother.

Most would agree that epidural analgesia given early can save the mother exhaustion in a trial of labour; she is then better able to withstand the stress of delivery by Caesarean section. With respiratory and cardiac disease minimal strain is placed on the mother's limited physical reserves, and under epidural analgesia she can conveniently be delivered by forceps as soon as the labour has reached the second stage. The safety of a premature or high-risk infant may be jeopardised by the conventional narcotic and inhalational agents. Properly managed epidural analgesia has no harmful effect on the fetus as long as aorto-caval occlusion is avoided (David and Rosen, 1976).

For a difficult vaginal operative delivery when the stomach is known to be full, a single dose epidural block is a safer alternative to a general anaesthetic. However, if a rapid onset of perineal analgesia is important, a saddle subarach-noid block may be preferred in these circumstances (Crawford, 1972). Consideration of the dangers of general anaesthesia in labour prompted Hellman (1965) to report on 26,127 cases in whom epidural analgesia was induced as a routine procedure only 15 minutes before the expected time of delivery.

The more controversial indications are those where epidural analgesia is given in compliance with the mother's expressed wishes. A hard-pressed anaesthetic service may not accept the prospect of an increase in requests for "unnecessary" epidurals and yet it is just on these willing and undistressed patients that one can train other anaesthetists to perfect their technique. Experience has shown that the more frequently epidural analgesia is practised in a maternity department, the less frequent are its complications and the more likely is the anaesthetist to be able to carry it out swiftly and accurately in the individual case.

There are some centres where the epidural service is particularly well-developed against the background of local enthusiasm and exceptionally plentiful staffing. Here it has become the accepted method of pain relief virtually to the exclusion of any other. Nevertheless, it should not be forgotten that some women are quite satisfied by the more conventional analgesic methods and may even wish to bear some pain in labour as long as it does not become excessive. These patients should not be pressed to accept epidural blockade in the absence of strong therapeutic indications.

Contra-indications to Epidural Analgesia

It has been stated that epidural analgesia may be offered to any patient in labour willing to accept it and in whom it is not contra-indicated. Absolute contra-indications are few but circumstances still exist in which the safety or desirability of the method are debatable. These are discussed as "Controversial Conditions".

Sepsis at the site of injection.—Skin infection could be transferred to the epidural space and might be followed by epidural cellulitis or abscess formation. Accidental dural puncture could carry infection to the subarachnoid space with ensuing meningitis (Bromage, 1954). However, a case has been reported of an epidural abscess occurring spontaneously in a parturient to whom an anaesthetist had refused to give an epidural because of the presence of septic spots on her back (Male and Martin, 1973).

Haemorrhagic disease or anticoagulant therapy.—Some vascular damage frequently occurs during the insertion of the epidural cannula. Normally this is of little consequence but in the presence of a bleeding tendency a slight ooze may continue indefinitely leading to the formation of a large haematoma in the epidural space and possible cord compression and paraplegia (Frumin and Schwartz, 1952; Gingrich, 1968).

Absence of consent.—While it should not be necessary to warn against the practice of any anaesthetic procedure without the consent of the patient, it should be recognised that there still exists a strong specific prejudice against epidural injections. Care should be taken not to press patients to accept this method of analgesia against their wishes, particularly if there is no clearly defined medical indication.

Absence of facilities.—Epidural analgesia should not be carried out in an environment where the appropriate equipment and personnel for the proper care of the patient are not readily available, unless the anaesthetist is prepared to supply them himself and is willing to exercise close personal supervision throughout the whole course of the labour.

Controversial Conditions

Previous Caesarean Section

The view that epidural analgesia may conceal the pain of a rupturing uterine scar is put into a different perspective by Case *et al.* (1971) who reported the relative infrequency of pain as a warning of scar rupture in the lower segment. Caesarean section was carried out in 20 cases because of pain in the scar which, at operation, was found to be intact in 14 and in only one case had it ruptured. They stated that a far more reliable indication of scar rupture was the appearance of a swelling on the anterior wall of the uterus. Meehan *et al.* (1972) advocated the periodic digital palpation of the scar through the cervix during labour under caudal epidural analgesia. A small-dose selective epidural block is unlikely to conceal pathological pain and in any event, the situation calls for vigilant supervision of the labour as, even without epidural analgesia, fetal distress and intra-uterine death may be the first indication of uterine rupture. Epidural analgesia may be a decisive factor in making vaginal delivery possible by relieving maternal distress and promoting normal uterine activity. Some feel that the use of oxytocin is contra-indicated, but others consider it justifiable but stress the need for particularly close supervision.

Breech Delivery and Multiple Pregnancies

It has hitherto been thought that epidural block risks the possibility of a difficult breech extraction in a labour which would otherwise have ended in an easy assisted breech delivery. However, if no attempt is made to anaesthetise the perineum too early the mother will retain her ability to push the presenting part down on to the perineum; the pressure of the soft breech causes minimal distress in contrast to that caused by the hardness of the head when the vertex presents. Only when the obstetrician is ready to deliver the infant should the perineum be anaesthetised by a top-up in the sitting position.

Breech labours with infants of low birth weight give the greatest cause for concern. The patient may experience an uncontrollable desire to push before full dilatation of the cervix and delivery tends to be precipitate. In these cases an early top-up in the sitting position will block the bearing-down reflex and a controlled delivery may be obtained (Crawford, 1974). It is in the context of breech labours that the small-dose or "selective" technique is seen to its best advantage; in fact, in many centres, breech delivery has become a positive indication for epidural analgesia (Darby et al., 1976).

It has been held in the past that general anaesthesia should be used in twin delivery to prevent the uterus clamping down on the second infant. The problem is not beyond solution by the adroit obstetrician who practises the more modern active management of twin labour. After delivery of the first twin, the second amniotic sac is artificially ruptured and the presenting part is drawn down thus preventing closure of the cervix. Analgesia and relaxation of the birth canal allow the expeditious delivery of the second twin which may be imperilled by the reduction in area of the placental site following the birth of the first twin (Crawford, 1975).

Aortocaval Occlusion (Supine Hypotensive) Syndrome

While the small degree of sympathetic blockade necessary to relieve pain may unmask the effects of aortocaval occlusion one might feel obliged to avoid epidural analgesia where supine hypotension is manifest before the injection is given. Such patients can safely be managed by giving half the intended dose of local anaesthetic while lying on one side and then injecting the other half-dose through the cannula, after a five-minute interval, with the patient lying on the opposite side. The mother should not be allowed to lie on her back unsupervised during labour and should be delivered on her side. If this is not practicable or if a forceps delivery is required, it is sometimes safe cautiously to turn the mother on to her back. Usually by the time that the fetus has moved lower down into the pelvis the uterus may not be exerting the harmful pressure on the inferior vena cava but, as an added precaution, the patient should be tilted to the left by a pillow placed under the right buttock and the uterus may be displaced to the left by hand.

Severe Shock, Hypotension and Hypovolaemia

These conditions must be treated effectively before epidural blockade is given and it follows that haemorrhage occurring during epidural analgesia must be energetically treated with the patient in the lateral posture. In any case, severe antepartum haemorrhage demands immediate delivery by forceps or by Caesarean section.

Previous Spinal Surgery

The main reason why previous spinal surgery might contra-indicate epidural block is that the anatomical disturbance might prevent the accurate identification of the epidural space and obstruct spread of the local anaesthetic to the sacral region. Laminectomy is most commonly carried out in the *lower* lumbar region; thus the 1st–2nd and 2nd–3rd lumbar interspaces are not usually involved. In the relatively few cases that the writer has dealt with, perfect analgesia was achieved by an injection at the 2nd–3rd lumbar interspace above the previous operation site and no difficulty has been experienced in achieving perineal analgesia when needed. However, if this were so, the caudal route of injection could be used or the obstetrician could give a pudendal block. Some difficulty may be experienced following posterior spinal fusion in the upper lumbar region. However, if the extent of the fusion is limited, uterine pain may be relieved by an injection through a cannula placed to block the lower thoracic segments and perineal pain through another cannula placed in the lumbosacral space or in the caudal canal to block the sacral roots. Previous surgery for anterior (intercorporeal) spinal fusion should not prevent a safe and successful epidural puncture.

Neurological Disease

The fear of an exacerbation of the symptoms of existing or suspected neurological disease may cause some reluctance to give epidural analgesia. In particular, women with existing bladder dysfunction may suffer urinary retention or incontinence following childbirth and the epidural may be suspected as being a contributory factor. In these circumstances it is advisable to obtain a signed statement from the patient that she recognises the risk and is prepared to accept it.

Epidural analgesia is strongly indicated in a patient with a cerebral tumour or in one who has had a subarachnoid haemorrhage because the rise of blood pressure due to experience of pain is prevented, the rise of intracranial pressure due to the bearing-down reflex can be controlled and effective analgesia is provided for elective forceps delivery.

THE CARE OF PATIENTS DURING EPIDURAL ANALGESIA

It is particularly important that midwives and others in attendance should be aware of the special needs of patients receiving epidural analgesia.

Records.—Detailed records should be kept of all local anaesthetic doses given to the mother together with their effect on blood pressure, pulse rate and fetal heart rate. The effect of the doses and the extent of the accompanying sensory blockade will help to determine the size of the subsequent doses required. The occurrence of side-effects and the progress of labour should also be recorded. The use of a purpose-designed record card has the advantage not only of imposing a discipline on the labour ward staff to ensure the proper care of the patients, but also of facilitating the hand-over should a change of clinical charge of the case be necessary.

Posture.—The most important single safety factor in the care of patients receiving epidural analgesia is the alertness of those in attendance for the signs and symptoms of the aortocaval occlusion syndrome (supine hypotension) which is discussed in greater detail in Chapter 43.

Ideally, the patient should be nursed on her side throughout labour but it must be accepted that obstetricians and midwives may feel obliged to turn her on to her back for abdominal palpation and auscultation, catheterisation of the bladder and vaginal examination. They should be aware that a pillow placed under the right hip will provide a reasonable postural compromise.

One of the advantages claimed for the small-dose or selective block is that the mother retains mobility on the labour-ward bed at least at first. In longer labours, when repeated doses have to be given, weakness and paresis of the legs may occur and, if not helped to change her position, the patient will lie passively and without complaint. She must be turned from one side to another at intervals. Scrupulous attention must be paid to smoothing out ridges in the bed linen which must be changed frequently when soiled. Duthie *et al.* (1968) have reported a pressure sore in a patient after 24 hours of epidural anaesthesia in spite of the retention of motor power in the legs.

Care of the bladder.—Care must be taken to ensure that the bladder does not become over-distended during labour as the desire for micturition is lost. The bladder should therefore be emptied before each top-up dose is given. The larger dose of local anaesthetic given for forceps delivery may cause prolonged loss of sensation in the immediate post-partum period and the bladder is liable to become over-filled owing to natural diuresis and the cessation of the anti-diuretic effect of synthetic oxytocin used in labour. A voluntary effort to micturate should be made despite the temporary absence of the desire to do so. If this fails there should be no hesitation in passing a catheter as overdistension of the bladder may result in prolonged dysfunction of micturition.

Diversion and nutrition.—Because the mother remains fully alert during labour some form of diversion is welcome including reading matter, portable radio and visits from close family relatives. Bland fluids may be given although the mother herself often refuses them. Occasionally she may be troubled by persistent nausea, which should be treated by intravenous perphenazine 2·5 mg. Larger doses are unnecessary and may cause undue sleepiness.

Topping-up.—The management of topping-up is based on the following standard instructions:

(*a*) For uterine pain give 7 ml bupivacaine 0·5 per cent with the patient lying horizontally.

(*b*) For perineal pain or forceps delivery give 8 ml bupivacaine 0·5 per cent with the patient sitting up and staying in this position for 5 minutes after completion of the injection.

It is particularly important that top-up doses be given as soon as contractions become painful; there is nothing to be gained by allowing the mother's morale to fail and she should be encouraged to draw attention to the first sign of returning discomfort. The provision of perineal anaesthesia for spontaneous or operative delivery must be anticipated by giving a top-up in the sitting position well in advance of need. It should also be emphasised that the top-up doses should continue to be given even though a decision may have been made to deliver by Caesarean section.

As a general rule uterine pain is associated with the first stage and perineal pain with the second stage of labour. Nevertheless top-ups should be given in the recumbent position for uterine pain and in the sitting position for perineal pain irrespective of the state of cervical dilatation. For example, if the fetal head is high in early labour, pressure on the sacral promontory may cause perineal or rectal discomfort and an injection in the sitting position would be required. Once the perineal pain is relieved the discomfort of uterine contraction may then demand relief by a top-up in the horizontal position. Similarly a top-up in the recumbent position may be required for the return of uterine pain in the second stage even though the perineum has already been anaesthetised by a previous injection in the sitting position.

In some departments there is a tendency to discontinue top-ups in the second stage in order to encourage voluntary expulsive efforts in the hope of improving the chances of spontaneous delivery. This results in the mother, who has been perfectly comfortable throughout the first stage of labour, then being allowed to experience severe labour pain, usually without any other form of analgesia. This practice is not to be encouraged.

Nevertheless, after prolonged epidural block the mother may not notice a change of sensation when labour has progressed to the second stage. She may feel the uterus contracting and be able to push spontaneously in concert with it, but on the other hand she may be totally unaware of the contractions and require constant reminders to bear down in compliance with her attendant's instructions. In multiparae, particularly with oxytocin stimulation, the fetal head may be discovered unexpectedly on the perineum, and while spontaneous delivery is unusual, those in attendance should be warned that periodic visual and manual examination is needed to assess progress of labour.

These instructions provide a logical framework for the management of epidurals but experience has shown that attendants sympathetic to this method of analgesia can achieve more effective results than those who are otherwise inclined.

After delivery.—Following delivery the epidural cannula is removed and checked to ensure that no portion has been sequestered and the puncture site is covered with a small adhesive dressing. The patient should be warned of the weakness of her legs which may persist for three to four hours following the last top-up, and she should be accompanied for her first few steps out of bed.

It has been noted that mothers who have been delivered under epidural anaesthesia appear to be unduly sensitive to the discomforts of the "after-pains" and of the sutured perineal wound. These require prompt and frequent relief with oral analgesics. It is possible that when labour pains have been endured with less effective analgesic methods the discomforts of the puerperium pale into relative insignificance. When labour and delivery have been free from pain the need to relieve "after-pains" and perineal discomfort assumes a disproportionate importance.

In short, mothers receiving epidural blockade require little more than the application of the proper standard of care expected in any well-run labour ward. Epidural anaesthesia merely demands that there should be no relaxation of these standards.

Epidural Analgesia and the Forceps Rate

A possible discouragement to the more frequent use of epidural analgesia has been the belief that it inevitably leads to the need for operative delivery (Moir and Willocks, 1967). While this impression persists it is not surprising that hospital obstetricians see in it a source of increased pressure of work, midwives a cause of deprivation of the opportunity to practise their art and train their pupils, and mothers the denial of the pleasure and satisfaction of parturition by their own unaided efforts.

The theoretical reasons why the use of epidurals should predispose to operative delivery are firstly, the abolition of the involuntary urge to bear down in the second stage of labour, and secondly, the paralysis of the muscles of the pelvic floor which may cause malrotation and incomplete flexion of the fetal head. However, the relief of maternal distress should eliminate one of the main indications for operative delivery.

Noble and de Vere (1970) reported that an increased use of epidural analgesia at the Westminster Hospital had not increased the rate of instrumental delivery. A satisfactory by-product of this policy was the virtual abolition of general anaesthesia for vaginal operative delivery.

In labours predominantly conducted by obstetricians, delivery by forceps may be elective and spontaneous parturition following epidural analgesia may be allowed to occur in only about 10 per cent of labours (Kandel *et al.*, 1966; de Vere, 1969). In other circumstances epidural analgesia may be used only in abnormal labours when assisted delivery would be anticipated irrespective of the type of pain relief employed.

From personal observation of the practice of several obstetricians, the writer has noted a considerable variability in the time that each allows his patients under epidural anaesthesia to remain undelivered in the second stage of labour. All patients in the care of one obstetrician were delivered within an average time of 30 minutes of full dilatation of the cervix. The overall forceps rate was 69 per cent, 95 per cent for primigravidae and 40 per cent for multigravidae. Another obstetrician was willing to await delivery without intervention for an average time of more than one hour in the second stage of labour; the overall forceps rate was 10 per cent, 19 per cent in primigravidae and 3 per cent in multigravidae.

It is suggested that epidural analgesia might be less frequently associated with forceps delivery provided that:

1. The technique is employed in normal as well as in abnormal labours;
2. The strength of uterine contraction is augmented if necessary by an oxytocin infusion;
3. A selective technique is used involving minimal doses of local anaesthetic directed at the nerve pathways by which the mother is feeling pain at the time of injection;
4. The mother is encouraged by her attendants to bear down in concert with the uterine contractions of which she may be unaware;
5. The attending obstetrician is willing to allow the mother time and opportunity to deliver herself without unduly hasty intervention (Doughty, 1969*b*).

It should be remembered that the practice of epidural analgesia is developing concurrently with the introduction of more sophisticated and reliable methods of monitoring, which provide earlier warning of possible hazard to the fetus. The awareness of increasing maternal and fetal acidaemia by many obstetricians has dictated the need to limit the length of the second stage of labour (Pearson and Davies, 1974). As a result, instrumental delivery is now carried out more frequently irrespective of the increasing use of epidural blockade. An epidural service facilitates the application of this trend in obstetrics as well as contributing to the greater comfort and safety of the patient during operative delivery.

PRACTICABILITY OF EPIDURAL ANALGESIA IN OBSTETRICS

While the practice of epidural analgesia is growing there are undoubted difficulties in establishing a service in many major obstetric units. In some the obstetricians would like to see the service established but the anaesthetists are unable to supply it; in some the anaesthetists are able to offer the service but their obstetrician colleagues are unconvinced of its value, while in others local opinion is satisfied with the existing methods of pain relief and sees no reason for any change particularly if it implies an increase in the work of a busy department.

In establishing the service the necessary skill must be available to provide epidural analgesia. The technique may be taught under general anaesthesia on the gynaecological operating list. However, the increasing practice of inserting the epidural cannula before the start of labour has enabled the initial teaching to be carried out in the labour ward, as it is only after the contractions have become painful that undue delay is intolerable.

Fear of the complications tend to have a deterrent effect. There are only four which assume practical importance. *First* is dural puncture, the frequency of which can only be reduced by conscientious teaching, meticulous technique and constant practice. *Second* is the unrecognised dural puncture followed by the injection of local anaesthetic into the subarachnoid space. This will cause a profound fall of blood pressure possibly leading to respiratory and cardiac arrest. No-one should attempt epidural analgesia unless prepared to take all precautions to avoid this complication (such as giving a test dose) and to treat it efficiently and promptly on the rare occasions that it occurs. A most important measure is the establishment of an intravenous infusion before the epidural is given. *Third* is the occasional fall of blood pressure due to the unmasking of the effects of aortocaval occlusion. It is of the utmost importance that the midwives in attendance on the patient should be trained to recognise and treat, by turning the mother on to her side, the early symptoms of supine hypotension which may follow the induction of epidural analgesia and the subsequent top-ups. *Fourth* is puncturing an epidural vein leading to the possibility of intravenous injection of the local anaesthetic and of an epidural haematoma forming a nidus for subsequent infection. (See also p. 1178 *et seq.*)

There has been a persistent suspicion that epidural analgesia may be responsible for neurological complications following parturition. The risks are minimal provided that the technique is managed with close attention to the precautions already described. It should not be forgotten that even normal labour without epidural anaesthesia may be followed by neurological damage (Chalmers, 1949). Bladder disturbances, headache, lumbo-sciatic pain and foot-drop are recognised as not uncommon sequelae of both normal and operative delivery without epidural block (Grove, 1973). One should, therefore, keep an open mind as to whether epidural analgesia does or does not add to these risks.

The key to setting up an epidural service is a corporate desire of midwives, obstetricians and anaesthetists to have it and to make it work. There must be facilities for the continual training of all concerned in the technical skills involved and a standard routine must be evolved so that epidural anaesthesia becomes accepted for what it is, a normal and effective method of pain relief in a modern maternity department.

CAUDAL EPIDURAL ANALGESIA

This technique for the relief of pain in labour was introduced by Hingson and Edwards in 1942. Local anaesthetic solution was injected through the sacral hiatus in quantities sufficient to rise within the epidural space to affect the sympathetic afferent pathways entering the central nervous system at the lower thoracic segments. In its passage up the epidural space the local anaesthetic also blocks the sacral roots producing perineal anaesthesia and relaxation of the muscles of the pelvic floor long before such a block might be indicated by the mother's need. The sacral block is reinforced with each successive top-up but the high rate of assisted delivery has been considered a small price to pay for the benefit of total relief of pain. In effect caudal analgesia is more specifically suited to operative delivery and relief of labour pain accrues as a secondary effect achieved by higher dosage.

Technique (Meehan, 1969; see also Chapter 35)

With the patient in the left lateral position and after full aseptic precautions the sacral hiatus is identified using the left thumb which then acts as a marker. The Hingson and Edwards malleable needle is inserted into the sacral hiatus at right angles to the skin. A distinct "give" is felt as the needle pierces the sacro-coccygeal ligament. The hub of the needle is then depressed towards the natal cleft so that the needle lies at an angle of 40° to the skin and the needle is gently advanced into the sacral canal. The stylet is withdrawn and an aspiration test carried out to ensure that the needle has not pierced the dura or a dural vein. A length of polyvinyl cannula is introduced through the needle which is then withdrawn over the cannula. A test dose of local anaesthetic is injected. If, after five minutes, the patient can still move her legs, inadvertent subarachnoid block can be excluded. The main therapeutic dose of 16 to 20 ml of local anaesthetic is then injected through the cannula and relief of pain becomes fully established within 10 to 20 minutes.

Difficulties

Some trouble may be encountered in identifying and penetrating the sacral hiatus owing to obesity, oedema or anatomical abnormalities. With the mother lying on her side gravity causes the soft parts to fall thus giving a false impression of the midline of the body. Moore (1961) overcame these problems by meticulous marking of the posterior superior iliac spines and the sacral cornua on the skin and inserting the caudal needle with the patient in the knee-elbow position.

Other difficulties arise from misplacement of the needle. Its point may lie superficially to the sacrum and injection will be seen to produce swelling under the skin. Subperiosteal injection will cause severe pain as the periosteum is stripped from the bone. More serious but rare complications have been reported due to the passage of the needle past the body of the 5th sacral vertebra into the rectum or even into the fetus (Finster *et al.*, 1965). When the needle is correctly placed in the sacral epidural space, injection of air or fluid should encounter no resistance.

COMPARISON OF THE TECHNIQUES OF LUMBAR AND CAUDAL EPIDURAL ANALGESIA

The two techniques have much in common. The indications for and contra-indications to their employment are identical. Similar side-effects and complications occur, and the same precautions should be taken in caring for the patient with either form of epidural analgesia.

However, important differences arise mainly because of the contrasted sites of injection. The sacrum is well known for its anatomical abnormalities; it may be bifid, or the sacral hiatus may be too small or obliterated by ossification of the sacro-coccygeal ligament. In these cases an attempt at caudal analgesia is likely to fail. Although rare, anatomical abnormalities occur in the lumbar spine, but the anaesthetist has a choice of lumbar interspaces through which he may attempt a second puncture if the first is unsuccessful. Similarly dural puncture through the caudal canal is usually regarded as a reason for abandoning the technique, while this same complication in the lumbar region need not preclude lumbar epidural anaesthesia being given through an adjoining interspace.

A patient in whom obesity or oedema prevents the ready identification of the sacral hiatus may nevertheless have easily palpable lumbar spines and thus present no difficulty with the induction of lumbar epidural analgesia.

A feature of descriptions of the technique of both caudal and lumbar epidural anaesthesia is the invariable recommendation to give a test dose through the cannula as a precaution against the effects of inadvertent dural puncture. Although the dural sac within the sacral canal may occasionally extend below the level of the body of the 2nd sacral vertebra, it is usually considered safe to advance the needle up to 5 cm without fear of dural puncture. In the lumbar region the epidural space may be from 3 to 9 cm from the surface and the distance from the ligamentum flavum to the dura is only 0·3 cm to 0·5 cm. One would expect a higher frequency of inadvertent dural puncture at the hands of the inexpert, yet in spite of this, practitioners of lumbar epidurals now regard this complication as an avoidable and culpable error of technique.

The site of injection for epidural block through the caudal canal also influences the size of the dose required to block the lower thoracic segments. Meehan's dosage (1969) of 16 to 20 ml of local anaesthetic solution is conservative in comparison with that of other authors yet even he mentions toxic reaction to local anaesthetics as one of the complications of the method. Lumbar epidural anaesthesia may be achieved with only 5 to 7 ml and toxic reactions are unlikely to occur unless injection is made directly into an epidural vein. A dose adequate to reach the lower thoracic segments is essential for total relief of labour pain. Small doses given caudally will produce perineal anaesthesia without necessarily relieving the pain of uterine contractions. Selectivity of block is impossible with caudal analgesia and a high frequency of assisted delivery has to be accepted.

Lastly, a caudal injection has to be made through a potentially unhygienic area, and whatever measures are taken to seal the site of entry of the cannula in the sacral hiatus the dressings are liable to become contaminated during the course of labour. Moore (1961) recognises this difficulty and maintains the hygiene of the site of injection by keeping the mother turned on to her side throughout labour. Lumbar epidural analgesia may be induced and maintained with a far higher standard of hygiene.

Whichever method is used will depend on the predilection and training of the practitioner. In the United Kingdom caudal epidural blockade has been practised mainly by obstetricians despite its difficulties and disadvantages (Yates and Kuah, 1968; Meehan, 1969). With a few exceptions (Cooper et al., 1972), lumbar epidural anaesthesia appears to be the preserve of the anaesthetist who would use the caudal route only if the lumbar approach were impracticable.

PARACERVICAL BLOCK

Paracervical block is a comparatively simple technique for the relief of the pain of uterine contractions in the first stage of labour. It may be given from 5 cm dilatation of the cervix and can be repeated provided that a rim of cervix is identifiable lateral to the fetal head. Local anaesthetic solution is injected into the pelvic cellular tissue at the base of the broad ligament where it spreads in the utero-vaginal plexus to block both the sympathetic and parasympathetic afferent pathways to the central nervous system (see Chapter 41). Its variable success may be due to the alternative afferent pathway from the fundus of the uterus via the tubo-ovarian vessels, well away from the site of injection.

Cooper and Chassar Moir (1963) used a specially constructed guard-tube 14 cm in length, the tip of which is manipulated to the top of each lateral vaginal fornix. A needle is inserted through the tube and is of such a length that it protrudes beyond it for not more than 7 mm. It should, therefore, just penetrate the vaginal wall; any further extension beyond the base of the broad ligament carries the risk of injection into the uterine vessels, the placental site and even into the fetus itself. The dose originally recommended was 10 ml 1 per cent lignocaine with adrenaline 1 in 200,000 on each side of the cervix; this has now been superseded by bupivacaine 0·5 per cent with adrenaline 1 in 200,000 which gives a longer period of action (Cooper et al., 1968). Yates (1969) found that lignocaine/adrenaline gave pain relief for a mean time of only 88 minutes as compared with a mean time of 144 minutes afforded by bupivacaine/adrenaline. Even so, this relatively short period of action is a disadvantage and a technique has been described for inserting Teflon cannulae into the paracervical tissues so that supplementary doses can be given with the waning of effect of the previous dose (Baggish, 1964). Although paracervical block may be used from 5-cm dilatation of the cervix, it is most useful towards the end of the first stage of labour as a means of removing the desire to bear down before the cervix is fully dilated. It will only relieve the pain of uterine contraction and if the patient complains of perineal discomfort, a pudendal nerve block should be performed to block the somatic afferent pathway from the sacral segments.

Some anxiety has been expressed concerning fetal bradycardia which has been noted shortly after the injection. Unexpected deaths in utero and the death of an infant—affected during labour—in the neonatal period have been reported (Stern *et al.*, 1969). Early speculation was that the adrenaline given with the local anaesthetic to reduce its toxicity and to prolong its action might be responsible for the effect on the fetus by reducing the blood supply to the placental site (Crawford, 1963). More recently it has been suggested that bradycardia is the direct effect of the local anaesthetic on the fetal myocardium. Cord blood studies have shown that the injected drug can rapidly reach the fetal circulation from the highly vascular paracervical tissues (Shnider *et al.*, 1968). They showed that normally the umbilical vein:maternal artery concentration ratio was about 1:2; in fetal-bradycardia cases the ratio tended to be reversed. This could be explained only by injection into or near the intervillous space and it was felt that fetal bradycardia was due more to technical errors than to the method itself. Gomez (1969) cites these errors as firstly, the alignment of the needle guide parallel with the vaginal wall on the side to be injected instead of at the correct inclination, and secondly the mistaken belief that the depth of injection is limited by the 7 mm of needle projecting from the tip of the guard-tube. Light pressure on a yielding fornix may carry it beyond the safety limits. He emphasises that a small dose (4–5 ml 1 per cent lignocaine) given by an accurate technique is quite sufficient to relieve pain and will help to avoid the dangers to the fetus. He also warns that fetal bradycardia ascribed to paracervical block may be due to associated obstetric causes.

The biochemical confirmation of fetal distress by Teramo (1969) leaves little doubt that paracervical block, unless it is properly carried out, imposes the greatest risk on the fetus of all the local anaesthetic techniques simply on account of the close proximity of the area of injection to the uterine vessels and to the placental site. Evidence that direct passage of the drug to the fetus is indeed a risk inherent in the technique is presented by Beazley *et al.* (1972).

Appendix to Chapter 42

OBSTETRIC ANALGESIA AND THE MIDWIFE

In the United Kingdom most women are delivered of their infants by midwives and it is customary for "medical aid" to be enlisted only when the management of the labour is beyond the midwife's competence. It follows that, in the past, it has been unusual for an anaesthetist to assume personal responsibility for the relief of pain in a labour that is being conducted by a midwife. It is against the background of midwife-managed obstetrics that a variety of methods of pain relief have been developed, the over-riding consideration being that they should be safe for the single-handed midwife to administer in the mother's own home without interfering with her main task—that of delivering the baby. Nevertheless, it must be regretted that this consideration has, until recently, resulted in a stultifying effect on the development of more effective methods of pain relief, particularly as over 90 per cent of mothers are now delivered in hospital where a wider range of analgesic methods should be available.

The midwife's activities in England and Wales* are regulated by the Central Midwives Board who prescribe her training, hold the examinations which she must pass before being allowed to practise and maintain the Roll of qualified midwives from which her name may be removed for serious breaches of professional conduct.

The anaesthetist has a part to play in the instruction of midwives concerning relief of pain and in the general supervision of the practice of analgesia in the labour wards of his hospital. The following extracts from the Handbook issued by the Central Midwives Board suggest the range of responsibility of the anaesthetist in the training and practice of the midwife:

Section B

Rule 18*b* During either the first or second period of training a pupil-midwife shall receive theoretical and practical instruction in anaesthesia and analgesia in midwifery practice as follows:
(i) 3 lecture demonstrations by a specialist anaesthetist;
(ii) the administration of an analgesic to at least 15 patients in labour by means of an apparatus or method approved by the Board under the general supervision of a specialist anaesthetist and under the detailed supervision of a midwife who is experienced in the use of the apparatus or method or of a resident medical officer who is similarly experienced.

Rule 23*b* An institution shall not be approved in respect of instruction in analgesia unless:
(i) the institution is one training pupils or medical students or is providing post-certificate courses for midwives or holding postgraduate courses for medical practitioners, or is otherwise considered by the Board as suitable for approval;
(ii) the institution has attached to it a specialist anaesthetist;
(iii) the resident medical officer or the midwife who would undertake the

*In Scotland and in Northern Ireland midwives are subjected to the regulations of separate authorities.

detailed supervision of the practical work is experienced in the use of the apparatus or method on which the instruction at the institution will be based.

Rule 39 The Second Examination shall be oral, clinical and practical. A candidate may be required to answer questions on the following subjects:

(a) practical midwifery;

(b) analgesia in childbirth;

(c) etc. . . .

Section E

Treatment Outside a Midwife's Province

Rule 5 (a) A practising midwife must not, except in an emergency, undertake any treatment which is outside her normal province. The question whether in any particular case such treatment was justified will be judged on the facts and circumstances of the case.

(b) A practising midwife must not on her own responsibility use any drug, including an analgesic, unless in the course of her training, whether before or after enrolment, she has been thoroughly instructed in its use and is familiar with its dosage and methods of administration or application.

(c) A practising midwife must not, except on the instructions and in the presence of a registered medical practitioner, administer an inhalational analgesic otherwise than by means of an apparatus which is of a type approved by the Board for use by midwives, and, where the Board so directs in relation to particular types of apparatus, has been inspected and approved by or on behalf of the Board, within such a period before the date of administration as the Board shall from time to time determine, as fit for use by midwives.

(d) A practising midwife must not, except on the instructions and in the presence of a registered medical practitioner, administer an inhalational analgesic by means of an apparatus which is required by this rule to have been inspected and approved within a specified period before the date of use unless there is in the possession of the body or person by whom the apparatus is held a certificate signed on behalf of the Board, certifying that the apparatus was inspected and approved by or on behalf of the Board on a date falling within the appropriate period, as fit for use by midwives.

(e) A practising midwife must not, except on the instructions and in the presence of a registered medical practitioner administer an inhalational analgesic unless:

(i) she has, either before or after enrolment received at an institution approved by the Board for the purpose, special instruction in the essentials of obstetric analgesia and has satisfied the institution or the Board that she is thoroughly proficient in the use of the apparatus; and

(ii) the patient has at some time during the pregnancy been examined by a registered medical practitioner who has signed a certificate that he finds no contra-indication to the administration of the analgesic by a midwife and, if any illness which required medical attention subsequently developed during pregnancy, the midwife obtained confirmation from a medical practitioner that the certificate remained valid; and

(iii) one other person, being any person acceptable to the patient, who in the opinion of the midwife is suitable for the purpose, is present at the time of the administration in addition to the midwife.

(f) Unless special exemption is given by the Board to enable particular institutions to investigate new methods, a midwife must not administer any anaesthetic otherwise than on the instructions and in the presence of a registered medical practitioner.

Lecture Course to Midwives

The Central Midwives Board offers the following suggestions as to the content of the prescribed lecture course:

First Lecture

Short history of the relief of pain in labour.

Definition of analgesia, amnesia and anaesthesia, and difference between sedation and analgesia.

Drugs commonly used in the first stage of labour, and methods of administration and dosage.

Effect of drugs on maternal and fetal condition, and on uterine contractions, and abnormal reactions which might occur.

Causes of failure to give relief.

Second Lecture

Inhalational analgesia or anaesthesia, with detailed description of approved apparatus maintenance of such apparatus.

Principles of local infiltration, pudendal block and epidural block.

Choice of analgesic method and contra-indications.

Statutory rules and regulations relating to the use of drugs and analgesic methods of midwives.

Third Lecture

Preparation of patients for anaesthetics required for operative deliveries.

Care of the unconscious patient after delivery under anaesthesia.

Emergencies of anaesthesia, including the treatment of cardiac arrest.

Prevention and treatment of Mendelson's syndrome.

Resuscitation of mother and/or baby.

Comments

While many anaesthetists may be involved in giving pupil midwives their three statutory lecture demonstrations (Section B, Rule 18b) it may come as a surprise to find that they are expected to maintain a general supervision of the administration of analgesia in the labour wards of their hospitals. This provides a salutary opportunity to assess the effectiveness of their teaching and in this way they can help to maintain the standard of labour analgesia. They should be able and willing to introduce improved techniques for the administration of the permitted methods, and they are likely to be familiar with new agents which become "approved" for use by the unsupervised midwife. Section E, Rule 5b implies that the professionally qualified midwife relies on them for appropriate instruction in the use of such agents, and in recent years the introduction of methoxyflurane, pentazocine and diazepam may be cited as cases in point.

In the ever-widening scope of subjects related to analgesia and anaesthesia one may wonder with some justification whether the three prescribed lecture demonstrations are sufficient, not only to acquaint pupil midwives with all they should know but also to make sure that they really understand the basic principles of relieving pain in labour (Section E, Rule 5*b*).

The Central Midwives Board obviously has in mind the likelihood of research into new methods of analgesia which might be given by the unsupervised midwife. Section E, Rule 5*f*, is a reminder that any such research involving the midwife's co-operation must have the Board's approval.

Epidural Analgesia and the Midwife

The availability of epidural analgesia has been revolutionised since the Central Midwives Board's approval of midwives assisting with the topping-up procedure. The "top-up" dose could be recognised as "any drug including any analgesic" permitted under Section E, Rule 5*b*. However, this rule should not be interpreted against the background of circumstances to which it was never intended to apply. Nevertheless, in 1971, the Central Midwives Board stated that while the injection of local anaesthetic substances into the epidural space was primarily the province of the doctor, the Board would not raise any objection to an experienced midwife undertaking the topping-up procedure (not the primary dose) provided the following safeguards were observed:

(i) The ultimate responsibility for such a technique should be clearly stated to rest with the doctor.
(ii) Written instructions as to the dose should be given by the doctor concerned.
(iii) In all cases the dose given by the midwife should be checked by one other person.
(iv) Instructions should be given by the doctor as to the posture of the patient at the time of injection, observation of blood pressure, etc. and measures to be taken in the event of any side-effect.
(v) The midwife should have been thoroughly instructed in the technique so that the doctor concerned is satisfied as to her ability.

A recent circular from the Central Midwives Board has modified the provisions of Section B, Rule 18*b*. It states that because of modern trends in obstetric analgesia, the current requirements for training of pupil midwives were no longer appropriate. In future a pupil midwife would no longer be required to administer inhalational analgesia to a specified number of patients. The approved teacher must now certify that she has received satisfactory training and experience to administer analgesia on her own responsibility *as well as to participate in advanced techniques carried out under the supervision of a registered medical practitioner*. Here one may see this not so much as the midwife taking over a procedure which should normally be carried out by a doctor, but more as the doctor placing in the hands of the midwife the means by which she may more effectively manage the patient's labour pains.

It would appear that midwives' participation in the maintenance of epidural analgesia has received the unqualified approval of the Central Midwives Board. Thus, it is reasonable to infer that any institution in which the technique is not practised might be regarded, in this respect, as defective in its capability of training pupil midwives. Equally, in departments where epidural analgesia is particularly well-developed almost to the exclusion of any other analgesic method, approved teachers might find difficulty in truthfully certifying pupil midwives as having received satisfactory training and experience in administering the simpler analgesics on their own responsibility.

It will be noted that, despite the participation of midwives in the technique of epidural analgesia, the responsibility for the safety of the procedure and the quality of the service provided remains entirely with the doctor concerned. The midwife's only responsibility is the meticulous observance of the instructions given by the anaesthetist. These ideals are best achieved by the use of a purpose-designed epidural record card and the distribution to all midwives of an instruction booklet which is accepted as "standing orders" for the procedure. The frequent presence of a senior anaesthetist in the maternity department ensures that high standards of care are maintained and that the constantly changing midwifery staff are kept informed of the special needs of patients receiving epidural analgesia.

REFERENCES

ABOULEISH, E., and DEPP, R. (1975). Acupuncture in obstetrics. *Anesth. Analg. Curr. Res.*, **54**, 83.

BAGGISH, M. S. (1964). Continuous paracervical block. *Amer. J. Obstet. Gynec.*, **88**, 968.

BARACH, A. L., and ROVENSTINE, E. Q. (1945). The hazards of anoxia during nitrous oxide anesthesia. *Anesthesiology*, **6**, 449.

BEAZLEY, J. M., LEAVER, E. P., MOREWOOD, J. H. M., and BIRCUMSHAW, J. (1967). Relief of pain in labour. *Lancet*, **1**, 1033.

BEAZLEY, J. M., TAYLOR, G., and REYNOLDS, F. (1972). Placental transfer of bupivacaine after paracervical block. *Obstet. and Gynec.*, **39**, 2.

BLUMBERG, H., DAYTON, H. and WOLF, P. (1966). Counteraction of narcotic antagonist analgesics by the narcotic antagonist naloxone. *Proc. Soc. exp. Biol. (N.Y.)*, **123**, 755.

BODLEY, P. O., MIRZA, V., SPEARS, J. R., and SPILSBURY, R. A. (1966). Obstetric analgesia with methoxyflurane. *Anaesthesia*, **21**, 457.

BOISVERT, M., and HUDON, F. (1962). Clinical evaluation of methoxyflurane in obstetrical anaesthesia: a report on 500 cases. *Canad. Anaesth. Soc. J.*, **9**, 325.

BONICA, J. J. (1972). *Obstetric Analgesia and Anesthesia*, p. 42. Berlin: Springer Verlag.

BRACKEN, A., BROUGHTON, G. B., and HILL, D. W. (1968). Safety precautions to be observed with cooled pre-mixed gases. *Brit. med. J.*, **3**, 715.

BRAHAM, J., and SAIA, A. (1958). Neurological complications of epidural anaesthesia. *Brit. med. J.*, **2**, 657.

BRIDENBAUGH, L. D., MOORE, D. C., BAGDI, P., and BRIDENBAUGH, P. O. (1968). The position of plastic tubing in continuous block techniques: an X-ray study of 552 patients. *Anesthesiology*, **29**, 1047.

BROMAGE, P. R. (1954). *Spinal Epidural Analgesia*. Edinburgh: E. & S. Livingstone.

BROMAGE, P. R. (1961). Continuous lumbar epidural analgesia for obstetrics. *Canad. med. Ass. J.*, **85**, 1136.

BROMAGE, P. R. (1975). Mechanism of action of extradural analgesia. *Brit. J. Anaesth.*, **47**, S 199.

CAMPBELL, D., MASSON, A. H. B., and NORRIS, W. (1965). The clinical evaluation of narcotic and sedative drugs. II: A re-evaluation of pethidine and pethilorfan. *Brit. J. Anaesth.*, **37**, 199.

CASE, B. D., CORCORAN, R., JEFFCOATE, N., and RANDLE, G. H. (1971). Caesarean section and its place in modern obstetric practice. *J. Obstet. Gynaec. Brit. Cwlth.*, **78**, 203.

CENTRAL MIDWIVES BOARD (1962). Handbook incorporating the *Rules of the Central Midwives' Board*, 25th edit. London: Spottiswoode Ballantyre & Co.

CHALMERS, J. A. (1949). Traumatic neuritis of the puerperium. *J. Obstet. Gynaec. Brit. Emp.*, **56**, 205.

CHANG, A., WOOD, C., HUMPHREY, M., GILBERT, M., and WAGSTAFF, C. (1976). The effects of narcotics on fetal acid-base status. *Brit. J. Obstet. Gynaec.*, **83**, 56.

COLE, P. V. (1964). Nitrous oxide and oxygen from a single cylinder. *Anaesthesia*, **19**, 3.

COOPER, K., and CHASSAR MOIR, J. (1963). Paracervical block. A simple method of pain relief in labour. *Brit. med. J.* **1**, 1372.

COOPER, K., GILROY, K. J., and HURRY, D. J. (1968). Paracervical nerve block in labour using bupivacaine (Marcain). *J. Obstet. Gynaec. Brit. Cwlth.*, **75**, 863.

COOPER, K., VELLA, P., and BROWNING, D. (1972). Lumbar epidural analgesia given by obstetricians. *J. Obstet. Gynaec. Brit. Cwlth.*, **79**, 144.

CRAWFORD, J. S. (1963). Paracervical nerve block. *Brit. med. J.*, **2**, 119.

CRAWFORD, J. S. (1972). *Principles and Practice of Obstetric Anaesthesia*, 3rd edit., p. 209. Oxford: Blackwell Scientific Publications.

CRAWFORD, J. S. (1974). An appraisal of lumbar epidural blockade in patients with a singleton fetus presenting by the breech. *J. Obstet. Gynaec. Brit. Cwlth.*, **81**, 867.

CRAWFORD, J. S. (1975). An appraisal of lumbar epidural blockade in labour in patients with multiple pregnancy. *Brit. J. Obstet. Gynaec.*, **82**, 929.

CRAWFORD, J. S., ELLIS, D. B., HILL, D. W., and PAYNE, J. P. (1967). Effects of cooling on the safety of premixed gases. *Brit. med. J.*, **2**, 138.

CRAWFORD, J. S., and TUNSTALL, M. E. (1968). Notes on respiratory performance in labour. *Brit. J. Anaesth.*, **40**, 612.

CREE, J., MEYER, J., and HAILEY, D. M. (1973). Diazepam in labour: its metabolism and effect on the clinical condition and thermogenesis of the newborn. *Brit. med. J.*, **4**, 251.

DARBY, S., THORNTON, C. A., and HUNTER, D. J. (1976). Extradural analgesia when the breech presents. *Brit. J. Obstet. Gynaec.*, **88**, 35.

DAVID, H., and ROSEN, M: (1976). Perinatal mortality after epidural analgesia. *Anaesthesia*, **31**, 1054.

DAVIDSON, J. A. (1962). An assessment of the value of hypnosis in pregnancy and labour. *Brit. med. J.*, **2**, 951.

DAVIES, A., SOLOMON, B., and LEVENE, A. (1958). Paraplegia following epidural anaesthesia. *Brit. med. J.*, **2**, 654.

DE VERE, R. D. (1969). Painful labour: modern methods of management. *Proc. roy. Soc. Med.*, **62**, 186.

DOUGHTY, A. (1969a). Painful labour: modern methods of management. *Proc. roy. Soc. Med.*, **62**, 189.

DOUGHTY, A. (1969b). Selective epidural analgesia and the forceps rate. *Brit. J. Anaesth.*, **41**, 1058.

DOUGHTY, A. (1974). A precise method of cannulating the lumbar epidural space. *Anaesthesia*, **29**, 63.

DOUGHTY, A. (1975). Lumbar epidural analgesia—the pursuit of perfection: with special reference to midwife participation. *Anaesthesia*, **30**, 741.

DUNDEE, J. W., and LOVE, W. J. (1963). Alterations in response to somatic pain with anaesthesia: XIV. Effects of subnarcotic concentrations of methoxyflurane. *Brit. J. Anaesth.*, **35**, 301.

DUNDEE, J. W., and MOORE, J. (1961). The myth of phenothiazine potentiation. *Anaesthesia*, **16**, 95.

DUTHIE, A. M., WYMAN, J. B., and LEWIS, G. A. (1968). Bupivacaine in labour. Its use in lumbar extradural analgesia. *Anaesthesia*, **23**, 20.

EPSTEIN, H. G., and MACINTOSH, R. R. (1949). Analgesia inhaler for trichlorethylene. *Brit. med. J.*, **2**, 1092.

EVANS, J. M., DAVID, H., ROSEN, M., REVILL, S., ROBINSON, J., McCARTHY, J., and HOGG, M. I. J. (1976). Patient-activated intravenous narcotic. *Anaesthesia*, **31**, 847.

FADL, E., and UTTING, J. E. (1969). A study of maternal acid-base state during labour. *Brit. J. Anaesth.*, **41**, 327.

FILLER, W. W., HALL, W. C., and FILLER, N. W. (1967). Analgesia in obstetrics: the effect of analgesics on uterine contractility and fetal heart rate. *Amer. J. Obstet. Gynec.*, **98**, 832.

FINSTER, M., POPPERS, P. J., SINCLAIR, J. C., MORISHIMA, H. O., and DANIEL, S. S. (1965). Accidental intoxication of the fetus with local anesthetic drug during caudal anesthesia. *Amer. J. Obstet. Gynec.*, **92**, 922.

FRUMIN, M. J., and SCHWARTZ, H. (1952). Continuous segmental peridural anesthesia. *Anesthesiology*, **13**, 488.

FRUMIN, M. J., SCHWARTZ, H., BURNS, J. J., BRODIE, B. B., and PAPPER, E. M. (1953). The appearance of procaine in the spinal fluid during peridural block in man. *J. Pharmacol.*, **109**, 102.

GALE, C. W., TUNSTALL, M. E., and WILTON-DAVIES, C. C. (1964). Pre-mixed gas and oxygen for midwives. *Brit. med. J.*, **1**, 732.

GINGRICH, T. F. (1968). Spinal epidural hematoma following continuous epidural anesthesia. *Anesthesiology*, **29**, 162.

GIRVAN, C. B., MOORE, J., and DUNDEE, J. W. (1976). Pethidine compared with pethidine-naloxone administered during labour. *Brit. J. Anaesth.*, **48**, 563.

GOMEZ, D. F. (1969). Paracervical block in obstetrics. *Lancet*, **1**, 1163.

GROVE, L. H. (1973). Backache, headache and bladder dysfunction after delivery. *Brit. J. Anaesth.*, **45**, 1147.

HELLMAN, K. (1965). Epidural anaesthesia in obstetrics. A second look at 26,127 cases. *Canad. Anaesth. Soc. J.*, **12**, 398.

HINGSON, R. A., and EDWARDS, W. B. (1942). Continuous caudal anesthesia during labor and delivery. *Anesth. Analg. Curr. Res.*, **21**, 301.

HOLDCROFT, A., and MORGAN, M. (1974). An assessment of the analgesic effect in labour of pethidine and 50 per cent nitrous oxide in oxygen (Entonox). *J. Obstet. Gynaec. Brit. Cwlth.*, **81**, 603.

HUCH, A., HUCH, R., LINDMARK, G., and ROOTH, G. (1974). Maternal hypoxaemia after pethidine. *J. Obstet. Gynaec. Brit. Cwlth.*, **81**, 608.

JONES, P. L., ROSEN, M., MUSHIN, W. W., and JONES, E. V. (1969a). Methoxyflurane and nitrous oxide as obstetric analgesics. I—a comparison by continuous administration. *Brit. med. J.*, **3**, 255.

JONES, P. L., ROSEN, M., MUSHIN, W. W., and JONES, E. V. (1969b). Methoxyflurane and nitrous oxide as obstetric analgesics. II—a comparison by self-administered intermittent inhalation. *Brit. med. J.*, **3**, 259.

KALLOS, T., and SMITH, T. C. (1968). Naloxone reversal of pentazocine-induced respiratory depression. *J. Amer. med. Ass.*, **204**, 932.

KANDEL, P. F., SPOEREL, W. E., and KINCH, R. A. H. (1966). Continuous epidural analgesia for labour and delivery: review of 1,000 cases. *Canad. med. Ass. J.*, **95**, 947.

KOCH, G., and WANDEL, H. (1968). The effect of pethidine on the postnatal adjustment of respiration and acid-base balance. *Acta obstet. gynec. scand.*, **47**, 27.

LA SALVIA, L. A., and STEFFEN, E. A. (1950). Delayed gastric emptying time in labor. *Amer. J. Obstet. Gynec.*, **59**, 1075.

LATTO, I. P., MOLLOY, M. J., and ROSEN, M. (1973). Arterial concentrations of nitrous oxide during intermittent patient-controlled inhalation of 50 per cent nitrous oxide in oxygen (Entonox) during the first stage of labour. *Brit. J. Anaesth.*, **45**, 1029.

LINDGREN, L. (1959). Influence of anaesthetics and analgesics on different types of labour. *Acta anaesth. scand.*, Suppl. **2**, 449.

McANENY, T. M., and DOUGHTY, A. (1963). Self-administered nitrous oxide/oxygen analgesia in obstetrics. *Anaesthesia*, **18**, 488.

MACGREGOR, W. G., BRACKEN, A., and FAIR, J. A. (1972). Piped premixed 50 per cent nitrous oxide and 50 per cent oxygen mixture (Entonox). *Anaesthesia*, **27**, 14.

MAJOR, V., ROSEN, M., and MUSHIN, W. W. (1966). Methoxyflurane as an obstetric analgesic: a comparison with trichloroethylene. *Brit. med. J.*, **2**, 1554.

MAJOR, V., ROSEN, M., and MUSHIN, W. W. (1967). Concentration of methoxyflurane for obstetric analgesia by self-administered intermittent inhalation. *Brit. med. J.*, **4**, 767.

MALE, C. G., and MARTIN, R. (1973). Puerperal spinal epidural abscess. *Lancet*, **1**, 608.

MALTAU, J. M., ANDERSON, H. T., and SKREDE, S. (1975). Obstetrical analgesia assessed by free fatty acid mobilisation. *Acta anaesth. scand.*, **19**, 245.

MATTHEWS, A. E. B. (1963). Double-blind trials of promazine in labour. *Brit. med. J.*, **2**, 423.

MEDICAL RESEARCH COUNCIL (1954). *The Use of Trilene by Midwives*. London: H.M.S.O.

MEDICAL RESEARCH COUNCIL (1970). Clinical trials of different concentrations of oxygen and nitrous oxide for obstetric analgesia. *Brit. med. J.*, **1**, 709.

MEEHAN, F. P. (1969). Painful labour: modern methods of management. *Proc. roy. Soc. Med.*, **62**, 185.

MEEHAN, F. P., MOOLGAOKER, A. S., and STALLWORTHY, J. (1972). Vaginal delivery under caudal analgesia after Caesarean section and other major uterine surgery. *Brit. med. J.*, **2**, 740.

MICHAEL, A. M. (1952). Hypnosis in childbirth. *Brit. med. J.*, **1**, 734.

MINNITT, R. J. (1934). Self-administered nitrous oxide and air. *Proc. roy. Soc. Med.*, **27**, 1313.

MOIR, D. D., and HESSON, W. R. (1965). Dural puncture by an epidural catheter. *Anaesthesia*, **20**, 373.

MOIR, D. D., and WILLOCKS, J. (1967). Management of inco-ordinate uterine action under continuous epidural analgesia. *Brit. med. J.*, **3**, 396.

MOIR, D. D., and WILLOCKS, J. (1968). Epidural analgesia in British obstetrics. *Brit. J. Anaesth.*, **40**, 129.

MOORE, D. C. (1961). *Regional Block*, 3rd edit., p. 349, Springfield, Ill.: Chas. C. Thomas.

MOORE, D. C., BRIDENBAUGH, L. D., BAGDI, P. A., and BRIDENBAUGH, P. O. (1968). Accumulation of mepivacain hydrochloride during caudal block. *Anesthesiology*, **29**, 585.

MOORE, J., CARSON, R. M., and HUNTER, R. J. (1970). A comparison of the effects of pentazocine and pethidine administered during labour. *J. Obstet. Gynaec. Brit. Cwlth.*, **77**, 830.

MOORE, J., McNABB, T. G., and GLYNN, J. P. (1973). The placental transfer of pentazocine and pethidine. *Brit. J. Anaesth.*, **45**, Suppl., 798.

NIMMO, W. S., WILSON, J., and PRESCOTT, L. F. (1975). Narcotics and analgesics and delayed gastric emptying during labour. *Lancet*, **1**, 890.

NOBLE, A. D., and DE VERE, R. D. (1970). Epidural analgesia in labour. *Brit. med. J.*, **2**, 296.

PAYNE, J. P. (1954). The effects of N-allylnormorphine on healthy subjects premedicated with morphine. *Brit. J. Anaesth.*, **43**, 837.

PEARSON, J. F., and DAVIES, P. (1974). The effect of continuous lumbar epidural analgesia upon fetal acid-base status during the first stage of labour. *J. Obstet. Gynaec. Brit. Cwlth.*, **81**, 971.

PHILLIPS, T. J. and MACDONALD, R. R. (1971). Comparative effects of pethidine, trichloroethylene and Entonox on fetal and neonatal acid-base and Po_2. *Brit. med. J.*, **3**, 558.

POPPERS, P. J. (1975). Evaluation of local anaesthetic agents for regional anaesthesia in obstetrics. *Brit. J. Anaesth.*, **47**, 322.

REYNOLDS, F. (1971). A comparison of the potential toxicity of bupivacaine, lignocaine and mepivacaine during epidural blockade for surgery. *Brit. J. Anaesth.*, **43**, 567.

REYNOLDS, F. (1972). The influence of adrenaline on maternal and neonatal blood levels of local analgesic drugs. *Proceedings of the Symposium on Epidural Analgesia in Obstetrics.* ed. Andrew Doughty. London: H. K. Lewis & Co.

REYNOLDS, F., HARGROVE, R. L., and WYMAN, J. B. (1973). Maternal and fetal plasma concentrations of bupivacaine after epidural block. *Brit. J. Anaesth.,* **45,** 1049.

REYNOLDS, F., and TAYLOR, G. (1970). Maternal and neonatal concentrations of bupivacaine: a comparison with lignocaine during continuous extradural analgesia. *Anaesthesia,* **25,** 14.

REYNOLDS, F., and TAYLOR, G. (1971). Plasma concentrations of bupivacaine during continuous epidural analgesia in labour: the effect of adrenaline. *Brit. J. Anaesth.,* **43,** 436.

ROBERTS, H., KANE, K. M., PERCIVAL, N., SNOW, P., and PLEASE, N. W. (1957). Effects of some analgesic drugs used in childbirth with special reference to variations in respiratory minute volume of the newborn. *Lancet,* **1,** 128.

ROMINE, J. C., CLARK, R. B., and BROWN, W. E. (1970). Lumbar epidural anaesthesia in labour and delivery: one year's experience. *J. Obstet. Gynaec. Brit. Cwlth.,* **77,** 722.

RORKE, M. J., DAVEY, D. A., and DU TOIT, J. H. (1968). Fetal oxygenation during Caesarean section. *Anaesthesia,* **23,** 585.

ROSEN, M., LATTO, P., and ASSCHER, A. W. (1972). Kidney function after methoxyflurane analgesia during labour. *Brit. med. J.,* **1,** 81.

ROSEN, M., MUSHIN, W. W., JONES, P. L., and JONES, E. V. (1969). Field trial of methoxyflurane, nitrous oxide and trichloroethylene as obstetric analgesics. *Brit. med. J.,* **3,** 263.

ROUGE, J. C., BANNER, M. P., and SMITH, T. C. (1969). Interactions of levallorphan and meperidine. *Clin. Pharmacol. Ther.,* **10,** 643.

SANCHEZ, R., ACUNA, L., and ROCHA, F. (1967). An analysis of the radiological visualisation of the catheters placed in the epidural space. *Brit. J. Anaesth.,* **39,** 485.

SCOTT, D. B. (1968). Inferior vena caval occlusion in late pregnancy and its importance in anaesthesia. *Brit. J. Anaesth.,* **40,** 120.

SHNIDER, S. M., ASLING, J. H., MARGOLIS, A. J., WAY, E. L., and WILKINSON, G. R. (1968). High fetal blood levels of mepivacaine and fetal bradycardia. *New Engl. J. Med.,* **279,** 947.

SIKER, E. S., WOLFSON, D., CICCARELLI, H. E., and TELAN, R. A. (1967). Effect of subanesthetic concentrations of halothane and methoxyflurane on pain threshold in conscious volunteers. *Anesthesiology,* **28,** 337.

SIKER, E. S., WOLFSON, D., DUBNANSKY, J., and FITTING, G. M. (1968). Placental transfer of methoxyflurane. *Brit. J. Anaesth.,* **40,** 588.

STERN, L., OUTERBRIDGE, E. W., and FAWCETT, J. S. (1969). Paracervical block in obstetrics. *Lancet,* **2,** 322.

TELFORD, J., and KEATS, A. S. (1961). Narcotic-narcotic antagonist mixtures. *Anesthesiology,* **22,** 465.

TERAMO, K. (1969) Fetal acid-base balance and heart rate during labour with bupivacaine paracervical block anaesthesia. *J. Obstet. Gynaec. Brit. Cwlth,* **76,** 881.

TORDA, T. A. G. (1963). The analgesic effect of methoxyflurane. *Anaesthesia,* **18,** 287.

TUNSTALL, M. E. (1961). Obstetric analgesia. The use of a fixed nitrous oxide and oxygen mixture from one cylinder. *Lancet,* **2,** 964.

URQUHART-HAY, D. (1969). Paraplegia following epidural analgesia. *Anaesthesia,* **24,** 461.

USUBIAGA, J. E., DOS REIS, A. JR., and USUBIAGA, L. E. (1970). Epidural misplacement of catheters and mechanism of unilateral blockade. *Anesthesiology,* **32,** 158.

VAUGHAN-WILLIAMS, C., JOHNSON, A., and LEDWARD, R. (1974). A comparison of CVP changes in the third stage of labour following oxytocic drugs and diazepam. *J. Obstet. Gynaec. Brit. Cwlth.,* **81,** 596.

WALLIS, K. L., SHNIDER, S. M., HICKS, J. S., and SPIVEY, H. T. (1976). Epidural anesthesia in the normotensive pregnant ewe. *Anesthesiology,* **44,** 481.

YATES, M. J. (1969). Painful labour: modern methods of management. *Proc. roy. Soc. Med.*, **62,** 183.

YATES, M. J., and KUAH, K. B. (1968). Bupivacaine caudal analgesia in labour. *J. Obstet. Gynaec. Brit. Cwlth.*, **75,** 749.

Chapter 43

ANAESTHESIA FOR OPERATIVE OBSTETRICS AND GYNAECOLOGY

INTRODUCTION

A woman in labour poses one of the most critical of all problems to the anaesthetist. The hazard to two lives has to be considered and either or both of these may already have been jeopardised by disease or abnormal labour. Some of the precautions usually taken before anaesthesia may be impracticable and the danger may be increased by the urgency of the obstetrical procedure, the unsatisfactory environment in which it takes place, the absence of proper equipment and the inadequacy of the assistance available to the anaesthetist. These facts are well-recognised yet avoidable maternal deaths due to the complications of anaesthesia continue to be reported. A maternal death, however infrequently it may occur, is a disaster, not only because of its tragic social consequences, but also because it is unexpected and frequently avoidable.

The most widely known feature of these deaths is their common association with aspiration pneumonitis following vomiting or regurgitation of stomach contents during anaesthesia. The frequency of this complication should be minimised by the appropriate skill of an experienced anaesthetist taking all the requisite precautions. If unhappily it should occur, the failure to treat pulmonary aspiration by intensive therapy may cost lives that might otherwise have been saved.

Anaesthesia and Maternal Mortality

The seven triennial Reports on Confidential Enquiries into Maternal Deaths in England and Wales give details of all the known causes of obstetric mortality over the 21 years from 1952 to 1972. Table 1 shows the remarkable fall not only in the number of deaths due to the complications of pregnancy or childbirth but also in those due to conditions and diseases associated with but unrelated to pregnancy. Unhappily, the progressive improvement in the safety of childbirth has not been matched by an improvement in the safety of obstetric anaesthesia. Following a period of diminishing anaesthetic mortality from 1952 to 1963 the number of deaths has risen sharply from 1964 onwards and the proportion of anaesthetic deaths within the total maternal mortality has more than doubled from 3·04 per cent in 1952/63 to 6·65 per cent in 1964/72.

During the years 1952 to 1954, when the overall maternal mortality was comparatively high, 49 deaths were attributed to the complications of anaesthesia. Of these, 32 were due to inhalation of stomach contents, and the remainder to various causes, including the effects of individual drugs such as chloroform, which accounted for 6 deaths (Ministry of Health, 1957). In the years 1955–57 there were 31 deaths due to anaesthesia, 18 of which were associated with vomited or regurgitated stomach contents (Ministry of Health, 1960). During 1958–60, 30 women died due to complications of anaesthesia, in 17 of whom vomiting or regurgitation accounted for death (Ministry of Health, 1963). Three others died after receiving chloroform, and two after halothane. Some of the remainder died following the use of muscle relaxants, but the actual cause of death was not clearly specified.

In the Report for 1961–63 (Ministry of Health, 1966) 28 deaths were considered to be due to complications of anaesthesia of which 16 were associated with inhalation of stomach contents. The Report specifically stated "failure to intubate the trachea seemed to be the commonest fault, though this procedure

43/TABLE 1

DEATHS ASSOCIATED WITH COMPLICATIONS OF ANAESTHESIA COMPARED WITH ALL
DEATHS IN THE ENQUIRY SERIES AND WITH TOTAL MATERNITIES

	Total maternities	Deaths		Deaths associated with complications of anaesthesia in the enquiry series	Rate per 1,000 maternal deaths in the enquiry series	Rate per million maternities
		Due to pregnancy or child-birth	Associated with pregnancy or childbirth			
1952–54	2,052,953	1,094	316	49	34·8	23·9
1955–57	2,113,471	861	339	31	25·8	14·7
1958–60	2,294,414	742	254	30	30·1	13·1
1961–63	2,520,420	692	244	28	29·9	11·1
1964–66	2,600,367	579	176	50	66·2	19·2
1967–69	2,457,444	455	243	50	70·2	20·3
1970–72	2,298,198	355	251	37	61·1	16·1

(Figures taken from successive Reports on Confidential Enquiries into Maternal Deaths in England and Wales)

alone is not an absolute safeguard. Sellick's manoeuvre (cricoid pressure) might have prevented regurgitation which occurred before intubation could be performed. Amongst 16 women whose death was either certainly or probably due to inhalation of stomach contents, in only 5 was it recorded that tracheal intubation was a planned procedure during the induction of anaesthesia". Concerning the acid aspiration (Mendelson's) syndrome the Report states: "this was often not treated energetically enough. In particular, the injection of hydrocortisone was often delayed until symptoms had appeared, by which time it appeared to be ineffective".

The Report for 1964–66 (Ministry of Health, 1969) showed a disturbing rise in the number of deaths associated with the complications of anaesthesia. 50 deaths were reported of which 26 were considered to be due to the inhalation of stomach contents. In contrast with the period 1961–63 there was no reported failure to intubate the trachea as a planned procedure although the technical difficulties of intubation were considered to have contributed to some maternal deaths. The Report states that the practice of inflating the lungs after paralysing the vocal cords is likely to encourage the entry of regurgitated material into the lung; and it concludes: "Patients with obstetric emergencies are gravely at risk and require the knowledge and the skill of an experienced anaesthetist who must be readily available".

The Report for 1967–69 (Department of Health and Social Security, 1972) gives details of 50 deaths said to be associated with the complications of anaesthesia of which two-thirds were considered to have been avoidable, that is, due to an error on the part of the anaesthetist; 26 (52 per cent) followed the pulmonary aspiration of stomach contents and as many as 36 (72 per cent) occurred during or after anaesthesia for Caesarean section. Viewed in another way, complications of anaesthesia accounted for 36 out of 124 (29 per cent) of all deaths associated with Caesarean section. This fact suggests that a substantial improvement in maternal mortality could be attained solely by focusing attention on improvements in the methods and facilities of anaesthetising patients for this operation.

The Report for 1970–72 (Department of Health and Social Security, 1975) shows a trend towards lowering the frequency with which the complications of anaesthesia were implicated in maternal deaths. There were 37 deaths in all, 16 (43 per cent) followed acid pulmonary aspiration and 19 (51 per cent) deaths were associated with anaesthesia for Caesarean section and these comprised only 17 per cent of the 111 deaths reported during and after the operation. The Report also lists cardiac arrest due to hypoxia often due to difficulties of intubation and failure or misuse of apparatus; it also cites the special dangers in coloured women in whom cyanosis may easily be overlooked. Attention is drawn to the fact that 22 out of the 37 deaths were avoidable and involved junior anaesthetic staff. The Report concludes: "Women suffering from obstetric emergencies are often gravely at risk and deserve the knowledge and skill of an experienced anaesthetist. Round the clock cover for anaesthesia should be readily available in all obstetric units and a senior anaesthetist should be available at all times for difficult cases."

Thus each successive triennial Report repeatedly stresses the need for competent obstetric anaesthesia, but in practice, it must be admitted that this important dictum does not appear to be sufficiently appreciated. Most fatalities can be attributed to a failure on the part of the anaesthetist rather than to any intrinsic danger in the drugs used. Evidence from the Reports show that while some avoidable deaths happen with specialist anaesthetists, the majority occur when an inexperienced anaesthetist is giving the anaesthetic. As the Report for 1964–66 states "The consultant anaesthetist must assume responsibility for errors made by junior members of his team unless they disobey his instructions, and for seeing that obstetric emergencies are not left to unsupervised members of his team." In addition to the expected lack of knowledge, dexterity and expertise of the inexperienced anaesthetist, he does not possess the authority or the determination to resist the pressure of obstetrical urgency to take time to ensure that all the anaesthetic apparatus is in working order ready for use, and that personal assistance is at hand at least for the period of induction of anaesthesia. A clearer and more sympathetic understanding of the anaesthetist's problems by all who work in the labour ward would be a major contribution to the safety of obstetrical anaesthesia.

It is worth noting that while figures are available concerning maternal mortality due to the complications of anaesthesia, little is known about the incidence of maternal morbidity or of neonatal mortality and morbidity following their occurrence. Thus pulmonary aspiration of stomach contents, while not always fatal to the mother, may result in permanent respiratory disability. The hypoxia caused by the acute episode may result in the birth of a dead or a severely handicapped infant. As our knowledge of such hazards increases, so possibly will the justification for an entirely specialised approach to obstetric anaesthesia.

EMERGENCY OBSTETRICS

ANAESTHESIA FOR OPERATIVE VAGINAL DELIVERY

Unless there are strong indications to the contrary, local analgesia should be used for operative vaginal delivery. Nevertheless, a patient may aspirate stomach contents when vomiting in the supine position even though fully conscious (Moya, 1960), and a heavily sedated patient in the same position must be at considerably greater risk. Local analgesia must be used when an experienced anaesthetist is not at hand or when an unsuitable environment or the inadequacy of the available equipment may prejudice the safety of general anaesthesia. On the other hand, local analgesia may be contra-indicated either because of the need for intra-uterine manipulation or because of the failure of the mother's co-operation. Occasions will always arise when a general anaesthetic is required and the safest policy is to ensure that those who anaesthetise obstetric patients are fully competent to do so. Even so, the choice of technique will be influenced by the availability of equipment because some essentials, such as a suction apparatus, which should always be found in the comparatively ideal circumstances of a hospital labour ward, would rarely be provided in domiciliary practice. There is a strong case for the mandatory admission to hospital of all domiciliary obstetric patients requiring a general anaesthetic. Where this is not possible reasonable safety depends on arrangements being made to transport all the necessary equipment to the patient's home in specially designed portable containers (Argent and Evens, 1961).

Local Anaesthesia for Operative Obstetrics

Simple infiltration or pudendal nerve block is employed for many obstetric procedures. Infiltration is suitable for episiotomy and the subsequent perineal repair. Pudendal nerve block enables the majority of forceps deliveries to be successfully performed, but where rotation of the head or difficulty in extraction is anticipated general or epidural anaesthesia will be required. The techniques of local analgesia are usually carried out by the obstetrician and the skill should be acquired by all doctors likely to practice obstetrics.

Transperineal pudendal nerve block.—The pudendal nerve can be blocked behind the ischial spine before it enters its canal in the wall of the ischio-rectal fossa. A skin weal is raised over the right ischial tuberosity, and through this a

10-cm (4-inch) needle is inserted. The fingers of the right hand are placed in the vagina and the needle guided through the ischio-rectal fossa until its point lies above and behind the ischial spine where 10 ml of 0·5 per cent lignocaine are injected. The injections must be repeated on the left side.

Transvaginal pudendal nerve block.—This technique is performed with a guarded needle similar to that used for paracervical block (see p. 1343) the tip of which is inserted just above and behind the ischial spine. The needle point is passed first through the vaginal mucous membrane and then through the sacrospinous ligament to the region of the pudendal nerve.

Pudendal nerve block by either route must be supplemented by perineal infiltration to block the endings of the perineal branch of the posterior cutaneous nerve of the thigh. In addition, infiltration of the labia majora will be required to block the labial branches of the ilio-inguinal and genito-femoral nerves.

Infiltration anaesthesia.—As an alternative to nerve block, the branches of the pudendal nerve may be more simply infiltrated as they pass near the ischial tuberosity (Fig. 1). A skin weal should be raised over the tuberosity and the

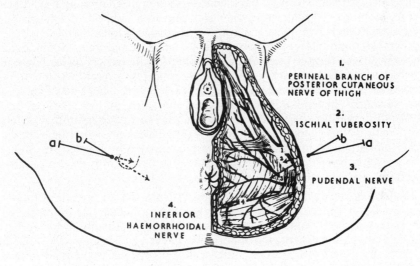

43/Fig. 1.—Diagram to illustrate nerve block of perineum and vulva.

needle advanced on to its inferior aspect, where about 5 ml of 0·5 per cent lignocaine solution should be injected to block the perineal branch of the posterior cutaneous nerve of the thigh. The needle is then passed medial to the tuberosity and, keeping close to the bone, into the ischio-rectal fossa for a distance of 2·5 cm (1 inch), where a further 10 ml of solution is placed so that it may diffuse around the inferior haemorrhoidal nerve and the termination of the pudendal nerve. The process is then repeated on the opposite side. Simple infiltration analgesia is suitable only for low "lift-out" forceps deliveries for which strong traction and intra-vaginal manipulations are not required.

The dangers of local analgesia are the inadvertent intravascular injection or overdosage of the local anaesthetic drug. The maximum advisable dose of lignocaine by infiltration is 200 mg, i.e. 40 ml of 0·5 per cent solution. There may be a strong temptation to use a 1 per cent solution to ensure a more rapid onset and greater certainty of effect. In these circumstances the admixture of adrenaline, 1 in 200,000, would raise the maximum advisable dose to 500 mg or 50 ml of 1 per cent lignocaine.

These techniques of local analgesia do not provide total block of all the sensation associated with forceps delivery and they do not relieve the pain of labour. To avoid undue traction on the ligaments supporting the uterus, particular care must be taken to ensure that the pull of the forceps is synchronised with the mother's own voluntary efforts during the uterine contraction. The whole procedure may be combined with inhalational analgesia, but as an alternative, a *slow* intravenous injection of a mixture 10 mg diazepam (Valium) with 30 mg pentazocine (Fortral) may be given until the mother becomes drowsy; the full dose may be sufficient to induce brief unconsciousness in some mothers and even a moderate dose may lead to depression of the glottic reflex with consequent danger of pulmonary aspiration should vomiting occur.

The fact that some form of supplementary general sedation and analgesia appears to be needed with pudendal block and local infiltration anaesthesia suggests that neither of these methods is adequate on their own to achieve comfortable conditions for forceps delivery. Scudamore and Yates (1966) found that only 36 per cent of pudendal nerve blocks achieved complete bilateral analgesia of the perineum and vulva and that of the two approaches, the transperineal route was far less reliable than the transvaginal. They concluded that many so-called "pudendal" blocks must depend solely on local perineal and vulval infiltration for their effect. For operations involving more than a low forceps delivery they favour other forms of regional block or general anaesthesia. If this limitation of pudendal block were more widely appreciated, many mothers would be spared unnecessary discomfort when relatively complicated procedures are attempted under inadequate anaesthesia.

Epidural or subarachnoid block.—Epidural block should provide complete anaesthesia for forceps delivery without the need to sedate the mother. The technique is relatively time-consuming and, in practice, the obstetric urgency rarely allows the anaesthetist the opportunity to carry out the injection with all the necessary aseptic precautions. Further delay is caused by the need to give the local anaesthetic time to act. The advantages of subarachnoid over epidural block are the speed of action and the greater ease and certainty with which it can be performed by the inexperienced anaesthetist. Using 1 ml of 0·25 per cent heavy cinchocaine in the sitting position, complete anaesthesia may be obtained in a little over five minutes from the time of injection (Crawford, 1972). The main disadvantage of a subarachnoid block is the incidence of headache which occasionally follows its use.

One of the attractive features of relieving labour pain by continuous epidural block is that the means of inducing anaesthesia for operative delivery is already present. The injection of a dose of local anaesthetic through a safely sited epidural cannula does not necessarily demand the presence of an anaesthetist. A wider use of the method simply for pain relief would diminish the frequency of the need for general anaesthesia.

GENERAL ANAESTHESIA FOR OPERATIVE OBSTETRICS

The problem might be summarised by saying that the anaesthetic technique, though comparatively simple in itself, is inevitably complicated by the need to guard against the aspiration of acid gastric contents into the lungs. The discussion of general anaesthesia for operative obstetrics centres round the numerous precautions which may be taken to reduce this risk.

Reduction of the quantity of gastric contents.—The decrease in gastric tone occurring in labour, particularly after the use of narcotic analgesics, results in delay in emptying of the stomach. Despite this fact it is not good practice to ignore the mother's need for nutrition and hydration. Those who are considered as unlikely to require a general anaesthetic may be given light and easily digested food when labour is imminent; when labour has started small quantities of sweetened fluids should be allowed. Those for whom there is a strong probability of delivery under a general anaesthetic should take nothing by mouth except small measured quantities of water and hydration should be maintained by an intravenous infusion of dextrose. These "high-risk" patients are those in labour with suspected cephalo-pelvic disproportion, breech or multiple pregnancy, pre-eclampsia, cervical dystocia or those whose infants are considered to be at risk.

Taylor and Pryse-Davies (1966) measured the quantity and pH of the gastric contents of 99 women who had been in active labour for at least 2 hours and who required general anaesthesia for obstetric surgery. In more than half of the patients the volume of gastric juice aspirated was in excess of 40 ml. The pH of the gastric contents even without artificial alkalinisation ranged from 1·25 to 8·20; neither the volume nor the pH of the gastric contents bore any relation to the length of labour. It follows that every woman needing an anaesthetic in labour must be assumed to have a full stomach of highly acid fluid contents.

To reduce the volume of gastric contents an attempt can be made to empty the stomach by the passage of a wide-bore oesophageal tube. Alternatively vomiting may be induced by the intravenous injection of 3 mg of apomorphine (Holmes, 1957). This dose should be diluted in 10 ml sterile water and injected slowly until just sufficient has been given to cause emesis. It is rarely necessary to use the full dose and once vomiting starts atropine 1 mg should be given intravenously. This not only antagonises the effect of apomorphine but conveniently premedicates the patient for the subsequent general anaesthesia.

Both these methods of attempting to empty the stomach have their advocates and one can respect the view of those who would use one or other on every patient needing general anaesthesia in labour as it is impossible to determine which patient is liable to regurgitate or vomit during the induction. The protest that forcible emptying of the stomach by tube or by apomorphine-induced vomiting is distasteful and distressing to an already distressed mother may quite reasonably be countered by a reminder that these are precautions taken to protect the mother from avoidable death.

Although individual circumstances and experience may occasionally suggest otherwise, it is not our practice to empty the stomach of an obstetric patient before anaesthesia, but rather to regard her as an exception to the general rule regarding emergency operations and rely upon the technique of anaesthesia and the skill of the anaesthetist to avoid the hazards of pulmonary aspiration.

Alkalinisation of the gastric contents.—Taylor and Pryse-Davies (1966) repeated in rats the experiments originally carried out by Mendelson on rabbits (1946). They showed that lesions in the lungs comparable with those seen in Mendelson's syndrome could be produced by the instillation of hydrochloric acid or gastric juice into the trachea. The most severe damage was seen where the pH of the material instilled was below 1·75. Hydrochloric acid or gastric juice with a pH higher than this tended to produce only slight histological changes or in many cases no changes at all. Similar experiments were carried out on rats with hydrochloric acid and gastric juice neutralised with antacids. Magnesium trisilicate appeared to prevent severe pulmonary lesions while colloidal aluminium hydroxide did not give the same degree of protection. The reason for the difference was that the latter formed a gel which caused some bronchial obstruction. In their investigations on emergency obstetric patients they found that in 42 per cent the pH of the gastric juice was less than 2·5 but that when given 14 ml of magnesium trisilicate mixture (B.P.C.) the pH remained above this level for about 2 hours. It was therefore recommended that all patients requiring obstetric surgery under general anaesthesia should be given an oral antacid before operation to reduce the incidence of acid pulmonary aspiration. A dose of 14 ml magnesium trisilicate mixture (B.P.C.) was shown to be suitable for this purpose and its administration was recommended as soon as the decision was made to give the anaesthetic.

More recently Crawford (1970, 1972) has recommended a more rigorous antacid discipline. Every woman should be given 15 ml magnesium trisilicate (B.P.C.) at *two-hourly intervals* in order to maintain the pH of the gastric contents above 2·5 throughout labour. It is considered a dangerous and potentially lethal practice to withold this prophylactic measure until the time that the patient requires to be anaesthetised. Those admitted as emergencies who have not received prophylactic antacid therapy should be given a double dose (30 ml) of magnesium trisilicate as soon as the decision to operate has been made. Alternatively, a dose of 15 ml 0·3 molar sodium citrate has been recommended in these circumstances (Lahiri et al., 1973).

Peskett (1973), like Taylor and Pryse-Davies, reported that 43·5 per cent of untreated patients presenting for Caesarean section had gastric contents with a pH of 2·5 or less. Unlike Taylor and Pryse-Davies they found that although, after one dose of magnesium trisilicate, many women had highly alkaline gastric juices, as many as 8·5 per cent had stomach contents with a pH below the danger level of 2·5 and were therefore still at risk of developing Mendelson's syndrome if pulmonary aspiration occurred. It was recommended that pre-operative emptying of the stomach should be combined with antacid therapy but this does not guarantee safety because of the continuous secretion of gastric juice. Thus the wisdom of continuous antacid therapy in labour is confirmed.

It should not be assumed that mere alkalinisation of the gastric contents renders their aspiration innocuous. The material may be solid and cause death by suffocation or to a lesser degree collapse of the lung, mediastinal shift and consolidation. Women delivered at the end of prolonged labour may have accumulated in the stomach large quantities of material with a high pH similar to that found in patients with bowel obstruction. Aspiration into the lungs may cause respiratory distress associated with severe endotoxaemic shock which may prove very difficult to treat successfully (Bosomworth and Hamelberg, 1962).

Anaesthetic technique and safety.—Faced with the problem of anaesthesia in a patient with a full stomach most anaesthetists instinctively turn to a technique which centres on the passage of a cuffed endotracheal tube to protect the lungs from the aspiration of gastric contents. It is therefore surprising that in the context of anaesthesia for emergency obstetrics the acceptance of an endotracheal technique is not universal especially in view of the criticisms made in the Reports on Confidential Enquiries into Maternal Deaths. However, Crawford (1965) states "We must soon seriously begin to question the applicability to newly developing countries of the methods of obstetric anaesthesia which we teach for 'home consumption' ". To some extent this counsel may apply more universally as long as experienced anaesthetists are not always available for emergency obstetrics. There may be circumstances where the occasional anaesthetist may be less dangerous using a simple technique rather than attempting to use methods which are safe only in the hands of the expert. The writer, while himself holding little brief for the avoidance of tracheal intubation, feels obliged to recognise that many responsible authors take an opposite view.

The safety of an intubation technique depends on three factors:

1. The prevention of regurgitation or vomiting of gastric contents.
2. The prevention of pulmonary aspiration.
3. The intubation of the trachea as soon as possible following loss of consciousness.

Unfortunately some of the precautions recommended are irreconcilable. While the theoretical and practical aspects of dealing with patients with a full stomach are dealt with in Chapter 37 their special application to women in labour is discussed in this chapter. Some repetition is therefore inevitable.

1a. *Prevention of regurgitation.*—The force of gravity can be enlisted as an aid in the prevention of the passive regurgitation of gastric contents. Following O'Mullane's (1954) observation that even when the stomach is distended with fluid the intragastric pressure does not rise above 18 cm (1·8 kPa) of water, Snow and Nunn (1959) calculated that a 40° tilt from the horizontal would raise the larynx a vertical distance of 19 cm above the cardio-oesophageal junction. This precaution presupposes that the patient is on a bed or operating table capable of being tilted to 40°. If regurgitation should occur the patient's safety depends on the table being tilted rapidly into the head-down position to enable the stomach contents to drain by gravity away from the larynx. Such tables have been designed by Wylie (1956) and Steel (1961), but in the absence of such facilities there may be a tendency to pay only lip service to the need for a foot-down tilt and any tilt less than 40° would encourage regurgitated stomach contents to enter the trachea far more readily than if the patient were horizontal.

Another factor which may raise the intragastric pressure is the lithotomy position where the flexed thighs press against the gravid uterus (Spence *et al.*, 1967). The anaesthetist may find the patient in this position after the obstetrician has failed to extract the baby under a local anaesthetic. Considerable persuasion may be required to get the mother taken down from the lithotomy position before the anaesthetic is started, but if not, and if regurgitation should occur, the delay involved in turning her on to her side may prove fatal.

An important factor in the prevention of passive regurgitation of gastric contents into the pharynx is the use of backward pressure on the cricoid cartilage to compress the upper oesophagus against the cervical spine; this manoeuvre is claimed to withstand reflux pressures of up to 100 cm H_2O (9·8 kPa) (Sellick, 1961). This implies the services of an assistant to apply the pressure while the anaesthetist is intubating the trachea. Unfortunately, in practice, there are occasions when this help is not readily forthcoming. The same assistant can contribute to the safety of the induction of anaesthesia not only by applying cricoid pressure with one hand but also by holding a working suction nozzle ready for use with the other.

Backward pressure on the cricoid cartilage has an incidental value in bringing the larynx into a better position for intubation, particularly in the patient with the more difficult oropharyngeal anatomy. However, if the manoeuvre is not correctly applied and the pressure is lateral rather than backward, intubation is made more difficult and the anaesthetist must guide the assistant's finger on the larynx into the position where it comes into view. Sellick has warned that should active vomiting occur during the manoeuvre the intra-oesophageal pressure may rise dangerously and tend to cause rupture of the oesophagus.

Suxamethonium given to facilitate intubation is a factor which also facilitates passive regurgitation. It is believed that the cardiac sphincter becomes incompetent towards the end of pregnancy, and in the recumbent position, the gastric contents are prevented from access to the pharynx solely by the tone of the cricopharyngeus muscle. Once this muscle relaxes there is no further obstruction to its flow into the pharynx. This fact underlines the importance of trained assistance to apply cricoid pressure, readily available suction and intubation without delay following the induction of anaesthesia when a relaxant technique is used.

It has been shown that the muscular fasciculations caused by suxamethonium during the initial period of its action could temporarily raise the intragastric pressure (Spence et al., 1967). Whether this would be a significant factor with the abdominal muscles well stretched by the gravid uterus is a matter for surmise.

1b. *Prevention of vomiting.*—Active vomiting of the stomach contents as distinct from their passive regurgitation is more frequently a hazard of the induction or recovery stage of inhalational anaesthesia without intubation. The anaesthetic agents, ether, trichloroethylene or cyclopropane, may be responsible as may the premature insertion of the oropharyngeal airway before the vomiting reflex has been suppressed. The anaesthetist's dilemma at this point in overcoming pharyngeal obstruction, is that the insertion of an oral airway may cause vomiting, coughing or laryngeal spasm during an inhalational induction, and yet the mother's nasal mucosa may be so congested as to block the airway through the nose. A shortened, well-lubricated nasopharyngeal tube of relatively small bore, say 5–6 mm, should be inserted as a temporary means of overcoming respiratory obstruction until the patient will tolerate an oral airway.

It must not be assumed that active vomiting on induction occurs solely with an inhalational non-relaxant technique. The hasty insertion of the laryngoscope into the pharynx before the relaxant has had time to become effective may also be responsible.

2. *Prevention of aspiration of gastric contents into the lungs.*—While a head-up tilt to 40° may help to prevent regurgitation, this same posture will facilitate the access of gastric contents to the trachea if they should rise to the pharynx. By the same token the head-down position would tend to encourage the drainage of the regurgitated or vomited stomach contents from the pharynx away from the glottis and safety would be improved if the patient were also on her side. Trained help for the anaesthetist and a working suction apparatus is of the greatest importance at this stage.

Another cause of aspiration of stomach contents is the practice of oxygenating the patient by positive pressure through a face-mask following induction of anaesthesia and neuromuscular block. Any regurgitated stomach contents would then be pushed into the trachea through the relaxed vocal cords. When a relaxant technique is used the patient should be given pure oxygen to breathe for three minutes before induction of anaesthesia. Her apprehension at having a mask held over her face may be dispelled by telling her that she is breathing oxygen for the benefit of her baby.

Deaths have occurred due to aspiration of stomach contents during recovery from the anaesthetic. To prevent this the passage of a wide-bore stomach tube during anaesthesia is recommended. The patient should recover from the anaesthetic on her side on a tilting bed and under the personal supervision of the anaesthetist or an experienced nurse armed with a suction apparatus. The endotracheal tube with inflated cuff should not be removed until return of consciousness. The shortening of the necessary period of close supervision of the patient is one of the advantages of a relaxant, intubation, nitrous oxide/oxygen method as distinct from a purely inhalational technique with more potent agents.

3. *Elimination of delay in intubation.*—The most dangerous period of an obstetric anaesthetic is that between loss of consciousness and intubation of the trachea. Indeed some authors continue to recommend an inhalational technique with a mask applied to the face and suggest that it is safe provided the patient is anaesthetised in the lateral position with the head down, that the obstetrician can be persuaded to apply the forceps in this position, that the mask is not strapped on to the face and that the anaesthetic is continued until the operation is completed. It may be true that this could be the safest course where the anaesthetist is unskilled but, in view of the criticisms implied in the Report on Confidential Enquiries into Maternal Deaths, it might be legally difficult for a specialist anaesthetist to defend this choice of technique in court.

Where an intubation technique is used it is essential to take all possible steps to minimise the interval between loss of consciousness and intubation. At this point the anaesthetist may consider whether the mother has anatomical abnormalities that may cause a dangerous delay of intubation as repeated unsuccessful attempts to pass the tube may result in greater hazard than a straightforward inhalational induction by mask alone. A short mandible, prominent teeth, high arched palate, a short, thick neck and the inability to extend the neck and open the mouth widely are warning signs of likely difficulty. Yet these are also signs which warn the anaesthetist of difficulty with the airway if a tube were not passed. Thus the patient with the well-recognised difficult anatomical features would give trouble with either method of anaesthesia, but once a tube is passed into the trachea and the cuff inflated, most of the difficulties are solved. The temptation to opt for intubation is therefore overwhelming but, when faced with obvious anatomical difficulty, the use of regional analgesia should be seriously considered in preference to giving a general anaesthetic without the safeguard of tracheal intubation.

To minimise the hazardous induction-intubation interval the patient should be given pure oxygen to breathe for three minutes before induction, a diaphragm needle fixed into a vein and atropine 0·6 mg followed by 100 mg methohexitone injected. Methohexitone is preferred to thiopentone because of its shorter recovery time. As soon as consciousness is lost suxamethonium 100 mg is given. The relatively large dose is required to ensure total relaxation and hence near perfect conditions for an easy intubation. One must be certain that the potency of the suxamethonium has not diminished as a result of being kept unrefrigerated.

If the patient is to be intubated with the minimum of delay she should be placed in a position most advantageous and familiar to the anaesthetist. A steep head-up position to prevent regurgitation, a head-down or lateral position to reduce the chance of aspiration of stomach contents, all tend to make a rapid intubation more difficult. The relaxation of the cricopharyngeus muscle with the patient in the head-down position may result in a flood of gastric contents which will occupy the anaesthetist's whole attention before intubation is possible. As speed of intubation is essential the patient should be in the horizontal position with the neck flexed and the head extended. Cricoid pressure should be applied and the laryngoscope inserted with the onset of muscular relaxation.

Selection of the correct size of tube is important for ensuring a rapid intubation. Owing probably to the retention of fluid in the tissues in late pregnancy, the size of the glottis appears to be reduced. While a 9-mm cuffed tube would be expected to pass through the vocal cords in the non-pregnant woman, attempts to pass a tube of this size in the parturient woman may only lead to dangerous delay. Accordingly an 8-mm tube should be selected initially and tubes of 7·5 mm and 7 mm size should be ready for use if the larger one will not pass.

The failure of the laryngoscope light at the moment of intubation may be a further cause of delay. It follows that the instrument should be tested before use, and a second tested laryngoscope should be immediately at hand. A further safety factor is the rapid inflation of the tube cuff as soon as possible after intubation so the tube should be passed with the inflating syringe attached.

If any anatomical abnormality is likely to prevent the rapid passage of the tube, a malleable stylet may be useful and should be ready for use.

In an attempt to reduce the induction-intubation time it has been suggested that the intravenous barbiturate and the suxamethonium should be mixed and injected together rather than in succession (Davies, 1963). Although there is no clinical evidence of loss of potency of the relaxant if the mixture is freshly prepared, this practice was not recommended because a small proportion of patients retained an unpleasant recollection of the muscle fasciculations caused by suxamethonium. Khawaja (1971*a*) reported the almost complete elimination of the memory of muscle fasciculations by a careful correlation of the dose of thiopentone in relation to body weight (4 mg/kg). Furthermore, the fasciculations could be abolished by a dose of 3 mg tubocurarine given 2 minutes before induction of anaesthesia (Khawaja, 1971*b*), but in the interests of safety this technique cannot be recommended for obstetric anaesthesia as even this small dose may adversely affect the depolarising action of suxamethonium.

Failed Intubation Drill

Despite the measures already discussed, it must be anticipated that occasionally the anaesthetist may embark upon a general anaesthetic and fail in repeated attempts at intubation. The patient is put at serious risk either on account of apnoeic hypoxia or because of her unprotected respiratory tract. Once the decision has been made to abandon further attempts at intubation a pre-arranged plan similar to that advocated by Tunstall (1976) should be put into action immediately.

Cricoid pressure should be maintained and the waiting obstetric team summoned to assist the anaesthetist. The patient must be turned on to her side and her head lowered. An oral airway is inserted, the pharynx aspirated if necessary and oxygenation established by gentle positive pressure through a face-mask. If obstruction to the airway persists the cricoid pressure should be cautiously released.

If the airway is not obstructed the patient should be ventilated with nitrous oxide, oxygen and a volatile agent to establish surgical anaesthesia by spontaneous ventilation when the effect of the suxamethonium has worn off. A wide-bore stomach tube should then be passed, the gastric contents aspirated and 30 ml magnesium trisilicate (B.P.C.) or 30 ml 0.3 molar sodium citrate instilled. The stomach tube is withdrawn and the pharynx aspirated. The table may now be levelled and the operation allowed to proceed under inhalational anaesthesia via the face-mask with the patient on her side.

If difficulty in maintaining a clear airway persists the effect of the suxamethonium should be allowed to wear off, the stomach is emptied through a wide-bore stomach tube, magnesium trisilicate or molar sodium citrate instilled and the patient allowed to awaken. Local or regional analgesia should then be carried out as a safer alternative to general anaesthesia.

Equipment

The obstetric anaesthetist is expected to be both safe and speedy but, under no circumstances, should he allow himself to be pressed into a hurried induction of anaesthesia without first taking time to check that the equipment is ready for use and that all the safety precautions have been observed. An assistant must be appointed to help the anaesthetist at least for the critical first few minutes of the anaesthetic. A purpose-designed anaesthetic trolley should be provided on which all the necessary drugs and equipment are displayed ready for use and a discipline should be established so that every anaesthetist using the equipment leaves it in a state of readiness for a subsequent anaesthetic.

Recommended Standard Technique for General Anaesthesia

It cannot be too strongly emphasised that safety in obstetric anaesthesia for vaginal delivery lies in the wider use of local analgesic techniques so that the dangers of general anaesthesia can be avoided. In most departments the need for general anaesthesia for forceps deliveries has been virtually eliminated, particularly where regional analgesia is practised for the relief of labour pain.

The diversity of sometimes irreconcilable opinions concerning general anaesthesia for forceps delivery is sufficient evidence that no single technique on its own can guarantee safety to the mother and baby. Nothing can substitute for the skill, judgement, experience and dexterity of the individual anaesthetist. Subject to these reservations and to sum up all the foregoing discussions, the following standard technique is recommended.

The patient, who has received magnesium trisilicate mixture two-hourly during labour, lies horizontally on a bed capable of being tilted head-down. Following a further dose of 15 ml magnesium trisilicate mixture the patient is given pure oxygen to breathe for three minutes. An assistant is at hand to apply cricoid pressure and to hold a working sucker nozzle ready for use. A diaphragm needle is inserted into a convenient vein. Intravenous atropine 0·6 mg is given followed by methohexitone 100 mg and refrigerated suxamethonium 100 mg. The assistant applies cricoid pressure as consciousness is lost. The patient is intubated with an 8-mm cuffed endotracheal tube and the cuff is inflated. Anaesthesia is maintained with nitrous oxide, oxygen and a trace of halothane. The patient is turned to her side at the end of the operation before anaesthesia is allowed to lighten. She recovers under close supervision and the cuffed tube is not removed until she regains consciousness.

Treatment of Pulmonary Aspiration (Mendelson's) Syndrome (McCormick, 1975)

Acid pulmonary aspiration should be suspected following any obstetric general anaesthetic if the patient shows symptoms similar to those of an acute asthmatic attack with cyanosis, tachycardia, tachypnoea and hypotension with wheezes, rales and rhonchi heard over the affected areas of the lungs. Should the symptoms have arisen following vomiting or regurgitation of stomach contents during anaesthesia the diagnosis is seldom in doubt, but severe symptoms requiring intensive therapy have been reported following an apparently uneventful anaesthetic (McCormick et al., 1966). The onset of symptoms may be immediate or may be delayed until some hours later when a sense of false security may have been induced.

The diagnosis may be confirmed radiographically; there is widespread infiltration of the lungs, more on the right than on the left, and more in the lower than in the upper lobes. Blood gas analysis reveals severe hypoxaemia despite a high inspired oxygen tension and, in severe cases, a low pH due to a combination of respiratory and metabolic acidosis.

Management of aspiration of stomach contents.—If pulmonary aspiration is suspected the patient should be placed head down on her right side to provide postural drainage. Following intubation with a sterile cuffed tube and rapid suction of the trachea and bronchi, the lungs should be ventilated with pure oxygen. Hydrocortisone 200 mg should be given intravenously followed by

100 mg 6-hourly intramuscularly for 48–72 hours and then tailed off to avoid the hazards of secondary infection.

If symptoms and signs are minimal, no further treatment is required beyond careful surveillance against the later development of severe respiratory distress. With the onset of more serious symptoms such as bronchospasm, semi-coma, persistent hypotension and peripheral cyanosis despite the inhalation of pure oxygen, the patient must be moved immediately to an intensive care unit, paralysed with pancuronium and mechanically ventilated with oxygen. Very high inflation pressures may be required owing to a greatly reduced lung compliance (Adams *et al.*, 1969). The patient's acid-base state must be assessed and any base deficit corrected with intravenous sodium bicarbonate. Bronchospasm is relieved by intravenous hydrocortisone and aminophylline. If pulmonary oedema develops it must be treated by aspiration and diuretics, but if hypovolaemia occurs as may be revealed by hypotension, low central venous pressure and a rising haematocrit, the loss of plasma volume should be replaced by plasma substitutes in preference to crystalloid solutions.

It is usually considered desirable to withhold prophylactic antibiotic therapy until bacteriological diagnosis and sensitivities are confirmed. Certainly ampicillin and the cephalosporins are unlikely to prevent the growth of the aerobes and anaerobes found in the mouth and upper respiratory tract which are so highly destructive when aspirated into the lungs. On the other hand, infection by these organisms can be controlled by a combination of gentamycin and penicillin G which must be given prophylactically in all cases of *severe* aspiration pneumonitis (Seeley and Smith, 1976). Clindamycin may be required later if bacteroides or resistant staphylococci predominate in the sputum cultures.

Bronchial suction.—There may be a temptation to aspirate gastric contents from the lungs by bronchoscopy. In unskilled hands this procedure is extremely hazardous in a hypoxic patient and in any case the amount of material which can be aspirated is small as any liquid matter will already have been absorbed from the bronchial lumen. Bronchoscopic aspiration is only indicated where the bronchi are obstructed by solid matter, that is when the hazards of the procedure are outweighed by the danger of its omission. Otherwise, endotracheal intubation and suction by catheter is safer because it can be performed more quickly and allows simultaneous oxygenation of the patient.

Pulmonary lavage.—Lavage of the lungs with large volumes of bicarbonate or saline to neutralise or dilute the acid was at one time recommended as a valuable therapeutic measure. However Hamelberg and Bosomworth (1964) believe that the spread of the acid is so rapid that it would not be neutralised by the subsequent lavage with an alkaline solution. Bannister *et al.* (1961) have shown that lavage, by increasing its volume, may further the spread of acid to areas of the lung hitherto unaffected causing even more tissue necrosis and breakdown of the capillary endothelium. Lavage with large volumes of fluid is therefore strongly contra-indicated.

ANAESTHESIA FOR CAESAREAN SECTION

General anaesthesia for Caesarean section involves consideration of both maternal and fetal welfare. A technique using an intravenous barbiturate, muscle relaxant and tracheal intubation followed by IPPV with nitrous oxide and oxygen is widely used. This method enjoys a well-merited popularity because it can provide light narcosis with minimal central depression and full oxygenation of the infant. Nevertheless over the past few years there have been reservations expressed concerning its uncritical, complacent and routine acceptance. Misgivings have arisen principally from an overwhelming concern for the welfare of the mother, especially in view of the continuing reports of deaths due to the aspiration of gastric contents during anaesthesia for the operation, which often must be performed as an emergency with little time to take all the necessary safety precautions. In these circumstances the fetus is so often at risk that the anaesthetic technique must be adjusted to cause minimal depression and maximal oxygenation of the infant. In so doing the anaesthetist's constant concern is the risk that the mother may return to consciousness during the course of the operation. Thus there is no room for complacency and with the introduction of new drugs, ideas and apparatus, techniques must be constantly reviewed to determine whether their employment would contribute to both the improvement of maternal and fetal welfare in Caesarean section.

The anaesthetic requirements are, for the mother, the highest possible standard of anaesthesia as for any abdominal operation together with the maintenance of adequate placental perfusion with maternal arterial blood; for the fetus, the satisfactory exchange of respiratory gases, the avoidance of metabolic acidosis, together with freedom from drug-induced central nervous depression. According to Crawford (1972) "Elective Caesarean section provides the set-piece of the obstetric anaesthetist's repertoire. His degree of expertise can most accurately be judged by reference to the quality and consistency of his results in this area."

Awareness during Anaesthesia

The occurrence of awareness under nitrous oxide-oxygen-relaxant anaesthesia for general surgery was reported by Hutchinson (1961). Enquiry was made of 656 patients and 8 appeared to have "dreams" connected with events in the operating theatre. Wilson and Turner (1969) reported factual recall by 3 out of 150 patients for elective and emergency Caesarean section. A larger number complained of disturbing dreams making a total of 26 who had an unpleasant recall of their experience. Hyperventilation did not reduce its incidence and oxygen "flushing" at the time of delivery surprisingly did not increase the frequency of unpleasant recall. The only significant factor was that it occurred more in the elective than in the emergency group. This was assumed to be because a high proportion of the emergencies had received an opiate during labour before the operation. It was concluded that potent premedication was still appropriate in patients undergoing nitrous oxide-oxygen-relaxant anaesthesia for Caesarean section. As respiratory depressant drugs are contra-indicated it was suggested that benzodiazepine drugs might be suitable although the same authors in a later publication showed that diazepam premedication appeared to increase the frequency of unpleasant recall (Turner and Wilson, 1969).

An alternative approach in preventing unpleasant recall is to make use of the amnesic effect of hyoscine as premedication instead of the traditional atropine and to supplement nitrous oxide with *very low* concentrations of more potent volatile anaesthetics such as trichloroethylene 0·2 per cent, methoxyflurane 0·2 per cent (Crawford *et al.*, 1976) or halothane up to 0·5 per cent (Moir, 1970). This would make more sure of the mother's unconsciousness during the early part of the operation particularly if oxygen-rich gas mixtures are given for the benefit of the fetus.

The Choice of Induction Agents

Thiopentone 4mg/kg or methohexitone 1·5 mg/kg have become established as acceptable intravenous barbiturate induction agents in anaesthesia for Caesarean section. The introduction of the non-barbiturate agents, propanidid, Althesin and ketamine has prompted investigations to determine whether these could supplant their well-tried predecessors.

Propanidid should possess an advantage over thiopentone as an induction agent on account of its rapid bio-degradation in the body and because of its mild analgesic effect. However, Mahomedy *et al.* (1976) reported that, in contrast to thiopentone, it was associated with marked maternal tachycardia, a higher degree of biochemical and drug-induced fetal asphyxia and a higher incidence of painful factual recall by the mother. Along with Bradford and Moir (1969) they concluded that, despite theoretical considerations, propanidid offered no marked advantage over thiopentone as an induction agent for Caesarean section.

Althesin, on theoretical grounds, might also have advantages over thiopentone on account of its rapid metabolism, its favourable acceptance by the patient and its freedom from serious sequelae. Downing *et al.* (1974) could find no positive advantages and showed that with Althesin, maternal and fetal acidosis was increased and maternal and fetal oxygenation was reduced despite similar inspired oxygen concentrations in the mother.

Ketamine, in a dose of 1 mg/kg, was compared with thiopentone 3 mg/kg by Peltz and Sinclair (1973) who found it to be associated with a greater degree of post-operative analgesia and a virtual absence of awareness during anaesthesia. They claimed that ketamine was particularly advantageous when the partial pressure of 60 per cent nitrous oxide was reduced by the low barometric pressures at relatively high altitudes. The condition of the infant, the tone of the uterus and the intra-operative blood loss was comparable in the two groups. However, Clark (1973) warned that, while ketamine in low doses given just before delivery may leave the neonate unaffected, larger doses given further in advance of delivery would allow time for greater fetal uptake and might result in the birth of an infant with marked muscular spasticity, which would interfere with the establishment of spontaneous ventilation.

The Choice of Muscle Relaxants

There is almost complete unanimity of opinion that intubation before Caesarean section should be facilitated by a dose of 100 mg suxamethonium. There is less agreement as to the choice of agent by which the subsequent muscle relaxation should be maintained; this lies between continuing with suxamethonium by intravenous infusion 1 mg/ml or by intermittent injection or by using any of the well-established non-depolarising relaxants.

Fazadinium (Fazadon) in a dosage of 1 mg/kg offers a speed of onset of relaxation equal to that of suxamethonium, the avoidance of muscle pains and fasciculations, a length of action sufficient for the performance of the operation and a ready reversibility by neostigmine at the end of the operation. In common with other relaxants it docs not cross the placental barrier in clinically significant amounts (Blogg *et al.*, 1973).

In reporting on its use in 29 Caesarean sections, Cane and Sinclair (1976) achieved a mean induction-intubation time of 29·7 seconds, all intubations being easy and atraumatic. Prompt reversal of the non-depolarising block by neostigmine was obtained in all but two cases. In these the residual "curarisation" was treated with an infusion of 1 g of calcium chloride in normal saline given over 15 minutes. The only side-effect of fazadinium was a marked maternal tachycardia lasting for the whole course of anaesthesia.

A possible disadvantage of fazadinium is that the safety of the "failed intubation drill" (Tunstall, 1976) depends on the short period of action of the relaxant used for the attempted intubation (see p. 1367). In this respect the rapid return to spontaneous ventilation following suxamethonium might continue to weigh heavily in its favour.

Fetal Oxygenation during Caesarean Section

Oxygenation of the infant is the most important single factor bearing on its well-being following delivery by Caesarean section. While it must be accepted that some degree of fetal hypoxia may on occasion be related to placental insufficiency, the anaesthetist must always maintain the optimum degree of maternal oxygenation during the critical induction-delivery interval.

The effect of varying concentrations of oxygen in the inspired mixture given to 34 women undergoing Caesarean section has been examined by Rorke *et al.* (1968). The patients were divided into three groups according to whether they received 33 per cent, 67 per cent, or 100 per cent oxygen with a muscle relaxant and IPPV technique. These inspired concentrations of oxygen resulted in mean maternal Po_2 levels of 135 mm Hg (18 kPa), 255 mm Hg (34 kPa) and 440 mm Hg (58·7 kPa) respectively. Unconsciousness was assured by adding 2 per cent ether or 0·3 per cent methoxyflurane to the gas mixture. The mean induction-delivery time was over 45 minutes. Samples of blood for oxygen and carbon dioxide tensions together with acid-base values were taken from the maternal radial artery, from the fetal scalp immediately before delivery and from the umbilical artery and vein immediately after delivery. The findings can be summarised as follows:

1. The umbilical vein Po_2 increased as the maternal Po_2 rose to 300 mm Hg (40 kPa). Further increase in maternal Po_2 resulted in a fall in the umbilical vein Po_2. This supports the findings in animal experiments by Dawes and Mott (1964) that an increase in maternal oxygen tension may alter the blood flow in the placental vessels in order to protect the fetus against excessively high oxygen tensions.

2. Despite ventilation of the mother at 12 litres/minute, the maternal Pco_2 only fell significantly from the pre-operative level in the group receiving 33 per cent oxygen in the inspired gases and then only by 4 mm Hg (0·53 kPa). This correlates with the opinions of Scott *et al.* (1969) that it is difficult to produce respiratory alkalosis by mechanical ventilation in obstetric patients.

3. Despite efforts to maintain comparable ventilatory control in all three

groups, the maternal P_{CO_2} rose with the percentage of oxygen in the inspired mixture. The rise of P_{CO_2} in the umbilical vein and artery rose disproportionately more than the maternal arterial P_{CO_2}. This suggests that very high oxygen tensions in the mother interfere with the elimination of carbon dioxide by the placenta.

4. The Apgar scores of infants born of mothers given 67 per cent oxygen were significantly higher than of those given 33 per cent. There was no further improvement in the state of the infants born of mothers given 100 per cent oxygen, in fact a reverse tendency was noted.

5. The umbilical vein P_{O_2} and the Apgar score improved with a rise of the maternal P_{CO_2} to an optimal level of 32–34 mm Hg (4·2–4·5 kPa), that is, approximately the pre-operative level. Above this level there was a decrease in the umbilical venous P_{O_2}.

The results of this work suggest that the ideal anaesthetic technique should attempt to achieve in the mother's arterial blood an oxygen tension of 300 mm Hg (40 kPa) and carbon dioxide tension of 32–34 mm Hg (4·3–4·5 kPa) and that as long as the anaesthetic gas mixture is rich in oxygen there is no merit in oxygen "flushing" before delivery. The best results are obtained when the maternal P_{CO_2} is near the pre-operative level so that hyperventilation is contra-indicated. Unconsciousness in the mother is assured by the addition of low concentrations of volatile agents which appeared to have no adverse effect on the infant despite a background of relatively slow surgery.

It is probable that high oxygen concentrations of the inspired gas mixtures may also be beneficial because they are necessarily accompanied by low concentrations of nitrous oxide. Marx (1973) noted that, with a nitrous oxide mixture containing only 33 per cent oxygen, the degree of depression of the infant was related to the duration of anaesthesia before delivery. Nitrous oxide is rapidly transmitted across the placenta and the umbilical artery-umbilical vein concentration ratio increased progressively with the duration of anaesthesia. It was concluded that prolonged nitrous oxide anaesthesia could cause neonatal depression not only by a high fetal brain concentration but also by diffusion hypoxia.

Hyperventilation and Fetal Welfare

Some doubt has been cast on the safety to the fetus of hyperventilation of the mother during anaesthesia for Caesarean section. Holmes (1963) found that spontaneous respiration was established more rapidly in babies born of mothers in whom the anaesthetic technique caused respiratory acidosis than of those on whom mechanical hyperventilation imposed a respiratory alkalosis.

Motoyama et al. (1966) observed that the umbilical vein P_{O_2} was significantly lower when the maternal P_{CO_2} was low than when it was raised. This finding was confirmed by experiments on pregnant sheep by direct comparison of maternal arterial P_{CO_2} against samples taken from the fetal carotid artery. Moya et al. (1965) confirm that moderate hyperventilation with slight lowering of the maternal P_{CO_2} can reduce the degree of fetal acidosis but this did not improve the condition of the infant as judged by the Apgar score. Increasing degrees of hyperventilation interfered with the exchange of blood gases across the placenta, producing severe fetal metabolic acidosis and thus adversely affecting the state of the baby at birth. They suggested that the critical level of maternal arterial P_{CO_2} is 17 mm Hg (2·27 kPa) and below this level fetal acidosis was likely to delay the onset of respiration.

Coleman (1967) questioned whether maternal hypocapnia was harmful to babies delivered by Caesarean section. Eighteen mothers in early labour were anaesthetised by a thiopentone, relaxant and hyperventilation technique. Immediately before delivery the mean maternal arterial pH was 7·6 and the mean arterial P_{CO_2} 15·7 mm Hg (2·1 kPa). The mean pH of the umbilical vein blood at delivery was 7·31 and the mean P_{CO_2} 36·3 mm Hg (4·8 kPa). In these cases therefore marked maternal respiratory alkalosis was not matched by a comparable fetal respiratory alkalosis. Three infants who were judged clinically to have respiratory depression at birth had blood values similar to those of their clinically normal fellows. It was concluded that there was no reason to forego the valuable technique of "hypocapnic enhancement" of nitrous oxide anaesthesia in obstetrics on the grounds of possible harm to the infant.

Scott et al. (1969), in seeking to reconcile these opposing views, found that while they could confirm that fetal acid-base status moved in the same direction as that of the mother, the high inflationary pressures required to produce hyperventilation during anaesthesia could cause a reduction in cardiac output by as much as 50 per cent. An additional factor in causing interference with placental circulation could be the effect of inferior vena caval occlusion, when a maintained maternal blood pressure would be accompanied by a reduced cardiac output. These very considerable changes in the circulation were likely to be of much greater importance than changes in maternal oxygen and carbon dioxide tensions.

It was concluded that, in spite of the theoretical dangers of a hypocapnic technique, the method appeared in practice to be free from deleterious effects on the infants. This could be due to the fact that adverse effects, if any, were not operating for a sufficiently long time to produce irreversible fetal hypoxia. Light general anaesthesia with controlled ventilation was a safe and useful method for Caesarean section, provided that excessive inflationary pressures were avoided, that the maternal P_{CO_2} did not fall below 20 mm Hg (2·7 kPa), that delivery of the child was not unduly delayed by slow surgery and that allowance was made for other forms of coincidental circulatory embarrassment.

Time, Posture and Caesarean Section

Depression of the newborn at Caesarean section is usually due to the combination in varying proportions of the effect of anaesthetic drugs and of biochemical changes due to utero-placental insufficiency. Recent publications have drawn attention to the close relationship between the state of the infant at birth, the induction-delivery interval and the posture of the mother at operation (Downing et al., 1974).

Ansari and his associates (1970) reported that the tilted posture was associated with a marked increase in the oxygen saturation of the umbilical arterial and venous blood particularly if the operation were carried out under spinal anaesthesia. This was attributed to the improvement in cardiac output consequent on relief of vena caval occlusion.

Crawford (1972) noted that infants born to a group of mothers who were tilted on the operating table were consistently less acidotic than those whose mothers had remained supine. The latter's infants showed a greater variability in their clinical and associated acid-base state which could be due to variations in the effect of posture on the individual mothers' inferior venae cavae and the varying patency of the collateral venous channels. The advantages of the lateral tilt were more evident with an increasing induction-delivery time (Crawford *et al.*, 1972). The infants born to non-tilted mothers became more acidotic while those born of mothers who were tilted at operation were less asphyxiated even with a longer induction-delivery interval. This suggests a gradual recovery from the ill-effects of the supine posture during transport from bed to anaesthetic room and underlines the protective nature of a lateral tilt against the deleterious effects of slow surgery; indeed, Crawford and Davies (1975) have shown that an induction-delivery interval of 30 minutes is consistent with fetal welfare as long as the time elapsing between the uterine incision and delivery of the infant is not unduly prolonged.

Following induction with hexobarbitone 250–300 mg and with all his patients tilted, Magno *et al.* (1975) showed that a short induction-delivery interval (mean 2·75 min) resulted in the birth of infants with higher oxygen tensions, less CO_2 retention and less metabolic acidosis than those delivered after a longer interval (mean 9 min). Unfortunately, with the shorter induction-delivery interval, the mothers had less time to become adequately anaesthetised by the nitrous oxide given for maintenance of unconsciousness and, months later, nearly half retained persistent unpleasant memories of their operation. On the other hand, an induction-delivery interval as long as 15 minutes might risk drug-induced depression as it would allow time for the fetal brain to become equilibrated with the maternal level of barbiturate remaining from the dose given for induction of anaesthesia. The optimum induction-delivery time was estimated to be about 8 minutes.

The work of these and other authors suggests that fetal welfare is best served by reasonably expeditious surgery and by delaying induction of anaesthesia until the surgeon is ready to begin the operation which should be carried out with the patient in the tilted posture at least until after delivery of the infant. It follows that she should be turned on to her side while awaiting operation and should remain so during transit to the operating theatre.

The lateral tilt is even more important if the operator is slow, particularly when Caesarean section is indicated by fetal distress. Nevertheless, surgeons may protest that the tilted posture may prolong induction-delivery time by increasing the technical difficulty of operating and it may also pre-dispose to surgical error by altering the normal anatomical relations in the lower abdomen.

Recommended Technique for General Anaesthesia—Summary

1. Left lateral tilt on the operating table.
2. Precautions against pulmonary aspiration of gastric contents.
3. Inspired oxygen concentration between 50 and 65 per cent.
4. Nitrous oxide anaesthesia supplemented by low concentrations of volatile agent to avoid awareness.
5. IPPV with avoidance of hyperventilation and high inflation pressures.
6. Prompt replacement of excessive blood loss.

Details: On arrival in the operating theatre, the anaesthetist should check that one litre of cross-matched blood has been placed in a nearby refrigerator and that devices for warming and accelerating the flow of transfused blood are in working order. A trained assistant should be in attendance with whom the anaesthetist will check all the apparatus to be used during the operation.

Following the precautions against the dangers of pulmonary aspiration of stomach contents detailed on p. 1361 *et seq.*, the patient is placed on the operating table with a wedge under her right side. Oxygen is given by mask for three minutes during which a diaphragm needle is inserted into a convenient vein. After an intravenous injection of hyoscine 0·4 mg and the application of cricoid pressure by the assistant, anaesthesia is induced with intravenous thiopentone 200–250 mg, followed by suxamethonium 100 mg. The mask is removed without positive-pressure inflation of the lungs and the trachea intubated as soon as possible after the onset of relaxation. The patient is ventilated mechanically at an expired minute volume of 6–8 litres/min with nitrous oxide/oxygen 50:50 per cent supplemented with 0·5 per cent halothane. An infusion of compound sodium lactate solution is set up as a convenient channel for rapid transfusion and for the administration of drugs. Apnoea is maintained with intermittent or continuous suxamethonium or a dose of non-depolarising relaxant. As the baby's head is delivered 0·5 mg ergometrine is given intravenously and once the cord is clamped 20 mg papaveretum is given to confer intra-operative and post-operative analgesia. The proportion of nitrous oxide to oxygen is adjusted to 75:25 per cent and halothane administration is discontinued. The anaesthetist may then resuscitate the infant if no paediatrician is in attendance. At this stage a blood loss of 300–500 ml may be accepted as normal and should not require replacement owing to the autotransfusion by the contracting uterus. If uterine retraction is inadequate 20 units oxytocin should be added to each 500 ml of infusion fluid. Undue alarm should not be taken at the quantity of bloody fluid in the sucker bottle as the major part of this is likely to be liquor amnii. On the other hand a massive blood loss must be restored by a massive transfusion with due regard to warming the transfused blood, central venous pressure monitoring, and replenishment of the loss of ionised calcium with calcium gluconate.

At the end of the operation the patient must recover under close supervision and the endotracheal tube removed only as consciousness is regained. Despite the administration of an intravenous analgesic during the operation she should be given prompt and frequent intramuscular pain-relieving injections for the first post-operative 24 hours.

Epidural Anaesthesia and Caesarean Section

The modern widespread practice of epidural block for relief of pain in labour has prompted a renewed interest in the use of the technique for Caesarean section in preference to general anaesthesia. At first sight the advantages are attractive such as the avoidance of the dangers of general anaesthesia, the absence of drug-induced fetal depression, reduced blood loss (Moir, 1970) and the facility for extending effective analgesia into the post-operative period. Practitioners with experience of both techniques declare that, correctly used, both appear to be safe for mother and child and that the anaesthetist may be guided by the mother's choice as to whether she wishes to be awake or asleep at delivery (Crawford, 1972; Milne and Lawson, 1973; Marx, 1973; Magno *et al.*, 1975 and 1976). However, general anaesthesia would be preferred if the urgency of the operation does not allow time for an epidural injection to become effective, if the patient is suffering from haemorrhagic shock or is particularly sensitive to the supine posture or if the fetus is seriously at risk. One might also hesitate to give epidural analgesia to a very nervous patient or to one whose morale is low after a long and anxious labour. The only occasion when the anaesthetist might feel compelled to choose regional in preference to general anaesthesia would be if serious difficulty with intubation were anticipated.

The fundamental problem posed by epidural block is that for the painless performance of the operation the block must extend to a level at which half the sympathetic outflow is interrupted; a tendency to hypotension is inevitable. In addition the effects of vena caval occlusion are not always abolished by a mere 15 per cent lateral tilt and furthermore, the circulation may be embarrassed by operative haemorrhage both before and after delivery. Unless measures are taken to prevent hypotension the infant is bound to suffer severe biochemical depression. *The remedy is the mandatory rapid pre-loading of the circulation with 1 litre of compound lactate solution given as the block is taking effect.* The blood pressure must be monitored throughout the operation which, as a matter of course, must be carried out with the patient in the tilted posture. Oxygen must be given by face-mask until delivery of the infant and blood loss must be promptly replaced.

Milne and Lawson (1973) reviewed 182 Caesarean sections performed under epidural anaesthesia. Epidural anaesthesia had been induced for the relief of labour pain in 120 cases and the block was given solely for the operation in 62 cases. Lignocaine 2 per cent with adrenaline 1:200,000 was preferred to bupivacaine 0·5 per cent because of its greater speed and reliability of action. In patients with an established block an increment of 8–12 ml lignocaine 2 per cent gave an adequate segmental level of anaesthesia. In patients receiving epidural block for the operation alone, a cannula was passed into the epidural space through which 14–16 ml lignocaine was injected.

Operating conditions were satisfactory in over 80 per cent of cases except for occasional retching or coughing, but in 7 patients general anaesthesia was given because of poor muscle relaxation or restlessness. It follows that none of the precautions which should be taken before general anaesthesia must be omitted even though the intention is to deliver under regional block. A number of other patients were given various sedatives and analgesics, some before and some after delivery. Despite fluid pre-loading of the circulation and the tilted posture of the patient, serious hypotension demanded the use of ephedrine on 15 occasions. Nausea and vomiting occurred frequently after the injection of ergometrine but these symptoms were almost completely eliminated when oxytocin was substituted. As parturient women are highly sensitive to the hypertensive effects of ergometrine it should certainly never be used in conjunction with ephedrine (Moodie and Moir, 1976).

Combination of General Anaesthesia and Epidural Analgesia

The writer is not attracted to the routine use of epidural block as the sole method of anaesthesia for Caesarean section. There are however advantages in combining the two techniques in patients coming to section with a block already established for labour pain relief.

The technique already recommended for general anaesthesia is carried out with intermittent suxamethonium and IPPV until delivery of the child. When major haemorrhage has ceased, when blood loss has been replaced and when the infant no longer requires the anaesthetist's attention, 15 ml bupivacaine 0·5 per cent is injected through the epidural cannula and spontaneous ventilation allowed to return. The operation continues under nitrous oxide and oxygen anaesthesia with perfect muscular relaxation; later the patient rapidly resumes consciousness totally free from discomfort.

ELECTIVE OBSTETRIC PROCEDURES

External Cephalic Version

Conversion of a breech presentation to a vertex is usually carried out between the 32nd and 36th week of pregnancy and is nearly always achieved without an anaesthetic provided that the mother is able voluntarily to relax her abdominal muscles. After the 36th week of pregnancy the uterus becomes increasingly irritable until the onset of labour. Irrespective of the mother's co-operation the increase in uterine tone may prevent the success of the procedure and so an anaesthetic is required. Even with an anaesthetic, attempts at version may not succeed owing to intra-uterine causes such as extended legs of the fetus, an unduly short cord, a large fibroid, septate uterus or deficient quantity of liquor.

The anaesthetist must be prepared to provide complete relaxation of the abdominal musculature and, if uterine contractions impede the obstetrician's efforts, to relax the uterus with deep general anaesthesia. After premedication with papaveretum-hyoscine the patient should lie on a bed with a 15° head-down tilt to help lift the breech out of the pelvis. Before induction of anaesthesia the obstetrician should check that the breech is still presenting and that a spontaneous version has not occurred. He may find that under the premedication version without anaesthesia may be possible. If not, anaesthesia is induced with methohexitone, suxamethonium and tracheal intubation. During the short period of skeletal muscle relaxation the obstetrician may attempt a version or he may decide that his efforts are frustrated by excessive uterine tone. Complete uterine relaxation is then provided by deep halothane or ether anaesthesia which may take as long as 10–15 minutes to attain if the uterus is particularly irritable.

Complications of external version include fetal distress or detachment of the placenta with antepartum haemorrhage. The anaesthetist should remain in the vicinity for a short while in case an emergency Caesarean section is indicated. Marcus et al. (1975) have reported that an attempted or a successful external cephalic version may cause significant feto-maternal haemorrhage in 6 per cent of cases. Thus it may be a cause of rhesus iso-immunisation and, in their view, should not be performed in a Rh-negative mother unless the father of the child is also Rh negative. If a version has been attempted, fetal cell counts should be made and Rh immunoprophylaxis administered if necessary.

Because of these considerations many obstetricians are unwilling to attempt external cephalic version unless it can be carried out easily and without an anaesthetic.

Induction of Labour

Simple amniotomy can be performed without an anaesthetic but the procedure can be made more comfortable for the patient by a prior slow intravenous injection of diazepam 10 mg and pentazocine 30 mg. The use of full general anaesthesia is justified if the obstetrician wishes to stretch the cervix and to "sweep" the membranes. If epidural analgesia is planned for the labour the cannula should be sited in advance of the obstetrician's arrival and 12 ml bupivacaine 0·5 per cent injected with the patient in the sitting position; uterine and perineal analgesia should be obtained within 30 minutes.

OPERATIVE OBSTETRICS AND HALOTHANE

In the early years of its use as an anaesthetic, halothane gained a reputation as a potent myometrial relaxant and neonatal depressant when used for operative obstetrics. Experience showed that the uterine response to ergometrine was abolished and postpartum haemorrhage was increased. Infants born following halothane anaesthesia were more depressed than those delivered following a nitrous oxide/oxygen-relaxant sequence (Montgomery, 1961). Further work by Crawford (1965) led to the dictum: "There is absolutely no justification, other than the desire to produce uterine relaxation, for administering halothane to an obstetric patient."

More recent experience has modified this opinion. Following their use of halothane-oxygen anaesthesia in elective Caesarean section, Johnstone and Breen (1966) showed that maternal narcotic requirements were well below the dose that would depress the contractility of the uterus or the fetal respiratory centre. This view is confirmed by Moir (1970) who found that anaesthesia for Caesarean section based on nitrous oxide/oxygen 50:50 with halothane 0·5 per cent was associated with livelier infants and no more operative blood loss than after an unsupplemented nitrous oxide/oxygen sequence.

A more tolerant attitude towards halothane in obstetrics may be associated with a more rational approach towards its employment. Those who described its undesirable effects tended to give it with the vaporiser setting at 1·5 to 2 per cent in contrast to Moir's more cautious dosage of 0·5 per cent.

The place of halothane in operative obstetrics remains primarily as a myometrial relaxant. For external version high vapour concentrations are used because the anaesthetist is concerned neither with the dangers of postpartum haemorrhage nor of neonatal depression but solely with achieving the optimum conditions for the obstetrician. For the relaxation of a constriction ring, the release of an infant from a tonic uterus at Caesarean section, at breech delivery, or for the second of twins, a concentration of 1·5 to 2 per cent is given only until the desired effect is obtained. Halothane is then discontinued and washed out with unsupplemented nitrous oxide and oxygen so that uterine tone is restored as soon as possible.

Anaesthesia for the removal of a retained placenta implies producing just sufficient myometrial relaxation to facilitate the obstetrician's work. If the placenta is detached but trapped in the cervix less halothane will be required than if the obstetrician has to introduce his hand into the uterine cavity to detach it from the placental site. In these circumstances the anaesthetist must be guided by his colleague as to the degree of relaxation he requires. Excessive myometrial flaccidity may make it difficult for him to define the plane of cleavage between the placenta and the uterine wall. Following removal of the placenta, halothane is discontinued and washed out with unsupplemented nitrous oxide and oxygen. Ergometrine is given and any excessive loss of blood volume is replaced.

Halothane 0·5 per cent may safely be given for its purely narcotic effect not only as a supplement to nitrous oxide and oxygen for Caesarean section but also for any of the various short but painful procedures in obstetrics such as perineal suture without fear of interfering with myometrial contractility.

PROBLEMS ASSOCIATED WITH OBSTETRIC ANAESTHESIA

1. The Aortocaval Occlusion Syndrome

Postural hypotension with fainting and nausea may occur in pregnant women approaching term when they lie on their backs. Wright (1962) found that of

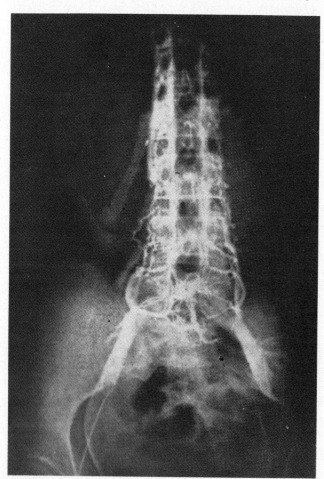

43/Fig. 2(a).—Inferior vena cavogram in the supine position immediately before Caesarean section. Little or no dye enters the inferior vena cava traversing instead the collateral circulation through the paravertebral veins.

100 women lying supine in the ninth month of pregnancy 47 showed a fall of 10 per cent in their normal systolic blood pressure and 6 showed a 30 per cent fall with nausea and faintness. The hypotension is associated with a rise of venous pressure in the iliac veins and is due to the compression of the inferior vena cava by the gravid uterus restricting the venous return to the heart; the hypotension is corrected and the symptoms relieved when the woman lies on her side. Until recently the condition has been known as the "supine hypotensive syndrome" but in view of the more extensive knowledge of the alteration in circulatory haemodynamics the term is now regarded as inappropriate.

Scott (1968) has shown radiologically that some degree of vena caval obstruction occurs in the majority of women in late pregnancy and yet comparatively few suffer severely from the effects. This is not to imply that the circulation is unaffected by vena caval occlusion. Admittedly, in some women an unimpaired venous return is provided by an adequate collateral circulation from the internal iliac vein through the ascending lumbar and paravertebral veins to the vena azygos (Figs. 2 and 3). A few are completely intolerant of the supine

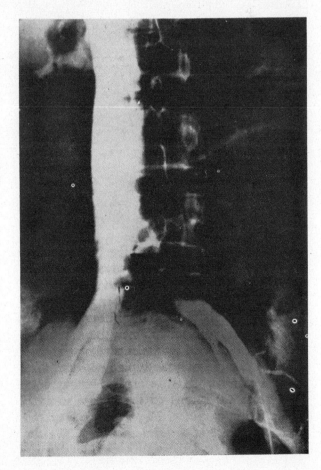

43/Fig. 2(b).—The same patient immediately following delivery. Virtually all the dye now travels up the inferior vena cava.

THE EFFECT OF CHANGE FROM THE LATERAL TO THE SUPINE POSTURE ON THE
HAEMODYNAMIC PATTERNS IN LATE PREGNANCY (after Scott 1968)

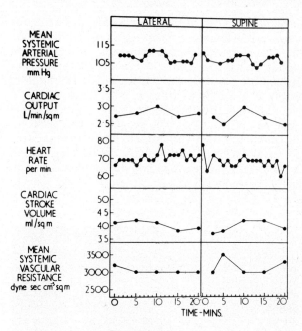

43/FIG. 3.—Arterial pressure, cardiac output and peripheral resistance were not affected by change of posture.

Caval occlusion caused no reduction of venous return possibly because of an adequate collateral venous circulation.

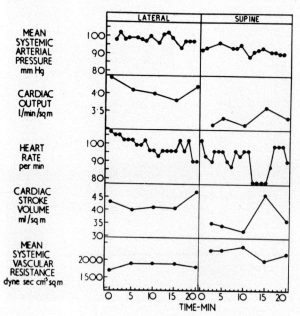

43/FIG. 4.—"Concealed" caval occlusion. The patient was symptom-free in the supine posture but with a reduced cardiac output and an increased peripheral resistance.

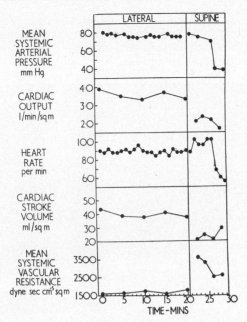

43/FIG. 5.—Patient exhibiting the typical "supine hypotensive syndrome". There was an immediate fall in cardiac output in the supine position but the arterial pressure was temporarily maintained by a rise in peripheral resistance. Then a sudden bradycardia occurred accompanied by
fainting and hypotension.

posture and represent those in whom the collateral circulation is very poorly
developed. In most women the venous return is reduced to a variable degree
and it is estimated that a fall in cardiac output up to 20 per cent is compatible
with their being symptomatically unaffected by the supine posture. This fall
is not necessarily accompanied by an alteration in mean arterial pressure or
in heart rate because of the compensatory increase in peripheral resistance by
which the systemic blood pressure is maintained at near normal levels. The
immediate effect of vena caval occlusion is thus *concealed* by a sympathetic
vasoconstrictor response to the lowered cardiac output (Fig. 4). The resulting
state of circulatory instability may be *revealed* by further diminution in cardiac
output as with a vasovagal attack (Fig. 5), a reduction in circulating blood
volume such as occurs with haemorrhage or dehydration, or by the loss of
vascular sympathetic tone accompanying epidural analgesia or light general
anaesthesia (Crawford *et al.*, 1972).

The clinical importance of the hazards of the supine position in late pregnancy and labour has been stated on many occasions in the preceding pages;
some points however are worthy of mention. Before induction of anaesthesia for
operative delivery the blood pressure should be measured in both the lateral and
then in the supine posture. A marked difference in the *pulse pressures* observed
in the two positions would suggest that anaesthesia might be more safely induced

with the patient laterally tilted. Even in the lateral posture some degree of caval compression may persist (Fig. 6). It is sometimes worth comparing the effect of turning the mother to one side and then on to the other; paradoxically, the left side is not always the most favourable.

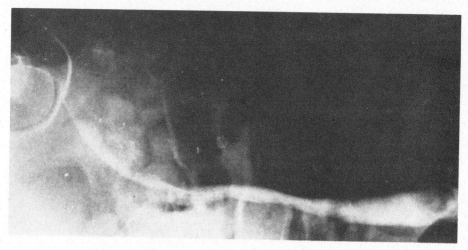

43/FIG. 6.—Cavogram (lateral view) of pregnant patient lying on her side. Despite the lateral posture a long segment of the inferior vena cava is seen to be partially compressed.

A woman who has been troubled by symptoms of caval occlusion in late pregnancy and early labour may sometimes be turned on to her back quite safely for delivery, as by this time the fetal head may have descended deeply into the pelvis so that the caval pressure has, to some extent, been relieved.

Patients severely shocked with antepartum haemorrhage may show a marked improvement after turning to the side because of the resulting increased venous return to the heart. It has been observed that fetal distress, as evidenced by bradycardia and lowered pH of blood samples, has been followed by a rapid return to normal as soon as the mother is turned laterally. If this simple expedient were tried in all cases of fetal distress, many mothers might be saved unnecessary operative interventions (Beard and Roberts, 1970).

If pregnant patients are anaesthetised in the supine position for Caesarean section, the lightest anaesthetic causes vasodilatation which effectively reduces the compensatory rise in peripheral resistance which maintains a normal arterial blood pressure when the cardiac output is diminished. The anaesthetist must be on guard against a sudden fall of blood pressure which is very simply avoided by tilting the patient to the left before induction of anaesthesia.

The limited degree of sympathetic blockade which accompanies obstetric epidural analgesia may unmask the effects of vena caval occlusion in at least 20 per cent of patients. Usually the mother complains of nausea or faintness before a measurable fall of blood pressure occurs. The symptoms must be treated immediately by turning the patient on to her side. Should the symptoms be neglected a severe fall of blood pressure and fetal distress may follow. This underlines the importance of keeping patients under close observation for a short time after the setting up of epidural anaesthesia and after each top-up injection. As a safety precaution, they should always be left lying in the lateral posture particularly if close supervision is not possible.

The use of vasopressors for the treatment of persistent hypotension is strongly contra-indicated. With the possible exception of ephedrine and mephentermine, they tend to cause diminution in placental perfusion by uterine arterial vasoconstriction without increasing cardiac output. They may also increase the risk of pulmonary oedema and arterial hypertension when the caval occlusion is released at parturition. The dangers to patients with cardiac disease or pre-eclampsia are evident. If change of posture fails to restore the fall in blood pressure, a rapid intravenous dextrose infusion should be given to increase the circulating blood volume.

The effect of *aortic* compression by the gravid uterus must also be taken into account. Bienarz *et al.* (1966) showed that, while brachial and femoral artery pressures are equal in supine normotensive pregnant women, the femoral systolic pressure falls 20 mm Hg (2·7 kPa) below the brachial when they are severely hypotensive. Thus compression of the aorta together with inferior vena caval occlusion may aggravate fetal distress by further reducing blood flow to the placenta.

Since more sensitive methods of fetal monitoring have been employed, there is now mounting evidence of the benefit to fetal welfare of the avoidance of vena caval and aortic compression during labour and at delivery. Weaver *et al.* (1975) suggest that not only should women under epidural analgesia be routinely nursed in the lateral position but also that the supine position should be avoided in *all parturients*. The implementation of this precept will require considerable effort in the education of midwives – and obstetricians – who have become accustomed to examining, auscultating, catheterising and delivering patients in the dorsal position. No doubt in time the benefits of the lateral or tilted posture will be better appreciated by all who manage patients in labour.

2. Amniotic Fluid Embolism

Amniotic fluid may reach the maternal circulation during labour or during normal or operative delivery. It is most likely to do so with very high intra-uterine pressures as may occur in a tumultuous labour or with an uncontrolled oxytocin infusion. It is traditionally believed that the fluid enters the uterine venous sinuses in the area of the utero-placental site but Shnider and Moya (1961) consider that entry via the endocervical veins is more probable. They postulate that the intra-myometrial pressure is high enough to minimise entry into the vessels of the upper uterine segment, but that the great intra-uterine pressure will force the amniotic fluid towards the cervix, the veins of which are lacerated even in normal labour. The liability to this rare complication increases with age and parity.

The clinical features of amniotic fluid embolism result from both an *embolic* and a *haemorrhagic* component. Entry of fetal material into the maternal blood stream precipitates a massive conversion of fibrinogen to fibrin which effectively blocks the pulmonary circulation while fibrinogen depletion of the blood causes uncontrollable haemorrhage due to coagulation failure.

A definitive diagnosis can only be made by the post-mortem findings of fetal squames, vernix or meconium in the lung capillaries. A presumptive diagnosis should be made on the symptoms of sudden onset of dyspnoea, cyanosis, tachycardia, pulmonary oedema and circulatory failure. A chest X-ray reveals perihilar mottling and the ECG shows right heart strain. The pulmonary artery and central venous pressures are raised. Coagulation failure is frequently but not invariably present, but when it occurs uncontrollable haemorrhage issues from the uterus, the urinary tract, into the skin and from the mucous membranes and the blood shed does not clot. The mortality is said to be over 80 per cent, the primary cause of death being the circulatory disturbance caused by blockage of the pulmonary capillary bed by fibrin deposition.

Immediate treatment is to combat acute hypoxia by ventilating the patient with 100 per cent oxygen and replacing the loss of blood volume by massive transfusion against central venous pressure monitoring. Low molecular weight dextran may be given in an attempt to improve pulmonary blood flow, but there is little agreement concerning further definitive treatment. Some recommend giving fresh blood, triple strength plasma or purified fibrinogen. Fibrinolytic inhibitors are available such as epsilonaminocaproic acid, a competitive inhibitor of the activator-plasminogen reaction, while aprotinin (Trasylol) in addition prevents the activation of prothrombin by thromboplastin and thus regulates the abnormal conversion of fibrinogen to fibrin. Others recommend the use of heparin to prevent the continued fibrinogen-fibrin conversion and progressive pulmonary vascular occlusion, believing that the giving of exogenous fibrinogen merely provides extra material to produce the fatal vascular obstruction in the lungs (Loeliger, 1966). Scott (1969) considers this a more rational approach, although when faced with acute obstetric collapse, severe haemorrhage and coagulation failure it requires courage to apply it. Success of this treatment is measured not so much by restoration of normal coagulation but by the return to normal of the pulmonary arterial and central venous pressures. The problem is that in some cases the fibrinogen deficiency may be life-saving; in others it may endanger life. The patient may, with suitable treatment, survive the pulmonary vascular occlusion but may succumb to continued and uncontrollable haemorrhage which may exhaust the available blood transfusion resources.

It is clear that the successful management of this rare complication would be difficult in a maternity unit isolated from the laboratory and intensive care facilities normally found only in a large general hospital (Willocks et al., 1966).

3. Pre-eclampsia

Pre-eclampsia is characterised by hypertension, oedema and albuminuria which may be complicated by eclampsia which is defined as the occurrence of fits in a pre-eclamptic patient. It appears to be a kind of hypertensive encephalopathy, the immediate effect of which is to produce localised arteriolar spasm, leading to cerebral anaemia and cerebral hypoxia. Eclamptic convulsions may occur without warning and without severe symptoms of pre-eclampsia, but they are most likely to be triggered by a sudden increase in the blood pressure due to muscular work or to any external stimulus. The manifestations of the disease are thought to be due to a widespread intravascular coagulation with deposition of micro-emboli in the brain, the lungs, the liver and the kidneys. There is a progressive diminution in placental efficiency due to deposition of fibrin on the maternal side of the fetal villi.

Treatment.—The essential treatment of pre-eclampsia is, of course, primarily the obstetrician's responsibility. It consists of complete rest, restriction of fluid intake, control of the blood pressure and the prevention of eclampsia. Attempts may be made to reduce the blood pressure with various hypotensive agents but their value remains unproven particularly in terms of fetal salvage. Termination of the pregnancy by induction of labour or Caesarean section may be considered. The obstetrician has to weigh the risk to the infant of prematurity against the risk of increasing placental insufficiency and the risk to the mother of eclampsia and permanent renal damage if the pregnancy is allowed to continue. It should be remembered that a fair proportion of cases of eclampsia occur in the puerperium.

For the prevention of eclampsia sedation with large doses of morphia is sometimes used, although this is criticised on the grounds that morphia stimulates the supra-optic nucleus and increases the output of antidiuretic hormone and hence fluid retention. Amylobarbitone and phenobarbitone may be considered more suitable sedatives in preventing the onset of convulsions, as may mixtures of phenothiazines with pethidine. Currently the most popular sedative appears to be diazepam given by intravenous infusion, although its possible effect on the neonate must be borne in mind (Chapter 42).

A method of preventing or treating eclampsia was described by Duffus *et al.* (1968) using the anticonvulsant chlormethiazole. It is given as an 0·8 per cent intravenous infusion and the patient is maintained in a state of light sleep from which she can easily be aroused, the rate of infusion being increased if she becomes restless or wakeful. In practice the minimum effective dose of chlormethiazole is difficult to judge even when the infusion rate is accurately controlled and patients may remain unconscious for longer than desired after delivery.

For the control of hypertension, hydrallazine (20 mg) or diazoxide (100 mg) are given intravenously as required and urinary output is maintained with frusemide.

The anaesthetist is likely to be involved in the management of eclampsia or pre-eclampsia to assist in controlling the convulsions, sedating the patient, lowering of blood pressure and in giving anaesthesia for delivery of the infant. In controlling the convulsions the minimum effective dose of thiopentone should be given possibly followed by suxamethonium as a muscle relaxant, and as a matter of course facilities for intubation and artificial ventilation must be at hand.

Continuous epidural analgesia is used as a supplementary method of lowering the blood pressure. An injection of 8–10 ml bupivacaine 0·5 per cent without adrenaline, is given at the 2nd–3rd lumbar interspace and should produce analgesia up to the 9th–10th dorsal dermatome. Further injections through the cannula are given until the desired fall of blood pressure has been attained. However, despite initial success, attempts to control hypertension with epidural analgesia over long periods are often disappointing as the blood pressure may continue to rise even though the sensory block has reached a level well above the costal margin. It has therefore no place in treatment before labour has begun. Given during labour it controls the rise of blood pressure due to the experience of pain and provides effective analgesia for an elective forceps delivery. The fetus, already at a disadvantage with prematurity and placental insufficiency, is given time to recover from the depressant drugs given to the mother and should stand a better chance of survival at birth. Nevertheless, the accumulation of anticonvulsant and hypotensive drugs may result in severe depression of the infant whose condition may require intensive therapy with intermittent positive-pressure ventilation.

ANAESTHESIA FOR GYNAECOLOGICAL OPERATIONS

Gynaecological operations in the lower abdomen present few problems different from those of general surgical procedures and the choice of anaesthetic should be made in accordance with the principles discussed in Chapter 37.

Reduction of Blood Loss in Vaginal Surgery

Operations for the repair of prolapse may require a reduction of congestion in the surgical field. While many surgeons are satisfied with a standard anaesthetic technique for pelvic floor repair, others will demand more complex techniques to reduce blood loss at the operation site especially in pre-menopausal patients in whom bleeding may be particularly troublesome. Induced hypotension with ganglionic blockade has been advocated; the head-down position helps to drain the blood from the site of operation and decreases the risk of an inadequate cerebral blood flow.

Epidural anaesthesia has been shown to provide the most effective and safe "bloodless field" in this area despite the maintenance of near normal blood pressure levels (Moir, 1968). With ganglionic blockade a comparably dry field can only be achieved by inducing hypotension. The aid of posture, an essential part of the technique, cannot be fully exploited unless the surgeon is prepared to perform the vaginal repair in the "jack-knife" position—an unusual and unlikely event.

Bond (1969) measured the blood loss on 45 patients undergoing major vaginal surgery some of whom had epidural analgesia with opiate sedation while others were given epidural analgesia with endotracheal halothane and oxygen. The fall of blood pressure was significantly less in those patients given an epidural with opiate sedation than in those who were given halothane anaesthesia in addition to the epidural. However the mean blood losses in the two groups were similar and there was no correlation between blood loss and the fall of blood pressure. The explanation is that an epidural affecting segments D10 to S3 causes sympathetic blockade only from D10 to L1, but because the pelvic viscera receive their vasomotor innervation from above the level of the epidural blockade, the baroreceptor response can produce a compensatory vasoconstriction at the site of operation and thus diminution of bleeding. If, in addition to the epidural, a general anaesthetic is given, the reflexly constricted vessels in the pelvic viscera become dilated. The blood pressure falls, no further reduction in bleeding is achieved and the impression of a blanched surgical field is lost.

The advantages of epidural anaesthesia in major gynaecological surgery are not confined to the reduction of blood loss. If the epidural cannula is left in place, effective post-operative analgesia may be maintained which can be of particular benefit to bronchitic patients in whom pain may hinder effective coughing.

The individual anaesthetist will decide for himself whether the benefits of epidural blockade outweigh the disadvantage of using a time-consuming technique on a lengthy operating list. One might reflect that the time may be well spent if it results in an increase in the number of anaesthetists competent to perform epidural techniques in circumstances where they are more clearly indicated.

LAPAROSCOPY

Laparoscopy involves the inspection of the abdominal cavity following the preliminary induction of a pneumoperitoneum by passing carbon dioxide or nitrous oxide through a Verrés needle. The laparoscope is then passed through the abdominal wall usually at the inferior margin of the umbilicus. The operation is most frequently carried out for the investigation of infertility or for tubal sterilisation, but it is also indicated for the diagnosis of early extra-uterine pregnancy or to seek causes for amenorrhoea, ovarian dystrophy, dysmenorrhoea, obscure pelvic pain, tuberculosis, endometriosis and acute and chronic pelvic disease.

The increase in the practice of laparoscopy has been accompanied by a growing concern over its possible complications. The Verrés needle may perforate the intestine or cause haemorrhage from perforation of the blood vessels of the abdominal wall. Introduction of even normal quantities of gas may cause parietal or omental emphysema; sudden death from gas embolism has been reported. The introduction of excessive quantities of gas has caused the aggravation of hernias, mediastinal emphysema, pneumothorax and rupture of the diaphragm.

While it is important that anaesthetists should be aware of the surgical hazards of laparoscopy, their main concern must be to provide safe and satisfactory anaesthesia for the procedure and to minimise its respiratory and circulatory effects.

Hodgson et al. (1970) described some of the cardiorespiratory effects of peritoneal insufflation of carbon dioxide at laparoscopy. When using a spontaneous breathing technique they noted hyperventilation, an irregular pulse and occasionally hypotension and cardiac dysrhythmias. When artificial ventilation was used a rise of Pa_{CO_2} still occurred, but this was to a lesser degree than in the spontaneously breathing patients and hence it was judged less likely to exceed the threshold for halothane dysrhythmias. In the artificially ventilated patients the decreased chest compliance due to the elevation of the diaphragm necessitated the increase of the inflation pressure by 15 to 20 cm (1·47 to 1·96 kPa) of water to maintain a constant minute volume of ventilation. It might be thought that this increase of inflation pressure might reduce venous return to the heart. However, as long as the intraperitoneal pressure did not become excessive, the central venous pressure rose and the cardiac output was not diminished. The rise in central venous pressure was considered to be due to enhanced sympathetic activity following the increase in Pa_{CO_2} and suggested the possibility of a hazard to a patient on the verge of congestive cardiac failure. An alternative explanation is that blood is squeezed out of viscera by the raised intra-abdominal pressure.

Scott (1970) reported that a marked resistance to spontaneous ventilation occurred with the raised intra-abdominal pressure but this was counteracted by the ventilatory drive due to accumulating endogenous and exogenous carbon dioxide. The rise of central venous pressure was considered to be due to the raised ventilatory pressure required to keep a constant inspired volume after the pneumoperitoneum had been induced. Cardiac dysrhythmias, usually coupled beats, occurred in 27 out of 100 patients. For maintenance of anaesthesia, nitrous oxide, oxygen and halothane by spontaneous ventilation was used, intubation was not carried out, thus post-operative sore throat and muscle pains were avoided. A device limiting the intraperitoneal pressure was regarded as an essential safety precaution and reference was made to two cases of cardiac arrest, attributable to gas embolism, occurring within seconds of switching on the gas flow to the peritoneal cavity.

Scott and Julian (1972) reported a far lower incidence of cardiac dysrhythmias when nitrous oxide rather than carbon dioxide was used as the inflating gas. The commonest dysrhythmia was ventricular extrasystole after the P wave fusing and coinciding with the normally conducted impulse. This was impossible to diagnose by palpation of the radial pulse and was not considered to be of serious significance even though halothane was used in the inhaled anaesthetic mixture. In assessing the relative merits of the two inflating gases they pointed out that the high solubility of carbon dioxide contributed to the more rapid absorption of the gas remaining in the peritoneal cavity and its comparative safety on accidental intravascular injection. Nitrous oxide, which has a plasma solubility 68 per cent that of carbon dioxide, caused fewer cardiac dysrhythmias and a smaller rise in Pa_{CO_2} and, with a lower respiratory drive, gave a quieter field for the surgeon.

Robinson et al. (1975) drew attention to the possibility of an explosion hazard if nitrous oxide were used as the inflating gas. Theoretically, hydrogen and methane could diffuse from the intestines into the peritoneal cavity and combustion would be supported if diathermy were used. However, no such accident was quoted, and no actual gas measurements have yet established the presence of an explosive mixture in the peritoneal cavity. In any case, apart from sterilisation, diathermy is used in relatively few laparoscopies (Corall et al., 1975; Drummond and Scott, 1976).

Kelman et al. (1972) reported some of the cardiovascular changes during laparoscopy. In artificially ventilated patients, a moderate rise in intra-abdominal pressure is accompanied by an increase in central venous pressure and cardiac output. Above a critical but variable intra-abdominal pressure (about 50 cm H_2O—4·9 kPa), central venous pressure and cardiac output fall. The rise of central venous pressure is greater in pregnant than in non-pregnant patients. There is also a significant difference in the rise of central venous pressure between the parous and nulliparous non-pregnant patients. This suggests a better tolerance of laparoscopy in the pregnant or parous patient than in nulliparous non-pregnant patients.

Comment

There is a considerable dispute as to the ideal anaesthetic technique for laparoscopy which must be considered against the choice as to whether carbon dioxide or nitrous oxide is employed as the insufflating gas. When carbon dioxide is used a technique involving total muscle relaxation and artificial ventilation continued for a few minutes beyond the end of the surgical procedure will provide adequate ventilation while the abdomen is distended and will ensure the rapid elimination of carbon dioxide absorbed into the blood stream from the peritoneal cavity. High inflation pressures should not be used for fear of depressing venous return and cardiac output. A close watch must be kept for the occurrence of cardiac dysrhythmias and bradycardia. The former can largely be prevented by the use of moderate hyperventilation whilst the heart rate can be regulated with small doses of atropine.

When nitrous oxide is used as the insufflating gas, a quieter operating field may be expected than with carbon dioxide and an anaesthetic technique involving spontaneous breathing may be used. Hypoxia due to excessive pressure on the diaphragm is unlikely as long as the inhaled anaesthetic mixture contains 37 per cent oxygen. As some post-operative hypoxia may be expected, particularly in patients with respiratory disease, supplementary oxygen should be given during the recovery period. Patients with serious diminution of lung function should always be artificially ventilated during laparoscopy (Corall *et al.*, 1974).

Whatever technique is used the patient must be carefully monitored throughout, and controlled ventilation would seem preferable. A device which limits intra-abdominal pressure to a maximum of 40 cm H_2O (3·9 kPa) should be incorporated in the apparatus delivering gas to the Verrés needle. The surgeon should be well aware that the sudden occurrence of bradycardia and hypotension demands the immediate reduction of the intraperitoneal pressure particularly in patients with impaired cardiac function. Special care is indicated in patients with ruptured ectopic gestation in whom the rate of insufflation and the total volume of insufflating gas should be reduced to minimise the effects of the procedure against the background of acute anaemia and hypovolaemia (Lenz *et al.*, 1976).

In short, while laparoscopy may be regarded as a relatively minor procedure by the gynaecologist, it can pose major problems for the anaesthetist.

THERAPEUTIC TERMINATION OF PREGNANCY

The prevention of excessive haemorrhage is the major preoccupation in termination of pregnancy and it is now well recognised that the critical factor influencing blood loss is the choice of anaesthetic agents and techniques. Cullen *et al.* (1970) noted a reduction in blood loss with reducing halothane concentrations and an even lower blood loss when halothane was omitted altogether from the inhaled anaesthetic mixture. Loung *et al.* (1971) entirely avoided inhalational anaesthesia for therapeutic abortion managed by vacuum aspiration by using intravenous diazepam 10 mg, pentazocine 30 mg, and methohexitone together with 0·5 mg ergometrine. Even so 30 per cent of 1,000 patients lost more than 200 ml blood of whom 61 required fluid replacement.

Dunn *et al.* (1973) recognising the disadvantages of halothane anaesthesia, compared the effects of four other anaesthetic techniques for termination of pregnancy by suction curettage.

(a) Thiopentone, nitrous oxide/oxygen with trichloroethylene.

(b) Thiopentone, suxamethonium, nitrous oxide/oxygen and intermittent positive-pressure ventilation.

(c) Intravenous ketamine and paracervical block with lignocaine 1 per cent.

(d) Intravenous pentazocine and diazepam, increments of methohexitone as required and paracervical block with lignocaine 1 per cent.

Anaesthesia with thiopentone, nitrous oxide, oxygen and trichloroethylene was associated with an unacceptably high average loss of 241 ml and was discontinued at the request of the surgeon. There was a considerably smaller blood loss with the other three techniques, the average ranging from 32–55 ml. Thiopentone, suxamethonium nitrous oxide/oxygen risked the added morbidity of intubation, the side-effects of suxamethonium and in addition nearly half the patients suffered post-operative nausea and vomiting. One-third of the patients given ketamine with paracervical block suffered unpleasant psychic disturbances either while under the anaesthetic or on awakening. The combination of diazepam, pentazocine, with increments of methohexitone followed by paracervical block was associated with low average blood loss (32 ml), no nausea and vomiting and minimal psychic disturbance. It was concluded that this was the technique of choice for therapeutic termination of pregnancy.

Thus will be seen the possibility of numerous variations in anaesthetic technique with the common theme of the need to prevent excessive blood loss by the avoidance of volatile inhalational agents. In view of the current trend towards carrying out terminations as day cases it is also important that patients should recover rapidly from anaesthesia with a minimum of post-operative sequelae.

REFERENCES

ADAMS, A., MORGAN, M., JONES, B. C., and McCORMICK, P. W. (1969). A case of massive aspiration of gastric contents during obstetric anaesthesia. *Brit. J. Anaesth.*, **41**, 176.

ANSARI, I., WALLACE, G., CLEMETSON, C. A. B., MALLIKARJUNESWARA, V. R., and CLEMETSON, C. D. M. (1970). Tilt Caesarean section. *J. Obstet. Gynaec. Brit. Cwlth*, **77**, 713.

ARGENT, D. E., and EVANS, M. D. (1961). Anaesthesia in domiciliary obstetrics. Experiences with a flying squad. *Lancet*, **1**, 994.

BANNISTER, W. K., SATTILARO, A. J., and OTIS, R. D. (1961). Therapeutic aspects of aspiration pneumonitis in experimental animals. *Anesthesiology*, **22**, 440.

BEARD, R. W., and ROBERTS, G. M. (1970). Supine hypotension syndrome. *Brit. med. J.*, **2**, 297.

BIENARZ, J., MAQUEDA, E., and CALDEYRO-BARCIA, R. (1966). Compression of aorta by the uterus in late human pregnancy. *Amer. J. Obstet. Gynec.*, **95**, 795.

BLOGG, C. E., SIMPSON, B. R., TYERS, M. B., MARTIN, L. E., BELL, J. A., ARTHUR, A., JACKSON, M. R., and MILLS, J. (1973). Placental transfer of AH8165. *Brit. J. Anaesth.*, **45**, 638.

BOND, A. G. (1969). Conduction anaesthesia, blood pressure and haemorrhage. *Brit. J. Anaesth.*, **41**, 942.

BOSOMWORTH, P. P., and HAMELBERG, W. (1962). Etiologic therapeutic aspects of aspiration pneumonitis. Experimental study. *Surg. Forum.*, **13**, 158.

BRADFORD, E. M. W., and MOIR, D. D. (1969). Anaesthesia for Caesarean section: A comparison of thiopentone and propanidid. *Brit. J. Anaesth.*, **41**, 274.

CANE, R. D., and SINCLAIR, D. M. (1976). The use of AH8165 for Caesarean section. *Anaesthesia*, **31**, 212.

CLARK, R. B. (1973). Analgesia during labor: effect on the fetus and neonate. In: *Parturition and Perinatology*, p. 148, Ed. by G. F. Marx. Philadelphia: F. A. Davis Co.

COLEMAN, A. J. (1967). Absence of harmful effect of maternal hypocapnia in babies delivered at Caesarean section. *Lancet*, **1**, 813.

CORALL, I. M., ELIAS, J. A., and STRUNIN, L. (1975). Laparoscopy explosion hazards with nitrous oxide. *Brit. med. J.*, **4**, 288.

CORALL, I. M., KNIGHTS, K., POTTER, D., and STRUNIN, L. (1974). Arterial oxygen tensions during laparoscopy with nitrous oxide in the spontaneously breathing patient. *Brit. J. Anaesth.*, **46**, 925.

CRAWFORD, J. S. (1965). *Principles and Practice of Obstetric Anaesthesia*, p. 171. 2nd edit. Oxford: Blackwell Scientific Publications.

CRAWFORD, J. S. (1970). The anaesthetist's contribution to maternal mortality. *Brit. J. Anaesth.* **42**, 70.

CRAWFORD, J. S. (1972). *Principles and Practice of Obstetric Anaesthesia*, p. 209. 3rd edit. Oxford: Blackwell Scientific Publications.

CRAWFORD, J. S., BURTON, M., and DAVIES, P. (1972). Time and lateral tilt at Caesarean section. *Brit. J. Anaesth.*, **44**, 477.

CRAWFORD, J. S., and DAVIES, P. (1975). A return to trichloroethylene for obstetric anaesthesia. *Brit. J. Anaesth.*, **47**, 482.

CRAWFORD, J. S., JAMES III, F. M., DAVIES, P., and CRAWLEY, M. (1976). A further study of general anaesthesia for Caesarean section. *Brit. J. Anaesth.*, **48**, 661.

CULLEN, B. F., MARGOLIS, A. L., and EGER, E. I. (1970). The effects of anaesthesia and pulmonary ventilation and blood loss during elective therapeutic abortion. *Anesthesiology*, **32**, 108.

DAVIES, J. A. H. (1963). Thiopentone and suxamethonium mixture. *Anaesthesia*, **18**, 511.

DAWES, G. S., and MOTT, J. C. (1964). Changes in O_2 distribution and consumption in fetal lambs with variations in umbilical blood flow. *J. Physiol. (Lond.)*, **170**, 524.

DEPARTMENT OF HEALTH and SOCIAL SECURITY (1972). *Report on Confidential Enquiries into Maternal Deaths in England and Wales 1967–1969*. London: H.M.S.O.

DEPARTMENT OF HEALTH and SOCIAL SECURITY (1975). *Report on Confidential Enquiries into Maternal Deaths in England and Wales 1970–1972*. London: H.M.S.O.

DOWNING, J. W., MAHOMEDY, M. C., COLEMAN, A. J., MAHOMEDY, Y. H., and JEAL, D. E. (1974). Anaesthetic induction for Caesarean section. Althesin versus thiopentone. *Anaesthesia*, **29**, 689.

DRUMMOND, G. B., and SCOTT, D. B., (1976). Laparoscopy explosion hazards with nitrous oxide. *Brit. med. J.*, **1**, 1531.

DUFFUS, G. M., TUNSTALL, M. E., and McGILLIVRAY, J. (1968). Intravenous chlormethiazole in pre-eclamptic toxaemia in labour. *Lancet*, **1**, 335.

DUNN, S. R., SECKER WALKER, J., ASTON, D. L., and CRIPPS, D. (1973). Effect of anaesthetic technique on blood loss in termination of pregnancy. *Brit. J. Anaesth.*, **45**, 633.

HAMELBERG, W. and BOSOMWORTH, P. P. (1964). Aspiration pneumonitis: experimental studies and clinical observations. *Anesth. Analg. Curr. Res.*, **43**, 669.

HODGSON, C., McCLELLAND, R. M. A., and NEWTON, J. R. (1970). Some effects of the peritoneal insufflation of carbon dioxide at laparoscopy. *Anaesthesia*, **25**, 382.

HOLMES, F. (1963). Neonatal respiration following abdominal delivery. *Brit. J. Anaesth.*, **35**, 433.

HOLMES, J. M. (1957). The prevention of inhaled vomit during obstetric anaesthesia. *Proc. roy. Soc. Med.*, **50**, 556.

HUTCHINSON, R. (1961). Awareness during surgery: a study of its incidence. *Brit. J. Anaesth.*, **33**, 463.

JOHNSTONE, M., and BREEN, P. J. (1966). Halothane in obstetrics: elective Caesarean section. *Brit. J. Anaesth.*, **38**, 386.

KELMAN, G. R., SWAPP, G. H., SMITH, I., BENZIE, R. J., and GORDON, N. L. M. (1972). Cardiac output and arterial blood gas tension during laparoscopy. *Brit. J. Anaesth.*, **44**, 1155.

KHAWAJA, A. A. (1971a). Thiopentone-suxamethonium mixture: a method for reducing the aspiration hazard during induction of anaesthesia. *Brit. J. Anaesth.*, **43**, 100.

KHAWAJA, A. A. (1971b). A rapid intubation technique for prevention of aspiration during induction of anaesthesia. *Brit. J. Anaesth.*, **43**, 980.

LAHIRI, S. K., THOMAS, T. A., and HODGSON, R. M. H. (1973). Single dose antacid therapy for the prevention of Mendelson's syndrome. *Brit. J. Anaesth.*, **45**, 1143.

LENZ, R. J., THOMAS, T. A., and WILKINS, D. G. (1976). Cardiovascular changes during laparoscopy. *Anaesthesia*, **31**, 4.

LOELIGER, E. A. (1966). *Coagulation Disorders in Obstetrics*, p. 89. Amsterdam: Excerpta Medica.

LOUNG, K. C., BUCKLE, A. E. R., and ANDERSON, M. M., (1971). Results in 1,000 cases of therapeutic abortion managed by vacuum aspiration. *Brit. med. J.*, **4**, 477.

McCORMICK, P. W. (1966). The severe pulmonary aspiration syndrome in obstetrics. *Proc. roy. Soc. Med.*, **59**, 66.

McCORMICK, P. W. (1975). Immediate care after aspiration of vomit. *Anaesthesia*, **30**, 658.

McCORMICK, P. W., HAY, R. G., and GRIFFIN, R. W. (1966). Pulmonary aspiration of gastric contents in obstetric patients. *Lancet*, **1**, 1127.

MAGNO, R., KJELLMER, I., and KARLSSON, K. (1976). Anesthesia for Cesarean section—III. Effects of epidural analgesia on the respiratory adaptation of the newborn in elective Cesarean section. *Acta anaesth. scand.*, **20**, 73.

MAGNO, R., SELSTAM, U., and KARLSSON, K. (1975). Anesthesia for Cesarean section II. Effects of the Induction-Delivery interval on the respiratory adaptation of the newborn in elective Cesarean section. *Acta anaesth. scand.*, **19**, 250.

MAHOMEDY, M. C., DOWNING, J. W., JEAL, D. E., and COLEMAN, A. J. (1976). Anaesthetic induction for Caesarean section with propanidid. *Anaesthesia*, **31**, 205.

MARCUS, R. G., CREWE-BROWN, H., KRAWITZ, S., and KATZ, J. (1975). Feto-maternal haemorrhage following successful and unsuccessful attempts at external cephalic version. *Brit. J. Obstet. Gynaec.*, **82**, 578.

MARX, G. F. (1973). Anesthesia for elective Cesarean section. Clinical anesthesia. In: *Parturition and Perinatology*. Ed. by G. F. Marx. Philadelphia: F. A. Davis Co.

MENDELSON, C. L. (1946). Aspiration of stomach contents into the lungs during obstetric anaesthesia. *Amer. J. Obstet. Gynec.*, **52**, 191.

MILNE, M. K., and LAWSON, J. I. M. (1973). Epidural analgesia for Caesarean section. *Brit. J. Anaesth.*, **45**, 1206.

MINISTRY OF HEALTH (1957). *Report on Confidential Enquiries into Maternal Deaths in England and Wales, 1952–1954*. London: H.M.S.O.

MINISTRY OF HEALTH (1960). *Report on Confidential Enquiries into Maternal Deaths in England and Wales, 1955–1957*. London: H.M.S.O.

MINISTRY OF HEALTH (1963). *Report on Confidential Enquiries into Maternal Deaths in England and Wales, 1958–1960*. London: H.M.S.O.

MINISTRY OF HEALTH (1966). *Report on Confidential Enquiries into Maternal Deaths in England and Wales, 1961–1963*. London: H.M.S.O.

MINISTRY OF HEALTH (1969). *Report on Confidential Enquiries into Maternal Deaths in England and Wales, 1964–1966*. London: H.M.S.O.

MOIR, D. D. (1968). Blood loss during major vaginal surgery. *Brit. J. Anaesth.*, **40**, 233.

MOIR, D. D. (1970). Anaesthesia for Caesarean section. *Brit. J. Anaesth.*, **42**, 136.

MONTGOMERY, J. B. (1961). The effect of halothane on the newborn infant delivered by Caesarean section. *Brit. J. Anaesth.*, **33**, 156.

MOODIE, J. E., and MOIR, D. D. (1976). Ergometrine, oxytocin and extradural analgesia. *Brit. J. Anaesth.*, **48**, 571.

MOTOYAMA, E. K., RIVARD, G., ACHESON, F., and COOK, C. D. (1966). Adverse effect of maternal hyperventilation on the fetus. *Lancet*, **1**, 286.

MOYA, F. (1960). Obstetric anesthesia: general principles. *Bull. Sloane Hosp. Wom. N.Y.*, **6**, 41.

MOYA, F., MORISHIMA, H. O., SHNIDER, S. M., and JAMES, L. S. (1965). Influence of maternal hyperventilation on the newborn infant. *Amer. J. Obstet. Gynec.*, **91**, 76.

O'MULLANE, E. J. (1954). Vomiting and regurgitation during anaesthesia. *Lancet*, **1**, 1209.

PELTZ, B., and SINCLAIR, D. M. (1973). Induction agents for Caesarean section. A comparison of thiopentone and ketamine. *Anaesthesia*, **28**, 37.

PESKETT, W. G. H. (1973). Antacids before obstetric anaesthesia. *Anaesthesia*, **28**, 509.

ROBINSON, J. S., THOMPSON, J. M., and WOOD, A. W. (1975). Laparoscopy explosion hazards with nitrous oxide. *Brit. med. J.*, **3**, 764.

RORKE, M. J., DAVEY, D. A., and DU TOIT, H. J. (1968). Foetal oxygenation during Caesarean section. *Anaesthesia*, **23**, 585.

SCOTT, D. B. (1968). Inferior vena caval occlusion in late pregnancy and its importance in anaesthesia. *Brit. J. Anaesth.*, **40**, 120.

SCOTT, D. B. (1970). Some effects of peritoneal insufflation of carbon dioxide at laparoscopy. *Anaesthesia*, **25**, 590.

SCOTT, D. B., and JULIAN, D. G. (1972). Observations on cardiac arrhythmias during laparoscopy. *Brit. med. J.*, **1**, 411.

SCOTT, D. B., LEES, M. M., DAVIE, I. T., SLAWSON, K. B., and KERR, M. G. (1969). Observations on cardiorespiratory function during Caesarean section. *Brit. J. Anaesth.*, **41**, 489.

SCOTT, J. S. (1969). Disordered blood coagulation in obstetrics, *Brit. J. hosp. Med.*, **2**, 1847.

SCUDAMORE, J. H., and YATES, M. J. (1966). Pudendal block—a misnomer. *Lancet*, **1**, 23.

SEELEY, H. F., and SMITH, R. G. (1976). Immediate care after aspiration of vomit. *Anaesthesia*, **31**, 800.

SELLICK, B. A. (1961). Cricoid pressure to control regurgitation of stomach contents during induction of anaesthesia: preliminary communication. *Lancet*, **2**, 404.

SHNIDER, S. M., and MOYA, F. (1961). Amniotic fluid embolism. *Anesthesiology*, **22**, 108.

SNOW, R. G., and NUNN, J. F. (1959). Induction of anaesthesia in the foot-down position for patients with a full stomach. *Brit. J. Anaesth.*, **31**, 493.

SPENCE, A. A., MOIR, D. D., and FINLAY, W. E. I. (1967). Observations on intragastric pressure. *Anaesthesia*, **22**, 249.

STEEL, G. C. (1961). A hydraulic-powered, foot-operated, tilting obstetric bed. *Brit. med. J.*, **1**, 963.

TAYLOR, G., and PRYSE-DAVIES, J. (1966). The prophylactic use of antacids in the prevention of the acid-pulmonary-aspiration syndrome (Mendelson's syndrome). *Lancet*, **1**, 288.

TUNSTALL, M. E. (1976). Failed intubation drill. *Anaesthesia*, **31**, 850.

TURNER, D. J., and WILSON, J. (1969). Effect of diazepam on awareness during Caesarean section under general anaesthesia. *Brit. med. J.*, **2**, 736.

WEAVER, J. B., PEARSON, J. F., and ROSEN, M. (1975). Posture and epidural block in pregnant women at term. *Anaesthesia*, **30**, 752.

WILLOCKS, J., MONE, J. G., and THOMPSON, W. J. (1966). Amniotic fluid embolism: case with biochemical findings. *Brit. med. J.*, **2**, 1181.

WILSON, J., and TURNER, D. J. (1969). Awareness during Caesarean section under general anaesthesia. *Brit. med. J.*, **1**, 280.

WRIGHT, L. (1962). Postural hypotension in late pregnancy. *Brit. med. J.*, **1**, 760.

WYLIE, W. D. (1956). Modified "Oxford" labour-ward bed. *Lancet*, **1**, 840.

Chapter 44

PLACENTAL TRANSFER OF RESPIRATORY GASES AND DRUGS

THE placenta provides the sole enduring means of communication between the mother and her fetus *in utero* which, like radiocommunication with astronauts, ceases on entry into the earth's atmosphere. It performs for the fetus the function of gastro-intestinal tract, lung, liver, kidney and endocrine gland (Marx, 1961). The human placenta is of the haemomonochorial type, indicating that at term only a single layer of fetal chorionic tissue (the syncytiotrophoblast) separates maternal blood from fetal capillary endothelium. Maternal blood in intervillous spaces or placental sinuses is thus in direct contact with fetal chorionic villi. These chorionic villi are covered with a continuous layer, the syncytiotrophoblast, with isolated remnants of cytotrophoblast beneath it. The fetal capillaries lie in chorionic connective tissue.

The syncytiotrophoblast is the active part of the placenta, performing several functions. (1) It produces placental hormones: chorionic gonadotrophin, placental lactogen, oestrogens, progesterone. (2) It produces enzymes for the active transport of certain essential requirements, and for the breakdown of a few pharmacologically active substances. (3) It has a brush border which can engulf macromolecules and plasma droplets (pinocytosis).

Damage to the syncytiotrophoblast is repaired by fibrin deposition from the maternal circulation. The aging or dysmature placenta may have a reduced area available for maternal-fetal exchange.

The placenta is supplied with maternal blood from the uterine vessels. The uterine blood supply is thus shared by the uterine muscle, the placenta and the fetus. Blood enters the maternal sinuses in jets from the open ends of the placental arterioles. Two umbilical arteries, arising from the fetal internal iliac arteries, carry fetal blood via the umbilical cord to the placenta, and a single umbilical vein returns it to the fetus.

Substances may cross the placenta in several ways:—
1. *By active transport processes*, which are available for the transport of such essential requirements as amino acids, vitamins etc, which are enabled to cross to the fetus against a concentration gradient. Such specialised processes involve the consumption of metabolic energy.
2. *By facilitated diffusion*, which transfers glucose for example down a concentration gradient but at a rate more rapid than simple physical laws would allow.
3. *By simple diffusion*, which occurs only down a concentration gradient and is a purely passive process governed by physical laws.
4. *By pinocytosis* or by leakage across porous defects.

Respiratory gases and drugs used by anaesthetists cross the placenta mainly by passive diffusion.

PLACENTAL TRANSFER OF RESPIRATORY GASES

In the placenta fetal blood is brought into close proximity with maternal blood in the placental sinuses (*vide supra*) and returned, oxygenated, to the fetus via the umbilical vein.

Respiratory gases pass across the placenta by passive diffusion. The placenta does not impose any barrier to diffusion of such small molecules which are said to be rather *flow* dependent than *permeability* dependent (Meschia, *et al.,* 1967).

The transfer of oxygen and carbon dioxide across the placenta is thus dependent upon three factors:—

1. Tension gradient, and relative affinities of maternal and fetal blood for gases.
2. The (a) maternal and (b) fetal blood flow.
3. The area of placental adhesion.

THE TENSION GRADIENT

The transfer of a gas across any biological barrier is dependent upon the tension gradient of the gas across that barrier. The oxygen and carbon dioxide tensions of maternal and fetal blood are given in Table 1.

An important factor which tends to preserve these concentration gradients and so enhance respiratory gas exchange is the difference between the dissociation curves of mother and fetus (see Fig. 1).

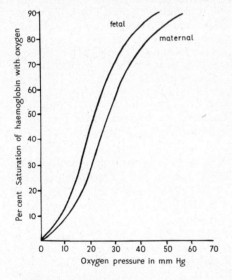

44/Fig. 1.—Oxygen Dissociation Curves of Human Infant at Birth (upper line) and Pregnant Woman (lower line).

Note the large difference in oxygen saturation of fetal and maternal blood at an oxygen pressure of 22 mm Hg (2·9 kPa).

Thus fetal blood shows a higher affinity for oxygen than does maternal blood.

Carbon dioxide.—The CO_2 dissociation curve is nearly linear and maternal and fetal CO_2 tensions are closely correlated over a wide range of values. Carbon dioxide is a highly diffusible gas and the difference in tension between fetal and maternal blood is usually remarkably constant, although Baillie (1970) found that the gradient was considerably increased in the presence of perinatal asphyxia. The double Haldane effect (see Chapter 3), analogous to the double

Bohr effect described below, promotes the passage of carbon dioxide from fetus to mother.

Oxygen. Many factors, however, influence the partial pressure and content of oxygen in maternal and fetal blood.

(a) *The shape of the curve.*—An increase in maternal Po_2 beyond the flat upper part of the dissociation curve increases the maternal oxygen content relatively little, and therefore little additional oxygen becomes available to the fetus. Rorke *et al.* (1968) showed that an increase in maternal Po_2 up to about 300 mm Hg (40 kPa) was accompanied by a related rise in fetal Po_2 but beyond this point no further increase in fetal Po_2 occurred, indeed in some cases the fetal Po_2 actually fell. It has been postulated that this fall could be due to a reduction in placental blood flow (*vide infra*).

44/TABLE 1

OXYGEN AND CARBON DIOXIDE TENSIONS IN MATERNAL AND FETAL BLOOD

	Maternal	Fetal	Tension Gradient
Oxygen	Arterial: 95 mm Hg (12·7 kPa) (96 per cent saturated) Venous: 33 mm Hg (4·4 kPa) (51 per cent saturated)	UA: 15 mm Hg (2·0 kPa) (26 per cent saturated) UV: 28 mm Hg (3·7 kPa) (64 per cent saturated)	80 mm Hg (10·7 kPa)
Carbon dioxide	Arterial: 33 mm Hg (4·4 kPa) Venous: 42 mm Hg (5·6 kPa)	UA: 55 mm Hg (7·3 kPa) UV: 40 mm Hg (5·3 kPa)	22 mm Hg (2·9 kPa)

UA = umbilical artery, i.e. "venous" blood
UV = umbilical vein, i.e. "arterial" blood

(b) *Fetal haemoglobin* has a higher affinity for oxygen than does maternal haemoglobin, as is shown in Fig. 1. Thus at a tension of 22 mm Hg (2·9 kPa) maternal blood is only 38 per cent saturated with oxygen whereas fetal blood reaches a value of 75 per cent saturation. With the progress of pregnancy, adult haemoglobin begins to appear, so that the concentration of this type rises from 6 per cent at the twentieth week to just over 20 per cent at birth. After birth, fetal red cells, and with them fetal haemoglobin, rapidly disappear, so that by the fourth month they can no longer be detected in the blood.

(c) *Increased fetal haemoglobin concentration.*—As pregnancy nears term the fetal PCV rises, while that of the mother is well below normal. At term the fetal haemoglobin concentration is 17–19 g per 100 ml (g/dl) blood, which may be almost double that in the mother.

(d) *The Bohr effect.*—The oxygen dissociation curves of fetal and adult haemoglobin are influenced by the acid-base state.

A "double Bohr" effect was described by Hauge (1969). The transfer of acids from the umbilical arteries into the maternal intervillous spaces causes the fetal pH to rise and increases the affinity of fetal blood to oxygen (Bohr shift to the left). At the same time the acids, passing to the maternal circulation, cause the maternal pH to fall, thereby reducing the affinity of maternal blood for oxygen (Bohr shift to the right), so further oxygen is released to the fetus.

The influence of the Bohr effect on fetal oxygen uptake has been demonstrated principally in sheep. Motoyama *et al.* (1966) studied the anaesthetised ewe and Levinson and his colleagues (1974) the conscious ewe. The latter's findings largely confirm those found in the anaesthetised animal. Their principal observation was that maternal hyperventilation with marked respiratory alkalosis caused hypoxia in the fetus (see Fig. 2). When the duration of maternal hypocapnia was prolonged, a metabolic acidosis could be detected in the fetus.

There may be several causes for the observed fetal hypoxia: Levinson *et al.* (1974) showed that uterine blood flow was reduced during periods of hyperventilation, even when the Pa_{CO_2} was kept within normal limits (by added CO_2), but even when uterine blood flow was reduced by hyperventilation, the fetal oxygen tension was only reduced during periods of maternal respiratory

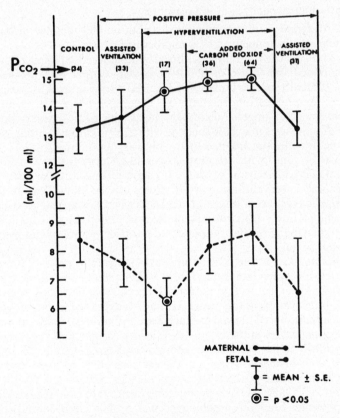

44/Fig. 2.—Changes from control values in mean maternal and fetal arterial oxygen content during five periods of positive-pressure ventilation. Mean maternal Pa_{CO_2} (mm Hg) during each period indicated at top of figure (From Levinson *et al.*, 1974).

alkalosis. The best explanation for this phenomenon was therefore the Bohr effect.

Ralston and his co-workers (1974) confirmed this hypothesis by showing that an infusion of sodium bicarbonate to produce a metabolic alkalosis in ewes did indeed cause a significant degree of fetal hypoxia.

MATERNAL PLACENTAL BLOOD FLOW

The uterine blood flow is distributed to the uterine musculature and to the placenta. The respiratory gases available for exchange with the fetus are contained in that portion of the uterine flow destined for the placenta, allowing for the metabolism of the placenta itself (see Table 2). The placental metabolic oxygen consumption has been found to be between 1 and 2 ml O_2 per minute for an average 0·5 kg placenta (Friedman et al., 1962).

Changes in placental blood flow depend upon:
  i.   The maternal cardiac output and its distribution.
  ii. The vasomotor tone of the uterine vessels.
  iii. The state of uterine contraction.
  iv. Pathological changes in the placenta.

i & ii. **Maternal cardiac output**, its distribution and the **tone of the uterine blood vessels** may be influenced by a number of factors.

Aortocaval occlusion in mothers nursed or anaesthetised supine is the most important remediable cause of a fall in cardiac output and uterine underperfusion. It readily results in fetal bradycardia implying fetal hypoxia. It may occur in any mother at or near term but decompensation is especially likely during epidural block or general anaesthesia, causing overt supine hypotension.

General anaesthesia may be associated with a fall in cardiac output, especially if halothane or enflurane are used in any but very low concentrations. A fall in maternal cardiac output may produce placental underperfusion as evidenced by a fall in fetal Po_2. Levinson et al. (1974) showed that both positive-pressure respiration and hyperventilation could reduce uterine blood flow, but that the effect on fetal oxygenation was more dependent on the maternal acid-base state than upon blood flow (*vide supra*). Bieniartz et al. (1969) suggested that the effect on the fetus of a fall in cardiac output could be offset to some extent by preferential placental flow.

Epidural blockade is free from ill effects upon the fetus unless it is associated with hypotension, when fetal bradycardia is likely. Hypotension, resulting from a block limited in extent to that required for pain relief in labour, is commonly due to decompensation in the presence of aorto-caval occlusion and as such is readily remediable by left uterine displacement. Epidural blockade, in preventing reflex vasoconstriction in the region supplied by the blocked sympathetic outflow, may mitigate the detrimental effect of aorto-caval occlusion on uterine blood flow. This beneficial effect may however be offset by hypotension itself, occurring in the supine position (Weaver et al., 1975).

Johnson and Clayton (1955) produced evidence that caudal epidurals could improve placental function in prolonged and dysfunctional labours. There is evidence that epidural blockade has little effect on uterine blood flow in the normal, though if adrenaline is used blood flow is reduced transiently (Wallis et al., 1976). A lot of workers have shown, however, that epidural analgesia in labour improves both the maternal and fetal acid-base status, and that the metabolic acidosis that usually occurs progressively throughout labour is much reduced in both mother and baby (Pearson and Davies, 1974; Thalme *et al.,* 1974). Moreover if epidural analgesia replaces pethidine, the rise in PCO_2 and fall in pH which may occur in the baby after delivery (even following small doses of pethidine) are avoided (Thalme *et al.,* 1974).

Maternal hyperventilation may reduce uterine blood flow. Hyperventilation can reduce cardiac output and blood pressure and a reduced maternal PCO_2 might theoretically produce uterine vasoconstriction. However, Levinson *et al.* (1974) suggest that in fact the effect of hyperventilation in reducing placental flow is mechanical and, moreover, has little effect *per se* on fetal oxygenation. A significant reduction in fetal oxygenation occurs only in the presence of maternal alkalosis, and is probably the result of the Bohr effect (*vide supra*). Motoyama *et al.* (1966) found that the production of very low maternal PCO_2 levels in ewes reduced *umbilical* blood flow and significant maternal-fetal circulatory mismatch reduced oxygen transfer to the fetus. Prolonged maternal hyperventilation could lead to severe fetal hypoxia and metabolic acidosis.

Provided maternal oxygenation remains constant, a maternal $PaCO_2$ of 30–34 mm Hg (4·0–4·5 kPa) is probably the optimum for fetal oxygenation (Rorke *et al.,* 1968) which falls only when the maternal PCO_2 is well below this level.

However, the combination of maternal hypotension, associated with hyperventilation, diminished uterine blood flow, and the shift of the oxygen dissociation curve may all impair placental transfer of oxygen and produce fetal hypoxaemia. The implication of this observation upon clinical practice is that *excessive* artificial ventilation of a patient anaesthetised at or near term, will tend to restrict the oxygen supply to the fetus. It is most unlikely that the cause of apnoea in a baby born in such circumstances is due to a low arterial CO_2 level. A more probable cause is hypoxia, and appropriate resuscitative measures should be instituted.

Maternal PaO_2.—The importance of the maternal PaO_2 lies in the direct effect it has upon the oxygen tension gradient across the placenta, and its effect on placental perfusion is unimportant. Very high levels, however, well above the optimum 300 mm Hg (40 kPa), may be associated with umbilical vein PO_2 values akin to those found when the mother breathes 21 per cent oxygen (Rorke *et al.,* 1968). This may be because some reduction in placental perfusion occurs at a very high oxygen tension.

Vasopressor drugs.—When a sympathomimetic drug with a predominantly α-stimulant action, such as methoxamine, is used to raise the blood pressure, it is likely to reduce tissue perfusion both because of local vasoconstriction in areas where α-receptors are numerous and also because of reflex cardio-depression (Forrest *et al.,* 1974). The detrimental effect is prominent in the uterine vessels whose α-receptors appear particularly sensitive (Wallis *et al.,* 1976). A sympathomimetic agent with mixed α and β effects, such as ephedrine, methylamphetamine and mephentermine, has a less detrimental effect on tissue perfusion and is to be preferred in obstetrics (Ralston *et al.,* 1974). However even adrenaline, a drug with pronounced *β* effects, has been shown to reduce uterine blood flow in sheep in the absence of hypotension (Rosenfeld *et al.,*

1976). Thus it is clear that in obstetrics no vasopressor should be used until the patient has been turned on her side, the legs have been raised, and plasma expanders tried, and yet a dangerous degree of hypotension is still present; then only a mixed α and β stimulant, such as ephedrine or mephentermine in minimal doses, should be used.

    iii. **Uterine contraction.**—Placental blood flow is appreciably impaired during uterine contractions. The response of a normal fetus to a contraction is a transient bradycardia corresponding to the peak of the contraction. This and other changes in fetal heart rate associated with increasing placental insufficiency are described in Chapter 41.

    iv. **Pathological changes in the maternal blood vessels** supplying the placenta, such as are associated with pre-eclampsia, may result in impaired placental blood supply and placental insufficiency leading to fetal hypoxia and acidosis.

44/TABLE 2

SUMMARY OF O_2 EXCHANGES ACROSS PLACENTA

Uterine arterial O_2 content (ml/100 ml)	15·8	17·0	Umbilical venous O_2 content (ml/100 ml)
Uterine venous O_2 content	10·8	7·0	Umbilical arterial O_2 content
O_2 released per 100 ml	5·0 ml	10·0 ml	Oxygen acquired per 100 ml
But uterine blood flow is 700 ml/min O_2 availability for uterus, placenta and fetus (5·0 ml/100 ml × 700)			But umbilical blood flow is 300 ml/min O_2 acquired *could* be (10 ml/100 ml × 300)
	35 ml/min	30·0 ml/min	

Assumptions

Maternal:

Hb	12 g/100 ml (g/dl)
PaO_2	95 mm Hg (12·7 kPa)
SaO_2	95 per cent
PvO_2	33 mm Hg (4·4 kPa)
SvO_2	55 per cent

Fetal:

Hb	19 g/100 ml (g/dl)
PvO_2	28 mm Hg (3·7 kPa)
SvO_2	64 per cent
PaO_2	15 mm Hg (2·0 kPa)
SaO_2	26 per cent

(from nomograms of Hellegers and Schruefer, 1961)

O_2 Balance Sheet

Uterine O_2 availability		35 ml/min
Fetal O_2 requirement (at term)	18 ml/min	
Uterine O_2 consumption	15 ml/min	
Placental O_2 consumption	1·5 ml/min	
Total debit	34·5	
Balance		+0·5 ml/min

FETAL UMBILICAL BLOOD FLOW

    The potential effect of the blood flow on the fetal side of the placental membrane on respiratory gas exchange should not be overlooked. Vasoconstriction could be caused by an excessively high P_{O_2} (hard to produce in practice), a reduced P_{CO_2} (Motoyama et al., 1966) and by vasopressor drugs. Cord compression during the second stage of labour may also reduce fetal placental blood flow.

Area of Placental Adhesion

Finally, the overall speed of placental gas exchange depends also upon the area of contact available for exchange between maternal and fetal blood. Abruptio placentae or varying degrees of placental separation may lead to fetal hypoxaemia.

Table 2 summarises factors involved in oxygen transfer across the placenta in an ideal "normal" case.

PLACENTAL TRANSFER OF DRUGS

The effects that drugs given to a woman in labour may have upon the fetus and neonate have increased in importance in recent years as graver dangers to the baby have diminished.

Drugs may affect the fetus either indirectly, by altering maternal physiology, or directly after passage across the placenta. When assessing the direct effect, it is useful to understand the factors that influence the extent to which a drug may cross the placenta.

Drugs used to relieve pain or to provide anaesthesia in labour cross the placenta by passive diffusion down a concentration gradient. In this respect, the placenta can be expected to behave like any other lipid membrane such as the blood-brain barrier or the cell membrane. Such a membrane allows the passage of lipid-soluble substances up to a molecular weight of 600–1,000 and of non-ionised water-soluble molecules up to 100. It is self-evident that drugs which act upon the nervous system and can cross the blood-brain barrier are certain to be able to cross the placenta. Inhalational anaesthetics, highly diffusible lipid-soluble molecules that are non-polar (unable to acquire a charge) cross the placenta with ease. Weak acids such as barbiturates and weak bases such as narcotic analgesics and local anaesthetics all cross the placenta readily in the non-ionised state. Fully ionised drugs, such as neuromuscular blocking drugs and other quaternary ammonium compounds, which do not readily cross other lipid barriers in the body, would in theory be expected to diffuse across the placenta only very slowly if at all. In this respect however the placenta does not always behave like other lipid barriers. Large particles, such as macromolecules and even fetal cells, that cannot diffuse across lipid membranes do cross the placenta, either by pinocytosis or across hypothetical porous defects.

Three aspects of placental transfer of drugs must be considered:—
1. The rate of transfer.
2. The fetal-maternal concentration ratio in equilibrium or steady state.
3. Factors that might upset this equilibrium.

The Rate of Placental Transfer

Both placental and drug characteristics influence the rate of passive diffusion.

(a) Placental Factors

(i) *The area and thickness of the membrane.* The reduction in area available for exchange in the aging placenta could theoretically retard net drug transfer and so delay equilibration. In practice this factor is probably less important in the context of drug transfer than it is to the supply of metabolic requirements.

(ii) *Maternal and fetal blood flow.* Blood flow on either side of the membrane maintains the concentration gradient of any substance that is not in equilibrium across the placenta, and so promotes its passage. Maternal placental flow may be reduced by a number of mechanisms which are of vital importance in the transfer of respiratory gases (see p. 1400), but the only factor of note concerned in drug transfer is the effect that transient reduction in blood flow during uterine contraction may have upon transfer of a drug injected by intravenous bolus.

(iii) *Placental enzymes.* The placenta contains numerous enzymes and there is evidence of some drug metabolism, for example of barbiturates, within the placenta (Kyegombe *et al.*, 1973).

(b) Drug Characteristics

Concentration gradient and lipid solubility are the salient drug factors influencing the rate of transfer (Seeds *et al.*, 1976). The route of administration affects the concentration gradient: a bolus intravenous injection may lead to a short-lived high maternal concentration and consequent massive transfer. Only the *free, non-ionised* drug is diffusible, thus high-protein binding and a high degree of ionisation can both reduce the effective concentration gradient. Drugs used for analgesia and anaesthesia in labour all possess molecular weights compatible with lipid diffusion, thus lipid solubility, itself partly dependent upon pKa, promotes rapid placental transfer. There is ample evidence, however, that inhalation anaesthetics and induction agents, and local and systemic analgesic drugs, all cross the placenta very rapidly (*vide infra*) as there is no barrier to diffusion of such lipid-soluble drugs. Because the fetus does not require or *consume* these drugs, as it does essential requirements such as oxygen, their *rate* of transfer is of no clinical importance. Fully ionised drugs such as quaternary ammonium compounds, on the other hand, would be expected to cross at a very slow rate.

The Fetal-Maternal Concentration Ratio

For local anaesthetic drugs and those acting upon the central nervous system, the fetal-maternal plasma concentration ratio is not, beyond the first few minutes, directly related to sampling time, as it would be if the rate of transfer were slow. In fact, there is a persistent and fairly consistent apparent gradient for a given drug even in the presence of a relatively steady maternal concentration.

Two drug characteristics influence this steady state ratio:

(i) **pKa** (see p. 734). This property determines the degree of ionisation at a given pH. There is normally a small pH gradient across the placenta; basic drugs are more ionised in the more acid fetus, while acidic drugs are more ionised in the mother. Only the non-ionised form diffuses across readily, and so the free concentration of a basic drug tends to be higher in the fetus (see Fig. 3), and that of an acidic drug higher in the mother. The stronger the base or acid, the more marked will be this disparity. A very weak acid or base—virtually non-ionised—would by contrast tend to have a fetal-maternal free concentration ratio near unity.

(ii) **Protein binding.** Disparity in protein binding between fetal and maternal plasma is probably the most important determinant of the equilibrium in fetal-maternal ratio (see Fig. 3). *In vitro* studies of the binding of a range of acidic drugs (Ehrnebo *et al.*, 1971) and of local anaesthetics (Tucker *et al.*, 1970; Thomas *et al.*, 1976) suggest more extensive binding by maternal than by fetal plasma. Mendenhall (1970) demonstrated a higher concentration of certain proteins, including albumin, in the umbilical cord than in the maternal circulation at vaginal delivery, and the reverse at Caesarean section. Levy *et al.* (1975)

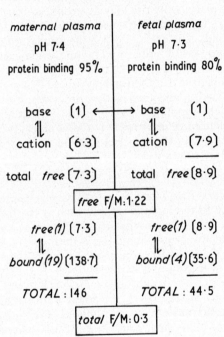

BUPIVACAINE, pK_a 8·2

44/FIG. 3.—Transplacental distribution of a basic drug such as bupivacaine with a pKa of 8·2. At equilibrium the concentration of *unbound, non-ionised* drug (free base), the diffusible component, is equal in maternal and fetal plasma. The top half of the figure shows how the distribution of *free* (unbound) drug is determined by the pH gradient and the pKa, relative concentrations of cation and base having been calculated from the Henderson-Hasselbalch equation. The lower half of the figure shows how disparities in protein binding alter the final total concentration in mother and fetus.

A pH gradient of 0·1 between maternal and fetal plasma is in accord with the findings of Thalme *et al.* (1974). Protein-binding figures are derived from Reynolds (1970). The figure for fetal plasma is higher than that reported by Tucker *et al.* (1970) of 65 per cent. This percentage may be artificially low because it was measured at a concentration much higher than that found clinically. The same balance was demonstrated by Thomas *et al.* (1976) who found a fetal-maternal ratio for bupivacaine of 0·24, and slightly lower fetal and maternal protein binding, demonstrating no gradient for free non-ionised bupivacaine.

found higher protein binding of salicylate in fetal than in maternal plasma, both *in vivo* and *in vitro*, not fully accounted for by higher fetal plasma protein concentration.

One can postulate, therefore, that except when maternal concentration of a drug is changing rapidly, there may actually be little or no gradient for *diffusible* (free, non-ionised) drugs between maternal and umbilical venous plasma. Drugs may continue to cross the placenta because of a gradient between maternal arterial and umbilical arterial plasma, accounting for a persistent gradient between umbilical artery and vein.

Factors That Might Upset the Equilibrium
(Levy and Hayton, 1973)

Any rapid rise or fall in maternal concentration of a drug is likely to recreate a gradient across the placenta. A rise may be produced by maternal inhalation or a bolus intravenous injection. The reverse occurs when stopping inhalation, because the fetus cannot exhale drugs as can the mother, or after a bolus when drug redistribution produces a more rapid fall in the maternal than in the fetal circulation.

The maternal rate of drug metabolism may exceed that of the fetus, especially for aromatic hydroxylation and conjugation processes, but the disparity may be less than one might suppose for the comparatively small load imposed by analgesic drugs. The fetus may be protected to some extent because a proportion of drug in umbilical venous blood is detoxicated in the liver before gaining access to the systemic circulation.

Total Dose of Drug Received by the Fetus

The absolute concentration of a drug in fetal plasma and tissues is, of course, of greater importance to the infant's welfare than is the fetal-maternal ratio. As this concentration is a product of maternal concentration and fetal-maternal ratio, the extent to which a drug accumulates in the maternal circulation may be crucial for the baby. Moreover, the longer the time that the baby is exposed to high concentrations of a drug and its metabolites, the more nearly will fetal tissues become saturated with the substances, and the longer it will take the fetus to eliminate them. Thus, Apgar scores, measured within minutes of birth, may fail to distinguish deleterious effects of cumulative depressant drugs, which could better be detected by later neuro-behavioural assessment (Brazelton, 1973; Brackbill *et al.*, 1974a).

PLACENTAL TRANSFER OF INDIVIDUAL DRUGS

Inhalational Anaesthetics

Inhalational anaesthetics diffuse rapidly across the placenta, and provided they are evenly distributed between cells and plasma (because of the difference between maternal and fetal haematocrits) one would expect the equilibrium whole blood fetal-maternal ratios to be near unity. Indeed, the solubility of inhalation agents in maternal and fetal blood is very similar; the greatest disparity has been observed with halothane, which is about 1·3 times as soluble in maternal as in fetal blood (Gibb *et al.*, 1975).

Yet it has long been remarked that babies frequently emerge awake from anaesthetised mothers, a phenomenon contributing to the impression of a placental "barrier". The presence of a barrier is a misconception. The fetus comprises a compartment that is "deeper" (Levy and Hayton, 1973) than maternal vessel-rich tissues and equilibrium may take longer than would be expected even for nitrous oxide (Marx et al., 1970). Marx and her co-workers found umbilical venous-maternal ratios of about 0·8 during nitrous oxide anaesthesia, with evidence of continued uptake in a persistent umbilical arterio-venous gradient, after maximum duration of administration of 19 minutes. Stenger et al. (1969) studied the effect of prolonged thiopentone/nitrous oxide anaesthesia, and after a mean of 36 minutes, uterine venous and umbilical venous nitrous oxide concentrations were nearly equal. The incidence of depressed infants increased with duration of anaesthesia.

The much more soluble methoxyflurane equilibrates even more slowly than nitrous oxide. Maternal and fetal plasma concentrations of methoxyflurane have been measured during both analgesia and anaesthesia and in both cases, umbilical venous-maternal ratios were about 0·7 with evidence of continuing uptake after 15 minutes of anaesthesia. The neonatal methoxyflurane levels and incidence of depression were higher when methoxyflurane anaesthesia succeeded analgesia, than when analgesia or brief anaesthesia were given on their own (Clark et al., 1970; Siker et al., 1968).

In a study of the distribution of radioactive halothane in maternal and fetal guinea-pig tissues, the concentration after 5 to 45 minutes was higher in all maternal than fetal tissues except the liver, in which fetal concentrations exceeded maternal (Geddes et al., 1972).

The likelihood of neonatal depression is clearly greater from anaesthetic than from analgesic doses of anaesthetics, yet for such cumulative agents as trichloroethylene and methoxyflurane, long duration of analgesia may often be detrimental. Phillips and Macdonald (1971) found lower Apgar scores in infants of mothers given trichloroethylene analgesia than in the control group, while nitrous oxide, a much less cumulative drug, had no such effect. The 50 per cent oxygen in Entonox may contribute an overall benefit. This is in contrast to the necessarily limited concentration of oxygen in nitrous oxide anaesthesia, which may contribute to the detrimental effect of prolonged nitrous oxide anaesthesia (Palahniuk et al., 1977).

Barbiturates

Barbiturates are weak acids whose pKa values are near or above the physiological pH range. They are, therefore, largely non-ionised and pass readily across the placenta by lipid diffusion. Protein binding may be more extensive in maternal than in fetal plasma (Ehrnebo et al., 1971), thus at equilibrium both free and total concentrations are higher in mother than in fetus. Bolus intravenous injection of the more highly lipid-soluble barbiturates produces early massive transfer and early peak fetal levels, with backwash occasionally producing levels transiently higher in fetus than mother. Cassano et al. (1967) showed that thiopentone administered intravenously to mice produced peak fetal levels in 10 minutes whereas the much less lipid-soluble phenobarbitone did not reach a maximum in the fetus until 30 minutes. Finster et al. (1966) found lower cord concentrations of thiopentone after vaginal delivery than after Caesarean section and suggested that cord compression limits transfer.

Kyegombe *et al.* (1973) found evidence of hexobarbitone metabolism by human placentae.

Large doses of barbiturates given to women in labour are recognised to produce neonatal depression and have been found to delay the establishment of breast feeding by as much as two days (Brazelton, 1961).

Narcotic Analgesics

Narcotic analgesic drugs, being amines, are bases and are more than 95 per cent ionised at physiological pH. Nevertheless the non-ionised fraction is of sufficient lipid solubility for rapid placental transfer by lipid diffusion. Shier *et al.* (1973) gave pethidine intravenously over 3 minutes to pregnant ewes and found that umbilical venous exceeded maternal arterial concentrations within a minute of the end of infusion, and thereafter remained higher, which is compatible with the pH gradient effect and an element of backwash. Clinical studies have demonstrated fetal-maternal pethidine ratios of usually less than unity (Apgar *et al.*, 1952; Crawford and Rudofsky, 1965), although always higher than those of pentazocine (Beckett and Taylor, 1967; Duncan *et al.*, 1969; Moore *et al.*, 1973). A fetal-maternal ratio of less than one can be accounted for by incomplete fetal-maternal equilibration, and indeed Caldwell and his associates (1977) found that at least two-and-a-half hours may elapse before the fetal concentration exceeded that found in the mother. The more marked accumulation of pethidine than pentazocine in mothers results in neonatal pethidine levels many times higher than pentazocine. The half-life of pethidine in the neonate may be more than 20 hours—greatly in excess of that found in the mother (Caldwell *et al.*, 1977).

Pethidine has long been known to produce neonatal sedation with respiratory depression that may not be reversed by the older narcotic antagonists (Roberts *et al.*, 1957). Even small doses impair the acid-base state (Thalme *et al.*, 1974), suckling and other neuro-behavioural responses (Brackbill *et al.*, 1974*b*). The detrimental effect has been found to be greatest when pethidine has been given 3 hours or more before delivery (Shnider and Moya, 1964; Morrison *et al.*, 1973) and has been attributed to the accumulation of metabolites (Stephen and Cooper, 1977; Morrison *et al.*, 1976).

Although pentazocine crosses the placenta less readily than pethidine, a difference in effect on the neonate has not been demonstrated (Duncan *et al.*, 1969). Moreover, pentazocine usually produces less effective pain relief than pethidine, albeit with fewer side-effects (Moore *et al.*, 1970).

Tranquillisers

Although phenothiazines are used extensively in labour and, as weak bases, are certain to cross the placenta, few studies of their placental transfer have been made. Promazine crosses the placenta rapidly, but fetal levels are lower than maternal (Crawford and Rudofsky, 1965). Chlorpromazine crosses the placenta readily but its conjugated metabolites (water soluble substances) do not, nor can the baby produce them (O'Donoghue, 1971). Chlorpromazine itself becomes concentrated in the fetal eye (Ullberg, 1973), a finding possibly associated with phenothiazine retinopathy.

In contrast to the phenothiazines, diazepam, during its short period of popularity for routine obstetrics, was quite extensively studied. It is a very poorly ionised base and an equal distribution between fetal and maternal plasma would be expected. Yet the fetal-maternal ratio appears quite consistently to be 2 (Idanpaan-Heikkila *et al.*, 1971; Erkkola *et al.*, 1973; Mandelli *et al.*, 1975) a finding that has been attributed to more extensive fetal than maternal protein binding. The concentration in the fetal heart is high, an interesting finding in view of the depression of cardiac autonomic control with which diazepam is associated. It causes loss of beat-to-beat variation of fetal heart rate, hypothermia and hypotonia in the neonate.

Local Anaesthetics

Local anaesthetics are weak bases that all cross the placenta readily but whose equilibrium fetal-maternal ratios vary greatly. They range from about 0·3 for bupivacaine and etidocaine, 0·55 for lignocaine, 0·7 for mepivacaine to >1 for prilocaine (Reynolds and Taylor, 1970; Poppers *et al.*, 1975; Lund *et al.*, 1977; Moore *et al.*, 1968; Morishima *et al.*, 1966; Epstein *et al.*, 1968). These fetal-maternal ratios appear to be related to protein binding, the most highly bound yielding the lowest ratios. Tucker *et al.* (1970), Reynolds (1970) and Thomas *et al.* (1976) demonstrated more extensive binding of local anaesthetics to maternal than to fetal plasma proteins. Thomas *et al.* (1976) found that there was actually no gradient for free non-ionised bupivacaine across the placenta. The effect of a high degree of maternal binding on the fetal-maternal ratio is explained in Fig. 3.

Bupivacaine and etidocaine used epidurally yield low maternal concentrations, consequently neonatal concentrations are very much lower than those of lignocaine and mepivacaine: both markedly cumulative when used for continuous epidural analgesia in labour. Prilocaine, although producing low maternal levels is little used in obstetrics because of the danger of methaemoglobinaemia.

There is evidence that the neonate can eliminate lignocaine much as can the mother (Shnider and Way, 1968*a*; Blankenbaker *et al.*, 1975). Brown *et al.* (1975) found a lignocaine half-life in the neonate of 3 hours, that is within normal adult limits (Aps *et al.*, 1976) but that of mepivacaine was 9 hours. Mepivacaine metabolism may be depressed in neonates (Meffin *et al.*, 1973). Caldwell *et al.* (1976) suggest that bupivacaine elimination may be delayed in the neonate.

Low Apgar scores associated with high plasma concentrations of local anaesthetics, have been reported after prolonged epidural analgesia with lignocaine (Shnider and Way, 1968*b*) and mepivacaine (Morishima *et al.*, 1966). No such association has been reported with bupivacaine. In a trial without random allocation of patients, infants born of mothers who had received epidural analgesia with lignocaine or mepivacaine, had lower scores for muscle strength and tone than the bupivacaine series, although other neuro-behavioural responses were similar (Scanlon *et al.*, 1974). The same workers found no such detrimental effect associated with bupivacaine (Scanlon *et al.*, 1976).

Neuromuscular Blocking Drugs

Neuromuscular blockers are all quaternary ammonium compounds, which are fully ionised, and therefore would be expected to diffuse across the placenta only very slowly. The delivery of a vigorous baby from a mother paralysed by a normal dose of a neuromuscular blocking drug provides familiar clinical evidence to support this theory. True neonatal neuromuscular blockade may occur only after prolonged curarisation. A case was reported of a curarised baby born at 28 weeks' gestation to a mother who had been given 245 mg of tubocurarine in the treatment of status epilepticus (Older and Harris, 1968).

Studies of small doses of alcuronium, pancuronium, dimethyltubocurarine and suxamethonium suggest that a bolus injection may force small quantities of these drugs across the placenta, but that in such circumstances, equilibrium distribution between fetus and mother does not occur and paralysing levels are not reached in the fetus (Thomas et al., 1969; Speirs and Sim, 1972; Kivalo and Saarikoski, 1976; Drabkova et al., 1973). Umbilical venous:maternal venous ratios as high as 0·4 have been reported for pancuronium after 20 minutes anaesthesia (Booth et al., 1977), but this compares a pre-mixed fetal level with a post-mixed maternal, and therefore does not represent anything approaching a clinically effective fetal dose.

Drabkova et al. (1973) state that the placenta does not break down suxamethonium, and they showed that fetal monkey plasma broke down suxamethonium more slowly than maternal. They therefore suggest that large successive doses to the mother and the administration of anticholinesterase to the baby, might cause neonatal paralysis.

Atropine and Neostigmine

Atropine, a weak base, crosses the placenta and, after intravenous injection to the mother causing a rapid rise in maternal heart rate, produces a slow rise in fetal heart rate (Schifferli and Caldeyro-Barcia, 1973). The fetal-maternal ratio has been found to rise rapidly to about 93 per cent at 5 minutes (Kivalo and Saarikoski, 1977). Neostigmine, which possesses a quaternary ammonium group, is unlikely to cross the placenta readily. Indeed, there is circumstantial evidence that it does not cross, since when given to the mother, it fails to reduce atropine tachycardia in the fetus.

REFERENCES

APGAR, V., BURNS, J. J., BRODIE, B. B., and PAPPER, E. M. (1952). The transmission of meperidine across the human placenta. Amer. J. Obstet. Gynec., 64, 1368.

APS, C., BELL, J. A., JENKINS, B. S., POOLE-WILSON, P. A., and REYNOLDS, F. (1976). Logical approach to lignocaine therapy. Brit. med. J., 1, 13.

BAILLIE, P. (1970). Acid-base balance at birth. Proc. roy. Soc. Med., 63, 78.

BECKETT, A. H., and TAYLOR, J. F. (1967). Blood concentrations of pethidine and pentazocine in mother and infant at time of birth. J. Pharm. Pharmacol., 19, Suppl., 50.

BIENIARTZ, J., YOSHIDA, T., ROMERO-SALINAS, G., CURUCHETE, B., CALDEYRO-BARCIA, R., and CROTTOGINI, J. J. (1969). Aorto-caval compression in late human pregnancy. Amer. J. Obstet. Gynec., 103, 19.

BLANKENBAKER, W. L., DIFAZIO, C. A., and BERRY, F. A. (1975). Lidocaine and its metabolites in the newborn. *Anesthesiology*, **42**, 325.

BOOTH, P. N., WATSON, M. J., and MCLEOD, K. (1977). Pancuronium and the placental barrier. *Anaesthesia*, **32**, 320.

BRACKBILL, Y., KANE, J., MANNIELLO, R. L., and ABRAMSON, D. (1974*a*). Obstetric premedication and infant outcome. *Amer. J. Obstet. Gynec.*, **118**, 377.

BRACKBILL, Y., KANE, J., MANNIELLO, R. L., and ABRAMSON, D. (1974*b*). Obstetric meperidine usage and assessment of neonatal status. *Anesthesiology*, **40**, 116.

BRAZELTON, T. B. (1961). Psychophysiological reactions in the neonate II. Effect of maternal medication in the neonate and his behaviour. *J. Pediat.*, **58**, 513.

BRAZELTON, T. B. (1973). Assessment of the infant at risk. *Clin. Obstet. Gynec.*, **16**, 361.

BROWN, W. U., BELL, G. C., LURIE, A. O., WEISS, J. B., SCANLON, J. W., and ALPER, M. H. (1975). Newborn blood levels of lidocaine and mepivacaine in the first postnatal day following maternal epidural anesthesia. *Anesthesiology*, **42**, 698.

CALDWELL, J., MOFFATT, J. R., SMITH, R. L., LIEBERMAN, B. A., CAWSTON, M. O., and BEARD, R. W. (1976). Pharmacokinetics of bupivacaine administered epidurally during childbirth. *Brit. J. clin. Pharmacol.*, **3**, 956P.

CALDWELL, J., WAKILE, L. A., NOTARIANNI, L. J., SMITH, R. L., LIEBERMAN, B. A., JEFFS, J., COY, Y., and BEARD, R. W. (1977). Transplacental passage and neonatal elimination of pethidine given to mothers in childbirth. *Brit. J. clin. Pharmacol.*, **4**, 715P–716P.

CASSANO, G. B., GHETTI, B., GLIOZZI, E., and HANSSON, E. (1967). Autoradiographic distribution study of "short-acting" and "long-acting" barbiturates: ^{35}S-thiopentone and ^{14}C-phenobarbitone. *Brit. J. Anaesth.*, **39**, 11.

CLARK, R. B., COOPER, J. O., BROWN, W. E., and GREIFENSTEIN, F. E. (1970). The effect of methoxyflurane on the foetus. *Brit. J. Anaesth.*, **42**, 286.

CRAWFORD, J. S., and RUDOFSKY, S. (1965). Placental transmission and neonatal metabolism of promazine. *Brit. J. Anaesth.*, **37**, 303.

DRABKOVA, J., CRUL, J. F., and VAN DER KLEIJN, E. (1973). Placental transfer of ^{14}C labelled succinylcholine in near-term Macaca Mulatta monkeys. *Brit. J. Anaesth.*, **45**, 1087.

DUNCAN, S. L. B., GINSBURG, J., and MORRIS, N. F. (1969). Comparison of pentazocine and pethidine in normal labor. *Amer. J. Obstet. Gynec.*, **105**, 197.

EHRNEBO, M., AGURELL, S., JALLING, B., and BOREUS, L. O. (1971). Age differences in drug binding by plasma proteins: studies on human foetuses, neonates and adults. *Europ. J. clin. Pharmacol.*, **3**, 189–193.

EPSTEIN, B. S., BANERJEE, S. G., and COAKLEY, C. S. (1968). Passage of lidocaine and prilocaine across the placenta. *Anesth. Analg. Curr. Res.* **47**, 223.

ERKKOLA, R., KANGAS, L., and PEKKARINEN, A. (1973). The transfer of diazepam across the placenta during labour. *Acta obstet. gynec. scand.*, **52**, 167.

FINSTER, M., MARK, L. C., MORISHIMA, H. O., MOYA, F., PEREL, J. M., JAMES, L. S., and DAYTON, P. G. (1966). Plasma thiopental concentration in the newborn following delivery under thiopental-nitrous oxide anesthesia. *Amer. J. Obstet. Gynec.*, **95**, 621.

FORREST, A. L., LAWSON, J. I. M., and OTTON, P. E. (1974). A non-invasive technique of comparing myocardial performance following epidural blockade and vasopressor therapy. *Brit. J. Anaesth.*, **46**, 662.

FRIEDMAN, E. A., LITTLE, W. A., and SACHTLEBEN, M. R. (1962). Placental oxygen consumption *in vitro*. *Amer. J. Obstet. Gynec.*, **84**, 561.

GEDDES, I. C., BRAND, L., FINSTER, M., and MARK, L. (1972). Distribution of halothane-^{82}Br in maternal and foetal guinea-pig tissues. *Brit. J. Anaesth.*, **44**, 542.

GIBB, C. P., MUNSON, E. S., and THAM, M. K. (1975). Anesthetic solubility coefficients for maternal and fetal blood. *Anesthesiology*, **43**, 100.

HAUGE, A. (1969). Gasvekslingen i placenta. *Nord. Med.*, **20**, 621.

HELLEGERS, A. E., and SCHRUEFER, J. J. (1961). Nomograms and empirical equations relating oxygen tension, percentage saturation, and pH in maternal and fetal blood. *Amer. J. Obstet. Gynec.*, **81**, 377.

IDANPAAN-HEIKKILA, J. E., JOUPPILA, P. I., POULAKKA, J. O., and VORNE, M. S. (1971). Placental transfer and fetal metabolism of diazepam in early human pregnancy. *Amer. J. Obstet. Gynec.*, **109**, 1011.

JOHNSON, T., and CLAYTON, C. G. (1955). Studies in placental action during prolonged and dysfunctional labours using radioactive sodium. *J. Obstet. Gynaec. Brit. Cwlth.*, **62**, 513.

KIVALO, I., and SAARIKOSKI, S. (1976). Placental transfer of ^{14}C-dimethyltubocurarine during caesarean section. *Brit. J. Anaesth.*, **48**, 239.

KIVALO, I., and SAARIKOSKI, S. (1977). Placental transmission of atropine at full-term pregnancy. *Brit. J. Anaesth.*, **49**, 1017.

KYEGOMBE, D., FRANKLIN, C., and TURNER, P. (1973). Drug-metabolising enzymes in the human placenta, their induction and repression. *Lancet*, **1**, 405.

LEVINSON, G., SHNIDER, S. M., LORIMER, A. A., and STEFFENSON, J. L. (1974). Effects of maternal hyperventiliation on uterine blood flow and fetal oxygenation and acid-base status. *Anesthesiology*, **40**, 340.

LEVY, G., and HAYTON, W. L. (1973). Pharmacokinetic aspects of placental drug transfer. In: *Fetal Pharmacology*, pp. 29–39. Ed. by L. Boreus. New York: Raven Press.

LEVY, G., PROCKNAL, J. A., and GARRETTSON, L. K. (1975). Distribution of salicylate between neonatal and maternal serum at diffusion equilibrium. *Clin. Pharmacol. Ther.*, **18**, 210.

LUND, P. C., CWIK, J. C., GANNON, R. T., and VASSALLO, H. G. (1977). Etidocaine for Caesarean section—effects on mother and baby. *Brit. J. Anaesth.*, **49**, 457.

MANDELLI, M., MORSELLI, P. L., NORDIO, S., PARDI, G., PRINCIPI, N., SERENI, F., and TOGNONI, G. (1975). Placental transfer of diazepam and its disposition in the newborn. *Clin. Pharmacol. Ther.*, **17**, 565.

MARX, G. F. (1961). Placental transfer and drugs used in anesthesia. *Anesthesiology*, **22**, 294.

MARX, G. F., JOSHI, C. W., and ORKIN, L. R. (1970). Placental transmission of nitrous oxide. *Anesthesiology*, **32**, 429.

MEFFIN, P., LONG, G. J., and THOMAS, J. (1973). Clearance and metabolism of mepivacaine in the human neonate. *Clin. Pharmacol. Ther.*, **14**, 218.

MENDENHALL, H. W. (1970). Serum protein concentrations in pregnancy III. Analysis of maternal-cord serum pairs. *Amer. J. Obstet. Gynec.*, **106**, 718.

MESCHIA, G., BATTAGLIA, F. C., and BRUNS, P. D. (1967). Theoretical and experimental study of transplacental diffusion. *J. appl. Physiol.*, **22**, 1171.

MIRKIN, B. L. (1973). Drug distribution in pregnancy. In: *Fetal Pharmacology*, pp. 1–26. Ed. by L. Boreus. New York: Raven Press.

MOORE, D. C., BRIDENBAUGH, L. D., BAGDI, P. A., and BRIDENBAUGH, P. O. (1968). Accumulation of mepivacaine hydrochloride during caudal block. *Anesthesiology*, **29**, 585.

MOORE, J., CARSON, R. M., and HUNTER, R. J. (1970). A comparison of the effects of pentazocine and pethidine administered during labour. *J. Obstet. Gynaec. Brit. Cwlth.*, **77**, 830.

MOORE, J., MCNABB, T. G., and GLYNN, J. P. (1973). The placental transfer of pentazocine and pethidine. *Brit. J. Anaesth.*, **45**, 798.

MORISHIMA, H. O., DANIEL, S. S., FINSTER, M., POPPERS, P. J., and JAMES, L. S. (1966). Transmission of mepivacaine hydrochloride (Carbocaine) across the human placenta. *Anesthesiology*, **27**, 147.

MORRISON, J. C., WHYBREW, W. D., ROSSER, S. I., BUCOVAZ, E. T., WISER, W. L., and FISH, S. A. (1976). Metabolites of meperidine in the fetal and maternal serum. *Amer. J. Obstet. Gynec.*, **126**, 997.

MORRISON, J. C., WISER, W. L., ROSSER, S. I., GAYDEN, J. O., BUCOVAZ, E. T., WHYBREW, W. D., and FISH, S. A. (1973). Metabolites of meperidine related to fetal depression. *Amer. J. Obstet. Gynec.*, **115**, 1132.

MOTOYAMA, E. K., RIVARD, G., ACHESON, F., and COOK, C. D. (1966). Adverse effect of maternal hyperventilation on the foetus. *Lancet*, **1**, 286.

O'DONOGHUE, S. E. F. (1971). Distribution of pethidine and chlorpromazine in maternal, foetal and neonatal biological fluids. *Nature (Lond.)*, **229**, 124.

OLDER, P. O., and HARRIS, J. M. (1968). Placental transfer of tubocurarine. *Brit. J. Anaesth.*, **40**, 459.

PALAHNIUK, R. J., SCATLIFF, J., BIEHL, D., WIEBE, H., and SANKARAN, K. (1977). Maternal and neonatal effects of methoxyflurane, nitrous oxide and lumbar epidural anaesthesia for Caesarian section. *Canad. Anaesth. Soc. J.*, **24**, 586.

PEARSON, J. F., and DAVIES, P. (1974). The effect of continuous lumbar epidural analgesia upon fetal acid-base status during the first stage of labour. *J. Obst. Gynaec. Brit. Cwlth.*, **81**, 971.

PHILLIPS, T. J., and MACDONALD, R. R. (1971). Comparative effect of pethidine, trichloroethylene and Entonox on fetal and neonatal acid-base and P_{O_2}. *Brit. med. J.*, **3**, 558.

POPPERS, P., COVINO, B., and BOYES, N. (1975). Epidural block with etidocaine for labour and delivery. *Acta anaesth. scand.*, Suppl. 60, 89.

RALSTON, D. H., SHNIDER, S. M., and LORIMER, A. A. (1974). Uterine blood flow and fetal acid-base changes after bicarbonate administration to the pregnant ewe. *Anesthesiology*, **40**, 348.

REYNOLDS, F. (1970). *Systemic toxicity of local analgesic drugs with special reference to bupivacaine.* M.D. thesis (Univ. of London).

REYNOLDS, F., and TAYLOR, G. (1970). Maternal and neonatal concentrations of bupivacaine: a comparison with lignocaine during continuous extradural analgesia. *Anaesthesia*, **25**, 14.

ROBERTS, H., KANE, K. M., PERCIVAL, N., SNOW, P., and PLEASE, N. W. (1957). Effects of some analgesic drugs used in childbirth with special reference to variation in respiratory minute volume of the newborn. *Lancet*, **1**, 128.

RORKE, M. J., DAVEY, D. A., and DU TOIT, H. J. (1968). Foetal oxygenation during Caesarean section. *Anaesthesia*, **23**, 585.

ROSENFELD, C. R., BARTON, M. D., and MESCHIA, G. (1976). Effects of epinephrine on distribution of blood flow in the pregnant ewe. *Amer. J. Obstet. Gynec.*, **124**, 156.

SCANLON, J. W., BROWN, W. U., WEISS, J. B., and ALPER, M. H. (1974). Neurobehavioural responses of newborn infants after maternal epidural anesthesia. *Anesthesiology*, **40**, 121.

SCANLON, J. W., OSTHEIMER, G. W., LURIE, A. O., BROWN, W. U., WEISS, J. B., and ALPER, M. H. (1976). Neurobehavioural responses and drug concentrations in newborns after maternal epidural anesthesia with bupivacaine. *Anesthesiology*, **45**, 400.

SCHIFFERLI, P-Y., and CALDEYRO-BARCIA, R. (1973). Effects of atropine and beta-adrenergic drugs on the heart rate of the human fetus. In: *Fetal Pharmacology*, pp. 259–278. Ed. by L. Boreus. New York: Raven Press.

SEEDS, A. E., STOLEE, A., and EICHHORST, C. (1976). Permeability of human chorion laeve to diazepam and meperidine. *Obstet. and Gynec.*, **47**, 28.

SHIER, R. W., SPRAGUE, A. D., and DILTS, P. V. (1973). Placental transfer of meperidine HCl. Part II. *Amer. J. Obstet. Gynec.*, **115**, 556.

SHNIDER, S. M., and MOYA, F. (1964). Effects of meperidine on the newborn infant. *Amer. J. Obstet. Gynec.* **89**, 1009.

SHNIDER, S. M., and WAY, E. L. (1968a). The kinetics of transfer of lidocaine (Xylocaine®) across the human placenta. *Anesthesiology*, **29**, 944.

SHNIDER, S. M., and WAY, E. L. (1968b). Plasma levels of lidocaine (Xylocaine®) in mother and newborn, following obstetrical conduction anesthesia. *Anesthesiology*, **29**, 951.

SIKER, E. S., WOLFSON, B., DUBNANSKY, J., and FITTING, G. M. (1968). Placental transfer of methoxyflurane. *Brit. J. Anaesth.*, **40**, 588.

SPEIRS, I., and SIM, A. W. (1972). The placental transfer of pancuronium bromide. *Brit. J. Anaesth.*, **44**, 370.

STENGER, V. G., BLECHNER, J. N., and PRYSTOWSKY, H. (1969). A study of prolongation of obstetric anesthesia. *Amer. J. Obstet. Gynec.*, **103**, 901.

STEPHEN, G. W., and COOPER, L. V. (1977). The role of analgesics in respiratory depression: a rabbit model. *Anaesthesia*, **32**, 324.

THALME, B., BELFRAGE, P., and RAABE, N. (1974). Lumbar epidural analgesia in labour I. Acid-base balance and clinical condition of mother, fetus and newborn child. *Acta obstet. gynec. scand.*, **53**, 27.

THOMAS, J., CLIMIE, C. R., and MATHER, L. E. (1969). The placental transfer of alcuronium. *Brit. J. Anaesth.*, **41**, 297.

THOMAS, J., LONG, G., MOORE, G., and MORGAN, D. (1976). Plasma protein binding and placental transfer of bupivacaine. *Clin. Pharmacol. Ther.*, **19**, 426.

TUCKER, G. T., BOYES, R. N., BRIDENBAUGH, P. O., and MOORE, D. C. (1970). Binding of anilide-type local anesthetics in human plasma: II Implications *in vivo*, with special reference to transplacental distribution. *Anesthesiology*, **33**, 304.

ULLBERG, S. (1973). Autoradiography in fetal pharmacology. In: *Fetal Pharmacology*, pp. 55–69. Ed. by L. Boreus. New York: Raven Press.

WALLIS, K. L., SHNIDER, S. M., HICKS, J. S., and SPIVEY, H. T. (1976). Epidural anesthesia in the normotensive pregnant ewe: effects on uterine blood flow and fetal acid-base status. *Anesthesiology*, **44**, 481.

WEAVER, J. B., PEARSON, J. F., and ROSEN, M. (1975). Posture and epidural block in pregnant women at term. Effects on arterial blood pressure and limb blood flow. *Anaesthesia*, **30**, 752.

Chapter 45

PAEDIATRIC ANAESTHESIA

Changes in Circulation That Take Place at Birth

THE fetal circulation is a complex one. The flow of blood in the inferior vena cava appears to move in two almost distinct streams. Oxygenated blood coming from the placenta via the umbilical vein and the ductus venosus passes along the inside track of the inferior vena cava and through the foramen ovale into the left atrium—via sinistra (Fig. 1.). The other stream, consisting of blood coming from the lower limbs and viscera, passes along the outside track of the inferior vena cava to join blood from the superior vena cava and pass to the right atrium —via dextra. This division of the vena cava into two streams is achieved by a ridge termed the crista dividens.

The blood flowing by the via sinistra to the left ventricle is more highly oxygenated and is distributed to the head and neck. The blood passing to the right ventricle by the via dextra is pumped into the pulmonary artery whence a varying proportion, usually at least 80 per cent, is bypassed into the aorta through the ductus arteriosus. This blood contains a large proportion of de-

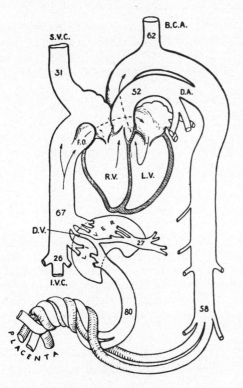

45/FIG. 1.—THE FETAL CIRCULATION IN THE LAMB.

I.V.C.: Inferior vena cava.
R.V.: Right ventricle.
D.V.: Ductus venosus.
D.A.: Ductus arteriosus.
S.V.C.: Superior vena cava.
L.V.: Left ventricle.
F.O.: Foramen ovale.
B.C.A.: Brachiocephalic artery.

The figures indicate the mean O_2 percentage saturation in samples of blood withdrawn simultaneously and averaged from estimations on six lambs.

N.B. The human circulation normally has only a single vein.

saturated blood from the head and neck and extremities and is distributed to the lower half of the body and the umbilical arteries.

The balance of the fetal circulation is upset at birth by the sudden cessation of placental (low-resistance) blood flow which produces an increase in the systemic vascular resistance.

At the same time the lungs become inflated and the pulmonary vascular resistance falls. The net result of these changes in balance between systemic and pulmonary resistance is an increased pulmonary blood flow. This, in turn, alters the differential pressure across the atrial septum. Once the pressure in the left atrium exceeds that in the right, the foramen ovale closes.

As most of the output of the right heart is now directed into the lungs, there is no further functional necessity for the ductus arteriosus and it undergoes muscular constriction. This is initiated by the postnatal increase in PaO_2 (Born et al., 1956). Anatomical closure is delayed for 2–3 weeks (Heymann and Rudolph, 1975). The process of alteration of the circulation from that of the fetus to the neonate, to the adult type (Fig. 2), involves changing from ventricles acting in parallel to acting in series (Dawes, 1968).

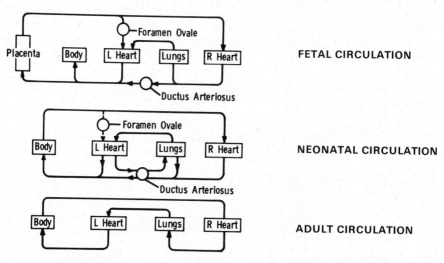

45/FIG. 2.—Diagrams of the fetal, neonatal and adult circulations.

Fetal Breathing

It is now clear that regular (episodic) respiratory movements can be detected in the fetus from an early gestational age. The movements increase in size and frequency as maturity of the fetus proceeds (Dawes et al., 1972). The periods of fetal breathing are increased in the presence of fetal hypercapnia and arrested during hypoxaemia (Boddy et al., 1973). Breathing movements have been detected by ultrasound in humans, and are apparently present for a large proportion of the time (Boddy et al., 1974).

Onset of Breathing at Parturition

It was previously thought that asphyxia and the effect of tactile stimuli during parturition were the stimuli necessary to initiate breathing (Barcroft, 1946). That explanation alone is inadequate.

Now the question that should be posed is why *episodic* antenatal breathing becomes established into *regular* breathing after birth?

The tension of oxygen in carotid blood rises at birth from 23 mm Hg (3·1 kPa) to more than 60 mm Hg (8·0 kPa) and the carbon dioxide level falls from 45 mm to 35 mm Hg (6·0–4·7 kPa). These changes do not explain the onset of regular breathing, as newborn lambs immediately immersed in water, failed to breathe when the cord was ligated (Harned *et al.*, 1970), but if similar lambs were allowed to breathe air through a tracheostomy tube, whilst immersed, regular breathing became established (Dawes *et al.*, 1975).

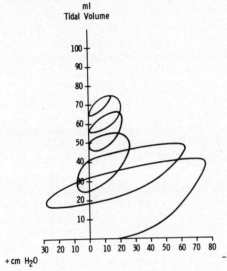

ml
Tidal Volume

45/Fig. 3.—Pressure-volume loops of a neonate's first five breaths. Note the large negative and positive swings during the first two breaths, and the gradual increase in residual volume until the lungs are filled.

It is possible that the onset of regular breathing is initiated and subsequently maintained by the use of the neonate's lungs for the first time as organs of gas exchange, accompanied by the altered response of chemoreceptors to the changes in arterial oxygen saturation which take place at birth.

The infant's first breath of air generates very considerable intrathoracic pressures which may drop to as much as 80 cm (7·8 kPa) of water below atmospheric. The first exhalations are also active, expelling liquor and material from the bronchial tree. Pressure-volume loops of the initial breaths (Fig. 3) show a rising residual volume which is increasing during the early hours of life. The residual volume may rise to 70–80 ml whilst the tidal volume falls from the initial breaths of 30–80 ml to 15–20 ml (5 ml/kg body wt.).

Fetal Lung Maturation

Most complicated pregnancies are allowed to proceed to a point where the risk of death from fetal immaturity no longer exceeds that of intra-uterine death due to placental insufficiency. In these cases it is important to be able to assess fetal maturation. Although many of the physiological functions of the neonate are precarious, the ability of a fetus to survive depends to a great extent on the capacity of the lungs to expand and exchange gases satisfactorily.

R. E. Pattle (1958) noted that the bubbles in pulmonary oedema fluid had "an altogether peculiar property". This property of low surface activity is now known to be due to surfactant action. Clements (1957) has shown that the surface tension of a film of lung washings decreased as the area of the film was decreased, corresponding to a fall in surface tension within the alveoli during expiration, preventing complete collapse. Pattle hypothesised that a deficiency of surfactant may be responsible for hyaline membrane disease and this was confirmed by Avery and Mead (1959).

The active constituents of surfactant are phospholipids—mainly lecithin which appears in the amniotic fluid towards term. Tests to assess fetal lung maturity involve the estimation of the amount of lecithin present. Gluck et al. (1971) showed that the terminal increase in lecithin in amniotic fluid is greatly in excess of syringomyelin (another surface-active phospholipid) and that observation is the basis for the test which estimates the lecithin/syringomyelin ratio. This has been shown to be an accurate indication of possible respiratory distress.

These advances in diagnosis enable the physician to initiate treatment to enhance surfactant production in premature fetuses.

There is ever-increasing evidence from animal and clinical studies that corticosteroids can enhance or accelerate fetal lung maturation (De Lemos et al., 1970; Liggins and Howie, 1972; Spellacy et al., 1973; Fargier et al., 1974; Nathan, 1975). The form of corticosteroid which is given is not important, but there is some evidence that betamethasone, not being protein-bound, will pass the placental barrier more easily, but dexamethasone, cortisol and prednisone have been used as well. Indirect evidence of the efficacy of steroid therapy in the prevention of Respiratory Distress Syndrome (RDS) is available from the British Perinatal Mortality Survey analysed by Fedrick and Butler (1972). They drew attention to the lower mortality from RDS of infants born by Caesarean section where the mother had been in labour compared with those whose mother had not gone into labour, the inference being that the stress of labour had initiated endogenous corticosteroid activity which, in turn, had accelerated the fetal lung to maturity.

Other substances known to promote fetal lung maturation are *thyroxin* (Wu et al., 1973), *heroin* (Glass et al., 1971) and *isoxsuprine*—a vasodilator with some β-sympathomimetic properties (Kero, 1973). From the accumulated evidence, it appears that if pre-term induction of labour is necessary on obstetric grounds (e.g. diabetes, rhesus haemolytic disease) or if premature labour can be delayed (by β-agonists such as salbutamol), considerable reduction in the incidence of RDS can be achieved by the administration of steroids at least 24 hours before delivery.

Management of Respiratory Distress Syndrome (RDS)

Such significant advances have been made in the last decade that this condition is no longer the principal cause of death in pre-term infants (Reynolds, 1975). Once the diagnosis has been clearly distinguished from other causes of respiratory distress, treatment may be instituted.

45/TABLE 1
OXYGEN THERAPY IN RESPIRATORY DISTRESS

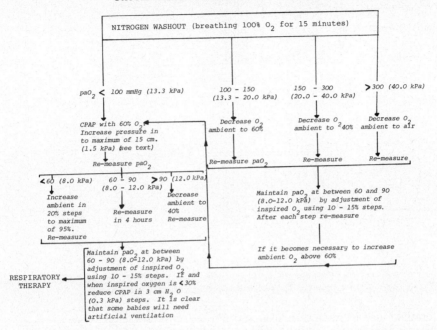

A rational approach to the treatment of RDS has been described by Davies *et al.* (1972)—see Table 1. The therapy required is appropriate to the severity of the disease. When oxygen therapy is indicated in the newborn, the danger exists of producing retinal damage by retrolental fibroplasia. It is known that this condition is caused by excessively high arterial oxygen tensions, rather than high inspired oxygen concentrations *per se* (Aranda *et al.*, 1971). Thus considerable emphasis is placed on regular, frequent analyses of the baby's arterial oxygen tension. On-line, continuous blood gas monitoring is becoming a practical procedure with intravascular probes (Parker and Souttar, 1975) but discrete samples may be obtained from indwelling umbilical arterial cannulae. The dangers of allowing umbilical arterial cannulae to remain *in situ* are sufficiently well-recognised to limit this mode of sampling to about 48 hours. Peripheral arterial samples may be taken from an accessible artery such as the radial. Alternatively, the heel or other parts of the skin may be arterialised and a capillary stab sample used.

Transcutaneous measurement of oxygen tension has been demonstrated (Huch *et al.*, 1972) but the technique is dependent upon adequate capillary perfusion. Parker and Souttar (1975) have suggested that intravascular PaO_2 monitoring may be necessary when peripheral perfusion is impaired, although transcutaneous monitoring correlates closely with intravascular measurements when the cardiovascular state is stable.

A less well-documented effect of high inspired oxygen concentration is that of bronchopulmonary dysplasia. In this condition there is destruction of the

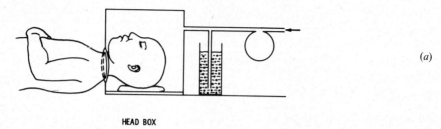

HEAD BOX

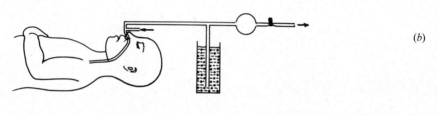

NASOTRACHEAL TUBE

45/FIG. 4(a) and (b).—Continuous positive airway pressure (CPAP) achieved using (a) a box surrounding the infant's head, and (b) an endotracheal tube.

terminal airways with dysplasia and fibrosis. It is associated with respiratory therapy in pre-term infants requiring raised inflation pressures and increased F_1O_2 (Reynolds and Taghizadeh, 1974).

Mild cases of RDS are treated by increasing the inspired oxygen concentration until the arterial oxygen tension reaches a level between 60 and 90 mm Hg (8·0–12·0 kPa). If this is not possible within an ambient oxygen concentration of 60 per cent, the effect of Continuous Positive Airways Pressure (CPAP) is tried. If the disease is too severe to respond to CPAP, intermittent positive-pressure ventilation (IPPV) is necessary.

Methods of Applying CPAP

CPAP is a logical method of treating the principal failure in RDS, i.e. that of the tendency of affected lungs to collapse. The method originally described by Gregory et al. (1971) involved placing the infant's head in a box with a seal around the neck, so that the pressure within the box could be maintained at a few cm H_2O above atmospheric (Fig. 4a).

Other methods are variations of the principle but employ different means of attachment to the infant. This may be done with the infant intubated (Fig. 4b), with bilateral nasopharyngeal catheters, or by close application of a face-mask. Another approach has been to lower the pressure surrounding the infant's trunk (as in the tank respirator or "iron lung"), thus raising the relative intra-pulmonary pressure.

Whilst there is no doubt of the efficacy of CPAP as a therapeutic procedure, there have been few controlled trials to compare it with other methods of treatment (Rhodes and Hall, 1973). The disadvantages of some methods of applying CPAP are difficult access to the patient for routine care (head-box), raised intracranial venous pressure causing possible cerebral haemorrhage (head-box neck-seal, and negative pressure tank) and interference with the circulation. A raised intrapulmonary pressure may cause an increase in pulmonary vascular resistance. This in turn will tend to restore the right-to-left shunt through the foramen ovale that existed antepartum.

An elegant modification of the T-piece circuit using a double lumen delivery/ expiratory tube has been described by Crew et al. (1975).

Respirator Treatment

If, despite application of CPAP, (1) the infant's Pao_2 cannot be raised above 30 mm Hg (4·0 kPa); (2) the infant is having apnoeic attacks; or (3) the $Paco_2$ becomes greater than 90 mm Hg (12·0 kPa), the use of intermittent positive-pressure ventilation (IPPV) is indicated.

The various types of ventilators available which are suitable for neonates fall into two types, pressure-limited devices and volume-limited devices. Reynolds (1974) has reviewed respiration therapy in RDS and favours pressure-limited devices which compensate for intentional air-leaks around the endotracheal tube. Moreover, it has been shown that bronchopulmonary dysplasia is due in part to excessive inflation pressures. A pressure-limiting facility will tend to minimise this type of lung damage.

Pressure-Limited Ventilators
Bird
Bennett PR2
Sheffield
Loosco
Drager Spiromat

Volumic-Controlled Ventilators
Engström
Cape (Universal attachment)
Servo

Reynolds (1974) considers the desirable facilities in a respirator to be used for artificial ventilation of neonates to be:

1. The ability to alter the inspiratory/expiratory ratio.
2. The ability to alter the wave-form to conform as closely as possible to a square wave.
3. The ability to limit inflation pressures.
4. The ability to apply positive end-expiratory pressure (PEEP).

No single ventilator available is able to fulfil all these criteria, but some (Drager Spiromat, Servo) can comply reasonably closely.

The Sheffield and Amsterdam Infant Ventilator (A.I.V.), Loosco Ventilator

These ventilators are described together as they embody a common working principle. There are T-tube occluders, that is, the method of cycling involves the intermittent occlusion of the expiratory limb of a basic T-piece anaesthesia circuit.

In the A.I.V. the rate is set electronically between 20 and 60/min and the inspiratory/expiratory time ratio varies from 1:1 to 1:3. The ventilator normally works as a volume-constant device. The gas flow rate required to produce a given minute volume is derived using a nomogram which takes into account the volume of gas "lost" during the expiratory phase. PEEP may be applied to the expiratory limb of the ventilator, which can also be used as a pressure-constant device by incorporating a pressure-limiting relief valve.

The Sheffield Ventilator

This is a similar device with an electronically-timed solenoid valve which occludes the expiratory limb (Fig. 5).

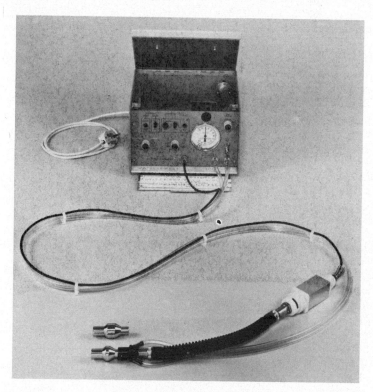

45/Fig. 5.—Sheffield ventilator.

The Cape Universal Attachment

This is a "bag-in-bottle" arrangement for ventilation of infants with small, accurate tidal volume. A full-sized ventilator is connected to the "bottle" and provides the motive force for compression of the inflating bellows. The weighted bellows refill passively. This is a volume-constant device.

The "bag-in-bottle" principle is employed in the Drager Spiromat with greater sophistication so that different inspiratory wave-forms can be produced.

LONG-TERM ENDOTRACHEAL INTUBATION

The complications of prolonged endotracheal intubation in children have been described in many series. These include blockage of the tube and displacement, but the most serious is the development of subglottic stenosis of the trachea (Allen and Steven, 1965; Jackson Rees and Owen Thomas, 1966).

In the continuation of their series, Allen and Steven (1972) report that experience gleaned from the initial 61 cases enabled them to reduce the incidence of complications by using the smallest possible diameter of tube that enabled the patient to breathe without obstruction. Their recommendations regarding tube diameter for the different age groups are considerably smaller than those normally suggested. It is possible that the smaller tubes were acceptable as very few of these patients underwent artificial ventilation.

45/TABLE 2

NASOTRACHEAL TUBE SIZES RECOMMENDED FOR LONG-TERM INTUBATION BY ALLEN AND STEVEN (1972)

Age	Tube size (internal diameter)
0–6 months	3·0 mm
6 months–2 years	3·5 mm
2 years–5 years	4·0 mm
5 years +	4·5 mm

In a recent review of cases treated at the Hospital for Sick Children, Great Ormond Street, London, Battersby and his co-workers (1977) report a very low incidence of complications following prolonged nasotracheal intubation. They attribute their success to meticulous attention to details of humidification, endobronchial toilet and loose-fitting, biologically inert PVC tubes. The diameter of tube selected should be such that an audible air leak is present during positive-pressure ventilation. Extubation stridor, when it occurred, was treated with systemic dexamethasone.

Tracheostomy is now reserved for selected cases, usually when intubation is anticipated to be necessary for longer than 2 weeks (Aberdeen, 1965).

Neonatal Asphyxia

Neonatal asphyxia may be due to a failure to breathe or due to an inability to expand the lungs. A failure to breathe may be due to respiratory centre depression caused by intra-uterine hypoxia or by narcotic or anaesthetic drugs. The depressant action of opiates is well known but diazepam has also been shown to produce neonatal depression when given in large doses (in excess of 30 mg) in the 24 hours prior to delivery (Cree, 1973). Asphyxia may also be caused by brain-stem injury due to cerebral haemorrhage. The lungs may not be able to expand if the infant is very premature or if the airway is obstructed by mucus or meconium.

After observing experimental animals subjected to birth asphyxia, Dawes (1968) described neonatal asphyxia in two phases, i.e. primary apnoea and terminal apnoea.

The sequence of events (as observed in animals) is as follows: After an initial period of distressed attempts at breathing, a period of apnoea occurs (*primary apnoea*). This is followed, after an interval, by a series of gasps increasing in frequency, but diminishing in effectiveness until all activity ceases (*terminal apnoea*). Unless active measures are taken very quickly, the heart will stop and the animal will be dead. There is every reason to believe that these observations apply equally to the human infant.

Primary Apnoea

An infant in this state will make active efforts to breathe at first, will be blue in colour and will respond to external stimuli, albeit weakly. Its tone will be weakly flexural, and its heart rate usually over 100/min. In other words, it will have an Apgar score of about 6.

Most cases of primary apnoea will respond to routine care (clearing the nasopharyngeal mucus and application of oxygen). "Lazy" babies will often gasp actively if expansion of the lungs is initiated by application of positive pressure (e.g. by mask and inflating bag).

If the period of asphyxia has been prolonged or severe, the baby will pass to a stage of *terminal apnoea*. It is important to recognise this state as urgent resuscitative measures are required to save the child.

In terminal apnoea, the baby will be white or pale and will make no attempt to breathe; it will be limp and will not respond to external stimuli, and its heart rate will be below 100, gradually becoming even slower. The Apgar score will be under 3.

The Apgar Score

A more objective method of evaluating the state of a newborn infant is by means of scoring, using five signs noted sixty seconds after birth, but disregarding the cord and placenta (Apgar, 1953; Apgar *et al.*, 1958). The signs are heart rate, respiratory effort, muscle tone, reflex irritability, and colour. Each sign is given a score of 0, 1 or 2. A total score of 10 shows that the infant is in the best possible condition. Active resuscitation is necessary below 5. Details of this Apgar score are given in Table 3.

45/TABLE 3
THE APGAR SCORE

Sign	Score		
	0	1	2
Heart rate	absent	slow (below 100)	over 100
Respiratory effort	absent	weak cry hypoventilation	good strong cry
Muscle tone	limp	some flexion of extremities	well flexed
Reflex irritability (response of skin stimulation to feet)	no response	some motion	cry
Colour	blue pale	body pink extremities blue	completely pink

A systematic approach to resuscitative intervention has been described by Gregory (1975) and is summarised in Table 4.

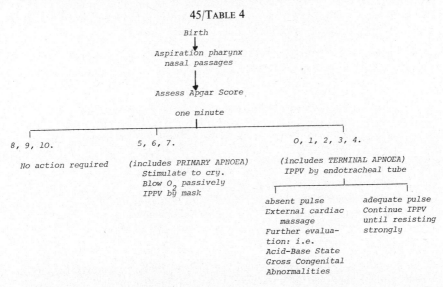

45/TABLE 4

In practice it is often difficult to distinguish between primary and terminal apnoea and little is lost, and a great deal gained, by early active treatment of apnoeic infants. The infant should be intubated and given artificial ventilation.

Artificial Respiration

This may be administered by mask (Mushin, 1967) but it is most readily and efficiently achieved by endotracheal intubation. Following initial aspiration, the lungs are inflated with regular short puffs (less than 0·5 s) of oxygen administered from an oxygen source incorporating a pressure-limiting device. A pressure of 80 cm H_2O (7·8 kPa) may be reached during the first inflation of collapsed lungs, but this is rarely necessary, and regular short puffs of 10–20 cm H_2O (1–2 kPa) are quite sufficient.

The technique of intubation involves the use of the straight-bladed laryngoscope (e.g. the Oxford Infant Blade). The tip of the blade of the laryngoscope is advanced into the posterior pharynx or upper oesophagus. The blade is then slowly withdrawn whilst maintaining pressure on the tongue anteriorly. The larynx will pop into view, whilst the epiglottis is retained anterior to the blade. A tube of size 12 FG (equivalent to 2·5 mm diameter) will be suitable for most neonates, although a 10 FG (2·0 mm) may be necessary for a small baby.

If intravenous drugs are to be given, they may be injected conveniently into the umbilical vein, but prolonged cannulation of the umbilical vein may lead to grave complications. Narcotic depression is best treated with naloxone 0·005–0·01 mg/kg.

Cardiac Arrest or Severe Bradycardia (< 30/min)

In such circumstances, external cardiac massage must be instituted to maintain a cardiac output. The technique is slightly different to that used on the adult. Pressure is applied over the upper sternum as there is danger of causing damage to the liver by depression of the lower sternum. Pressure is applied with two fingers only or, alternatively, the upper thorax is held with both hands and pressure applied to the upper sternum with both thumbs.

THE NEONATE

Some average values for the neonate are shown in Table 5.

45/TABLE 5
SOME AVERAGE VALUES FOR A NEONATE WEIGHING 3·4 kg

Respiratory rate	30–40/min
Tidal volume	17 ml
Alveolar ventilation	460 ml/min
Pulse rate	120–160/min
Mean blood pressure	65 mm Hg (8·7 kPa)
Haemoglobin concentration	17–19 g/100 ml (g/dl)
Urinary output	17–85 ml/24 hours
Fluid requirement	100–170 ml/24 hours

A neonate will lose weight from the time of birth, but generally the birth weight will be regained in ten days. A normal child can then be expected to double its birth weight in five months.

General Management

Thermal regulation.—It has long been recognised that the newborn baby is vulnerable to changes in his environmental temperature and the pre-term and low birth weight baby particularly so. There have been attempts in the past to nurse babies in low temperatures but Silverman *et al.* (1963) showed the reduction in infant mortality that could be achieved by regulation of the thermal environment. When low birth weight infants (< 1·5 kg) were nursed in incubators maintained at 31·7° C, instead of 28·9° C, as previously employed, mortality was reduced by 40 per cent.

Most healthy babies can increase their metabolic heat production but rarely shiver. It is thought that much of any increase in heat output is achieved by oxidation of brown adipose tissue (Hey, 1972). These responses to cold stimuli are muted at birth and only develop in the first week of life. A baby will also respond to an over hot environment by a cutaneous vasodilatation, even in very early life. The ability to sweat is present in newborn babies but only initiated when rectal temperature rises by 1° C.

The set point around which babies respond to changes in their environment appears to be much the same as in later life. Between environmental temperatures that provoke an increased heat production or cutaneous vasodilatation and sweating, there lies an environmental temperature within which a baby maintains a constant deep body temperature. This is known as the *Thermoneutral Zone* (Hey, 1972). This thermoneutral zone differs according to age and weight, but it is possible to determine the optimum environmental temperature for any given infant. The newborn baby in the delivery room is particularly vulnerable to cold stress as its response is muted, it is wet and subject to evaporative heat losses, and this may lead to metabolic acidosis (Gandy *et al.*, 1964).

The use of aluminised melamine swaddlers, a blanket or overhead radiant heaters (Fig. 6) will reduce inevitable heat losses. However, considerable heat losses can occur during resuscitative procedures, if attention is not paid to the foregoing remarks.

Neonatal water and electrolyte requirements.—The normal neonate excretes between 5 and 25 ml/kg of urine each 24 hours; add to this an insensible loss of 25–30 ml per kg/24 hours and the basic water requirement is about 30–50 ml/kg/24 hours. However, in post-operative conditions, this requirement may be

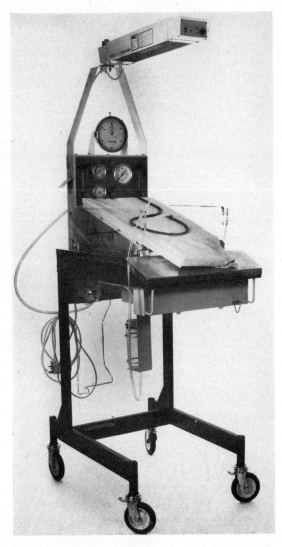

45/FIG. 6.—Vickers Resuscitaire. A resuscitation trolley for neonates, incorporating an overhead radiant heater.

reduced by as much as half as a result of fluid retention and nursing in high humidity incubators.

Thus the post-operative fluid requirement in a neonate may be very small and has lead some authorities to advocate a policy of minimal or no intravenous fluids until oral feeding is recommenced (Nixon, 1972).

Neonatal water and electrolyte replacement.—Rickham and Johnstone (1969) advocate restriction of intravenous fluids in the early post-operative period to 40 ml/kg/24 hours rising to 60–80 ml/kg/24 hours by 7 days of age when the urinary output may have increased fourfold (120–150 ml/kg/24 hours). The fluid may be given as 10 per cent dextrose solution, or as 4·3 per cent dextrose in 0·18 per cent saline if there are appreciable electrolyte losses in aspiration or secretions. Diluted human plasma is a useful source of protein.

Hypoglycaemia.—It is becoming increasingly clear that hypoglycaemia is a common condition occurring in the neonatal period, particularly in a baby suffering from a condition requiring surgical correction, and this will influence the outcome. Hypoglycaemia of the newborn is defined as a blood glucose of less than 20 mg/100 ml (1·1 mmol/l). The introduction of Dextrostix has enabled the physician to check the neonate's blood sugar very rapidly on a heel prick.

A baby with a blood sugar under 20 mg/100 ml (1·1 mmol/l) will require calories either by mouth, if it has not developed symptoms (apnoeic attacks, convulsions, jerky movements of limbs, etc.) or does not require immediate surgery; or intravenously, as a 10 per cent dextrose infusion (65 ml/kg/24 hours). Hypothermia may be a cause of a low blood glucose.

SURGICAL EMERGENCIES: NEONATAL

The following conditions are amenable to surgery:

Diaphragmatic Hernia

This condition, where the abdominal contents herniate through an incompletely formed diaphragm can produce acute respiratory distress. There is an obvious deficiency of the abdomen which is often scaphoid in contour and the mediastinal contents are moved to the right (in 80 per cent of cases). If gas is blown or swallowed into the stomach the respiratory distress is increased and endotracheal intubation is the only safe means of ventilation. A nasogastric tube is passed to deflate the stomach and diminish the pressure of the abdominal contents upon the thoracic viscera. An X-ray will confirm the diagnosis, showing loops of bowel within the chest. Survival depends upon the extent to which the lung on the affected side is developed. Many cases of diaphragmatic hernia present with hypoplastic lungs and the infant will probably require ventilatory support post-operatively (Lewis and Young, 1969). Recent reports of the use of CPAP are encouraging.

Lobar Emphysema

Lobar emphysema is a condition due to congenital weakness of the bronchial cartilages and consequent over-distension of a lobe of the lung. The distension may be considerable and cause collapse of surrounding normal lung. Paradoxically, efforts at resuscitation by endotracheal inflation may exacerbate the respiratory embarrassment.

Congenital lung cysts present a very similar clinical picture.

Choanal Atresia

Failure of the posterior nares to develop properly may produce acute respiratory distress. Immediate relief is obtained by placing an oropharyngeal airway in the mouth.

Tracheo-Oesophageal Fistula (Fig. 7)

This malformation may be suspected when the pregnancy has been complicated by hydramnios. Fistulous communication can exist between the oesophagus and trachea, or alternatively there may be a failure in the development of the oesophagus; other intestinal abnormalities are frequently present (Lloyd and Clatworthy 1958).

The baby may present with respiratory distress and discharging quantities of clear mucus from its mouth. The abdomen is often distended with gas if the fistula exists between the trachea and lower oesophagus. If a nasogastric tube cannot be passed into the stomach, the diagnosis is confirmed.

Anaesthetic management of tracheo-oesophageal fistula.—There is frequently "spill-over" of oesophageal or gastric contents into the trachea. If the abnormality is of the commonest variety, the blind-ending pouch of the upper oesophagus must be kept aspirated with a Replogle's tube.

Difficulties may be encountered with positive-pressure respiration due to inflation of the stomach through the fistula. This can only be minimised by either allowing the infant to breathe spontaneously until the chest is opened, or by limiting inflation pressures to prevent excessive gastric inflation.

The post-operative management depends largely upon the severity of pulmonary involvement, and positive-pressure ventilation may be necessary to

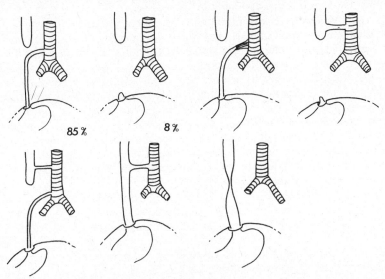

45/Fig. 7.—Varieties of tracheo-oesophageal fistulae or atresia. The incidence of the common types is also indicated.

maintain satisfactory oxygenation. It would seem logical to apply continuous positive airway pressure (CPAP) in suitable cases, although reports of this method of treatment have not yet appeared.

Mandibular Retrognathia

This is the "Pierre Robin" syndrome of mandibular retrognathia associated with cleft palate. The condition usually presents at birth with respiratory distress as the tongue falls backwards and into the palatal cleft. Difficulties are often experienced when intubation is attempted.

Intestinal Obstruction

Vomiting in a neonate is a serious symptom and the nature of the vomit is important. Clear vomiting or regurgitation may be a symptom associated with oesophageal atresia. Yellow vomit may be due to carotene from the maternal milk. Bile-stained vomit has a green colour and, occurring in the first 24 hours of life, indicates the necessity for investigation of obstruction.

Duodenal atresia.—This condition is frequently associated with Down's syndrome (mongolism). X-rays reveal the presence of two distinct gas bubbles in the stomach and in the duodenum. Gas is not seen in distal loops of the bowel, which remain collapsed. Occasionally a maldevelopment of the bile duct and pancreas cause an obstruction of the duodenum. Atresias or stenosis occur in the ileum and jejunum, but these are rarely associated with Down's syndrome.

Malrotation.—This failure of the midgut to rotate and fix properly, gives rise to obstruction in two ways. Firstly the midgut becomes prone to volvulus and, secondly, peritoneal bands ("Ladd's bands") pass across the duodenum and may also cause compression and obstruction.

Meconium ileus.—This is a manifestation of the condition known as fibrocystic disease or mucoviscidosis. The mucus secreted by mucosal cells is viscid and thick. The abnormal intestinal mucus becomes inspissated and forms a mechanical obstruction within the gut. The gut wall is often hypertrophied and may twist forming a volvulus or may perforate, with grave consequences.

Hirschsprung's disease.—Vomiting is a later symptom in this disease, the first presentation being an increasing abdominal distension combined with absence of meconium in the stools. The obstruction is caused by a segment of bowel failing to contract normally due to the absence of a normal autonomic plexus. The distended loop of bowel is normal and proximal to the diseased segment. The disease does not invariably cause complete obstruction and the passage of meconium may only be delayed.

Necrotising enterocolitis.—This is a complication of Hirschsprung's disease which is probably an ischaemia of the mucosa. It also occurs following a difficult delivery with fetal distress or following exchange transfusions.

Functional intestinal obstruction.—This, as the name implies, is an obstruction which is not primarily due to an organic cause. It responds to conservative treatment and often resolves within 10 days.

Imperforate anus.—Complete imperforate anus is a rare condition, as there is often a pinhole orifice and meconium may be seen. Imperforate anus is frequently associated with other gut malformations such as oesophageal or duodenal atresia.

Exomphalos and gastroschisis (para-umbilical defect).—Exomphalos can occur in differing degrees of severity. The greater the deficiency of the abdominal wall, the greater the difficulty in effecting a primary closure, and the greater the mortality.

Other conditions which may present for surgery in early life are strangulated inguinal hernias and pyloric stenosis, usually in the first four to six weeks.

Anaesthetic management of intestinal obstruction.—An attempt must be made to diminish the risk of aspiration of gastric contents and a nasogastric tube should be inserted and the stomach emptied. As with most neonatal surgery, if intubation of the trachea is indicated, this is probably safest performed with the infant awake.

Paralysis and controlled ventilation with nitrous oxide and oxygen using a Rees modified Ayre's T-piece provides good operating conditions.

Spina Bifida

The failure of the bony vertebral canal to close produces the abnormality of spina bifida. In 10 per cent of cases there is an associated simple meningocele which, if closed, should lead to a normal life. However, in 90 per cent there is involvement of cord, nerve roots and meninges. It is this group in which closure may be associated with a wide range of neurological disabilities. A large number of meningomyeloceles are either associated with hydrocephalus at birth, or will develop the condition shortly afterwards (the Arnold-Chiari syndrome).

Hydrocephalus

Hydrocephalus is not necessarily associated with meningomyelocele but may be due to aqueduct closure, stenosis of the foramen of the fourth ventricle, etc. In either case, surgical relief of the hydrocephalus may be performed by inserting a valved tube to drain CSF from the lateral ventricle to the superior vena cava or right atrium.

Tumours

Renal fibroma (Wilm's tumour) may achieve considerable proportions and even complicate delivery. It should be distinguished from giant hydronephrosis and polycystic disease. Neuroblastoma is another tumour frequently presenting in the neonatal period in which complete removal has the prospect of a good prognosis. These tumours often secrete catecholamines which may complicate the anaesthetic management.

A sacrococcygeal teratoma causes a characteristic "duck-bottomed" deformity; the prognosis is good if removal is early and complete.

Cardiovascular Abnormalities

There are a few congenital abnormalities which require urgent correction within the first few days of life, but these are dealt with elsewhere (see Chapter 14).

Hare-Lip and Cleft Palate

As previously mentioned, this condition may be associated with retrognathia

(Pierre Robin syndrome) and difficulty may be experienced with intubation. Another difficulty in patients with cleft palates is that the laryngoscope blade tends to fall into the cleft. A hare-lip deformity is usually corrected at the age of about 3 months and an anterior palatal deficiency at the same time. A posterior or soft palatal deformity is repaired between the ages of 12 and 18 months.

The anaesthetist should choose an anaesthetic technique that ensures rapid recovery of pharyngeal reflexes. Endotracheal intubation is mandatory, although an oral tube may be used in conjunction with the commonly employed Dott mouth-gag. Care should be taken to check the patency of the tube after insertion of the gag as the lumen may be occluded by pressure of the gag on the mandible. An Oxford tube is most suitable. The pharynx must be packed to prevent aspiration of blood. Blood loss may be considerable and the patient should have blood cross-matched before surgery.

It is fairly common practice to insert a strong suture in the tongue post-operatively to facilitate the maintenance of a clear airway in an emergency.

TECHNIQUES OF ANAESTHESIA

Premedication

In the neonate.—Sedative premedication is not desirable in the neonate, although antisialogogue drugs are indicated, as even a little mucus in a small airway can cause respiratory embarrassment. Hyoscine is poorly tolerated in the very young as the cerebral excitant action may predominate. Atropine should be given, 0·2 mg for the average neonate, and 0·1 mg for the small-for-dates baby. If the baby is pyrexial or the environmental temperatures are high, atropine may increase the pyrexia and therefore should only be used with extreme caution.

In older children.—Up to the age of 6–9 months, atropine only is given as premedication. Over the age of 9 months, some form of sedative premedication is desirable. This may be given by injection or given orally. Although few children welcome injections, it is occasionally the only certain way in which medication may be given.

Preparations

Trimeprazine (Vallergan) elixir.—This is a phenothiazine derivative with antihistaminic actions, but given principally for its sedative effect. The dose is 2–4 mg/kg and the elixir is available either in a concentration of 7·5 mg/5 ml or 30 mg/5 ml (Forte).

Triclofos elixir (Tricloryl syrup).—Trichloroethyl phosphate is an acceptable form of chloral prepared in a suitably flavoured vehicle in a concentration of 500 mg/5 ml. It produces satisfactory sedation in the majority of children given in a dose of 75 mg/kg (maximum 1600 mg). Post-operative vomiting is common.

Barbiturates.—Short-acting barbiturates will induce sleep in children when given in a dose of 7 mg/kg (maximum 200 mg). The disadvantages of barbiturates are:

1. The possibility of respiratory depression.

2. A bitter taste.

3. Post-operative restlessness.

This latter action can be controlled with the addition of opiates.

Diazepam elixir (Valium syrup).—Many investigators have examined the use of diazepam 0·2 mg/kg as a paediatric premedication and it appears to be a suitable agent. It is available in a concentration of 2 mg/5 ml. Some workers have found that salivary secretions are inadequately suppressed and the addition of atropine may be considered prudent.

Rectal premedication.—Thiopentone may be given rectally either as a 5 per cent or 10 per cent solution in water (40 mg/kg) or in suspension. Suppositories are available in increments of 125 mg. A child given rectal premedication must be closely observed as the depth of sedation produced is not predictable.

I.M. methohexitone.—2 per cent methohexitone may be given by intramuscular injection (6 mg/kg). The same precautions apply as for rectal thiopentone.

Anaesthesia

Induction of anaesthesia in a child is a controversial subject. Some anaesthetists prefer to premedicate their patients sufficiently for them to be asleep on arrival in the anaesthetic room whilst others deliberately sedate their patients only lightly and induce anaesthesia in a somnulent but conscious patient. A co-operative parent, accompanying his or her child to the anaesthetic room, can often smooth a potentially difficult induction.

If an inhalational induction is to be given, since all the commonly used anaesthetic gases and vapours are heavier than air, the technique employed should take advantage of this property. Either cyclopropane and oxygen or nitrous oxide and oxygen with halothane are suitable.

If an intravenous induction agent is preferred, thiopentone, methohexitone or Althesin may be used, but it should be noted that methohexitone may cause intense pain when given into small veins in children.

Ketamine can be given either intravenously or intramuscularly (see also Chapter 22). The intramuscular route is particularly useful in an unco-operative child and given in a dose of 8–10 mg/kg will produce complete anaesthesia (I.V. dose 2–4 mg/kg). The undesirable side-effects of this agent are not observed in small children, certainly emergence delirium is not evident, but postoperative vomiting is relatively common. Some caution must be exercised when using ketamine as an induction agent in very small infants or neonates. By its very nature, this agent does not inhibit to any marked extent the protective reflexes and, should intubation be performed following induction of anaesthesia with ketamine, difficulty may be experienced during extubation when recurrent laryngeal spasm can occur. In addition, spontaneous movements unrelated to the surgical stimulus are much commoner in the very small child under ketamine anaesthesia. It would appear that despite its convenient mode of induction, ketamine is unsuitable for the neonate and the very small child. It is, however, a most useful agent in the age group 1–5 years.

Paediatric Anaesthetic Systems

Elimination of apparatus dead space and minimal resistance to respiration are the most important factors to be considered. Any addition to the normal dead space of a small child can seriously hamper the adequacy of pulmonary exchange. This becomes evident when one considers that the tidal volume of a full-term normal neonate is about 20 ml, and that the physiological dead space is one-third this amount, alveolar ventilation therefore amounting only to some 14 ml. The addition of only a few ml of apparatus dead space therefore represents a large proportional increase in the newborn baby.

45/TABLE 6

GUIDE TO ENDOTRACHEAL TUBE SIZE

(Keep and Manford, 1974; Penlington, 1974).

Age	Size (equals internal diam. mm)	
Small neonate	2·5–3·0	*FORMULA*
Average neonate	3·5	$\dfrac{Age}{3} + 3\cdot5$
6 months	4·0	
1 year	4·0	
2 years	4·0	
3 years	4·5	
4 years	5·0	
5 years	5·0	
6 years	5·5	
7 years	6·0	$\dfrac{Age}{4} + 4\cdot5$
8 years	6·5	
9 years	6·5	
10 years	7·0	

45/TABLE 7

GUIDE TO ORAL ENDOTRACHEAL TUBE LENGTH

(Levin, 1958)

Age	Length of Oral Tube (cm)	
		FORMULA
6 months	12·0	$\dfrac{Age}{2} + 12$ cm
1 year	12·5	
2 years	13·0	
3 years	13·5	
4 years	14·0	
5 years	14·5	
6 years	15·0	
7 years	15·5	
8 years	16·0	
9 years	16·5	
10 years	17·0	

Masks.—Even a small mask adds to the dead space of the anaesthetic system, and in proportion to the small tidal and alveolar ventilation of a child becomes a factor of importance. A good mask for small babies must be designed to reduce apparatus dead space to a minimum and also to suit the flat contour of the face which is normal at the start of life. The most suitable mask at present available is that described by Rendell-Baker and Soucek (1962). The nominal dead space in the size intended for mature neonates is 4 ml.

Endotracheal tubes.—A guide to the selection of an endotracheal tube for an infant is given in Tables 6 and 7.

Mattila *et al.* (1971) have derived a formula for calculating the distance from the external nares to the carina:—

$$0.16 \times \text{height of child (cm)} + 4.5 \text{ cm}$$

A nasotracheal tube should be 2 cm shorter than this.

The figures given above for endotracheal tube sizes are intended only as a

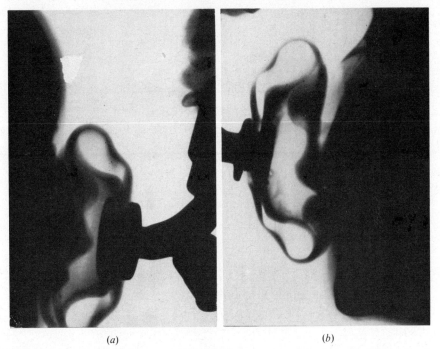

(a)   (b)

45/FIG. 8.—X-ray pictures showing the difference in contour of the face of an infant (a) and a 4-year-old child (b). This illustrates the need for a special type of mask for the infant.

guide. In terms of diameter, tubes one size larger and smaller than the selected tube should be immediately available. As far as the length of the tube is concerned, endobronchial intubation must be excluded by ensuring that movements and breath sounds on the two sides of the chest are similar; radiographic confirmation of the tube's position is advisable in cases of prolonged intubation, so that if the tube is impinging upon the carina it can be shortened.

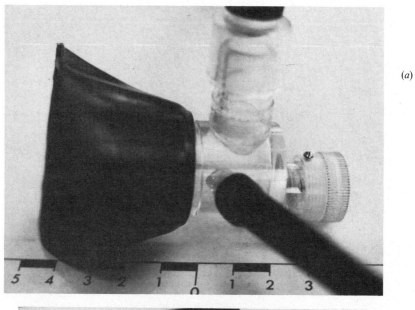

(a)

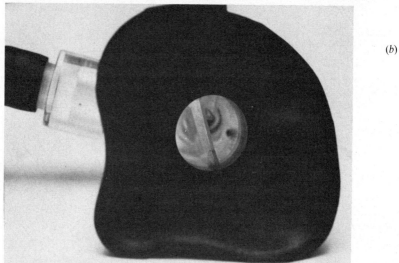

(b)

45/Fig. 9.—(a) and (b).—The Rendell-Baker paediatric anaesthetic apparatus.
See text for details. The scale is in centimetres.

Apparatus.—Paediatric anaesthetic equipment should offer the least possible dead space and resistance to respiration for the child to contend with. It should also be light and easily managed. In this country two systems are most commonly used.

(1) *The Rendell-Baker apparatus.*—This equipment is excellent for mask

anaesthesia with spontaneous respiration, and can be adapted for use during controlled ventilation (Fig. 9). It consists of a partitioned mask adaptor fitted with an inlet tube and a light expiratory valve on one side of the partition, and a large port on the other side onto which an open-ended bag can be attached. Fresh gases are directed by the partition so that they flow over the child's face, and therefore the apparatus dead space is almost nil. The apparatus can be assembled in two ways. Fresh gases can be introduced into the side-arm on the partitioned adaptor, passing down over the child's face and out of the large port into the open-ended bag. Used like this it acts as a type of Ayre's T-piece. Alternatively gases can be led in through the open-ended bag, expiration taking place via the expiratory valve. Fresh gas flows should exceed twice the minute volume of the child.

(2) *Ayre's T-piece.*—This equipment is used for endotracheal anaesthesia with either controlled or spontaneous respiration. Ayre (1956) has summarised the approximate gas flow rates and sizes for the expiratory limb of a T-piece.

At present it is customary to deliver a generous gas flow to the side-arm of the T-piece (at least twice the minute volume of the child) and to use only one size for the expiratory limb. An open-ended bag may be attached to the expiratory limb in order to monitor spontaneous respiration, or to manually control ventilation, as suggested by Jackson Rees.

Age	Rate of flow of fresh gases (litres/minute)	Capacity of expiratory limb (ml)
0–3 months	3–4	6–12
3–6 months	4–5	12–18
6–12 months	5–6	18–24
1–2 years	6–7	24–42
2–4 years	7–8	42–60
4–8 years	8–9	60–72

Other types of apparatus (one-way valves, and both to and fro' and circle absorber systems) have been designed for paediatric use, but have not achieved popularity in this country. When used for neonatal anaesthesia they often have too large a dead space, present too high a resistance to respiration, or are difficult to fix alongside the small head of a baby. They are unnecessarily complicated where simple equipment is extremely satisfactory.

Drugs for Maintenance of Anaesthesia

The relaxant drugs are dealt with elsewhere and are most suitable for use in the neonate and older child (see Chapter 26).

The neonate is very tolerant to the relaxant action of suxamethonium (2 mg/kg) but displays marked sensitivity to the muscarinic side-effects of the drug. For this reason, an adequate quantity of atropine (0·05 mg/kg) must be given parenterally beforehand. The neonate is sensitive to non-depolarising muscle relaxants and the correct dose may be difficult to assess. A practical approach is to give incremental doses of 0·25 mg *d*-tubocurarine until satisfactory conditions are achieved.

In older children, the non-depolarising relaxants are well tolerated. Nightingale and Bush (1973) compared *d*-tubocurarine (0·8 mg/kg) and pancuronium (0·13 mg/kg) and found both satisfactory in children aged 2–15 years. *d*-Tubocurarine had a slightly longer duration of action in their series. Non-depolarising relaxants are reversed with atropine (0·02–0·04 mg/kg) and neostigmine (0·08–0·1 mg/kg) either mixed together or given sequentially.

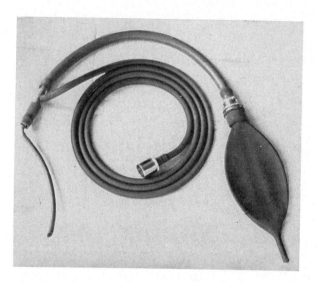

45/Fig. 10.—T-piece system for paediatric anaesthesia.

Artificial ventilation may be maintained with nitrous oxide and oxygen using the Rees/Ayre's T-piece. It should be noted that artificial ventilation using such a circuit can produce very marked falls in Pa_{CO_2} and this occasionally may be critical in low-output states (Prys-Roberts *et al.*, 1968).

Halothane is a most satisfactory anaesthetic agent for children, being rapidly absorbed and eliminated and giving excellent operating conditions. In the Mayo Clinic in 1970 it was used as a general anaesthetic agent in 91 per cent of patients under 10 years of age (Carney and Van Dyke, 1972).

In the very nature of many paediatric conditions, repeated general anaesthetics are necessary, either for investigation or for minor procedures or surgical adjustments, where sedation would suffice in adults. In spite of recent alarm, halothane is probably still the safest drug for these procedures in children. In the National Halothane Study there was no report of jaundice ascribed to halothane in a child under the age of 10 years.

Carney and Van Dyke (1972), in an extensive search of the literature could find only 9 cases of children developing jaundice with the remote possibility of halothane involvement. It would be unwise to suggest that post-halothane jaundice does not occur in children, but it is clear that the incidence, if it occurs, is very low (Sherlock, 1976), and many frequently repeated administrations are witness to the safety of halothane (Solosko *et al.*, 1972).

Routine Monitoring During Anaesthesia

Conventional adult methods of monitoring are not readily applicable to the small infant. Peripheral pulses are not easily accessible and the simplest method of monitoring both circulation and respiration entails the use of either a precordial or an oesophageal stethoscope (Fig. 11). With either of these instruments the pulse rate and respiratory rate may be monitored, while the breath sounds provide some indication of tidal volume.

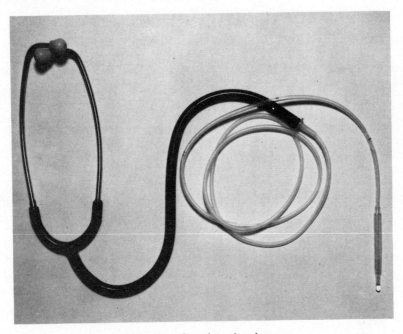

45/Fig. 11.—Oesophageal stethoscope.

The sphygmomanometer method of determining blood pressure in a neonate or small child is difficult due to inaudibility of the Korotkoff sounds. The width of the occluding cuff must cover at least two-thirds of the arm above the elbow and surround at least three-quarters of the limb. It should be remembered that a crying baby can raise its blood pressure as much as 30–50 mm Hg (4·0–6·7 kPa).

The recommendations of the American Heart Association (1967) include the use of oscillometry or the "flush" method (total limb exsanguination and observation of the pressure at which "flushing" occurs). In practice, blood pressure is rarely measured in a neonate or small child because of the difficulty of obtaining reliable readings. Instead, reliance is placed on monitoring the pulse rate and observing the colour and temperature of the skin.

As the temperature of a neonate or small child is subject to changes in the environment, a means of continuously recording the child's temperature is essential. This is conveniently done by placing a thermistor probe in the rectum or oesophagus. Temperature conservation may be achieved by wrapping the limbs and trunk or abdomen in aluminium foil, or supplementary heat provided from a low-temperature heating pad or water blanket.

Blood Replacement

The blood volume of a neonate is relatively greater than an adult and may be estimated at 88 ml/kg. Although the haemoglobin level of the neonate may be very high, this consists of both fetal and adult type, the former in rapid decline. Thus any blood losses at operation which are not replaced, on the basis of a pre-existing high haemoglobin, will contribute to an excessive physiological decline. A blood loss in excess of 10 per cent of the blood volume should be replaced with whole blood. As the blood volume of an average neonate is 300 ml this means that a blood loss of only 30 ml should be replaced. Conventional methods of estimating blood loss are not sufficiently accurate to measure such small amounts. If swabs are to be weighed, they must be kept wet to counter losses incurred by drying. An accurate scale is balanced with a dish containing water on each side. If the soiled swabs are then submerged in one dish and balanced with identical swabs in the other dish, quite small amounts of blood may be weighed accurately. In addition, it should be noted that a significant amount of blood may be overlooked in a length of suction tubing unless a measuring trap is inserted.

Small amounts of blood to be transfused may be given conveniently from a syringe. It should be warmed, and this may be done in the anaesthetist's hand. The blood should be fresh, when the potassium content is lower. Certain types of infusion apparatus are quite unsuitable for blood transfusion. Some sets with calibrated burettes do not have a filter proximal to the drip chamber. In consequence, larger particles in the blood tend to occlude the lumen of the drip orifice. These types of infusion sets should be reserved for aqueous infusions for which they are eminently suitable.

REFERENCES

ABERDEEN, E. (1965). Tracheostomy and tracheostomy care in infants. *Proc. roy. Soc. Med.*, **58**, 900.

ALLEN, T. H., and STEVEN, I. M. (1965). Prolonged endotracheal intubation in infants and children. *Brit. J. Anaesth.*, **37**, 566.

ALLEN, T. H., and STEVEN, I. M. (1972). Prolonged nasotracheal intubation in infants and children. *Brit. J. Anaesth.*, **44**, 835.

APGAR, V. (1953). Proposal for new method of evaluation of newborn infant. *Anesth. Analg. Curr. Res.*, **32**, 260.

APGAR, V., HOLADAM, D. A., JAMES, L. S., WEISBROT, I. M., and BERRIEN, C. (1958). Evaluation of the newborn infant; second report. *J. Amer. med. Ass.*, **168**, 1985.

ARANDA, J. V., SAHEB, N., STERN, L., AVERY, M. E. (1971). Arterial oxygen tension and retinal vasoconstriction in newborn infants. *Amer. J. Dis. Child.*, **122**, 189.

AVERY, M. E., and MEAD, J. (1959). Surface properties in relation to atelectasis and hyaline membrane disease. *Amer. J. Dis. Child.*, **95**, 517.

AYRE, P. (1956). The T-piece technique. *Brit. J. Anaesth.*, **28**, 520.

BARCROFT, J. (1946). *Researches on Pre-natal Life.* Vol. 1. Oxford: Blackwell Scientific Publications.

BATTERSBY, E. F., HATCH, D. J., and TOWEY, R. M. (1977). The effects of prolonged naso-endotracheal intubation in children (a study in infants and young children after cardiopulmonary bypass). *Anaesthesia*, **32**, 154.

BODDY, K., DAWES, G. S., and NATHANIELS, Z. (1973). In: *Fetal and Neonatal Physiology*. London: Cambridge University Press.

BODDY, K., DAWES, G. S., and ROBINSON, J. S. (1974). In: *Modern Perinatal Medicine*. Chicago: Year Book Medical Publishers.

BORN, G. V. R., DAWES, G. S., MOTT, J. C., and RENNICK, B. R. (1956). The constriction of the ductus arteriosus caused by oxygen and by asphyxia in newborn lambs. *J. Physiol. (Lond.)*, **132**, 304.

CARNEY, F. M. T., and VAN DYKE, R. A. (1972). Halothane hepatitis: a critical review. *Anesth. Analg. Curr. Res.*, **51**, 135.

CLEMENTS, J. A. (1957). Surface tension of lung extracts. *Proc. Soc. exp. Biol. (N.Y.)*, **95**, 170.

CREE, J. E., MEYER, J., HAILEY, D. (1973). Diazepam in labour: its metabolism and effect on the clinical condition and thermogenesis of the newborn. *Brit. med. J.*, **4**, 251.

CREW, A. D., WALL, E., and VARKONYI, P. I. (1975). Continuous positive airway pressure breathing (CPAP). *Anaesthesia*, **30**, 67.

DAVIES, P. A., ROBINSON, R. J., SCOPES, J. W., TIZARD, J. P. M., and WIGGLESWORTH, J. S. (1972). In: *Medical Care of Newborn Babies*. London: Spastics International Medical Publication.

DAWES, G. S. (1968). *Fetal and Neonatal Physiology*. Chicago: Year Book Medical Publishers.

DAWES, G. S., FOX, H. E., and RICHARDS, R. T. (1972). Variations in asphyxial gasping with fetal age in lambs and guinea-pigs. *Quart. J. exp. Physiology*, **57**, 131.

DAWES, G. S., JOHNSON, P., and ROBINSON, J. S. (1975). Foetal breathing. *Brit. med. Bull.*, **31**, 3.

DeLEMOS, R. A., SHERMATA, D. W., KNELSON, J. H., KOTAS, R., and AVERY, M. E. (1970). Acceleration of the appearance of surfactant in fetal lamb by administration of corticosteroids. *Amer. Rev. resp. Dis.*, **102**, 459.

FARGIER, P., SALLE, B., BAUD, M., GAGNAIRE, J. C., ARNAUD, P., and MAGNIN, P. (1974). Prévention du syndrome de détresse respiratoire chez le prémature intérêt du traitement antepartum par les glucorticoides. *Nouvelle Presse méd.*, **iii**, 1595.

FEDRICK, J., and BUTLER, N. R. (1972). British Perinatal Mortality Survey. *Lancet*, **2**, 768.

GANDY, G., ADAMSONS, K., CUNNINGHAM, N., SILVERMAN, W. A., and JAMES, L. S. (1964). Thermal environment and acid/base homeostasis in human infants during the first few hours of life. *J. clin. Invest.*, **43**, 751.

GLASS, L., RAJEGOWDA, B., and EVANS, H. E. (1971). Absence of respiratory distress syndrome in premature infants of heroin-addicted women. *Lancet*, **2**, 685.

GLUCK, L., KULOVICH, M. V., BORES, R. C., BRENNER, P. H., ANDERSON, G. G. and SPELLACY, W. N. (1971). Diagnosis of respiratory distress syndrome by amniocentesis. *Amer. J. Obstet. Gynec.*, **109**, 440.

GREGORY, G. A. (1975). Resuscitation of the newborn. *Anesthesiology*, **43**, 225.

GREGORY, G. A., KITTERMAN, J. A., PHIBBS, R. H., TOOLEY, W. H., and HAMILTON, W. K. (1971). Treatment of the idiopathic respiratory distress syndrome with continuous positive airway pressure. *New Engl. J. Med.*, **284**, 1333.

HARNED, H. S., HERRINGTON, R. T., and FERREIRO, J. I. (1970). The effects of immersion and temperature on respiration of newborn lamb. *Pediatrics*, **45**, 598.

HEY, E. (1972). Thermal regulation in the newborn. *Brit. J. hosp. Med.*, **5**, 51.

HEYMANN, M. A., and RUDOLPH, A. M. (1975). Control of the ductus arteriosus. *Physiol. Rev.*, **55**, 62.

HUCH, R., LUBBERS, D. W., and HUCH, A. (1972). Quantitative continuous measurement of partial oxygen pressure on the skin of adults and newborn babies. *Pflügers Arch. ges. Physiol.*, **337**, 185.

JACKSON REES, G., and OWEN THOMAS, J. B. (1966). A technique for pulmonary ventilation with a nasotracheal tube. *Brit. J. Anaesth.*, **38**, 901.

KEEP, P. J., and MANFORD, M. L. M. (1974). Endotracheal tube sizes for children. *Anaesthesia*, **29**, 181.

KERO, P., HIRVONEN, T., and VALIMAKI, I. (1973). Letter: Prenatal and postnatal isoxsuprine and respiratory-distress syndrome. *Lancet*, **2**, 198.

LEVIN, J. (1958). Endotracheal tubes in children. *Anaesthesia*, **13**, 40.

LEWIS, M. A. H., and YOUNG, D. G. (1969). Ventilatory problems with congenital diaphragmatic hernia. *Anaesthesia*, **24**, 571.

LIGGINS, G. C., and HOWIE, R. N. (1972). A controlled trial of antepartum glucocorticoid treatment for prevention of respiratory distress syndrome in premature infants. *Pediatrics*, **50**, 515.

LLOYD, J. K., and CLATWORTHY, H. W. (1958). Hydramnios as an aid to the early diagnosis of congenital obstruction of the intestinal tract: a study of the maternal and fetal factors. *Pediatrics*, **21**, 903.

MATTILA, M. A. K., HEIKEL, P. E., SCUTARINEN, T., and LINDROSS, E. L. (1971). Estimation of a suitable nasotracheal tube length for infants and children. *Acta anaesth. scand.*, **15**, 239.

MUSHIN, W. W. (1967). A neonatal inflating-bag. *Brit. med. J.*, **1**, 416.

NATHAN, D. M. (1975). The respiratory distress syndrome and glucortoid treatment: the case for enzyme induction. *Mt. Sinai J. Med. (N.Y.)*, **42**, 50.

NIGHTINGALE, D. A., and BUSH, G. H. (1973). A clinical comparison between tubocurarine and pancuronium in children. *Brit. J. Anaesth.*, **45**, 63.

NIXON, H. H. (1972). Neonatal emergency surgery. *Brit. J. hosp. Med.*, **8**, 73.

PARKER, D., and SOUTTAR, L. P. (1975). *In vivo* monitoring of blood P_{O_2} in newborn infants. In: *Oxygen Measurements in Biology and Medicine*, p. 269. Eds. Payne, J. P., and Hill, D. W. London: Butterworth & Co.

PATTLE, R. E. (1958). Properties, function and origin of the alveolar lining layer. *Nature (Lond.)*, **175**, 1125.

PENLINGTON, G. N. (1974). Endotracheal tube sizes for children. *Anaesthesia*, **29**, 494.

PRYS-ROBERTS, C., KELMAN, G. R., GREENBAUM, R., KAIN, M. L., and BAY, J. (1968). Haemodynamics and alveolar/arterial P_{O_2} differences at varying PA_{CO_2} in anaesthetised man. *J. appl. Physiol.*, **25**, 80.

RENDELL-BAKER, L., and SOUCEK, D. H. (1962). New paediatric face-masks and anaesthetic equipment. *Brit. med. J.*, **1**, 1960.

REYNOLDS, E. O. R. (1974). Pressure waveform and ventilator settings for mechanical ventilation in severe hyaline membrane disease. *Int. Anesthesiol. Clin.*, **12**, 259.

REYNOLDS, E. O. R. (1975). Management of hayline membrane disease. *Brit. med. Bull.*, **31**, 18.

REYNOLDS, E. O. R., and TAGHIZADEH, A. (1974). Improved prognosis of infants mechanically ventilated for hyaline membrane disease. *Arch. Dis Childh.*, **49**, 505.

RHODES, P. G., and HALL, R. T. (1973). Continuous positive airway pressure delivered by face mask in infants with the idiopathic respiratory distress syndrome. *Pediatrics*, **52**, 1.

RICKHAM, P. P., and JOHNSTONE, J. H. (1969). In: *Neonatal Surgery*. London: Butterworth & Co.

SHERLOCK, S. (1976). Personal communication.

SILVERMAN, W. A., AGATE, F. J., and FERTIG, J. W. (1963). A sequential trial of the non-thermal effect of atmospheric humidity on survival of newborn infants of low birth weight. *Pediatrics*, **31**, 719.

SOLOSKO, D., FRISSELL, M., and SMITH, R. B. (1972). 111 halothane anaesthesias in a paediatric patient. A case report. *Anesth. Analg. Curr. Res.,* **51,** 706.

SPELLACY, W. N., BULII, W. C., RIGGALL, F. C., and HOLSINGER, K. L. (1973). Human amniotic fluid lecithin/sphingomyelin ratio changes with estrogen or glucocorticoid treatment. *Amer. J. Obstet. Gynec.,* **115,** 216.

WU, B., KIKKAWA, Y., ORZALES, I. M., MOTOYAMA, E. K., KAIBARA, M., ZIGAS, C. J., and COOK, C. D. (1973). The effect of thyroxine on the maturation of fetal rabbit lungs. *Biol. Neonat. (Basel),* **22,** 161.

Section Seven

HISTORY

Chapter 46

AN OUTLINE OF THE DEVELOPMENT OF ANAESTHETIC APPARATUS

IT is not easy to trace the development of anaesthetic apparatus. Different anaesthetists and manufacturers have often worked on similar lines but achieved dissimilar results and unless their ideas were published they had little impact on future apparatus.

This outline will endeavour to trace the use of drawover inhalers for ether and chloroform, the use of blown air as a vehicle, the introduction of nitrous oxide leading to its use with oxygen and the development of the continuous flow machine, intermittent flow machine and the closed circuit. For those who are stimulated to delve deeper into the subject, Barbara Duncum's *Development of Inhalation Anaesthesia* and *The Development of Anaesthetic Apparatus* by K. Bryn Thomas can be thoroughly recommended, whilst the two slim volumes of W. Stanley Sykes, *Essays on the First Hundred Years of Anaesthesia* make delightful light reading.

Ether Inhalers

The first successful public administration of an anaesthetic for major surgery was administered by William Thomas Green Morton (1819–1868) on October 16th, 1846 at the Massachusetts General Hospital, Boston, U.S.A. Morton used sulphuric ether (di-ethyl ether) on a sponge in a glass sphere with an inlet and outlet (Fig. 1). For subsequent administrations he incorporated leather flap valves in the brass tube leading to the patient.

The first anaesthetic in England was given by Dr. Boott at his home, 24 Gower Street, London, on December 19th, 1846, for dental extraction on a Miss Lonsdale. Two days later Mr. William Squire anaesthetised Frederick Churchill for the amputation of his right leg. This was performed through the thigh by Robert Liston at University College Hospital. The latter is usually said to be the first major operation to be performed under anaesthesia in the United Kingdom. However, Sykes (1960) produced evidence that on December 19th, 1846, Dr. William Scott used ether for an operation, the nature of which is unknown, at Dumfries and Galloway Royal Infirmary (see also Baillie, 1966). The early inhalers were made of glass and were modifications of chemical apparatus in general use (Fig. 2).

John Snow (1813–1858), the first physician anaesthetist, realised early in 1847 that glass was not a good conductor of heat (caloric as he called it) and that the cooling of the ether lowered the inspired concentration of the anaesthetic. He then designed four inhalers and performed many experiments on animals to ascertain the quantity of ether to produce the various stages of anaesthesia. These he described in his book *On Chloroform and Other Anaesthetics* which he was writing when he died in 1858 and which was published posthumously.

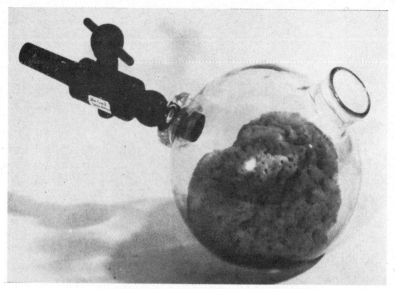

46/Fig. 1.—Morton Ether Inhaler (1846)

This is a photograph of a replica of the device used by Morton on 16th October, 1846. By the following day he had incorporated valves into a brass mouthpiece inserted into the globe.

46/Fig. 2.—Squire's Ether Inhaler

Used by Robert Liston on 21st December, 1846, at University College Hospital.

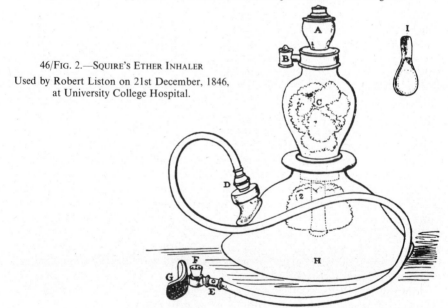

A. The Urn with its stopper, into which the ether is poured.
B. Valve which admits the air.
C. Contains sponge saturated with ether.
D. Valve which opens at each inspiration, and closes at each expiration.
E. Ferule for regulating the quantity of atmospheric air admitted.
F. Valve for the escape of expired air.
G. Mouth-piece.
H. Lower vase.
I. Spring for closing the nose.

His final model (Fig. 3a and b) was described in *On the Inhalation of the Vapour of Ether in Surgical Operations* (September, 1847). It was based on an inhaler designed for therapeutic use by Mr. Julius Jeffreys and had been in use for three months. The apparatus consisted of a japanned tin or plated copper box "of the size and form of a thick octavo volume", to serve as a carrying box and also as a water bath with a capacity of over 100 cubic inches (1·6 l) "which will supply, however, the caloric necessary to the conversion of one or two ounces of ether into vapour without being much reduced in temperature". The ether chamber, also of metal, was nearly 6 in (152 mm) in diameter and $1\frac{1}{4}$ in (32 mm) in depth with two orifices in the top, one peripheral and one central. It could be filled (or emptied) via the peripheral orifice into which a brass tube was screwed. In John Snow's words "merely for preventing a trifling loss of ether which would arise from evaporation into the apartment . . . and offer less resistance to the ingress of air than the most delicately balanced valve". The air entering by the tube was directed in a spiral course to the centre hole by a metal baffle of five turns, fixed to the top of the chamber with a gap of 1/16 in (1·6 mm) between it and the bottom plate. From the central hole a three-foot flexible pipe of $\frac{3}{4}$ in (19 mm) internal diameter led the ether-laden air to Snow's modification of F. Sibson's (1814–1876) face-piece. The face-piece, which he first used in May 1847, was made of metal with inlet and outlet valves of vulcanised india-rubber. The expiratory flap-valve was arranged to pivot so that air could be admitted to dilute the ether vapour.

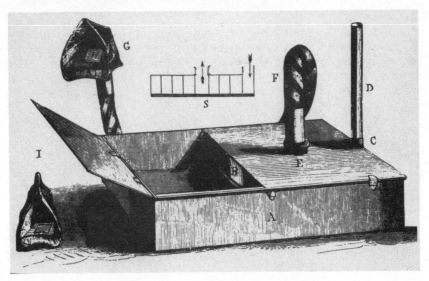

46/FIG. 3(a).—SNOW'S ETHER INHALER (1847)

A = Container/water bath
B = Ether chamber
C = Opening to ether chamber
D = Tube to prevent loss of ether
E = Connection to . . .
F = Flexible pipe
G = Face-piece
H = Inspiratory valve
I = Compressed face-piece

S = Section of ether chamber with arrows showing air flow.

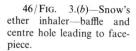

46/Fig. 3.(*b*)—Snow's ether inhaler—baffle and centre hole leading to face-piece.

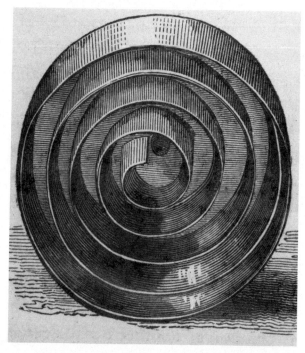

All the dimensions of the device were the results of experiments and Snow felt them all to be significant, as the following excerpt from his book shows: "The breathing tube ought to be so capacious as to offer no impediment to the most rapid inspiration, and to meet this requirement it must be wider than the trachea to compensate for the resistance arising from friction of the air against the interior of the tube. It is therefore $\frac{3}{4}$ in (19 mm) in internal diameter. The pipe for the admission of air to the ether is but $\frac{5}{8}$ in (16 mm) in diameter, but that is amply sufficient, since it has to give passage to a much smaller volume of fluid than the elastic tube: for the air expands to nearly twice its bulk, in passing over the ether, by the vapour it takes up". Thus John Snow, even at this early date, was aware of many of the problems to be overcome in the design of anaesthetic apparatus, especially those due to resistance to respiration and to the temperature change of a liquid when it vaporises.

Epstein (1958) found that with a minute volume of 9 l/min a respiratory rate of 27/min and the water temperature initially 62° F (16·6° C) this inhaler produced the following concentrations of ether (in vols. per cent) at the following times:

Time in min.	0·5	1	2	4	8
Concentration (Vols. per cent)	20	15	14	13	12

In 1877, Joseph Thomas Clover (1825–1882) described his portable regulating ether inhaler and this apparatus soon became very popular (Fig. 4). It consisted of a metal sphere on half of which was soldered a cylinder as a water jacket, the whole rotating on a central tube which, in the original model, was fashioned as two whistle-tips but in later versions was made with ports and baffles. The disadvantage of this inhaler was that the baffle narrowed the central tube, thus increasing the resistance to respiration. Various modifications were described, the first being Wilson Smith of 1899, but this was overlooked when Frederick Hewitt (1901) described his modification with a wider bore and, in later versions, without the water compartment—this modification of the Clover inhaler was in use as late as the early 1950s (for the others see Galley and King, 1948).

On the Continent, the inhaler described by Louis Ombrédanne (1871–1956) in 1908 was preferred and has been used until very recently in those parts of the world under French influence. The inhaler is a sphere originally containing a sponge but in later models a felt-pad was preferred. The air inlet and the bag are attached to the control tube which is at right angles to the filling orifice and the opening for the mask. The mask is made of metal and has a finger ring on either side. Ombrédanne particularly noted the effect of carbon dioxide retention in increasing the respiration.

In 1921, Stanley Rawson Wilson (1882–1927) and Kenneth Bernard Pinson (b. 1890) described the "ether bomb" which produced 100 per cent ether vapour and was independent of either bellows for air or the use of nitrous oxide (Fig. 5). The amount of ether could be accurately controlled by a needle valve and as the bomb was placed in hot water the issuing vapour was warm. In fact, the temperature under the mask was found to be between 90° F and 98° F (32° C–37° C).

In 1939, Dabrick Joseph Flagg (1886–1970), in the 6th edition of his book *The Art of Anaesthesia* described a simple ether vaporiser "the Flagg Can" which Sir Robert Macintosh had, in fact, used in 1938 under war conditions in Spain. It consisted of an ether tin with holes punched in its top for the admission of air, connected by a rubber tube from the filling hole to either a face-mask, pharyngeal airway or endotracheal tube.

The need for simple and safe vaporisers for use by hurriedly-trained anaesthetists in wartime conditions led Macintosh to design the Oxford Vaporiser in 1941. In this vaporiser the ether chamber was kept at 30° C by the melting and crystallization of calcium chloride. Concentrations of up to 25 vols per cent of ether could be obtained. A spring-containing bellows incorporated on top of the apparatus provided an indication of the respiration of the patient, and by gently pressing this bag with the hand, the patients lungs could also be inflated.

In 1952, Lucien Morris introduced the copper kettle (Vernitrol) vaporiser for ether but it proved so useful that it was soon being used for the vaporisation of halothane and other volatile anaesthetic agents. This most versatile of vaporisers is based on the principle of using a highly conductive material in manufacture. When firmly attached to a table top of an anaesthetic machine of similar conductivity, a large heat reservoir is created that prevents the temperature of the liquid falling much below room temperature. Provided the vapour pressure of the liquid in the chamber is known, then, when a specified quantity

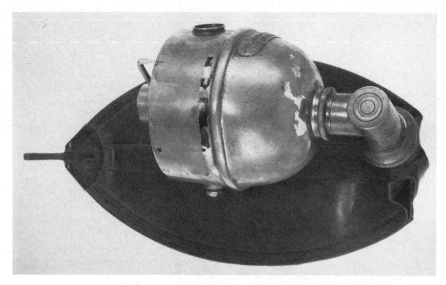

46/Fig. 4.—Clover's Portable Regulating Ether Inhaler (1877)
(for description, see text).

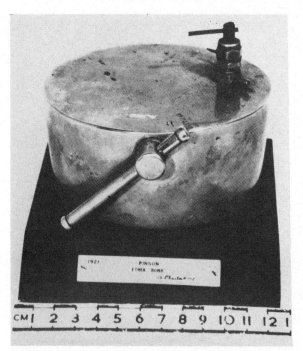

46/Fig. 5.—The Pinson Ether Bomb (1921)

A strong cast-steel vessel in which the ether was placed, the whole immersed in warm water, so that pure ether vapour could be delivered when the valve was opened.

of oxygen is "bubbled-through" the vaporiser and added to 5 litres of nitrous oxide and oxygen, the concentration of the contained anaesthetic vapour can be easily calculated (see Chapter 7).

In 1956, Epstein and Macintosh developed the E.M.O. inhaler (Fig. 6). This was designed to deliver a required concentration of anaesthetic vapour irrespective of variations in the temperature of the liquid anaesthetic throughout the range likely to be met in clinical practice. The apparatus incorporates a water-bath which surrounds the vaporising chamber and, by acting as a heat buffer, prevents sudden marked changes in the temperature of the liquid anaesthetic.

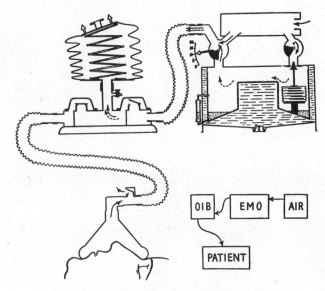

46/Fig. 6.—Epstein, Macintosh, Oxford (E.M.O.) Inhaler
With Oxford Inflating Bellows (OIB) unit arranged for ether and air inhalation.

An ether-containing, bellows-type thermostat automatically ensures that a constant vapour concentration of anaesthetic leaves the inhaler. The E.M.O. inhaler must be calibrated to suit the particular volatile anaesthetic used in it.

Divinyl ether (Vinesthene).—Many other ethers were tried as anaesthetics; the only one which found favour, albeit for only a short time, and led to the design of special vaporisers, was divinyl ether (Vinesthene), the anaesthetic properties of which were discovered in 1930 by Leake and Chen (see Chapter 7). It was only used for brief procedures as prolonged anaesthesia with this agent caused liver damage. Goldman (1936) (Fig. 7) described a metal inhaler containing a sponge together with a simple rotating control attached to a bag. This was improved by Boston and Salt at Oxford in 1940, by the addition of a valve to allow the entry of air when the bag was empty and the control was modified to produce a smoother increase of concentration. Goldman also used a simple drip vaporiser which, unlike those used for diethyl ether, did not require a water-jacket because the divinyl ether was more volatile than diethyl ether and only two drops of the former were needed per inspiration.

46/Fig. 7.—Goldman's Divinyl Ether (Vinesthene)
Inhaler

The metal drum attached to the face-piece contains a
sponge which is impregnated with divinyl ether. The control
tap on the top of the drum has three positions "Fill", "On"
and "Off". In the "On" position the patient breathes the
divinyl ether mixture.

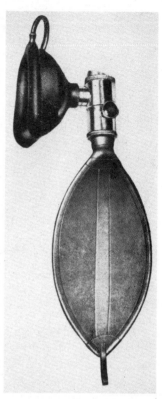

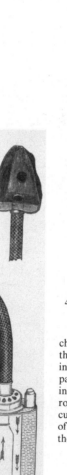

46/Fig. 8.—Snow's Chloroform
Inhaler

Sectional view of the vaporising
chamber showing the water jacket,
the chloroform level gauge and, in the
inner cylinder, the roll of blotting
paper supported on wires and dipping
into the liquid chloroform. The arrows indicate the direction of the
current of air drawn through the ring
of holes around the tube leading to
the face-piece.

Chloroform Inhalers

In 1847, following a suggestion of David Waldie (1813–1889) (a Liverpool chemist), Sir James Young Simpson (1811–1870) of Edinburgh successfully administered chloroform as an anaesthetic. As this new agent lacked the irritant properties of ether its popularity spread rapidly throughout the United Kingdom. Simpson preferred the use of a towel on which to vaporise the chloroform, whilst others designed inhalers. For example, Edward William Murphy (1802–1877) described a very small inhaler for use in obstetrics (1848) containing a sponge which was charged with three-quarters of a drachm (2·5 ml) of chloroform.

It only covered the mouth; the nose was closed until the effects of the chloroform appeared, then it was released. It would appear that the state of unawareness produced was really analgesia, although it was not known by that name at the time.

In 1853, John Snow described his chloroform inhaler (Fig. 8) which he had been using for some years. It consisted of a double metal cylinder, the outer space of which was a water-jacket, the inner being the vaporising chamber for the chloroform which was absorbed on to two coils of stout "bibulous paper". It was in this year (1853) that he successfully administered chloroform to Her Majesty Queen Victoria at the birth of Prince Leopold, but in this particular instance he dropped the chloroform on to a handkerchief.

John Snow's principle of adding a measured quantity of chloroform to a known volume of air to produce a mixture of the required concentration was used by Clover in 1862. Although this method provided sufficient air and chloroform for a number of patients, it was clumsy in that it required a large bag to be slung over the shoulder of the anaesthetist. The mixture was diluted by admitting air with a valve on the face-piece. In the same year, Thomas Skinner developed a simple drop-bottle for chloroform to be used in conjunction with a metal-framed mask covered with lint or gauze. This was the first collapsible mask to be produced and it was small enough to be carried in a top hat. Many such devices were then introduced of which the best known is that described by Kurt Schimmelbusch (1860–1895) in 1890. Walter Tyrrell (1852–1931), anaesthetist to St. Thomas' Hospital, in 1898 described his rigid mask, the centre support of which was hollow and perforated so that oxygen could be administered and it also had the added advantage in that it could be connected to a Junker's inhaler (see below). Chloroform, at an early date, was used with ether and even alcohol. Robert Ellis described his improved inhaler in 1866, which would administer all three vapours. He used wicks and capillary attraction to increase the vaporisation of the liquids.

Although the inhaler developed by F. A. Junker (1828–1901) in 1867 is not a drawover inhaler, it is worth mentioning here (Fig. 9). This was first used for bichloride of methylene, a mixture of chloroform and methyl alcohol. Air was blown from a rubber bulb through the chloroform by a tube dipping into the eight drachms (27 ml) of liquid which were placed therein and flowed out via a short tube to be delivered, by narrow tubing, to a vulcanite face-piece. It was thus possible, by connecting the rubber tubes to the pipe of the inhaler to blow liquid chloroform at the patient, inevitably with fatal results. Even as late as 1927, a death occurred from this cause despite many modifications to prevent

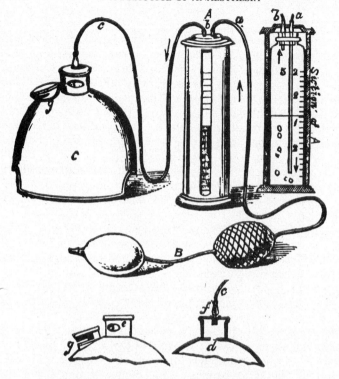

46/FIG. 9.—JUNKER CHLOROFORM INHALER (1867)

Air is blown from the double bellows (B) to the chloroform jar (A) via the pipe (a). The vapour then passes by the pipe (b and c) to the face-mask (C). The latter has an inlet valve (e) to allow the patient to breathe in air and expire through a rubber flap expiratory valve (see lower sectional diagram).

this tragedy (e.g. Dudley Buxton in 1890; Carter Braine in 1892; Frederick Hewitt in 1901; and the incorporation of a one-way valve by M. Rigby in 1917).

An ingenious inhaler for delivering a known percentage of chloroform (Fig. 10) was brought into being in 1903 by Augustus George Vernon Harcourt (1814–1919). The chloroform bottle was tapered, to help compensate for the lowering of the level of the liquid as the chloroform evaporated, and two beads were placed in the chloroform as a temperature indicator. Thus, if the temperature fell below 16° C, both beads would float whilst if it rose above 18° C, both would sink. Incorporated into this device were two metal unidirectional valves, one on the chloroform side and the other on the air inlet side of the mixing chamber. As the whole apparatus was portable, it could be positioned either on a stand (one version of which had a candle-stand to enable the correct temperature to be maintained) or suspended from the neck of the anaesthetist.

Goodman Levy (1856–1954) designed his inhaler in 1905 to deliver known concentrations of chloroform, with a water bath and thermometer. Thus he introduced the principle of manual thermo-compensation into the design of anaesthetic devices (Fig. 11). In 1911, he demonstrated the fact that adrenaline caused ventricular fibrillation in cats lightly anaesthetised with chloroform.

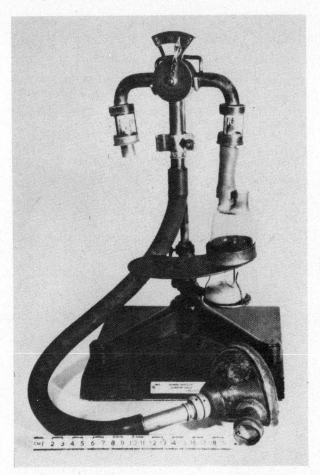

46/FIG. 10.—VERNON HARCOURT CHLOROFORM INHALER (1903)

Air is drawn through two unidirectional metal flap valves in glass cylinders on the side-arms, one connected to the chloroform-containing bottle. The two streams are controlled and mixed in the drum in the centre and then drawn by the patient down the centre tube to the face-mask.

This led the Committee on Anaesthesia of the American Medical Association of 1912 to state that "the use of chloroform for major operations is unjustifiable". However, its use continued in Scotland for many years after this.

In 1933, Zebulon Mennell (1876–1939) modified the "Junker" chloroform bottle for the production of analgesia for obstetrics (Fig. 12). The advantage of this modification was that, as it was necessary to invert the inhaler before filling, the pipes could be so positioned that the chamber could not be overfilled. This also meant that it was impossible to blow liquid chloroform at the patient. The two tubes on the top were connected by a small by-pass which limited the strength of chloroform vapour that could be produced.

In 1943, The E.S.O. Chloroform Vaporiser was introduced for the use of

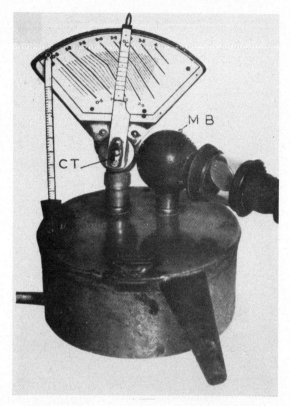

46/Fig. 11(a).—Regulating Chloroform Inhaler designed by Levy in 1905.

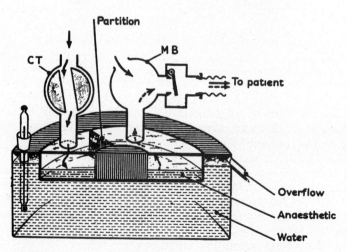

46/Fig. 11(b).—Schematic section of Levy's chloroform inhaler of 1905.

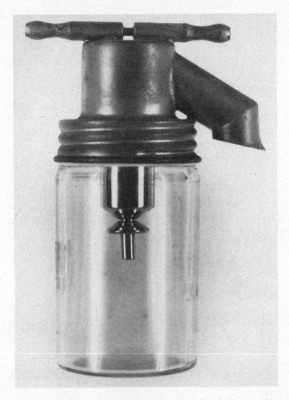

46/FIG. 12.—Mennell's Chloroform Bottle (see text)

airborne troops because pilots did not wish to carry highly inflammable ether on board. Concentrations of chloroform between 0·5 per cent and 4·5 per cent could be obtained with this apparatus.

Trichloroethylene Inhalers

Trichloroethylene was introduced by Langton Hewer and Hadfield in 1941. Initially this agent was used in the chloroform bottle of the Boyle's machine, but in 1942, Marrett described a drawover apparatus consisting of two bottles with wicks and controls for the production of anaesthesia using trichloroethylene and/or ether. In 1943, Freedman based his inhaler on that of Mennell's modified Junker bottle but as it was a drawover inhaler, the gas pathways were enlarged. It was intended primarily for producing analgesia in childbirth. However, performance of this device was very variable thus enabling the concentration of trichloroethylene to be increased sufficiently to produce the second stage of anaesthesia. For this reason it never won the approval of the Central Midwives Board as a suitably safe apparatus for patient self-administration in labour. An automatic temperature-activated compensatory device was clearly required and therefore a variety of patterns were then produced.

Hill (1944) described an inhaler for delivering trichloroethylene vapour on demand for self-administered analgesia in dentistry. This device was similar to the Mennell but contained a wick as trichloroethylene has a lower vapour pressure than chloroform.

Following much work in the Nuffield Department of Anaesthesia at Oxford, Epstein and Macintosh in 1949 developed the first Emotril inhaler in which the temperature compensation was manually operated as in the E.S.O. inhaler. The following year, however, the Anaesthetics Committee of the Medical Research Council added the specification that the thermo-compensation should be automatic, i.e. over a wide range of external temperatures the output of the apparatus must remain constant. The redesigning of the Emotril took eighteen months and the final model used a mercury filled thermostat. There was a simple additional air inlet so that the inhaled mixture could be diluted from 0·5 per cent to 0·3 per cent.

The Airlene inhaler made by Airmed, was a small hand-held inhaler using a bimetallic helix as the temperature compensatory mechanism. The dilution control could be locked in place with a key, so that the patient could not vary the concentration of trichloroethylene that was to be delivered.

Cyprane in the Tecota Mk I (Fig. 13, a prototype of the late 1940s) used a

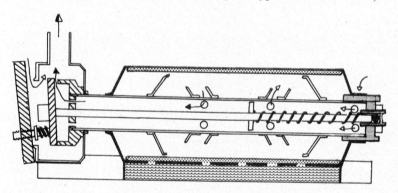

46/Fig. 13.—Section of Tecota Mk I Trilene Inhaler

On the right side air (→) is drawn into the vaporising chamber and collects trichloroethylene vapour (→). This is then mixed with air (→) on the left side of the diagram and the mixture (→) then passes to the face-mask. The central metal bar runs from one end of the inhaler to the other and is spring-loaded so that the dilution of the trichloroethylene vapour can be adjusted.

long metal bar, the expansion and contraction of which altered the position of a spring-loaded plate and would thus vary the amount of air passing through the vaporising chamber. This and other versions were all prototypes until the Mk 6 was marketed in 1955. On this machine, the thermo-compensatory device is a bimetallic strip which, whilst opening and shutting an orifice, controls the amount of trichloroethylene vapour saturated air that leaves the vaporising chamber.

The mechanism is the same as that used in the Fluotec (see below) for halothane and the Cardiff Penthrane Inhaler for methoxyflurane (Jones *et al.*, 1971) but, in the latter, two bimetallic strip valves are used. Burns (1954) designed the Burns Benson inhaler for the self-administration of trichlorethylene in labour. It was unique, as it used the carburetter principle.

Halothane

Following the introduction of halothane in 1956, it was administered in a Boyle's bottle, but this, in spite of modifications, did not give a sensitive enough control. Cyprane produced the Fluotec Mk I in 1957 (McKay, 1957; Brennan, 1957) which was calibrated for up to 3 per cent halothane. The Mk II was of similar shape but calibrated to 4 per cent, whilst the Mk III, introduced in 1969 (Paterson *et al.*) although acting on the same principle of a bimetallic strip altering a valve from the vaporising chamber, has an easier, rotating disc control instead of a rotating bar. This is more accurate at low flows and with varying pressures, and is calibrated to 5 per cent halothane. It is also less likely to stick (see p. 285).

B.O.C. produced the Halox vaporiser (Young, 1966) based on a variation of the Copper Kettle principle, but requiring calculations to obtain the delivered concentration, while the concentration delivered by the Foregger "Fluomatic" is read from a scale similar to that on the Levy's chloroform vaporiser.

As the design of thermo-compensated vaporisers was taking place, Goldman described the first version of his modified McKesson 965 vaporiser in 1959 and the improved model in 1962 (see p. 286). This simple device used an AC petrol-pump bowl to contain the halothane and delivered no more than 2·3 per cent. It had a low resistance and thus could be placed inside a circle system, or used as a drawover inhaler.

To speed the induction of anaesthesia with ether delivered from the E.M.O., the Oxford team developed the simple halothane induction unit in 1964 (Bryce-Smith). After four years' work, Parkhouse, in 1966, described the performance of the Oxford miniature vaporiser which is primarily designed as a drawover unit for induction of anaesthesia, although it functions safely with continuous flow. It is not thermo-compensated but has a small sealed water-filled compartment in its base which acts as a heat reservoir and buffer. Blease produced a Universal vaporiser which, by changing the controller, could be used to vaporise ten different anaesthetics or mixtures.

The Abingdon vaporiser was first marketed in 1970 with a vapour-filled temperature compensator which was altitude sensitive. In 1973 this was modified with a similar temperature compensator to that in the E.M.O. based on the expansion of liquid ether inside flexible metal bellows within a capsule.

The Promedica Research and Development Corporation produced the Vaporex vaporiser which works on the drip-feed principle, dropping the liquid halothane on to a vaporising surface. The scale attached to the flowmeter is calibrated so that the percentage of halothane entering the system in relation to the flow rate of the carrier gas can be read directly. The Vaporex produces up to 4 per cent halothane.

Nitrous Oxide

Nitrous oxide was discovered in about 1772 by Joseph Priestley, who called it "dephlogisticated nitrous air". Humphry Davy prepared it, inhaled it, noted its intoxicating properties and renamed it Nitrous Oxide or "Laughing gas". He investigated its other properties and in 1800 published his important book *Researches Chemical and Philosophical, Chiefly Concerning Nitrous Oxide or Dephlogisticated Nitrous Air and its Respiration*, in which he wrote:

"As nitrous oxide in its extensive operation appears capable of destroying physical pain, it may probably be used with advantage during surgical operations in which no great effusion of blood takes place."

This remark was not acted upon and inhalation of nitrous oxide became part of the shows demonstrated by itinerant chemists, particularly in the United States.

At one of these, given by Gardner Quincy Colton (1814–1898) in Hartford, Connecticut on December 10th, 1844, Horace Wells (1815–1848), a dentist, noticed that one of the audience injured his leg badly whilst under the influence of nitrous oxide without feeling any pain. He arranged for Colton to administer nitrous oxide to himself while Mr. Rigg removed a tooth—a procedure he found quite painless. Wells then arranged a demonstration at the Massachusetts General Hospital, Boston, before the students of John Collins Warren, an old student of Astley Cooper and of Dupuytren, which was a total fiasco. Wells was jeered and booed by the students as he left the hospital, but Morton had been there and this set him on the road to the events of October 16th, 1846.

Nitrous Oxide Cylinders

Nitrous oxide was originally made and stored in gasometers of which one of the earliest was described by Humphry Davy in his book. It was transferred to bags made from animal bladders or oiled silk for inhalation. T. W. Evans (1823–1897), an English dentist practising in Paris, having seen a demonstration by G. Q. Colton in 1867, came to England in 1868 with a record of hundreds of cases. He gave a demonstration at the Dental Hospital which stimulated such interest that a Committee of Investigation into Nitrous Oxide was formed by members of the Odontological Society and the Dental Hospital in London.

Messrs. Coxeter and Messrs. Barth, in about 1865, made bulky cylinders of brass bound copper to contain the nitrous oxide under pressure. These were replaced by iron in 1870 by S. S. White of Philadelphia and, finally, by molybdenum steel, the modern light-weight cylinders. An iron cylinder of approximately 9 in × 3 in (23 cm × 8 cm) weighed 6 lb (2·7 kg) when empty and contained 9 oz (136 l) of nitrous oxide when full.

Nitrous Oxide Apparatus

In 1868, Clover described his face-piece with inspiratory and expiratory valves and an opening for the attachment of a rebreathing bag if required. The figure shows the great difficulties that anaesthetists must have had in those days to obtain a good fit of the face-piece (Fig. 14).

A piece of apparatus which proved successful for fifty years or more was designed by Hewitt, later Sir Frederick Hewitt (1857–1916), in 1893. This was a cylinder stand with foot-operated control and valved stopcock for the administration of nitrous oxide and air (Fig. 15). In 1897 he improved it by the addition of a cylinder of oxygen and two conjoined bags, regulating stopcock and mixing chamber but as the pressure in the bags was not identical, the concentration of oxygen delivered was unreliable.

Alfred Coleman, H. J. Paterson and Harvey Hilliard all described different methods of administering the nitrous oxide by the nasal route in 1898, including the use of a nasal catheter passed into the pharynx.

The S.S.White Dental Manufacturing Co. produced a nitrous oxide-oxygen apparatus in the late 1890s, using a modern yoke system, for the mixing and delivery of the gases. In the 1903 catalogue the "gauge plate" which controlled the oxygen was described as "especially designed to enable the operation to follow Dr. Hewitt's method. It must be understood, however, that exact and predetermined percentages are neither practical nor desirable".

In 1910 approximately, A. C. Clark Co. of Chicago produced a nitrous oxide and oxygen machine for analgesia or anaesthesia consisting of a four-yoke cylinder stand without reducing valves but with a mixing chamber, the mixture of nitrous oxide and oxygen being controlled by a single handle. The gases were passed into two rubber bags contained within string bags in an attempt to equalise the pressures. In 1909, Arthur Ernest Guedel (1883–1956) devised the

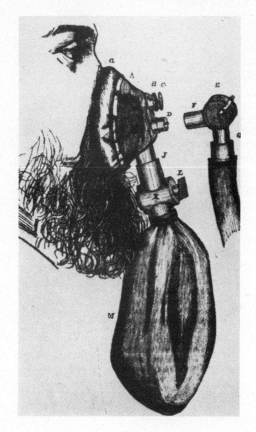

46/Fig. 14.—Clover's Face-piece

A = Metal face-piece body.
a = Rubber pad.
B = Expiratory valve, very lightly spring-loaded ivory plate.

C = Expiratory valve cover.
D = Inspiratory valve.
E = 3-way tap with connection F to fit over D and G, to wire-wound hose H, which leads to Cattlin bag.

J = Connection to tap K and thus to rebreathing bag M.

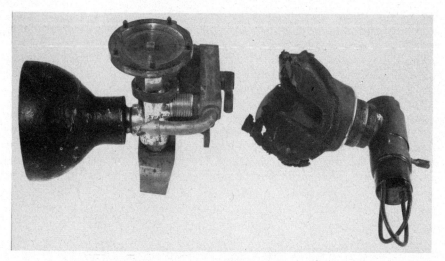

46/Fɪɢ. 15.—Hᴇᴡɪᴛᴛ's Vᴀʟᴠᴇ Sᴛᴏᴘᴄᴏᴄᴋ ᴀɴᴅ Cʏʟɪɴᴅᴇʀ Sᴛᴀɴᴅ

On the left of the picture are shown one of the two nitrous oxide cylinders, the studded foot-key control, and the gas outlet. The nitrous oxide then passed by rubber tubing to the rebreathing bag (not shown) and face-piece (shown on right). The control lever (far right) could be adjusted so that the patient breathed either room air or pure nitrous oxide. By repeatedly manipulating the lever the patient could be made to inspire air and then expire into the rebreathing bag. For practical purposes induction usually took place with total rebreathing of nitrous oxide and this was followed by an inspiration of air every 3 or 4 breaths to provide a very inadequate oxygen intake.

technique of self administration of nitrous oxide for obstetrics and minor surgical operations, but it needed constant attention to the cylinder key to keep the bag inflated.

In 1910, Elmer Isaac McKesson (1881–1935) whilst still an intern in Toledo, devised the first "intermittent" flow nitrous oxide and oxygen apparatus with an accurate percentage control and in 1911 he introduced the principle of fractional rebreathing. The McKesson apparatus was developed into its present form in 1930.

Jay Albion Heidbrink (1878–1957) following dissatisfaction with a nitrous oxide/oxygen machine shown him by Charles Teter of Cleveland in 1903, designed his own using commercially available reducing valves. His first commercial model was produced in 1912. F. J. Cotton and W. M. Boothby described their "perfected" apparatus in 1912 containing a method of making the flow of gases "visible so that the proportions may be approximately estimated at a glance"—the first of the anaesthetic flowmeters.

Nitrous Oxide Analgesia Apparatus (Dental and Obstetric)

The Walton I (produced in 1925) was the first British *intermittent* flow machine designed for the use of nitrous oxide/oxygen anaesthesia in dentistry. It used a simple but effective system whereby a metal bar (applied to the outside of a rubber bag) moved as the bag filled to control a pinchcock acting on the tubing admitting the fresh gas from the cylinder. As the design also incorporated reducing valves on the gas cylinders, the relatively low pressures used allowed the gas tubing to be easily compressed. When the patient inspired, the bag partially emptied and the pinchcock then allowed more gas to flow in again. There was a bag for nitrous oxide and another one using the same principle for oxygen. Finally, the incorporation of a mixing chamber enabled the anaesthetist to vary the concentration of the two gases. The other models culminated in the Model V which was produced in 1958.

Robert James Minnitt (1889–1974) and A. Charles King adapted the McKesson machine to produce 35 per cent nitrous oxide in air for analgesia in obstetrics in 1934 (Fig. 16). The Queen Charlotte's version of this apparatus was produced in 1936 in which the reducing valve was an Adams' with a bag-operated pinchcock—this delivered 50 per cent nitrous oxide in air. In 1937, a device to

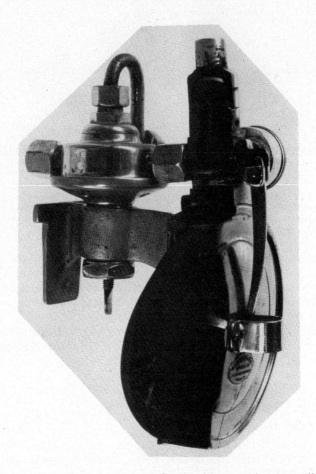

46/FIG. 16.—MINNITT'S GAS/AIR ANALGESIA APPARATUS (1933)

The nitrous oxide flows at 60 p.s.i. (414 kPa) from the McKesson reducing valve (on left) into the rubber bag within the metal can. As the bag expands so the lever compresses the inlet until it is finally occluded. The nitrous oxide flows up past a check valve and comes in contact with an air-inlet for dilution before passing to the patient. Once emptied the bag refills again.

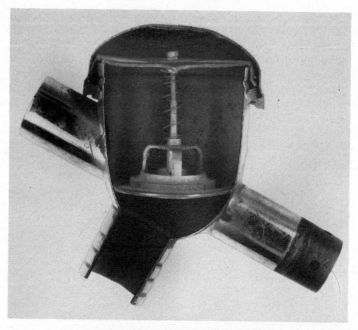

46/FIG. 17.—THE C.M. ATTACHMENT

The apparatus is fitted to enable the patient to receive 3 breaths of 100 per cent nitrous oxide before reverting to the pre-selected mixture. The nitrous oxide enters the attachment through the small holes seen on right of picture and then flows up under the diaphragm to the reservoir bag attached to bottom tube. When filled the negative pressure created by inspiration opens the diaphragm and the contents of the bag pass to the patient via the port on left side of picture.

enable the patient to take three breaths of 100 per cent nitrous oxide at the beginning of each pain was produced, namely the C.M. attachment (Fig. 17). However, this rendered the machine unsuitable for use by unsupervised midwives. The Minnitt machine was not superseded until the production of safe inhalers for trichloroethylene were introduced in the 1950s.

Bracken (1963) demonstrated the possibility of mixing 50 per cent nitrous oxide and 50 per cent oxygen in one cylinder (marketed by B.O.C. as "Entonox"). The production of the small two-stage reducing valve is the latest item in the analgesia story, providing a safe apparatus for use by midwives or paramedical personnel (e.g. ambulance drivers). The Central Midwives Board approved the mixture in 1963 and the apparatus in 1965.

Nitrous Oxide and Anaesthetic Vapours

In 1876, Clover recorded his nitrous oxide and ether apparatus which he had used successfully in 2,000 cases but in 1877 it was superseded by his portable regulating inhaler (see Fig. 4).

James Taylor Gwathmey (1863–1944) used the water-sight feed flowmeter in his anaesthetic machine of 1912 which incorporated a holder for a spirit lamp below the nitrous oxide control to prevent freezing and a heater below the water bottle of the flowmeter. It was the meeting of Henry Edmund Gaskin Boyle

(1875–1941) of St. Bartholomew's Hospital with Gwathmey at a Congress in 1912 that led the former to produce the first Boyle machine in 1917. Prior to this, in 1915, Sir Geoffrey Marshall of Guy's had devised his nitrous oxide-oxygen-ether apparatus which he did not describe in print until 1920 (Fig. 18).

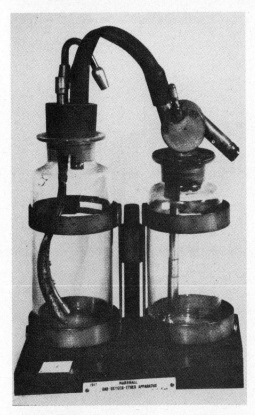

46/FIG. 18.—MARSHALL'S GAS-OXYGEN-ETHER APPARATUS (1917)

The bottle on the left is a water-sight flowmeter and on the right an ether vaporiser. The gases enter the flowmeter bottle and depending on the flow emerge from one of the holes under the water. They then pass by the wide-bore tubing to the vaporiser. The amount of gases entering this bottle could be controlled by the ON/OFF lever.

The first Boyle machine was very similar to the Marshall and was first shown publicly at the Royal Society of Medicine in 1918. The flowmeter and ether bottle were mounted on an upright, attached to a wheeled stand, containing four nitrous oxide cylinders with reducing valves warmed by spirit lamps, and one oxygen cylinder (Fig. 19). The gases were delivered to a Cattlin bag, a Hewitt stopcock and face-mask. 1926 saw the addition of a second vaporising bottle, 1927 the addition of a tube for carbon dioxide to the flowmeter and in 1930 plungers were added to the vaporisers. Coxeter produced the dry bobbin flowmeter in 1933, at first with no controls but later needle valves were incorporated. In 1937, Rotameters superseded the less accurate dry bobbin flowmeter and the machine has virtually remained the same ever since. Variations to the above general plan are fairly common—in the collection of apparatus at St. Thomas' Hospital there is a Coxeter Boyle's machine with a three gas water-sight flowmeter, no plungers, but needle valves on the flowmeter. Harold Norris Webber (1881–1954) in 1920 produced his modified Boyle's bottles in which the chloroform and ether bottle were placed in parallel to prevent contamination of the liquid in the second bottle when both were used together.

Flowmeters

Apart from Cotton and Boothby's water-sight flowmeter that Gwathmey and Boyle used in their machines (see above), other devices were being produced. Karl Connell (d. 1941) was concerned with the accurate measurement of gas flows and employed kinetic flowmeters of the piston principle in 1908, which he

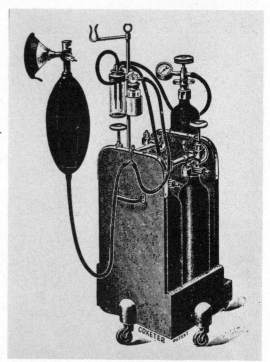

46/Fig. 19.—Boyle Apparatus as set up.

changed to a rotating vane type in 1911. In 1934, he patented his two-ball flowmeter. The glass tubes containing the two balls are of a complex design so that it is possible to measure both low and high flows with a great degree of accuracy. The scale beside the tubes can be rotated so that the same tube can be used to deliver more than one gas. The apparatus was also mounted with a soda-lime canister, drip-feed vaporiser and one-way valves, and a rebreathing bag, all set on a stainless-steel trolley—an early date for the use of such materials.

In the Heidbrink flowmeter the tube containing a float is made of metal, which makes machining to an exact form easier. On top of the float is a light-weight rod which rises in a glass tube so that it can be seen and the flow rate measured.

The Foregger flowmeters are of the water-depression type, the increased pressure being produced by a small fixed orifice. The disadvantages of this type of flowmeter are that dirt in the orifice leads to a much lower flow than that indicated and the scale is crowded at the lower flows.

Reducing Valves

In England the first reducing valve used in anaesthesia was that designed by A. A. Beard in 1899 for the production of a constant pressure of oxygen and acetylene for the "lime light" used for stage illumination. It consisted of a rubber bellows, the expansion of which, acting via lazy tongs, prevented the further passage of the gas. On the top of the bellows was a spring. The bellows, piston and spring were enclosed in a metal case with a hole to allow the outside of the bellows to be at atmospheric pressure. F. H. Adams, a mechanic in the

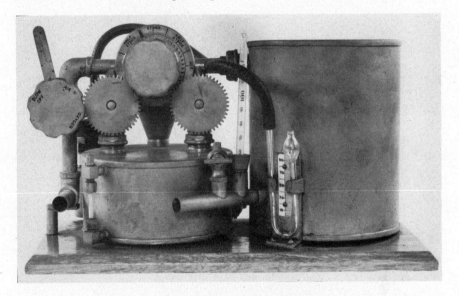

46/Fig. 20.—Mennell's Endotracheal Insufflation Apparatus

The amount of air which passes over the ether (left tank) is controlled by the three cogwheels and the resulting mixture flows through a coil in the water bath (right tank) and thence to the gum elastic catheter. There is a thermometer and a mercury manometer. Oxygen could be added to the air blown by an electrically driven pump (not shown).

workshop of Coxeter Ltd., patented his improved version in 1921. The Adams valve which reduced the pressure to 5–10 lb f in^{-2} (34–69 kPa) was more sturdily built and the bellows were replaced by a sheet of thicker rubber. The compression of the spring could be varied and there was an additional small spring acting in a contrary direction to the first to prevent juddering. All reducing valves act on the principle that the product of the high pressure from the cylinder times the small area of the orifice through which the gas flows, equals the product of the lower pressure times the larger area of the diaphragm plus the pressure exerted by the spring. The other British reducing valve was the Endurance in which the lazy tongs linkage between the diaphragm and the valve seating was replaced by a rigid bar, as in the McKesson and Heidbrink reducing valves, but in the latter two the diaphragm was made of metal and the outlet pressure was 60 lb f in^{-2} (414 kPa).

The Adams and Endurance valves were replaced by the B.O.C. 60 M and 120 M valves in 1965, in which the diaphragm is made of plastic and the high-pressure orifice is closed by a needle plunger pressed on to the diaphragm by a small spring.

INTRATRACHEAL INSUFFLATION

Samuel Meltzer and John Auer, working at the Rockefeller Institute,

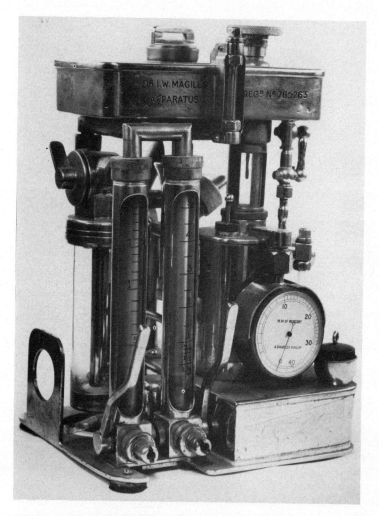

46/Fig. 21.—Dr. I. W. Magill's Apparatus

This consists of flowmeters for oxygen and nitrous oxide, a bottle for vaporising chloroform and an ether drip-feed. There is a Sparklet and small flowmeter for the addition of carbon dioxide. There is also a pressure gauge and release valve.

demonstrated in 1909 that intratracheal insufflation would maintain life in curarised animals. C. A. Elsberg (1911) described its application to man. Sir Robert Ernest Kelly (1879–1944), Professor of Surgery at Liverpool University, introduced the method into England in 1912. Air from an electric blower was passed over ether and then through a coil immersed in warm water to an endo-tracheal gum elastic catheter. The amount of air passing over the ether was controlled by a three-cogwheel control. The pressure was set between 10 and 30 mm Hg (1·3–4·0 kPa). In 1913, Sir Francis Shipway and Mennell (Fig. 20) produced modified versions of this apparatus. In 1916, Sir Francis Shipway described his simple warmed ether apparatus which would also administer chloroform. Later in 1925 he improved his model by vaporising the ether using a drip-feed device.

Following the development of endotracheal anaesthesia by Magill and Rowbotham during the 1914–18 war, machines were developed with wide-bore outlets. Sir Ivan Whiteside Magill devised a series of these between 1921 and 1932 culminating in his very compact machine (Fig. 21), which shows similarities to that described by Ivor Nicholas Lewis (1900–1932) of St. George's Hospital.

CARBON DIOXIDE ABSORPTION

D. E. Jackson in 1915 advocated carbon dioxide absorption but only used his apparatus on animals. He used an electrically driven pump to circulate the gases; the carbon dioxide was absorbed by a strong aqueous solution of sodium and calcium hydroxide.

Ralph M. Waters, in 1924, reported on two-and-a-half years of work on the principle of carbon dioxide absorption, culminating in his simple to-and-fro' system using a canister of soda-lime. This technique was a major advance in the development of anaesthesia and led to the introduction of the circle anaesthetic system. In 1930, Brian C. Sword described his closed-circuit circle system apparatus which he developed with Richard V. Foregger. This idea crossed the Atlantic in 1933 and the first circle machine, in England, was made for Frankis Evans (1900–1974). Many variations were made of which that described by Gillies in 1938 was the most compact.

The Coxeter Mushin circle was produced in 1941 and its main features include a two-way flow through the soda-lime canister, a wickless ether vaporiser and a handle for manual assistance of respiration. Metal canisters have now been replaced by clear plastic ones so that with the aid of a dye-indicator the activity of the soda-lime can be observed (see Chapter 3).

REFERENCES

BAILLIE, T. W. (1966). *From Boston to Dumfries. The First Surgical Use of Anaesthetic Ether in the Old World.* Dumfries: Robert Dinwiddie & Co.

BOSTON, F. K., and SALT, R. H. (1940). An improved Vinesthene inhaler. *Lancet*, **2**, 623.

BRENNAN, H. J. (1957). A vaporiser for Fluothane. *Brit. J. Anaesth.*, **29**, 332.

BRYCE-SMITH, R. (1964). Halothane induction unit. *Anaesthesia*, **19**, 393.

BURNS, T. H. S. (1954). A constant strength trichloroethylene inhaler utilising a new principle. *Brit. med. J.*, **1**, 329.

CLOVER, J. T. (1868). On the administration of chloroform in dental operations. *Brit. J. dent. Sci.*, **11**, 123.

CLOVER, J. T. (1876). An apparatus for administering nitrous oxide gas and ether, singly or combined. *Brit. med. J.*, **2**, 74.

CLOVER, J. T. (1877). Portable regulating ether inhaler. *Brit. med. J.*, **1**, 69.

DAVY, H. (1800). *Researches, Chemical and Philosophical, chiefly concerning nitrous oxide or dephlogisticated nitrous air and its respiration.* London: J. Johnson. Facsimile edition, Butterworth (1972).

ELLIS, R. (1866). On the safe abolition of pain in labour and surgical operations. London: Hardwickes.

ELSBERG, C. A. (1911). Anaesthesia by the intratracheal insufflation of air and ether. *Ann. Surg.*, **53**, 161.

EPSTEIN, H. G. (1958). Principles of inhalers for volatile anaesthetics. *Brit. med. Bull.*, **14**, No. 1, 18.

EPSTEIN, H. G., and MACINTOSH, R. R. (1949). Analgesia inhaler for trichloroethylene. *Brit. med. J.*, **2**, 1092.

FREEDMAN, A. (1943). Trichlorethylene air analgesia in childbirth. An investigation with a suitable inhaler. *Lancet*, **2**, 696.

GALLEY, A. H., and KING, A. C. (1948). Modifications of the Clover's ether inhaler. *Anaesthesia*, **3**, 147.

GOLDMAN, V. (1936). Vinyl ether, a new method of administration. *Brit. med. J.*, **2**, 122.

GOLDMAN, V. (1959). Fluothane in dental surgery. *Anesth. Analg. Curr. Res.*, **38**, 192.

GOLDMAN, V. (1962). The Goldman vaporiser Mk II. *Anaesthesia*, **17**, 537.

HEWER, C. L., and HADFIELD, C. F. (1941). Trichlorethylene as an inhalation anaesthetic. *Brit. med. J.*, **1**, 924.

HEWITT, F. W. (1893). *Anaesthetics and their Administration.* London: Charles Griffin & Co.

HEWITT, F. W. (1897). *The Administration of Nitrous Oxide and Oxygen for Dental Operations.* London: Ash.

JACKSON, D. E. (1915). A new method for the production of general analgesia and anaesthesia with a description of the apparatus used. *J. Lab. clin. Med.*, **1**, 1.

JONES, P. L., MOLLOY, M. J., and ROSEN, M. (1971). The Cardiff Penthrane inhaler. *Brit. J. Anaesth.*, **43**, 190.

JUNKER, F. E. (1867). Description of a new apparatus for administering narcotic vapours. *Med. Tms Gaz.*, **2**, 590.

KELLY, R. E. (1911). Intratracheal anaesthesia. *Brit. J. Surg.*, **1**, 90

LEWIS, I. N. (1931). Apparatus for anaesthesia. *Lancet*, **2**, 1304.

MACKAY, I. M. (1957). Clinical evaluation of Fluothane with special reference to a controlled percentage vaporizer. *Canad. Anaesth. Soc. J.*, **4**, 235.

McKESSON, E. I. (1911). Nitrous-oxide oxygen anaesthesia with a new apparatus. *Surg. Gynec. Obstet.*, **13**, 456.

MARSHALL, G. (1920). Two types of portable gas-oxygen apparatus. *Proc. roy. Soc. Med.*, **13**, (1), 18.

MELTZER, S. J., and AUER, J. (1909). Continuous respiration without voluntary movements. *J. exp. Med.*, **11**, 622.

MENNELL, Z. (1933). Modified Junker bottle for maternal analgesia. *Practitioner*, **130**, 519.

MINNITT, R. J. (1934). A new technique for the self-administration of gas-air analgesia in labour. *Lancet*, **1**, 1275.

MORRIS, L. E. (1952). A new vaporiser for liquid anaesthetic agents. *Anesthesiology*, **13**, 581.

MURPHY, E. W. (1848). *Chloroform in the Practice of Midwifery.* London: Harveian Society.

OMBRÉDANNE, L. (1908). Un appareil pour l'anesthésie pour l'ether. *Gaz. Hôp. (Paris)*, **81**, S, 10095.

PARKHOUSE, J. (1966). Clinical performance of the O.M.V. inhaler. *Anaesthesia*, **21**, 498.

PATERSON, G. H., HULANDS, G. H., and NUNN, J. F. (1969). Evaluation of a new halothane vaporiser. The Cyprane Fluotec Mk 3. *Brit. J. Anaesth.*, **41**, 109.

RIGBY, M. (1917). A modification of the Junkers inhaler. *Lancet*, **2**, 862.

SHIPWAY, F. (1916). The advantages of warm anaesthetic vapours and an apparatus for their administration. *Lancet*, **1**, 70.

SIMPSON, J. Y. (1847). *Account of a New Anaesthetic Agent as a Substitute for Sulphuric Ether in Surgery and Midwifery*. Edinburgh: Sutherland and Knox.

SKINNER, T. (1862). Anaesthesia in midwifery, with a new apparatus for its safer induction with chloroform. *Brit. med. J.*, **2**, 108.

SNOW, J. (1847). *On the Inhalation of the Vapour of Ether in Surgical Operations*. London: Churchill.

SNOW, J. (1858). *On Chloroform and other Anaesthetics*. London: Churchill.

SWORD, B. C. (1930). The closed circle method of administration of gas anaesthesia. *Curr. Res. Anesth.*, **9**, 198.

SYKES, W. S. (1960). *Essays on the first Hundred Years of Anaesthesia*, Vol. 1, p. 50. Edinburgh: Livingstone.

VERNON HARCOURT, H. G. (1903). Special chloroform committee. *Brit. med. J.*, **2**, Suppl. 142.

WATERS, R. M. (1924). Clinical scope and utility of carbon dioxide filtration in inhalation anesthesia. *Curr. Res. Anesth.*, **3**, 20.

WILSON, S. R., and PINSON, K. B. (1921). A warm ether bomb. *Lancet*, **1**, 336.

WILSON-SMITH, T. (1899). Improved ether inhaler. *Lancet*, **1**, 1005.

YOUNG, J. V. (1966). The practical use of the "Halox" vaporiser. *Anaesthesia*, **21**, 557.

FURTHER READING

ARMSTRONG DAVISON, M. H. (1965). *The Evolution of Anaesthesia*. Altrincham: John Sherratt.

BRYCE-SMITH, R., MITCHELL, J. V., and PARKHOUSE, J. (1963). *The Nuffield Department of Anaesthetics, Oxford, 1937–1962*. London: Oxford Univ. Press.

BRYN THOMAS, K. (1975). *The Development of Anaesthetic Apparatus*. Oxford: Blackwell Scientific Publications.

DUNCUM, B. M. (1947). *The Development of Inhalation Anaesthesia with Special Reference to the Years 1846–1900*. London: Oxford Univ. Press.

KING, A. CHARLES (1946). *The History and Development of Anaesthetic Apparatus*. *Brit. med. J.*, **2**, 536.

SYKES, W. S. (1960). *Essays on the First Hundred Years of Anaesthesia*, 2 Vols. Edinburgh: Livingstone.

Appendix I

CARE AND STERILISATION OF ANAESTHETIC EQUIPMENT

Too little consideration is generally given to the cleanliness and sterility of apparatus used in anaesthesia, and particularly to those parts which indirectly or directly come into contact with the air passages. Absolute sterility is not always essential, since the upper air passages are in constant contact with the atmosphere but there is evidence that infections have been spread from patient to patient through the use of contaminated anaesthetic or respiratory apparatus. This has been shown to occur with the use of ventilators (see Chapter 10). For this reason those parts of the anaesthetic system through which rebreathing takes place, and apparatus such as an endotracheal tube, face-mask and laryngoscope which actually comes into direct contact with the patient, must be thoroughly washed after use and either sterilised, disinfected or at least kept clean until required again. If the equipment has been used for a patient suffering from a known infection then washing *must* be followed by sterilisation.

Constant washing and sterilisation of apparatus, particularly of rubber or plastic components, leads to some wear, but a more potent cause of deterioration is to be found in the use of lubricants containing Vaseline or greasy bases. The use of these, rather than repeated sterilisation, is the commonest cause of deterioration of cuffed tubes (Buckley, 1952). The lubricants should always be non-greasy and either alone or incorporated with local anaesthetic; for example, K.Y. jelly and topical lignocaine 4 per cent jelly.

Lubricants can harbour organisms, so that they are best dispensed in small tubes which can be discarded daily before they become infected.

DISINFECTION AND STERILISATION

A. *Disinfection* is the term used to signify the removal of most vegetative organisms which are easy to kill whilst spores may survive. There are four methods available for anaesthetic apparatus (where applicable):

  (i) *Boiling water*—immersion for five minutes kills all vegetative bacteria and *some* spores.

  (ii) *Low-temperature steam* (subatmospheric at 80° C)—kills all vegetative bacteria but no spores.

  (iii) *Glutaraldehyde (2·5 per cent; Cidex)*—soaking for 30 minutes kills all vegetative bacteria and *some* spores. Automatic disinfecting machines using this agent are available.

  (iv) *Chlorhexidine and spirit (70 per cent)*—soaking for 30 minutes kills all vegetative bacteria but *no* spores.

B. *Sterilisation* is the term used to signify the destruction of all vegetative organisms *including* spores. The principal methods available are:

  (a) *Autoclaving*—the most commonly recommended routine is
$$134° \text{ C at } 32 \text{ lb/sq in (221 kPa) for 3 minutes.}$$

  (b) *Gas Sterilisation*—two principal methods are available:

(i) Low-Temperature Steam (i.e. subatmospheric at 80° C) plus Formaldehyde is probably the most satisfactory method available to create spori-
cidal conditions and can be used for most anaesthetic equipment such
as laryngoscopes, bronchoscopes, endotracheal tubes, etc. It is faster
and cheaper than ethylene oxide and has the added advantage that it is
devoid of toxic by-products that can be isolated from rubber and plastic
materials after ethylene oxide (Clinical Anaesthesia Conference, 1969).

(ii) Ethylene Oxide—requires slightly longer exposure and is more toxic
if either patients or attendants come into contact with the vapour.
Sykes *et al.* (1976) recommend that ethylene oxide or liquid disinfec-
tants should not be used for endotracheal tubes because they may leak
out and cause tissue irritation (Rendell-Baker, 1972).

Sterilisation of Anaesthetic Apparatus

Airways.—Ideally these are available in a disposable plastic. Expense may
necessitate recycling in which case the rubber airway is more suitable. Great
care must be taken to see that each airway is thoroughly washed in soap and
water, both internally and externally, then dried and finally sterilised. Autoclaving is satisfactory for these items.

Endotracheal tubes.—Plastic disposable tubes are the most satisfactory
(minimal irritation to laryngeal and tracheal mucosa) and are particularly
important for those patients who may have to undergo prolonged ventilation.
If recycling is essential then (as with airways) autoclaving is sufficient. Should
ethylene oxide be used for sterilisation, particular care must be taken to ensure
that none of the gas is retained in rubber endotracheal tubes which might leak
out *in situ.*

Face-masks are usually thoroughly washed in soap and water, dried and
re-used. Unfortunately, they will not survive frequent autoclaving.

Laryngeal sprays are a potential source for the introduction of infection.
Casewell and Dalton (1977) report on six women who underwent general
anaesthesia and later developed clinical evidence of respiratory tract infection.
The common source was traced to a Forrester laryngeal spray which was found
to be infected with *Pseudomonas aeruginosa.* All laryngeal sprays should be made
of materials that can be *sterilised* frequently.

Anaesthetic circuits.—All corrugated tubing should be thoroughly washed
and dried after every case. Ideally it should also be sterilised but frequent autoclaving causes damage to the material.

Ventilators.—See Chapter 10.

Sterilisation of Plastic Materials

The introduction of plastic materials into clinical practice was largely
brought about by the desire to control cross-infections in hospital by using
disposable items. Also, many plastics are non-irritating to mucous membranes
and therefore are to be preferred to red rubber when left in contact with the
mucosa of the trachea or urethra for any prolonged period. In their disposable
form, plastic items avoid all the problems of re-sterilisation, but rising costs
have led some anaesthetists to reconsider the whole problem. It is essential to
have some knowledge of the plastic materials available and their response to
the various methods of sterilisation (see Table 1).

Polyvinyl Chloride (PVC) is the most widely used material, particularly for endotracheal and tracheostomy tubes. The great advantage of PVC is its flexibility so that with various additives (plasticisers) a wide range of hardness can be obtained.

Methods of Sterilisation of PVC

Gamma radiation.—(i) *Endotracheal tubes.*—Some degree of discolouration or yellowing will usually occur and this becomes more pronounced with prolonged storage. The colour change is due to the partial dechlorination of the PVC but the mechanical and functional properties of the material are not significantly affected. Repeated doses are not recommended as they lead to pronounced discolouration with undesirable changes in the pH of the aqueous extract and a perceptible stiffening of the material.

(ii) *Tracheostomy tubes.*—These are also made of PVC and therefore the same conditions apply as with endotracheal tubes. However, other parts (using different plastics) are often fitted to these tubes. For example, the Portex tracheostomy has a collar (made of acetyl polymer) attached to facilitate its use with swivel connectors. In these circumstances, the tracheostomy tube is not suitable for gamma radiation sterilisation.

Steam sterilisation.—This requires the high-speed vacuum process which is operated at 136° C. When autoclaving PVC it is particularly important to avoid any stress during the process (such as heavy weights from packing) because at autoclave temperatures PVC softens and can become permanently altered in shape.

Multiple autoclaving cycles can lead to a perceptible stiffening and discolouration of the material.

Ethylene oxide.—Sterilisation processes are usually operated at, or below, 55° C in order to avoid damage to heat-labile materials. Considered solely from the standpoint of possible damage to the product this is the best method available as it can be undertaken repeatedly without any perceptible effect on the PVC endotracheal and tracheostomy tubes. However, particular attention must be paid to adequate batch-by-batch biological monitoring of the efficacy of the sterilisation and also to the need for adequate post-sterilisation aeration of the product to avert hazards arising from ethylene oxide residues.

Other methods, such as the low-temperature steam/formalin process, are available but are considered less suitable because of the difficulty of ensuring the complete absence of any residual formalin. In conclusion, although re-sterilisation may be considered desirable on a cost basis, it must be remembered that with the unused sterilised manufactured product, provided the package is undamaged and if storage conditions are satisfactory, there is only one chance in one million of finding a product which is non-sterile (Vincent, 1976; Portex Ltd—personal communication).

Further details of the effect of sterilisation and disinfection processes are shown in Table 1.

APPENDIX I/TABLE 1

THE EFFECT OF STERILISATION AND DISINFECTION PROCESSES ON MEDICAL AND SURGICAL PLASTICS

Material	Autoclaving	Dry heat	High-energy irradiation	Ethylene oxide	Boiling water	Liquid chemicals	Comments
PVC (a) Flexible	Tubing satisfactory up to 136° C. Mouldings may distort. Avoid external loading while hot.	Unsuitable	Satisfactory up to 2·5 Mr. at higher doses discolours with liberation of hydrogen chloride.	Satisfactory	Satisfactory. Avoid external stress while hot. Mouldings may distort.	Not recommended. Attacked by some chemicals, in particular phenolic agents.	Flexible film and sheeting usually distorts on autoclaving. PVC tends to become opaque or cloudy in hot water or steam. Clarity restored on drying at R.T. more rapidly at 60° C.
(b) Rigid	Unsuitable because of deformation. Softens above 60° C.	Unsuitable	Medical grades usually unsatisfactory because of discolouration.	Satisfactory	Usually unsatisfactory because of dimensional changes. Thick sections less affected. Protect from external stresses.	Usually satisfactory. Phenolic agents should be avoided.	As for flexible PVC
Polyethylene Low density (L.D.) High density (H.D.)	Unsuitable L.D. softens at 80–100° C. H.D. softens at 120–130° C	Unsuitable	Satisfactory. Polyethylene becomes progressively harder and tougher above 2·5 Mr. and up to 25 Mr.	Satisfactory. Highly permeable to gases. Film may be used for packaging.	Usually satisfactory for H.D. polythene but L.D. polythene not satisfactory above 80° C.	Satisfactory	
Polypropylene	Satisfactory—mouldings may distort.	Unsuitable—softens at 145–150° C.	Not usually suitable. Some grades said to be more resistant. Oxidative degradation can occur especially on storage with subsequent embrittlement.	Satisfactory	Satisfactory	Satisfactory	

REFERENCES

BUCKLEY, R. W. (1952). Danger from endotracheal tubes. *Brit. med. J.*, **2**, 939

CASEWELL, M. W., and DALTON, M. T. (1977). Forrester laryngeal sprays as a source of pseudomonas respiratory tract infection. *Brit. med. J.*, **2**, 680.

CLINICAL ANAESTHESIA CONFERENCE (1969). Hazards associated with ethylene oxide sterilisation. *N.Y. St. J. Med.*, **69**, 1319.

RENDELL-BAKER, L. (1972). "Ethylene oxide. II Aeration". In: Infections and sterilisation problems. Ed. R. B. Roberts. *Int. Anesthesiol. Clin.*, **10**, 101.

SYKES, M. K., McNICOL, M. W., and CAMPBELL, E. J. M. (1976). *Respiratory Failure*, p. 172. Oxford: Blackwell Scientific Publications.

FURTHER READING

CRUIKSHANK, R., DUGUID, J. P., MARMION, B. P., and SWAIN, R. H. A. (1973). *Medical Microbiology*, Chap. 5. Edinburgh: Churchill Livingstone.

LENNETTE, E. H., SPAULDING, E. H., and TRUANT, J. P. (1974). *Manual of Clinical Microbiology*, p. 852. Washington: Amer. Soc. Microbiol.

LOWBURY, E. J. L., AYLIFFE, G. A. J., GEDDES, A. M., and WILLIAMS, J. D. (1975). *Control of Hospital Infection*, Chap. 10. London: Chapman and Hall.

Appendix II

USEFUL FACTS

SI UNITS

THE SI system of units (Système International d'Unités) has been developed in an endeavour to reduce the enormous number of units in current use to a relatively small number of internationally acceptable units with standard symbols.

There are seven *base units* (Table 1),

APPENDIX II/TABLE 1
THE SI BASE UNITS

Physical quantity	Name of SI Unit	Symbol for SI Unit
Length	metre	m
Mass	kilogram	kg
Time	second	s
Electric current	ampere	A
Thermodynamic temperature	kelvin	K
Amount of substance	mole	mol
Luminous intensity	candela	cd

which may be combined by multiplication or division to produce *derived units* (Table 2).

APPENDIX II/TABLE 2
SOME DERIVED SI UNITS

Physical quantity	Name of SI Unit	Symbol	Definition of SI Unit
Volume	cubic metre	—	m^3
Force	newton	N	$kg\ m\ s^{-2} = J\ m^{-1}$
Pressure	pascal	Pa	$kg\ m^{-1}\ s^{-2} = N\ m^{-2}$
Work	joule	J	$kg\ m^2\ s^{-2} = N\ m$
Power	watt	W	$kg\ m^2\ s^{-3} = J\ s^{-1}$
Surface tension	pascal metre	—	$Pa\ m = N\ m^{-1} = kg\ s^{-2}$
Periodic frequency	hertz	Hz	s^{-1}

There are in addition *supplementary units* such as the radian and *special non-SI units* such as litre (l), day (d), hour (h), minute (min).

By attaching appropriate prefixes, decimal multiples and fractions of these units can be formed.

APPENDIX II/TABLE 3
SI PREFIXES AND THEIR SYMBOLS

Fraction	SI prefix	Symbol	Multiple	SI prefix	Symbol
10^{-1}	deci	d	10	deca	da
10^{-2}	centi	c	10^2	hecto	h
10^{-3}	milli	m	10^3	kilo	k
10^{-6}	micro	μ	10^6	mega	M
10^{-9}	nano	n	10^9	giga	G
10^{-12}	pico	p	10^{12}	tera	T
10^{-15}	femto	f			
10^{-18}	atto	a			

The Mole

The quantity of a substance of known molecular weight is expressed in moles, where

$$\text{Number of moles (mol)} = \frac{\text{Weight in g}}{\text{Molecular Weight}}$$

and the units of concentration are therefore mol/l, mmol/l, μmol/l, etc. For univalent ions such as Na^+, K^+, HCO_3^- Cl^-, millimoles and milliequivalents are numerically equal. In the case of a divalent ion such as Ca^{++} the number of milliequivalents must be divided by 2 (the valency) to convert to millimoles. To convert results previously expressed as mg/100 ml to mmol/1 the figure should be divided by the molecular weight of the substance concerned (to convert mg to mmol) and multiplied by 10 (to convert from 100 ml to 1 litre).

Example: to convert 90 mg/100 ml glucose to mmol/l:

$$\frac{90 \times 10}{180 \text{ (molecular weight of glucose)}} = 5 \text{ mmol/l}$$

(when considering amount of substance, rather than concentration,

$$90 \text{ mg glucose} = \frac{90}{180} = 0\cdot5 \text{ mmol})$$

In the case of some substances the molecular weight is not known, for example the globulin fraction of plasma protein consists of a mixture of proteins of different molecular weights, so for these substances *mass concentration* is used (kg/l, g/l, mg/l, etc.). It has not yet been decided whether the molecular weight of haemoglobin will be calculated for the monomer (Hb) or tetramer (Hb$_4$), so haemoglobin concentration will continue to be reported in g/100 ml or g/dl.

Volume

In 1964, the litre which had previously been defined in terms of the volume of 1 kg of pure water under standard conditions, was redefined as being equal

| | | | Conversion factors | |
Quantity	SI Unit or multiple	Other Units	Other Units to SI Units multiply by	SI Units to Other Units multiply by:
Length	metre (m)	inch	0·0254	39·37
		foot	0·305	3·281
Mass	kilogram (kg)	ounce	0·0284	35·27
		pound	0·454	2·205
Force (mass × acceleration)	newton (N)	dyne (cm g s⁻²)	0·00001	100,000
		poundal (ft lb s⁻²)[1]	0·138	7·233
		pound-force (lbf)	4·448	0·225
Pressure[2] (force ÷ area)	kilopascal[3] (kPa)	mm Hg \} Torr	0·1333	7·501
		kg f cm⁻²	98·07	0·0102
		cm H_2O	0·0981	10·20
		Std atmosphere	101·3	0·00987
		lbf in⁻²	6·895	0·145
		bar	100	0·01
Work or Energy[4] (force × distance or, pressure × volume)	kilojoule[5] (kJ)	kilocalorie	4·184	0·239
Surface tension	pascal metre (Pa m)	dynes/cm	0·001	1,000
Compliance	litres per kilopascal (1 kPa⁻¹)	l/cm H_2O	10·20	0·0981
Resistance to flow	kilopascals × litres⁻¹ × seconds (kPa l⁻¹ s)	cm H_2O l⁻¹ sec	0·0981	10·20
Transfer factor	millimoles × minutes⁻¹ × kilopascals⁻¹ (mmol min⁻¹ kPa⁻¹)	ml min⁻¹ mm Hg⁻¹	0·335	2·986

[1] This is a technical unit of force, where the mass (lb) is multiplied by the standard acceleration due to gravity (9·8 m s⁻²).
[2] Most pressure gauges read zero when the actual pressure = atmospheric pressure; so gauge pressures are pressures referred to atmospheric pressure, whereas absolute pressures are pressures referred to true zero pressure or vacuum.
[3] The kilopascal has been given rather than the pascal, since in medical practice the kPa will be more commonly used.
[4] Movement of gas in response to a pressure gradient.
[5] The kilojoule has been given rather than the joule since in medical practice the kJ (and MJ) will be more commonly used.

to 1 cubic decimetre (1 l = 1 dm³). The SI unit of volume is the cubic metre (m³), but for medical purposes the litre will continue to be used.

$$1 \text{ pint} = 0.568 \text{ l}$$
$$1 \text{ litre} = 1.760 \text{ pt}$$
$$1 \text{ gallon (U.K.)} = 1.201 \text{ gal (U.S.)} = 4.546 \text{ l}$$
$$1 \text{ gallon (U.S.)} = 0.833 \text{ gal (U.K.)} = 3.785 \text{ l}$$

Temperature

The SI unit is the kelvin (K), but for everyday use the degree Celsius (formerly called Centigrade) will be retained. The Fahrenheit scale is no longer used.

$$0° \text{ C} = 273.15 \text{ K} = 32.0° \text{ F}$$
$$\text{Celsius to Kelvin: K} = °\text{C} + 273$$
$$\text{Kelvin to Celsius: } °\text{C} = \text{K} - 273$$
$$\text{Celsius to Fahrenheit: } °\text{F} = °\text{C} \times \tfrac{9}{5} + 32$$
$$\text{Fahrenheit to Celsius: } °\text{C} = (°\text{F} - 32) \times \tfrac{5}{9}$$

SPECIAL SYMBOLS*

For Gases

PRIMARY SYMBOLS
(Large Capital Letters)

V = gas volume

$\dot{V}$ = gas volume/unit time

P = gas pressure

$\bar{P}$ = mean gas pressure

F = fractional concentration in dry gas phase

f = respiratory frequency (breaths/unit time)

D = diffusing capacity

R = respiratory exchange ratio

EXAMPLES

V_A = volume of alveolar gas

$\dot{V}_{O_2}$ = O_2 consumption/min.

$P_{A_{O_2}}$ = alveolar O_2 pressure

$P_{C_{O_2}}$ = mean capillary pulmonary O_2 pressure

$F_{I_{O_2}}$ = fractional concentration of O_2 in inspired gas

D_{O_2} = diffusing capacity for O_2 (ml O_2/min/mm/Hg)

R = $\dot{V}_{CO_2}/\dot{V}_{O_2}$

SECONDARY SYMBOLS
(Small Capital Letters)

I = inspired gas

E = expired gas

A = alveolar gas

T = tidal gas

D = dead space gas

B = barometric

EXAMPLES

$F_{I_{CO_2}}$ = fractional concentration of CO_2 in inspired gas

V_E = volume of expired gas

$\dot{V}_A$ = alveolar ventilation/min

V_T = tidal volume

V_D = volume of dead space gas

P_B = barometric pressure

— Dash above any symbol indicates a *mean* value.

. Dot above any symbol indicates a *time derivative*.

* This list of special symbols with examples is reproduced from *The Lung* by the kindness of Professor Julius H. Comroe and the Year Book Medical Publishers, Incorporated.

For Blood

PRIMARY SYMBOLS (Large Capital Letters)	EXAMPLES
Q = volume of blood	Qc = volume of blood in pulmonary capillaries
$\dot{Q}$ = volume flow of blood/unit time	$\dot{Q}c$ = blood flow through pulmonary capillaries/min.
C = content of gas in blood phase	Ca_{O_2} = ml O_2 in 100 ml arterial blood
S = per cent saturation of Hb with O_2 or CO	$S\bar{v}_{O_2}'$ = saturation of Hb with O_2 in mixed venous blood

SECONDARY SYMBOLS (Small Letters)	EXAMPLES
a = arterial blood	Pa_{CO_2} = partial pressure of CO_2 in arterial blood
v = venous blood	
$\bar{v}$ = mixed venous blood	$P\bar{v}_{O_2}$ = partial pressure of O_2 in mixed venous blood
c = pulmonary capillary blood	Pc_{CO} = partial pressure of CO in pulmonary capillary blood

For Lung Volumes

VC = Vital Capacity	= maximal volume that can be expired after maximal inspiration
IC = Inspiratory Capacity	= maximal volume that can be inspired from resting expiratory level
IRV = Inspiratory Reserve Volume	= maximal volume that can be inspired from end-tidal inspiration
ERV = Expiratory Reserve Volume	= maximal volume that can be expired from resting expiratory level
FRC = Functional Residual Capacity	= volume of gas in lungs at resting expiratory level
RV = Residual Volume	= volume of gas in lungs at end of maximal expiration
TLC = Total Lung Capacity	= volume of gas in lungs at end of maximal inspiration

Average Values for Adult Male

For further information about lung function tests see Cotes (1975).[*]

Vital capacity	4,800 ml
Functional residual capacity	2,400 ml
Residual volume	1,200 ml
Total lung capacity	6,000 ml
Tidal volume	600 ml
Respiratory frequency	12/min

[*] Cotes, J. E. (1975). *Lung Function*, 3rd edit. Oxford: Blackwell Scientific Publications.

Minute volume.................................. 6 1/min
Dead space (Upright position)
    anatomical................................. 150 ml (2 ml/kg)
    physiological.............................. 190 ml (VD/VT < 0·3)
Alveolar ventilation............................ 4·2 1/min
Oxygen consumption (at rest)..................... 240 ml/min (10·7 mmol min^{-1})
Carbon dioxide output (at rest).................. 192 ml/min (8·6 mmol min^{-1})
Respiratory exchange ratio (RQ).................. 0·8
Peak expiratory flow rate (PEFR)................. 500 1/min
[1]FEV per cent.................................. 85 per cent
Diffusing capacity (transfer factor) for carbon monoxide 30 ml min^{-1} mm Hg^{-1}
    (Dco)..................................... (10 mmol min^{-1} kPa^{-1})
Compliance
    lungs..................................... 0·2 1 cm H$_2$O^{-1}
        (2·04 1 kPa^{-1})
    thorax.................................... 0·2 1 cm H$_2$O^{-1}
        (2·04 1 kPa^{-1})
    total..................................... 0·1 1 cm H$_2$O^{-1}
        (1·02 1 kPa^{-1})
Airway resistance............................... 1·0 cm H$_2$O 1^{-1} sec
        (0·1 kPa 1^{-1} s)

1. FEV per cent = forced expiratory volume measured over 1 second (FEV 1·0) expressed as a percentage of the forced vital capacity (FVC).

Composition of Dry Air (Vol per cent)[1]

Nitrogen	78·08
Oxygen	20·95
Argon	0·93
Carbon dioxide	0·03
Other gases	trace amounts

GAS TENSIONS IN INSPIRED AIR, ALVEOLAR GAS AND BLOOD

	Inspired air		Alveolar gas		Arterial blood		Mixed venous blood	
	mm Hg	(kPa)	mm Hg	(kPa)	mm Hg	(kPa)	mm Hg	(kPa)
Nitrogen	590	(78·6)	564	(75·2)	567	(75·6)	567	(75·6)
Oxygen	158	(21·1)	102	(13·6)	99	(13·2)	40	(5·3)
Carbon dioxide	[0·2	(—)]	40	(5·3)	40	(5·3)	46	(6·1)
Water vapour	5	(0·7)	47	(6.3)	47	(6·3)	47	(6.3)
Total (excluding argon)	753	(100)	753	(100)	753	(100)	700	(93)[2]

Note: 1. Partial pressure (kPa) and per cent composition of gas (at sea level) are numerically similar.
2. The sum of the partial pressures of gases in venous blood is considerably smaller than that in arterial blood.

Conversion of Gas Volumes

1. To convert ml of gas/100 ml into mmol/l and vice versa:

$$mmol/l = \frac{ml/100\ ml}{2\cdot24}\ ^*$$

$$ml/100\ ml = 2\cdot24 \times mmol/l$$

2. Temperature and pressure corrections

  ATPS = ambient temperature and pressure, saturated.
  BTPS = body temperature and ambient pressure, saturated.
  STPD = standard temperature (0° C) and pressure (760 mm Hg), dry.

Gas volumes may be measured under various conditions of temperature, pressure and saturation with water vapour. In the field of respiratory physiology, these volumes are usually corrected to BTPS. Conversions are made using the combined gas equation:

$$\frac{P_1V_1}{T_1} = \frac{P_2V_2}{T_2}$$

  P = pressure minus the water vapour pressure
  V = volume of gas
  T = absolute temperature (K), = °C + 273

BIOCHEMICAL VALUES

For many of these values there is considerable variation in the "normal range" quoted by different laboratories.

	Old Units	SI Units	Conversion factors Old Units to SI Units Multiply by:	SI Units to Old Units Multiply by:
Amylase	70–300 Int. Units/l	70–300 Int. Units/l	—	—
Bicarbonate	23–30 mEq/l	23–30 mmol/l	—	—
Bilirubin	0·3–1·2 mg/100 ml	5–20 μmol/l	17·1	0·0585
Calcium	90–102 mg/l	2·25–2·55 mmol/l	0·025	40·1
Chloride	95–110 mEq/l	95–110 mmol/l	—	—
Cholesterol	100–240 mg/100 ml	2·6–6·2 mmol/l	0·0258	38·7
Cortisol	8–26 μg/100 ml	0·22–0·71 μmol/l	0·0276	36·3
Creatinine:				
Men	0·6–1·2 mg/100 ml	53–106 μmol/l ⎫	88·4	0·0113
Women	0·5–1·0 mg/100 ml	44–88 μmol/l ⎬		
Fasting Blood Glucose:				
Under 30 years	55–85 mg/100 ml	3·1–4·7 mmol/l ⎫	0·056	18·0
Over 30 years	60–105 mg/100 ml	3·3–5·8 mmol/l ⎬		
Iron	67–150 μg/100 ml	12–27 μmol/l	0·179	5·59

* (The molar volume of an *ideal* gas at 0° and 760 mm Hg is 22·414 l. In the case of CO_2, the molar volume is 22·257 l).

Iron Binding				
Capacity	224–420 µg/100 ml	40–75 µmol/l	0·179	5·59
Lead	10–50 µg/100 ml	0·5–2·4 µmol/l	0·0483	20·7
Magnesium	1·5–2·4 mg/100 ml	0·6–1·0 mmol/l	0·411	2·43
Phosphatase:				
Acid	1–5 KA Units/ 100 ml	1–5 KA Units/dl	—	—
Alkaline	4–13 KA Units/ 100 ml	4–13 KA Units/dl	—	—
Phosphate	2·4–4·3 mg/100 ml	0·8–1·4 mmol/l	0·323	3·10
Protein-bound				
Iodine	4–8 µg/100 ml	320–640 nmol/l	78·8	0·0127
Protein:				
Albumin	4·0–5·5 g/100 ml	40–55 g/l		
Globulin	1·5–3·0 g/100 ml	15–30 g/l	10	0·1
Fibrinogen	0·2–0·5 g/100 ml	2–5 g/l		
Total	6·0–8·0 g/100 ml	60–80 g/l		
Sodium	134–143 mEq/l	134–143 mmol/l	—	—
Thyroxine (T4)	4·8–10·3 µg/100 ml	62–133 nmol/l	12·9	0·078
Triglyceride				
(fasting)	60–160 mg/100 ml	0·7–1·8 mmol/l	0·0113	88·5
Urate (Uric Acid)				
Men	3·6–8·0 mg/100 ml	0·21–0·48 mmol/l	0·0595	16·8
Women	2·1–6·0 mg/100 ml	0·13–0·36 mmol/l		
Urea	18–41 mg/100 ml	3·0–7·0 mmol/l	0·167	6·01

(Transaminases have not been included because of the very different "normal ranges" quoted by various laboratories).

HAEMATOLOGICAL VALUES

	Old Units	SI Units
B.12 (serum)	180–1,000 pg/ml	180–1,000 ng/l
Folate (red cell)	160–640 ng/ml	160–640 µg/l
Erythrocyte Sedimentation Rate (ESR)-Westergren	2–12 mm in 1 hour	2–12 mm in 1 hour
Haemoglobin:		
Men	14–18 g/100 ml	14–18 g/dl
Women	12–16 g/100 ml	12–16 g/dl
At Birth	17–20 g/100 ml	17–20 g/dl
Haematocrit (PCV or packed cell volume)		
Men	42–52 per cent	0·42–0·52
Women	37–47 per cent	0·37–0·47
Platelets	150,000–400,000/mm³	150–400 × 10^9/l
Reticulocytes	0·2–2·0 per cent	0·2–2·0%
White Cells	4,000–10,000/mm³	4·0–10·0 × 10^9/l
Neutrophils	40–75 per cent	
Lymphocytes	20–50 per cent	
Monocytes	2–10 per cent	
Eosinophils	1–6 per cent	
Basophils	0–1 per cent	

CEREBROSPINAL FLUID

	Old Units	SI Units
Cells	$<5/mm^3$	$<5 \times 10^9/l$
Chloride	120–130 mEq/l	120–130 mmol/l
Glucose	50–75 mg/100 ml	2·8–4·2 mmol/l
Pressure	70–180 mmH$_2$O	0·7–1·8 kPa
Protein, total	15–45 mg/100 ml	15–45 mg/100 ml

URINE

	Old Units	SI Units
Calcium	100–250 mg/24 hours	2·5–6·2 mmol/24 hours
Creatinine	0·8–1·8 g/24 hours	7–16 mmol/24 hours
Potassium	25–100 mEq/24 hours	25–100 mmol/24 hours
Sodium	130–260 mEq/24 hours	130–260 mmol/24 hours
Urea	10–30 g/24 hours	170–500 mmol/24 hours
Vanillylmandelic acid (VMA)	1–7 mg/24 hours	5–35 µmol/24 hours

BODY WATER

Body water expressed as percentage of body weight:

	Adults		Infants
	Men	Women	Infants
Total body water	60	50	75
Intracellular	40	30	40
Extracellular	20	20	35
a) Intravascular	4	4	5
b) Interstitial	16	16	30

Water *intake* (Adult) per 24 hours
As liquid........ 1,500 ml
As food .... 1,000 ml (including 300 ml water of oxidation)

Total........ 2,500 ml

Water *elimination* (Adult) per 24 hours
Skin.................. 500 ml
Lungs.................. 400 ml
Faeces.................. 100 ml
Urine.................. 1,500 ml

Total............... 2,500 ml

GASTRIC SECRETION

Fasting juice
Volume............. 20–100 ml
pH.................. 0·9–1·5
Emptying time....... 3–6 hours

INDEX